The Battle of the Bulge

A History of Obesity Research

THE BATTLE OF THE BULGE

A History of Obesity Research

by

George A. Bray, M.D.

DORRANCE PUBLISHING CO., INC.
PITTSBURGH, PENNSYLVANIA 15222

The opinions expressed herein are those of the author, who assumes complete and sole responsibility for them, and do not necessarily represent the views of the publisher or its agents.

ISBN: 978-0-8059-7094-4
Library of Congress Control Number: 2005933069

Printed in the United States of America

First Printing

For more information or to order additional books, please contact:
Dorrance Publishing Co., Inc.
701 Smithfield Street, Third Floor
Pittsburgh, Pennsylvania 15222
U.S.A.
1-800-788-7654
www.dorrancebookstore.com

Dedication

This book is dedicated to my wife and children, and to my many professional colleagues who have energized my interest in the battle of the bulge.

Contents

Preface

The Battle of the Bulge refers to a famous military battle of World War II. For us, however, it refers to the current epidemic of obesity. Although body weight and body fat have been increasing for more than one hundred years, these changes have mostly reflected improved nutrition and resulted in taller people. However, in the last twenty years of the twentieth century something changed. The number of overweight people increased significantly. As a result, interest in the problem posed by corpulence and increasing adiposity likewise increased. This occurred at the political level and on the part of the public in general. This book adds a perspective to this problem that cannot readily be achieved from the other books that are available about obesity.

The seeds for this book were sown many years ago. One of the lucky transitions for me was the selection of an internship at the Johns Hopkins Hospital where the spirit of Sir William Osler (1849–1919) still walked the halls and the medical wards. The impact of this giant in medicine on that institution and on its graduates—and indeed on the entire medical profession—is immense. Among his other legacies is a rich literature in the medical history. His biographical sketches and essays are a pleasure to read and his impact on me is evident from my pursuit of the history of obesity as found in the annals of the history of medicine.

These early seeds began to germinate when I spent a year at the National Institute for Medical Research in London in 1961–62. Although more than a decade after the end of World War II, the scars of the war were still evident along the streets of London. To be immersed in a culture where history was measured in centuries added to my interest in the history of medicine. It was here I first began to explore the rich medical heritage of London and to visit the museum started by Sir Henry Wellcome that was housed at that time in the Wellcome Institute in London. This period also saw the germination of my interest in collecting books related to medicine.

My focus on obesity, which is the basis for this historical book, began right after returning to the United States. The molecular basis for several diseases such as galactosemia, phenylketonuria, and sickle cell anemia had been identified in the 1950s and 1960s. Watson and Crick had proposed the helical structure of DNA in 1957. When I went to work with Dr. Edwin B. Astwood (1920–1974), a famous endocrinologist, at the Tufts-New England Medicine Center in Boston, MA, in 1961, he had acquired a strain of animals that inherit obesity. They were fat unless we deprived them of food, and even then they remained fat but lighter in weight. Dr. Astwood suggested that it would be a valuable research program to pursue the genetic basis for the obesity in these animals. From this experimental starting point, I developed a research program in which the basic scientific advances needed to understand how obesity developed were evaluated in human beings as well as in animals. This research program has been the basis of my scientific work.

Obesity is not a new problem. This became evident as I began to explore its origins. Statues from the old Stone Age more than twenty thousand years ago were examples of obesity in humans, predominantly women, which show that obesity has been around for more than twenty thousand years. The ancient origins of obesity and my historical interests stimulated early in my career made an easy transition to this project of putting the scientific and cultural basis of obesity together in a historical perspective.

In this book I have divided the record of obesity into three parts. The first part is the prehistorical materials coming largely from the Paleolithic and Neolithic ages about forty thousand to thirty-five hundred years ago. The second part contains the recorded information about obesity from the time written languages first appeared at the dawn of civilization some five thousand years to three thousand years ago, before the Common Era [BCE] up to A.D. 1500. I have selected A.D. 1500 as a dividing line since this was just after the introduction by Gutenberg of printing using movable type. This revolution in the communication of information was as profound as the discovery of written languages and the introduction of computers in the late twentieth century.

The third part includes descriptions of the key discoveries that have guided the battle of the bulge. After each of these discoveries are the scientific articles that provide the basis for these advances. I hope that this volume will provide a source of information and enjoyment for students, scholars, and interested individuals who want a more detailed picture of the growth of the field of obesity than can be obtained in scientific monographs, journal articles, or from the popular press.

The preparation of this book has been a labor of love. It has enabled me to search the libraries of the world for materials of relevance. Professor Hans Berthoud and Scott Houghton helped with some of the translations. I am particularly grateful to the New York Academy of Medicine, the National Library of Medicine, The Wellcome Library, the British Library, the

Countway Library, the Philadelphia College of Physicians and Surgeons, the Johns Hopkins Medical Institutions, Institute of the History of Medicine, and the Welch Library for the wonderful collections that they have and that I have been privileged to use. Their library staff members have been most helpful in this endeavor. The information specialist Ms. Lori Steib, at the Pennington Biomedical Research Center, has been an invaluable asset in finding older materials. My very able editor and technical writer, Ms. Heather Miller, has devoted countless hours to editorial work on this book for which I am deeply grateful. Finally I want to thank my wife, Marilyn, for her encouraging me to collect books on the history of medicine that ignited my interest in the subject and led to this volume. She has also been a devoted critic and provided many helpful comments during the editing of the manuscript.

—George A. Bray, M.D. January 2006

Introduction

The goal of historical scholarship is to reconstruct the past, but the only past available for reconstruction is that which we can see from the present. The nature of science as an analytical discipline, involved at one and the same time in the uncertainties of discovery and in the accumulation of a body of objective knowledge, raises some special problems of historical reconstruction.

— Crombie[1]

We are bombarded, day after day, with headlines telling us that more and more people are becoming overweight or obese. We are told that we have an epidemic, that obesity is a worldwide problem with more than three hundred million people in trouble, that the costs of this problem can bankrupt health care systems by leading to more diabetes, heart disease, high blood pressure, and cancer. What are we to do?

Is this epidemic due to our genes? Is it due to the food we eat? What can we do about it? Answers to these questions are not yet in, but we do have a large reservoir of knowledge that can guide decisions. This book uses important published scientific papers about obesity to guide our understanding of the problem. Although we are surrounded by an epidemic of obesity, it may (or may not) be comforting to know that the problem has been with us for more than twenty thousand years. It is not new. It has engaged medical and scientific minds since the beginning of recorded history. As with most other areas of human endeavor, understanding doesn't come immediately or easily.

Crombie [1] admirably summarizes the challenge of preparing a history on the battle of the bulge. I will tell the story of battle of the bulge using the published record provided by scientific papers that I consider to be important. They tell us about obesity "as an analytical discipline...and the accumulation of a body of objective knowledge." In this book I will explore the historical framework in which this accumulation of knowledge has occurred.

Up front I must admit that I am not a historian and thus lack the perspective of someone trained in this field. Rather, I do biomedical research and use my historical reading to understand the processes of experimental science and to help improve my own science. Many historical milestones in this story of the battle of the bulge were included in a series of articles about important papers relating to obesity appearing in the journal *Obesity Research*[2]. This book will build on these earlier contributions and attempt to place them in a broader historical context[2-33].

As we explore the battle of the bulge together, we need a plan for where we are going. In the first part of the book I will try to convince you that the battle of the bulge began in prehistoric times and continues to the present. There are three chapters that will trace the history of the battle from prehistoric times to the twenty-first century. The first chapter will review the problem as told in the prehistoric Stone Age carvings. The second chapter will consider the battle of the bulge from the beginning of recorded history (ca. 3600 B.C.) to the onset of the scientific era (ca. A.D. 1500). This will be the first time that we see consistent efforts to tackle this problem by medical practitioners. The third chapter will cover the battle to prevent adiposity in the scientific era from A.D. 1500 to 2000. You will see that this battle has been a long one and that by the beginning of the twentieth century we had only made a modest amount of progress. The explosive growth of biomedical science during the twentieth century offers hope that the battle will be won in the twenty-first century.

Following this overview of the war on obesity that has been waged for twenty thousand years, I will provide more detailed descriptions of the various battles that have been waged and how they have contributed to the current state of affairs. This is done in twenty-eight chapters that cover topics ranging from basic scientific ideas about how to win the war on obesity to the application of these ideas to individual patients. I have selected one or more scientific papers that have opened each field up to further investigation or led to a new concept in our fight. The choice of papers is my own, but they provide a framework of commentary on classic papers that will be useful in exploring further the field of obesity.

Clearly there were many important scientific and mathematical advances before 1500[34, 35]. However, the advent of printing with movable type and the appearance of the scientific method led to an accelerating rate of scientific advance in the battle of the bulge after A.D. 1500. Observations in clinical medicine related to obesity antedate 1500, but the impact of many early discoveries on scientific medicine was delayed until the beginning of the nineteenth century. If one wanted a demarcation line for the beginning of modern medicine, it might well be at the time of the American and French Revolutions (1776–1789)[36, 37].

This book on the battle of the bulge has some important lessons for all of us. For physician scientists who become interested in this important problem, I would suggest that they heed the words of Ivan Pavlov (1849–1936) quoted below. Pavlov was one of the great Russian scientists who applied his immense intellect to the problem of food intake. I have provided this quote here. Although Pavlov intended this advice for the youth of his country, it applies just as well to the rest of the world's young scientists and is as valid today as when he wrote it nearly a century ago:

> This is the message I would like to give to the youth of my country (Russia) [The rest of the world's young scientists could also benefit from it]. First of all, be systematic, I repeat, be systematic. Train yourself to be strictly systematic in the acquisition of knowledge. First study the rudiments of science before attempting to reach its heights. Never pass on to the next stage until you have thoroughly mastered the one on hand. Never try to conceal the defects in your knowledge even by the most daring conjectures and hypotheses. Practice self-restraint and patience. Learn to do the drudgery of scientific work. Although a bird's wing is perfect, the bird could never soar if it did not lean upon the air. Facts are the air on which the scientist leans. Without them you will never fly upward. Without them your theories will be mere empty efforts. However, when studying experiments, or observing, try not to remain on the mystery of the origin. Search persistently for the laws which govern them. The second important requisite is modesty. Never at any time imagine that you know everything. No matter how highly you are appreciated by others, have the courage to say to yourself "I am ignorant." Do not let pride possess you. The third thing that is necessary is passion. Remember that science demands of a man his whole life. And even if you could have two lives they would not be sufficient. Science calls for tremendous effort and great passion. Be passionate in your work and in your search for truth[38].

In this book, I have tried to incorporate some of the passion that Pavlov identifies. His caution of being modest certainly applies to my efforts in this book. I will almost surely overlook important contributions and give some of the ones I select an importance that others would disagree with. I accept these limitations and admit my limitations.

References

1. A.C. Crombie (ed). *Scientific Changes: Historical Studies in the Intellectual, Social and Technical Conditions for Scientific Discovery and Technical Investigation, from Antiquity to the Present.* Ed. New York: Basic Books, 1963.
2. Bray, G.A. Commentary on paper by Chambers. *Obes Res.* 1 (1993): 85–6
3. Bray, G.A. Commentary on Banting Letters. *Obes Res.* 1 (1993): 14–152.
4. Bray, G.A. Commentary on Atwater Classic. *Obes Res.* 1 (1993): 223–227.
5. Bray, G.A. Commentary on Classics of Obesity 4. Hypothalamic Obesity. *Obes Res.* 1 (1993): 325–328.
6. Bray, G.A. Commentary of Classics of Obesity. 5. Fat Cell Theory and Units of Knowledge. *Obes Res.* 1 (1993): 403–407.
7. Bray, G.A. Commentary on Classics of Obesity 6. Science and Politics of Hunger. *Obes Res.* 1 (1933): 489–493.
8. Bray, G.A. Commentary on Classics of Obesity 1. Quetelet: Quantitative Medicine. *Obes Res.* 2 (1994): 68–77.
9. Bray, G.A. Commentary on Classics of Obesity. Lavoisier and Scientific Revolution: The Oxygen Theory Displaces Air, Fire, Earth, and Water. *Obes Res.* 2 (1994): 183–188.
10. Bray, G.A. Commentary on Classics of Obesity. Amphetamine: The Janus of Treatment for Obesity. *Obes Res.* 2 (1994): 282–285.
11. Bray, G.A. Commentary on Classics of Obesity. What's in a Name? Mr. Dickens's "Pickwickian" Fat Boy Syndrome. *Obes Res.* 2 (1994): 380–383.
12. Bray, G.A. Commentary on Classics of Obesity. Harvey Cushing and the Neuroendocrinology of Obesity. *Obes Res.* 2 (1994): 482–485.
13 Bray, G.A. Commentary on Classics in Obesity. The Inheritance of Corpulence. *Obes Res.* 2 (1994): 601–605.
14. Bray, G.A. Commentary on Classics in Obesity. Life Insurance and Overweight. *Obes Res.* 3 (1995): 97–99.
15. Bray, G.A. Commentary on Classics in Obesity. From Very-Low-Energy Diets to Fasting and Back. *Obes Res.* 3 (1995): 207–209.
16. Bray, G.A. Commentary on Classics in Obesity. Measurement of Body Composition: An Improving Art. *Obes Res.* 3 (1995): 291–293.
17. Bray, G.A. Commentary on Classics in Obesity. Laurence, Moon, Bardet, and Biedl: Reflections on a Syndrome. *Obes Res.* 3 (1995): 383–386.
18. Bray, G.A. Commentary on Classics in Obesity. Luxuskonsumption—Myth or Reality? *Obes Res.* 3 (1995): 491–495.
19. Bray, G.A. Commentary on Classics in Obesity. The Tide Shifts Again: The Ebb and Flow of History. *Obes Res.* 3 (1995): 605–608.
20. Bray, G.A. Commentary on Classics in Obesity. Hereditary Adiposity in Mice: Human Lessons from the Yellow and Obese (ob/ob) Mice. *Obes Res.* 4 (1996): 91–95.

21. Bray, G.A. Commentary on Classics in Obesity. Body Fat Distribution and the Distribution of Scientific Knowledge. *Obes Res.* 4 (1996): 189–192.
22. Bray, G.A. Commentary on Classics in Obesity. Obesity and Surgery for a Chronic Disease. *Obes Res.* 4 (1996): 301–303.
23. Bray, G.A. Commentary on Classics in Obesity. Eat Slowly—from Laboratory to Clinic; Behavioral Control of Eating. *Obes Res.* 4 (1996): 397–400.
24. Bray, G.A. Commentary on Classics in Obesity. Static Theories in a Dynamic World: A Glucodynamic Theory of Food Intake. *Obes Res.* 4 (1996): 489–492.
25. Bray, G.A. Commentary on Classics in Obesity. Methods and Obesity Research: The Radioimmonoassay of Insulin. *Obes Res.* 4 (1996): 579–582.
26. Bray GA. Commentary on Classics in Obesity. Energy Expenditure Using Doubly Labeled Water: The Unveiling of Objective Truth. *Obes Res.* 5 (1997): 71–77.
27. Bray, G.A. Commentary on Classics in Obesity. Archeology of Mind—Obesity and Psychoanalysis. *Obes Res.* 5 (1997): 153–156.
28. Bray, G.A. Commentary on Classics in Obesity. Growth of a Molecular Base for Feeding: The Mind-Body Dualism. *Obes Res.* 5 (1997): 271–274.
29. Bray, G.A. Commentary on Classics in Obesity. Amino Acids, Protein, and Body Weight. *Obes Res.* 5 (1997): 373–376.
30. Bray, G.A. Commentary on Classics in Obesity. Anorexia Nervosa and Socio-Economic Status. *Obes Res.* 5 (1997): 489–491
31. Bray, G.A. Temperature, Food Intake and Internal Milieu. *Obes Res.* 5 (1997): 638-640.
32. Bray, G.A. "Obesity: Historical Development of Scientific and Cultural Ideas." *Int J Obes.* 14 (1990): 909–926.
33. Bray, G.A. "Historical Framework for the Development of Ideas About Obesity." *Handbook of Obesity*. Ed. G.A. Bray, C. Bouchard, and W.P.T. James. New York: Elsevier, 1998.
34. Needham, J. *Science and Civilization in China*. Cambridge: Cambridge University Press, 1988.
35. Singer, C., E.J. Homyard, A.R. Hall, T.L. Williams. *A History of Technology*. New York: Oxford University Press, 1954–1958.
36. Ackerknecht, E.H. *Medicine at the Paris Hospital*. Baltimore: Johns Hopkins University Press, 1967.
37. Foucault, M. *The Birth of the Clinic. An Archeology of Medical Perceptions*. New York: Vintage Books, 1973.
38. Babkin, B.P., *Pavlov: A Biography*. Chicago: University of Chicago Press, 1949.

PART I.

Changing Methods of Communication during the Battle of the Bulge

Chapter 1

The Bulge Begins in the Stone Age—The Battle Comes Later

> *We do not live in our own time alone; we carry our history within us.*
>
> —Gaarder [1]

A. The Stone Age

Imagine your surprise when your spade comes upon a small statue of a fat woman when you are digging for a construction project on the outskirts of a small town. A curious mind would want to know more about this statue and about the times from which it came. The statue I am referring to is called the Venus of Willendorf [2] after the town in Austria where it was found in 1908 during excavations along the Danube River. It is a small limestone statuette measuring a little over 4 inches (11 cm) in height.

The arms are small, there are no feet or facial features, but there is clear-cut abdominal obesity and pendulous breasts. You might wonder was this the only statue of its kind? What did it represent? What was its role in this culture and how did the people live when it was made? These and many other questions have been the subject of research since the statue was found about one hundred years ago and add a fascinating perspective to the battle of the bulge. First, this statue tells us that obesity has been a human issue for a very long time. Second, it has raised boundless speculation about whether this statue represented some kind of good or bad omen or whether it was a part of a fertility rite.

Learning about disease and medicine prior to written history can only be done using artifacts such as the Venus of Willendorf or other artistic representations, skeletal finds, and related objects found in archeological excavations. From these artifacts it is clear that our forefathers and mothers suffered many illnesses, including obesity, and that they tried to do something about them. Treatment in prehistoric times was aimed at the relief of fevers and burns and attempts to relieve pain, to stop bleeding, and to repair broken bones. Injury, burns, fevers, and infections took a major human toll before our era of antibiotics and modern medicine. Indeed, it is hard to imagine life in the times before anesthesia, antibiotics, anti-sera, and automobiles.

One of the most interesting ancient surgical techniques is trepanning, or drilling holes in the skull. This procedure was practiced in many parts of the world. The reasons for drilling holes in the skull at a time before there was anesthesia to relieve pain or antisepsis to reduce infections are unknown, but there is much speculation. These operations may have been intended to let out "evil spirits," to treat epilepsy or convulsions, or to relieve skull fractures. Whatever the reason, this procedure of drilling holes in the skull of conscious people was practiced in many parts of the world up to the nineteenth century.

The medicine man and the relation of magic and religion to healing and disease are prominent features of prehistoric medicine and are present in many cultures even today. Explorers have found a wide distribution of Stone Age statues, showing that obesity was present long before recorded history and that, like the present epidemic, it was worldwide[3,4]. One explanation for the Venus of Willendorf and these other statues is that they represented a fertility cult. Let's examine what we have learned about some of these early Stone Age statues that depict obesity. They have been found both in the Old Stone Age and in the New Stone Age. They are widely distributed, meaning either that there was a spontaneous need for what these statues represented arising in many peoples at similar times or that there was communication across a broad land mass about these art forms.

B. Paleolithic Statues

It is interesting that almost all of the statues of obesity from the Paleolithic Stone Age are women[5,6]. These artifacts were found in Europe from Southwestern France to north of the Black Sea in Russia as well as in the Middle East[7,8]. The Eurasian locations in which they were found and the appearance of some of these Venuses, as they are often called, is shown in Figure 1–1. Most of these figures were produced during a fairly narrow period some twenty-three thousand to twenty-five thousand years ago (this period was called the Upper Perigordian or Gravettian part of the Paleolithic Era)[9]. A two thousand-year period (two millennia) may be an accurate estimate of the time during which they were created, or it may reflect the limits in our ability to date objects more precisely. These statues are distributed over more than 5000 km (3000 miles) from west to east and have been found either by lucky individuals or as part of systematic archeological excavations. In the Stone Age, the artisans' tools were stone, which limited the types of materials used for these statues, which were mainly composed of ivory, limestone, or baked clay (terra cotta).

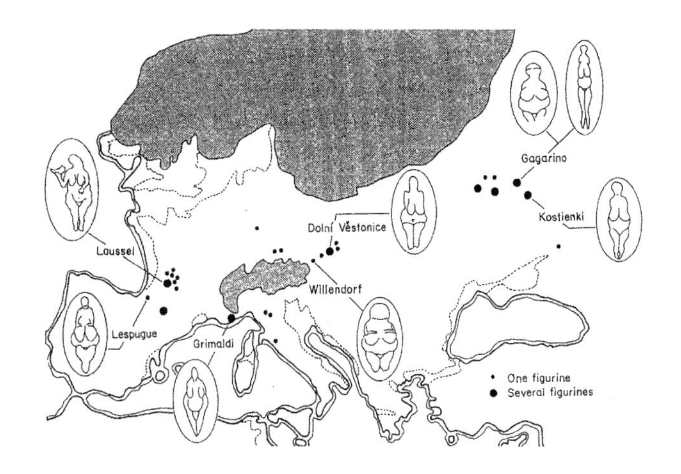

1-1 Geographc distribution across Europe of Venus-like figurines from the Old Stone (Paleolithic) Age. Handbook of Obesity, © 2005 George A. Bray, MD.

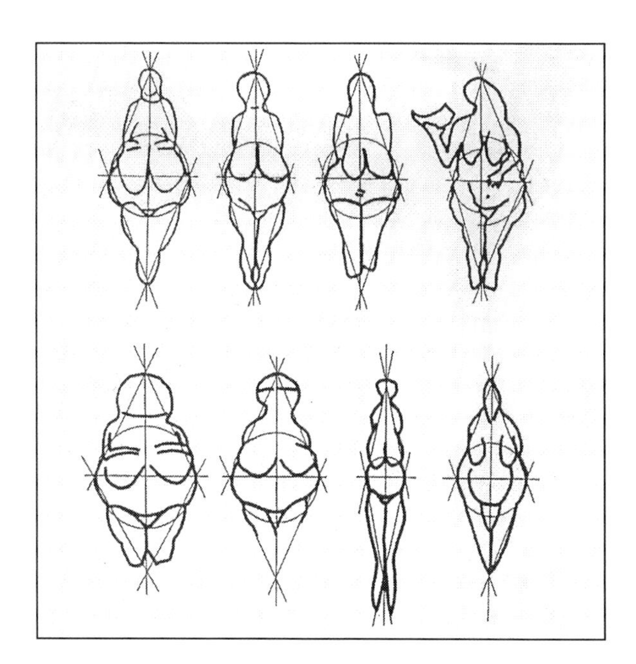

1-2 Similarity in features of several Paleolithic statuettes dating from 20,000 to 25,000 years ago that show obesity. Handbook of Obesity, © 2005 George A. Bray, MD.

Table 1-1. Paleolithic statuettes dating from 20,000 to 25,000 B.C.E. that show obesity

Name	Composition	Height(cm)	Location
Venus of Willendorf	Limestone	11	Austria
Venus of Lespugue	Ivory	14.7	Haute Garonne, France
Venus of Kostienki	Ivory	15.5	River Desna, Ukraine
Dolni Vestonice	Clay & ground bone	11	Moravia-Czech Republic
Venus of Laussel	Limestone relief		Dordogne, France
La Marche	Stone relief	42	Vienne, France (12,000)
Savignano	Serpentine marble	22.9	Savignano, Italy

One of these statuettes was found in southern France (Lespugue), two in Italy at Savignano, three in what was the Austro-Hungarian Empire (Dolni Vestonice[9], Moravany, and the Venus of Willendorf), and two in the Ukraine (Kostienki and Eliseevici). The similarity in design of these statues as shown in Figure 1-2 suggests that there may have been communication across Europe during the Ice Age in the Paleolithic period.

The height of these statues varies from about 1 inch (2 cm) to more than 10 inches (25 cm). The Venuses called Gagarino and Kostienki were found along the Volga River[8]. Both the Venus of Willendorf (Figure 1-3) and the Dolni Vestonice (Figure 1-4) were found along the Danube River in middle Europe.

The five limestone reliefs discovered at Laussel in the southern (Dordogne) region of France depict four obese women, one of whom is shown in Figure 1-5, and one obese man[5].

Several of these female statues had an additional feature; they have very large buttocks, also called *steatopygia*. This feature is more prominent here than in other statues from this period. At Brassempouy in France, three carved ivory statues were found in 1892 showing obese or steatopygic women. The statuettes carved in soapstone found at Grimaldi near Menton were also obese and steatopygic[5]. The Venus of Lespugue, made of ivory found near Haute Garonne in France in 1922, is one of the most perfect of this group[5].

The most distant member of this group is a fat plaster figure found at Tin Hinan in the Sahara Desert in Tunisia[5].

The meaning of these statues to their owners and to the cultures in which they lived has been the subject of intense controversy[5,6,10]. A French physician, Dr. Stephen-Chauvet, suggested that these obese figures with prominent buttocks might be "clinical" illustrations of endocrine, or glandular, disease that was present in Stone Age people[5]. Hautin, another Frenchman writing in 1939[3], interpreted these statues differently. He concluded that they proved the existence of obesity in Paleolithic times and that they also symbolized the expression and possible esthetic ideals of the period. Beller, in a much more recent book titled *Fat and Thin*, agrees with Hautin. She says, "The women immortalized in Stone Age sculpture were fat; there is no other word for it...[O]besity was already a fact of life for Paleolithic man—or at least for Paleolithic woman"[4].

Beller[4] also reached three other conclusions about obesity in Paleolithic times. First, the genes necessary for the development of corpulence were already present in the Paleolithic period of human development when the major event was likely to be hunger rather than surfeit. For people who had to hunt and gather their food, obesity could be an advantage in allowing them to store up food energy as fat for times when food was in short supply. In contrast, obesity would be a disadvantage for nomadic tribes who had to move from one place to another. The burden of carrying extra weight as fat slows an individual down and limits the amount she can carry and the distance she can carry it. Second, the wide geographic distribution of these figurines shows that adiposity could develop in many different regions of the world that had quite different diets derived from different plant and animal sources. This means that development of obesity did not require special foods or an agricultural society. Finally, the absence of corpulent male figures would fit with the present-day difference in the prevalence of corpulence in women as compared to men.

Another view of both the Paleolithic and Neolithic female figurines is as primordial female deities, reflecting the "bounty of the earth"[6,11,12]. In modern parlance, they are part of the view of obesity as a "feminist issue"[13]. This view of these "goddesses" has several proponents, including Melaart[14] and Gimbutas[6,15]. Their central idea is that a peaceful, goddess-centered culture existed in many places in the distant past and especially in "old Europe," Greece, Malta, Egypt, and the Near East. The end of the story tells of the takeover of her matriarchal society by warlike Indo-European males (ca. 3500 B.C.) and carries a strong moral subtext with women as the "goodies" and men as the "baddies"[6]. Lumping together the Paleolithic figures listed in Table 1-1, which were primarily located across middle Europe and separated by fifteen thousand years from the Neolithic figures (which are described below and located primarily in the Middle East), requires a major simplification that may lose important contexts for new interpretations of the data. These contrasting views are nicely summarized in a recent book of contributions to this problem by female archeologists[10]. Although there is clear evidence that obesity existed in the Old (Paleolithic) Stone Age, there is no evidence of how or if there was any effort to control obesity or whether it was looked at as a survival advantage.

C. The Battle of the Bulge in the New (Neolithic) Stone Age and Bronze Age

After an interval of nearly fifteen thousand years, a new wave of sculptures again appeared depicting obesity. This was in the New (Neolithic) Stone Age. Why this long interval? Did climatic and survival conditions eliminate corpulent individuals, thus removing the "model" for the artists? Did artistic preference change, or have examples from this period just not been found? We do not have the answer to these questions. However, in the Neolithic Stone Age, which spans the time from 8000 B.C. to approximately 5500 B.C., the battle of the bulge resumes as shown in corpulent figures from around the globe.

People in the Neolithic period introduced agriculture and established the first human settlements in Europe, Asia, and Meso-America. The Neolithic Age, along with the Copper (Chalcolithic) Age which continued to 3000 B.C., were notable for numerous corpulent statues or artifacts, often labeled as "Mother Goddesses"[6, 11, 12, 14]. One famous New Stone Age figure is made of clay and is called "Pazardzik." This figure was found in Thrace and dates from about 6000 B.C. (Figure 1-6).

She has a very large abdomen and hips and is sitting on a throne. Other artifacts showing obesity were found around the Mediterranean region, and particularly in Anatolia (currently Turkey) and Malta[2,16]. Finally, examples of corpulent figures from Meso-American cultures indicate that obesity or corpulence was worldwide even before the New World was discovered by Columbus in 1492.

1. Anatolia.

The region of Anatolia covers much of modern Turkey and has some of the richest finds of fat artifacts[17–20]. Probably the best-known finds were from the excavations at Çatalhöyük and the later ones from nearby Hacilar. These two cities were inhabited from about 6500 to 5600 BCE[14]. The thirty-two acres of excavations at Çatalhöyük make it one of the largest in Turkey. Most of the figurines found there are made of clay (terra cotta), but a few are made of limestone or alabaster (Figures 1-7 and 1-8).

Their corpulence is evident in the pendulous breasts and large fat deposits on the abdomen and hips.

These statues cover a wide range of sizes. Some are as short as 2.5 cm (1 inch), others are more than 24 cm (10 inches) tall, but most are in the middle. Probably the most famous is from Çatalhöyük, standing about 9 inches (20 cm) tall, which shows a woman sitting on a throne with two lions serving as her arm rests (Figure 1-8)[17, 19]. It is a very powerful image of a large imperial woman surrounded by two lions. Most of the figurines from this period show exaggerated hips, belly, and breasts.

The genital area is typically indicated by a triangular decoration, symbolizing motherhood and womankind.

One interpretation of these figures is that they are mother goddesses representing a matrilineal society. This proposition has been expounded in detail by Gimbutas[6].

Additional findings in the Çatalhöyük area in the 1990s have softened this interpretation. First, the places where these figures have been found are generally not in buildings associated with rituals. Second, whether these figures are women or men is often in doubt. There is also recent evidence that the hunter-gatherer role was more important in this culture than previously had been recognized. That is, the agricultural transition continued to depend in significant measure on hunting and gathering of food. Thus, the one clear conclusion that we can draw from these Neolithic Age figures is that obesity was evident in the New Stone Age culture as it had been in the Paleolithic Age fifteen thousand years earlier. This implies, as Beller noted earlier, that the genes needed for development of obesity were present from the earliest human history. From the available evidence it is not possible to establish a religious or "goddess" identity for these statues since they were distributed throughout villages with and without religious reference[17].

2. Malta

The settlers of Malta arrived from Sicily about 5000 B.C.E. and contact continued for up to fifteen hundred years[20]. Corpulent figurines from Malta are abundant and occur in several sizes. The smaller clay figures appear to be related to family units. Larger, almost life-sized, figures of clay or stone measuring up to 2 meters (6 feet) in height were found in public areas and were clearly intended for some visible function in the society. However, we don't yet know what the nature of the relationship of these statues to society was. The small sleeping woman from Malta is shown in figure 1-9.

Many of these are larger than the earlier ones found in Turkey and the Middle East. Stone is a common material used in their sculpture[20]. Making such large figures took a great deal of time and effort since the tools they used were also stone or copper and suggests that they were important to the culture in some as yet poorly understood way.

3. Eastern Mediterranean

The Neolithic period in Crete has left us with a number of examples of corpulent women. As with most of the other New Stone Age cultures, we have no clear idea of whether these figures were secular or religious in origin.

4. Middle East

Neolithic period pottery from around ten thousand years ago near the Tigris and Euphrates Rivers has left many examples of obesity. The settlement at Ain Ghazal near Amman, Jordan, produced pottery statuettes of obese women, standing about 6 inches (15 cm) tall[21]. They do not appear to represent pregnancy nor have they been associated with the cult of the female goddesses[22]. Other Stone Age statues, such as the one from the museum at Aleppo representing a corpulent woman from the latter part of the Neolithic Age, indicate the wide dissemination of the idea of obesity but do not help us to discern its precise cultural meaning.

The widespread distribution of the Eurasian artifacts showing obesity again allows us to conclude that obesity has been part of the human condition for many eons. The women whose bodily features are preserved in the statues reflect the interaction of a genotype that is capable of storing fat and a society where surpluses of food were frequent enough for them to store the fat that could help them survive the times of inadequate food. A genetically thrifty phenotype was at work. This phenotype had particular value during most of human history when famines occurred and when the nomadic existence where obesity is a disadvantage was exchanged for the agricultural existence that depended on raising crops.

5. Indus River Civilizations of South Asia

The Neolithic Age in the Indus Valley, in what is now Pakistan, also shows the presence of obesity in clay figures. Wheeler describes the makers of these obese terra-cotta figurines as "enjoying a sense of humor." In his book there is a picture of a "fat woman" with a large abdomen and hips[23]. The interpretation of obesity as a humorous subject has been a recurring one. Whether these early cultures disapproved of obesity, or disliked the people who were obese, is unknown. This important issue and the artistic representation of obesity in more modern times are examined later in this book. There is no record of what, if anything, was done to fight the battle of the bulge during Neolithic times.

6. Meso-American Neolithic Artifacts

Prior to the "discovery" of the New World by Columbus in 1492, there were three high cultures in the Meso-American world[24–26]. The Incas occupied the highlands along the west coast of what is now Peru in South America. The Mayan culture occupied the Yucatan Peninsula and surrounding areas of Central America, and the Aztecs controlled the high plateaus of Central America. When Columbus, Cortez, Pizarro, and their fellow explorers arrived in the New World, they brought several devastating diseases, including measles, smallpox, and chicken pox, which were more lethal than the military might of the invaders. The pre-Columbian Americans were still "Stone Age" cultures. However, they were highly sophisticated in their knowledge of mathematics, astronomy, written language, and medicine. The New World proved to be a rich source of new foods and medicines for Europe. Columbus and other explorers brought back corn, tomatoes, potatoes, and useful plants for treating disease. These included *Cinchona* bark, the source of quinine that was used to treat fevers, including malaria. At this time, diseases were believed to be caused by the supernatural and magical, and treatment was directed at these natural and supernatural causes. Sculptured artifacts are one of the sources of information about disease in pre-Columbian societies. These figurines represent malnutrition, deformity, and physical illness. As well as suffering from various diseases including spinal defects, endemic goiter, eye diseases, and skin ailments, they also suffered from obesity.

In Meso-America the major evidence for obesity comes from pottery statues from the so-called "Formative" or "Preclassic" period (1600 B.C. to A.D. 200). By the beginning of this period agriculture was widespread. Small, sedentary, and self-sufficient communities were well established. Human skeletal remains from this period show that the average man was short, with the average man being only 5 foot 4 inches, (164 cm) tall and an average woman being even shorter at 5 feet (153 cm). Numerous pottery finds from the early Preclassic Mayan culture show marked enlargement of the thighs, what we would call lower segment or pear-shaped obesity. Women with abdominal fat are also abundantly represented.

Other examples are found in other cultures. The Gulf Coast Olmec and Huasteca cultures produced many examples of corpulence. From the preclassic Olmec period an 18-cm pottery figurine referred to as "baby face" has fat legs and a fat abdomen. The Huasteca culture also provided several examples of obesity in pottery figures that are about the size and shape of the Venus of Willendorf (4–75 cm tall). There are also several examples of women with large thighs standing 4–10 cm tall.

What these Meso-American figurines tell us is that both central (apple-shaped) and peripheral (pear-shaped) forms of obesity were well known in the sedentary agricultural societies at the beginning of the cultural expansion in Central America. Even in the classic period of Mayan culture, dating from A.D. 650–800, obesity is evident.

In the classic period, arts reached a high level. A statue from this period in the Art Institute of Chicago shows an obese, round-bellied man. The statue is beautifully sculpted with headdress and ornaments. The bare bulging belly and the lifelike features suggest that it may be a portrait in pottery of one of the higher-level individuals, in whom we might expect more obesity because food was more available (Figure 1-10).

D. Conclusions

We have traveled from the Old Stone Age more than twenty thousand years ago when the Venus of Willendorf was made down through the New Stone age and Copper Age ending in the agricultural communities of early pre-history. In addition to showing that corpulence has a history as long as mankind, this survey of obesity in the Old and New Stone Ages also shows some other important things. First, almost all of the figures were either female or their sex could not be identified. Only two males, one from Laussel in France, and the one above were noted in this survey. Although these figures have been touted as examples of "mother goddesses," there is another interpretation proposed by Dr. Stephen-Chauvet who suggested that they are examples of glandular or endocrine disease evident before recorded history. Beller goes further, suggesting that these figures tell us that human beings knew about obesity and that the genetic basis for its development, independent of the type of diet, was present in early human cultures. Finally, these figures are distributed worldwide and in all cultures except Africa. The reason for the lack of such figures from Africa is unknown. It could be that obesity didn't appear in the culture for climatic reasons of increased heat; it may be that artists had other things to represent. We just don't know. The high prevalence of "obesity" in the Pre-Columbian statues from Central and South America is consistent with the high prevalence of this problem among the descendants of these pre-Columbian peoples of North and South America. In careful surveys, the prevalence of obesity in Latinos, many of whom are descendants of these early indigenous American peoples, is higher than in those of European ancestry. Although this survey shows us that the "battle of the bulge" has a long history, we have no information on how or if it was treated in these early periods. We will now turn to the historical record, where there is abundant evidence that obesity has been a medical and health concern as long as medicine has been practiced.

References

1. Gaarder, J. *Sophie's World. A Novel about the History of Philosophy.* Transl. P. Moller. London: Phoenix House, 1995.
2. Angell, W. *Die Venus von Willendorf.* Wien: Editions Wien. 1989.
3. Hautin, R.J.R. *Obésité. Conceptions actuelle. Thèse pour le Doctorat en Médecine.* Bordeaux: Imprimerie Bier, 1939.
4. Beller, A.S. *Fat & Thin: A Natural History of Obesity.* New York: Farrar, Straus and Giroux, 1977.
5. Stephen-Chauvet. *La médecine chez les peuples primitifs.* Paris: Librairie Maloine, 1936.
6. Gimbutas, M. *The Living Goddesses.* Ed. M.R. Dexter. Berkeley: University of California Press, 1999.
7. Bray, G.A. "Obesity in Historical Perspective." In *Handbook of Obesity.* Ed. G.A. Bray, C. Bouchard. New York: Elsevier, 2004.
8. Clark, G. *The Stone Age Hunters.* London: Thames and Hudson Ltd., 1967.
9. Gamble, C. *The Paleolithic Settlement of Europe.* Cambridge: Cambridge University Press, 1986.
10. Goodison, L.C. Morris. "Beyond the Great Mother: The Sacred World of the Minoans." In *Ancient Goddesses: The Myths and the Evidence.* London: British Museum, 1998.
11. Husain, S. *The Goddess. An Illustrated Guide to the Divine Feminine.* London: Duncan Baird Publishers, 1997.
12. Neumann, E. *The Great Mother. An Analysis of the Archetype.* 2nd edition. Transl. R. Manheim. Princeton: Princeton Bollinger, 1972.
13. Ohrbach, S. *Fat Is a Feminist Issue: The Anti-Diet Guide to Permanent Weight Loss.* New York: Paddington Press Ltd., 1978.
14. Melaart, J. *Earliest Civilizations of the Middle East.* London: Thames and Hudson, Ltd., 1965.
15. Gimbutas, M. *The Language of the Goddess.* London: Thames & Hudson. 1989.
16. *The Golden Age of Chinese Archeology: Celebrated Discoveries from the People's Republic of China.* Washington, D.C.: National Gallery of Art, 1999.
17. Kulacoglu, B. *Museum of Anatolian Civilizations. Gods and Goddesses.* Transl. J. Ozturk. Ankara: Museum of Anatolian Civilizations, 1992.

18 Seton, L. *Early Highland Peoples of Anatolia.* London: Thames and Hudson Ltd., 1967.

19. Meskell, L. "Twin Peak: The Archaeologies of Çatalhöyük." In *Ancient Goddesses: The Myths and the Evidence.* Eds. Goodison, C., L. Morris. London: British Museum, 1998.
20. Malone, C. "God or Goddess: The Temple Art of Ancient Malta." In

Ancient Goddesses: The Myths and the Evidence. Ed. Goodison, L., C. Morris. London: British Museum, 1998.

21. *Treasures from an Ancient Land: The Art of Jordan*. Ed. P. Bienkowski. Gloucestershire: Alan Sutton Publishing, 1991.
22. Westenholz, J.G. "Goddesses of the Ancient Near East 3000-1000 BC." *In Ancient Goddesses: The Myths and the Evidence*. Eds. Goodison, L., C. Morris. London British Museum Press, 1998.
23. Wheeler, M. *Civilizations of the Indus Valley and Beyond*. London: Thames and Hudson Ltd., 1966.
24. Moll, R.G., M.S. Cuesta. *Tlatilco de muheres bonitas, hombres y dioses*. Mexico: Circolo de Arte, 1998.
25. Bernal, I. *The Mexican National Museum of Anthropology*. Transl. C.B. Czitrom. Panorama Editorial S.A., 1999.
26. *The Olmec World: Ritual and Rulership*. Princeton: The Art Museum, 1995.

Chapter 2

The Bulge before Printing (3000 B.C. to A.D. 1500)

He who cannot draw on three thousand years is living from hand to mouth.

—Goethe[1]

When you are "sick" you want help. When you "bulge" you want help. For us this means calling the doctor, going to an emergency room, seeking information on the Internet, or getting advice from myriad popular magazines. It has not always been so. Although medical traditions have developed in all cultures, we know much more than our ancestors, even those living ten and twenty years ago[2-5]. To understand how the battle of the bulge has been waged at various times in history, we need to have some understanding of these various medical traditions. Several of them are described in the following pages, along with evidence that people were aware of the bulge more than three thousand years ago.

We find obesity in all medical traditions and geographic regions, except possibly Africa, which suggests that, independent of diet, the potential to turn food into fat evolved even before we have an historical record documenting this fact[6-8].

The development of agriculture, metallurgy, writing systems, and political structures all influence the level of sophistication within each culture. Several of the most sophisticated cultures have developed between two great river systems, and this has given rise to the "two rivers" hypothesis of cultural development. This hypothesis implies that we should look for higher levels of cultural sophistication where two rivers parallel each other. Some of these pairs of rivers are the Yellow River and the Yangtse River in China, the Ganges and Indus rivers in India, the Amu Darya and Syr Darya rivers in Central Asia, and the Tigris and Euphrates rivers in the Fertile Crescent, which includes Iraq, in the Middle East. In all of these regions there have been many examples of the "bulge" and of efforts to battle it.

A. Mesopotamian Medicine

The Tigris and Euphrates river basin was the land of healers and astrologers. Cuneiform writing, libraries, sanitation, and medical knowledge were evident by 3600 B.C. Of the thirty thousand clay tablets with cuneiform writing that were recovered in the library at Nineveh from approximately 2000 B.C., eight hundred are related to medical matters. The medical armamentarium of Sumerian physicians consisted of more than one hundred twenty minerals and two hundred fifty herbs, including cannabis, mustard, mandragora, belladonna, and henbane[9]. In this advanced culture, we find one of the best-known examples of a corpulent figure, which is shown in Figure 2-1. It was so popular that many copies were made.

Several other examples will serve to make the point that the bulge, and possible early efforts to battle it, were well recognized in the Babylonian-Sumerian Period (3000–1500 B.C.). A clay statuette showing enormously fat thighs and arms is another example of the problem we are fighting.

B. Egyptian Medicine

Paralleling the Mesopotamian medical tradition was the tradition of Egyptian medicine (3000–1000 B.C.). The physicians in Egypt were often priests, and many priests were physicians. For example, Imhotep, who became the god of healing, began as a vizier, or trusted adviser, to King Zoser in 2900 B.C. Imhotep was a man of great accomplishment who, in addition to being a physician, was also an architect, a poet, and a statesman. Two major archeological finds, the Edwin Smith papyrus[12] written between 2500 and 2000 B.C. and the Ebers papyrus written approximately 1550 B.C., provide our major knowledge about medicine in Egypt. The bulge was known to the Egyptians, and there may well have been attempts to battle it, particularly among the ruling classes. A study of royal mummies showed that both stout women (queens Henut-Tawy and Inhapy) and stout men were not uncommon in Egypt among the upper classes. Culturally, "obesity was regarded as objectionable"[13] since the ideal depicted in their art was the thin stylized body. Several examples of obesity are also seen in the stone reliefs, which were the principal artistic medium: a doorkeeper in one temple of Amon-Ra Khor-en-Khonsu complex; a cook in another tomb of Ankh-ma-Hor complex (Sixth Dynasty of the Middle Kingdom 2613–2181 B.C.)[14]; a fat man enjoying food presented to him by his lean servants in Mereruka's tomb; the local yeoman, the famed Sheikh et Balad[13]; and the grossly obese harpist playing before the prince Aki at the time of the Middle Kingdom[15]. Studies of the skin fold thickness of mummies using x-rays showed that Amenophis III and Ramses III were fat[15].

Several statues are carved in black granite. One of the most interesting figures is that of the Queen of Punt from the temple of Queen Hatshepsut, Deir el-Bahri (Eighteenth Dynasty). She has markedly prominent buttocks (steatopygia) and appears to have shortening of the lower extremities, suggesting *dyschondroplasia* or dislocated hips[13-16].

One example of this is type of deformity is shown in this Cypriot representation of the Egyptian god Bes from the sixth century B.C. (Figure 2-2)

C. Chinese and Tibetan Medicine

The early Chinese believed that disease was sent by the gods or by demons. From the examination of bone fragments from Chinese graves, we know that the Chinese suffered from leprosy, typhoid fever, cholera, and plague. Although anatomic dissection was not permitted in China because of ancestor worship, the Chinese nonetheless developed a vigorous medical tradition. Herbal medicines were very important to the ancient Chinese. Their physicians could select from at least 365 herbal medicines. The principal source of early medical teachings was the *Yellow Emperor's Inner Canon (Hung Tu Hei Ching),* which dates from 200 B.C. and is a dialogue on bodily functions and disease. The father of Chinese medicine is Zhang Zhongjing, who is considered the Chinese equivalent of the Greek Hippocrates in Western civilization. Zhang described symptoms and treatment for many diseases. Hua Toh (third century A.D.) is the only known surgeon from early China. Acupuncture, the art of treatment by inserting sharp needles into the body, was developed in China and reached its zenith there. An acupuncture site on the earlobe is said to reduce appetite and may have been a treatment in the battle of the bulge.

Obesity was common among the upper classes in the Tang Dynasty (618–907 A.D.). During the first half of the Tang Dynasty, the female courtesans were physically active and were particularly skillful on horseback. During the second half of this dynasty, they lost interest in physical activity, and horseback riding by the women was largely abandoned. Corpulence followed. This is nicely illustrated in a series of beautiful porcelain figures of women at court[18]. These figures stand nearly 20 inches (50 cm) tall. These elegantly painted porcelain figures clearly show "portly" or "plump" women dressed in long flowing gowns with well-coiffed hairstyles (Figure 2-3).

The Tibetan offspring of the Chinese medical tradition is beautifully illustrated in the seventeenth century treatise titled *The Blue Beryl,* composed by Sangye Gyamtso, the scholar and regent of Tibet. It is an erudite yet practical commentary on the ancient text entitled *The Four Tantras*[19]. In this text, the bulge is described as a condition requiring catabolic treatment (breakdown of fat tissue), documenting that in this medical tradition there was a battle against the bulge:

> [O]vereating...causes illness and shortens life span. It is a contraindication to the use of compresses or mild enemas. For treatment of obesity two suggestions are made...The

> vigorous massage of the body with pea flour counteracts phlegm diseases and obesity...The gullet hair compress and flesh of a wolf remedy [treat] goiters, dropsy and obesity[19].

D. Indian Medicine

A fourth great medical tradition is that of India[17]. In the sacred medical texts of Ayurvedic medicine, sin was viewed as the cause of disease and medical knowledge was closely interwoven with religion and magic. The *Caraka Samhita* was the first book on Indian medicine and the *Susruta Samhita* was the second great medical Indian Sanskrit text. These texts describe many aspects of medical practice. For example, the *Caraka Samhita* describes 20 sharp and 101 blunt instruments used in surgery, as well as an operating table. For non-surgical treatment, at least five hundred drugs are listed along with seven hundred medical herbs. Included in this list are cinnamon, borax, castor oil, ginger, and sodium carbonate. A tactic in the battle of the bulge is mentioned in the *Ayurveda* and consists of administrating testicular tissue (organotherapy) as a cure for impotence as well as a treatment for obesity[20].

The Indian sculpture has many corpulent figures that demonstrate the presence of obesity. One of the most impressive is the representation of a laughing Buddha lounging on his right arm (Figure 2-4).

E. Greco-Roman Medicine

From the vantage point of Western civilization, Greco-Roman medicine has been the major source of our medical tradition. Greco-Roman medicine also provides lessons for the battle of the bulge. The health hazards associated with obesity were clearly noted in the medical writings of Hippocrates. He stated that "sudden death is more common in those who are naturally fat than in the lean"[21]. The Greeks also noted that obesity was a cause of infertility in women and that the frequency of menses was reduced in the obese.

Sleep apnea is a condition with snoring at night that obstructs breathing with occasional periods with no breaths and a compensatory sleepiness during the daytime. Sleep apnea is particularly likely to occur as a complication of the bulge. The first descriptions of this complication associated with obesity date from Roman times. Dionysius, the tyrant of Heracleia of Pontius who reigned about 360 B.C., is one of the first historical figures afflicted with obesity and somnolence. When this enormously fat man frequently fell asleep, his servants would insert long needles through his skin and fat to the muscle beneath to jolt him into wakefulness. Kryger cites a second case of Magas, King of Cyrene, who died in 258 B.C. He was a man "weighted down with monstrous masses of flesh in his last days; in fact he choked himself to death"[22,23].

Artistic representations show the similarity of the Greco-Roman culture to those of its neighbors and predecessors with respect to corpulence. The first is a clay figure from Boetia showing an obese woman sitting in a chair. We have seen a similar example in the Neolithic period from the excavations at Çatalhöyük in modern-day Turkey.

The final example comes from the Palmyran culture, which was between Rome and the Persian Sassanids to the east along the Tigris River. For the wealthy, the tops to the funeral coffins were carved with likenesses of the owners. One of these in Palmyra, Syria, shows the owner with a clear abdominal paunch. This is one of the few men showing obesity that I have found, and in this instance it is a reflection of the wealth of the individual and the associated opportunities to stress the old genetic machinery geared for times of starvation with a culinary experience of surfeit.

Galen was the leading physician of Roman times. His influence on medicine and medical teaching lasted more than one thousand years. He identified two types of obesity; one he called "moderate" and the other "immoderate." The former is regarded as natural and the other as morbid. By this he meant it was associated with the development of other serious diseases.

Being overweight was often associated with the upper classes in Roman culture, as it has been in other cultures throughout history. A letter written to the Roman historian Tacitus by Pliny the Younger describing the eruption of Mount Vesuvius that destroyed erupted Pompeii in A.D. 79 describes both his uncle, Pliny the elder who was admiral of the fleet, and his mother as fat.

> ....Mount Vesuvius was blazing in several places with spreading and towering flames, whose refulgent brightness the darkness of the night set in high relief. But my uncle [Pliny the Elder, admiral of the fleet], in order to soothe apprehensions, kept saying that some fires had been left alight by the terrified country people, and what they saw were only deserted villas on fire in the abandoned district. After this he retired to rest, and it is most certain that this rest was a most genuine slumber: for his breathing, which, as he was pretty fat, was somewhat heavy and sonorous, was heard by those who attended at his chamber-door.

This sonorous and heavy breathing might be interpreted as a precursor to the respiratory problem of sleep apnea that is discussed in Chapter 23. Further on Pliny the Younger says about his mother as she urged him to flee:

> My mother began to beseech, exhort, and command me to escape as best I might: a young man could do it: she, burdened with age and corpulence, would die easy if only she

> had not caused my death. (Melmoth-Hutchinson translation, quoted in Wolfgang Leppmann's *Pompeii in Fact and Fiction*, London, 1968).

The approach of the physician to the battle of the bulge can be traced to Greek and Roman times. From the time of Hippocrates twenty-five hundred years ago[24] and Clarissimus Galen (A.D.131-201) at the height of the Roman Empire[25] in the prescientific era, diet and exercise were an integral part of the therapeutic regimen for obese patients. Hippocrates, the "Father of Medicine," (Figure 2-5) suggested in the fifth century B.C. that

> [o]bese people and those desiring to lose weight should perform hard work before food. Meals should be taken after exertion and while still panting from fatigue and with no other refreshment before meals except only wine, diluted and slightly cold. Their meals should be prepared with sesame or seasoning and other similar substances and be of a fatty nature as people get thus satiated with little food. They should, moreover, eat only once a day and take no baths and sleep on a hard bed and walk naked as long as possible[24].

Galen, nearly two thousand years ago, outlined his approach to treatment of the obese as follows:

> I have made any sufficiently stout patient moderately thin in a short time, by compelling him to do rapid running, then wiping off his perspiration with very soft or very rough muslin and then massaging him maximally with diaphoretic inuctions, which the younger doctors customarily call restoratives, and after such massage leading him to the bath after which I give him nourishment immediately but bade him rest for a while or do nothing to which he was accustomed, then lead him to a second bath and then gave him abundant food of little nourishment so as to fill him up but distribute little of it to the entire body[25].

F. Arabic Medicine

With the decline of Roman influence after A.D. 400 scholarly activity shifted from Rome to Byzantium and then to the broader Arabic world following the rise of Islam in the seventh century. One of the leading figures of this medical tradition was Abu Ali ibn Sina, or Avicenna in its Westernized form. Like Galen he was an influential scholarly author who published more than

40 medical works and 145 works on philosophy, logic, theology, and other subjects. Obesity was well known to this Arabic physician.

From the Greco-Roman beginning, dietary treatment in the battle of the bulge can be traced to the Arabic tradition in medicine. In the first book of Avicenna's five-volume *Canon*, he describes how to reduce the overweight individual:

> The regimen which will reduce obesity. (1) Produce a rapid descent of the food from the stomach and intestines, in order to prevent completion of absorption by the mesentery. (2) Take food which is bulky but feebly nutritious. (3) Take the bath before food, often. (4) Hard exercise....[26]

As we can see, the idea of diet and exercise as the bulwarks in the battle of the bulge have an ancient history. Had they accomplished what their authors intended, we would have effective strategies, and the current quest might not have been needed. However, the fact that we have an epidemic of obesity today that is covering the globe suggests that the strategically simple ideas of eating less and exercising more, ideas that require commitment and personal involvement by the individual, have not been very successful. As we move forward in trying to understand the battle of the bulge, we need to be alert to strategies and tactics that may not require individual motivation and commitment—history has shown that they do not work well.

In this chapter we have explored obesity and some of its treatments from the beginning of written language through the time when printing was introduced. We can conclude that obesity was worldwide from the earliest recorded medical traditions. Quantitatively we are ahead, but the problem still existed five thousand years ago and earlier. Changes in diet and exercise were major recommendations. The early descriptions of obesity reinforce the conclusions of Beller cited earlier. As she noted, obesity has been present in both historic and prehistoric times. It has developed in cultures eating widely divergent diets, meaning that specific foods are neither necessary nor preventive. Finally, the genes for enlargement of fat cells that predispose us to a battle of the bulge were present in the earliest Stone Age cultures and continued through the period of written history.

Biosketch

Clarissimus Galen A.D. 131–201 was one of the most influential physicians of Western history. He was born in Pergamon on the western coast in what is now modern Turkey, probably in A.D. 131.

This was at the height of the Roman Empire, and Galen became its most famous physician. Osler captured his lofty medical standing in these words:

> No other physician has ever occupied the commanding position of Cl[arissimus] Galen. For fifteen centuries he dominated medical thought powerfully as did Aristotle in the school of the day. Not until the Renaissance did daring spirits begin to question the infallibility of this medical Pope. He was the last, and, in many ways, the greatest of the Greeks—a man very much of our own type, who, could he visit this country today, might teach us many lessons[27].

Galen was born into an affluent family at a time of relative peace in the Roman Empire. His father spared no expense on his son's education, sending him to study in Greece at the School of the Stoics, at the School of the Academicians, at the School of the Peripatetics, and finally with the School of the Epicureans. He had many of the famous physicians of his time as his mentors, but he outshone all of them. He was appointed physician to the gladiators, which provided him with considerable clinical exposure to traumatic wounds. He spent at least two periods of his life in Rome. Periodically he returned to Pergamon, the city of his birth in Turkey. His published output was prodigious and speaks to an unquenchable internal drive to write. We can account for more than four hundred works on medicine, and there were books on other subjects as well. However, only eighty-three works survive[2].

Galen could be called a "teleologic dogmatist" since he believed that "Nature acts with perfect wisdom and does nothing uselessly"[2]. Although he did many experiments, his teleologic approach to understanding medicine left no experimental heritage for the future.

His ego matched his scholarly output. As Professor Selwyn-Brown observed about Galen in his book on great medical personalities,

> His style was forceful and persuasive, but it was also pugnacious...Galen's enthusiasm and conceit led him to class all writers who disagreed with him as fools, and this unfortunate capacity for making enemies kept him continually embroiled with his fellow doctors[28].

Another medical historian, Castiglioni, noted that "[h]e often magnified in exaggerated terms his diagnostic and therapeutic successes"[2]. He is reputed to have said, "No one before me has given the true method of treating diseases." Galen considered himself the greatest of all physicians, just as his contemporary the Emperor Trajan considered himself the greatest of all Roman emperors. Galen's scholarly impact is clear from the fact that his work was still used in European medical education into the seventeenth century.

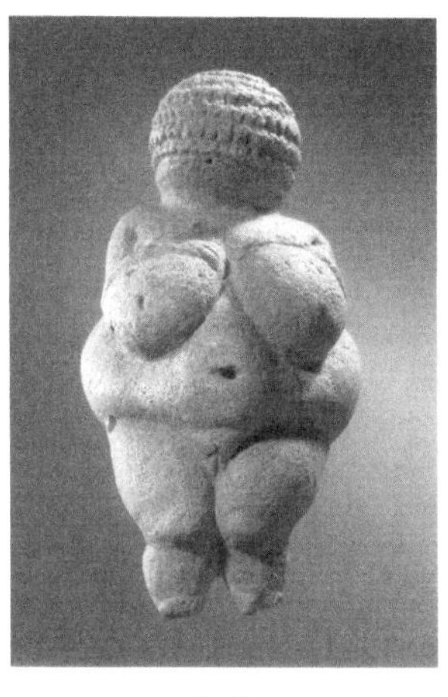

1-3

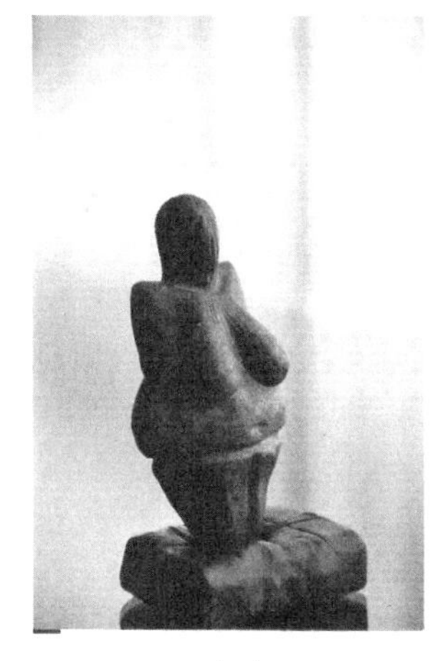

1-4

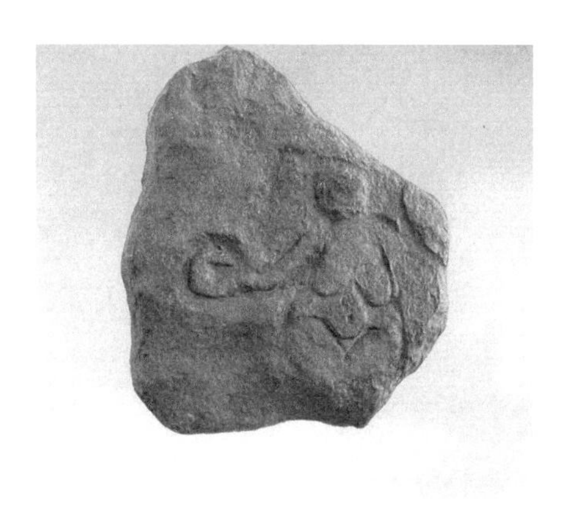

1-5

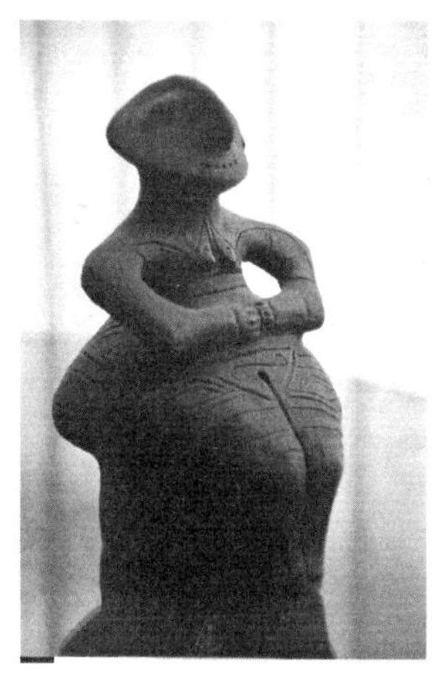

1-6

1-3 Copy of the Venus of Willendorf. This small Paleolithic statuette was unearthed in Willendorf, Austria, approximately 20,000 to 25,000 years ago. The original is in the Vienna Museum of Natural History. From the collection of the author.

1-4 Copy of the Venus of Dolni Vestonice. From the collection of the author.

1-5 Venus of Laussel. Bas-relief found in Dordogne in southern France. Courtesy of Museum für Vor-und Frühgeschichte der Staatlichen Museen zu Berlin.

1-6 Copy of the Venus of Padzarzik, a Copper Age clay statue from the mid-5th millennium found in Pazardzik, and thus called the Pazardzik Venus. From the collection of the author.

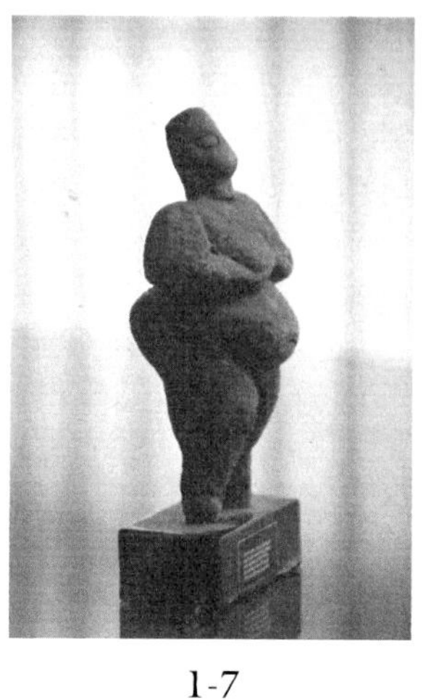

1-7

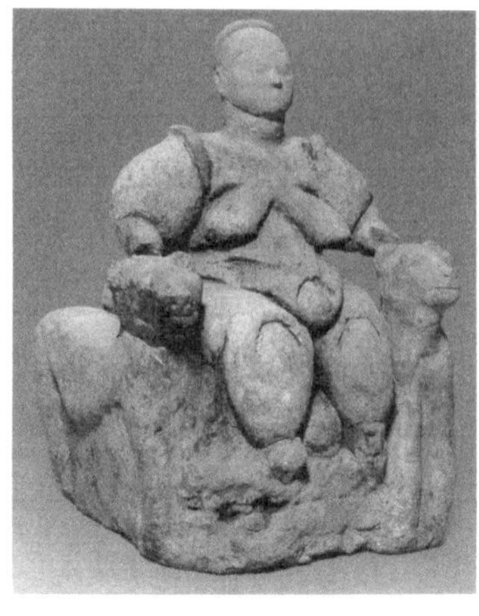

1-8

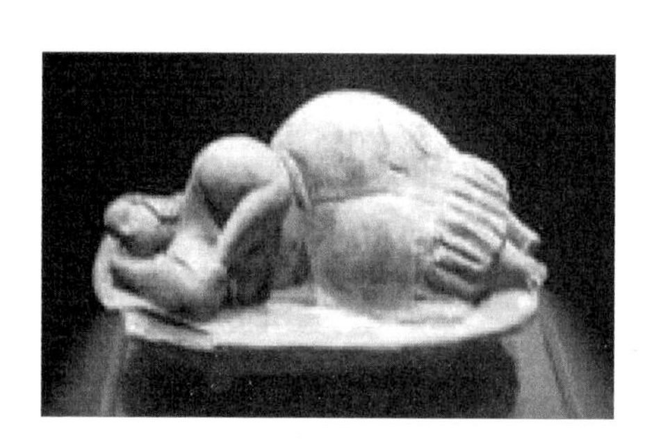

1-9

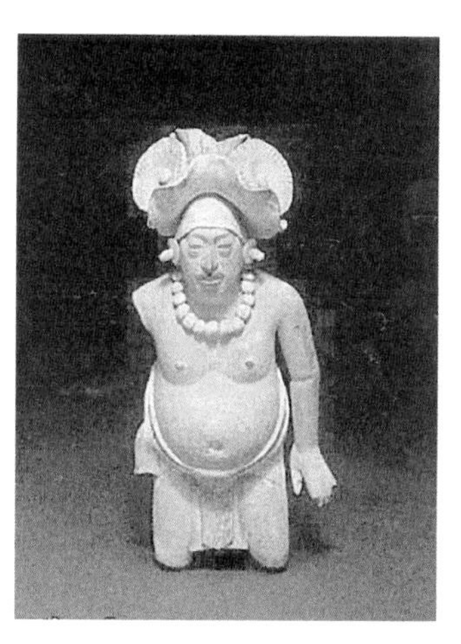

1-10

1-7 Copy of a Venus statuette from Hacilar made in the late Neolithic stone age about 6000 BCE. From the collection of the author.

1-8 Copy of a baked clay statuette of an overweight goddess flanked by 2 lions from 5750 BCE. From the collection of the author.

1-9 Sleeping woman from Malta. From the collection of the author.

1-10 Kneeling male Mayan figure from the Classic period. Courtesy of The Art Institute of Chicago.

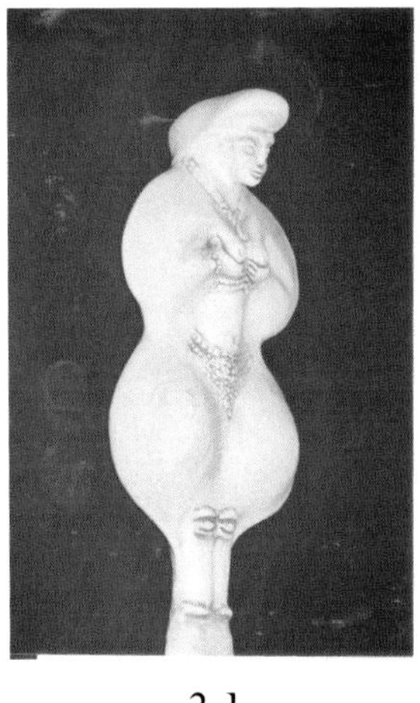

2-1

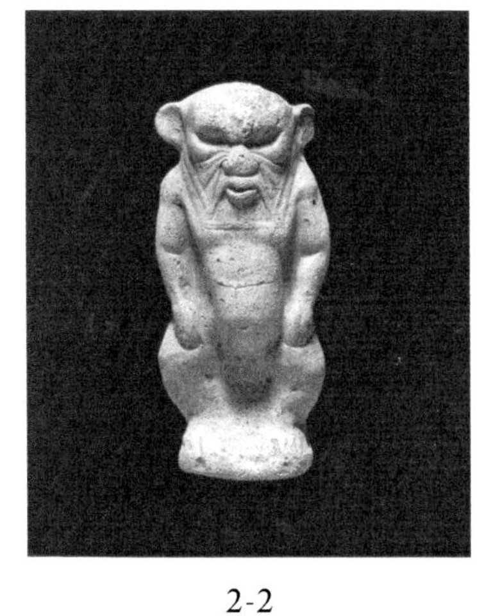

2-2

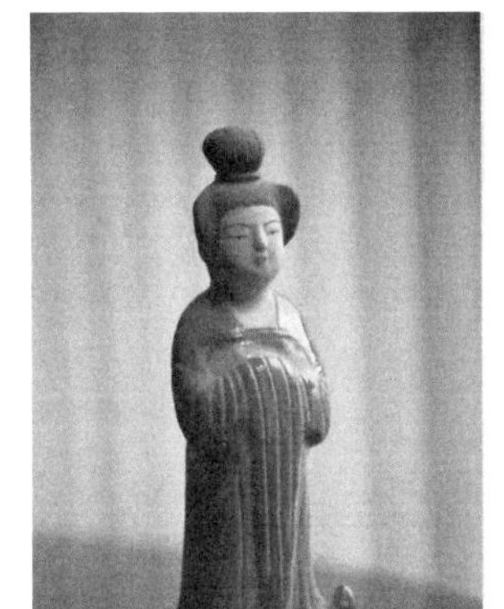

2-3

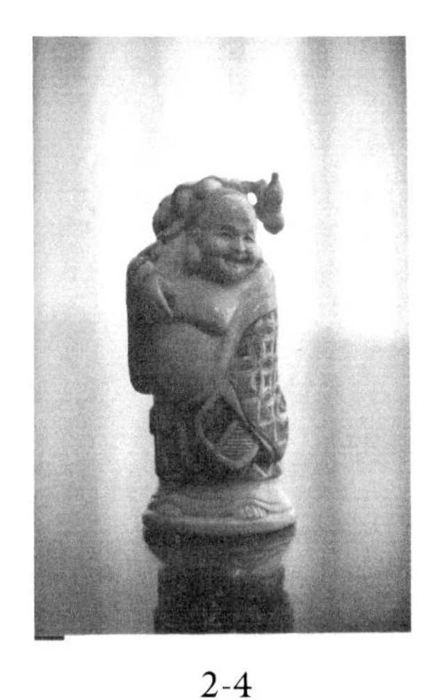

2-4

2-1 Copy of a nude female figurine from Ur in Mesopotamia. From the collection of the author.

2-2 Goddess Bes. Courtesy of Musée de Louvre.

2-3 Copy of a figure from the Tang Dynasty in China. From the collection of the author.

2-4 Laughing Buddha. From the collection of the author.

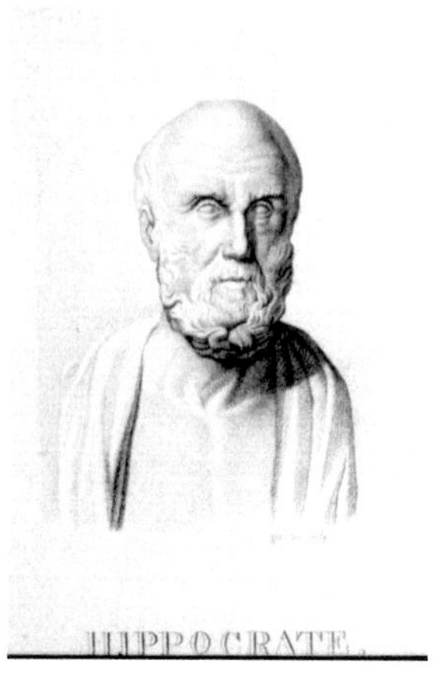

2-5

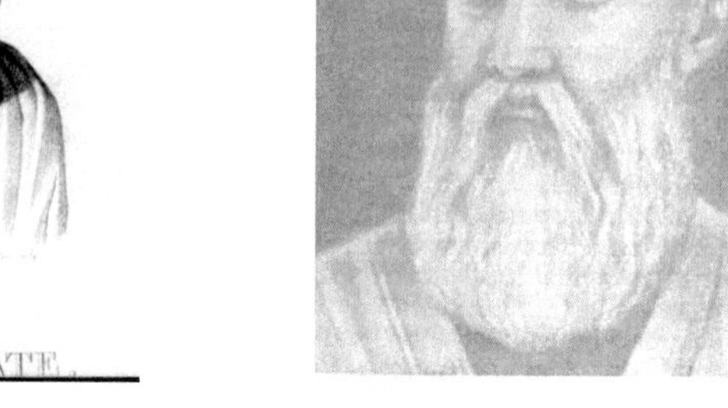

2-6

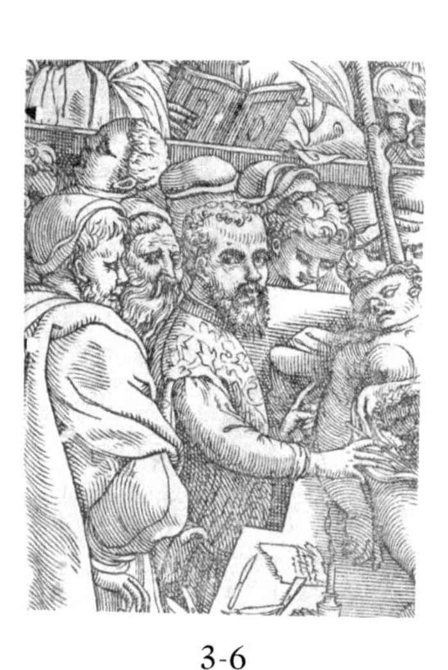

3-6

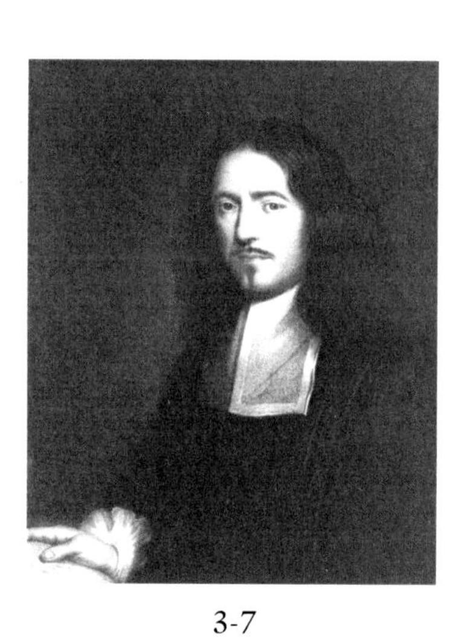

3-7

2-5 Hippocrates. Courtesy of the National Library of Medicine.

2-6 Abu-Ali al-Husayn ibn-Abd-allah ibn-Sina (Avicenna). Courtesy of the National Library of Medicine.

3-6 Andreas Vesalius from frontispiece of the 1555 edition of *De Humani Corporis Fabrica*. From the collection of the author.

3-7 Marcello Malphighi (1628-1694). Courtesy of the National Library of Medicine.

Galen's system of disease evolved from the humoral ideas of Hippocrates and the four elements—fire, air, earth, and water. Bleeding was important in the therapeutic armamentarium of Galen. Galen also believed strongly in the use of diet as an approach to treating obesity [Chapter 20][25].

Biosketch

Abu- 'Ali al-Husayn ibn-'Abd-allah ibn-Sina (Latinized as Avicenna) (980–1037) was born in Afshana near Bokhara in what is now the central Asian country of Uzbekistan. The Arab lands of those days extended from Spain in the west to central Asia in the east. The time of Avicenna's birth was one of intellectual ferment in Bokhara that saw a flowering of talent in many fields. (Figure 2-6)

According to Avicenna's "self-conscious autobiography" written at the age of 18, he had memorized the Koran by age 10 and was a practicing doctor by age 16. He is alleged to have successfully treated Amir Nuh ibn-Mansur Al-Samani, prince of Khorasan, the ruler of Bokhara. His success gave him access to the Amir's library, which was reputed to be the second best in the world. Avicenna's scholarship extended into many areas, including religion, law, metaphysics, mathematics, astronomy, and medicine. The instability of the local governments in central Asia led him to take up arms to fight in military campaigns. His military life resulted in riotous living followed by a long severe illness and his eventual death at the age of fifty-seven in 1037.

Avicenna's masterpiece is his five-volume work on medicine called the *Canon* on medicine (*Kitab al-Qanun*) that was translated into Latin in the eleventh century by Gerard of Cremona and used in Western medical education until at least the seventeenth century. The *Canon* contains no personal experiences and no new ideas, but rather was a summary of existing knowledge. The first book deals with theoretical medicine, including physiology, etiology, symptomatology, disease classification (nosology), and the principles of therapy. The second book is largely about hygiene and hygienic matters. The third book is on localized diseases and their treatment, and the fourth book is about generalized diseases and their treatment. The final book deals with herbal treatments called *materia medica* and is a dispensary and an apothecary's book.

Avicenna surpassed both Aristotle and Galen in his dialectical subtlety[29,30]. By some estimates he published more than one hundred medical books, as well as many volumes in other areas. Avicenna's attempt to reconcile the doctrines of Galen with those of Aristotle is similar to the effort of the intellectual Catholic scholar St. Thomas Aquinas to reconcile these authors with the teachings of the Roman Catholic Church some two centuries later. The influence of the *Canon* on Western medicine was on the whole bad, for "it confirmed physicians in the pernicious idea that the use of syllogisms and logic is a better way to solve problem than first-hand observation and investigation" of nature[9]. Albrecht van Haller in the eighteenth century referred to the *Canon* as a "Methodic Inanity." Fielding Garrison, the twentieth century historian of medicine, called Avicenna's *Canon* "a huge, unwieldy storehouse of learning."

With increasing trade and travel in the twelfth to the sixteenth centuries, European culture gradually reestablished contact with Arabian medicine and the Roman traditions which it absorbed. Both the Crusades in the Middle Ages and the invasions by the Arabs of the Peloponessus and southern Spain brought an infusion of classical knowledge from which came the Renaissance and the beginning of the scientific era in the fifteenth and sixteenth centuries[2, 30].

References

1. Gaarder, J. *Sophie's world: A novel about the History of Philosophy.* Transl. P. Moller. London: Phoenix House, 995.
2. Castiglioni, A. *A History of Medicine.* Transl. E.B. Krumbhaar. New York: Alfred A. Knopf, 1941.
3. Sigerist, H.E. *A History of Medicine.* New York: Oxford University Press, 1961.
4. Major, R.H. *A History of Medicine.* Springfield, IL: Charles C. Thomas, 1954.
5. Garrison, F. *An Introduction to the History of Medicine.* Philadelphia: W.B. Saunders and Co., 1929.
6. Martinie, J. *Notes sur l'histoire de l'obésité. Thèse de Paris 1934.* Paris: Les Presses Universitaires de France, 1934.
7. Hautin, J.R. *Obésité: Conceptions actuelle. Thèse pour le Doctorat en Médecine.* Bordeaux: Imprimerie Bier, 1939.
8. Bray, GA. "Obesity: Historical Development of Scientific and Cultural Ideas." *Int J Obes.* 14 (1990): 909–926.
9. Garrison, F.H. *An Introduction to the History of Medicine with Medical Chronology, Bibliographic Data, and Test Questions.* Philadelphia: W.B. Saunders Co., 1914.
10. Contenau, G. *La médecine en Assyrie et en Babylonie.* Paris: Librairie Maloine, 1938.
11. E Spycket, A. "Kassite and Middle Elamite Sculpture." In: *Later Mesopotamia and Iran. Tribes and Empires 1600–538* B.C. London: British Museum Press, 1995.
12. Smith, E. *The Edwin Smith Surgical Papyrus. Published in Facsimile and Hieroglyphic Transliteration with Translation and Commentary in Two Volumes by James Henry Breasted. Classics of Medicine,* Special Edition, 1984. Chicago: University of Chicago Press, 1930.
13. Darby, W.J., P. Ghalioungui, L. Grevetti. *Food: The Gift of Osiris.* London: Academic Press, 1977.
14. Nunn, J.F. *Ancient Egyptian Medicine.* London: British Museum Press, 1996.
15. Reeves, C. *Egyptian Medicine.* London: Shire Publications Ltd., 1992.
16. Filer, J. *Egyptian Bookshelf, Disease.* London: British Museum Press, 1995.
17. Alphen, J.V., A. Aris. *Oriental Medicine: An Illustrated Guide to the Asian Arts of Healing.* Boston: Shambhala, 1996.
18. Archeological catalogue of China.
19. "Tibetan medical paintings." *Illustrations to the Blue Beryl Treatise of Sangye Gyamtso. (1635–1705).* New York: Henry N. Abrams Inc., 1992.
20. Lason, A.H. *The Thyroid Gland in Medical History.* New York: Frobin Press, 1946.

21. *Hippocrates. Oeuvres complètes d'Hippocrate: traduction nouvelle avec le texte grec en regard, collationné sur les manuscrits et toutes les éditions; accompagnée d'une introduction,...suivie d'une table générale des matières / par É. Littré.* Paris: J.B. Balliere, 1839.
22. Kryger, M.H. "Sleep Apnea: From the Needles of Dionysius to Continuous Positive Airway Pressure." *Arch Intern Med.* 143 (1983): 2301–2303.
23. Kryger, M.H. "Fat, Sleep and Charles Dickens: Literary and Medical Contributions to the Understanding of Sleep Apnea." *Clin Chest Med.* 6 (1985): 555–562.
24. Precope, J. *Hippocrates on Diet and Hygiene.* London: Zeno, 1952.
25. Green, R.M. *A Translation of Galen's Hygiene (De Sanitate Tuenda).* Springfield, IL: Charles C. Thomas, 1951.
26. Gruner, O.C. *A Treatise on the Canon of Medicine of Avicenna Incorporating a Translation of the First Book.* London: Luzac, 1930.
27. Osler, W. *The Evolution of Modern Medicine.* New Haven: Yale University Press, 1921.
28. Selwyn-Brown, A. *The Physician throughout the Ages.* New York: Capehard-Brown Co. Inc., 1928.
29. Campbell, D. *Arabian Medicine and Its Influence on the Middle Ages.* London: Kegan Paul, Trench, Trubner & Co. Ltd., 1926.
30. Ullmann, M. *Islamic Medicine.* Edinburgh: University Press, 1978.

Chapter 3

Battle of the Bulge in the Age of Science (A.D. 1500 to 2000)

Religions dissipate like fog, kingdoms vanish, but the works of scientists remain for eternity.

—Ulug Beg[1]

The history of truth is neither linear nor monotone.

—Canguilhem[2]

This part of the story begins with Gutenberg, that famous German who invented movable type and used it to print Bibles in the middle of the fifteenth century. Thus began the third revolution in communication: the first was the spoken language; the second was the written language; and the third the printed language. At the end of the twentieth century we entered the fourth revolution in communication: the electronic and Internet revolution.

Printing has been a driving force in the expansion of knowledge since the sixteenth century. It provided a rapid means of communicating new ideas from A.D. 1500 to the present. It has informed us of our progress and our failures. It has helped scientists communicate and it has provided a way for good and bad advice to be distributed widely. The electronic age has dramatically changed the way in which scientific information is communicated, retrieved, and distributed as surely as the printed word did five hundred years ago. All of these revolutions in communication have impacted our understanding of the problem of obesity and have provided ever more rapid means of disseminating knowledge about how to battle it.

In the fifty years following the development of the printing press in A.D. 1450 printing presses and printing shops gradually spread throughout Europe. By 1500 large numbers of classical texts from Greek and Roman times had been printed and widely circulated and a smattering of original books began to appear in print as well. From a scientific point of view, two of the most important books published in the first century of printing were the sixteenth century books by Nicholas Copernicus (1473–1543) on the heliocentric theory of the solar system titled *De Revolutionibus Orbium Colestium. Libri VI* and the anatomical work on the human body by Andreas Vesalius (1514–1564) titled *De humani corporis fabrica*. Both books were published in 1543.

Most of the major contributions to science and our knowledge about obesity in the sixteenth and seventeenth centuries appeared in the form of monographs, syllabuses, pamphlets, and textbooks. As the number of scientists increased during the seventeenth century, early scientific societies were formed in England, France, and Italy. These scientific societies became a focal point for meetings and correspondence about new scientific discoveries.

The revolution in communication provided by printing ushered in the age of anatomy at the beginning of the sixteenth century. Before the sixteenth century, the writings of Galen in Roman times and the *Canon* of Avicenna from Arabic medicine in the tenth century had been the main source of information about anatomy, physiology, and clinical medicine. These sources had come down through handwritten texts. Although there is no clear evidence that either Galen or Avicenna ever dissected a human cadaver, their influence over the teaching of anatomy was diminished only by the application of direct dissection and dissemination of these findings in printed books.

As the amount of scientific literature has grown since Gutenberg, so have the complaints about it. The frustration engendered by the steady and rapid growth of scientific books and journals has been reflected in quotations from scholars over many centuries. Following are a few examples of these complaints:

A seventeenth century comment:

> One of the diseases of this age is the multiplicity of books; they doth so overcharge the world that it is not able to digest the abundance of idle matter that is every day hatched and brought forth into the world. (Barnaby Rich; 1613[4])

From the great eighteenth century encyclopedist Diderot we have the following statement of the problem:

> The number of books will grow continually, and one can predict that a time will come when it will be almost as difficult to learn anything from books as from the direct study of the whole universe. It will be almost as convenient to search for some bit of truth concealed in nature as it will be to find it hidden away in an immense multitude of bound volumes. (Diderot, originally published 1755[4])

In the nineteenth century a leading physician made these comments about the problem:

> You must needs hang your heavy head, and roll your blood shot eyes over thousands of pages weekly. Of their contents at the week's end you will know about as much of a district through which you have been whirled night and day in the mail coach. (Beddoes, 1802[6])

In the twentieth century as the volume of scientific literature about the battle of the bulge has increased, even more concerns have been raised:

> Scientists have always felt themselves to be awash in a sea of scientific literature that augments in each decade as much as in all times before. (Price, 1963[4])
>
> Like beach bums, new journals appear in crops overnight...There are too many of them, they are published too often, they stare from the racks and reproach us for sloth. (Weissmann, 1990[7])
>
> ...it has been apparent for the past couple of centuries, that like books, the making of journals is endless. (Bynum and Wilson, 1992[8])
>
> Today, when the excessive number of medical journals is a common source of complaint it is salutary to realize that even by the end of the eighteenth century some were voicing the same concern. (Loudon and Loudon, 1992[9])

The modern scientific tradition is one of experimentation. The scientist has a question, for example, how do we become obese? He designs an experiment to ask whether an animal or a human being can become obese when food intake is limited. The results of this experiment will either support or not support the original idea. As Hans Popper, one of greater philosophers of the scientific method, has defined it, experimentation is a method of verification and falsification[10]. That is, progress was made by designing experiments to test hypotheses and applying mathematical analysis, where appropriate, to the results. The fruitfulness of this tradition is everywhere around us. Witness cellular telephones, the Internet, and the new drugs to fight human disease, including obesity.

Application of the experimental method to obesity and the battle of the bulge has come, as it has come to all other areas, but progress has been slow. From the beginning of the "scientific era" (A.D. 1500) to the beginning of "modern medicine" (around A.D. 1800), only a small number of scientific dissertations or theses resulting from academic scholarship with obesity as the subject matter had been published[11–17]. In general these early scholarly theses reflected the medical traditions that originated more than one thousand years earlier in the writings of Hippocrates, Galen, or Avicenna.

The writings of Newton and Galileo in the seventeenth century provided a new mechanical basis for interpreting bodily functions. William Harvey, who discovered the circulation of the blood, capitalized on this mechanical view when he showed that the heart was a pump circulating blood through the arteries and veins. This mechanical view of the world was applied to interpreting medical phenomena by the eighteenth century as a medical-mechanical (iatro-physical) view of health and disease. As chemistry came of age, a medical-chemical (iatro-chemical) view of the world provided a second broad new approach to thinking about medical illness. As interest in obesity increased, a much larger number of theses with obesity as their subject were published in the nineteenth century[18–51], as well as the first books devoted entirely to obesity[29, 52]. Table 3-1 is a list of most English, French, and German books about obesity that were published before 1950[53–71].

Table 3-1 List of Monographs on Obesity Written between 1700 and 1950 in English, French and German.

English	French	German
18th Century		
Short[181]		
Flemyng[182]		
19th Century		
Wadd[39, 230]	Maccary[149]	Kisch[235]
Chambers[231]	Dancel[233]	Ebstein[189]
Harvey, J.[232]	Worthington[234]	
Harvey, W.[185]	Regneller[252]	
20th Century		
Williams[236]	Leven[244]	Von Noorden[249]
Christie[237]	Heckel[245]	Pfaundler[250]
Rony[216]	Le Noir[246]	Gries, Berchtold and Berger[251]
Rynearson and Gastineau[238]	Boivin[247]	
Craddock[239]	Creff and Herschberg[248]	Bray[116]
Bruch[240]	Louvet[253]	
Mayer[241]		
Garrow[242]		
Stunkard[243]		

From these beginnings there has been a steady logarithmic growth in knowledge and information. The epidemic of obesity expands around us, as does the scientific literature from which solutions will eventually come. To provide some order for the journey through the increasing scientific knowledge and to provide a picture of the battlefield, I have developed a series of five timelines. For the five centuries covered by this chapter, I have prepared timelines beginning in 1500. Clearly there were many important scientific and mathematical advances before 1500[41, 42]. However, the advent of printing with movable type and the appearance of the scientific method led to an accelerating rate of scientific advance after A.D. 1500, thus the timelines only encompass the past five centuries. Each timeline consists of eleven separate lines. They show the developments in science and technology, anatomy and histology, physiology, chemistry/biochemistry, genetics, pharmacology, neuroscience, and clinical medicine. If one wanted a demarcation line for the beginning of modern medicine, it might well be the time of the American and French Revolutions (1776–1789)[43, 44]. To these timelines, I have added the American presidents beginning with George Washington in 1789.

These timelines provide a framework for relating the medical and scientific advances in each century to some of the key historical events that were occurring at the same time. These other events are intended to anchor the scientific achievements in a broader historical framework. The rate of scientific progress over these five centuries is evident from the increasing number of entries in each category. The rapidity of scientific progress is particularly clear from the beginning of the nineteenth century (Figure 3-4) through the twentieth century (Figure 3-5). I will highlight a few of these events. The sixteenth century (Figure 3-1) set the groundwork, primarily in physics and mathematics. The major biological publication of the sixteenth century was the anatomical masterpiece of Andreas Vesalius. The year 1543 also marked the time that Copernicus[34] published his book on the solar system, arguing that planets revolved around the sun.

In the seventeenth century (Figure 3-2), the work of William Harvey[11] (1578–1657) led to his discovery of the circulation of the blood. Although Harvey published his theory on the circulation of the blood in 1628, this important discovery didn't impact clinical medicine for another two hundred years. The discovery of oxygen by Joseph Priestley (1733–1804)[12] and Wilhelm Scheele (1742–1786)[13] and the introduction of the oxygen theory of metabolism by Antoine Lavoisier (1743–1794)[14] were key events in the eighteenth century. They provided the beginnings for the modern study of metabolism (Figure 3-3). When the American and French Revolutions ended at the close of the eighteenth century, the stage was set for a rapid expansion in chemical sciences. If the sixteenth and seventeenth centuries were the centuries of physics and mathematics, the eighteenth and nineteenth centuries were the centuries of chemistry and biology. With the dawn

TIMELINE 1500 - 1600

Science and Technology	1543 - Copernicus - Heliocentric Theory of the solar system; 1589-Galileo's Law of Falling Bodies
Anatomy and Histology	1543 Vesalius - Human Anatomy published; 1549 - Anatomic Theater built in Padua
Physiology	1540 - Servetus describes pulmonary circulation
Chemistry / Biochemistry	
Genetics	
Pharmacology	1526 - Paracelsus Founds 'Chemotherapy'
Neuroscience	
Clinical Medicine	1505 - Royal College of Surgeons - Edinburgh; 1518 - Royal College of Physicians - London; 1524 - First Hospital in Mexico City; 1530 - Frascatorius Poem on Syphilis; 1544 - St. Bartholomew's Hospital-London; *1595- First Thesis on Obesity*
	1500 1510 1520 1530 1540 1550 1560 1570 1580 1590
Presidents of the U.S.	
Events	1492 - Columbus Discovers America; 1517-1521 - Luther Reformation; 1519-1522 - Magellan Circumnavigates the globe; 1545-1563 - Council of Trent; 1558 - 1603 - Reign of Queen Elizabeth I; 1564-1616 - Shakespeare; 1588-Spanish Armada Destroyed; 1589-Reign of Henry IV of France; 1598- Edict of Nantes

3-1 16th Century Timeline © 1996 George A. Bray.

TIMELINE 1600 - 1700

Science and Technology	1620 - Bacon's *Organum Novum*; 1662-Descartes De Homine; 1662-Newton & Leibniz develop calculus; 1665 - Newton's Law of Gravity; 1687-Newton's *Principia*
Anatomy and Histology	1610-Galileo devises Microscope; 1658 - Swammerdam describes red corpuscles; 1661-Malpighi publishes *Pulmonary Circulation*; 1665 Hooke's *Micrographia*; 1672-DeGraaf ovarian follicle; 1675 Leeuwenhoek protozoa
Physiology	1614 Santorio, father of Metabolic Obesity, describes metabolic scale, pulse counting, thermometer.; 1628 Harvey publishes *Circulation of Blood*; 1665 - Lower - transfuses blood in dogs
Chemistry / Biochemistry	1661 Boyle - defines Chemical Element; 1674 - Mayow-Animal heat in muscles.
Genetics	
Pharmacology	
Neuroscience	
Clinical Medicine	1639 - 1st hospital in Canada; 1642 - Jacob Bontius describes beri-beri; 1650 - Glisson describes rickets; 1656 - Wharton publishes *Adenographia*; 1659 Willis describes Puerperal Fever; 1670 - Willis describes "sweet" urine in diabetes; 1683- Sydenham treatise on gout
	1600 1610 1620 1630 1640 1650 1660 1670 1680 1690
Presidents of the U.S.	
Events	1607 Jamestown, VA, settled; 1618-1648 - 30 Years War; 1620 Plymouth, MA, settled; 1636 Harvard College founded; 1640-1688- Reign of Frederick the Great Elector; 1642-1661 English Civil War & Cromwell Rule; 1654-1715 Reign of Louis XIV; 1660-1689 Reign of Charles II of England; 1666-London Fire; 1682-1725-Reign of Peter the Great of Russia; 1690- Locke publishes *On Human Understanding*; 1692- Salem Witch-Hunt

3-2 17th Century Timeline © 1996 George A. Bray.

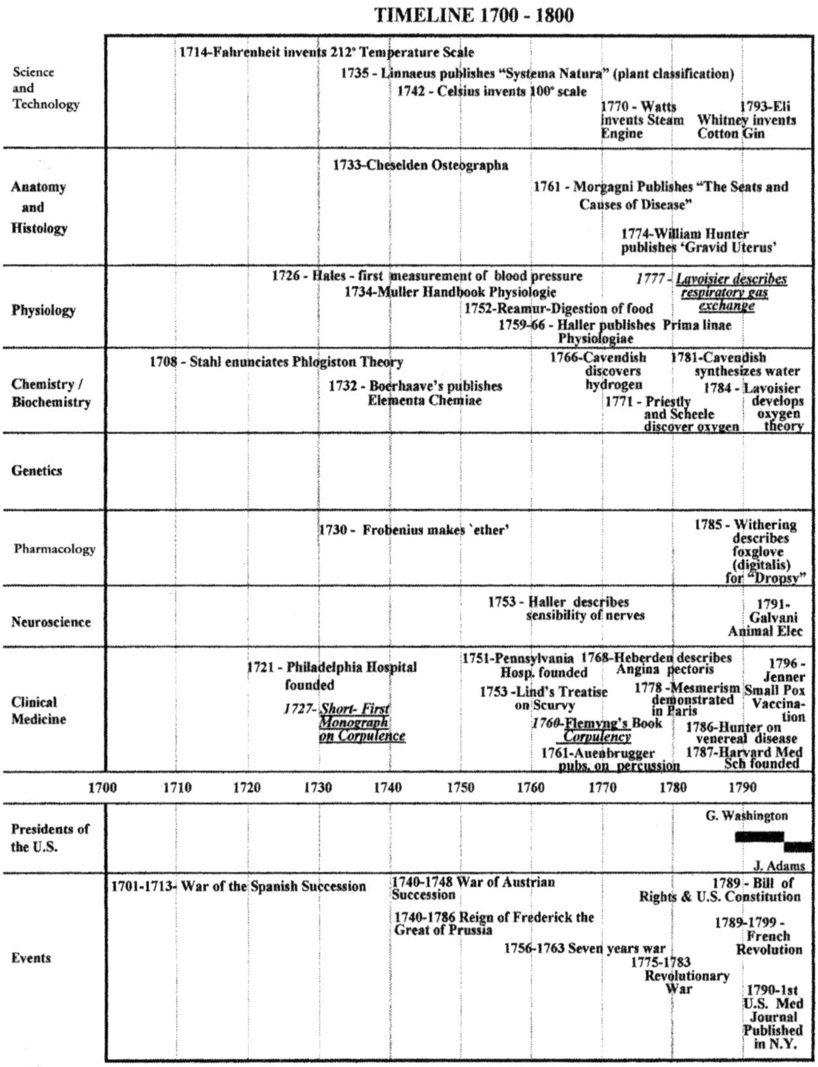

TIMELINE 1700 - 1800

Science and Technology
- 1714-Fahrenheit invents 212° Temperature Scale
- 1735 - Linnaeus publishes "Systema Natura" (plant classification)
- 1742 - Celsius invents 100° scale
- 1770 - Watts invents Steam Engine
- 1793-Eli Whitney invents Cotton Gin

Anatomy and Histology
- 1733-Cheselden Osteographa
- 1761 - Morgagni Publishes "The Seats and Causes of Disease"
- 1774-William Hunter publishes 'Gravid Uterus'

Physiology
- 1726 - Hales - first measurement of blood pressure
- 1734-Muller Handbook Physiologie
- 1752-Reamur-Digestion of food
- 1759-66 - Haller publishes Prima linae Physiologiae
- *1777 - Lavoisier describes respiratory gas exchange*

Chemistry / Biochemistry
- 1708 - Stahl enunciates Phlogiston Theory
- 1732 - Boerhaave's publishes Elementa Chemiae
- 1766-Cavendish discovers hydrogen
- 1771 - Priestly and Scheele discover oxygen
- 1781-Cavendish synthesizes water
- 1784 - Lavoisier develops oxygen theory

Genetics

Pharmacology
- 1730 - Frobenius makes 'ether'
- 1785 - Withering describes foxglove (digitalis) for "Dropsy"

Neuroscience
- 1753 - Haller describes sensibility of nerves
- 1791- Galvani Animal Elec

Clinical Medicine
- 1721 - Philadelphia Hospital founded
- *1727- Short- First Monograph on Corpulence*
- 1751-Pennsylvania Hosp. founded
- 1753 -Lind's Treatise on Scurvy
- *1760-Flemyng's Book Corpulency*
- 1761-Auenbrugger pubs. on percussion
- 1768-Heberden describes Angina pectoris
- 1778 -Mesmerism demonstrated in Paris
- 1786-Hunter on venereal disease
- 1787-Harvard Med Sch founded
- 1796 - Jenner Small Pox Vaccination

1700 1710 1720 1730 1740 1750 1760 1770 1780 1790

Presidents of the U.S.
- G. Washington
- J. Adams

Events
- 1701-1713- War of the Spanish Succession
- 1740-1748 War of Austrian Succession
- 1740-1786 Reign of Frederick the Great of Prussia
- 1756-1763 Seven years war
- 1775-1783 Revolutionary War
- 1789 - Bill of Rights & U.S. Constitution
- 1789-1799 - French Revolution
- 1790-1st U.S. Med Journal Published in N.Y.

3-3 18th Century Timeline © 1996 George A. Bray.

TIMELINE 1800 - 1900

Science and Technology	1800-Electrical Cell; 1803 - Fulton's Steamboat; 1814 - First Locomotive; 1825 - Erie Canal; 1827 - First Photograph; 1834 - Babbage's "Analytical Engine"; 1860-Internal Combustion Engine; 1876-Telephone; 1877-Phonograph; 1880-Edison Electric Light; 1886-Kodak Camera; 1887- Arrhenius- Ion Theory; 1895 - Motion Picture Camera
Anatomy and Histology	1800-Bichat's Tissue Pathology; 1801-Bell System of Anatomy; 1830-Lister-Achromatic microscope; *1835*-Quetelet describes body mass index; 1838-Schwann and Schleden propose cell theory; *1849*-Hassall *Fat Cell*; 1858-Virchow publishes Cellular Pathology; 1858-Gray's Anatomy
Physiology	1821-Magendie- Food Absorption; 1833- Beaumont on digestion; 1833-Muller's Physiology Text; 1842-Mayer conservation of energy; 1846-Bernard-Digestive function of pancreas; 1847-Ludwig-Kymograph; 1849-Ludwig-Urinary secretion; 1867-Helmholtz Physiological optics
Chemistry / Biochemistry	1825-Wohler synthesizes urea; 1847-Helmholtz -*Conservation of Energy*; 1848-Bernard isolates glycogen; 1863-Voit & Pettenkoffer- Metabolism; 1896- Atwater makes calori- meter
Genetics	1859-Darwin-Origin of the Species; 1865-G. Mendel - Plant breeding genetics
Pharmacology	1805 - Pelletier isolates Morphine; 1819-Pelleter & Caventon isolate Quinine; 1822-Magendie's Pharmacopoeia; 1833-Atropine isolated; 1834 - Chloroform discovered; 1856 - Cocaine Extracted; 1893- Thyroid to treat Obesity
Neuroscience	1811-Bell spinal nerve function; 1854 - Bernard vasodilator nerves; 1863-Helmholtz - *Book of Hearing*
Clinical Medicine	1809-McDowell-Ovariotomy; 1819 - Laennec Stethoscope; *1826 - Wadd on Corpulence*; 1840- Basedow Goiter; 1846-Ether Anesthesia; 1847-Semmelweis- Puerperal Fever; 1849-Addison & Pernicicus Anemia & suprarenal disease; *1850 - Chambers on Obesity*; 1851 - Helmholtz-Opthalmoscope; 1854 - Laryngoscope; 1863-Banting *"Letter On Corpulence"*; 1865 - Antiseptic Surgery; *1866*-Russel - *sleep apnea*; 1873-Gull-Myxedenia; 1882-Koch isolate tubercle bacillus; 1895 - Roentgen Discovers x-rays
(Years)	1800 1810 1820 1830 1840 1850 1860 1870 1880 1890
Presidents of the U.S.	T.Jefferson; J.Madison; J.Monroe; J.Q.Adams; Jackson; Van Buren; W. Harrison; Tyler; Polk; Taylor; Fillmore; Pierce; Buchannon; Lincoln; Johnson; U.Grant; Hays; Garfield; Arthur; Cleveland; Harrison; Cleveland; McKinley
Events	1804-1815-Napoleon Emperor; 1805-Battle of Trafalgar; 1812 - War of 1812; 1830-Reign of Louis Phillipe; 1839-R. Hill-Postage stamps introduced; 1848 - 1849 - California Gold Rush; 1848 - 1852-Second French Republic; 1861-1865-Civil War; 1863 - Emancipation Proclamation; 1866-Seven weeks war; 1870-1871-Franco-Prussian War; 1886 - Statue of Liberty; 1898- Spanish- American War

3-4 19th Century Timeline © 1996 George A. Bray.

TIMELINE 1900 - 2000

Science and Technology	1903 - Wright Brother's Flight; 1915 - Theory of Relativity; 1926 - Liquid Fueled Rocket; 1927 - Lindbergh's Flight; 1933 - Television demonstrated; 1939 - DDT Synthesized; 1939 - Polyethylene invented; 1945 - Atomic Bomb dropped; 1947 - Transistor invented; 1956 - Birth control pill tested; 1957 - Sputnik launched; 1969 - Armstrong walks on moon; 1975-Wilson-Sociobiology; 1980-Transgenic mouse; 1989-Human genome project
Anatomy and Histology	1928-Ramon y Cajal; 1932-Knoll & Ruskin-Electron microscope; 1951-*Hyperplastic Obesity*; 1973-*CT Scan*; 1982-*CT of Viseral Fat*
Physiology	1902-Bayliss - secretin; 1912-*Cannon & Carlson-Gastric contraction & hunger*; 1918-Starling-Law of the Heart; 1929-Haymans-Carotid sinus reflex; 1932-Cannon-Wisdom of the body; 1946-*Hydrostatic Weight*; 1946-*Fat cells metabolize*; 1949-*Lipostatic Theory*; 1953-*Glucostatic Theory*; 1963-*Doubly-labelled water*; 1975-*Fat cells cultured*; 1978-*BAT/SNS*; 1978-*Adrenalectomy prevents obesity*; 1982-*NPY Stimulates F.I.*
Chemistry / Biochemistry	1912-Hopkins -Vitamins; 1921-Banting isolates insulin; 1928-Warburg broken cells respire; 1937 Krebs - Citric acid cycle; 1946-Lippmann - Coenzyme; 1953-Insulin sequenced; 1958-Sutherland Cyclic Amp; 1960-RIA for Insulin; 1965-Holley transfer RNA; 1972-*Releasing factor*; 1995-*Cpe-gene Leptin-receptor gene*
Genetics	1909-Garrod-Inborn Errors; 1924-*Davenport - Familial Association of Obesity*; 1944-Avery-DNA; 1950-*Obese mouse described*; 1953-Watson & Crick Double Helix; 1956-*Prader-Willi syndrome*; 1992-*Yellow gene cloned*; 1994-*Leptin gene cloned*
Pharmacology	1901 - Adrenaline Isolated; 1909-Ehrlich invents Salvarsan; 1912 - Vitamin Coined; 1922 - Insulin Therapy; 1928 - Fleming Discovers Penicillin; 1932-Domagk discovers Sulfonamide; 1937-*Lesses & Myerson-Amphetamine to treat obesity*; 1944 - Quinine Synthesized; 1954 - Salk Polio Vaccine; 1973-*Fenfluramine approved*; 1992-*Weintraub Combined Rx*
Neuroscience	1900-1901-*Frohlich-Babinski syndrome*; 1902-Pavlov-Conditioned reflexes; 1912-*Cushings Syndrome*; 1940-*Hetherington VMH Lesion*; 1953-Eccles-Nerve transmission; 1962-*ME stimulates feeding*; 1967-*Behavior Modification*; 1992-*Glucocorticoid Obesity transgene*
Clinical Medicine	1901-*Life Insurance Companies show Risk of Obesity*; 1903 - Electrocardiograph-Einthoven; 1928-*Very-low-calorie diets*; 1947 - *Risk of Peripheral Fat*; 1951 - Heart-Lung Machine; 1953-*Bypass surgery for obesity*; 1963-*Socio-economic status & obesity*; 1968-*Vermont overfeeding study*; 1978 - First Test Tube Baby; 1981 - First AIDS Diagnosis; 1986-*Twin overfeeding study*
	1900 · 1910 · 1920 · 1930 · 1940 · 1950 · 1960 · 1970 · 1980 · 1990
Presidents of the U.S.	T. Roosevelt; W. Taft; Wilson; Harding; Coolidge; Hoover; F. D. Roosevelt; Truman; Eisenhower; Kennedy; L.B. Johnson; Nixon; Ford; Carter; Reagan; Bush; Clinton
Events	1914-1918 - W.W.I; 1919-Prohibition; 1920 - U.S. Women get to vote; 1929-The Great Depression; 1939-1945-W.W.II; 1941 - Pearl Harbor Attack; 1945-United Nations Founded; 1950-1953-Korean conflict; 1961-Berlin Wall; 1962 - Cuban Missile Crisis; 1962-1976 Vietnam War; 1963 - Kennedy Assassinated; 1968 - MLK Assassinated; 1974 - Nixon Resigns; 1989-Berlin Wall Falls; 1991-Desert Storm; 1991-Soviet Union Dissolves

3-5 20th Century Timeline © 1996 George A. Bray.

of the twentieth century (Figure 3-5), scientific medicine came into its own, highlighted by the revolution in genetics and the helical model for deoxyribonucleic acid (DNA).

The French Revolution of 1789, like the slightly earlier American Revolution of 1776, was a watershed for our battle of the bulge. During the French Revolution, the existing system of medical education was destroyed along with the monarchy. The citizens' government in France believed that all citizens could be their own doctors and that medical education in the classical sense was no longer needed[16]. With the military campaigns that followed the ascent of Napoleon as first consul and then emperor, it became clear that the care of military casualties required trained physicians, and medical schools were reborn.

These medical schools were radically different from those in France prior to the revolution. Two important changes were introduced that altered the future of medical education. First, medicine and surgery were brought together in the same medical faculty, ending forever the barber-surgeon status of surgery. Second, medical teaching shifted from the lofty atmosphere of amphitheaters to the hospitals where the sick and injured awaited care.

From this period of enormous excitement with the restructuring of medical education arose a ferment in France that led to a period of unprecedented medical and scientific advances, with major new contributions stemming from clinical medicine. A young man named François Xavier Bichat (1771–1802)[17] expounded a pathology of disease based in tissues. This was the beginning of the overthrow of the concept of a humoral-based pathology of disease in which an imbalance in one of the four humors (fire, air, water, and earth) was thought to cause disease. In the second half of the eighteenth century (1861), an Austrian named Leopold Auenbrugger (1722–1809) discovered the concept of clinical diagnosis by percussion[18]. Like so many other important discoveries, this one was not widely recognized for more than forty years after it was published. Recognition of the importance of percussion came from the translation of Auenbrugger's work into French by Corvisart (1755–1821) in 1808[19]. Similarly, René Théophile Hyacinthe Laennec (1781–1826)[20] in 1816 invented the stethoscope, a key instrument for clinical diagnosis for nearly two centuries. Using the clinical discoveries he made with the stethoscope, Laennec wrote the first modern textbook of medicine where diseases of the chest were diagnosed by percussion and auscultation.

France in the early years of the nineteenth century was the center of scientific and medical discovery. During this period of excitement in French medicine, morphine was isolated and quinine was extracted from *Cinchona* bark. Physiologic science expanded through the genius of Francois Magendie (1783–1855)[21], the teacher of the famous Claude Bernard

(1813–1878)[22]. Thus "Paris Medicine," as it has been called because of its focus on clinical diagnosis at the bedside, was the center for teaching of clinical medicine in the first part of the nineteenth century. The stagnation of French medicine later in the nineteenth century stemmed in part from the failure of French scientists to recognize the importance of the microscope as a tool to investigate nature and the failure to pursue chemical and laboratory medicine.

However, Paris Medicine had an important impact on British and American medicine, since many of the clinicians in this period were trained in Paris. The list includes many of the nineteenth century luminaries such as Thomas Hodgkin (1798–1866)[23] who described the lymphatic tumors known as Hodgkin's disease; Richard Bright (1789–1858)[24] who identified the form of kidney disease called Bright's disease; Thomas Addison (1793–1860)[25] who identified failure of the adrenal glands, so-called Addison's disease, as the basis for a wasting disease; and William Jenner (1749–1823)[26] who introduced vaccination for smallpox at the end of the eighteenth century. All of these men were steeped in the clinical tradition being taught in Paris.

If the first half of the nineteenth century can be described as the French Clinical School with Paris Medicine as its center, the second half of the nineteenth century belongs to the German Laboratory School or German Laboratory Medicine, so called for the numerous contributions to chemical and laboratory studies. The date for the transition between the French Clinical School and the German Laboratory School can be set at 1850. The German Laboratory School of Medicine grew in large measure from two eminent scientists, Johannes Müller (1801–1858)[27] and his students and Justus Liebig (1803–1873)[28] and his followers. Müller recognized the importance of the microscope as a tool for studying life and, unlike his French colleagues, encouraged his students to use it. Liebig established the first laboratory for chemistry and agricultural science.

The idea that cells were the basic biological unit of life, the so-called "Cell Theory," was conceived in 1838 by Theodor Schwann and Matthias Schleiden, two students of Johannes Müller. The Cell Theory had an impact on the way in which diseases were viewed. As the young Bichat in France in the first half of the nineteenth century had shifted the focus for the study of disease from organs to the tissues that make up these organs, so Virchow (1821-1902)[29] in the second half of the nineteenth century, using microscopic techniques, shifted the focus for the study of diseases from tissues to the cells that composed these tissues.

Müller also trained students as physiologists to explore the function of the human body. Hermann von Helmholtz (1821–1894) was among his most famous of these students.[30] He invented the ophthalmoscope, which allows physicians to probe the back of the eye to gain clues about the diseases that might be occurring in blood vessels, including consequences of obesity. He also described the idea that energy is neither made nor lost—the conservation of energy, which is referred to as the First Law of Thermodynamics and is a central dogma for understanding the battle of the bulge. Other outstanding members of the German School were Robert Koch (1843–1910)[31] who discovered the bacteria as causes of specific diseases, and Wilhelm Roentgen (1845–1923)[32] who discovered x-rays in 1895. As we shall see, x-rays have played an important role in the battle of the bulge in the latter part of the twentieth century.

The status of obesity and the battle of the bulge up to the middle of the nineteenth century has been summarized for us by Thomas King Chambers (1817–1889)[15] in a lecture he presented to the Royal College of Physicians in London in 1849 called the Gulstonian Lecture. This important battle plan was published simultaneously in *The Lancet* and as a book in 1850. In his lecture, Dr. Chambers presents a picture of the science of corpulence in the middle of the nineteenth century. The book by Chambers marks a dividing line in the history of obesity and contains a number of important ideas about this field, some of which are fundamental for obesity as a science. These included a table of average body weights for a given height, the idea that obesity was more common in some families than in other families, and that the old remedies of eating less and exercising more were still applicable.

The small book by Thomas King Chambers titled *On Corpulence,* published in 1850[15], can conveniently serve as a dividing line between Paris Medicine (1800–1850) and German Laboratory Medicine (1850–1920). In his Gulstonian Lecture, he describes the changing knowledge about the basis of fat deposition at a time when the Cell Theory of biology had just come into existence. He said, "For the formation of fat it is necessary that the materials be digested in a greater quantity than is sufficient to supply carbon for respiration."[15]. This early statement of the concept of a positive energy balance as the basis of adiposity has been amply confirmed.

Chambers goes on to note that the overweight individual

> is prone to heart disease, to apoplexy [stroke] and congestions. While if a person is much above or below the standard weight, it is not necessary to discover any other bad symptom to pronounce the insurance of his life as "above the ordinary risk"[15].

This insurance approach to assessing risk in relation to obesity has been a major stimulus to the study of this field from the time of Chambers through most of the twentieth century. Chambers's book goes farther and provides a table of weights in relation to height that had only been published three years earlier.

The hereditary disposition to obesity, which has become a major focus for research in the battle of the bulge at the beginning of the twenty-first century, can clearly be dated as far back as Chambers in 1850. He points to the familial basis of obesity through a series of thirty-eight cases in which he notes the strong familial history; it would become clear that we need to initiate our battle of the bulge within the family. Chambers was also the first to note that "obese girls often menstruate at an unusually early age[15]. He noted the predisposing effects of sedentary occupations, of marriage and of decreased exercise as important components in the increase of fat as individuals age. "Birth of a first child appears as a proximate cause" of obesity for many women (15). Thus, in his understanding of the natural history and development of obesity, Chambers is a truly modern physician.

His admonitions on treatment for obesity, however, follow a long tradition dating from the time of Hippocrates. "The first thing indicated in all cases, is to cut off as far as possible, the supply of material [food]. Fat, oil and butter should be rigorously interdicted in the diet." He goes on to say that "Very light meals should be taken at times most favorable to rapid digestion," and he then proceeds to describe a number of components of meals[15].

Chambers also noted the importance of physical activity for overweight people. He said,

> As respects exercise, a distinction requires to be made. The young and vigorous, whose obesity does not prevent their use of their legs, cannot employ them more usefully than in walking as long as they are able. The greater number of hours per diem that can be devoted to this exercise, the quicker will be the diminution of bulk[15].

This is a very modern notion indeed—the more you exercise the more quickly you will lose weight, providing that your joints hold up. He also notes, "It is very convenient for a patient to wear a band round the abdomen which may be tightened gradually"[15]. The concept of using a band to reflect changes in weight thus has a long tradition. A similar strategy has been tried with some success in modern times. Many fashion models have used such bands around the waist to help them keep control of their size.

In contrast to these relatively modern pronouncements about obesity, Chambers's discussion of treatment for our battle of the bulge is far less modern; rather, it is steeped in the traditional scientific base of the mid-nineteenth century and earlier, including bleeding, purging, and the use of soap or vinegar. It is, however, his insights into pathogenesis, physiology, and pathology that make his book the first truly modern document in the field of corpulence and thus in my judgment a "classic" in the field.

The growth of science through the nineteenth century (Figure 3-4), and particularly the twentieth century (Figure 3-5), has been characterized by specialization. This is one obvious consequence of the rapid and logarithmic growth of scientific knowledge and the limited capacity of any one scientist to encompass it all. Corpulence as we know it has been studied by many of these subspecialty disciplines. As new areas of specialization develop, they will add further dimensions in our battle of the bulge. Each of the major biomedical disciplines related to our ideas about corpulence is described briefly in the next few pages.

A. Anatomy

The year 1543 is a major milestone in the story of anatomy. That was the year when Andreas Vesalius (1514–1564) published his treatise on human anatomy[3], the first modern book on anatomy based on dissections performed by the author. Andreas Vesalius was only twenty-eight years old when he published his masterpiece (Figure 3-6).

In his accurate and careful dissections, Vesalius showed that the human body could be directly explored by dissection rather than reading from Galen's anatomy, a book that had been written fifteen hundred years earlier in Roman times and which was based more on anatomy learned from treatment of wounded soldiers and from animal dissections than from human dissections. Vesalius applied the concept of direct verification and experimental manipulation to identify a number of inaccuracies in the earlier anatomical teachings of Galen, including the idea of a seven-lobed liver, the horned uterus, the seven-segmented sternum, the double bile duct, and the presence of interventricular pores[34].

The first anatomical dissections of obese individuals are attributed to Théophile Bonet (1620–1689)[35]. Other descriptions appear in the publications by Giovanni Morgagni (1682–1771) (see Chapter 20)[36], by Albrecht van Haller (1708–1777)[37, 38], and most particularly by William Wadd[39].

Wadd's fascinating little book describes a number of autopsy examinations where enormous accumulations of fat were found. This is the first instance of a monograph devoted solely to obesity that contained anatomical dissections (see Chapter 20).

B. Microscopic anatomy (Histology)

The invention of the microscope in the seventeenth century moved anatomy to the next level. Three great anatomists working in England, The Netherlands, and Italy—countries that were at the heart of the Renaissance and the Religious Reformation—might be described as "three who made a revolution." In the middle decades of the seventeenth century, early microscopists began to publish the results of their investigations using simple microscopes. Their pictures were breathtaking. The important initial observations by Robert Hooke (1635–1703)[40], Antoni Leeuwenhoek (1632–1723)[41] Marcello Malpighi (1628–1694)[42], identified the pulmonary circulation, the fine structure of small animals and red blood cells, and sperm, among others. (Figures 3-7 and 3-8)

Gradually, the sophistication of the microscope improved and the first simple lenses were replaced by complex ones. The introduction of the compound microscope with two lenses was a big step forward. This was followed by the introduction of achromatic lenses in the early nineteenth century, which made microscopes sufficiently powerful to define the structures inside cells. It was the combination of the achromatic microscope, which allowed sufficient resolution to distinguish the multiple structures inside cells, coupled with the intellectual genius of Theodor Schwann (1810–1882)[43] and of Matthias Schleiden (1804–1881)[44] that recognized the unifying principles of the cell wall, nucleus, and an area of structures surrounding this nucleus as the basic elements of cell biology. Shortly afterwards, the first substantial textbooks of microscopic anatomy were published[45, 46]. A few years later the fat cell was recognized as a member of this group. A description of the growth and development of fat cells was published in 1879 by Hoggan and Hogan[47]. In his early observations on the development of the fat vesicle, Arthur Hassall[48] suggested that certain types of obesity might result from an increased number of fat cells. It was more than a century later that the work of Per Bjurulf[49], of Jules Hirsch (1929–)[50], and of Per Bjorntorp (1931–2003)[51] elaborated this important concept as the "hyperplastic" form of obesity in individuals with an increased number of fat cells. Within the twenty years following the formulation of the cellular theory of biology[43, 44], Rudolf Virchow (1821–1902)[29, 52] provided a cellular interpretation of disease processes. The next advance in microscopic anatomy was the introduction of the electron microscope by Knoll and Ruska in 1932[53], which has provided an even more detailed look at the interior of the fat cell and other cells.

C. Physiology

The discovery by William Harvey (1578–1657) that blood circulated in the body was one of the leading physiological discoveries of the seventeenth century. He applied experimental methods to the demonstration that blood must circulate, rather than ebb and flow from the liver as Galen had suggested. William Harvey first announced his discovery in 1616[11] and published it in 1628. His theory is monumental in the way that experimental observations and human reasoning were brought together. His theory of the circulation of the blood was published before the capillaries that connect the arterial and venous circulation had even been described[42]. While in medical school in Padua, Italy, Harvey had seen his professor, Fabricius ab Aquapendente (1537–1619), demonstrate the presence of valves in the veins that only allowed blood to flow one way. At some point between his graduation from Padua in 1596 and his anatomic dissections at the Royal College of Physicians in London in 1616, he realized the importance of these valves in the veins. They meant that blood could only flow one way because the valve would prevent it from flowing the other way. From the limited quantity of blood in the body, he argued, therefore, that the blood must circulate and be reused. He presented his revolutionary discovery to the Royal College of Physicians in 1616 to a ho-hum reception[54] (Figure 3-9).

Gradually, the importance of the discovery and of the method by which he argued its cogency became apparent. It was, however, not for another fifty years that capillary circulation was demonstrated by Marcello Malpighi using one of the early simple microscopes[42], confirming one requirement of Harvey's theory.

The early physiological studies by Harvey on the circulation of the blood set the stage for further work in physiology. Two of these themes are particularly relevant to our study of the battle of the bulge. The first is digestion, the way the body converts food you eat into chemicals that can be absorbed into the body. The second is metabolism, the study of how the body uses the chemicals from digested food for energy or storage. If you store too much, you may be called on to fight your own battle of the bulge. The man who began the study of metabolism, and thus might be called "Father of Metabolic Obesity," is Santorio Santorio (1561–1636), who was a contemporary of William Harvey at the University of Padua.

In 1614 Santorio Santorio (see Chapter 4) described his metabolic balance[55, 56] that consisted of a platform on which he could sit, counterbalanced by a beam to which weight could be added or subtracted to record changes in his weight related to bodily functions. With this system, he could measure his food intake and his excretory losses.

In more recent times, Louis Newburgh and his colleagues working at the University of Michigan in the 1930s[57] used a similar method to record the loss of water with respiration and showed that the energy involved in vaporizing water in the lungs accounted for about 24 percent of the heat produced by the body.

The other group of physiological studies that relate to obesity describe how the gastrointestinal tract digests and absorbs food. In 1752 Rene-A-F Reamur (1683–1757)[58] succeeded in isolating the gastric juice from his pet bird by putting a sponge into the stomach attached to a string that he could withdraw. When he put the gastric juices that he withdrew with his sponge in contact with food, the juices digested the food. Later in the eighteenth century, Abate Lazaro Spallanzani (1729–1799)[59, 60] showed that gastric juice outside the body would both digest food and prevent putrefaction.

Occasionally an experiment of nature provides an opportunity to make new discoveries. This was true for the American military surgeon William Beaumont (1785–1853)[61]. He made significant advances in understanding the working of the human stomach by directly observing it through a fistula, or hole, into the stomach in a patient who survived a gunshot wound (Figure 3-10).

Alexis St. Martin suffered a bullet wound in his abdomen that did not completely heal, leaving him with the fistula that allowed Dr. Beaumont to observe the stomach and its contents. One of the most intriguing findings was the way the lining of the stomach changed color in relation to the patient's emotional state of anger or happiness. When angry, the stomach became red and engorged, this faded when he was not angry. Two French physiologists, Francois Magendie (1783–1855) and his distinguished pupil Claude Bernard (1813–1878), demonstrated that substances produced by the pancreas digested food and that the liver contained glycogen, a complex of glucose molecules that was the source of blood sugar (glucose) between meals[62].

These eighteenth- and nineteenth-century observations on digestion were followed in the early twentieth century by the seminal and long-lasting theory that hunger resulted from gastric contractions. This theory was based on direct measurements of the association of gastric contraction with hunger by A.L. Washburn and Walter Cannon[63] and independently by Anton Carlson[64]. These ideas are expanded in more detail in Chapter 15.

D. Chemistry and Biochemistry

Modern chemistry might be traced to the seventeenth century and the work of Robert Boyle (1627–1691), who established the concept of chemical elements[65]. By the late seventeenth century, Boyle and his students recognized that when a lighted candle went out in a bell jar, a mouse living in the same jar rapidly died[66]. It was clear that some important element was present in the air that was essential for life and for a candle to burn. At the beginning of the eighteenth century, Georg Stahl (1660–1734)[67] postulated that this substance was phlogiston. It was not until the work of Joseph Priestley (1733–1804)[12] and of Carl Wilhelm Scheele (1742–1786)[13], who simultaneously discovered what we now call oxygen, and particularly of Antoine-Laurent Lavoisier (1743–1794)[14] (Chapter 10), that the Phlogiston Theory was replaced by the Oxygen Theory of Combustion (Figure 3-11).

Lavoisier's Oxygen Theory recognized that oxidation meant combining with oxygen. His experimental work showed that metabolism was similar to a slow combustion. Lavoisier's death at the hands of Revolutionary French government in 1794 deprived humanity of one of its great intellects[68].

The eighteenth century legacy of Lavoisier and the development of the laws of the conservation of mass and energy[69] in the middle of the nineteenth century formed the basis for the work on metabolism during the latter half of the nineteenth century, which is central to understanding how our bulge developed and what we need to do about it. Max Rubner (1854–1932)[70, 71], a member of the German Laboratory School, formulated the Law of Surface Area based on the observation of a straight-line relationship between metabolic expenditure of animals of many sizes and their surface area, determined as [body weight]$^{0.7}$. Two other Germans, Carl Voit (1831–1908) and Max Pettenkofer (1818–1901)[72], along with Rubner, began the studies that ultimately demonstrated that the Law of Conservation of Energy proposed by Helmholtz applied to animals. The final piece of this important work was done by Wilbur Atwater (1849–1907)[73, 74] who, along with the physicist Edward B. Rosa, constructed the first functional human calorimeter at Wesleyan College in Middletown, Connecticut, in 1896. This instrument served as a tool for extensive studies on metabolic requirements during food intake and on the effects of starvation by Atwater and by Francis Benedict (1870–1957)[75, 76] (Chapters 11 and 28).

Following the work of Atwater and Benedict in the early twentieth century, studies using metabolic chambers languished until after World War II. The earliest of these post-World War II chambers were built in Paris and at the National Institutes of Health in Bethesda, Maryland. However, it was a chamber built in Lausanne, Switzerland, by Eric Jequier[77] and the ones built in London[78] and Phoenix, Arizona[79], that have provided the most extensive and continuing series of studies on energy expenditure in human subjects in the post-World War II period. They have shown that for human beings fat-free mass, or body weight from which the amount of body fat has been subtracted, provides a slightly better relationship between energy expenditure and body weight than the surface area concept developed by Rubner almost a century earlier[78]. Utilizing these metabolic room-sized chambers, several predictors of obesity have been found, including a low metabolic rate[79], a high rate of carbohydrate oxidation (as indicated by a high respiratory quotient [RQ], the ratio of the carbon dioxide produced to the oxygen used during metabolism), and sensitivity to insulin.

One of the major findings of the last quarter of the twentieth century was that human beings were notoriously unreliable in reporting the amount of food they ate. This insight came from the study of energy expenditure in human beings in the past two decades following the introduction of doubly labeled water. This is a technique for measuring total energy expenditure over a period of several days in free-living people[80]. Doubly labeled water measures energy expenditure by following the way the body metabolizes the two parts of the water molecule, hydrogen (as its heavy form, deuterium) and oxygen (as its heavy form oxygen-18 [^{18}O]) through the metabolic pathways in the body. Deuterium can only be excreted as water, while ^{18}O can be excreted as water or as carbon dioxide through the lungs following metabolism of carbon-containing compounds to carbon dioxide. Over several days the ratio of hydrogen and oxygen (deuterium to ^{18}O ratio) gradually diverges following the administration of these two isotopes of water. The rate of this change can be used to calculate energy expenditure (Chapter 13).

Applying the technique of doubly labeled water to human beings has produced startling results. Both overweight and normal weight people under-report what they eat. That is, the most careful records of food eaten usually do not account for the energy the body needs. Not surprisingly, overweight people underestimate their dietary intake more than normal weight people[81]. This new tool has provided a way to assess energy needs with accuracy. The under-reporting of food intake by both normal and overweight individuals questions the validity of data obtained from dietary records. These findings make it all the more difficult to use reports of food intake to help bulging individuals in their battle to lose weight.

The term *biology* as the study of living things with the cell as its basic unit was a nineteenth-century concept. Biological chemistry or biochemistry is also a nineteenth-century concept. Friedrich Wöhler (1800–1882) performed a key experiment in 1828 that broke down the barrier between the world of the inorganic, such as rocks and chemicals, and the world of the organic, found in living creatures[82]. He showed that urea, an organic molecule that is used by the body to excrete nitrogen in the urine, could be produced from inorganic molecules. As the importance of this insight grew, the field of biological chemistry and then biochemistry emerged to take a major place at the table of biological sciences.

Biological chemistry in the mid-nineteenth century was dominated by three main figures. The first was François Magendie (1783–1855)[21] in France at the beginning of the nineteenth century. He was a leader in the application of the experimental method to the study of living animals (Figure 3-12). He was succeeded by his outstanding pupil Claude Bernard (1813–1878)[22] in the middle of the nineteenth century in France. Bernard also discovered liver glycogen as the source of blood glucose[22] and showed that damage (*piqure*) to the hypothalamus could produce loss of glucose in the urine or glycosuria. Bernard's scientific philosophy was one of "gradualism," that is, that scientific theory would naturally lead to step-by-step progress, a concept that was a dominant element in the nineteenth century philosophy of science[83]. Gradualism could also be viewed as the best strategy in the battle of the bulge. This concept of gradualism is in sharp contrast to the concept of paradigm shifts and scientific revolutions[84] and correspondingly to the use of surgical treatments for obesity which produce profound weight loss.

Justus von Liebig (1803–1873)[28] was the third giant of biochemistry. He was born in Darmstadt, Germany, and headed one of the most productive laboratories on chemistry, food chemistry, and agricultural chemistry in the nineteenth century. His ultimately flawed concept that the carbohydrates, proteins, and fats were all that were needed for human nutrition served as the basis for nutritional science during much of the nineteenth century. The discovery of vitamins at the turn of the twentieth century gave birth to a new and broader concept of nutrition[85]. This "new nutrition" occupied the first half of the twentieth century and was centered on the discovery and function of vitamins. This era of vitamin discovery closed in 1948 with the chemical structure of vitamin B_{12}. With the focus no longer on vitamins, the macronutrients fat, carbohydrate, and protein returned to center of the nutritional stage as the recognition of the role of dietary fats and obesity in the development of cardiovascular disease grew[86].

The twentieth century has seen an explosion in the application of chemical and biochemical techniques to the study of obesity and its health implications. The study of body composition is one of these areas. Chemical analysis of human cadavers was conducted in the nineteenth and early twentieth centuries, and the fat in adipose tissue was found to be primarily triglyceride. Sophistication in the measurement of body components has greatly expanded, allowing us to measure body fat accurately in living human beings. The work by Behnke, Feen, and Wellman[87] (Chapter 6) during World War II showed how to use the weight of the body in and out of water, or body density, to measure the fat and non-fat parts of the body. Even better methods appeared after World War II when radioactive isotopes were used to study body composition[88, 18]. The introduction of ultrasound, a method similar to sonar, for measuring fat thickness below the skin; the use of computed tomographic (CT) scans and magnetic resonance imaging (MRI) scans to measure fat inside body cavities; the use of low-energy x-rays (dual-energy x-ray absorptiometry), which allows a computer to tell us how much fat is in the body; and the use of whole-body neutron activation have all provided sophisticated techniques for accurate and detailed determination of body composition of living people[90].

E. Genetics and Molecular Biology

The biological revolution of the last quarter of the twentieth century had its roots in the mid-nineteenth century. The publication by Charles Darwin (1809–1882) of *On the Origin of Species*[91] and by Gregor Mendel (1822–1884)[92] of the notion of inheritable traits, subsequently called genes, was a bombshell that is still reverberating in scientific circles and is clearly relevant to the battle of the bulge (Figure 3-13). In the early twentieth century, Archibald Garrod (1857–1936)[93] suggested the concept of "metabolic" disorders, which was the forerunner of the interest in the genetic basis for changes in metabolism.

Gradually, genetic material was traced to deoxyribonucleic acid (DNA) in the nucleus of the cell. A new field of molecular biology was born in 1953 from the seminal work of James Watson (1927–) and Francis Crick (1917–2004)[94], who proposed the double-helix model for the structure of

DNA. This led to the cracking of the genetic code, the development of the tools for molecular biology, and the translation of genetic information into protein structures. With these techniques it became possible to identify and isolate the genes underlying the rare forms of inherited obesity in animals. The Human Genome Project has now completed the sequencing of all of the genes in several species, including human beings. When we read the book of life in the genetic code, we will have new tools in the battle of the bulge (Figure 3-14).

The first genetic breakthrough in the study of obesity came in 1992 with the identification by Woychick and his colleagues of the genetic defect in the yellow obese mouse and the coat color gene that produced a yellow coat color and obesity[95] (Chapter 8). This gene provides information to the cell on how to make a peptide with 133 amino acids. In the yellow obese mouse, the abnormal gene is expressed in many tissues where it is not normally found. The protein produced by this gene competes in a lock-and-key manner with receptors that are pivotal to the control of food intake and coat color. Through this mechanism this protein can account for the yellow coat color, hyperphagia, and obesity present in these animals.

In 1994, Jeffrey Friedman (1954-) and his colleagues at the Rockefeller University in New York City reported the discovery of the genetic defect in a mouse that is born to be fat (the obese or ob/ob mouse)[96]. The gene in this mouse is altered so that it stops making its protein after 105 amino acids have been assembled, rather than completing the entire 167 amino acid protein. This shortened protein is rapidly destroyed, whereas the normal 167 amino acid protein, called leptin, is secreted from fat cells. Leptin is produced almost exclusively in fat cells. After release from the fat cell, leptin circulates in the blood where it can enter the brain. Once inside the brain, leptin influences a number of important biological molecules that control eating. Thus, leptin is a message from fat that can, by its concentration in the blood, tell the brain about the state of peripheral fat stores and their adequacy for reproduction. Leptin is also involved in modulating a number of other important biological functions including regulation of food intake, energy expenditure, and function of cells in the bone marrow. In the obese (ob/ob) mouse, and in the rare human beings who do not make leptin, treatment with leptin will reverse obesity and correct the other defects.

The third obesity gene to be discovered (cloned) was the gene for the recessively inherited FAT mouse[97]. The nature of this gene defect was suspected from the high levels in these animals of pro-insulin, the molecule that is split to form insulin. Cleavage or splitting of proinsulin to form insulin requires the enzyme carboxypeptidase-E. The gene for this enzyme is defective in a mouse called FAT and results in defective synthesis of hormones and neuromediators that require an enzyme to split them into an active and inactive part.

Some human beings, too, inherit genes that make them obese. Understanding genetic susceptibility for human obesity has also benefited from advances in experimental genetics and molecular biology[98]. Beginning with the work of Charles Davenport (1866–1944)[99] on the inheritance of size and body weight in families, and the work of von Verscheuer on identical twins[100] ever more data argue that important components of total body fat and fat distribution are inherited and controlled by genes[101, 102] (Chapter 24). More than one hundred different genes have been implicated in human obesity[98, 103, 104].

F. Pharmacology

Pharmacology, the study of drugs and their biological effects, grew from a base in chemistry[105]. Its early successes in the first half of the nineteenth century included the isolation from various plants of morphine, strychnine, emetine, and quinine and the publication in 1822 by François Magendie (1783–1855) of the first pharmacopeia of drugs for use by physicians[106]. The discovery of anesthesia in the middle of the nineteenth century was one of the major advances in pharmacology and surgery. It was discovered almost simultaneously by three Americans. Crawford Long (1815–1878)[107] was a native of Georgia. He first used ether anesthesia to remove a tumor in 1842, but did not publish this finding until many years later. William Thomas Green Morton (1819–1868)[108] and Horace Wells (1815–1848)[109] were both dentists. Wells pioneered the use of nitrous oxide or laughing gas in anesthesia, but when he demonstrated his technique during surgery at the Massachusetts General Hospital in Boston, it failed because the patient was not adequately anesthetized. Morton got attention with the first successful public demonstration of the use of ether anesthesia. It occurred in October 1846 in a room now appropriately called the "Ether Dome" at Massachusetts General Hospital. At the end of the operation, the elderly but distinguished surgeon John Warren (1778–1856) said, "This is no humbug." Morton's patient had remained unconscious throughout the surgical procedure. The subsequent publication of this event brought anesthesia to worldwide attention[110] (Figure 3-15).

The risk of infection is a major hazard during surgery, and this was all the more so before sterile techniques were introduced. Shortly after the discovery of anesthesia and the introduction of the ideas that "germs" could cause disease, Joseph Lister (1827–1912) in 1865 introduced the use of carbolic acid sprays in the operating room to reduce infection during surgery[111,112].

There are always people eager to make money with "shady" remedies. For people who are overweight, the associated stress prompts many people to try shady treatments if they promise successful treatment in their battle of the bulge. The nineteenth century saw its share of shady remedies as the patent medicine man plied his wares. Among these were the use of hydrotherapy and various laxatives and purgatives. Thyroid extract was also initially used to treat obesity in 1893 as the nineteenth century was drawing to a close.

The aniline dyes used in dyeing fabrics had a major impact on the entire field of pharmacology in the late nineteenth and twentieth centuries[113]. Developed by the chemical industry, aniline served as the base for synthesizing numerous drugs in the twentieth century and for the "magic bullet" concept of Paul Ehrlich (1854–1915)[114]. Ehrlich reasoned that there should be a molecular structure like a key that would fit into a lock and be an effective treatment for syphilis, a sexually transmitted disease that was a scourge of the day. His discovery of salvarsan, a moderately effective compound, bore out his concept.

Imagine eating all you wanted and not gaining weight because your body was burning off those "unwanted" calories. Dinitrophenol, for a fleeting time, offered such a promise. This drug was one of the aniline dye products that was used to treat obesity. This interlude provides important lessons in translating discoveries in the laboratory into effective treatments in the battle of the bulge. Dinitrophenol was introduced for treatment of obesity when weight loss was noted in chemical workers who handled dinitrophenol. It was used with limited testing in animals and was subsequently abandoned after it produced cataracts and diseases of the nerves[115]. This tragedy of treatment shows the need for careful clinical evaluation of drugs before they are made available for general clinical use[116].

Amphetamine was a second product of the synthetic organic chemical industry that was used for treatment of obesity. In the 1930s, dextroamphetamine, which was synthesized in 1887, was shown to produce weight loss in individuals being treated for narcolepsy[117]. Because amphetamine is addictive, it fell into disrepute and led to a negative view of all so-called "amphetamine-like" drugs with a similar chemical structure. However, the similarity of chemical structure on paper proved misleading pharmacologically. Drugs work in a lock-and-key fashion. Changing the design of the key will change the lock it opens. This analogy applies to this and other groups. The β-phenethylamine chemical structure is the backbone of amphetamine (alpha-methyl β-phenethylamine). Amphetamine affects two brain chemicals or neurotransmitters, dopamine and norepinephrine. Modifying the β-phenethylamine structure can completely change the effect on these neurotransmitters. Phentermine is a β-phenethylamine cousin of amphetamine which affects primarily norepinephrine. Fenfluramine, another β-phenethylamine cousin of amphetamine, is pharmacologically so different as to be unrelated to amphetamine, since it only affects serotonin release.

G. Neuroscience

The brain has become a central arena in the battle of the bulge; it is where leptin, the hormone from fat, acts. It is where information from various sense organs is integrated into decisions about eating and other activities. A neural basis for some kinds of obesity became evident at the beginning of the twentieth century. Two widely known case reports, one by Joseph Babinski (1871–1953)[118] and the other by Alfred Frohlich (1857–1932)[119] described single individuals who developed obesity due to a tumor at the base of the brain. This important clinical finding opened a new field of research and heralded the development of techniques to produce obesity in experimental animals by damaging specific areas at the base of the brain by injection of a toxic material, such as chromic oxide[120], or more specifically by localized passage of an electric current or application of heat to specific nests of hypothalamic brain cells or nuclei[121, 122]. These studies showed that there were two different types of hypothalamic centers. In one center (the ventromedial hypothalamus) damage would produce an increase in food intake and obesity. The other center was located a small distance away (the lateral hypothalamus) and damage here decreased food intake[123]. The presence of these two regions with different effects on food intake led in 1954 to the proposal of the dual center hypotheses by Elliot Stellar (1919–1993)[124]. The idea that an increase or decrease in food intake was controlled by different areas of the hypothalamus in the brain served as the basis for thinking about hunger and satiety for the next twenty years.

It soon became clear that overeating, or hyperphagia, was not essential for the development of obesity after a hypothalamic lesion[125] or in genetically obese mice[126]. A supplemental explanation for the development of obesity was provided by the autonomic hypothesis[127]. This hypothesis was based on the observation of increased activity of the vagal parasympathetic nervous system[128] and reduced activity of the sympathetic nervous system[129]. The diminished activity of the sympathetic nervous system reduced heat generation in small animals and suggested that beta-adrenergic drugs that produced heat might be potential agents for treating obesity[130].

The discovery of a number of peptides that are present in both the brain and in the gastrointestinal tract has brought together the areas of neuroscience and gastrointestinal physiology in the control of body fat and obesity. Secretin was the first GI hormone discovered[131]. Subsequently, cholecystokinin was found to stimulate contraction of the gall bladder and to reduce food intake[132]. Of the many peptides now known, neuropeptide-Y, polypeptide-YY, ghrelin, and glucagon-like peptide-1 are among the more interesting because they are potent stimulators (NPY, PYY, ghrelin) or inhibitors (GLP-1) of food intake[133].

H. Clinical Medicine and the Battle of the Bulge

Each era has its own clinical scholars[134]. I have chosen several of them to illustrate the broad sweep of their contributions. Thomas Willis (1621–1675)

(Figure 3-16)[135] and Thomas Sydenham (1624–1689) were seventeenth century physicians (Figure 3-17)[136]. Willis is noted particularly for his work on the nervous system. It is the circulatory connection between the right and left half of the brain that carries his name, the Circle of Willis. Willis also detected the "sweetness" of urine from diabetic patients. Sydenham, on the other hand, is noted for his clinical acumen[136]. He believed that direct observation by the physician was the primary basis for knowledge of disease. Direct clinical observation was the basis for the important work by Richard Morton (1635–1698) who described anorexia nervosa[137] (Chapter 18).

The eighteenth century (Figure 3-3) saw a transition in medical dominance from Italy and France, where schools at Padua and Montpellier had been preeminent, to countries in northern Europe. The seat of greatness in medicine shifted to Leiden in the first half of the eighteenth century, where Hermann Boerhaave (1668–1738)[138] attracted students from all over Europe. His eminence as a teacher was expanded by the introduction of hospital beds that were specially assigned for teaching. With Boerhaave's death, the center for clinical medicine moved to Edinburgh in the last half of the eighteenth century, where many American physicians studied. William Cullen (1712–1790), one of the leading clinicians in Edinburgh, is important in this volume for his work on classifying diseases including obesity[139] (Figures 3-18 and 3-19).

As had happened before, the clinical hospitals and universities for medical education and leadership moved again in the nineteenth century with the changing times. From Edinburgh in the eighteenth century, it moved to France in the first half of the nineteenth century and then to Germany in the last half of the nineteenth century. The collection of outstanding clinicians and scientists in Paris during the early years of the nineteenth century has been referred to as "The Paris School" by historian Erwin Ackerknecht. The early nineteenth century in Paris was the first time that surgery and medicine had been taught together in the same curriculum. The emphasis was on teaching medicine and surgery at the bedside. Like Edinburgh before it, Paris was the center for medical education for many young American physicians. Among the leading physicians in Paris Medicine were Pierre-Charles-Alexandre Louis (1787–1872)[140] the founder of medical statistics, and René-Théophile-Hyacinthe Laennec[20], who invented the stethoscope. This is relevant to the battle of the bulge because he conceived the idea during the examination of an obese patient. He was having difficulty hearing her heart when his ear was next to her chest because of the thick layer of adipose tissue. When he rolled up a newspaper and put one end on her chest and the other to his ear, he could hear her heart beat, thus inventing the first stethoscope (Figure 3-20).

At mid-century as the Paris Clinical School was declining in importance, the German Laboratory or Experimental School was on the ascendancy. Many eminent German physician-investigators developed during this period. Robert Koch (1843–1910)[141] was one of the leaders in the new field of infectious disease. He identified the germ that causes tuberculosis and directed attention toward bacteria as the cause of wound infections. Hermann von Helmholtz (1821–1894) was another giant intellect from the German Laboratory School of the late nineteenth century. He described the First Law of Thermodynamics, which tells us that energy is conserved. For the science of obesity, his contribution means that when you eat more energy in your food than you need, you will store it as fat. Helmholtz early came under the influence of Johannes Müller (1901–1858)[27] in Berlin who attracted and trained many of the premier minds who collectively are described as the German Laboratory School. In addition to describing the First Law of Thermodynamics, Helmholtz invented the ophthalmoscope[142] which allows doctors to look in the back of the eye, and he provided a modern theory of how we hear and see (Figure 3-21).

Well before the scientific era, which I have dated as beginning in A.D. 1500, individuals with massive obesity have been noteworthy. Cases of massive obesity have been noted since antiquity[135, 143, 44, 145, 146]. In the nineteenth century, Dubourg[147] discussed twenty-five such cases, Schindler[148] identified another seventeen individuals, and Maccary described eleven more[149]. Individual cases of very overweight individuals have also been reported by many other authors[150–159]. These individuals were frequently noted for their "odd" or "monstrous" appearance. The outlook for this group was particularly bleak, both from a clinical and social perspective.

These case reports beg a very important question that we have only begun to answer recently. That is, are all cases of obesity the same? Classification of obesity is part of the more general efforts to classify diseases. Although many classifications of disease exist, one of the most interesting was the effort to classify disease based on the binary classification of plants and animals introduced by Karl von Linne (Linnaeus) (1707–1778)[160]. His system involved giving each individual a genus and species name and categorizing the genera into classes, orders, and phyla.

Although Thomas Sydenham (1624–1689)[136] began such a systematic classification of disease, the two best-known efforts to classify diseases in this way were published by Bossier de Sauvages (1706–1767)[161] in France and William Cullen (1710–1790) in Edinburgh[139]. In both of them obesity was called *polysarcie*, meaning "too much tissue." In the English translation of Cullen's work, *polysarcie* (Obesity) is in Class III, called the *Cachexieas*, which refers to changes in body composition. It is listed under the second order called *Intumescentiae* (swelling) with a genus name of *Polysarcia* (*Corporis pinguedinosa intumescentia molesta*). *Obesity*, as a word to describe increased fatness, gradually replaced *polysarcie*, the French word *embonpoint*, and the English word *corpulence* during the nineteenth century.

A small monograph written by the surgeon William Wadd titled *Cursory Remarks on Corpulence: By a Member of the Royal College of Surgeons*[39] describes clinical cases of obese individuals and how they fit into the ideas of obesity. In the last edition of this book, published in 1829, Wadd described several cases, and using his skills as a draftsman drew graphic pictures of some of them. Most of the cases in this last book were from his medical correspondence, a characteristic way of evaluating patients by consulting physicians since the physical examination was not a part of the usual medical evaluation in the early 1800s. Of the twelve cases in his book, all but one were men. Weights were noted in five cases and ranged from 106 kg (16 st 10 lb or 234 pounds) to 146 kg (23 st 2 lb or 324 pounds). Two of the cases examined at post-mortem had enormous accumulations of fat. Although autopsy observations of obese individuals had been made previously, this is the first instance in which it is included in a monograph devoted to obesity and leanness (Chapter 20).

Wadd[39] notes that sudden death is not uncommon in the corpulent, thus validating Hippocrates. Wadd states, "A sudden palpitation excited in the heart of a fat man has often proved as fatal as a bullet through the thorax." In several of Wadd's cases, corpulent patients had asked for pills to treat their obesity although nothing of value was available then. Wadd makes a distinction between the therapeutic activists and those favoring less aggressive therapy, with the homeopathists being at the far extreme with minimal dosage of medication. As Wadd said, "Truly it has been said—some Doctors let the patient die, for fear they should kill him; while others kill the patient, for fear he should die" (Chapter 20).

One important lesson from the study of massively obese individuals was the association of obesity with sleep apnea, a disease often referred to as the Pickwickian Syndrome[162], referring to Joe, the fat boy, in *The Pickwick Papers* by Charles Dickens. Patients with this syndrome snore at night and have periods when breathing briefly stops. During the daytime they are often sleepy[144, 145]. The earliest published medical report of sleep apnea and the hypoventilation and its consequences was that of Russell in 1866[146] and is described in more detail in Chapter 23.

Other clinical subtypes of obesity, in addition to the massively obese and those with sleep apnea, have been gradually defined. In the early part of the twentieth century, Cushing recognized[163] that obesity was associated with tumors of the pituitary gland (basophilic adenomas)[164] (Chapter 26). Cushing's syndrome can also be caused by medication with adrenal steroids. A number of other drugs, including anti-psychotics, some antidepressants (amitriptyline), some anti-convulsants (valproate), anti-serotonin drugs, and anti-diabetic drugs, can also cause weight gain. Other endocrine diseases such as hypogonadism and isolated growth hormone deficiency are also associated with increased amounts of body fat. Several rare genetic disorders cause obesity or have obesity as a finding[98]. Finally, a sedentary lifestyle and a high-fat diet are associated with obesity.

Besides the lessons from individual patients provided by these case reports, there are the lessons that come from evaluation of collective data. In the mid-nineteenth century, Lambert-Adolph-Jacques Quetelet (1796–1874)[165] was one of the leaders in developing mathematical methods to evaluate populations. He developed the concept of the "average man" and used the ratio of weight divided by the square of stature (height) (kg/m^2) as a measure of an individual's fatness. This unit, the body mass index, might be termed the Quetelet Index (QI) in honor of the man who developed what has become a widely used way of evaluating weight status (Chapter 5).

The life insurance industry has extended the population-based view of obesity[166]. As early as the mid-nineteenth century, data began to appear showing that both excess amounts of weight and central distribution of this weight shortened life expectancy. Because of the financial need to relate risk of mortality to the costs of life insurance, the life insurance industry has continued to provide data showing these relationships (Chapter 21). This data was responsible for stimulating evaluation of the association of weight status with mortality risks in several population-based studies[167–172]. In all of these studies, the risk of death or disease increases in a curvilinear fashion with rising weight or body mass (Quetelet) index.

Although the relationship of fat located on the trunk to increased mortality could be discerned in these early insurance studies, it remained for Jean Vague[172] to bring this concept of increased health risk from central adiposity to the attention of health professionals. Although Vague's data is clear, the adipo-muscular ratio that he used to measure fat distribution was complex, and it remained for the simpler measurement of the waist circumference or the ratio of the circumference of the waist divided by the hip circumference (the WHR) to provide the wide recognition that the risk to health is greater with centrally located fat than with fat on the hips or thighs. With better methods of measuring fat distribution with CT and MRI scans, it is now clear that increased fat inside the abdomen, or visceral fat, is an important component of the health risks associated with obesity (Chapter 22).

The twentieth century has seen an explosion of scientific knowledge that we can use in the battle of the bulge. The publication by Sir William Osler (1869–1919) in 1892 of his *Principles and Practice of Medicine*[173] stands as a milestone in medical education. Osler was born in 1869 and was educated at McGill University in Montreal. He then came to the United States where he was successively professor of medicine at the University of Pennsylvania and the first professor of medicine at the newly founded Johns Hopkins Medical School from 1889 to 1905. While there he set a tone for the clinical practice of medicine that continued throughout the twentieth century. His professional career was capped by appointment as Regius Professor of Medicine at the University of Oxford in 1905. His textbook of 1892, republished in various forms throughout most of the twentieth century, provides us with a glimpse in the battle of the bulge from a century ago:

> Corpulence, and excessive development of the bodily fat, is a condition for which the physician is frequently consulted, and for which much may be done by judicious arrangement of the diet[173].

With this introduction, I will turn to the historical use of diet in the battle of the bulge.

I. Treatments for the Battle of the Bulge

Diet and exercise have been the cornerstones for treatment of obesity since the time of Hippocrates and Galen more than two thousand years ago. They were central parts of both the Greco-Roman and Arabian treatments in the battle of the bulge (see Chapters 1 and 2). As the centuries passed, many new ideas have been added, some reasonable, some "quackery." Our current epidemic indicates that none of these ideas has cured obesity, although from time to time there have been some dramatic successes. One of these is from the tenth century. It is the story of King Sancho I, also called Sancho the Fat[174]. Sancho I became king of León in Spain in A.D. 958, but his reign was short because his fatness became an impediment to his rule, and his noblemen deposed him. The physicians in Leon were unsuccessful in helping Sancho lose weight, so he sought the help of a brilliant and learned Jewish physician named Hisdai ibn Shaprut, physician to the caliph in the southern Spanish city of Cordoba. In a day when "house calls" were still in fashion, Shaprut traveled several hundred miles from Cordoba to Pamplona to evaluate Sancho. Shaprut agreed to take Sancho as a patient, but advised him that it would be a long treatment requiring him to relocate to Cordoba. The medicine that Shaprut prescribed was *Theriaca*, a mixture that probably contained opiates and that was often taken with wine and oils. Over time Sancho gradually lost weight. When he returned to León as a lean man, he returned to his throne. Thus was introduced a "medicine" in addition to the diet and exercise of old.

1. Sixteenth Century

From the twelfth century onward, the *Regimen Sanitatis*[175], written in the School of Medicine at Salerno, Italy, provided guidance for the use of diet and nutrition for achieving and maintaining good health. Although it went through many editions over several hundred years, the *Regimen* did not specifically provide advice for treating obesity, which was relatively infrequent during the Middle Ages. Chaucer, the great fourteenth century poet, echoed the advice of Hippocrates two thousand years earlier when he said against gluttony the remedy is abstinence, or in his Middle English, "Agonys glotonye, the remedie is abstinence."

The discovery of the New World by Columbus in 1492 brought tobacco and many other products back to Europe. As we will see, tobacco soon appeared in the treatment of the battle of the bulge. Daily doses of vinegar were also used as a treatment that has resurfaced time and again between A.D. 1500 and 1900. Finally, soap and other purgatives were common recommendations.

2. Seventeenth Century

The seventeenth century was the century of physics and mathematics with Galileo, Newton, and Kepler. Their ideas about the physical laws of nature formed the basis for one theory about diseases. This medico-physical (iatrophysical) approach to describing the function of the body and disease began to replace the four humors that had dominated medical thinking since the time of the Greeks. In one textbook from this period, there is a description of five approaches to treating "obesitas or corpulency," as it was called. I have cited these below from this textbook of 1682 by Théophile Bonet because they give a flavor of the kinds of things that were used for the individual who had a major problem with obesity.

Under the section called "Obesitas or corpulency" Bonet says:

a. Chiapinius Vitellius, Camp Master-General, a middle aged man, grew so fat, that he was forced to sustain his belly by a swath, which came about his neck. On observing that he was every day more unfit for the Wars than other, he voluntarily abstained from Wine, and continued to drink vinegar as long as he lived; upon which his belly fell, and his skin hung loose, with which he could wrap himself as with a doublet. It was observed that he lost 87 pounds of weight.
b. Lest any great mischief should follow, we must try to subtract by medicine, what a spare diet will not; because it has been observed, that a looseness either natural, or procured by Art, does not a little good. But this must be done by degrees and slowly, since it is not safe to disturb so much matter violently, lest it should come all at once. Therefore the best way of Purging is by Pills, of Rheubarb, Aloes each 2 drachms, Agarick 1 drachm, Cinnamon, yellow Sanders, each half a drachm. Make them up with Syrup of chicory. They must be taken in this manner: First 1 scruple must be

given an hour and a half before meal; then two or three days afterwards, take half a drachm or two scruples before Meal. Thus purging must be often repeated at short intervals, till you think all the cacochymie is removed.

c. A certain Goldsmith, who was extremely fat, so that he was ready to be choked, took the following Powder in his Meat, and so he was cured; Take of Tartar two ounces, Cinnamon three ounces, Ginger one ounce, Sugar four ounces. Make a Powder.

d. Horstius found the things following to take down fat men; especially onions, Garlick, Cresses, Leeks, Seed of Rue, and especially Vinegar or Squills: Let them purge well: Let them Sweat and purge by Urine; Let them use violent exercise before they eat: Let them induce hunger, want of Sleep and Thirst: Let them Sweat in a Stove and continue in the sun. Let them abstain from Drink between Dinner and Supper: for to drink between meals makes men fat.

e. I knew a Nobleman so fat, that he could scarce sit on Horse-back, but he was asleep; and he could scarce stir a foot. But now he is able to walk, and his body is come to it self, only by chewing Tobacco Leaves, as he affirmed to me. For it is good for Phlegmatick and cold Bodies.

f. Let Lingua Avis, or Ash-Keyes be taken constantly about one drachm in Wine. According to Pliny it cures Hydropical persons, and makes fat people lean[35].

Diets have been around since the battle of the bulge first began. The use of a "stringent diet" was popularized again in the seventeenth century by an Italian layman named Luigi Cornaro (c. 1475–1566)[176]. In a short book he championed dietary moderation after he successfully conquered his own obesity. At the beginning of his book he says:

> O wretched, miserable Italy! Does not though plain see, that gluttony deprives [us] of more soul years, than either war, or the plague itself could have done?

Cornaro's doctor's advice was to eat or drink nothing that was not wholesome and that only in small quantities. With this advice Cornaro lost his excess weight and then became a zealot for moderation in dieting (Figure 3-22).

3. Eighteenth Century

George Cheyne M.D. (1671–1743) was one of the most interesting medical figures in the eighteenth century for our story. He was born in Scotland

and obtained a medical degree from Edinburgh. Along with many others at the turn of the century, he made his way to London where he arrived in 1701. Over the ensuing few years his profligate living and familial tendency to corpulence led his weight to increase to 448 pounds[177]. In 1705 he had a medical and emotional crisis. He returned to Scotland and then migrated to Bath and to Bristol in the west of England. He developed a spiritual side of his life that became an important part of his medical practice. With continuing efforts, he brought his weight under control with periodic ups and downs over the rest of his life. Two books, *The Essay of Health and Long Life* published in 1724[178] and *The English Malady* published in 1733[179] are the most relevant to this story. In *The English Malady*, Cheyne includes a number of medical cases, including his own medical biography and battle of the bulge. Moderation was the key. In his dietary approach, Cheyne replaced meat, particularly red meat, with milk. Temperance and exercise were important and he recommended two pints of water and one of wine in twenty-four hours[177]. In *The English Malady* he elaborated on his themes of the relationship between mind, body, and spirit. The success of these two books is evident from the fact that they went through a number of editions and were translated into other languages.

J. Tweedie, in his book titled *Hints on Temperance and Exercise, Shewing their Advantage in the Cure of Dyspepsia, Rheumatism, Polysarcia, and Certain States of Palsy*, has provided one summary of dietary treatment for obesity from the eighteenth century (note that in the late eighteenth century, *polysarcia* and *corpulency* were used more often than the word *obesity*).

> In attempting its cure, when the habit is threatened with any morbid effects, from the plethora existing either in the head or lungs, this must be removed by a bleeding or two; and as corpulent people do not bear blood-letting well, purging is most to be depended upon for the removal of the plethora[180].

He also says,

> The diet should be sparing. They [the overweight] should abstain from spirits, wines and malt liquors, drinking in their stead, either spring water, toast and water or else water agreeably acidulated by any pure vegetable acids[180].

Finally, Tweedie recommends a gradual increase in exercise.

The eighteenth century also witnessed publication of the first two English books dealing exclusively with obesity. In each book, the author proposed a new way of treating obesity. The first book was by Thomas Short, published in 1727[181]. He begins by saying, "I believe no age did ever afford more instances of corpulency than our own." This is an amazing statement. We believe that we have an epidemic of obesity, yet more than two hundred fifty years ago Dr. Short was aware of a surge of obesity in England.

After a discussion of the pathology of obesity as he viewed it, Short proposed the following approaches to treatment. From Short's perspective, treatment of obesity required restoring the natural balance and removal of the secondary causes. If possible one should pick a place to live where the air is not too moist or too soggy and one should not reside in flat, wet countries or in the city or the woodlands. He thought that exercise was important and that the diet should be "moderate spare and of the more detergent kind"[181].

The second eighteenth century book was by Malcolm Flemyng, a graduate of the medical school in Edinburgh[182]. His approach to treatment of obesity was based on the results with a patient that he presented to the Royal Society in London in 1757 and subsequently published in 1760. His book listed four causes of corpulency[182].

The first cause is "the taking in of too large a quantity of food, especially of the rich and oily kind." He went on to note that not all obese people were big eaters. The second cause of obesity is "too lax a texture of the cellular or fatty membrane...whereby its cells or vesicles are liable to be too easily distended." The third cause was an abnormal state of the blood, which facilitated the storage of fat in the vesicles. Finally, defective evacuation was also an important cause. Since Flemyng believed sweat, urine, and feces all contained "oil," he believed that the treatment for obesity was to increase the loss of "oil" by each of these three routes. Thus, laxatives, diuretics, and sweating could be used for treatment.

4. Nineteenth Century

The nineteenth century began the proliferation of books about obesity and how to treat it. One of the best known and most interesting is a book titled *The Physiology of Taste, or Meditations on Transcendental Gastronomy* by Jean Anthelme Brillat-Savarin (1755–1826), published in 1826 and republished and translated many times. One of the most attractive versions of this masterpiece has been illustrated by Wayne Thibeault, a California artist whose paintings of food look so good that you think you could eat them right off the page[183]. Brillat-Savarin attributes obesity to two causes:

> The first is the natural temperament of the individual...The second principal cause of obesity lies in the starches and flours which man uses as the base for his daily nourishment...A double cause of obesity results from too much

> sleep combined with too little exercise...The final cause of obesity is excess, whether in eating or drinking[183].

From this, Brillat-Savarin moves to treatment. He says, "Any cure of obesity must begin with the three following and absolute precepts: discretion in eating, moderation in sleeping, and exercise on foot or on horseback"[183]. Having said this much he goes on to say, "Such are the first commandments which science makes to us: nevertheless I place little faith in them"[183]. He then goes on to recommend a diet low in grains and starches. The book by Brillat-Savarin covered not only obesity but many other areas of taste and food as well. It has continued to be a best seller, but never in the sense of the popular diet books that began only a few years later.

The first "popular" diet book appeared as recently as 1863. It was written by an undertaker and was based on his own experiences. The first edition of this small, twenty-one-page pamphlet titled *A Letter on Corpulence Addressed to the Public* was published privately by Mr. William Banting (1797–1878) in 1863[184]. The demand for this pamphlet was so great that a second and third edition were published within one year. In this pamphlet, Mr. Banting recounted his successful weight loss experience using a diet prescribed by his ear surgeon, Dr. William Harvey[184], who was no relation to the William Harvey who discovered the circulation of the blood two hundred years earlier. Why an "ear surgeon," you might ask? Mr. Banting had become so heavy, weighing more than 200 pounds, that at his age of sixty he had begun to lose his hearing and his sense of balance and was forced to come downstairs backwards, lest he fall. He tried the diet recommended by Dr. Harvey and during the course of one year lost more than 50 pounds (23 kg). The immediate success of this pamphlet led to reprinting worldwide and a popularization of the term "Bantingism" as a reference to dieting (Chapter 27).

Mr. Banting's diet consisted of the following:

> Breakfast, 8 A M.: 150 to 180 gm (5 to 6 oz.) meat or broiled fish (not a fat variety of either); a small biscuit or 30 gm (1 oz.) dry toast; a large cup of tea or coffee without cream, milk or sugar.
>
> Dinner, 1 P.M.: Meat or fish as at breakfast, or any kind of game or poultry, same amount; any vegetable except those that grow under ground, such as potatoes, parsnips, carrots, or beets; dry toast, 30 gm. (1 oz.); cooked fruit without sugar; good claret, 300 c.c. (10 oz.). Madeira or sherry.
>
> Tea, 5 P.M.: Cooked fruit, 60 to 90 gm (2 to 3 oz.); one or two pieces of zwieback; tea, 270 c.c. (9 oz.) without milk,

cream or sugar.

Supper, 8 P.M.: Meat or fish, as at dinner, 90 to 120 c.c. (3 to 4 oz.); claret or sherry, water, 210 c.c. (7 oz.).

Fluids restricted to 1050 c.c. (35 oz.) per day.

From these humble beginnings, diet books by professionals, self-styled professionals, and lay people have continued to appear, particularly as the concerns about obesity as a health and cosmetic problem have increased in the latter half of the twentieth century[5]. I have summarized three diets from the early twentieth century to show the approaches that were used at that time[186].

5. Twentieth Century

Three dietary themes have occupied the last one hundred fifty years. The first is the low-carbohydrate diet in various degrees of carbohydrate deprivation that begin with Banting's diet. The second is the low-calorie or balanced-deficit diet in which total calories are reduced and all of the macronutrients are reduced. The third theme is the low-fat diet that comes in both low-fat, about 25% of energy from fat, and very-low-fat, where the goal is 10% of energy from fat. Below are examples of these diets from the beginning of the twentieth century provided by leading medical experts. In addition to these examples, there are a very large number of popular diet books that have been published for use by the general public.

a. Treatment with Diet and Exercise.

In America there are fewer cures for obesity undertaken than abroad...because...there are fewer obese people here. –Carter[187]

This statement was made in 1917, but with time, the tides of obesity have overcome America, which is now the fattest country in the world, and the epidemic of obesity in America shows no signs of slowing down[188].

Von Noorden's Diet

Carl von Noorden (1853–1944) was one of the leading scholars of obesity at the beginning of the twentieth century, and he based his dietary approach on an estimate of an individual's caloric requirement. Basal calorie needs were estimated from ideal weight. For this he assumed that a 70-kg (154-pound) individual would require 37 kcal/kg or 2,590 calories. If the individual weighed 100 kg (220 pounds), he would need 1,110 extra calories to feed this extra 30 kg. Von Noorden's first-degree reduction diet reduced energy to 80% of the basal needs, or for the 70-kg individual to 2,000 kcal/day. His second-degree reduction diet reduced intake to 60% or 1,500 kcal/d for the individual requiring 2,500 kcal/day. His third-degree reduction, which was only infrequently used, lowered calories to 40% or 1,000 kcal/d. His dietary approach also reduced fat to 30 grams per day. His protein allowance was 120–180 g/d with carbohydrates in the neighborhood of 100 g/d. His menu plan, adapted from Carter et al[187], is summarized below:

	Minimal	Maximal
Protein	120 gm. (4 oz.) 492 cal.	180 gm. (6 oz) 738 cal.
Fat	30 gm. (1 oz.) 280 cal.	30 gm. (1 oz.) 280 cal.
Carbohydrate	100 gm. (3 1/3 oz) 410 cal.	120 gm. (4 oz) 492 cal.
Totals	1182 cal.	1510 cal.

A sample of the von Noorden Diet is shown below:

Breakfast:	Lean meat, 80 gm. (2 2/3 oz.); bread, 25 gm. (1 oz.); tea, one cup with milk, no sugar.
Midmorning:	One egg.
Luncheon:	Soup, 1 small portion; lean meat, 160 gms. (5 1/3 oz.); potatoes, 100 gms. (3 1/3 oz.); fruit, 100 gms. (3 1/3oz.).
Afternoon:	3 P.M. Cup of black coffee.
Snack:	4 P.M. Fruit, 200 gm. (6 2/3 oz.) 6 P.M.. Milk, 250 c.c. (8 oz.)
Dinner:	Meat, 125 gm. (3 1/6 oz.); bread (graham), 30 gm. (1 oz.); fruit, small portion as sauce without sugar; salad, vegetable or fruit, radishes, pickles.

Ebstein's Diet[189]

At the other extreme is the high-fat diet illustrated by Ebstein's diet. Ebstein modified existing diets by allowing a considerable amount of fat and restricting the carbohydrates by forbidding all sugar, sweets, and potatoes, but allowing 180 to 210 gms. (6 or 7 oz.) of bread. Vegetables that grow above ground are allowed and all sorts of meat, especially fatty meat is permitted. Fats are allowed, 120 to 180 gms. (4 to 6 oz.) per day. He used a three-meal plan with the largest meal at midday.

Breakfast:	One large cup of black tea, without cream or milk, or sugar; white or brown bread, 60 gms. (2 oz.) with plenty of butter.
Dinner:	2 P.M. Clear soup, meat 120 to 180 (4 to 6 oz.) with gravy and fat meat is especially recommended; vegetables in abundance

	(as noted above); small amount of fresh or stewed fruit (without sugar) or salad; two or three glasses of light white wine. Shortly after dinner a cup of tea is allowed with sugar or milk.
Supper:	7:30 P.M. Large cup of tea, without sugar or milk; one egg with or without a small portion of meat, preferably fat. Occasionally a little cheese or fresh fruit.
Total values:	Protein, 100 gm. (3 1/3 oz.); fat, 85 gm. (3 oz.); carbohydrate, 50 gm. (2 2/3oz.).

These two themes, the low-fat, high-protein, high-carbohydrate diet and the high-fat, low-carbohydrate diet, have been repeating throughout the twentieth century, but their origins were in the late nineteenth century. Had either of the low-carbohydrate or the low-fat approach "cured" obesity as their proponents hoped, there would have been no need for the continual supply of new diets that we have seen throughout the twentieth century.

Starvation Diets

Total starvation has been used occasionally to treat obesity. As a prelude to its clinical application, the metabolic consequences of starvation were explored by Francis Benedict using metabolic chambers[75, 76]. He found that human beings adapt to starvation by lowering energy expenditure and conserving protein and sodium and excreting water and potassium. At the same time the suggestion that calories could be dissipated by "burning them off," termed *luxuskonsumption*, was promoted by Gulick[190] and by Neumann[191] based on studies they conducted on themselves. This idea did not go unchallenged, and the debate about whether we can dissipate unneeded calories through changes in metabolism has been a recurring theme during the twentieth century[192] (Chapter 12).

Just before the beginning of the Great Depression in 1929, Evans[193] showed that a very-low-calorie diet had potential benefits for people needing to lose weight. Although Evans continued to publish on semi-starvation with a very-low-calorie diet as an approach to losing weight until the beginning of World War II, this idea was lost sight of until fasting was reintroduced as a treatment for obesity by Bloom in 1959[194]. Following his enthusiastic report, the use of liquid formula diets spread rapidly, but with an ultimate disaster. Liquid formula diets were initially popularized by the famous Rockefeller University in New York. Their use began gradually and then rapidly increased until seventeen deaths occurred in patients using a formula diet whose major protein was gelatin[195]. Although the nineteenth-century Gelatin Commission in France had concluded that gelatin was an inadequate protein to support life, this lesson was re-learned with lethal results in the 1970s[196, 197]. New liquid formula diets using high-quality protein replaced the gelatin based diets, and sales reached another peak in the late 1980s. When the U.S. Government raised concerns about these diets and other "commercial weight control" programs in 1989[198], there was a rapid and sudden decrease in public interest and a loss of commercial profitability.

b. Behavior Modification

Behavior therapy is one of the central developments in the treatment of obesity in the twentieth century. The psychoanalytic movement spearheaded by Sigmund Freud and his colleagues[199] provided several theories suggesting that obesity might result from "personality" disorders. These were carefully tested and found to be inadequate explanations for obesity[200]. That obesity had important social components, however, became clear from studies relating the prevalence of obesity to socio-economic status[201]. The prevalence of corpulence is much higher in people from lower socio-economic groups than in people from higher social and economic groups (Chapter 18).

Although psychoanalytic techniques were unsuccessful in treating obesity, other avenues of behavioral treatment were effective. One of these stems from the work on conditioned reflexes by Pavlov and his followers[202] and from the work on operant conditioning by Skinner[203, 204]. These latter techniques were used by Stuart[205] in his classic study in 1967. Stuart treated eleven patients, eight of whom were available for follow-up at the end of one year. In this group, weight losses were among the highest reported with any technique. He succeeded by helping his patients monitor their food intake and manipulating the environment in which the food was eaten. Subsequent to this seminal work, the principles of behavior modification have been widely applied to the treatment of obesity (Chapter 29).

c. Pharmacotherapy.

As the understanding of how drugs worked in the human body has increased, so too has its application to the treatment of obesity. Although one might call William Withering, who discovered the value of extracts of the foxglove plant for treating heart failure in 1785, the father of pharmacology[206], the first chemical work on drug isolation and purification came in the early nineteenth century during the important period of French Clinical Medicine[16]. A summary of nineteenth-century treatments for obesity can be found in a textbook from the late 1800s by Sajous[207]. The following is an excerpt:

> Besides the familiar dietetic treatment, thyroid gland to enhance catabolism, but not in the large doses usually pre-

> scribed, which provide hypercatabolism and greatly weaken the patient. From 2 to 3 grains (120–180 mg of levothyroxin) t.i.d. are enough to increase gradually the lipolytic power of the blood. Potassium iodide in increasing doses can be used instead, when thyroid extract cannot be obtained. Hyoscine hydrobromate 1/100 grain t.i.d. assists the reducing process by increasing the propulsive activity of the arterioles and causing them to drive an excess of blood into the fat-laden areas. Carlsbad, Homburg, and Marienbad waters owe their virtues mainly to the alkaline and purgative salts they contain, especially sodium sulphate. As a beverage alkaline Vichy water is advantageous to enhance the osmotic properties of the blood and facilitate the elimination of wastes[207].

Shortly after the discovery of endocrine glands in the nineteenth century, extracts were prepared and used for the treatment of obesity as early as the 1890s[207]. As Sajous says,

> The fact that thyroid preparations in sufficient doses promote the rapid combustion of fats has caused them to be used extensively in this disorder...In large doses (thyroid gland)... imposes hyperoxidation upon all cells...we behold gradual emaciation beginning with the adipose tissues, which are the first to succumb. Hence the use of thyroid preparations in obesity.

Sajous goes on to say that small doses (66 mg or 1 grain) are indicated in all cases to begin with.

> Briefly, in all cases of obesity in which thyroid gland is rationally indicated, the feature to determine is whether directly or indirectly hypothyroidia underlies the adiposis[207].

Sajous also describes the use of testicular extracts: "Testicular preparations, including spermine, have been recommended in a host of disorders, particularly...obesity... but others again have failed to obtain any favorable results"[207].

We now move to the last part of the twentieth century. Realizing that both serotonergic and noradrenergic receptors were involved in modulating food intake, Weintraub et al. in 1992 published a four-year study showing that combining a noradrenergic drug (phentermine) with a serotonergic drug (fenfluramine) might be better than monotherapy[208]. This classic series of papers opened a whole new pharmacologic approach to obesity that came to an abrupt end in 1997 when valvular heart disease (aortic insufficiency) was reported[209], leading to withdrawal of fenfluramine and dexfenfluramine from the market.

d. Surgery

Surgical intervention for excess fat can be dated at least from the Talmudic days, even though there was no anesthesia available at the time. According to Preuss[210], a corpulent rabbi named Eleazar was given a sleeping potion and taken into a marble chamber, where his abdomen was opened and many basketfuls of fat were removed. Plinius also describes a very similar "heroic cure for obesity:" "the son of the Consul L. Apronius had fat removed and thus his body was relieved of a disgraceful burden. More recently, in A.D. 1190 A.D., a surgeon cut open the abdomen of Count Dedo II of Groig in order to remove the excessive fat from him[210]. Following the advent of anesthesia in 1846, this procedure has been revived (Chapter 31).

The historical view of gastro-intestinal function in relation to obesity may be perceived to have reached its zenith (or nadir, depending on one's perspective) with the introduction of gastro-intestinal operations for obesity. Three operative approaches have been developed to treat obesity. The first procedure reported by Kremen[211] was a jejuno-ileal bypass on a single patient. Believing that if weight were lost patients would be able to maintain the weight loss, Payne and DeWind performed a series of eleven jejuno-colic anastamoses, which produced significant diarrhea and weight loss[212] When the patients were reanastamosed, they all regained weight. Realizing that this surgery had not "cured" obesity, procedures were designed for long-term use. The first of these long-term procedures was the jejuno-ileal bypass operation. These were associated with overwhelming and unacceptable metabolic and infectious complications, and this operative procedure for obesity was discontinued in the late 1970s.

An alternative long-term approach to altering gastro-intestinal function as a treatment for obesity was developed by Mason and Ito[213], who performed the first gastric reduction operation. These procedures have now become the dominant operative procedures for the treatment of obesity. Whether one or another of the currently used procedures is better than the others is part of a major clinical trial in Sweden. This study, called the Swedish Obese Subjects (SOS) study, has operated on two thousand patients and has a matched control group of two thousand unoperated patients who are being followed for the effects of the operation on health and social issues[214]. At the time of this writing, the balance of benefit appeared to be somewhat on the side of surgical intervention, but the final answers are not yet in.

J. Public Health and the Battle of the Bulge

With the advent of the twentieth century, concerns about the relation of obesity to the health risks gradually replaced concerns about being underweight[215]. During the twentieth century, four themes have coalesced to form the basis for a modern science of obesity. These include the behavioral or psychological aspects of obesity, the physiological approach to a controlled system of food intake, the cellular basis for obesity centered in the growing diversity of cellular functions for the fat cell, and the genetic and molecular biological approaches to understanding the problem.

Just as 1850 provided a watershed for medicine and obesity in the nineteenth century, so the beginning of World War II provides such a demarcation point in the twentieth century. The first American book devoted solely to obesity was published in 1940 by Rony[216]. It marks this transition. After World War II, there was a dominance of American politics, science, and medicine.

The period after World War II saw a dramatic growth in the scientific industry—and in obesity as well. The growth of the National Institutes of Health in the United States has served as a major stimulus for research in all fields of biology, including obesity[217]. An emphasis on obesity has become an imperative as the epidemic of obesity has spread worldwide. The World Health Organization and the National Institutes of Health have both recognized this burgeoning problem. The result has been an effort to focus research through establishing centers with concentrations of scientists interested in this problem. These obesity research centers are now located in a number of leading American universities and bode well for the future of research into the problem posed by obesity.

As the field of obesity matured, a number of things happened. First, groups of scientists interested in obesity began to form local organizations to promote interest in the problem of obesity. The first of these was in the United Kingdom. The Association for the Study of Obesity held its first meeting in 1968[218]. This was followed in 1973 by the first NIH Conference on Obesity held in Washington, D.C.[219]. One year later the First International Congress on Obesity was held in London[220]. Following these congresses, it was clear that a journal devoted to papers dealing specifically with obesity was needed, and the *International Journal of Obesity* was founded. Publication began in 1976 under the editorship of Dr. Alan Howard and Dr. George Bray. Subsequent international congresses were held in 1977 in Washington, D.C.[221]; in 1980 in Rome[222]; in 1983 in New York City[223]; in 1986 in Jerusalem[220]; in 1990 in Kobe, Japan[225]; in 1994 in Toronto[226]; in 1998 in Paris[227]; and in 2002 in Sao Paulo[228].

In 1986 the International Association for the Study of Obesity was formed under the leadership of Dr. Barbara Hansen. As growth continued, a second journal appeared in 1980 under the title *Obesity and Weight Regulation*. This journal, like so many others, succumbed in part because it was not part of one of the national associations. *Obesity Surgery* was the third journal to be founded and was followed in 1993 by *Obesity Research*, published by the North American Association for the Study of Obesity. This rapid growth of scientific journals surrounding a scientific discipline is characteristic of developments that have sprung up throughout the scientific sphere to provide a way of focusing the activities of scientists in a manageable way.

For some as yet unexplained reason, the last twenty years of the twentieth century saw a remarkable rise in the prevalence of obesity. As we begin the next sections of this book, the two maps from the U.S. Centers for Disease Control and Prevention depict the magnitude of this problem as it developed in the last decade of the century and millennium (Figure 3-23).

Biosketch

Thomas Short (?1690–1772), physician, was born in the south of Scotland and, after graduating in medicine, settled in practice at Sheffield. In 1713 one William Steel communicated to him the secret of making cerated glass of antimony a cure for dysentery, which he afterwards published. He made several journeys to visit the mineral springs of Yorkshire and of other parts of England. He published in 1725 "A Rational Discourse on the Inward Uses of Water" and in 1730 "A Dissertation upon Tea," In 1750 he published "New Observations on the Bills of Mortality" in which he adds something to the remarks of Graunt and Sir William Petty, and treats the whole subject in relation to a book published anonymously by him the year before, *A General Chronological History of the Air* in two volumes, dedicated to Dr. Mead. He spent eighteen years on these works. In 1750 he also issued "Discourses on Tea, Sugar, Milk, made Wines, Spirits, Punch, Tobacco &c" and in 1751 *Medicine Britannica*, an interesting and lucid herbal for the use of general readers. His "Treatise on Different Sorts of Cold Mineral Waters in England" appeared in 1766, and is an original work showing careful observations. A further "Discourse on Milk" appeared in 1766 and in 1767 he published *A Comparative History of the Increase and Decrease of Mankind,* in which he advocates early marriages, denounces alcohol "as a Stygian poison," and collects much historical and medical information. All of his books were published in London. He died in 1772[229].

Biosketch

The date of birth of Malcolm Flemyng (?–1764) is unknown but was in the early eighteenth century. There is also little information about Flemyng's early life. He received his medical education at Leyden, where he was a student of Hermann Boerhaave. He returned to Scotland and began medical practice around 1725 but shortly afterward moved to Hull. In 1751 he moved to London with his three children when the life of a country practitioner had taken a toll on his health. He taught one course of physiology lessons in 1751–52 but then moved to Brigg in Lincolnshire. From his correspondence we know he was hopeful of teaching physiology at Oxford or Cambridge. Flemyng was both an experimenter and a clinician. His contribution relevant to our book is *On Corpulency*, which was read to the Royal Society in 1757 and published 1760. It was translated into German by J.J. Plenk at Vienna in 1769 and reprinted in London as late as 1810. Flemyng continued to practice medicine in Lincolnshire until his death on March 7, 1764.

Biosketch

Thomas King Chambers (1817–1889) was the fifth son of Robert Joseph Chambers. He received his medical training at Christ Church, Oxford, where he graduated with honors in classics. He studied medicine at St. George's Hospital in London and received his bachelor of medicine in 1842 from Oxford. He became one of the first physicians at St. Mary's Hospital, London, and later a consulting physician to the Lock Hospital. As a result of a popliteal aneurism, one of his legs was amputated. Dr. Chambers was a censor with the Royal College of Physicians and delivered the Gulstonian Lectures in 1850, the Lumleian Lectures in 1863, and the Harveian Oration in 1871. He was one of the earliest advocates of medicine as a career for women. One of his chief hobbies was painting in watercolors. He was also an accomplished woodcarver[33].

Biosketch

Sir William Osler (1849–1919) was born in Bond Head, Ontario, Canada, in 1849. After finishing his education at Trinity College in Weston, where his scientific interests were awakened by William Johnson, he entered the University of Toronto, where he began his study of medicine. His last two years of medicine were completed at McGill University in Montreal where he graduated in 1872. His medical course was greatly influenced by Palmer Howard, professor of medicine. Following two years in Europe, Osler returned to McGill as professor and spent ten years teaching and actively engaged in pathological studies. From 1884 he spent five years as professor of medicine at the University of Pennsylvania before moving to Johns Hopkins University as the first professor of medicine in 1889. During the next fifteen years his department at Johns Hopkins pioneered clinical teaching. In 1892 Osler published the *Principles and Practice of Medicine*, the last great textbook of medicine to be written by a single author. This textbook was instrumental in the philanthropic efforts in New York, leading to the establishment of the Rockefeller Institute of Medical Research. In 1904 Osler accepted appointment to the Regius Professor of Medicine at Oxford University. In this setting, his interest in classic books in medicine and in the historical aspects of this field blossomed. Osler's humanity and personality remained strong at Johns

Hopkins throughout the twentieth century as a towering figure for younger students. He died in Oxford in 1919, at the age of seventy (Figure 3-24).

Biosketch

James D. Watson was born in Chicago, Illinois, in 1928. All of his early education was in Chicago. He entered the experimental four-year college at the University of Chicago in 1943 and received his bachelor's degree in 1947. His graduate work was done at the University of Indiana, where he received his Ph.D. in 1950 for work on x-ray studies of bacteriophage multiplication under the tutelage of S.E. Luria. His first post-doctoral experience in Copenhagen was followed by a second one at the Cavendish Laboratory in Cambridge, England, where he moved to study DNA. It was here that he met Francis Crick, who was also interested in DNA. They thought it should be possible to establish a model for the structure of DNA, and after their first effort was a failure, they returned with a second successful double-helix structure in 1953. It was for this work the two of them received the Nobel Prize in 1962 (Figure 3-14).

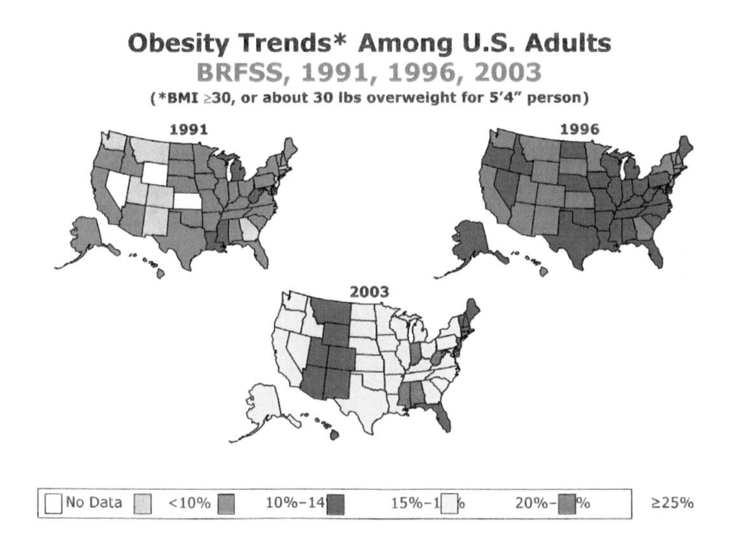

3-23 Maps showing the prevalence of overweight based on the telephone surveys conducted by Departments of Health in the 50 states under the supervision of the Centers for Disease Control and Prevention, Atlanta, GA. Courtesy of the Centers for Disease Control and Prevention.

References

1. Macleod and Mayhew. *In. Uzbekistan*, p. 170
2. Canguilhem, G. *Ideology and rationality in the history of the life sciences.* Trans. A. Goldhammer. Cambridge, MA: The MIT Press, 1988.
3. Beaujouan, G. "Motives and Opportunities for Science in the Medieval Universities." In *Scientific Change: Historical Studies in the Intellectual, Social and Technical: Conditions for Scientific Discovery and Technical Invention, from Antiquity to the Present.* A.C. Crombie, ed. New York: Basic Books, 1963.
4. Diderot, D. The Encyclopedia. In *Rameau's Nephew and Other Works.* Trans. Barzun, J., R.H. Bowen. Garden City, New York: Doubleday 1956: 277-307.
5. Beddoes, T. *Hygëia: or Essays Moral and Medical, on the Causes Affecting the Personal State of Our Middling and Affluent Classes.* Bristol J. Mills; 1802.
6. Price, D.J. de Solla. *Little Science, Big Science.* New Haven: Yale University Press, 1963.
7. Weissmann, G. *The Doctor with Two Heads and Other Essays.* New York: Alfred Knopf, 1990.
8. Bynum, W.F., and J.C. Wilson. "Periodical Knowledge: Medical Journals and their Editors in Nineteenth-century Britain." In Bynum, W.F., S. Lock, R. Porter eds. *Medical Journals and Medical Knowledge: Historical Essays.* New York. Routledge 1992: 29-48.
9. Loudon, J. and I. Loudon. Medicine, politics and the medical periodical 1800-1850. In: Bynum, W.F., S. Lock and R. Porter. eds. *Medical Journals and Medical Knowedge: Historical Essays.* New York: Routledge 1992: 798-69.
10. *Popper Selections.* Ed D. Miller. Princeton: Princeton University, Press; 1985.
11. Harvey, W. *The Anatomical Exercises of Dr. William Harvey. De Motu Cordis 1628: De circulatione sanguinis 1649: The First English Text of 1653 Now Newly Edited by Geoffrey Keynes.* London: Nonesuch Press, 1928.
12. Priestley, J. *Experiments and Observation on Different Kinds of Air.* London: J. Johnson, 1775.
13. Scheele, C.W. *The Discovery of Oxygen Part 2.* Edinburgh: William F. Clay, 1894. Alembic Club Reprint No. 8. From *Chemische Abhandlung von der Luft und dem Feuer,* Uppsala and Leipzig, 1777.
14. Lavoisier, A. L. *Traité élémentaire de chimie, présenté dans un ordre nouveau et d'aprés les découvertes modernes.* Paris: Chez Cuchet, 1789.
15. Chambers, T.K. "The Gulstonian Lectures on Corpulence." *Lancet* 2 (1850): 11–19, 342–350, 437–445.
16. Ackerknecht, E.H. *Medicine at the Paris Hospital.* Baltimore: Johns Hopkins University Press, 1967.

17. Bichat, X. *Anatomie générale, appliquée à la physiologie et à la médecine*. Paris: Chez Brosson, Gabon et Cie, 1801.
18. Auenbrugger, L. *Inventum novum ex percussione thoracis humani et signo abstnisos*. Vindobonae: J. T. Trattner, 1761.
19. Corvisart, J.-N. *An Essay on the Organic Diseases and Lesions of the Heart and Great Vessels*. Bound with: Auenbrugger, *On Percussion of the Chest*. Birmingham: Classics of Medicine Library, 1984.
20. Laennec, R.-T.-H. *De l'Auscultation Médiate, ou Traité du Diagnostic des Maladies des Poumons et du Coeur*. Paris: J.-A. Brosson J.-A. et J.-S. Chaudei, 1819.
21. Magendie, F. *Precis élémentaire de physiologie*. Paris: Mequignon-Marvis, 1816.
22. Bernard, C. *Sur le mécanisme de la formation du sucre dans le foie. C R Acad Sci.* 41 (1855): 461–469.
23. Hodgkin, T. On Some Morbid Apparances of the Absorbent Glands and Spleen. *Med Chir Trans.* 17 (1832): 68–114.
24. Bright, R. *Reports of Medical Cases, Selected with a View of Illustrating Symptoms and Cure of Diseases by a Reference of Morbid Anatomy*. London: Longmans, 1827-1831.
25. Addison T. *On the Constitutional and Local Effects of Disease of the Suprarenal Capsules*. London: Samuel Highley, 1855.
26. Jenner, E. *An Inquiry into the Causes and Effects of the Variolae Vaccinae, a Disease Discovered in Some of the Western Counties of England, particularly Gloucestershire, and Known by the Name of Cow Pox*. London: D.N. Shury, 1801.
27. Müller, J. *Handbuch der Physiologie des Menschen*. vol. Coblenz: J. Holscher, 1834–40.
28. von Liebig, J. *Chemistry in Its Application to Agriculture and Physiology*. Transl. Lyon Playfair. London: Taylor and Walton, 1842.
29. Virchow, R. *Cellular Pathology*. Transl. from the 2nd edition by F. Chance. London: J. Churchill, 1860.
30. von Helmholtz, H. *Beschreibung eines Augen-spiegels zur Untersuchung der Netzhaut im lebenden Auge*. Berlin: A. Forstnersche Verlagsbuchhandlung, 1851.
31. Koch, R. "Die Aetiologie der Tuberkulose." In *Mittheilungen aus dem Kaiserlichen Gesundheitsamte*. 2nd vol. Berlin: August Hirschwald, 1884.
32. Roentgen, W. "Eine neue Art von Strahlen." *Sitz Wurz Physik Med Gesellschaft*. (1895): 3–12.
33. Munks. *Rolls: Lives of the Fellows of the Royal College of Physicians of London, 1826–1925*. Compiled by Brown, OH, Litt, MAB. London: Published by the College 4 (1955):48–49, 1826, 1925.
34. Garrison, F. *An Introduction to the History of Medicine*. Philadelphia:

W.B. Saunders, 1912.

35. Bonetus, T. *Sepulchretum, sive anatomia practica, ex cadaveribus morbo denatis, proponens historias omnium humani corporis affectum.* Genevae: Sumptibus Cramer & Perachonv, 1700.
36. Morgagni, G.B. *De sedibus, et causis morborum per anatomen indagatis libriquinque.* Venetiis: typog. Remordiniana, 1761.
37. Haller A. "Corpulence Ill Cured; Large Cryptae of the Stomach" (etc). *Path Observ.* (1756): 44–49.
38. Haller, A. *Elementa physiologiae corporis humani.* Lausanne: Marci-Michael Boursquet & Sociorum, 1757.
39. Wadd, W. *Comments on Corpulency.* London: John Ebers & Co., 1829.
40. Hooke, R. *Micrographia, or Some Physiological Descriptions of Minute Bodies Made by Magnifying Glasses; with Observations and Inquiries Thereupon.* London: J. Martyn & J. Allestry, 1665–67.
41. Leeuwenhoek van, A. *The Select Works of Antony van Leeuwenhoek, Containing His Microscopial Discoveries in Many of the Works of Nature, translated from the Dutch and Latin editions published by the author Samual Hoole.* London: G. Sidney, 1800.
42. Malpighi, M. *Opera omnia.* Londini: R. Scott, 1686.
43. Schwann, T. *Mikroscopische Untersuchungen über die Übereinstimmung in der Struktur und dem Wachstum der Thier und Pflanzen.* Berlin: Sanders, 1839.
44. Schleiden, M.J. "Beiträge zur Phytogenesis." *Arch Anat Physiol Wiss Med.* (1839): 137–176.
45. Henle, F.G.J. *Allgemeine Anatomie.* Leipzig: L. Voss, 1841.
46. Hassall, A. *The Microscopic Anatomy of the Human Body, in Health and Disease.* London: Samuel Highley, 1849.
47. Hoggan, G., F.E. Hogan. "On the Development and Retrogression of the Fat Cell." *J R Microscop Soc.* (1879): 353.
48. Hassall, A. "Observations on the Development of the Fat Vesicle." *Lancet.* i (1849): 63–64.
49. Bjurulf, P. "An Therosclerosis and Body Build with Special Reference to Size and Number of Subcutaneous Fat Cells." *Acta Med Scand.* 66 (1959): Suppl 349: 99.
50. Hirsch, J., J.L. Kittle. "Cellularity of Obese and Nonobese Human Adipose Tissue." *Fed Proc.* 29 (1970): 1516–1521.
51. Bjorntorp, P., L. Sjostrom. "Number and Size of Adipose Tissue Fat Cells in Relation to Metabolism in Human Obesity." *Metabolism.* 20 (1971):703–713.
52. Virchow, R. *Die Cellularpathologie in ihrer Begrundung auf physiologische and pathologische Gewebelehre.* Berlin: August Hirschwald, 1858.
53. Knoll, M., E. Ruska. "Beitrag zur geometrischen Electronenoptik."

Ann Physik. 12 (1932): 607–661.
54. Osler, W. *The Evolution of Modern Medicine.* New Haven: Yale University Press, 1921.
55. Santorio, S. *Medicina statica: or, Rules of Health, in Eight Sections of Aphorisms. English'd by J.D.* London: John Starkey, 1676.
56. Santorio, S. *Medicina Statica: Being the Aphorisms of Sanctorius, translated into English with large explanations. The second edition. To which is added Dr. Keil's Medicina statica Britannica, with comparative remarks and explanations. As also medic-physical essays...by John Quincy.* London: W. and J. Newton, A. Bell, W. Taylor,and J. Osborne, 1720.
57. Newburgh, L.H., M.W. Johnston. *The Exchange of Energy between Man and the Environment.* Springfield, IL: Charles C. Thomas, 1930.
58. Reamur, R.A.F. "Sur la digestion des oiseaux." *His Acad Roy Sci.* (1756): 266–307, 461-495.
59. Spallanzani, L. *Opusculi di fisica animale e vegetabile.* Moedena: Soc. Tipografica, 1776.
60. Spallanzani, L. *Dissertations Relative to the Natural History of Animals and Vegetables.* Transl. from the Italian. London: J. Murray and S. Highley, 1796.
61. Beaumont, W. *Experiments and Observations on the Gastric Juices and the Physiology of Digestion.* Plattsburgh: F.P. Aller, 1833.
62. Bernard, C. "De I'origine du sucre dans I'économie animale." *Arch Gen Med.* 18 (1848): 303–319.
63. Cannon, W.B., A.L. Washburn. An Explanation of Hunger. *Am J Physiol.* 2 (1912): 441–454.
64. Carlson, A.J., *The Control of Hunger in Health and Disease.* Chicago: University of Chicago Press, 1916.
65. Partington, J.R. *A Short History of Chemistry.* 2nd edition. London: Macmillan and Co. Ltd., 1951.
66. Boyle, R. *The Works of the Honourable Robert Boyle.* London: A. Millar, 1764.
67. Stahl, G.E. *Theoria medica vera. Physiologiam & pathologiam.* Halae: Literis Ophanotrophei, 1708.
68. Lavoisier, Antoine Laurent in *Dictionary of Science Biography* ed. Charles Gillespie New York: Charles Scribner Sons, 1970–1980. pp. 66–71.
69. Helmholtz, H.L.F. *Über die Erhaltung der Kraft, eine physikalische Abhandlung.* Berlin: G. Reimer, 1847.
70. Rubner, M. *Die Gesetze des Energieverbrauchs bei der Ernahrung.* Leipzig: Franz Deuticke, 1902.
71. Rubner, M. *The Laws of Energy Consumption in Nutrition.* New York: Academic Press, 1982.
72. Pettenkofer, M.J., C. Voit. "Untersuchungen über die Respiration." *Ann Chem Pharm* (Heidelberg). Suppl2 (1862–63): 52–70.

73. Atwater, W.O., E.B. Rosa. "Description of a new respiration calorimeter and experiments on the conservation of energy in the human body." U.S. Department of Agriculture Office of the Experimental Station (1899): 63.
74. Atwater, W.O., F.G. Benedict. "Experiments on the Metabolism of Matter and Energy in the Human Body. 1900–1902." Washington: Government Printing Office, 1903. Office of the Experiment Station–Bulletin no.136.
75. Benedict, F.G. "A Study of Prolonged Fasting," 1915. Washington: Carnegie Institution of Washington. Report Num. 203.
76. Benedict, F.G., W.R. Miles, P. Roth, H.M. Smith. *Human Vitality and Efficiency Under Prolonged Restricted Diet.* Washington, D.C.: Carnegie Institution of Washington, 1919.
77. Jequier, E., Y Schutz. "Long-term Measurements of Energy Expenditure in Humans Using a Respiration Chamber." *Am J Clin Nutr.* 38 (1983): 989–998.
78. Garrow, J. *Energy Balance and Obesity in Man.* 2nd edition. Amsterdam: Elsevier/North Holland Biomedical Press, 1978.
79. Ravussin, E., B.A. Swinburn. "Pathophysiology of Obesity." *Lancet.* 340 (1992): 404–408.
80. Schoeller, D.A., E. Van Santen, D.W. Peterson, W. Dietz, J. Jaspan, P.D. Klein. "Total Body Water Measurement in Humans with ^{18}O and ^{2}H Labeled Water." *Am J Clin Nutr.* 33 (1980): 2686–2693.
81. Lichtman, S.W., K. Pisarska, E.R. Berman, et al. "Discrepancy between Self-reported and Actual Caloric Intake and Exercise in Obese Subjects." *N Engl J Med.* 327 (1992): 1893–1898.
82. Wohler, F. "Ueber kunstliche Bildung des Harnstoffs." *Ann Phys Chem (Leipzig).* 12 (1828): 253–256.
83. Bernard, C. *Introduction a l'étude de la médicine experimentale.* Paris: J.B. Bailliere et fils, 1865.
84. Kuhn, T.S. *The Structure of Scientific Revolutions.* Chicago: University of Chicago Press, 1962.
85. McCollum, E.V. *A History of Nutrition. The Sequence of Ideas in Nutrition Investigations.* Boston: Houghton Mifflin, 1957.
86. Select Committee on Nutrition and Human Needs (hearing) of the United States Senate 95th Congress. Diet Related to Killer Diseases. Washington, DC: U.S. Government Printing Office, 1977. Volume VI–VII (2VI, 2VII).
87. Behnke, A.R. Jr., B.G. Fenn, W.C. Welham. "The Specific Gravity of Healthy Men: Body Divided by Volume as an Index of Obesity." *JAMA.* 118 (1942): 495–498.
88. Hevesy, G. *Radioactive Indicators. Their Application in Biochemistry, Animal Physiology and Pathology.* New York: Interscience Publishers,

1948.

89. Moore, F.D., K.H. Olesen, J.D. McMurrey, H.V. Parker, M.R. Ball, C.M. Boyden. *The Body Cell Mass and Its Supporting Environment.* Philadelphia: W.B. Saunders and Co., 1963.
90. Wang, Z, R.N. Pierson, S.B. Heymsfield. "The Five-level Model: A New Approach to Organizing Body Composition." *Am J Clin Nutr.* 1 (1992): 19–28.
91. Darwin, C. *On the Origin of Species by Means of Natural Selection or the Preservation of Favored Races in the Struggle for Life.* London: John Murray, 1859.
92. Bateson, W. *Mendel's Principles of Heredity: A Defence.* London: Cambridge University Press, 1902.
93. Garrod, A.E. "Inborn Errors of Metabolism." The Coonian Lectures Delivered before the Royal College of Physicians of London, in June, 1908. London: Henry Frowde, Hodder & Stoughton, Oxford University Press, 1909.
94. Watson, J.D., F.H. Crick. "Molecular Structure of Nucleic Acids: A Structure for Deoxyribose Nucleic Acid." *Nature.* 171 (1953): 737–738.
95. Bultman, S.J., E.J. Michaud, R.P. Woychik. "Molecular Characterization of the Mouse Agouti Locus." *Cell.* 71 (1992): 1195–1204.
96. Zhang, Y.Y., R. Proenca, M. Maffei, M. Barone, L. Leopold, J.M. Friedman. "Positional Cloning of the Mouse Obese Gene and Its Human Homolog." Nature. 372 (1994): 425–432.
97. Naggert, J.K., L.D. Fricker, O. Varlamov, et al. "Hyperproinsulinaemia in Obese Fat/fat Mice Associated with a Carboxypeptidase-e Mutation Which Reduces Enzyme-Activity." *Nature Genet.* 10 (1995): 135–142.
98. Snyder, E., B. Wafts, L. Perusse, Y.C. Chagnon, S.J. Weisnagel, T. Rankinen, C. Bouchard. "The Human Obesity Gene Map: The 2003 Update." *Obes Res.* 12 (2004): 369–439.
99. Davenport, C.B. "Body Build and Its Inheritance." The Carnegie Institution. 329 (1923): 37.
100. Verschuer, O. Von. *Die Verebungsbiologische Zwillingsforschung. Ihre Biologischen Grundlagen. Mit 18 Abbildungen. Ergebnisse der Inneren Medizin and Kinderheilkunde.* 31st ed. Berlin: Verlag Von Julius Springer, 1927.
101. Vogler, G.P., T.I. Sorensen, A.J. Stunkard, M.R. Srinivassen, D.C. Rao. "Influences of Genes and Shared Family Environment on Adult Body Mass Index Assessed in an Adoption Study by a Comprehensive Path Model." *Int J Obes.* 19 (1995): 40–45.
102. Bouchard, C., J. Despres, P. Mauriege. "Genetic and Nongenetic

Determinants of Regional Fat Distribution." *Endocr Rev.* 1 (1993): 72–93.
103. Warden, C.H., J.S. Fisler, S.M. Shoemaker, et al. "Identification of 4 Chromosomal Loci Determining Obesity in a Multifactorial Mouse Model." *J Clin Invest* 95 (1995): 1545–1552.
104. West, D.B., J. Goudey-Lefevre, B. York, G.E. Truett. "Dietary Obesity Linked to Genetic-Loci on Chromosome-9 and Chromosome-15 in a Polygenic Mouse Model." *J Clin Invest.* 94 (1994): 1410–1416.
105. Paracelsus. *Wunder artzney, vonn allerley leibs gebruchen, und zu fallende Krankheiten, ohn sondere Beschwerung, Unlust unnd Verdrusz, kurtzlich zu heilen, unnd die Gesundheit widerumb mit geringem Kosten zun Wegen zubringen....* Basel: Sebastian Henricpetri, 1573.
106. Magendie, F. *Formulary for the Preparation and Employment of Several New Remedies, Namely, Resin of Nux Vomica, Strychnine, Morphine, Hydrocyanic Acid, Preparations of Cinchona... (Translated from the Formulaire of M. Magendie, published in Paris, October 1827).* London: T. and G. Underwood, 1828.
107. Long, C.W. "An Account of the First Use of Sulphuric Ether by Inhalation as an Anesthetic in Surgical Operations." *South Med Surg* 5 (1849): 705–713.
108. Warren, E. *Some Account of the Letheon: Or, Who Is the Discoverer of Anesthesia.* Boston: Dutton and Wentworth, 1847.
109. Wells, H. *A History of the Discovery of the Application of Nitrous Oxide Gas, Ether, and Other Vapors to Surgical Operations.* Hartford: J. Gaylord Wells, 1847.
110. Bowditch, N.L. *The Ether Controversy. Vindication of the Hospital Report of 1848.* Boston: John Wilsory, 1848.
111. Lister, J. "On the Effects of the Antiseptic System of Treatment upon the Salubrity of a Surgical Hospital." *Lancet.* 1 (1870): 4–6, 40–42.
112. Lister, J.B. *The Collected Papers of Joseph, Baron Lister. Member of the Order of Merit, Fellow and Sometime President of the Royal Society, Knight Grand Cross of the Danish Order of the Danebrog Knight of the Prussian Order pour le Mérite Associé Étranger de l'Institut de France.* Oxford: Clarendon Press, 1909.
113. Canguilhem G. *Ideology and Rationality in the History of the Life Sciences.* Transl. A Goldhammer. Cambridge: MIT Press, 1988.
114. Ehrlich, P., S. Hata. *Die experimentelle Chemotherapie der Spirillosen.* Berlin: Julius Springer, 1910.
115. Tainter, M.L., A.B. Stockton, W.C. Cutting. "Use of Dinitrophenol in Obesity and Related Conditions." *JAMA.* 101 (1933): 1472–1475.
116. Bray, G.A.. *The Obese Patient.* 9th ed. Philadelphia: W.B. Saunders Co., 1976.
117. Lesses, M.F., A. Myerson. "Human Autonomic Pharmacology XVI:

Benzedrine Sulfate as an Aid in the Treatment of Obesity." *N Engl J Med.* 218 (1938): 119–124.
118. Babinski, M.J. "Tumeur du corps pituitaire sans acromégalie et avec de développement des organes génitaux." *Rev Neurol.* 8 (1900): 531–533.
119. Frohlich, A. "Ein Fall von Tumor der hypophysis cerebri ohne akromegalie." *Wiener Klin Rdsch.* 15 (1901): 883–886.
120. Smith, P.E. "The Disabilities Caused by Hypophysectomy and Their Repair. The Tuberal (Hypothalamic) Syndrome in the Rat." *JAMA.* 88 (1927): 159–161.
121. Mohr, B. "Hypertrophie der Hypophysis cerebri and dadurch bedingter Druck auf die Hirngrundflache, insebesondere auf die Sehnerven, das Chiasma derselben und den linkseitigen Hirnschenkel." *Wschr ges heilk.* 6 (1840): 565–571.
122. Hetherington, A.W., S.W. Ranson. "Hypothalamic Lesions and Adiposity in the Rat." *Anat Rec.* 78 (1940): 149–172.
123. Anand, B.K., J.R. Brobeck. "Hypothalamic Control of Food Intake in Rats and Cats." *Yale J Biol Med.* 24 (1951): 123–146.
124. Stellar, E. "The Physiology of Motivation." *Psychol Rev.* 5 (1955): 22.
125. Han, P.W. "Hypothalamic Obesity in Rats without Hyperphagia." *N Y Acad Sci.* 30 (1967): 229–242.
126. Coleman, D.L. "Obese and Diabetes: Two Mutant Genes Causing Diabetes-Obesity Syndromes in Mice." *Diabetologia.* 14 (1978): 141–148.
127. Powley, T.L., C.A. Opsahl. "Ventromedial Hypothalamic Obesity Abolished by Subdiaphragmatic Vagotomy." *Am J Physiol.* 226 (1974): 25–33.
128. Bray, G.A., D.A. York. "Hypothalamic and Genetic Obesity in Experimental Animals: An Autonomic and Endocrine Hypothesis." *Physiol Rev.* 59 (1979): 719–809.
129. Nishizawa, Y., G.A. Bray. "Ventromedial Hypothalamic Lesions and the Mobilization of Fatty Acids." *J Clin Invest.* 61 (1978): 714–721.
130. Rothwell, N.J., M.J. Stock. "A Role for Brown Adipose Tissue in Diet-Induced Thermogenesis." *Nature.* 281 (1979): 31–35.
131. Bayliss, W.M. *Principles of General Physiology.* 2nd edition. London: Longmans, Green and Co., 1918.
132. Gibbs, J., R.C. Young, G.P. Smith. "Cholecystokinin Elicits Satiety in Rats with Open Gastric Fistulas." *Nature.* 245 (1973): 323–325.
133. Stanley, B.G., S.E. Kyrkouli, S. Lampert, S.F. Leibowitz. "Neuropeptide Y Chronically Injected into the Hypothalamus: a Powerful Neurochemical Inducer of Hyperphagia and Obesity." *Peptides.* 7 (1986): 1189–1192.
134. Celsus, A.A.C. *De Medicina with an English translation by W.G.*

Spencer. London: Heinemann, 1935–1938.
135. Willis, T. *Opera Omnia*. Leiden: Joannis Antonij Juguetan & Co., 1681.
136. Sydenham, T. *Observationes medicae circa morborum acutorum historiam et curationem*. Londini: G. Kettilby, 1676.
137. Morton, R. *Phthisologia seu excertitationes de Phthisi tribus libris comprehensae*. Londini: Samuel Smith, 1689.
138. Boerhaave, H. *Opera omnia medica, quorum sries post praefationem*. Venetiis: Laurentium Basilium, 1757.
139. Cullen, W. *First Lines of the Practice of Physic, by William Cullen, M.D. late professor of the practice of physic in the University of Edinburgh, and including the definitions of the nosology; with supplementary notes chiefly selected from recent authors, who have contributed to the improvement of medicine by Peter Reid, M.D.* Edinburgh: Abernethy and Walker, 1810.
140. Louis, P.C.A. *Recherches anatomico-pathologiques sur la phthisie*. Paris: Gabon of Cie, 1825.
141. Koch, R. "Zur Untersuchung von pathogenen Organismen." In *Mitthelungen aus dem Kaiserlichen Gesundheitsamte*. Berlin: Norddeutsches Buchdruckerei, 1881.
142. von Helmholtz, H. *Beschreibung eines Augen-spiegels zur Untersuchung der Netzhaut im lebenden Auge*. Berlin: A. Forstner'sche Verlagsbuchhandlung, 1851.
143. Gould, G.M., W.L. Pyle. *Anomalies and Curiosities of Medicine*. 1896. New York: Julian Press, 1956.
144. Kryger, M.H. "Sleep Apnea. From the Needles of Dionysius to Continuous Positive Airway Pressure." *Arch Intern Med*. 143 (1983): 2301–2303.
145. Kryger, M.H. "Fat, Sleep, and Charles Dickens: Literary and Medical Contributions to the Understanding of Sleep Apnea." *Clin Chest Med*. 6 (1985): 555–562.
146. Russell, J. "A Case of Polysarka, in Which Death Resulted from Deficient Arterializations of the Blood." *Br Med J*. i (1866): 220–221.
147. Dubourg, L. *Recherches sur les causes de la polysarcie*. Paris: A. Parent, 1864.
148. Schindler, C.S. "Monstrose Fettsucht." *Wiener Med Presse*. 12 (1871): 410–412; 436-439.
149. Maccary, A. *Traité sur la polysarcie*. Paris: Gabon, 1811.
150. Glais, J. *De la grossesse adipeuse*. Paris: A. Parent, 1875.
151. Dupytren. "Observation sur un cas d'obésité, suivie de maladie du coeur et de la mort." *J Med Chir Pharm*. 12 (1806): 262–273.
152. Anonymous. *The Life of That Wonderful and Extraordinarily Heavy Man, Daniel Lambert, from His Birth to the Moment of His Dissolution; with an account of men noted for their corpulency, and*

other interesting matter. New York: Samuel Wood & Sons, 1818.

153. Barkhausen. "Merkwürdige allgemeine Fettablagerung bei einem Knaben von 5 Jahren." *Hannov Ann f ges Heilk.* 8 (1843): 200–203.
154. Coe, T. "A Letter from Dr. T. Coe, Physician at Chelmsford in Essex, to Dr. Cromwell Mortimer, Secretary R.S. Concerning Mr. Bright, the Fat Man at Malden in Essex." *Phil Trans.* 47 (1751–1752): 188–193.
155. Don, W.G. "Remarkable Case of Obesity in a Hindoo Boy Aged Twelve Years." *Lancet.* 47 (1859): 363.
156. Eschenmeyer. "Beschreibung eines monstrosen fett Mädchen, das in einem Alter von 10 Jahren starb, nach dem es eine hohe von 5 Fuss 3 Zoll und ein Gewicht von 219 Pfund erreicht hatte." *Tubing BI f Naturw u Arznk.* 1 (1815): 261–285.
157. Gordon, S. "Art. XV—Reports of Rare Cases. IV. Case of Extensive Fatty Degeneration in a Boy 14 Years of Age. Death from Obstructed Arterial Circulation." *Dublin Q J Med Sci.* 33 (1862): 340–349.
158. McNaughton, J. "Cases of Polysarcia Adiposa in Childhood." *New York Medical and Physical Journal* No. XXX, July 1829. New Series—No. II. New York: C.S. Francis.
159. Wood, T. "A Sequel to the Case of Mr. Thomas Wood, of Billericay, in the Country of Essex, by the Same." *Med Trans (College of Physicians, London).* 3 (1785):309–318.
160. Linnaeus, Cv. *Species plantarum.* Stockholm: Salvius, 1753.
161. Sauvages, F.B. *Nosologia methodica sistens morborum classes juxta Sydenhami menten and botanicorum ordinem.* Amstelodami: Fratrum de Tournes, 1768.
162. Burwell, C.S., E.D. Robin, R.D. Whaley, A.G. Bickelman. "Extreme Obesity Associated with Alveolar Hypoventilation: A Pickwickian Syndrome." *Am J Med.* 21 (1956): 811–818.
163. Cushing, H. *The Pituitary Body and Its Disorders. Clinical States Produced by Disorders of the Hypophysis Cerebri.* Philadelphia: J.B. Lippincott, 1912.
164. Cushing, H. "The Basophil Adenomas of the Pituitary Body and Their Clinical Manifestations. Pituitary Basophilism." *Bull Johns Hopkins Hospital.* 14 (1932): 137–195.
165. Quetelet, A. *Sur l'homme et le développement de ses facultés, ou essai de physique sociale.* Paris: Bachelier, 1835.
166. Society of Actuaries. Build Study of 1979. City Recording and Statistical Corp, 1980.
167. Dawber, T.R. *The Framingham Study: The Epidemiology of Atherosclerotic Disease.* Cambridge: Harvard University Press, 1980.
168. Keys, A., C. Aravanis, H.W. Blackburn, et al. "Epidemiological Studies Related to Coronary Heart Disease: Characteristics of Men Aged 40-

59 in Seven Countries." *Acta Med Scand Suppl.* 460 (1966): 1–392.
169. Lew, E.A., L. Garfinkel. "Variations in Mortality by Weight Among 750,000 Men and Women." *J Chronic Dis.* 32 (1979): 563-576.
170. Waaler, H.T. "Height, Weight and Mortality: The Norwegian Experience." *Acta Med Scand.* 679 (198.4): 1–56.
171. Manson, J.E, W.C. Willett, M.J. Stampfer, et al. "Body Weight and Mortality among Women." *N Engl J Med.* 333 (1995): 677–685.
172. Vague, J. "La differenciation sexuelle. Facteur déterminant des formes de l'obésité." *Presse Med.* 55 (1947): 339–340.
173. Osler, W. *The Principles and Practice of Medicine.* New York: D. Appleton, 1892.
174. Hopkins, K.D., E.D. Lehmann. "Successful Medical Treatment of Obesity in 10th Century Spain." *Lancet.* 346 (1995): 452.
175. Harington. J. *The School of Salenum Regimen Sanitatis Salernitanum.* New York: Paul Hoeber, 1920.
176. Cornaro, L. *Sure and Certain Methods of Attaining a Long and Healthful Life: With Means of Correcting a Bad Constitution.* London: D. Midwinter, 1737.
177. Guerrini, A. *Obesity and Depression in the Enlightenment.* Norman: University of Oklahoma Press, 2000.
178. Cheyne, G. *The Essay of Health and Long Life.* 1724.
179. Cheyne, G. *The English Malady.* 1733.
180. Tweedie, J. *Hints on Temperence and Exercise, Shewing Their Advantage in the Cure of Dyspepsia, Rheumatism, Polysarcia, and Certain States of Palsy.* London: T. Rickaby, 1799.
181. Short, T. *A Discourse Concerning the Causes and Effects of Corpulency Together with the Method for Its Prevention and Cure.* London: J. Roberts, 1727.
182. Flemyng, M. *A Discourse on the Nature, Causes, and Cure of Corpulency. Illustrated by a Remarkable Case. Read before the Royal Society November 1757.* London: L. Davis and C. Reymers, 1760.
183. Brillat-Savarin, J.A. *The Physiology of Taste or, Meditations on Transcendental Gastronomy.* Transl. M.F.K. Fisher; drawings and color lithographs by Wayne Thiebaud. San Francisco: Arion Press, 1994.
184. Banting, W. *A Letter on Corpulence Addressed to the Public.* London: Harrison and Sons, 1863.
185. Harvey, W. *On Corpulence in Relation to Disease: With Some Remarks on Diet.* London: Henry Renshaw, 1872.
186. von Noorden, C. *Obesity. The Indications for Reduction Cures Being Part I of Several Clinical Treatises on the Pathology and Therapy of Disorders of Metabolism and Nutrition.* Bristol: John Wright & Co., 1903.
187. Carter, H.S., P.E. Howe, H.H. Mason. *Nutrition and Clinical Dietetics.* Philadelphia: Lea and Febiger, 1917.

188. Flegal, K.M., M.D. Carroll, R.J. Kuczmarski, C.L. Johnson. "Overweight and Obesity in the United States: Prevalence and Trends, 1960–1994." *Int J Obes Relat Metab Disord.* 22 (1998): 39–47.
189. Ebstein, W. *Die Fettleibigkeit (Korpulenz) und ihre Behandlung nach physiologischen Grundsätzen.* Wiesbaden: Bergmann, 1882.
190. Gulick, A. "A Study of Weight Regulation in the Adult Human Body During Over-Nutrition." *Am J Physiol.* 60 (1922): 371–395.
191. Neumann, R.O. "Experimentelle Beiträge zur Lehre von dem taglichen Nahrungsbedarf des Menschen unter besonderer Berucksichtigung der notwendigen Eiweifsmenge." *Arch Hyg.* 45 (1902): 1–87.
192. Wiley, F.H., L.H. Newburgh. "The Doubtful Nature of Luxuskonsumption." *J Clin Invest.* 10 (1931): 733–744.
193. Evans, F.A. "A Radical Cure of Simple Obesity by Dietary Measures Alone." *Atlantic Med J.* 30 (1926): 140–141.
194. Bloom, W.L. "Fasting as an Introduction to the Treatment of Obesity." *Metabolism.* 8 (1959): 214–220.
195. Sours, H.E., V.P. Frattali, C.D. Brand, R.A. Feldman, A.L. Forbes, R.C. Swanson, A.L. Paris. "Sudden Death Associated with Very Low Calorie Weight Reduction Regimens."*Am J Clin Nutr.* 34 (1981): 453–461.
196. Magendie, F. *"Rapport fait à l'Académie des Sciences au nom de la Commission dite de la gélatine." C R Acad Sci (Paris).* (1841): 237–283.
197. Carpenter, K.F. *Protein and Energy: A Study of Changing Ideas in Nutrition.* Cambridge: Cambridge University Press, 1994.
198. U.S. House of Representatives. Hearing before the Subcommittee on Regulation, Business Opportunities, and Energy of the Committee on Small Business. Deception and Fraud in the Diet Industry, Part I of II. Washington, D.C.: U.S. Government Printing Office, 1990.
199. Freud, S. *The Interpretation of Dreams.* New York: Macmillan, 1913.
200. Stunkard, A.J., M. Mendelson. "Obesity and the Body Image. I. Characteristics of Disturbances in the Body Image of Some Obese Persons." *Am J Psychiatr.* 123 (1967): 1296–1300.
201. Moore, M.E., A.J. Stunkard, L. Srole. "Obesity, Social Class, and Mental Illness." *JAMA.* 181 (1962): 962–966.
202. Pavlov, I.P. *Conditioned Reflexes: An Investigation of the Physiological Activity of the Cerebral Cortex.* Transl. by G.V. Anrep. London: Oxford University Press, 1928.
203. Skinner, B.F. *Science and Human Behavior.* New York: McMillan, 1953.
204. Ferster, C.B., J.I Nurenberger, E.B. Levitt. "The Control of Eating." *J Math.* 1 (1962): 87–109.
205. Stuart, R.B. "Behavioral Control of Overeating." *Behav Res Ther.* 5 (1967): 357–365.

206. Withering, W. *An Account of the Foxglove and Some of Its Medical Uses: with Practical Remarks on Dropsy and other Diseases.* Birmingham: M. Swinney, 1785.
207. Sajous, C.E, de M. *The Internal Secretion and the Principles of Medicine.* 7th edition. Philadelphia: F.A. Davis Co., 1916.
208. Weintraub, M., P.R. Sundaresan, B. Schuster, et al. "Long Term Weight Control: The National Heart, Lung and Blood Institute Funded Multimodal Intervention Study. I–VII." *Clin Pharmacol Ther.* 51 (1992): 581–646.
209. Connolly, H.M., J.L. Crary, M.D. McGoon, D.D. Hensrud, B.S. Edwards, W.D. Edwards, H.V. Schaff. "Valvular Heart Disease Associated with Fenfluramine-phentermine." *N Engl J Med.* 337 (1997): 581–588.
210. Preuss, J. *Biblical and Talmudic Medicine.* Transl. and ed. F. Rosner, M.D. New York: Hebrew Publishing Co., 1978.
211. Kremen, A.J., J.H. Linner, C.H. Nelson. "Experimental Evaluation of Nutritional Importance of Proximal and Distal Small Intestine." *Ann Surg.* 140 (1954): 439–448.
212. Payne, J.H., L.T. DeWind, R.R. Commons. "Metabolic Observations in Patients with Jejunocolic Shunts." *Am J. Surg.* 106 (1963): 273–289.
213. Mason, E.E., C. Ito. "Gastric Bypass." *Ann Surg.* 170 (1970): 329–339.
214. Sjostrom, C.D., L. Lissner, H. Wedel, L. Sjostrom. "Reduction in Incidence of Diabetes, Hypertension and Lipid Disturbances after Intentional Weight Loss Induced by Bariatric Surgery: The SOS Intervention Study." *Obes Res.* 5 (1999): 477–484.
215. Schwartz, H. *Never Satisfied. A Cultural History of Diets, Fantasies & Fat.* New York: Free Press, 1986.
216. Rony, H.R. *Obesity and Leanness.* Philadelphia: Lea and Febiger, 1940.
217. Harden, V.A. *Inventing the NIH: Federal Biomedical Research Policy, 1887–1937.* Baltimore: Johns Hopkins University Press, 1986.
218. Baird, I.M., A.N. Howard. *Obesity: Medical and Scientific Aspects.* Edinburgh: E. & S. Livingstone Ltd., 1969.
219. Bray, G.A. *Obesity in Perspective.* Fogarty International Center Series on Preventive Medicine Washington, D.C.: U.S. Government Printing Office. Publication #75–708. DHEW Publication 1976; 2, Parts 1 and 2.
220. Howard, A.N. ed. *Recent Advances in Obesity Research. Proceedings of the 1st International Congress on Obesity.* London: Newman Publishing, 1975.
221. Bray, G.A. *Recent Advances in Obesity Research: II. Proceedings of the 2nd International Congress on Obesity 23–26 October 1977, Washington, D. C.* London: Newman Publishing Ltd., 1978.
222. Bjorntorp, P., M. Cairella, A.N. Howard eds. *Recent Advances in*

Obesity Research: Ill. Proceedings of the 3rd International Congress On Obesity. London: John Libbey, 1981.

223. Hirsch, J., T.B. Van Itallie eds. *Recent Advances in Obesity Research: IV Proceedings of the 4th International Congress on Obesity 5–8 October 1983, New York, USA*. London: John Libbey, 1985.
224. Berry, E.M., S.H. Blondheim, E. Eliahou, E. Shafrir eds. *Recent Advances in Obesity: V. Proceedings of the 5th International Congress on Obesity*. London: John Libbey, 1987.
225. Oomura, Y., S. Tarui, S. Inoue, T. Shimazu. *Progress in Obesity Research 1990*. London: John Libbey, 1991.
226. Angel, A., H. Anderson, C. Bouchard, D. Lau, L. Leiter, R. Mendelson. *Progress in Obesity Research*: 7. London: John Libbey, 1996.
227. Guy-Grand, B., G. Ailhaud. *Progress in Obesity Research: 8*. London: John Libbey, 1999.
228. Medeiros-Neto, G., A. Halpern, C. Bouchard. *Progress in Obesity Research: 9*. London: John Libbey, 2003.
229. Short, T. In *Dictionary of National Biography*.
230. Wadd, W. *Cursory Remarks on Corpulence; or Obesity Considered as a Disease: with a critical examination of ancient and modern opinions, relative to its causes and cure*. London: J. Callow; 1816.
231. Chambers, T.K. *Corpulence; Or, excess of fat in the human body; its relation to chemistry and physiology, its bearings on other diseases and the value of human life and its indications of treatment*. London: Longman, Brown, Green and Longmans, 1850.
232. Harvey, J. *Corpulence, its diminution and cure without injury to health*. London: Smith; 1864.
233. Dancel, J.F. *Traité théorique et pratique de l'obésité (trop grand embonpoint). Avec plusieurs observations de guérison de maladies occasionées ou entretienues par cet état anormal*. Paris: J.B. Bailliere et fils, pp. 1-357, 1863.
234. Worthington, L.S. *De l'obésité. Étiologie, thérapeutique et hygiene*. Paris: E. Martinet, pp. 188, 1875.
235. Kisch, E.H. *Die Fettleibigkeit (lipomatosis universalis). Auf gurndlage Zahlreicher beobachtungen klinisch Dargestellt*. Stuttgart: Ferdinand Enke, 1988.
236. Williams, L.L.B. *Obesity*. London: Milford;1926.
237. Christie, W.F. *Obesity: A Practical Handbook for Physicians*. London: William Heinemann, 1937.
238. Rynearson, E.H., Gastineau, C.F. *Obesity*. Springfield, IL: Charles C. Thomas, 1949.
239. Craddock, D. *Obesity and Its Management*. Edinburgh and London: E. and S. Livingstone, 1969.
240. Bruch, H. *The Importance of Overweight*. New York: W.W. Norton

and Co., Inc., 1957.
241. Mayer, J. *Overweight: Causes, Cost and Control.* Englewood Cliffs, NJ: Prentice-Hall, 1968.
242. Garrow, J.S. *Treat Obesity Seriously. A Clinical Manual.* Edinburgh and London: Churchill Livingstone, 1981.
243. Stunkard, A.J. *The Pain of Obesity.* Palo Alto: Bull Publishing Co., 1976.
244. Leven, G. *Du obésité.* Paris: G. Steinheil, 1901.
245. Haeckel, F. *Grandes et petites obésités.* Cure Radicale. Paris: Masson et Cie, 1911.
246. LeNoir, P. *L'obésité et son traitement.* Paris: J.B. Bailliere et Fils, 1907.
247. Boivin, F. *La cure physiologique de l' obésité.* Paris: Jules Rousset, 1911;1-191.
248. Creff, A.F., Herschberg, A.D. *Abrege d' obésité.* Paris: Masson, 1979.
249. von Noorden, K. *Die Fettsucht.* Vienna: Holder, 1910.
250. Pfaundler, M. *Korpermass-studien an Kindern.* Berlin: Springer, 1916.
251. Gries, F.A., Berchtold, P., Berger, M. *Adipositas, Pathophysiologie, Klinik und Therapie.* Berlin: Springer-Verlag, 1976.
252. Regneller, G.D. *Traité complet de l'obésité et de la maigreur, de leurs causes et de leur guérison.* Paris: pour Bohaire, Gosseline et Ledoyen, 1814 XIme edition, probably 1839.
253. Louvet, L. *Contribution a l'étude de l'obésité dans la grande enfance et pendant la puberté.* Paris: Louis Arnette, 1934.

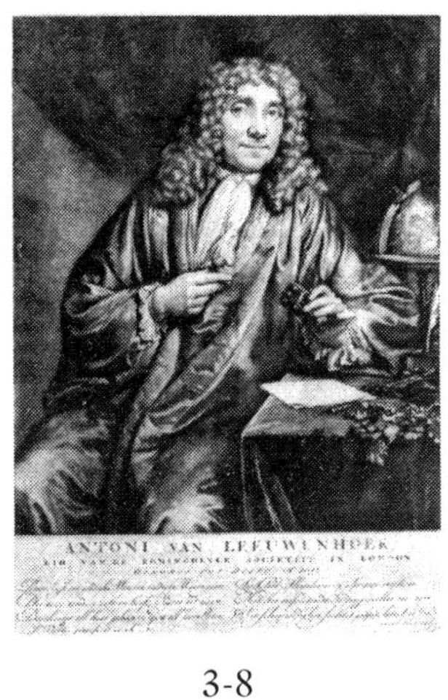

3-8

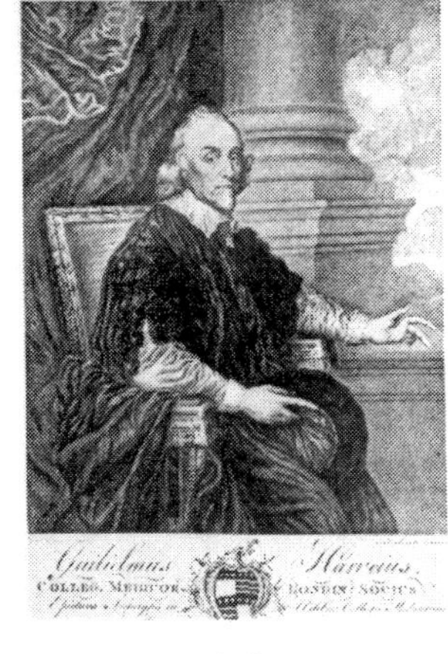

3-9

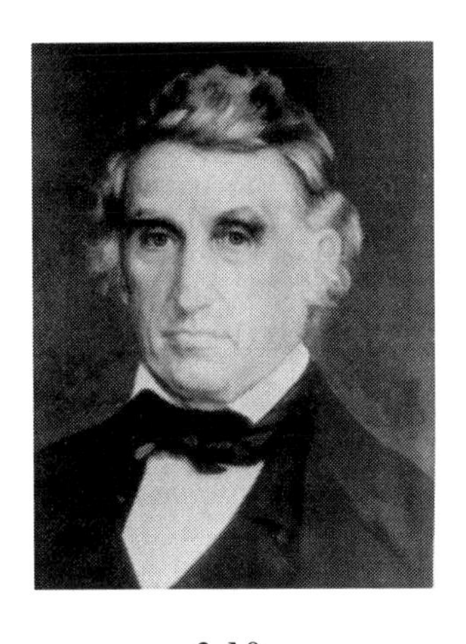

3-10

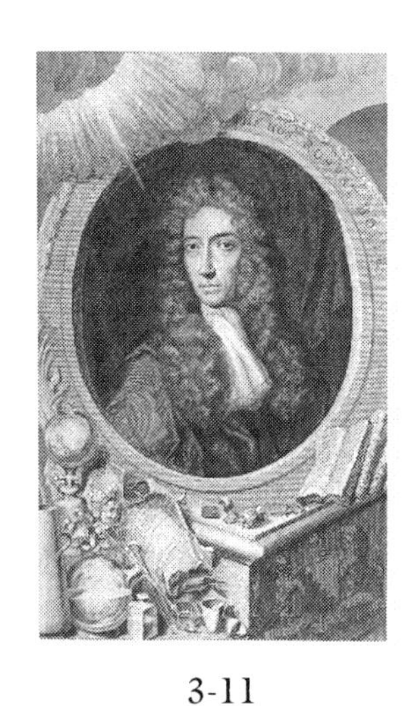

3-11

3-8 Antoni van Leeuwenhoek (1632-1723). Courtesy of the National Library of Medicine.

3-9 William Harvey (1578-1657). Courtesy of the National Library of Medicine.

3-10 William Beaumont (1785-1853). Courtesy of the National Library of Medicine.

3-11 Robert Boyle (167-1691). Courtesy of the National Library of Medicine.

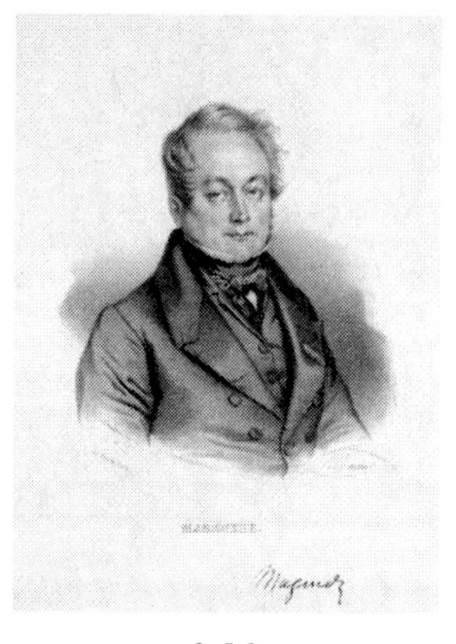

3-12

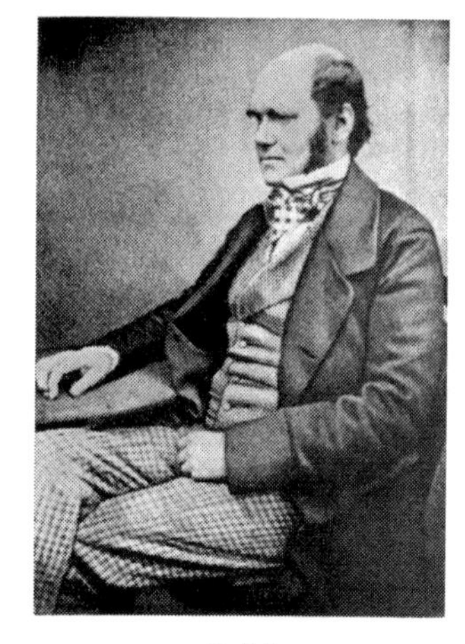

3-13

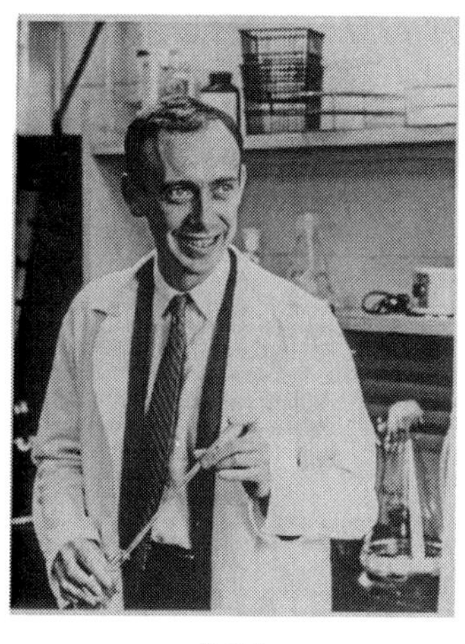

3-14

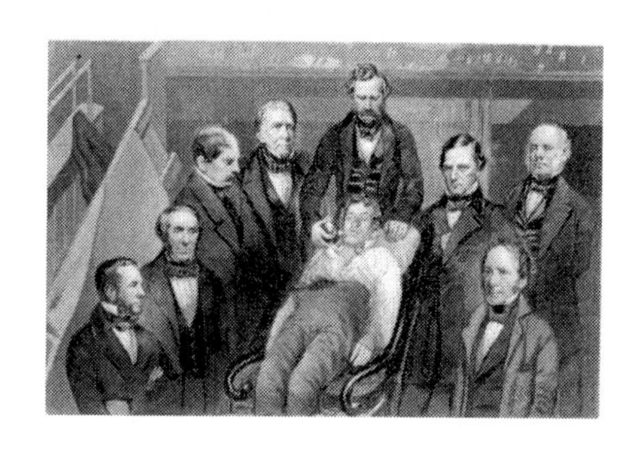

3-15

3-12 Francois Magendie (1783-1853). Courtesy of the National Library of Medicine.

3-13 Charles Robert Darwin (1809-1882). Courtesy of the National Library of Medicine.

3-14 James Dewey Watson (1927-). Courtesy of the National Library of Medicine.

3-15 Ether Operation at Massachusetts General Hospital, Boston, MA.

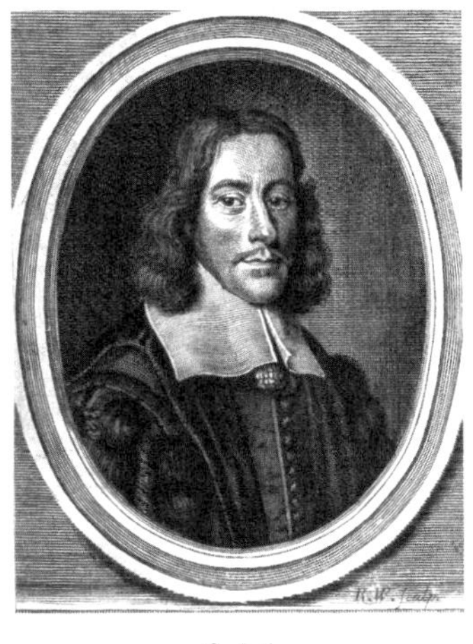

3-16

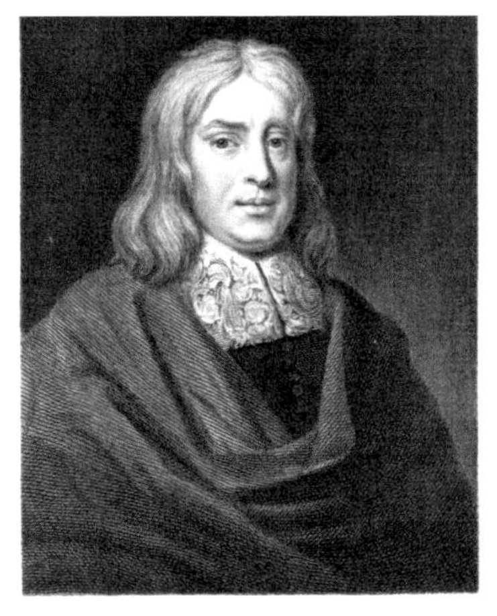

3-17

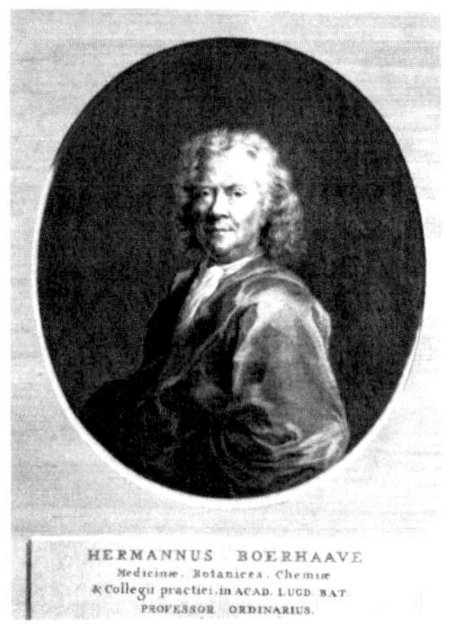

3-18

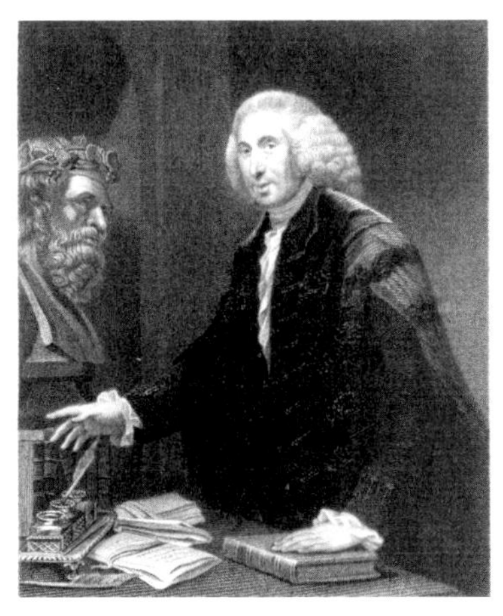

3-19

3-16 Thomas Willis (1621-1675). Courtesy of the National Library of Medicine.

3-17 Thomas Sydenham (1624-1675). Courtesy of the National Library of Medicine.

3-18 Herman Boerhaave (1668-1738). Courtesy of the National Library of Medicine.

3-19 William Cullen (1712-1790). Courtesy of the National Library of Medicine.

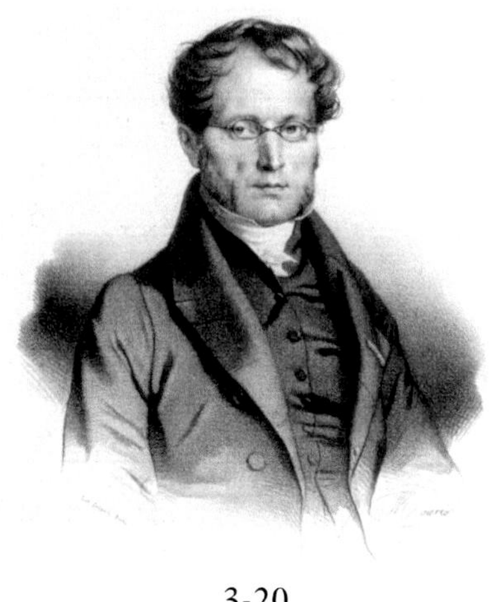

3-20

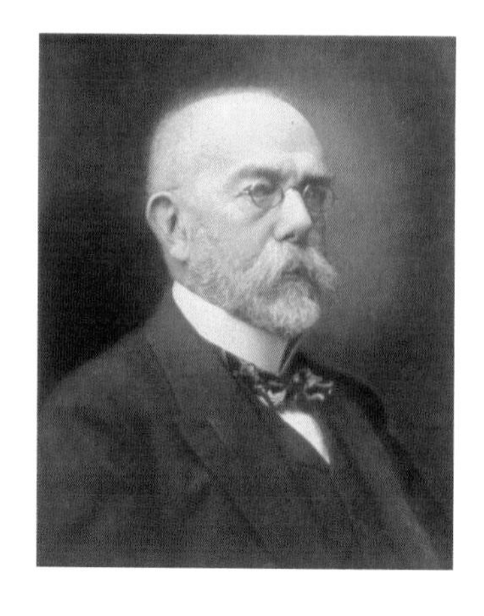

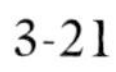

3-21

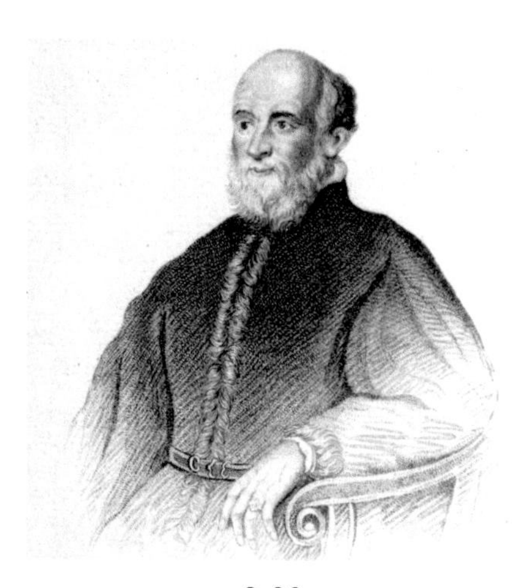

3-22

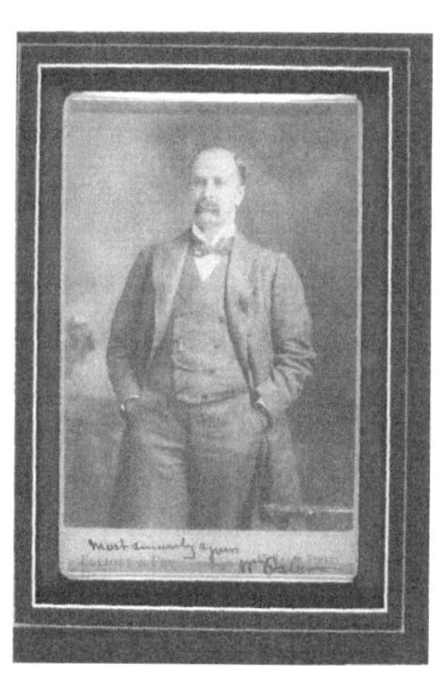

3-24

3-20 Pierre-Charles-Alexandre Louis (1787-1872). Courtesy of the National Library of Medicine.

3-21 Robert Koch (1843-1910). Courtesy of the National Library of Medicine.

3-22 Luigi Cornaro (1475-1566). Courtesy of the National Library of Medicine.

3-24 Sir William Osler (1849-1919). Courtesy of the National Library of Medicine.

PART 2.

Measurement of the Bulge: How Fat Are We?

CHAPTER 4

Santorio Santorio—The Father of Metabolism: Beginnings of Quantitative Methods

> *The tale of the seventeenth century is rather sadly full of many fine beginnings which faded away because contemporary opinion was not ready for them.*
>
> —Poynter & Keele, *A Short History of Medicine*[1]

Although he is the hero of this section, the work of Santorio Santorio[2] or by his Latin name Sanctorius, falls in the category of "many fine beginnings" described by Poynter and Keele[1]. It would be more than three hundred years before the insights of Santorio would be applied to an important problem in our discussion of the battle of the bulge (see Chapter 13).

Among the seventeenth century scientific giants were Galileo Galilei[3], the physicist; Robert Boyle, the chemist[4]; William Harvey, the physician who discovered the circulation of the blood[5]; Stephen Hales, the minister who first measured blood pressure[6]; Richard Lower, the scientist who first transfused blood; Robert Hooke[7], the technician who was one of the earliest microscopists; and Thomas Sydenham[8], a leading physician of his age. These men contributed to all areas of science that are relevant to the battle of the bulge, but in many instances their contributions were too far ahead of their time and fell on infertile soil.

But I am getting ahead of the story. The transition from the tradition of humoral medicine bequeathed to us by Galen in Roman times to the experimental method of the sixteenth century took a long time[9–11]. The synthesis of medical knowledge in the tenth century by Avicenna[12] from Latin and Arabic translations of Hippocrates, Aristotle, and Galen served only to provide a dialectical framework that kept on hold the probing of nature for answers. Avicenna's *Canon* was one of the leading texts in medical schools for the next several centuries until experimental and clinical approaches took over. It would take more than five hundred years (from A.D. 1000 to 1500) for the worldview exemplified by Avicenna and based on ancient Greek thought to be transformed into a worldview based on experimentation and observation.

The concept that experimental exploration of nature was a better strategy to advance human understanding than armchair reasoning took a long time to develop. The developments began slowly even before the thirteenth century. The key to the revival was the rediscovery of classics from the golden age of Greek science. This occurred first in areas where Arab, Greek, Jewish, and Latin cultures intersected, probably in Spain and Sicily. Steeped in the solid base of Christian doctrine, scholars of the day, most notably St. Thomas Aquinas and his mentor St. Albertus Magnus, attempted to harmonize the Greek philosophical system epitomized in the writings of Aristotle with the teachings of the Roman Church. The beginnings for discovery of new facts can be dated to the work of three men in the thirteenth century, St. Albert, Peter Peregrine, and Roger Bacon, who is probably the closest of these men to an experimental scientist. Bacon may even have had a laboratory at Oxford, where he may have done experiments with lenses[13]. Lenses and compasses were among the most important inventions of the late Middle Ages. Bacon's description of these lenses gives us insight into the level of science he practiced:

> And when we wish, things far off can be seen as near, and vice versa, so that at an incredible distance we might see grains of sand and small letters and the lowest things may appear very high, and vice versa and hidden things be seen openly and open things be hidden, and one thing may be seen as many and vice versa, so many suns and moons may be seen by the artifice of this kind of geometry....[13]

Bacon's comment about changing perspectives presages the changes that were to come during the early modern period beginning around A.D. 1500.

In spite of important contributions by individual men, the late Middle Ages A.D. 1200–1400 remained mired in the past. The view of the world was still based on the science of Aristotle and the medicine of Hippocrates. The universe was a sphere. Everything was matter and form. The elements air, earth, fire, and water could be transformed into one another. Balance between the four humors in human beings gave good health; imbalance, illness. However, historical changes between 1450 and 1600 redirected the efforts of early scientists away from contemplation of ancient precepts and toward the experimental confrontation of nature.

The period between 1450 and 1600 bridged the beginnings of science that occurred in the thirteenth century, through the great plague of 1347, which may have killed one-third of the European population, with the quantitative period of the seventeenth century. The earlier date, 1450, corresponds with the introduction by Gutenberg of printing using movable type. A major step forward came from the art world with the development of diminishing perspective, the ability to make a flat surface appear to have three dimensions by using one- or two-point perspective. The painter Giotto in the early fourteenth century was far along on this path when the Plague swept through Europe, wiping out a generation of creative minds. By the time of the Italian painter Masachio in the fifteenth century, diminishing perspective had been perfected. This was also the time when the clock and magnetic compass were developed[14]. Possibly most important in the final step in this process was the introduction of printing using movable type by Gutenberg, who in the middle of the fifteenth century published his now famous Bibles using this technique and opened a revolution in communication.

The Greek, Roman, and Arabic classics could now be widely disseminated in accurate printed copies. Once this happened, printing began to be used to disseminate opinions at a more rapid rate. By the early sixteenth century, publication of new and original documents began to spread widely, including the ninety-five theses of Luther that led to the Protestant Reformation, the work of Copernicus on the heliocentric theory of the solar system, and the first modern anatomy of the human body by Vesalius[15].

The revival of direct observation of nature can be traced to three sources. The first was the promulgation of learning from ancient Greece and the stimulus to learning that it provided. The second was the desire to expand knowledge of the geographical world as travel expanded. This was vastly accelerated by discovery of the New World by Christopher Columbus in 1492 and the search for gold and spices. The third, which followed on the heels of this geographical interest, was the gradual growth of industry and the technical needs that this demanded. Among these areas were metallurgy, mining, and the development of gunpowder and pyrotechnics. This industrial growth fueled the rise of wealthy and powerful families in cities across Europe.

Observational science and astronomy also grew in this period. As Taylor notes[13], the astronomers of the fifteenth and sixteenth centuries, of whom Copernicus is the most famous, showed three characteristics that we would recognize in modern scientists. First, they observed for themselves. Second, they abandoned preconceptions about the nature of the universe. And third, they kept accurate records of what they observed and converted these records into published findings.

Anatomy and astronomy grew together as observational sciences. Although Leonardo da Vinci had dissected some thirty bodies in the fifteenth century, his inverted writings could not be easily read and his anatomical work was not influential in his lifetime[16]. When Andreas Vesalius[15] published his anatomic dissections in the famous *De Humani Corporis Fabrica (On the Fabric of the Human Body)* in 1543, it opened the observational science of anatomy. Although Vesalius carried out an experiment demonstrating that there was a connection between the functioning of the vocal cords of an animal and the recurrent nerves in the neck, the field of physiology, or how things function, remained dominated for another two hundred years by the teachings of Galen, as it had been for the previous fifteen hundred years.

The period from 1450 to 1600 thus saw practical improvements in many areas of human knowledge. Experimentation, i.e., "doing things to see what happened" and recording the results, would not appear until the beginning of the seventeenth century. Galileo[3] was one of the first to apply experimental methods to find out what happened. According to Taylor, "The stimulating and creative idea of the new order was born...in the mind of Galileo"[13]. Indeed, he notes that "Galileo Galilei...was the first to employ the modern scientific method in its fullest"[13]. Galileo is particularly important for our story about Santorio because he was a professor at the University of Padua where Santorio Santorio was professor of medicine and where William Harvey[5] from England, who discovered the circulation of the blood, was a medical student.

Galileo established the field of mechanics. He was a man of great intellectual ability who was an able experimental scientist and who also knew how to write well. Galileo was at the center of the intellectual ferment that was part of the University of Padua. This was the university where Vesalius (1514–1564) had done the dissections for the monumental anatomy book of 1543; where Gabriele Fallopio (1523–1562) was professor of anatomy and discoverer of the fallopian tubes in the reproductive system; and where Hieronymous Fabricius ab Aquependante (1537–1619), also professor of anatomy, taught William Harvey about the valves in the veins that only allowed blood to move in one direction. Earlier, Matteo Realdo Colombo (1516–1559), another professor at Padua and anatomical dissector for Vesalius, discovered the pulmonary circulation — the flow of blood from the big veins through the lungs into the heart. Galileo was completing his work on the heliocentric nature of the solar system when he was put under house arrest by the Pope because of his heretical ideas. Galileo also introduced the telescope into Italy and set the stage for using magnification to examine the celestial universe and the microscopic examination of the invisible universe[3].

William Harvey was one of the many foreign students who came to Padua from England because of Padua's renown as an educational center[18] and received his doctorate in 1602. During his years at the University of Padua, the young Harvey learned anatomy from Hieronymous Fabricius ab Aquependante, who had been a student of Vesalius when Vesalius wrote his famous anatomy book, the first truly modern anatomy. During the anatomy lessons, Fabricius ab Aquependante had demonstrated the valves in the veins and showed the young William Harvey that they would only allow blood to pass in one direction. As Harvey pondered this finding, perhaps some time after his return to England at the end of 1595, he realized that these valves meant that blood could only travel in one direction around the circulatory system[5]. This revolutionary physiological idea overturned the Galenic system which proposed that blood ebbed and flowed from the liver. However, like so many other discoveries of the seventh century, the impact of this revolutionary idea was met with lukewarm reception when he first presented it in 1616[19].

The development of physics[3] and chemistry[4] in the seventeenth century were applied to interpreting medical findings. The opinion leaders of the time could be divided into two groups. Some men, of whom Santorio Santorio was one, believed that the human body and disease could be understood best in mechanical terms and were called "iatrophysicists." The mechanical properties of the muscles moving bone to make the body work were easily included in the iatrophysicists' frame of reference. The circulation of the blood described by Harvey also clearly fit into an iatrophysical concept of the world. Digestion of food, on the other hand, was not easily encompassed in the mechanical sphere of the iatrophysicist, except for the grinding functions of the stomach. Opposing the iatrophysicists in the seventeenth century were "iatrochemists." These men espoused a chemical basis for biological phenomena and interpreted human disease and function in chemical terms[9-11, 16]. The digestion of food and putrefaction of wounds were better explained in these iatrochemical terms than in mechanical or iatromechanical terms.

The iatrophysical and iatrochemical views of the world provided two frameworks for viewing health and disease and they began to undermine the old system of health as a balance between the four humors. The practical men of the seventeenth century who investigated nature in a reasonable and scientific way may not have been aware of the importance of their breakthroughs, but they did seem to understand that the way forward was "to do things and see what happened." Englishman Francis Bacon (1561–1626), who was a lawyer, Chancellor of the Exchequer, and landed gentleman, did realize the framework in which the new discoveries were being made. In the *Novum Organum*[20] he developed his ideas about the basis for the experimental method. Bacon rejected the armchair approach of rational thought that had been used to derive much of "ancient knowledge" associated with Greek science. Taylor[13] outlines the strategies Bacon recommended:

1. To collect reliable tested information especially by means of experiments.
2. To classify this material by tables of invention so that all the instances of the phenomenon could be compared.

3. From these tables, arrive at theorems or rules, and by comparing these rules arrive at general scientific laws.
4. These scientific laws must point out new instances of the phenomenon being studied.

This is not far from the modern scientific method. One major difference is that modern scientists use their judgment to decide what information to collect rather than aim to collect all information. Equally important, most scientists today tend to use numerical data handled mathematically rather than tables summarizing all experiments.

Descartes[21] was a French contemporary of Bacon who differed from him in several fundamental ways. Again according to Taylor,

> Bacon gave too much attention to gathering facts and little or none to mathematical reasoning about them: Descartes made precisely the opposite error. The practical scientists of the subsequent decades found out the happy mean; and such men as Boyle and Newton were able to treat Bacon's observations and experiments by Descartes' mathematical reasoning with the greatest success[13].

Santorio Santorio, or Sanctorius to use his Latin name, was professor of theoretical medicine at the University of Padua at the same time as Galileo, and he must have been influenced by this famous contemporary. Sanctorius began to apply some of Galileo's ideas of quantitative measurement to the study of medicine. As Castiglione observed: "To Sanctorius...belongs the glory of being the founder and initiator of that school which inaugurated the era of exact experimental research in physiology"[22].

Sanctorius is best known for his balance beam (Figure 4-1)[23].

He apparently spent much of his professional career measuring himself and others on this beam. Like so many early seventeenth century innovations, it was another two centuries before this invention and others resurfaced in medicine. Sanctorius introduced the concept of insensible fluid losses, that is, the losses that occur as evaporation of water in the lungs or as perspiration from the skin. Using his scale he was able to measure his own insensible perspiration as he sat on one side of this scale. Rather than describe the details of his experimental methods, his book contains a series of aphorisms that he believed were the practical lessons to be learned from his experiments in living on his scale. In the introduction to his book, Sanctorius says:

> It is a new and unheard of thing in Medicine that anyone should be able to arrive at an exact measurement of

> insensible perspiration. Nor has anyone either Philosopher or Physician dared to attack this part of medical inquiry. I am indeed the first to make the trial, and unless I am mistaken I have by reasoning and by the experience of thirty years brought this branch of science to perfection, which I judged more advisable than to describe all the details of my inquiry[18].

Sanctorius had pioneered a new approach to learning about how the human body functions in health and disease. With his balance beam he obtained new insights, but more important, he applied quantitative methods to medicine.

Sanctorius was a true experimenter who could apply the brilliant physical ideas of Galileo to medicine. In addition to his whole-body balance scale, he developed several other medical instruments that were well ahead of their times. It was not until more than three hundred years later in the nineteenth century that his ideas were reduced to everyday clinical practice and used in the battle of the bulge. He developed a mechanical bed that could be used in six different positions[22] (Figure 4-7). He also developed a type of body bag for giving patients a bath while in bed (Figure 4-2)[24].

Called the "balneatorium," this device was a leather bag which had an opening at the top for the patient to slide through. Once in the bag, warm or cool water could be poured in at the top and drained out at the bottom[23, 24]. He constructed a klyster (a tube and plunger for giving enemas) and pincers for extracting renal calculi[22]. In his book commenting on the work of Avicenna, the tenth century Arab physician[24], Santorio described four *pulsilogia,* or mechanical devices, for measuring the pulse.

The concept of using the swinging pendulum as a way to measure time was developed by Galileo, but it was Santorio who applied it to the measurement of the pulse with his *pulsilogium* (Figure 4-3).

He also described three thermometers for measuring body temperature. Galileo was probably the developer of the thermoscope for measuring temperature, but it was Santorio who applied the principle to measuring body temperature[24]. One of his thermometers had a large bulb to be held by the hand. A second type was put in the mouth (Figure 4-4).

Unfortunately, Santorio's observations had little impact on contemporary medicine, and thermometers did not come into clinical use until the nineteenth century, nearly three hundred years later. His inventions were regarded as interesting toys, and it remained a long time before his ideas were put into daily medical practice[10]. Of interest is that the drawings of these instruments were not published in his original book of aphorisms in 1614. Rather, they were published in 1625 in a book that was a critique of the writings of Avicenna, the tenth-century Muslim physician-scholar whose *Canon* was a major textbook until the time of another great physician-teacher,

Hermann Boerhaave who lived in Leyden, the Netherlands, in the eighteenth century[25].

In his introduction to the 1663 work, Santorio gives the reader a sense of the frustration he faced from the opposition other physicians had to the new ideas that he was teaching. This is not infrequently the case when new concepts disrupt the old order. This quote is from the Introduction to the 1663 edition, published fifty years after his original one[23].

> Only let us admonish the courteous Reader of one thing, in regard it is the custome among men rather to oppose new Inventions with envy, than to study to promote them. We know that not only many Vulgar people, but some also of the learned Gang, that love not truth, but being buz'd by ambition, or the vain lust of contradiction, or spurred by envy, will oppose this new Art [Santorio's scale], and highly detract from its worth, though they never before heard so much as the Name of it. But if they desire to follow truth, we shall so satisfie them that they will not onely perceive naked truth by their understandings, but they shall see her with their eyes, and feel her with their hands; if they please seriously to weigh and consider what we have said in this Book of the weight of insensible perspiration, of the reason and causes of the same, of the time, profit, and disprofit, excess and defect: of the Air, Meat and Drink, and other of the fix things not natural, that hinder or further perspiration, and whatsoever is here mentioned besides.
>
> In the first section we speak of the weight of the insensible perspiration. In the second section. Of Air and Water. In the third section. Of Meat and Drink. In the fourth section. Of sleep and waking. In the fifth section. Of exercise and rest. In the sixth section. Of venery. In the seventh section. Of the passions of the mind. In the last section. There is an answer to the arguments written against this famous art.
>
> The Aphorismes contained in our Book of Ballance Physick are approved to be true by the use of this Chair printed before this book.
>
> From which we find two benefits: first how much the insensible perspiration of breathing of our body is everyday; which thing if not rightly considered, Physick is vain: for all diseases come from too much or too little perspiration.
>
> Secondly, sitting in this chair while we eat, we easily perceive when we have eaten and drunk enough; for too

much or too little doth hurt.

The Chair printed before the Book is made as in this Figure appears, in which the Ballance or Scale is placed above the roof of the Dining-room privately, for people of Honor, that the Room may not be cumbered and unseemly, and that the unlearned to whom all things unusual are ridiculous, may not be offended. This Chair is lifted the breadth of a finger from the floor so that it may not easily be shake.

Therefore when by eating, we come to the due weight prescribed, then the end of the Scale is a little lifted up, and the Chair descends a little. And then we are presently admonished that he that sits therein hath eaten enough.

Now what quantity of weight of wholesome meat is fit for everybody, and how much the insensible perspiration ought to be, which is known by the Chair, every man may easily gather from this our Book of Balance Physick.

Sanctorius was a man ahead of his time. He provided important insights into the problem of energy balance, yet the idea of metabolism, energy balance, and heat loss were not to be realized for several hundred years. Nonetheless, he showed what is needed in a leader in the field. He was dedicated. He was committed. He was focused, and he recorded what he found. He can be a model for current physician-scientists who want to help solve the battle of the bulge.

Following are a sample of Santorio's Aphorisms:[28]

Of insensible perspiration, as it appears by weight.

Aphorism 1. If there daily be an Addition of what is wanting, and a subtraction of what abounds, in due Quantity and Quality, lost Health may be restor'd, and the present preserved.

Aphorism 2. If a Physician, who has the Care of another's Health, is acquainted only with the sensible Supplies and Evacuations, and knows nothing of the Waste that is daily made by insensible Perspiration, he will only deceive his Patient, and never cure him.

Aphorism 3. He only who knows how much, and when the Body does more or less insensibly perspire, will be able to discern, when, and what is to be added or taken away either for the Recovery or Preservations of Health.

Aphorism 4. Insensible Perspiration alone, discharges much more than all the servile Evacuations together.

Aphorism 5. Insensible Perspiration is either made by the Pores of the Body, which is all over perspirable, and cover'd with a Skin like a Net; or it is performed by Respiration through the Mouth, which usually, in the Space of one Day, amounts to about the Quantity of half a Pound, as may plainly be made appear by breathing upon a Glass.

Biosketch

Galileo Galilei (1564–1642) was born in Pisa, the town of the Leaning Tower, and received his education there (Figure 4-5). It was also there that he began his career by showing that a half-pound ball dropped as fast from the Leaning Tower as did a 100-pound cannon ball. However, contemporary reverence for Aristotle and the past was stronger than the desire to know the truth, a fact that eventually led Galileo to a confrontation with the pope and the Catholic Inquisition. Preceding this was his introduction of the "Dutch" telescope to explore the heavens and to make observations that supported the heliocentric theory of Copernicus. With his telescope, Galileo observed sun spots, which allowed him to show that the sun spun on its axis. In addition to his monumental astronomical observations, Galileo worked out the laws of falling bodies and showed that bullets followed a parabolic path. His observation of a swinging chandelier resulted in the formulation of the laws of pendular motion and their use for clocks. He also invented the first thermometer and attempted to measure the velocity of light. It was his work with pendulums and thermometers that was adapted by Santorio to clinical use[26].

Biosketch

Santorio Santorio (1561–1636), or Sanctorius in Latin, was born March 29, 1561, in Capodistria, the capital of Istria[22, 27]. He and his brother and two sisters were raised in an aristocratic family (Figure 4-7).

After his initial education in Capodistria, his father took him to Venice, where he was tutored by many of the best minds of his time. In 1575 he began his university education in Padua at age fourteen. After seven years of education he received his medical degree in 1582 at the age of twenty-one. After graduation he practiced medicine in Poland for fourteen years before returning to Venice, where he practiced medicine and joined the intellectual circle that included Galileo, Fabricio ab Aquapendente, and Fra Paolo Sarpi. His first book, *Methodus vitandorum errorum omnium qui in ante medica contigunt*, was published in Venice in 1602 (age forty-one) and nine years later he was invited to be professor of theoretical medicine in Padua from 1611 to 1624. He left academic medicine to practice medicine in Venice. His most famous work is *Ars de Statica medicina,* published in 1614.

This work was translated into Italian, English, German, and French and went through twenty-eight editions. Santorio Santorio never married and died in Venice in 1636. In the copy of his work that he presented to Galileo he claims to have studied more than ten thousand subjects in the span of twenty-five years, but sadly the records of these studies have been lost. Although the idea of insensible perspiration had been recognized by the Greeks and by Galen, it was Sanctorius who brought the concept of quantization and experimentation to this problem. His work on insensible perspiration probably began about 1582 when he graduated from medical school.

As one of the leading figures of the early scientific revolution, with many imaginative inventions to his credit, Sanctorius might appropriately be called the Father of Metabolic Obesity.

References

1. Poynter, F.N.L., K.D. Keel. *A Short History of Medicine*. London: Mills and Boon, 1961.
2. Santorio, Santorio. *Ars...de statica medicina a phorismorum sectionibus septum comprehensa. Accessit Statico Mastrix, sive ejusdem artis demolitio Hippolyti Obicii*. Leipzig: Gregor Ritsch für Zacharia Schurer und Mathias Gotzen, 1624.
3. Galilei, G. *Dialogue Concerning the Two Chief World Systems*. Transl. S. Drake. Berkeley: University of California Press, 1953.
4. Boyle R. *The Works of the Honourable Robert Boyle*. London: A. Millar. p. 1744.
5. Harvey, W. *The Anatomical Exercises of Dr. William Harvey. De Motu Cordis 1628: De circulatione sanguinis 1649: The first English text of 1653 now newly edited by Geoffrey Keynes*. London: Nonesuch Press, 1928.
6. Hales, S. *Statical Essays: Containing Haemstatics; or, an Account of Some Hydraulic and Hydrostatical Experiments Made on the Blood Vessels of Animals*. 3rd edition. London: Wilson and Nicol, 1769.
7. Hooke, R. *Micrographia, or Some Physiological Descriptions of Minute Bodies Made by Magnifying Glasses; with Observations and Inquiries Thereupon*. London: J. Martyn & J. Allestry, 1665–67.
8. Sydenham, T. *The Works of Thomas Sydenham, M.D. translated from the Latin Edition of Dr. Greenhill with a life of the author by R.G. Latham*. London: Sydenham Society, 1848.
9. Garrison, F.H. *An Introduction to the History of Medicine*. Philadelphia: W.B. Saunders Co., 1914.
10. Major, R.H. *A History of Medicine*. Vol. 1. Springfield, IL: Charles C. Thomas, 1954.
11. Duffin, J. *History of Medicine: A Scandalously Short Introduction*. Toronto: University of Toronto, 1999.
12. Avicenna. *The Canon of Medicine of Avicenna*. Ed. O. Cameron Gruner. London: Luzac and Co., 1930.
13. Taylor, F.S. *A Short History of Science and Scientific Thought with Readings from the Great Scientists from the Babylonians to Einstein*. New York, W.W. Norton & Co., 1963.
14. Boorstin, D. *The Discoverers. A History of Man's Search to Know His World and Himself*. New York: Random House, 1983.
15. Vesalius, A. *De Humani Corporis Fabrica*. Basileae: ex off. Joannis Oporini, 1543.
16. Boas, M. *The Scientific Renaissance 1450–1630*. New York: Harper Torchbooks, 1962.
17. Castiglione, A. *A History of Medicine*. Transl. E.B, Krumbhaar, MD.

New York: Alfred A. Knopf, 1941.

18. Foster, M. *Lectures on the History of Physiology during the Sixteenth, Seventeenth and Eighteenth Centuries.* Cambridge: University of Cambridge Press, 1901.
19. Osler, W. *The Evolution of Modern Medicine.* New Haven: Yale University Press, 1921.
20. Bacon, F. *Francisci de Verulamio Novum Organum Instauratio Magna.* 1620.
21. Descartes, R. *De honime figuris et latinitate donatus a Florentio Schuy, inclytae urbis sylvae ducis senatore, & ibidem philosophiae professore.* Leiden: Leffen and Moyardum, 1662.
22. Castiglioni, A. "Life and Work of Sanctorius." Transl. E. Recht. *Medical Life.* 1931.
23. Santorio, S. *A New Art of Physick. Contained in eight sections of aphorisms, concerning insensible perspiration; being a vapor of breathing from the body. Plainly shewing that health and sickness is best discerned by weighing the body. Being found true after thirty years experience and practise thereof. Transl. by Abdiah Cole Doctor of physick.* London: Peter Cole, 1663.
24. Santorio. S. *Commentaria in primam fen primi libri Canonis Avecennae....cum triplice indice, uno quetionum, altero instrumentorum, tertio terum notibium.* Venice: Marc-Antonio Brogiolo, 1646. 2nd ed.
25. Singer, C. *A Short History of Scientific Ideas.* Oxford: Clarendon Press, 1959.
26. Darrow, F.L. *Masters of Science and Invention.* New York: Harcourt, Brace and Co., 1923.
27. Eknoyan, G. "Santorio Sanctorius (1561–1636). Founding father of Metabolic Balance Studies." *Am J Nephrol.* 19 (1999): 226–233.
28. Stubbs, S.G.B, E.W. Bligh. *Sixty Centuries of Health and Physick.* New York: Paul B. Hoeber Inc., 1931.

CHAPTER 5

The Body Mass Index Invented by Quetelet

> *The more advanced the sciences have become, the more they have tended to enter the domain of mathematics, which is a sort of center towards which they converge. We can judge of the perfection to which a science has come by the facility more or less great, which it may be approached by calculation.*
>
> —*Hankins*[1]

Why the body mass index? How does it help us with the battle of the bulge? It is a term used for comparing your body weight and mine. It is the term used to define the current epidemic of obesity. However, it has only come into its own in the past few years and is still not widely used by most people. I became aware that it was becoming accepted when I overheard a conversation among a group of teenagers at the airport the other day. They had a copy of the local newspaper that described the body mass index. The kids were comparing their body mass index findings among themselves. Awareness of the body mass index is the first step in using it.

But why do we want to use the body mass index as a way to describe the current epidemic and to mark our successes in battling the bulge? Don't we have weight tables? Of course we do, but the widely used ones come from life insurance companies based on health statistics for the people who are insured. But the people who chose to buy insurance are not necessarily representative of all of us, so the search began for a better index. After a search that lasted more than a quarter of a century, the body mass index emerged.

The body mass index, or BMI as it is usually called, is not new. It originated more than a century ago, and this is a story about its beginnings, and why it is important to us today.

Lambert-Adolphe-Jacques Quetelet (1796–1874) introduced the concept of the body mass index as a tool to assess differences among human

SUR L'HOMME

ET LE

DÉVELOPPEMENT DE SES FACULTÉS,

OU

ESSAI DE PHYSIQUE SOCIALE;

PAR A. QUETELET,

Secrétaire perpétuel de l'Académie royale de Bruxelles, Correspondant de l'Institut de France, de la Société royale astronomique de Londres, des Académies royales de Berlin, de Turin, etc.

> Appliquons aux sciences politiques et morales la méthode fondée sur l'observation et sur le calcul, méthode qui nous a si bien servi dans les sciences naturelles.
>
> LAPLACE, *Essai ph. sur les probabilités.*

TOME PREMIER.

PARIS,

BACHELIER, IMPRIMEUR-LIBRAIRE,

QUAI DES AUGUSTINS, N° 55.

1835

5-1 Title page from Quetelet's book titled *Sur l'homme et le développement de ses faculties, ou Essai de physique sociale* (On the development of man and his faculties, published in 1835). From the collection of the author.

beings. His classic work titled *On the Development of Man and His Faculties (Sur l'homme et le développement de se facultés, ou Essai de physique sociale)*[2] was published in 1835 when he was age thirty-nine. This work made Quetelet famous throughout Europe (Figure 5-1).

A second edition of this volume was published in 1869[3], five years before his death.

The BMI introduced by Quetelet provides the basic unit for measuring the current epidemic of obesity and our successes in battling it. Obesity is one end of the distribution of body weight and thus the extreme weights for the "average man" are a central concept for Quetelet. The introduction and first two chapters in Part 2 of an English translation[4] of his classic are reproduced below. In summarizing the accomplishments of Quetelet, Freudenthal[5] says:

> With Quetelet's work of 1835, a new era in statistics began. It presented a new technique of statistics or, rather, the first technique at all. The material was thoughtfully elaborated, arranged according to certain pre-established principles, and made comparable. There were not very many statistical figures in the book, but each figure reported made sense. For every number, Quetelet tried to find the determining influences, its natural causes, and the perturbations, caused by man. The work gave a description of the average man as both a static and dynamic phenomenon[5].

This concept of the "average man" originated with Quetelet and is one of his seminal contributions.

To make progress beyond the descriptive phase of any phenomenon requires quantitative or mathematical approaches. This is where Quetelet's contribution stands tall. As the old medicine, dating back to the Roman period and influenced by Hippocrates[6] and Galen[7] , gave way to a first wave of modern medicine at the beginning of the nineteenth century, quantitative methods were required.

At the bedside, P.C.A. Louis[8], a master of clinical teaching during the peak of the Paris School in the first quarter of the nineteenth century[9], began to apply his numerical method to the study of disease. Quetelet, with his mathematical background, vastly expanded this area and took statistical methods into new arenas. He was a pioneer in the application of statistics to human biology, anthropology, and criminology, and, as Walker points out, Quetelet had a tremendous influence on the subsequent work of Sir Francis Galton, who discovered the individuality of fingerprints, and Florence Nightingale, the pioneer in nursing education[10].

Quetelet was interested in the underlying factors that were responsible for and determined the distribution of such events as births, marriages, deaths, and the prevalence of various types of crime. In his work he noted the seasonal distribution of births, deaths, and marriages. He also noted a seasonal distribution of crime and that crimes against property appeared more frequently in cold months and crimes against the person were more common in the summer. In commenting on the constancy of crimes from year to year he said,

> Thus we pass from one year to another with the sad perspective of seeing the same crimes reproduced in the same order and calling down the same punishments in the same proportions. A sad condition of humanity...[1]

Fortunately we have been able to change this apparent constancy by education, laws, and better government.

Much of the work in the volume *Sur l'homme* deals with means and distributions of the measurements he made. Quetelet is also known for his contributions to binomial distribution which are the essentials to understanding games of chance, such as poker. It was not until a later publication in 1845 in the *Bulletin de la Commission de Statistique (de Belgique)* that he dealt with the concept of the binomial distribution in detail. In his work, Quetelet spent a significant amount of space on the issue of height and weight and it is in that context that his work is of interest to the battle of the bulge. (Appendix)

To quote from chapter 2 of *Sur l'homme*, Quetelet says,

> If man increased equally in all his dimensions, his weight at different ages would be as the cube of his height. Now, this is not what we really observe. The increase in weight is slower, except during the first year after birth; then the proportion which we have just pointed out is pretty regularly observed. But after this period, and until near the age of puberty, the weight increases nearly as the square of the height. The development of the weight again becomes very rapid at the time of puberty, and almost stops at the 25th year. In general, we do not err much when we assume *that, during development, the square of weight at different ages are as the fifth powers of the height;* which naturally leads to this conclusion, in supposing the specific gravity constant, that the transverse growth of man is less than vertical[4].

These insights into the change of height and weight as we grow were central to the idea of the body mass index and its usefulness in assessing overweight.

> However, if we compare two individuals who are fully developed and well-formed with each other, to ascertain the relations existing between *the weight and stature, we shall find that the weight of developed persons, of different heights, is nearly as the square of the stature.* Whence it naturally follows, that a *transverse section, giving both the breadth and thickness, is just proportioned to the height of the individual.* We furthermore conclude that, proportion still being attended, width predominates in individuals of small stature[4].

These two paragraphs summarize the concept of the body mass index and Quetelet's rationale for developing it. The Quetelet (or body mass) index of an individual is the mass divided by stature squared [$Wt/(Ht)^2$].

Over the past quarter century, the BMI (it might also be called the Quetelet index or QI) has been widely used in epidemiologic studies. How valid is this index of weight and stature as a surrogate for obesity?

It has been suggested that "efforts should be made to develop uncomplicated indices that correlate better with body fat content than the Quetelet (Body Mass) Index does"[11]. But how well does this index correlate with body fatness? The QI has been embraced by some[12–16] but not by others[17–20] Strong support for use of the QI was provided by Keys et al[16], who evaluated three indices of weight [the Wt/Ht, $Wt/(Ht)^2$, and $Ht/\sqrt[3]{Wt}$ (Ponderal index)] against skinfold thicknesses or body density as estimates of body fat. Of these three, the BMI was slightly better correlated with fatness than Wt/Ht. The Ponderal Index was clearly worse.

Benn reopened the question[17]. He showed that a simple index of Wt/Ht^p could be derived for each population in which *p* was a power where weight had the lowest relation to height for that population. For most populations this number is between 1 and 2. The ratio which Quetelet proposed in 1835[2] had a power of 2 [$(Wt/(Ht)^2)$]. In an effort to apply a weight/height index to a variety of populations living in Hawaii, Lee, Kolonel, and Hinds[21] found different indices useful for ranking the different populations. However, these authors did not measure fatness, and since all of these weight-to-height indices are strongly related to weight[22], their data are unhelpful in resolving the value of the Quetelet or body mass index versus the Benn index as estimates of fat. Keys et al.[16] examined the relationship of weight-to-height indices in twelve populations. The best correlations with body fat as estimated from skinfolds were found with $Wt/(Ht)^2$. He found that the body mass or Quetelet index had correlations ranging between 0.611 and 0.850 when related to skinfold thickness. In a detailed evaluation of four large study populations, Garn and Pesick[22] showed a strong correlation between any index and weight which approximated r=0.90. In this study, the population-specific indices, or p as proposed by Benn $[(Wt/(Ht)^p)]$, ranged between 1.18 to 1.83. These population-specific indices provided *no* advantage over the $Wt/(Ht)^2$ when related to skinfolds.

Garrow and Webster[14] have also examined the QI as a measure of fatness in a group of obese subjects. Fat was measured by three separate techniques including densitometry, measurement of total body water, and measurement of total body potassium using γ-emission from naturally occurring radioactive potassium (^{40}K). As Garrow and Webster point out, there is considerable variation in estimating fat between the methods that they selected for this study. The accuracy for measuring fat was greater for men than for women by all methods used by Garrow and Webster. The standard deviations for estimating fat by the QI, however, were only slightly larger than those for density, body water, and body potassium. The relationship of $Fat/(Ht)^2$ plotted against $Wt/(Ht)^2$, yielded very similar slopes for men (0.715) and for women (0.713). This means that men and women of similar height differ in weight by the weight of a "tissue" that is approximately 71% fat and 29% non-fat. In their data analysis there was an important difference in the fatness between men and women such that a woman with 0 (zero) body fat would have a QI of 13.7 kg/m^2; whereas a man with 0 body fat would have a QI of 16.9 kg/m^2. Garrow and Webster thus conclude that "Quetelet's Index has been underrated as a measure of obesity in adults. It...provides a measure of fatness not much less accurate than specialized laboratory methods"[14]. The body mass or Quetelet index estimates fat better in fatter than leaner children[23]. As they point out, this index can be applied over the entire weight range, while such measurements as skinfold thickness are severely limited in obese individuals and nearly useless in very obese individuals.

An additional feature of the QI is the similarity of the mortality and morbidity curves plotted against QI for men and women. Whether related to excessive deaths or to morbidity from various disease entities, the minimum QI is similar for both sexes at comparable ages. Yet at all ages, the quantity of body fat in women is higher than in men for any given height/weight combination. This implies that the extra fat in women (the difference in BMI at zero-fat 16.9 minus 13.7 = 3.2 kg/m^2) is not associated with increased risk of excess morbidity or mortality. A similar conclusion, ushering in the era of studies in body fat distribution[5], suggests that for comparable increases in risk indices such as blood pressure, women required approximately 20 kg more fat than men[24].

The relationship between height and weight ($Wt/(Ht)^2$) proposed by Quetelet in 1835 has stood the test of time. That is why the BMI has replaced life insurance tables as the basis for examining overweight. Although life insurance tables were the basis for determining desirable weight during most of the twentieth century, they have recently been replaced by the BMI. We are currently in the midst of an epidemic of obesity, with rates that have increased 50 to 100% in recent decades. The BMI has provided a valuable tool to follow the progress of the battle of the bulge. In tribute to his contribution and its validation from a number of sources, it would be appropriate to refer to the BMI as the Quetelet index or QI and replace the frequently used body mass index or BMI with this new nomenclature.

Biosketch

Lambert-Adolf-Jacques Quetelet (1796–1874) (Figure 5-2) was born in Belgium in 1796 and died in Brussels in 1874[5]. Following his graduation from the Lycée in Ghent, he worked for a year as a teacher. In 1815, at the age of nineteen, he was appointed professor of mathematics at the college in Ghent and in 1819 received a doctorate from the newly established University of Ghent, with a dissertation on geometry. In the same year as he received his doctoral degree, Quetelet was appointed as professor of *mathématiques élémentaires* at the Athénée in Brussels. Although the work we have described by Quetelet focuses on statistics, he was a man of many talents. He wrote an opera with his friend G.P. Dandelin and also published poems and essays. He was a teacher of mathematics, physics, and astronomy and a major force in the development of the Belgian Observatory. His interest in probability theory may well be due to the influence of the French scientists LaPlace and Fourier. From 1832 onward he lived at the Observatory where his work on meteorology, astronomy, and geophysics was conducted with its strong statistical focus. Following publication of his famous work *Sur l'Homme*[2] he achieved international stature throughout Europe and spent a great deal of his activity organizing international cooperative activities in astronomy, meteorology, geophysics, and statistics. He was the driving force of the first International Statistical Congress that met in Brussels in 1853[10], and he was a member of more than one hundred learned societies. He wrote prodigiously, and his subjects covered the gamut from astronomy and meteorology to anthropometry and morals. In 1855, at the age of fifty-nine, he suffered a stroke, which impaired his subsequent work. He died in 1874 and his work has not been republished since[5]. Quetelet's contributions to mathematical statistics have been captured in this closing quote:

> "Statistics will not make any progress until it is trusted to those who have created profound mathematical theories."—Fourier[10]

Quetelet was one of the creators of profound theories.

References

1. Hankins, F.H. *Adolphe Quetelet as Statesman.* New York: Columbia University, 1908.
2. Quetelet, L.A.J. *Sur l'homme et le développement de ses facultés, ou Essai de physique sociale.* Paris: Bachelier, 1835.
3. Quetelet, L.A.J. *Physique sociale; ou, Essai sur le développement des facultes de l'homme.* Bruxelles: C. Marquardt, 1869.
4. Quetelet, L.A.J. *A Treatise on Man and the Development of His Faculties.* Edinburgh: William and Robert Chambers, 1842. In *Comparative Statistics in the Nineteenth Century.* Farnborough: Gregg International Publishers, 1973.
5. Freudenthal, H. "Lambert-Adolphe-Jacques Quetelet." In Gillespie. C.C. ed. *Dictionary of Scientific Biography.* New York: Charles Scribner's Sons, 1975.
6. Hippocrates. *Oeuvres complètes d'Hippocrate: traduction nouvelle avec le texte grec en regard, collationné sur les manuscrits et toutes les éditions ; accompagnée d'une introduction, de commentaires médicaux, de variantes et de notes philologiques; suivie d'une table générale des matières /par É. Littré.* Paris: J.B. Bailliere, 1839–1861.
7. Galen. *Opera, iam recens versa.* Basileae, Ex Aedibus And. Cratandri, 1531.
9. Louis, P.C.A. *Recherches anatomico-pathologiques sur la phthisie.* Paris: Gabon et Cie, 1825.
9. Ackerknecht, E. *Medicine at the Paris Hospital.* Baltimore: Johns Hopkins University Press, 1967.
10. Walker, H. *Studies in the History of Statistical Method.* Baltimore: Williams and Wilkins Co., 1929.
11. Simopolous. A.P., T.B. van Itallie. "Body Weight, Health and Longevity." *Ann Intern Med.* 100 (1984): 285–295.
12. Bardeen C.R. "General Relations of Sitting Height to Stature and of Sitting Height and Stature to Weight." *Am J Phys Anthrop* 6 (1923): 355–388.
13. Davenport, C.H. *Body-build and Its Inheritance.* Washington, D.C.: Carnegie Institution of Washington, 1923.
14. Garrow, J.S., J.D. Webster. "Quetelet's Index (Wt/Ht^2) as a Measure of Fatness." *Int J Obes.* 9 (1985): 147–153.
15. Kaup, J. "Bedeutung des Normbegriffes in der und experimentelle Beitrage zur Frage der Beeinflussung des Zahlenverhältnisses der Geschlechter." *Zeitschr. f. menschl. Vererb.-u. Konstitutionslechere.* 19 (1935): 213–252.
16. Keys, A., F. Fidanza, M.M. Karvonen, N. Kimura, H.L. Taylor. "Indices of Relative Weight and Obesity." *J Chron Dis* 25 (1972): 329–343.

17. Benn, R.T. "Some Mathematical Properties of Weight-height Indices Used as a Measure of Adiposity." *Br Prev Soc Med.* 25 (1971): 42–50.
18. Livi, D.R. *Antropoinetria Militare.* Roma: Presso IL Giornale Medico Del Regio Esercito, 1896.
19. Pirquet. "Eine einfache Tafel zur Bestimmung von Wachstum and Ernährungzustand bei Kindern." *Zs. f. Kinderh.* 6 (1913): 253–262.
20. Sheldon, W.H., S.S. Stephens, C.B. Tucket. *The Varieties of Human Physique: An Introduction to Constitutional Psychology.* New York: Harper, 1940.
21. Lee, J., N. Kolonel, M.W. Hinds. "The Use of an Inappropriate Weight-Height Derived Index of Obesity Can Produce Misleading Results." *Int J Obes.* 6 (1982): 233–239.
22. Garn, S.N., S.D. Pesick. "Comparison of the Benn Index and Other Body Mass Indices in Nutritional Assessment." *Am J Clin Nutr.* 36 (1982): 573–575.
23. Bray, G.A., J.M. DeLany, D.W. Harsha, J. Volaufova, C.C. Champagne. "Evaluation of Body Fat in Fatter and Leaner 10-year-old African-American and White Children in the Baton Rouge Children's Study." *Am J Clin Nutr.* 73 (2001): 687–702.
24. Krotkiewski, M., P. Bjorntorp, L. Sjostrom, U. Smith. "Impact of Obesity on Metabolism in Men and Women. Importance of Regional Adipose Tissue Distribution." *J Clin Invest.* 72 (1983): 1150–1162.
25. Mailly, L. "Essai sur la vie et les ouvrages de Quetelet." *Annuaire de l'academie royale des sciences, des lettres et des beaux-arts de Belgique, 28.* Brussels, 1875.

Chapter 6

How Fat Are We? Improving on Archimedes

Anatomy is to physiology, as geography to history; it describes the theater of events.

—Jean Fernel

You now know how to find your body mass index. You also know what it means and where this idea came from. But the physicians and scientists working to beat the bulge often need more accurate and precise estimates of body fat than are provided by the body mass or Quetelet index. The past century has greatly expanded the ability to measure how much fat you have, where the fat is, and whether it makes a difference to you. After all, if you are going to battle the bulge, you want to have all the information about your problem that you can get.

Advances in theory and methodology have both been important for progress in all areas of scientific research, including the battle of the bulge. These have been particularly important as the epidemic of obesity rages around us. An ancient principle discovered by the illustrious Greek mathematician Archimedes was used to calculate whether his king's gold crown had been adulterated with silver or lead. The amount of gold in the king's crown was determined from its density, that is, how much it weighed relative to water. This principle has been applied to provide a reproducible and accurate measurement of body fat. It is an example of how a method from another scientific discipline, in this case physics, can be applied to improving the measurement of body composition, that is, to answering the question of how fat we are.

Archimedes is attributed with the discovery of a concept known as "specific gravity" when he was trying to determine whether lead had been mixed with gold in the king's crown. When an object is placed in water, it will occupy a volume of water equal to the volume of the object placed in the water. The weight of a pure substance has a constant relationship to the weight of the water that it displaces. This is called "specific gravity." By finding out how much water the crown displaced, Archimedes could tell whether it was pure gold or whether the gold had been mixed with some other metal. It was pure gold. Whether the story is true or not, Archimedes understood the principles of specific gravity, as is shown in his book on floating bodies[2].

Table 6-1 High, Intermediate and Low specific Gravity Group Values in Relation to Weight and Circumference Measurements *

Category of Specific Gravity	Average Specific Gravity	Range of Specific Gravity	Average Weight (kg)	Average Height (cm)	Average Circumference (cm)	
					Chest	Abdomen
Low	1.081 (38)	1.075-1.097	67.8	177.0	89.7	75.2
Intermediate	1.066 (33)	1.060-1.074	71.2	173.5	90.9	77.2
High	1.056 (28)	1.021-1.059	80.0	175.3	95.5	86.1

* Adapted from Behnke et al JAMA 118(1942):495-8 () = number of men in group

The principle of specific gravity discovered by Archimedes is but one of many principles of physics that have been applied to the study of the human body and to our battle of the bulge. In this section I will discuss the application of Archimedes' principle and the use of x-rays to study how much fat there is in our body, where it is distributed, and what makes us bulge. X-rays were discovered by Roentgen more than two thousand years after Archimedes. The principle of using density to calculate body fat is older than x-rays but has been partly replaced by x-rays, which provide an easier method to peer inside the human body.

A number of efforts have been made to apply the principle of Archimedes to estimating body fat. The paper that I have chosen is one that appeared during World War II. It was the most successful of these efforts because the method was reproducible and could be applied to healthy human beings. This paper, "The Specific Gravity of Healthy Men: Body Weight Divided by Volume as an Index of Obesity" by Behnke, Feen, and Welham, applied Archimedes' principle to the study of human body composition. Their study was based on measurements in ninety-nine healthy male subjects aged twenty to forty years. Although not the first to apply this method, the precision of their work makes it a landmark in the way we measure body fat[3].

The history of the use of density to estimate fat goes back to 1757, when Robertson apparently made the earliest measurements of specific gravity of human beings[4]. He reported on ten volunteers who submerged themselves in a tank that measured 78 inches long, 30 inches wide, and 30 inches deep. This report and other early scientific publications measured specific gravity or density by the method of water displacement[4]. This can be done either by actually measuring the water displaced by the subject or by weighing the individual out of water and again when completely submerged. Living subjects as well as cadavers were studied. One limitation to this method is the amount of air in the lungs, since air is very light relative to other parts of the body. To reduce this error, lung volumes in this study were in maximal inspiration, maximal expiration, and at the usual level of respiration while they were submerged, thus allowing Robertson to estimate the contribution of lung air to the weight of his subjects and the water they displaced.

In a detailed review of the publications on this subject up to 1933, Boyd[5] identified 787 individual values for specific gravity of human subjects ranging from a fetus two months of age all the way up to an adult sixty years of age. Water displacement was used to measure specific gravity in 598 of these individuals, and hydrostatic weighing, i.e., the difference in weight between submersion and out of water, was used with 189 individuals. There were 205 cadavers and 582 living subjects in these studies[5]. He drew several conclusions from these earlier studies. First, specific gravity in all respiratory phases increased linearly with both age and height (stature). Second, the variability in these measurements was very large. Third, specific gravity increases with age in adults. However, about 18 percent of normal infants have values within the middle two-thirds of the range for adults. As we have learned since methods have improved, infants and children have a higher percentage of water in their tissues than do adults.

The wide range of estimates of specific gravity in Boyd's review[5] was undoubtedly due to the buoyancy of air in the lungs, which was not measured in most reports. The addition of a measurement of lung volume by Behnke et al.[3,6] improved this technique from a semi-quantitative to a quantitative one. By so doing, he established a gold standard for measuring body fat that lasted for more than fifty years.

Behnke and his group began their work as World War II was beginning. Behnke was in the U.S. Navy and working at the Naval Medical Center. His work was of importance to the war effort as a way to establish the degree of fatness in military personnel. To quote from the description by Behnke et al.[3]

> The essential measurement is that of body volume, which, based on Archimedes' principle, can be conveniently determined by the method of hydrostatic weighing, i.e., equivalent volume weight in air—weight in water[3].

Thus, a gold standard for measuring body fat was born—not the gold in the crown of Archimedes' king, but the intellectual gold that makes for important scientific advances.

Behnke and his team weighed their subjects underwater on two separate occasions to check the accuracy of their procedure. The air remaining in the lungs, called the "residual air," was determined separately by a technique called "helium dilution." This allowed them to obtain a direct measure of the unexpired air remaining in the lungs (residual volume), which set their approach apart from the earlier ones. After calculating the specific gravity of the ninety-nine men by this method, they divided the sample into three groups of nearly equal numbers according to their average specific gravity[3]. (See Appendix)

It is clear from this table that as body weight increased, the amount of body fat also increased (i.e., there was a decrease in average specific gravity). Thus, the heavier men had a lower specific gravity, implying more fat. In addition, body weight was directly related to the circumference of both the chest and waist, suggesting that heavier men had more fat in their abdomen and more air or fat in their chest.

Before turning to a consideration of the way one method is replaced by another, it would be important to summarize a few of the features of the "gold standard" for body fat provided from this important work of Behnke et al. Of the body constituents, fat and bone are most likely to be the chief determinants of the specific gravity. The method of hydrostatic weighing proposed by Behnke and his colleagues became the gold standard for *in vivo* measurement of body fat for nearly fifty years[3, 7–9] The principal limitations of this method have been the higher hydration of body tissues in infants and children and the higher bone density in some populations. Using appropriate conversions, the specific gravity can be converted into percent body fat. Based on their studies, Behnke et al.[3] drew the following conclusions:

1. The fundamental biological characteristics of body density can be accurately measured usually within 0.004 units by the method of hydrostatic weighing, provided a correction is made for the air in the lungs.
2. Values of specific gravity for healthy men ranging between 20 and 40 years of age were between 1.021 and 1.097.
3. Low values for specific gravity indicate obesity and conversely high values denote leanness.
4. Individual loss in weight through exercise and a restricted diet is associated with an increase in specific gravity.
5. Difference in the circumferential measurements of chest and abdomen serve as a criterion of obesity and can be correlated with specific gravity.
6. Variation in the percentage of bone in relation to body weight, excluding excess fat, is not expected to produce deviation of more than 0.013 units in comparable values.[3]

The important issues summarized above set the stage for the next advance. One limitation of body density is that it is difficult to weigh some people underwater. It requires cooperation, and for infants this is particularly difficult. In addition, some people don't like to submerge themselves. Finally, you have to have facilities for changing clothes into something suitable for the procedure and you need to have an appropriate tank of water. All of these limitations stimulated the search for a better method to measure body fat in the battle of the bulge.

Methods for determining body composition continue to advance as new techniques are discovered[10, 11]. Among the newer methods that have challenged hydrostatic or underwater weighing as the gold standard are the techniques for measuring total body water and procedures for measuring total body potassium. If you know how much water is in the body, about 73%, you can calculate how much potassium there is. Since potassium is a major mineral constituent (ion) inside of cells, knowing how much potassium there is in the body, you can also calculate the amount of cell mass and thus indirectly how much is fat[12]. The most promising new methods, however, are based on the use of x-rays.

The x-ray was originally discovered in 1895 by Roentgen[13]. He did this accidentally one day when he put his hand between a piece of film and a tube that was emitting radiation. These unknown "rays" were designated x-rays but have often been called Roentgen rays after their discoverer.

The use of x-rays to identify disease and to study the human body advanced rapidly during the last years of the nineteenth century. In the early twentieth century, x-rays were applied to the study of body composition to measure the fat thickness in the forearm[14]. Because of the risk of developing cancer and producing damage to reproductive tissues, the wider use of x-rays in the study of body composition had to wait until the last quarter of the twentieth century. It was the development of computed axial tomography (CT)[8] in 1973 and the introduction of dual-energy x-ray absorptiometry (DXA)[15] in 1970 that revolutionized the measurement of body composition and ousted underwater weighing as the gold standard for measuring body fat in the battle of the bulge.

Both computed tomography (CT) and the related technique of magnetic resonance imaging spectroscopy (MRI), along with dual-energy x-ray absorptiometry (DXA), have vastly increased the ease and accuracy of measuring body fat. CT scans have been applied with great success in telling us how much fat we have in various parts of the body[16]. For example, using CT scanning we can separate the fat that is under the skin from the fat which lies within various parts of the body. Doing this has helped us to understand that fat inside the body cavities, such as the abdomen, can have much worse consequences for health than fat under the skin. The so-called "apple-shaped" individual with an increased amount of fat inside the abdomen has a higher risk of diabetes, high blood pressure, heart disease, and cancer than another person with less fat inside the abdomen. DXA scanning (dual-energy x-ray absorptiometry) has made it possible to measure how much of the body is fat, how much lean tissue, and how much is bone. This latter measurement has been particularly important for people who have a risk for osteoporosis or bone-thinning[11]. Just as Behnke's contribution in 1942[3] was a milestone and gold standard, so these newer techniques derived from physics that have been applied to measuring body composition have provided new gold standards on the path of scientific methodology for measuring body fat in the battle of the bulge.

Figure 6-1 shows the different compartments into which the body can be divided, depending on the goals of the research. The human body can be analyzed from many perspectives. These five levels reflect improvements over the past five centuries in the methods of examining the human body. The initial studies of the human body during the Renaissance were done for artistic purposes, which required studies of the underlying anatomic structure. The anatomical studies of Leonardo da Vinci served this purpose but did not contribute to medical anatomy since they were not published. However, the anatomist Vesalius published the first modern anatomy of the human body in 1543.

With the invention of the microscope in the seventeenth century, the tissue (Level II) and cellular levels (Level III) of the human body were available for study and the veil of ignorance was gradually pulled back.

This was followed in the nineteenth and twentieth centuries by improvements in chemistry and physics that allowed for a molecular (Level IV) and atomic (Level V) understanding of body composition. A similar progression occurred in pathology: Organ pathology preceded tissue pathology, which in turn preceded cellular and molecular pathology.

Whole Body (Level I)

The first level of analysis of body composition is the whole body (Level I). Wang et al. identified at least ten different measurable components, including stature (height), length of limbs, various circumferences including waist and hips, skinfold thickness at various sites (e.g., triceps, subscapular), body surface area, body volume, BMI, and body density.

Tissue and Organ Composition (Level II)

The division of the body into organs and tissues is obvious. Five major tissues are shown in Figure 6-1, including skeletal muscle, adipose tissue, skeleton, blood or hematopoietic tissues, and all others. The amount and location of adipose tissue are most important. As much as 80% of body fat is subcutaneous; however, fat also surrounds many organs and accumulates around the abdominal organs. Fat in this latter category is most difficult to measure accurately except with expensive imaging techniques.

Cellular Composition (Level III)

A third level in the analysis of body composition is the cellular components. The body is composed of cells in all tissues and organs, which have intracellular fluid and are surrounded by extracellular fluids and solids. Figure 6-1 lists two major cellular categories. These include connective-tissue cells, neural cells, muscle cells, epithelial cells, and the fat cells that are the major cause of the bulge that we are battling. One technique for measuring body cell mass uses the naturally occurring radioactive isotope of potassium (^{40}K). Because more than 95% of potassium is intracellular, the ability to measure an isotope of potassium provides an index of body cell mass. ^{40}K is a naturally occurring isotope of potassium, and its abundance can be determined with whole-body radiation counters. Total body weight is the sum of all tissues, including muscle cells, connective tissue cells, epithelial cells, and neural cells. The metabolically active tissues, such as bone, adipose tissue, blood cells, and muscle, make up about 75% of body weight.

Molecular Composition (Level IV)

This part of the model is most widely used in clinical medicine. Water constitutes 60% or more of the weight in males and 50% in females. Of this 60%, approximately 26% is extracellular and 34% intracellular. Lipids range from less than 10% of body weight in well-trained athletes to nearly 50% in obese patients. Two percent to 3% of these lipids are essential structural lipids, and the remainder are nonessential stores. Protein constitutes 15% of normal body composition, and minerals constitute 5.3%. Thus, water, lipid, protein, and minerals account for 99.4% of the molecular constituents of the body.

Biosketch

Wilhelm Konrad Roentgen (1845–1922) discovered x-rays in 1895. His discovery provided a fundamental technique that has made current quantitative study of body composition so precise. Born to a German farmer and a Dutch mother, he was only a modest student during his education at Utrecht.

His path was set when he met Clauisius, whom he accompanied to Würzburg. It was during his studies at Würzburg in 1895, while working with the radiation from a Crooke's tube, that he discovered a greenish fluorescent light would be produced on a distant barium screen with platinum. These rays passed through most substances, particularly soft tissue so that the bones of the hand were easily visible. His discovery was published in 1895 and he won the Nobel Prize in 1901. He was troubled by the World War and died in relative isolation in 1922[17] (Figure 6-2).

Biosketch

Albert R. Behnke, Jr. (1903–1992) (Figure 6-3) was born in Chicago in 1903 and received his M.D. from Stanford University in 1930.

He served his internship at the U.S. Naval Hospital of Vallejo, California, following which he was a research fellow in the Department of Physiology in the Harvard School of Public Health from 1932 through 1935. Most of Behnke's career was spent in the U.S. Naval Medical Service, which he entered in 1929. He was an instructor from 1937 to 1942, scientific director of the Naval Medical Research Institute from 1943 to 1950, and medical director at the U.S. Navy Radiological Defense Laboratory from 1953 to 1959, when he retired from active service in the navy. After his military retirement, Behnke did extensive work on body composition and worked for a while at the University of California School of Public Health in Berkeley. He died in January 1992[18].

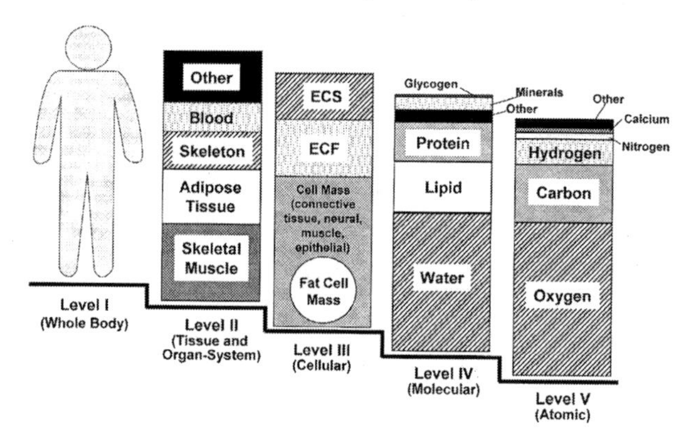

6-1 Five perspectives on body composition. The human body is classified into increasingly general categories, from the atomic level through the molecular, cellular, tissue-system, and whole-body levels. Each perspective is characterized by a set of unique components that define its measurement parameters. Adapted from Wang et al *Am J Clin Nutr* 1992;56(1):19-28.

References

1. Sherrington, C. *The Endeavor of Jean Fernel.* Cambridge: Cambridge University Press, 1906.
2. Singer, C.J. *A History of Biology to About the Year 1900: A General Introduction to the Study of Living Things.* 3rd ed. New York: Abelard-Schuman, 1959.
3. Behnke, A.R., B.G. Feen, W.C. Weiham. "The Specific Gravity of Healthy Men." *JAMA.* 118 (1942): 495–498.
4. Robertson, J. "An Essay Towards Ascertaining the Specific Gravity of Living Men." *Philos Trans R Soc Lon [Biol].* No 1. 50(1757):80-35.
5. Boyd, E. "The Specific Gravity of the Human Body." *Hum Biol.* 5(1933): 646–672.
6. Behnke, A.R., J.H. Wilmore. *Evaluation and Regulation of Body Build and Composition.* Englewood Cliffs, NJ: Prentice-Hall, 1974.
7. Brozek, J. *Human Body Composition: Approaches and Applications.* Oxford: Pergamon Press, 1965.
8. Hounsfield, G.M. "Computerized Transverse Axial Scanning (Tomography)." *Br J Radiol.* 46(1973): 1016–1022.
9. Moore, F.D., K.H. Olesen, J.D. McMurrey, H.V. Parker, M.R. Ball, C.M. Boyden. *The Body Cell Mass and Its Supporting Environment.* Philadelphia: W.B. Saunders and Co., 1963.
10. Lukaski, C. "Methods for the Assessment of Human Body Composition: Traditional and New." *Am J Clin Nutr.* 46(1987): 537–556.
11. Wang, Z., R.N. Pierson, S.B. Heymsfleld. "The Five-Level Model: a New Approach to Organizing Body Composition." *Am J Clin Nutr.* 56 (1992): 19–28.
12. Forbes, G.B. *Human Body Composition: Growth, Aging, Nutrition, and Activity.* New York: Springer-Verlag, 1987.
13. Röntgen, W.C. "Ueber eine neue Art von Strahlen. (Vorlaufige Mittheilung.)" *Sitzber a Phys Med Ges Würzburg.* 1895: 132–141.
14. Garn, S.M. "Comparison of Pinch-Caliper and X-ray Measurements of Skin Plus Subcutaneous Fat." *Science.* 124(1956): 178–179.
15. Mazess, R.B., J.R. Cameron, J.A. Sorenson. "Determining Body Composition by Radiation Absorption Spectrometry." *Nature.* 229(1970): 771.
16. Kvist, H., L. Sjostrom, U. Tylen. "Adipose Tissue Volume Determinations in Women by Computed Tomography: Technical Considerations." *Int J Obes.* 10(1986): 53–67
17. Garrison, F.H. *The History of Medicine.* Philadelphia: W.B. Saunders, 1912.
18. *Directory of Medical Specialists.* Evanston, IL: American Board of Medical Specialities, 1989–90.

Chapter 7

Measurements in Research: Insulin, Hormones, and Drugs

> *Measure what can be measured and make measurable what cannot be measured.*
>
> —Galileo[1]

Diabetes is a two-faced disease. In some people it is a disease that results from destruction of the cells in the pancreas that produce insulin. This type of diabetes is found in maybe 10% of all diabetics. The other type of diabetes, called Type 2 diabetes, is a disease of surfeit. As the epidemic of obesity roars ahead, an epidemic of Type 2 diabetes is right behind. In times of famine or starvation, Type 2 diabetes is almost nonexistent. Thus, diabetes is a clear marker of our success in the battle of the bulge. As the epidemic of obesity that we are battling increases, diabetes goes along hand in hand.

Diabetes of both types has been a scourge of mankind for centuries. This human plague was first recorded in a clinical description of the disease by Araetaeus more than two thousand years ago. He said,

> Diabetes is a wonderful affection, not very frequent among men, being a melting down of the flesh and limbs into urine. The patients never stop making water, but the flow is incessant, as if the opening of aqueducts. Life is short, disgusting and painful, thirst unquenchable; excessive drinking, which, however, is disproportionate to the large quantity of urine, for more urine is passed; and one cannot stop them either from drinking or making water; Or, if for a time they abstain from drinking, their mouth becomes parched and their body dry; the viscera seems as if scorched up; they are affected with nausea, restlessness and burning thirst; and at no distant term they expire.[2]

The sweet character of the urine from diabetics was identified by Thomas Willis (1622–1675)[3], a leading physician of the seventeenth century, nearly two millennia after the disease had been described by Araetaeus. To quote Willis,

> What, however, most authors assert, is far from being the truth, namely that too little is returned of what is drunk (or nothing unchanged), because the urine in all of those I ever knew (and I believe that this is so in all of them), is much different from the usual, because it is strangely sweet, partly from the drink imbibed, partly from the fluid created anywhere in our body.[4]

The sweetness of urine was shown to be sugar by Dobson (d. 1784)[5] in 1776, a date which corresponds to the beginning of the American Revolution. Dobson also reported that the serum from his patients was sweet, and thus became the first to demonstrate increased blood sugar or "hyperglycemia" in this disease.

Early efforts at treatment of diabetes were focused on diet, since that was essentially all that was available. Some of these diets were those high in meat, some high in fat, and some were calorie-restricted[6-8]. However, the plight of patients with diabetes was pitiful, as their flesh melted into urine.

An important step forward was a quantitative test for urine sugar that was introduced by Fehling[9] in the nineteenth century, making it easier to diagnose the disease. The next important step in understanding the cause of diabetes occurred in the late nineteenth century when von Mering and Minkowski (1858–1931) successfully produced diabetes in dogs by removing the pancreas[10]. By the time of the First World War, the idea or hypothesis that diabetes was due to lack of an internal secretion produced in the pancreas by the islets of Langerhans had become widely accepted, and the words *insuline*[11] or *insulin*[12] had been introduced as the name for this secretion.

In the year prior to the discovery of insulin, Macleod et al.[13] and Starling[14], two leading medical scientists of the time, had declared,

> We do not yet know how the pancreas affects sugar production or utilization in the normal animal. It is generally assumed that it secretes into the blood stream a hormone, which may, according to the view of the nature of diabetes which we adopt, pass to the tissues and enable them to utilize sugar or to pass to the liver and inhibit the sugar production of this organ. A very small portion of the pancreas is sufficient for this purpose, but we have been unable to imitate the action of the pancreas still in vascular connection

> with the body, by injection or administration of extracts of this organ.

It was at this juncture that Fred Banting, a surgeon in practice in London, Ontario, Canada, went to Professor Macleod asking for space to test his ideas about isolating insulin[15]. This was the right juncture of people since Macleod had been actively working in related areas for many years. Macleod assigned Charles Best, a medical student, to work with Banting during the summer of 1921[16]. At the end of the summer the progress was sufficient for Macleod, who had returned from a fishing vacation in Scotland, to provide additional support. By the end of the year, the work in the laboratory of J.J.R. Macleod had successfully isolated a crude version of insulin and provided what many hoped would be the cure for diabetes. Although credit for the isolation of insulin is given to Banting and Best, there is a body of literature that argues that Paulesco in Romania had actually isolated insulin earlier and published his data in 1921[17,18]. This discovery was apparently not known to Banting and Best when they carried out their monumental work[15]. (See Appendix)

Unraveling the two faces of diabetes required at least one more step. It required a way to measure the insulin that Banting and Best had isolated. The publication by Yalow and Berson titled "Immunoassay of Endogenous Plasma Insulin in Man"[19] provided this major step. From the time insulin was discovered until their work, it had not been possible to measure insulin with any accuracy. Their new method for measuring insulin in plasma opened the whole field for measuring hormones at very low levels in blood and other tissue. Prior to the introduction of the radioimmunoassay for insulin, bioassays for the response to insulin using either the diaphragm or adipose tissue were the principal techniques in use. The lower sensitivity, difficulty of performance, biological variability, and greater expense of these bioassays led to their rapid replacement by radioimmunoassays. Their work illustrates particularly well the words of Galileo cited above: "Measure what can be measured, and make measurable what cannot."

By the time of Berson and Yalow, two different types of diabetes had been established. The first occurred in young individuals who faded away and died within months to a few years without treatment using insulin. The second group were adults, usually overweight adults, who benefited from insulin, but who did not fade away and die without it. Using imprecise methods, most people believed that the young individuals with diabetes did not make insulin whereas the adults with diabetes had an excess amount of insulin but responded poorly to it.

Berson and Yalow developed a sensitive method for measuring insulin, which had previously been measurable only by slow and variable bioassay methods. A key component of their assay method was radioactive iodine.

Radioactivity is a property of natural or manmade molecules that makes them able to release one of several "particles." After the discovery of radioactivity by Marie and Pierre Curie at the end of the nineteenth century, the basic physics and biological meaning of this physics gradually emerged. Like the measurement of body composition using physical principles of density and x-radiation, the use of radioactive isotopes by Berson and Yalow was another adaptation of physics to medicine.

From the end of the nineteenth century until the beginning of the Second World War, there was steady progress in isolating radioactive elements. A brief look at this history is essential for understanding the progress in this area. In 1903 Marie and Pierre Curie[20] reported the discovery of radium because an ore containing radium exposed photographic plates even though they had not seen any light. Gradually the isotopic variants of other natural elements were described. By the beginning of World War II, radioisotopes had been introduced into biomedical research, and by 1945 they had been introduced into the treatment of clinical diseases[21]. One of the earliest was radioiodine, which was used for treatment of thyroid diseases[6]. In their early work Berson and Yalow had examined the metabolism of radioiodine by the human thyroid gland located in the neck. Their papers on the uptake and release of iodine-labeled compounds from the thyroid are classics in their own right[22]. During these studies they examined the effects of other substances that had radioactive iodine attached to them. It was during these studies that they made their discovery that radioactively labeled compounds such as insulin could be used to measure the amount of insulin in the blood.

The discovery of insulin lulled physicians and patients alike into believing that the problem in treating diabetes had been solved[23]. As Mirsky said in 1952 in the discussion of his paper "The Etiology of Diabetes Mellitus in Man,"

> Clinical experience during the past twenty-nine years has confirmed much of what was anticipated when insulin was discovered. With insulin, the patient with diabetes can now be assured of a fairly long life expectancy for he no longer need die from the acute complications and nutritional defects which killed him before 1922. The complacency induced by such beneficial therapeutic results with insulin was shattered when it became evident that insulin permits the patient with diabetes to live but only to develop retinopathy, neuropathy, arteriosclerosis, hypertension, glomerucosclerosis, and other vascular disturbances[23].

This paper by Mirsky was a key intellectual link for Berson and Yalow. In reviewing the reasons for the development of diabetes mellitus in man,

Mirsky had presented an important paper at the prestigious Laurentian Hormone Conference in Canada on the eve of work by Berson and Yalow. This idea was important in directing their studies[24]. Mirsky noted that a decrease in insulin secretion alone was sufficient to produce diabetes, but that many forms of diabetes were more severe than could be accounted for by complete removal of the pancreas and all endogenous insulin. He went on to suggest that "[a]n insufficiency of insulin may be due to an increased activity of those factors which are responsible for the destruction of insulin"[23].

Berson and Yalow set out to test this idea, or hypothesis by using insulin that had a molecule of radioactively labeled iodine (^{131}I) attached. They prepared ^{131}I labeled insulin and injected it into diabetic and non-diabetic subjects. To their surprise, they found that the radio-labeled insulin disappeared more slowly from the circulation of diabetics or individuals treated with insulin[25, 26]. This was contrary to the predictions of Mirsky[23]. Berson and Yalow suspected that the slowed rate at which insulin was removed might result from the presence of antibodies to insulin. At this time no one would accept the idea that antibodies could be made to such small naturally occurring molecules as insulin. Their original manuscript describing these studies was initially rejected by major scientific journals, including the *Journal of Clinical Investigation*[27] and the journal *Science* published by the American Association for the Advancement of Science, and only accepted after the words "insulin antibody" were deleted from the paper[24].

The difficulty that Berson and Yalow experienced in getting their initial publications accepted is all too common in science. Semmelweis in the nineteenth century[28] was ridiculed for his idea that washing one's hands after working in the autopsy room would reduce the spread of agents from the autopsy room to the labor room and thus reduce or prevent the development of puerperal fever that killed many mothers after delivery of their babies. Arrhenius's proposal that "ions" were produced when salt dissolved in water and that these ions were responsible for the flow of electricity (electrical conductivity) through the salt solutions was also ridiculed[29]. A quote from the great English writer Jonathan Swift who wrote *Gulliver's Travels* says, "When a true genius appears in the world, you may know him by this sign, that the dunces are all in confederacy against him." This aptly fits the problem that geniuses such as Semmelweis, Arrhenius, and Berson and Yalow encountered in their publications. Yalow made the same point when she said,

> Our use of techniques for studying the primary reaction of antigen with antibody and analyzing soluble complexes initiated a revolution in theoretical immunology in that it is now generally appreciated that peptides as small as vasopressin and oxytocin (with 8 amino acids) are antigenic in

> some species and that the equilibrium constants for the antigen-antibody reaction be as great as 10^{14} liters per mole, a value up to 10^{8} greater than the highest value predicted by Pauling's theory of 1940[24].

Using the interaction of antibodies with insulin, they then proceeded to develop the radioimmunoassay for insulin.

The introduction of the radioimmunoassay for insulin by Berson and Yalow[19, 26] was followed by other radioimmunoassays from their laboratory that measured adrenocorticotrophic hormone (ACTH)[30], growth hormone[31], gastrin[32], and cholecystokinin[33]. In a few short years the entire field of endocrinology and clinical laboratory medicine had been transformed with powerful new tools for measurement of hormones and other small molecules.

Close on the heels of the radioimmunoassay were a number of other competitive binding assays using naturally occurring proteins such as thyroxine binding globulin[34-36]. Competitive binding methods were also developed for receptor assays and enzyme-linked immunosorbent assays (ELISA). Following introduction by Berson and Yalow of the radioimmunoassay for insulin, the fields of endocrinology and clinical medicine were never the same.

The development of a sensitive and rapid method for measurement of insulin has also changed the tactics in the battle of the bulge. Shortly after the publication of the radioimmunoassay for insulin, Karam et al.[37] showed that overweight patients produced excess amounts of insulin. The presence of high levels of insulin and normal glucose levels was interpreted as "insulin resistance," or an ineffectiveness of insulin to stimulate the entry of glucose into cells. Insulin resistance is a hallmark of corpulence. This concept of insulin resistance was subsequently enlarged to the metabolic syndrome in which a variety of defects including hyperlipidemia, hypertension, central adiposity, and hyperinsulinemia were linked together. Although insulin is consistently elevated in corpulent individuals as a function of the degree of extra fat[38], it is still unclear how this occurs.

The introduction of the radioimmunoassay by Berson and Yalow has thus changed not only endocrinology but also the way most small molecules are measured. Since their methodologic advance, many new hormones have been identified and methods rapidly developed for their measurement. It would be fair to use the words of Winston Churchill in describing the contribution that these two investigators have made to the study of endocrinology and obesity: "Never in the field of human conflict was so much owed by so many to so few."[39]

Biosketch

Frederick Grant Banting (1891–1941) was the co-discoverer of insulin (Figure 7-1). He was born in Alliston, Ontario, into a farming family that instilled in him the love of animals. He received his medical training at the University of Toronto where he graduated in 1916 in the middle of World War I.

He served in the Canadian Army Medical Corps from 1917 to 1919, mostly in Europe. With a year's post-doctoral training in orthopedic surgery at the Sick Children's Hospital in Toronto, he opened a medical practice devoted largely to orthopedic surgery in London, Ontario. Beginning a new practice was difficult then and can be difficult now. Banting was not making a go of it. In 1920 he took a position as demonstrator in the Department of Physiology in London, Ontario. Stimulated by the findings in a scientific paper by Moses Barron on insulin, Banting returned to Toronto and approached J.J.R. Macleod, chairman of the Department of Physiology, about obtaining space and dogs to pursue his idea of isolating insulin. Macleod was intrigued by the possibility and assigned a medical student named Charles Best to work with him over the summer while Macleod went on a fishing vacation to Scotland. When Macleod returned, the progress had been more than expected, and Macleod provided more space and support, which led to the isolation of a crude insulin extract by December 1921. As the work progressed Banting feared that Macleod might steal his work. With the help of J.B. Collipp, a biochemist who was on leave at Toronto, a more purified preparation was prepared and tested in animals and then in humans. But this collaboration only heightened the animosity between Banting and Macleod. For this work Banting and Macleod received the Nobel prize in 1923. Macleod shared his prize money with Collipp, and Banting shared his prize money with Best. The animosity between Banting and Macleod continued throughout their lives. Banting was killed in an airplane crash at the beginning of World War II[4].

Biosketch

Professor John James Richard Macleod (1872–1935) was born in Scotland and received his medical education from the University of Aberdeen (Figure 7-2). Prior to coming to the United States in 1903 as professor of physiology at the Western Reserve University in Cleveland, Ohio, Macleod had trained in Germany and was a lecturer in biochemistry at the London Hospital School. He moved from the United States to become professor of physiology at the University of Toronto in 1918. Macleod was already well known for work on carbohydrate metabolism and had published *Diabetes: Its Pathological Physiology* in 1913. It was three fateful years after coming to Toronto when he was approached by Fred Banting about space and dogs with which Banting might try to isolate the substance from the pancreas, insulin, that could cure diabetes. With the help of Charles Best, a medical student assigned by Macleod, the Nobel Prize-winning work began. As it progressed, Macleod continued to offer advice, support and visibility. The animosity that grew up between Banting and Macleod was capped when they were both named to receive the Nobel Prize in 1923. Macleod left Toronto to become Regius Professor at the University of Aberdeen. The story of the discovery of insulin and the enmity that developed between Macleod and Banting is told brilliantly by Bliss in his book *The Discovery of Insulin*[15].

Biosketch

Solomon Berson, M.D., (1918–1972) (Figure 7-3) was born in 1918 in New York City and received his medical degree from New York University in 1945 at the end of World War II.

Following an internship at the Boston City Hospital and service in the Medical Corps of the U.S. Army, he returned to be medical resident at the Bronx Veterans Administration Hospital from 1948–50. He subsequently became chief of the Radioisotope Service, a position that he held until he became professor and chairman of the Department of Medicine at the Mount Sinai School of Medicine in 1968. By the time of his untimely death in 1972, he had published 231 scientific papers[40, 41].

Biosketch

Rosalyn Yalow, Ph.D., (1921–) (Figure 7-3) was born in 1921 in New York City and graduated from Hunter College in 1941 and married Aaron Yalow in 1943.

She received her Ph.D. from the University of Illinois in 1945, but returned to New York to teach at Hunter College. In 1950 she moved to the VA Hospital full time to become chief of the Radioisotope Service[40]. This was a critical point in her career, because it brought her in contact with Solomon Berson, with whom she developed a long-term working relationship. This continued until his death in 1972. From the time she received her Ph.D. in 1945, until 1972 when Dr. Berson died, these two had added significantly to the understanding of iodine metabolism in human disease and developed a new and highly sensitive method for measuring small amounts of hormones in biological fluids that revolutionized endocrinology and clinical diagnosis.

References

1. Rothshuh. K.E. *History of Physiology.* Trans. and ed. G.B. Risse. Huntington, NY: Krieger Publishing Co., 1973.
2. Araetaeus. *On Diabetes. In His Extant Works.* Trans. and ed. F. Adams. London: Syndenham Society, 1856.
3. Willis, T. *Pharmaceutice Rationalis Sive Diatriba de Medicamentorum Operationibis in Humano Corpore.* London: R. Scott, 1674–1675. English trans., 1679.
4. Medvei, V.C. *A History of Endocrinology.* Lancaster: MTP Press Ltd., 1982.
5. Dobson, M. "Experiments and Observations on the Urine in Diabetes." *Med Obs Inqu.* 5(1776): 298–316.
6. Allen, F.M. *Studies Concerning Glycosuria and Diabetes.* Cambridge: Harvard University Press, 1913.
7. Naunyn, B. *Der diabetes mellitus.* Wien: Alfred Holder, 1898.
8. Rollo, J. *Cases of Diabetes Mellitus; with the Results of the Trials of Certain Acids, and Other Substances in the Cure of the Lues Venera.* London: J. Callow, 1809.
9. Fehling, C. "Quantitative Bestimmung des Zuckers im Harn." *Arch Physiol Heilk.* 7(1848): 64–73.
10. von Mering, J., O Minkowskii. "Diabetes mellitus nach pancreasextirpation." *Arch Exp Path Pharmak.* 26(1890): 371–387.
11. Meyer, J. "Sur la relation entre la sécrétion intern du pancréas et la fonction glycogenique du foie." *Arch lnt Physiol.* 9(1910): 1
12. Sharpey-Schaefer, E.A. *The Endocrine Organs.* An Introduction to the Study of the Internal Organs. London: Longman-Greens. 1916.
13. Macleod, J.J.R., R.G. Pearce, A.C. Redfield, N.B. Taylor. et al. *Physiology and Biochemistry in Modern Medicine.* 3rd ed. St Louis: CV Mosby, 1920.
14. Starling, E.H. *Principles of Human Physiology.* 3rd ed. Philadelphia: Lea & Febiger, 1920.
15. Bliss, M. *The Discovery of Insulin.* Chicago: University of Chicago Press, 1982.
16. Banting, F.G., C.H. Best. "The Internal Secretion of the Pancreas." *J Lab Clin Med.* 7(1922): 251–266.
17. Murray, I. "Paulesco and the Isolation of Insulin." *J Hist Med.* 26(1971): 150–157.
18. Paulesco, N.C. "Recherches sur le role du pancréas dans l'assimilation nutritive." *Arch lnt Physiol.* 17(1921): 85–109.
19. Yalow, R.S., S.A. Berson. "Immunoassay of Endogenous Plasma Insulin in Man." *J Clin Invest.* 39(1960): 1157–1175.
20. Curie, M. *Traité de radioactivity.* Paris: Gauithier-Villars, 1910.

21. Hevesy, G. *Radioactive Indicators. Their Application in Biochemistry, Animal, Physiology, and Pathology.* New York: Interscience Publishers Inc., 1948.
22. Berson, S.A., R.S. Yalow, Sorrentino et al. "The Determination of Thyroidal and Renal Plasma 1131—Clearance Rates as a Routine Diagnostic Test of Thyroid Dysfunction." *J Clin Invest.* 1(1952): 141.
23. Mirsky, I.A. "The Etiology of Diabetes Mellitus in Man." *Recent Prog Horm Res.* 1(1952): 437–461.–
24. Yalow, R.S. "The Nobel Lecture in Immunology." *Scand J Immunol.* 35(1992): 1–23.
25. Berson, S.A, R.S. Yalow. "Kinetics of Reaction between Insulin and Insulin-binding Antibody." *J Clin Invest.* 36(1957): 873.
26. Berson, S.A., R.S. Yalow. "Quantitative Aspects of Reaction between Insulin and Insulin-binding Antibody." *J Clin Invest.* 38(1959): 1996–2016.
27. Berson, S.A., R.S. Yalow. "Species-specificity of Human Anti-beef Pork Insulin Serum." *J Clin Invest.* 38(1959): 2017–2025.
28. Semmelweis, I.P. "Höchst wichtige Erfahrungen über die Aetiologie der in Gebäranstalten epidemischen Puerperalfieber." *Zkk Ges Aerzte Wien.* 4(1848): 242–244.
29. Arrhenius, S.A. "Ueber die Dissociation der in Wasser gelosten Stoffe." *Z Physikal Chem.* 1(1887): 631–648.
30. Berson, S.A., R.S. Yalow RS. "Radioimmunoassay of ACTH in Plasma." *J Clin Invest.* 47(1968): 2725.
31. Roth, J., S.M. Glick, R.S. Yalow, S.A. Berson. "Hypoglycemia: A Potent Stimulus to Secretion of Growth Hormone." *Science.* 140(1963): 987.
32. Yalow, R.S., S.A. Berson. "Radioimmunoassay of Gastrin." *Gastroenterology* 58(1970): 1–14
33. Straus, E., J.E. Muller, H-S Choi, F. Paronetto, R.S. Yalow. "Immunohistochemical Localization in Rabbit Brain of a Peptide Resembling the C-terminal Cholecystokinin Octapeptide." *Proc Nat Acad Sc USA.* 74(1977): 3033–3034.
34. Ekins, R.P. "The Estimation of Thyroxine in Human Plasma by an Electrophoretic Technique." *Clin Chim Acta.* 5(1960): 453–459.
35. Herbert, V., Z. Castro, L.R. Wasserman. "Stoichiometric Relation Between Liver-Receptor, Intrinsic Factor and Vitamin B12." *Proc Soc Exp Biol Med.* 104(1960): 160–164
36. Murphy, B.E.P. "Application of the Property of Protein-binding to the Assay of Minute Quantities of Hormones and Other Substances." *Nature.* 201(1964): 679–682.
37. Karam, J.H., G.M. Grodsky, P.H. Forsham. "Excessive Insulin Response to Glucose in Obese Subjects as Measured by Immunochemical Assay." *Diabetes.* 12(1963): 197.

38. Bagdade, D., L. Bieirman, D. Poirte. "The Significance of Basal Insulin Levels in the Evaluation of the Insulin Response to Glucose in Diabetic and Non-Diabetic Subjects." *J Clin Invest.* 46(1967): 1549–1557.
39. Churchill, W.S. "Tribute to the Royal Air Force." Address to House of Commons, August 20, 1940.
40. "Rosalyn S. Yalow and Solomon A. Berson." *J Nucl Med.* 10(1987): 1637–1639.
41. Samols, E., "Solomon A. Berson—A Brief Biography." *Seminars in Nuclear Medicine.* No. 3 9(1979): 173.

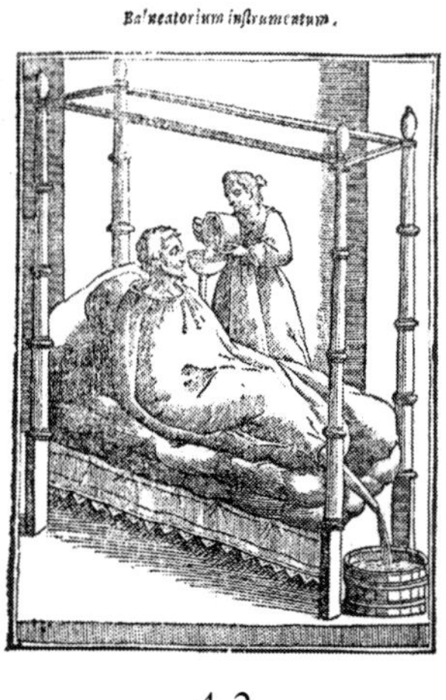

4-2

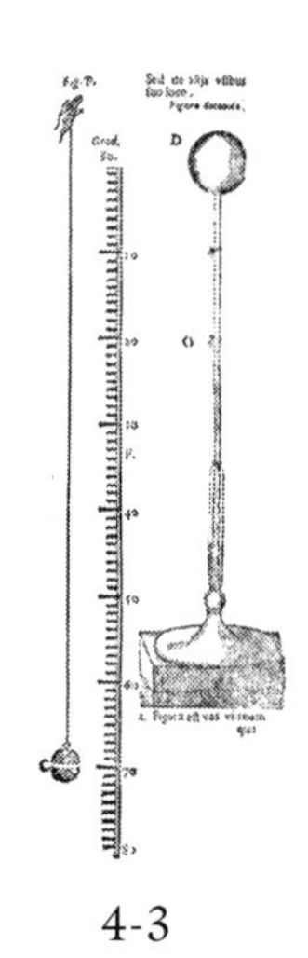

4-3

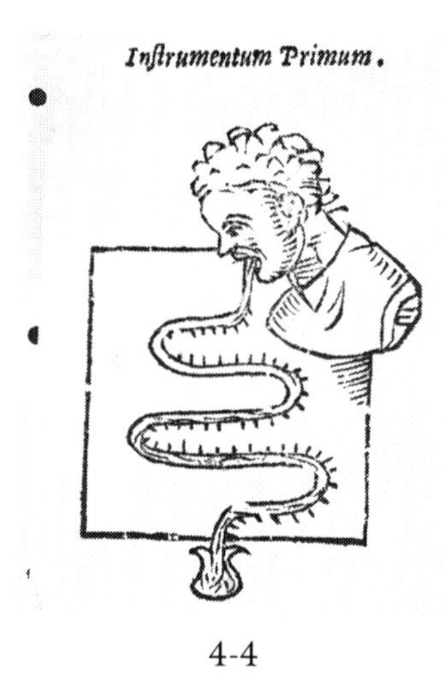

4-4

4-2 Bathing bag designed by Sanctorius to give patients a bath. Water was poured in at the top and drained from the bottom. From the collection of the author.

4-3 Sanctorius's pulsilogium based on the pendulum concept of Galileo. It was used to measure the pulse. From the collection of the author.

4-4 Sanctorius' thermometer based on the the thermoscope concept of Galileo. Santorius applied it to measure temperature of his patients. From the collection of the author.

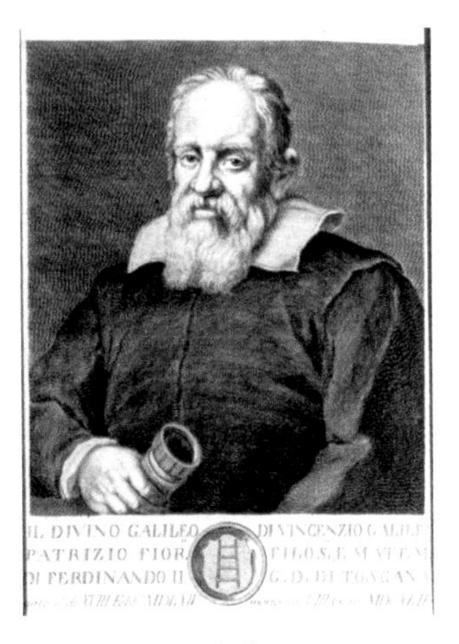

4-5

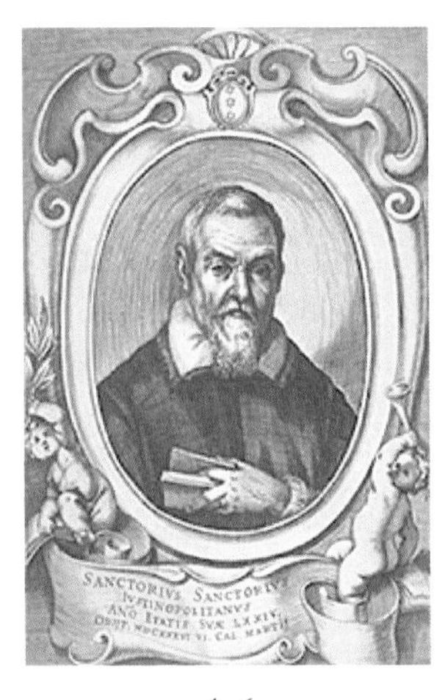

4-6

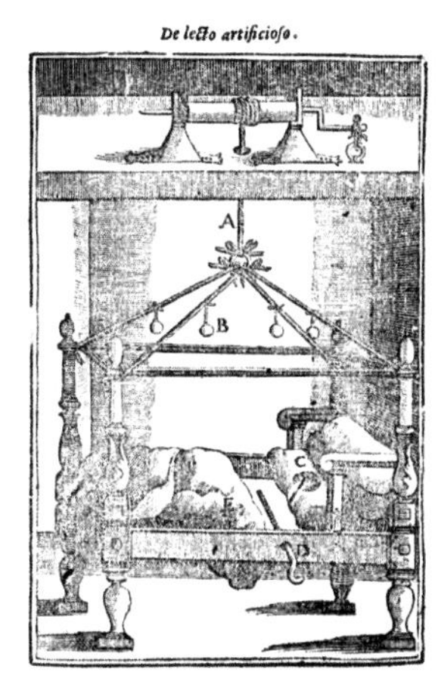

4-7

4-5 Galileo Galilei (1564-1642). Courtesy of the National Library of Medicine.

4-6 Santorio Santorio called Sanctorius (1561-1636). Courtesy of the National Library of Medicine.

4-7 Hospital bed with frame for lifting it off the floor. From the collection of the author.

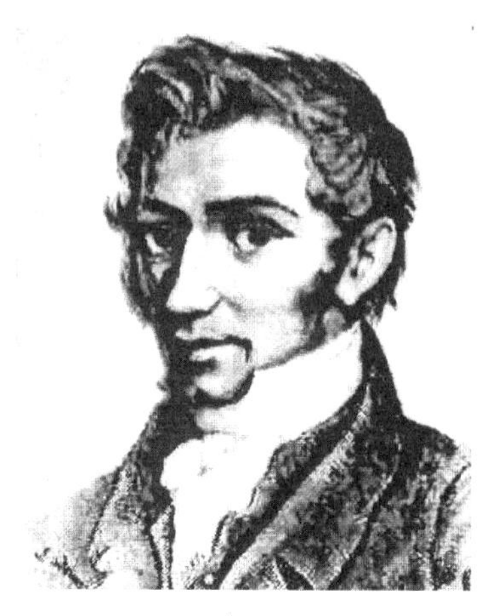

5-2

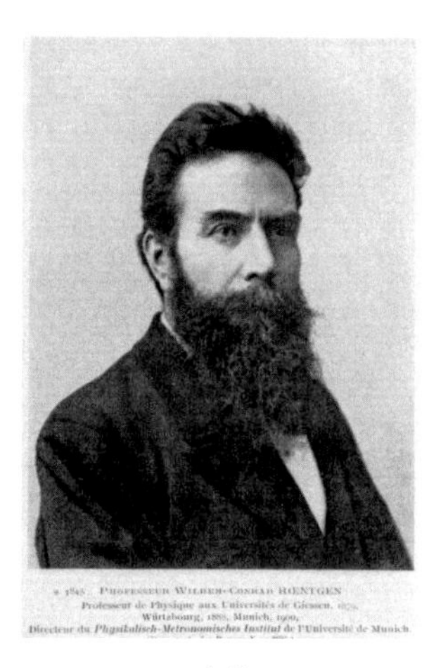

6-2

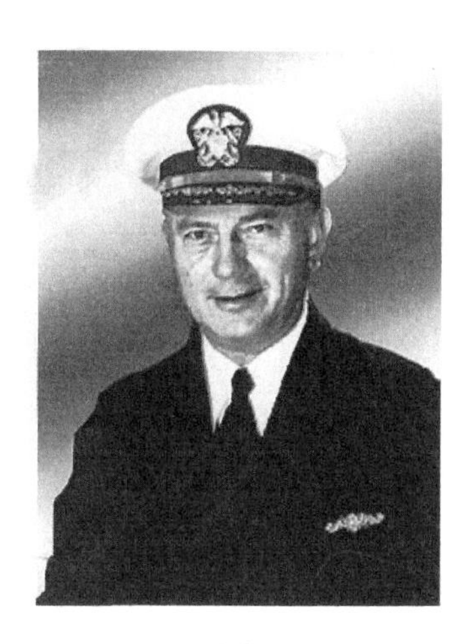

6-3

5-2 Lambert-Adolf-Jacques Quetelet (1796-1874) http://www-history.mcs.st-and.ac.uk/history/PictDisplay/Quetelet.html

6-2 Wilhelm Conrad Roentgen (1845-1922). Courtesy of the National Library of Medicine

6-3 Albert Richard Behnke, Jr. (1903-1992). Courtesy of *Military Medicine: International Journal of AMSUS.*

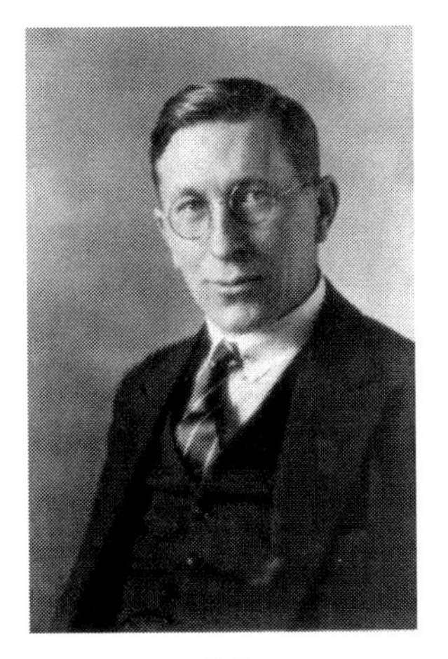

7-1

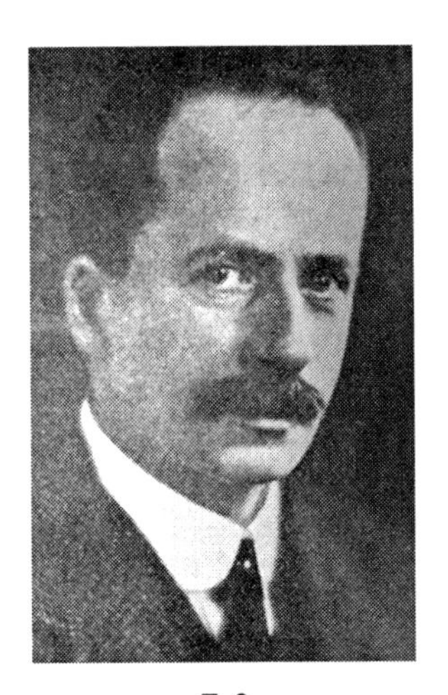

7-2

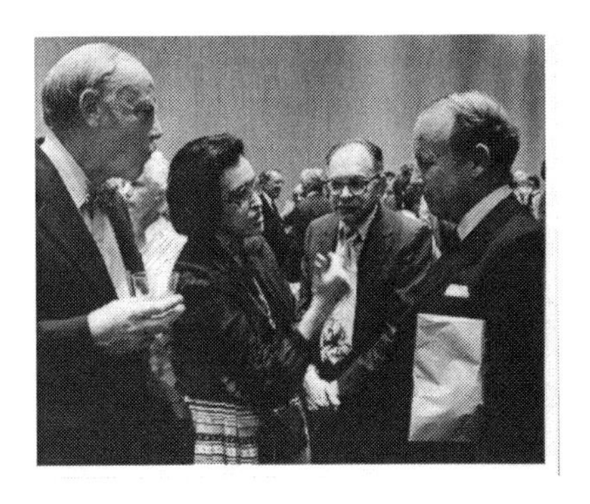

7-3

7-1 Sir Frederick Grant Banting (1891-1941). Courtesy of the National Library of Medicine.

7-2 John James Richard Macleod (1872-1935). Courtesy of the National Library of Medicine.

7-3 Solomon Aaron Berson (1918-1972) & Rosalyn Sussman Yalow (1921-) in the middle, Donald Frederickson on the right. Courtesy of the National Library of Medicine.

PART 3.

The Causes of the Bulge: How Did We Get That Way?

Chapter 8

Human Lessons from Overweight Mice

When we say that science is essentially progressive this does not mean that in his quest of truth man follows always the shortest path. Far from it, he beats about the bush, does not find what he is looking for but finds something else, retraces his steps, loses himself in various detours, and finally after many wanderings touches the goal.

—Sarton[1]

Genetics provides one of the most promising approaches to winning the battle of the bulge. If we can identify the genes that underlie the risk for obesity, there is great promise that we can find ways of modifying the effects of these genes. The last decade of the twentieth century saw remarkable progress in our understanding of genetics as they apply to the problem of adiposity. As our understanding grows, we can expect an ever increasing number of new weapons to use in our battle of the bulge.

The story of genetics goes back well over a century. It was a friar named Gregor Mendel (1822–1884) who, in the latter half of the nineteenth century, set the field in motion. Working with peas, Mendel showed that traits for short peas or tall peas and yellow peas or green peas could be transmitted in what appeared to be unitary fashion. That is, the number of green and yellow or short and tall plants occurred in defined numbers. This work was published only a few years after the momentous publication in 1859 of *On the Origin of Species* by Charles Darwin (1809-1882). This towering book describing the consequences of the survival of the fittest became one of the central biological doctrines of the nineteenth and twentieth centuries. The work of Mendel on the idea that characteristics of plants and animals could be inherited and transmitted as units, now called genes, was only recognized at the beginning of the twentieth century. It is this unitary nature of genetic traits that has now become the central doctrine of the molecular biological revolution.

I have selected three papers that chronicle the beginnings of the study of genetic obesity in animals. The first of these, by Danforth, is titled "Hereditary Adiposity in Mice" and was published in 1927; it is the only paper in this group that was published before World War II[2]. The second paper, published by Ingalls, Dickie, and Snell from the Jackson Laboratories in 1950, is the initial description of the obese (ob/ob) mouse[3]. As I will show, these two mice have played a critical role in our current understanding of the genetic and molecular basis of obesity. The third paper, by Zucker and Zucker, describes the fatty rat[4]. All three of these papers provide insight into strategies of scientific discovery. They also illustrate the paradigm shift that has occurred as our understanding increases, and they illustrate some aspects of the relationship of genetics to adiposity. I will deal briefly with each of these issues. (See Appendix for these 3 papers.)

The animal in our study of techniques to fight the battle of the bulge was the fat or obese yellow mouse, which had originally been described by Cuenot in 1905[5].

The first detailed study of this mouse was not done for more than twenty years and was published by Danforth in 1927[2]. The gene that produces the fat yellow mouse is dominantly inherited. Expression of this gene is independent of both the growth hormone and thyrotropin, since crossing the yellow mouse with the dwarf mouse that lacks a growth hormone produced the yellow coat color and adiposity. The adiposity in the fat yellow mouse appears at the time of puberty in a fashion similar to fatness in many people. Fat accounts for 90% of the extra weight, and these animals are, if anything, larger than normal, being both fatter and longer than their lean siblings. It was recognized early that the yellow coat color and degree of adiposity were related, thus suggesting an important relationship with melanocyte-stimulating hormone (MSH), the hormone that stimulates the melanocyte in the skin to produce black pigment and thus the black hair color, and also produces obesity[6]. This action of MSH is similar to a lock and key. The MSH attaches to a molecule (receptor) on the cell and provides information for the cell to respond. MSH is produced from a larger peptide called proopiomelanocortin (POMC). With this information at hand, it should have been possible to suggest that the yellow mouse resulted from failure of MSH to be produced, or a failure of the cellular receptors both peripherally and in the brain to respond to MSH. This lack of effect could occur because the receptors were defective or because there was some inhibitor to the MSH key fitting into the receptor (Figure 8-1).

In spite of many physiological clues, the genetic basis for the yellow mouse was only solved when molecular biological methods were applied. Using the genomic approach, Bultman and colleagues successfully isolated the defective gene, called agouti, that causes the obesity and yellow coat color. The gene produces a peptide having 133 amino acids[7]. This small protein is

Gene	Mutations	Chromosome
Pro-opiomelanocortin (POMC)	G701T and C deletion at nt 7133 exon 3 C3804A exon 2	2p23
Melanocortin 4-Receptor	More than 25 mutations have been reported to date with variable penetrance	18q21.3
Leptin	Deletion at codon 133 C to T Codon 105 Exon 3	7q31
Leptin Receptor	G to A Exon 16	1p31
Prohormone Convertase-1	G483R A to C Intron 5	5q15-q21
Peroxisome Proliferator-Activated Receptor-γ	P115Q	3p25
Thyroid hormone receptor-β	C434Stop C to A Exon 10	3p24.1-p22

Table 8-1 Lessons on human obesity from the single genes identified in animals to produce obesity.

produced in many tissues of the yellow mouse, in contrast to the limited expression in the black mouse. In the fat yellow mouse, this ubiquitous protein interferes with the lock-and-key mechanism for the melanocyte-stimulating hormone, the hormone that makes pigment cells in the hair follicle turn black and which inhibits food intake. By interfering with this lock-and-key receptor system in the pigment cell and in the brain, the mouse develops a yellow coat color and increased food intake[8] that produces obesity. The isolation of the gene for this defect is an example of the power of the molecular approach to unravel a key problem in the battle of the bulge where the physiological approaches had been previously unsuccessful.

In a second model of genetic adiposity, the so-called FAT mouse, physiological reasoning led to the discovery of the genetic defect[9]. These mice were found to have very high levels of proinsulin, the precursor from which insulin is made. This suggested that there might be a defect in the enzyme, called carboxypeptidase, that breaks the larger proinsulin molecule into insulin. In the FAT mouse, the defective gene led to one amino acid being substituted for another in this enzyme, a change that produced a defective form of the enzyme, carboxypeptidase E. The defective enzyme could not convert proinsulin to insulin nor could it convert a variety of other prohormones, the form in which the body makes them, into their active forms. The shortage of active hormones could thus account for the obesity in these mice.

The second paper in this section is the initial description of the obese mouse (gene symbol ob) by Ingalls, Dickie, and Snell in 1950[3]. The approach to solving this problem was similar to that for the yellow mouse, one in which molecular cloning provided a successful solution to the problem that had not been solved by the physiological approach[10]. Unraveling this genetic problem has also provided a paradigm shift in the understanding of adiposity.

Although the ob/ob mouse was described more recently than the yellow mouse, a substantially larger number of studies have been published using the ob/ob mouse as a subject[10] (Figure 8-2). A second mouse with the gene symbol db and called diabetes was described shortly after the ob/ob mouse[11]. The fatty rat described by Zucker and Zucker[4] is a third member of this type of obesity that occurs when each parent provides a defective copy of the gene—a so-called autosomal defect. Phenotypically, the obese (ob/ob) and diabetes (db/db) mouse and the fatty (Zucker) rat cannot be identified at weaning, but studies on body temperature, insulin, and adipocyte cell size have shown that defects are present as early as seven days of age. Enlargement of adipocytes, increased body fat, and decreased thermogenesis all appear prior to the development of hyperphagia and hyperglycemia. More than 90% of the increase in weight of these animals results from the accumulation of fat, and it is on the fat cell that a wide variety of studies have been focused.

Among the earliest explanations for the development of obesity in obese mice was that they ate too much. However, it soon became clear that hyperphagia was neither an early event nor a necessary feature[12]. In fact, the hyperphagia does not appear until twenty-five to thirty days of age, a time when the animals are already obese. Moreover, when these genetically obese mice are given identical amounts of food as their lean brothers or sisters, the genetically obese mouse becomes heavier and fatter on an identical food intake than its lean littermate.

A second group of explanations for the obese mice centered around defects in the way fat is stored. These could either be problems with the formation or synthesis of fat or impaired fat breakdown. Careful study of the fat cells revealed that in most instances the proposed defects in fat storage could be explained by differences in food intake and in the size of fat cells. The most critical studies were those of Meade et al.[13] who showed that transplantation of fat cells from obese mice to lean animals and vice versa resulted in the fat cells adopting the characteristics of the host rather than the donor. That is, large fat cells from the obese mice became smaller, and small fat cells from the lean animals became larger.

A third major group of explanations focused around hyperinsulinemia and insulin resistance[10, 14]. Hyperinsulinemia occurs early and appears to precede insulin resistance[15]. Hyperinsulinemia may well be related to hyperglycemia and to adrenal glucocorticoid effects because adrenalectomy will largely reverse hyperinsulinemia and completely reverse insulin resistance.

A fourth group of explanations revolved around the idea that the mice might have a defective heat-producing system. This could lower body temperature, and there might be a problem with increasing heat production in the cold. If these mice produced less heat, they could store more of the food energy they ate as fat and thus become obese[10]. In small animals, as well as in newborn human babies, heat production to keep them warm occurs by stimulating a heat-producing tissue called brown adipose tissue[16]. This tissue is named because it appears reddish brown. It is located in several parts of the body, but the largest collection of these brownish cells is between the shoulder blades. A second way to conserve energy for making fat would be to use less energy for the daily needs of life. This includes such things as pumping blood, maintaining the integrity of the body's cells, and reducing the activity of bodily processes that need energy. However, none of these defects appeared to be responsible for the obesity in these mice. Rather the changes in heat conservation appeared to reflect changes in the amount of hormones produced by the adrenal glands. Removal of the adrenal glands and the hormones they produce restored body temperature to normal and corrected the bodily functions essentially to normal[10].

A fifth and highly fruitful explanation for the obesity in the obese mouse was proposed by Coleman[6]. He suggested that these mice failed to produce a "satiety" signal telling them they had eaten enough. This was supported by the molecular studies of Zhang et al.[17] described below, who isolated this "satiety" signal and called it leptin.

Like the solution to the defect in the yellow mouse, the genetic defect in the obese mouse was solved by use of a molecular biological technique called positional cloning, which resulted in the isolation of a defective gene in the obese mouse[17]. One of the striking observations from the genomic information was that the gene was only expressed in adipose tissue. It rapidly became clear that the message, as well as the circulating peptide produced by the message, were directly related to the amount of fat tissue[18]. Corpulent humans have higher levels of leptin than do normal weight people. The observation of a peptide produced in adipose tissue and not in the brain, as had been widely suggested, led to a complete revolution in thinking about the battle of the bulge. As anticipated, this peptide lowers food intake when injected into obese mice but has only minor effects in lean animals[19–21]. The surprise from these findings is that the gene for leptin, the protein missing in the obese mouse, is produced almost exclusively in adipose tissue. None of the hypotheses for the obese mouse developed prior to the findings of Zhang et al.[17] had implicated adipose tissue alone[10]. Leptin deficiency has now been described in a few families as a rare cause of human obesity. In these individuals, leptin is successful in winning the battle of the bulge. A family tree for one of these families is shown in Figure 8-3. As might be expected, treatment of these individuals with leptin abruptly reduced their hunger and produced weight loss.

It has been known for some time that the female reproductive cycle in humans and animals only begins when the body has adequate amounts of fat. This concept was originally proposed by Frisch and Revelle in 1971[22] . Leptin may well be the message from adipose tissue that tells the brain about the relative nutritional status of the animal. As the size of the adipose tissue deposit increases, the quantity of leptin produced increases until the quantities are sufficient to initiate changes in brain chemistry that allow the reproductive system to initiate reproductive activity. As the degree of adiposity increases, higher levels of leptin may produce the irregularities in the reproductive system that plague some overweight women. Indeed many overweight women have problems becoming pregnant.

As Canguilhem said, "A theory is woven of many strands, some of which may be quite new while others are borrowed from older fabrics"[23].

This concept applies admirably to the intellectual revolution and tactical shift that is associated with the identification of leptin and the battle of the bulge. The old themes were the studies by Douglas Coleman of mice who shared their blood circulation, suggesting that there was a factor circulating in the mouse which produced satiety. With this focus, the initial studies on leptin (ob protein) showed that it decreased food intake as predicted[19–21]. Transferring this success to the broader battlefield in the war against obesity was less successful. In a clinical trial with leptin, there was a small amount of body weight lost when the peptide was injected, but there were unpleasant side effects that made the overall response unsatisfactory. Another skirmish lost.

A second important change occurred after the discovery of leptin and the ob gene. With this discovery, it became front-page news that some people were "born to be fat" and that there were chemicals that could produce, and thus possibly prevent, obesity. This changed the concept of obesity in some people's minds from a problem resulting because they didn't push themselves away from the table to a problem with a chemical basis. Leptin helped to reduce the stigma associated with obesity. The stigma that corpulent people confront everyday has been eloquently described by Allon:

> You are a glutton. Your physician has probably told you so. Or you have read a magazine article by some "expert" who demolished all those "myths" concerning frame size, metabolism, and heredity. About the only thing your physician or expert is willing to concede is that there are some psychological factors involved: you lack willpower, i.e., strength of

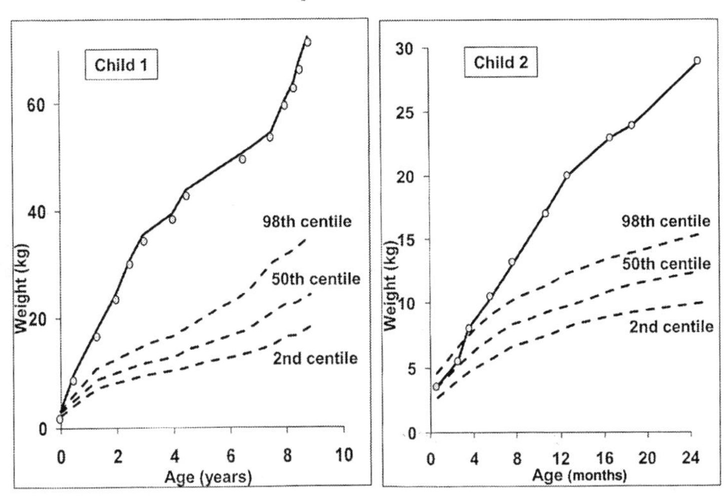

8-3 Growth curves for the first two children identified to have leptin deficiency. Redrawn by the author from Montague et al Nature 1997.

> character. You are a weakling. You are also, into the bargain, anti-social at best, suicidal at worst. You are an emotional mess as manifested by the fact that you are a physical slob.[24]

This deprecation of the corpulent people is also carried through to the low status accorded to the professionals who are the troops in the trenches in the battle of the bulge. This was described by Dr. Arthur Frank in an article from the *Journal of the American Medical Association* based on his personal experience:

> Medical professionals systematically avoid the problem of obesity. They send the obese patient to a dietitian who reinforces a recurrent litany of menu planning that has been therapeutically unsuccessful for the patient's last 30 years...The insidious image of sleaze pervades and discourages physicians who might choose to take on the challenge of the problem of treating obesity. It is an orphan disease of monumental size that does not fit neatly into the classification schemes of medical education. No one trains in

> obesity as one might in gastroenterology or psychiatry. No one is willing to take the professional risk[25].

The demonstration that molecular biology can unravel a form of obesity has raised to a new level of acceptability both the individuals who are overweight and those who study this important problem. There is now more enthusiasm for scientists and physicians to join in the search for strategies to help win the battle of the bulge.

Animal models with obesity have proven invaluable tools for understanding the rare forms of human obesity, as shown in Table 8-1. Several individuals have a deficiency in leptin or the leptin receptor. These people are massively overweight from early in life since the defect is present from conception. Failure to make proopiomelanocortin (POMC), the precursor for melanocyte-stimulating hormone (MSH) that inhibits food intake, produces a recognizable type of obesity. The child has reddish hair because MSH that stimulates darkening of hair follicles is absent, and they have defects in other glandular systems as well. The most common genetic defect that has been reported is in the melanocortin receptor system on which MSH acts. Unlike children who lack POMC and thus have reddish hair, the melanocortin receptor defects that lead to obesity are not the ones that control hair and skin color. Thus, individuals with melanocortin receptor defects and obesity cannot be detected by clinical observations. Table 8-1 also shows several other examples that are similar to the animals' defects. Of these, both the defect in the peroxisome proliferator-activated receptor and in the melanocortin receptor are the only ones that may play a significant role in the epidemic of human obesity.

Biosketch

Gregor Mendel (1822–1884) is the founder of genetics through his work on the hybridization of plants in the monastery where he was a priest. He was born in Heinzendorf, Austria. His talent was observed during his early years in school. When his time ended at the gymnasium, the high school equivalent of today, he was admitted to the Augustinian house of St. Thomas in Brunn. He was ordained a priest in 1847 but shortly afterward was given time and expenses from 1851 to 1853 for further education at the University of Vienna in mathematics, physics, and natural science (Figure 8-4).

From the time of his novitiate, he began work on the hybridization of plants. Mendel carried out his work on the transmissions of traits in plants between 1856 and 1864. These results were communicated to the Brunn Society in 1865 and published in 1866 but were unheeded for nearly forty years until rediscovered by Bateson. His scientific work was reduced after he became abbot of the Konigskloster in 1868. The intriguing question of why his work was not noticed for so long remains unsolved. Bateson thinks it lies in the general neglect of the experimental study of the problem of species, which supervened on the general acceptance of the Darwinian doctrines in the latter half of the nineteenth century. Whatever the cause, the unitary transmission of traits was the single-handed work of this now famous priest[37].

From the time of Mendel's discovery until 1900 when they were rediscovered, the "Darwinians," including Darwin, had been searching in vain for the mechanism by which natural selection could work. With the rediscovery of the concept of transmission of traits by genes, this problem was solved. It took another half century to begin to unravel the nature of genes at the chemical level and to apply them to the biological revolution known as molecular biology in the latter quarter of the twentieth century. Whether an earlier discovery of Mendel's concept of genetic transmission would have hastened this transformation is unclear, because other methods were necessary before the proposal of the double helix by Watson and Crick was possible[38]. Nonetheless, it is evident that publication of a revolutionary new concept in an obscure journal may delay its acceptance.

Biosketch

George D. Snell (1903–1996) (Figure 8-5) was born in Bradford, Massachusetts, and was the recipient of the 1980 Nobel Prize in medicine and physiology for his work on immunogenetics. Dr. Snell received his undergraduate education at Dartmouth College and continued his graduate studies at Harvard University with a thesis on genetic linkage. Following a teaching position in zoology at Brown University, Snell left teaching to concentrate on research at the University of Texas in Austin, where he explored the genetic effects of x-rays on mice. After a one-year position as assistant professor at Washington University, he and six other scientists moved to the newly formed Roscoe B. Jackson Memorial Laboratory in Bar Harbor, Maine, in 1935. His research work shifted from x-ray-induced mutations to studies on the role of heredity in the process of tissue rejection of transplants. It was his developments in this area that led to his award of the Nobel Prize in 1980. Among the animals he was studying were varieties of mice; his colleagues Ingalls and Dickie published with him the description of the ob/ob mouse cited below[39].

Biosketch

Charles Haskell Danforth (1883–1969) (Figure 8-6) was born in Oxford, Maine, and received his education in Boston. He received his bachelor's degree from Tufts University and his doctoral degree from Washington University in St. Louis in 1912.

Following teaching positions at the Harvard Medical School and Washington University, Danforth moved to Stanford University in the Department of Anatomy, where he rose to professor and executive head of the department until his retirement in 1949. His research work dealt with problems of inheritance and such topics as the mechanism and heredity of human twinning, mutation frequencies in man, and genetic-endocrine balance in birds and mammals. He was instrumental in a study of American soldiers discharged from the U.S. Army at the end of World War II, which catalogued basic anthropometric measures in 104,000 soldiers[40].

References

1. Sarton, G. *The History of Science and the New Humanism.* New York: Henry Holt and Co., 1931.
2. Danforth, C.H. "Hereditary Adiposity in Mice." *J Hered.* 18(1927): 153–162.
3. Ingalls, A.M., M.M. Dickie, G.D. Snell. "Obese, New Mutation in the Mouse." *J Hered.* 41(1950): 317–318.
4. Zucker, T.F., I.M. Zucker. "Fat Accretion and Growth in the Rat." *J Nutr* 80(1963): 6–20.
5. Cuenot, L. "Pure Strains and Their Combinations in the Mouse." *Arch Zoo Exptl.* Gen Ser. 4. no. 3 122(1905): 123. (French).
6. Shimizu, H. N. Shargill, G. Bray, T. Yen T, P. Gesellchen. "Effects of MSH on Food Intake, Body Weight and Coat Color of the Yellow Obese Mouse." *Life Sci.* 6 45(1989): 543–552.
8. Tsujii, S., G.A. Bray. "Acetylation Alters the Feeding Response to MSH and Beta-Endorphin." *Brain Res Bull.* 23(1989): 165–169.
9. Nagger, J.K., L.D. Fricker, O. Varlamov, et al. "Hyperproinsulinaemia in Obese Fat/fat Mice Associated with a Carboxypeptidase E Mutation Which Reduces Enzyme Activity." *Nat Genet.* no. 2 10(1995): 135–142.
10. Bray, G.A., J.S. Fisler, D.A. York. "Neuroendocrine Control of the Development of Obesity: Understanding Gained from Studies of Experimental Animal Models." *Front Neuroendocrinol* no. 2 11(1990): 128–181.
11. Coleman, D.L. "Obesity and Diabetes: Two Mutant Genes Causing Obesity-Obesity Syndromes in Mice." *Diabetalogia.* 14(1978): 141–148.
12. Coleman, D.L. "Effects of Parabiosis of Obese with Diabetes and Normal Mice." *Diabetologia* 9(1973): 194–298.
13. Meade, C.J., M. Ashwell, C. Sowter. "Is Genetically Transmitted Obesity Due to an Adipose Tissue Defect?" *Proc R Soc Lond (Biol)* no. 1160 205(1979): 395–410.
14. Renold, A.E., D.P. Cameron, M. Amherdt, et al. "Endocrine-Metabolic Anomalies in Rodents with Hyperglycemic Syndromes of Heredity and/or Environmental Origins." *Israel J Med Psycho.* 8(1972): 189–206.
15. Jeanrenaud, B. "Central Nervous System and Peripheral Abnormalities—Cues to the Understanding of Obesity and NIDDM." *Diabetologia.* No.52 37(1994): S169–178.
16. Himms-Hagen, J. "Neural Control of Brown Adipose Tissue Thermogenesis, Hypertrophy, and Atrophy." *Front Neuroendocrinol.* 1(1991): 38–93.

17. Zhang, Y.Y., R. Proenca, M. Maffei, M. Barone, L. Leopold, J.M. Friedman. "Positional Cloning of the Mouse Obese Gene and Its Human Homolog." *Nature.* 372(1994): 425–432.
18. Considine, R.V., E.L. Considine, C.J. Williams, et al. "Evidence Against Either a Premature Stop Codon or the Absence of Obese Gene mRNA in Human Obesity." *J Clin Invest.* 95(1996): 2986–2988.
19. Campfield, L.A., F.J. Smith, Y. Guisez, R. Devos, P. R. Burn. "Recombinant Mouse ob Protein: Evidence for a Peripheral Signal Linking Adiposity and Central Neural Networks." *Science.* 269(1995): 546–549.
20. Halaas, J.L., K.S. Gajiwala, M. Maffei, et al. "Weight Reducing Effects of the Plasma Protein Encoded by the Obese Gene." *Science.* 269(1995): 543–546.
21. Pelleymounter, M.A., M.J. Cullen, M.B. Baker, et al. "Effects of the Obese Gene Product on Body Weight Regulation in ob/ob Mice." *Science.* 269(1995): 540–543.
22. Frisch, R.E., R. Revelle. "Height and Weight at Menarche and a Hypothesis of Menarche." *Arch Dis Child.* no. 249 46(1971): 695–701.
23. Canguilhem, G. *Ideology and Rationality in the History of the Life Sciences.* Trans. A. Goldhammer. Cambridge, MA: MIT Press, 1988.
24. Allon, N. "The Stigma of Overweight in Everyday Life." In Bray, G.A., ed. *Obesity in Perspective.* Fogarty International Center Series on Preventive Medicine, vol. 2, part 2, page 83–110, Washington, D.C.: DHEW; Publication No. (NIH) 75–708.
25. Frank, A. "Futility and Avoidance: Medical Professionals in the Treatment of Obesity." *JAMA.* 269(1993): 2132–2133.
26. Krude, H., H. Biebermann, W. Luck, R. Horn, G. Brabant; and A. Gruters. "Severe Early-Onset Obesity, Adrenal Insufficiency and Red Hair Pigmentation Caused by POMC Mutations in Humans." *Nat Genet.* 19(1998): 155–7.
27. Vaisse, C., K. Clement, B. Guy-Grand, P. Froguel. "A Frameshift Mutation in Human MC4R Is Associated with a Dominant Form of Obesity." *Nat Genet.* 20(1998): 113–4.
28. Yeo, G.S.H., I.S. Farooqi, S. Aminian, D.J. Halsall, R.G. Stanhope. "A Frameshift Mutation in MC4R Associated with Dominantly Inherited Human Obesity." *Nat Genet.* 20(1998): 111–112.
29. Hinney, A., A. Schmidt K. Nottebom, O. Heibult I. Becker, A. Ziegler, G. Gerber, M. Sinan, T. Gorg, H. Mayer, W. Siegfried, M. Fichter, H. Remschmidt, J. Hebebrand. "Several Mutations in the Melanocortin-4 Receptor Gene Including a Nonsense and a Frameshift Mutation Associated with Dominantly Inherited Obesity in Humans." *J Clin Endocrinol Metab.* 84(1999): 1483–1486.

30. Montague, C.T., I.S. Farooqi, J.P. Whitehead, M.A. Sopos, H. Rau, N.J. Wareham, C.P. Sewter, J.E. Digby, S.N. Mohammed, J.A. Hurst, C. H. Cheetham, A.R. Earley, A. H. Barnett, J.B. Prins, S. O'Rahilly. "Congenital Leptin Deficiency is Associated with Severe Early-Onset Obesity in Humans." *Nature.* 387(1997): 903–8.
31. Strobel, A., T. Issad, L. Camoin, M Ozata, A. D. Strosbert. "A Leptin Missense Mutation Associated with Hypogonadism and Morbid Obesity." *Nat Genet.* 18(1998): 213–215.
32. Ozata, M., C. Ozdemiel, J. Licino. "Human Leptin Deficiency Caused by a Missense Mutation: Multiple Endocrine Defects, Decreased Sympathetic Tone, and Immune System Dysfunction Indicate New Targets for Leptin Action, Greater Central Than Peripheral Resistance to the Effects of Leptin, and Spontaneous Correction of Leptin-Mediated Defects." *J Clin Endocrinol Metab.* 84(1999): 3686–3695.
33. Clement K., C. Vaisse, N. Lahlou, S. Cabrol, V. Pelloux, D. Cassuto, M. Gourmelen, C. Dina, J. Chambaz, J.M. Lacorte, A. Basdevant, P. Bougneres, Y. Lebouc, P. Froguel, and B. Guy-Grand. "A Mutation in the Human Leptin Receptor Gene Causes Obesity and Pituitary Dysfunction." *Nature.* 392(1998): 398–401.
34. Jackson, R.S., J.W.M. Creemers, S. Ohagi, M.L. Raffin-Sanson, L. Sanders, C.T. Montague, J.C. Hutton, S. O'Rahilly. "Obesity and Impaired Prohormone Processing Associated with Mutations in the Human Prohormone Convertase 1 Gene." *Nat Genet.* 16(1997): 303–6.
35. Ristow, M., D. Muller-Wieland, A. Pfeiffer, A. Krone, C. Kahn. "Obesity Associated with a Mutation in a Genetic Regulator of Adipocyte Differentiation." *N Engl J Med.* 339(1998): 953–959.
36. Behr, R., D.M. Ramsden, J. Loos. "Deoxyribonucleic Acid Binding and Transcriptional Silencing by a Truncated c-erbA β–1 Thyroid Hormone Receptor Identified in a Severely Retarded Patient with Resistance to Thyroid Hormone." *J Clin Endocrinol Metab.* 82(1997): 1081–1087.
37. Bateson, W. *Mendel's Principles of Heredity.* Cambridge: University Press, 1909.
38. Watson, J.D., F.H.C. Crick. "Molecular Structure of Nucleic Acids; A Structure of Deoxyribose Nucleic Acid." *Nature.* 171(1953): 737–738.
39. Brown, M. "George D. Snell." *In The Nobel Prize Winners: Physiology and Medicine.* Vol. 3. Ed. F.N. Magill. Pasadena, CA: Salem Press, 1991.
40. Pursell, C. "Charles Haskell Danforth." In *Dictionary of Scientific Biography.* Ed. C.C. Gillespie. New York: Charles Scribner's Sons, 1971.

Chapter 9

The Heritage of Corpulence: Lessons from Human Genetics

> *When a subject is rapidly advancing it is interesting and often instructive to look back and reread some of the early contributors, where ideas which now seem commonplace were first formulated.*
>
> —Harry Harris[1]

Ask anyone and they will tell you that genes are an important cause of obesity. But how important? Where do genetic factors versus environmental ones fit into the cause of our epidemic, and how can they contribute to the battle of the bulge? We now believe that between 30% and 70% of the cause of obesity is genetic. But it has not always been so. When the problem of a bulge in the population began to confront us more than a century ago, knowledge about genes was rudimentary. In this chapter, I will explore the early information pointing to the importance of genetic factors in human obesity. I have highlighted this in the title of this chapter: In his 1962 presidential address to the Endocrine Society, Professor Edwin B. Astwood, one of my most important mentors, used "The Heritage of Corpulence" as the title for his speech[2].

In exploring this problem of genetics versus environment in the cause of obesity, I have heeded the advice of Harris and looked back at two early papers on the heritage of corpulence to understand the earliest ideas about the role of human genetics in the development of obesity that is now exploding around us.

The two selections that are printed in the appendix are from the first quarter of the twentieth century and deal with early studies on genetics and obesity. The first one is by Charles Davenport and examines the familial aspects of body build, another way of getting at the idea of obesity. The selection from Otmar von Verschuer is the first study of corpulence in twins. Twins make an ideal subject for the study of genetic factors, since identical (monozygotic) twins have the same set of genes, whereas non-identical (dizygotic) twins have the same distribution of genes as other brothers and sisters within a family.

What was the state of our knowledge about the heritage of corpulence in the early part of the twentieth century when these two papers were published? In the English literature, Thomas Chambers, writing on obesity in 1850, had noted that obesity tended to run in families[3]. Sir William Osler, in his classic textbook first published in 1892, says:

> Corpulence, and excessive development of the bodily fat, is a condition for which the physician is frequently consulted, and for which much may be done by judicious arrangement of the diet. The tendency to polysarcia or obesity is often *hereditary*, and is apt to be manifest after the middle period of life. It may, however, be seen early and in this country it is not very uncommon in young girls and young boys[4] (italics mine).

At the beginning of the twentieth century, Garrod gave impetus to the field of "inborn errors of metabolism" with his Croonian Lecture[1]. In this small book, he focused on the way some diseases seemed to result from disordered metabolism that was "inherited" or inborn. This perspective provided an important focus to the study of metabolic disease, which has been so productive in the last one hundred years.

We get another view of the importance of familial factors in the onset of obesity from the large five-volume work titled *Endocrinology and Metabolism*, edited by Lewellys F. Barker in 1922. Unfortunately, Tileston, who wrote the chapter on obesity, concludes that obesity is not inherited. In his comments, he says the following:

> A history of obesity in other members of the family is obtained in about seventy per cent of the cases. Since, however, the metabolism is normal, it is evident that the obesity is not inherited, and a careful inquiry will show that family habits of eating, possibly combined with the inheritance of a phlegmatic disposition, account for the condition[5].

His comment that "since...metabolism is normal...obesity is not inherited" was clearly wrong from our vantage point. His chapter was published before the landmark study by Davenport. By 1940, when Rony published the first American monograph devoted wholly to obesity [6], Davenport's classic observations were well known.

In contrast with the English literature, the French literature had included a discussion of the hereditary aspects of obesity from the latter quarter of the nineteenth century onward. Worthington, an American born in Cincinnati who had gone to Paris to study, wrote in 1875 in his monograph that a number of earlier authors had suggested that obesity was hereditary[7]. Among others he cites cases reported by Maccary[8], Dancel[9] and Wadd[10]. In spite of these allusions to the heritage of corpulence (or polysarcie, as Worthington refers to it), there were no significant systematic studies known to Worthington in the nineteenth century. This may in part be due to the strength of Francis Galton's ideas about heredity, and the fact that the work of Mendel on genetic transmission of traits did not come to wide attention until the early twentieth century. The study of continuous variables, of which weight and height are examples, showed that the variables may be transmitted as particulate traits, but it was widely believed that segregation of genes was not possible. This disagreement with the particulate transmission of the Mendel school was finally put to rest by the demonstration that continuous and discontinuous variations could be explained by segregation of independent genes[11]. With this problem settled, the door was open for progress in the study of segregation of human traits, including body build and corpulence. By 1911, when the Frenchman Heckel wrote his book titled *Petites et Grandes Obésités,* a discussion of familial components of obesity was incorporated as part of the chapter on the causes or etiology of corpulence[12].

In addition to the French, German physicians sensed that constitutional factors might be important. Among these German physicians, Carl von Noorden was the giant in the study of metabolic diseases[13]. In the English translation of his important three-volume monograph titled *Metabolism and Practical Medicine* he says,

> It is the general opinion of both physician and layman that there are obese persons whose condition is to some extent independent of overeating or deficient physical exercise, and is rather the result of a "constitutional tendency." Expressed in the language of metabolism, this would denote that their corpulence was due to a slowing in the processes of metabolism, or, in other words, to an abnormal cellular activity inherited or acquired in after-life[13].

What was needed at this point were more definitive studies of the variation among members of families with a wide range of difference in body build or fatness.

As the idea of a familial relationship for obesity or corpulence was gaining acceptance in the latter part of the nineteenth and early twentieth centuries, the first of a group of experimental animals with inherited obesity was described in 1883 (see Chapter 8)[14]. This animal, called the yellow obese mouse, was found to inherit obesity as a dominant trait. Thus on the animal side there was clear-cut evidence that Mendelian-type inheritance could produce obesity[15]. Similarly, in animal husbandry it was quite clear that breeding could make important differences in the amount and location of body fat.

In the paper by Davenport, titled "Body-Build and Its Inheritance," this animal experience is brought into the reasoning he used for studying the inheritance of fatness. He notes the difference in milk production between different breeds of cattles and goes on to note:

> Indeed, it is easily appreciated that steers of the beef and dairy types of cattle should metabolize differently when we consider the marked difference in the milk production of cows of these two types. The cow of the highest dairy type is capable of manufacturing 10 kilograms of milk containing 1.2 kilograms of butterfat in one day, or 6 percent. The cow of the meat type, of larger size, produces up to 30 kilograms of milk, and this contains, perhaps, 1.3 kilograms of butterfat per day, or only 4.3 percent. There is here obviously a difference in the metabolic processes in the cows and this is reflected in the steers also. There is an internal biochemical difference as well as a difference in feeding instinct. The latter is not merely a matter of family tradition, of the family economics or mores; it is a physiological phenomena as much as internal metabolism[16].

Against this background, Davenport conducted his classic study of the relation of variations in body build among members of families. It was the first study of the relation of "nature versus nurture" in the field of obesity

The strategy that Davenport took was summarized when he says, "Our problem is not what are all the causes of this diversity of build, but rather in how far do genetic factors play a part in this diversity"[16]. As a criterion to assess the differences between individuals in the families that he studied, Davenport selected the body mass index—the same formula developed by Quetelet one hundred years earlier and one now widely used in epidemiological studies of obesity. Using this index Davenport identifies five standard classes of body build or degrees of fatness.

Larger families, on the average, were derived from fleshy parents more often than from slender parents. That is, mating between two fleshy individuals, those with the higher body mass index, yielded 2.3 times as many children, on the average, per mating as the mating of two slender people"[16].

From an analysis of the regression of weights of progeny from various matings, Davenport concludes that:

> fleshy parents carry all sorts of gametes [genes] for build, slender parents carry a preponderance of gametes of their

> own kind... This suggests that the slender parents from various classes of parental mating are more nearly homozygous than the fleshy parents[16].

Davenport then says:

> Fleshy build results from the action of several positive (dominant) factors that make for stoutness, while slenderness results from the absence of one or more of such factors, or is due to recessive factors. Fleshy parents may, and frequently do, carry gametes which lack the "fleshy" or carry the "slender" factor, while in slender parents for the most part the gametes carry only the slender factor, hence the gametes of slender parents are more nearly homogeneous.

The data that Davenport published provide strong support for his ideas. A brief summary table from his work will make this clear[16].

Table 9-1 Body mass index (BMI) of adult offspring from various weight categories of parental mating. Adapted from Davenport 1924.

Parental mating	N offspring	VS	S	M	F	VF
VS X S	20	20	60	10	10	
SXS	51	10	69	21		
M X M	332	1	12	60	25	2
F X F	159		9	39	38	14
VF X VF	37			40	27	33

From an analysis of his data, Davenport reached a number of important conclusions that sound very modern:

- That, in adult life, changes in body build (BMI) vary among families
- that, in individuals characterized by slender body build (low BMI), there is typically little change during adult life; that those with a fleshy build (higher BMI), on the other hand, typically show progressive increase in weight up to age fifty years or more
- that, although there are numerous exceptions, a fleshy adult build is foreshadowed by a plump build in childhood
- that the fleshy parents, i.e., those with higher body build, have on average larger family size than slender parents
- that since regression toward the mean is less striking in the offspring of slender than of fleshy parents, Davenport concludes that fleshy parents

carry not only genes for fleshiness but also for slenderness, whereas parents who are slender carry genes for fleshiness with a lower frequency
- that the genetic effect on body build is controlled by multiple factors, with those for fleshiness tending to dominate slightly over those for thinness
- that slender parents are apparently of two kinds, those carrying only one kind of factor for fleshy build and the other two such gametic factors
- that the offspring of the slender parents are only slightly variable in weight while those carrying two changes in gametes are more variable
- that matings of slender and fleshy parents (mixed group) produce offspring which are variable in weight
- that the mode of body build in this mixed group is closer to that of two fleshy parents than in between the fleshy and lean ones, thus showing partial dominance of the traits for fleshiness
- that when matings of two heterozygous F1 parents occurs the offspring are exceptionally variable
- that the parents of medium build have one or two independent factors modulating body build; the progeny from these families are often strikingly invariable
- that variations in body build cannot be accounted for merely by variations in intake and outgo of calories; there must also be endogenous factors that determine the "economy of nutrition" (***nutrient partitioning*** or ***nutrient channeling*** in current terminology) or the cost of energy of adding an additional kilogram of weight to the body
- finally, that the number of factors involved in very fleshy build in some cases includes at least three independent ones.

Some of Davenport's ideas are buttressed by the second selection on the heritage of corpulence in twins. This is an extract and translation from a paper by von Verschuer ("Die Verebungsbiologische Zwillingsforschung. Ihre Biologischen Grundlagen")[18]. In this work von Verschuer expresses differences between pairs of twins as a percentage and then compares the percentage differences between monozygotic and dizygotic twins. The study compares 102 monozygotic twins who have the same genes and 45 dizygotic twins of the same-sex twins who have the variability of brothers or sisters and of different sex under a variety of circumstances. Several points are worth noting about the twins that von Verschuer measured.

Body weight was among the most variable differences between these twins. The variability among 80 pair of monozygotic twins is almost half as great as among 38 pair of same-gender dizygotic twins. This is shown in his Table 8 where he compares the number of twins with a difference that is greater than their average amount of variability. For the monozygotic twins this is 33% and for the dizygotic twins it is 69%.

The variability of monozygotic and dizygotic twins raised in the same or different environments was also examined. Among monozygotic twins who have the same genes, the mean percent deviation in body weight for those raised in the same environment was 1.39% compared to 3.60% for those raised in a different family environment. Among dizygotic twins with genetic diversity there was essentially no difference whether they were raised in the same family environment or in different families (4.7% vs. 4.2%). von Verschuer also noted, interestingly, that the percent deviation in body weight was much smaller for monozygotic twins having the same occupation as opposed to monozygotic twins having different occupations. For those with the same occupation, the mean percent deviation of body weight was 1.89% vs. 4.50% for monozygotic twins having different occupations.

The difference in birth weight was also reflected in variability in the adult weight of the twins. Where the difference in birth weight was less than 250 grams, monozygotic twins showed a mean percent deviation of 1.85% vs. 2.85% when the birth weight was greater than 250 grams. For dizygotic twins the percent deviation of body weight for those less than 250 grams was 2.90% and for those above 250 grams it was 6.40%. Finally, von Verschuer noted differences in the percent deviation waned as a function of age for both monozygotic and dizygotic twins.

Since the 1920s when these papers were published, there has been a rapidly growing scientific literature using family studies and studies of identical twins to separate the effects of nature from nurture in the development of obesity. In their 1937 book titled *Twins: A Study of Heredity and Environment*[19], Newman, Freeman, and Holzinger, in addition to confirming the findings of von Verschuer on the greater difference in weight between dizygotic and monozygotic twins, also compared body weights of monozygotic twins who had been reared together with those who had been reared apart. In confirmation of von Verschuer, they noted that the twins reared apart had a greater difference in body weights than those reared together. This technique has found subsequent productive use by many investigators[20–24].

From these early studies at the beginning of the twentieth century we have moved to the era of the double helix and molecular biology. Application of genetic technique to the study of inheritance of some forms of obesity has made great progress as later chapters will demonstrate. However, these early studies are the seminal backbone for the continuing efforts to understand the full impact of genetic factors in the development of obesity and how we will win the battle of the bulge.

Biosketch

Sir Archibald Edward Garrod (1857–1936) was the fourth son of a well-known zoologist[25]. He was educated at Oxford and received his medical training at St. Bartholomew's Hospital, London. After rising through the ranks at St. Bartholomew's, and participating in World War I, he returned to England to be named Regius Professor at Oxford, following Sir William Osler. He is probably best remembered for his 1908 Croonian Lecture titled "Inborn Errors of Metabolism," which was published in revised form in 1909. This work focused on measurements of metabolic products as a reflection of inborn errors of metabolism and was a precursor to modern genetic biochemistry[25]. (Figure 9-1)

Biosketch

Charles Benedict Davenport was born in Stamford, Connecticut, in 1866. Davenport's father was a key figure in his early development. The father, a founder and teacher in a private academy in Brooklyn, New York, taught his son at home until the age of thirteen and was a demanding, and some say harsh, puritanical and tyrannical father. At thirteen, this mainly solitary youth entered the Polytechnic Institute of Brooklyn and was soon at the head of his class despite his previous unorthodox schooling. After completion of his civil engineering degree in 1886, he entered Harvard College where he majored in zoology, receiving an AB degree in 1889 and a Ph.D. in 1892. In 1899, Davenport left Harvard where he was an instructor to become an assistant professor at the University of Chicago, where he advanced to associate professor in 1901. He left the University of Chicago in 1904 following establishment by the Carnegie Institution of the Cold Spring Harbour Station for Experimental Evolution. Shortly afterwards, he established and directed the Eugenics Record Office at the same location[26]. He was elected to both the American Philosophical Society and the National Academy of Sciences. The rediscovery of Gregor Mendel's results in 1900 turned many scientists toward genetic studies directed at a variety of organisms[26, 27]. As one Davenport biographer notes, "From 1907 Davenport's interest turned to human heredity and eugenics, a shift sparked at least partly by his wife"[26]. Davenport published more than four hundred communications. The great majority of these were without coauthor. Davenport became a "staunch advocate of an improved race of man...and urged great care in the selection of marriage partners, large families for those who had thus selected, a ban on racial mixing and the excluding of undesirable immigrants from the United States"[26]. (Figure 9-2)

Biosketch

Dr. Otmar Freiherr von Verschuer (1896–1969) was born in 1896. He completed his high school education during World War I and at the end of the war began medical school, where he specialized in internal medicine at Munich and at Tübingen. His longtime interest in twin research began during his time in Tübingen. By 1927, when the paper on twins cited here was published, he was appointed to direct a research group at the Kaiser Wilhelm

Institute for Anthropology in Human Genetics in Berlin. Following World War II, he moved to Munster to head the newly founded Institute of Human Genetics. During his active and productive scientific career he published more than two hundred seventy papers, primarily in the field of twin research. In 1934 von Verschuer was elected to be a member of the German Academy of Natural Sciences, and he subsequently received honorary membership in the Italian Society of Medical Genetics (1953), honorary member of the Viennese Society of Anthropology (1955), honorary member of the Japanese Society for Human Genetics (1956), and corresponding member of the Austrian Academy of Sciences (1959). He died on August 8, 1969, following an automobile accident nearly twelve months earlier. (Figure 9-3)

Biosketch

Edwin Bennett Astwood (1909–1976) (Figure 9-3) was born in Bermuda. He attended medical school in Loma Linda, California, and at McGill University in Montreal. Following completion of his training, he took a Ph.D. with Professor Hisaw at Harvard University, where many of the eminent endocrinologists of the 1920–30s were trained. He then joined the faculty at the Peter Bent Brigham Hospital, only to move later to the New England Medical Center as chief of endocrinology. He remained there conducting research on a broad array of endocrine topics, including ACTH and the adrenal gland, growth hormone and the pituitary gland, parathyroid hormone, reproductive hormones, adipose tissue, and obesity. The title of his address to the Endocrine Society when he was president is "The Heritage of Corpulence." I had the privilege of being one of Dr. Astwood's students during the 1960s. He retired from medicine in 1970 and returned to Bermuda.

References

1. Harris, H. *Garrod's Inborn Errors of Metabolism.* London: Oxford University Press, 1963.
2. Astwood, E.B. "The Heritage of Corpulence." *Endocrinology.* 71(1962): 337.
3. Chambers, T.K. "The Gulstonian Lectures—On Corpulence." *Lancet.* 2(1850): 11–19, 342–350, 438–445.
4. Osler, W. *The Principles and Practice of Medicine.* New York: D. Appleton, 1892.
5. Tileston, W. "Obesity." *In Endocrinology and Metabolism Presented in Their Scientific and Practical Clinical Aspects by Ninety-Eight Contributors.* Ed. L.F. Barker. Vol. 4. New York: D. Appleton and Co., 1922–24.
6. Rony, H.R. *Obesity and Leanness.* Philadelphia: Lea and Febiger, 1940.
7. Worthington, L.S. *De l'obésité, étiologie, therapeutique, et hygiene.* Paris: Martinet, 1875.
8. Maccary, A. *Traité sur la polysarcie.* Paris: Gabon, 1811.
9. Dancel, F. *Traité théorique et pratique de l'obésité (trop grand embonpoint). Avec plusieurs observations de guérison de maladies occasionées ou entretienues par cet état anormal.* Paris: J.B. Bailliere et fils, 1863.
10. Wadd, W. *Comments on Corpulency: Lineaments of Leanness, Mems on Diet and Dietetics.* London: John Ebers & Co., 1829.
11. Froggatt P., N.C. Nevin. "The Law of Ancestral Heredity and the Mendelian-Ancestrian Controversy in England, 1899–1906." *J Med Genet.* no. 1 1(1971): 1–36.
12. Heckel, F. *Grandes et Petites Obésités; Cure Radicale.* Paris: Masson, 1911.
13. von Noorden CH. Metabolism and Practical Medicine. Vol. 3. London: Heinemann, 1907.
14. Bray, G.A., D.A. York. "Hypothalamic and Genetic Obesity in Experimental Animals: an Autonomic and Endocrine Hypothesis." *Physiol Rev.* no. 3. 59(1979): 719–809.
15. Bateson, W. *Mendel's Principles of Heredity: A Defense.* Cambridge: Cambridge University Press, 1902.
16. Davenport, C.B. *Body-Build and Its Inheritance.* Washington: Carnegie Institution of Washington, 1923.
17. Bray G.A. "The Inheritance of Corpulence." In *The Body Weight Regulatory System: Normal and Disturbed Mechanisms.* Ed. L.A. Cioffi, W.P.T. James, T.B. Van Itallie. New York: Raven Press, 1981.
18. von Verschuer, O. "Die Verebungsbiologische Zwillingsforschung. Ihre Biologischen Grundlagen. Mit 18 Abbildungen." *Ergebnisse der Inneren Medizin und Kinderheilkunde.* Berlin: Verlag von Julius

Springer, 1927.

19. Newman, H.H., F.N. Freeman, K.J. Holzinger. *Twins: A Study of Heredity and Environment.* Chicago: University of Chicago Press, 1937.
20. Shields, J. *Monozygotic Twins Brought Up Apart and Brought Up Together; An Investigation into the Genetic and Environmental Causes of Variation in Personality.* London: Oxford University Press, 1962.
21. Stunkard, A.J., T.I. Sorensen, C. Hanis, et al. "An Adoption Study of Human Obesity." *N Engl J Med.* 314(1986): 193–198.
22. Stunkard, A.J., J.R. Harris, N.L. Pedersen, et al. "The Body-Mass Index of Twins Who Have Been Reared Apart." *N Engl J Med.* 322(1990): 1483–1487.
23. Bouchard, C. ed. *The Genetics of Obesity.* Boca Raton, FL: CRC Press, 1994.
24. Bouchard, C., L. Perusse, C. Leblanc, A. Tremblay, G. Theriault. "Inheritance of the Amount and Distribution of Human Body Fat." *Int J Obes.* 12(1988): 205-212.
25. Rolleston, J.D. "Sir Archibald Edward Garrod (1857–1936)." In *Dictionary of National Biography 1931–1940.* Ed. L.G. Wickham Legg. London: Oxford University Press, 1949.
26. MacDowell, E.C. "Charles Benedict Davenport, 1866–1944: A Study of Conflicting Influences." *Bios.* 17(1946): 3–50.
27. Mendel, G.J. "Versuch über Pflanzen-Hybriden." *Verb. naturf. Vereins Brunn.* 4(1866): 3–47.
28. Bateson, W. *Mendel's Principles of Heredity.* 2nd printing. Cambridge: Cambridge University Press, 1909.

Chapter 10

Metabolic Rate—The Oxygen Theory Displaces Air, Fire, Earth, and Water

Science is for those who study it a source of exultation. It is as if a force outside ourselves, say an angel, pulled us away from our previous level to a higher level in an indescribably, incomprehensible manner.

— Pais[1]

New methods are one of the cornerstones for advances in science. The discovery of the microscope, the introduction of radioactive isotopes into clinical medicine, and the development of the radioimmunoassay for hormones are but three in a long list that have provided tools for our battle of the bulge. This paper is about another method that was originally developed in animals and then applied to the study of energy expenditure in human beings with substantial new discoveries. This instrument was the calorimeter, which serves to measure heat production or heat loss either directly or indirectly. Calorimeters were revolutionary in their day, and with their use, Antoine-Laurent Lavoisier (1743–1794) shifted the paradigm for thinking about human metabolism. He started a scientific revolution that provided basic tools and ideas for our battle of the bulge.

Lavoisier's simple calorimeter measured the melting of ice by the heat generated from a guinea pig, which is a way of measuring the heat that is produced. But the impact was immense. He showed that metabolism was equivalent to a slowly burning candle. (See Appendix)

There are a number of different ways of measuring this heat, and thus a number of different instruments that are now available, but at the time of Lavoisier, just before the French and American revolutions, there was no such thing as a calorimeter.

The first two calorimeters were those of Lavoisier and Laplace[3] in Paris and Crawford in England[4]. Crawford measured the increase in temperature of water surrounding an animal's cage as the way of determining the heat given off by his guinea pigs. In contrast, Lavoisier and LaPlace used the melting of ice surrounding the cage of their guinea pigs to determine heat production. Page 514 is a picture of their calorimeter[3]. Some of the subsequent calorimeters have used this principle of direct measurement of heat loss, but most of them have measured energy expenditure indirectly by measuring oxygen consumption and carbon dioxide production. This indirect method became the method of choice, once the equivalence of heat loss and the uptake of oxygen had been demonstrated.

The revolution that Lavoisier began for obesity was as significant as the French Revolution—the revolution that took Lavoisier's life—was for liberty. It consisted in showing that the heat produced by the guinea pig was equivalent to the heat produced by a candle when it used the same amount of oxygen (at the time he did this work, oxygen as such was not yet identified or named).

The oxygen theory of combustion that resulted from Lavoisier's work provided the basis for understanding metabolism, the processes by which all living creatures get their energy. Among his scientific "firsts," Lavoisier conducted the first study of human metabolism by measuring the oxygen consumption of his assistant, Sequin. Their study showed that more oxygen was consumed when Sequin was in the cold at 12°C (54°F) than at room temperature of 26°C (79°F). Lavoisier also found that food digestion increased the use of oxygen and that the highest oxygen uptake was observed when Sequin exercised. Mendelsohn summarized this by saying:

> To the historian, the achievement of Lavoisier, and to a lesser extent of Crawford, in founding the oxidation theory of combustion and animal heat is the single most important innovation in the long history of attempts to account for the warmth of animals. It was only after the experimental successes of Lavoisier that one could look back and "rediscover" the combustion theory of Mayow and recognize the conceptual similarity between it and the oxygen theory of Lavoisier[5].

Lavoisier initiated a scientific revolution that overthrew the phlogiston theory. As Goodfield notes in his study of the history of physiology, "Lavoisier's contributions to the biological sciences were as great as his better-known contributions to chemistry. In both cases the key point was his emphasis on quantitative methods of study"[6]. The Oxygen Theory that Lavoisier spelled out was the final nail in the coffin of a cosmology of air, fire, earth, and water that dated back to a time before the great physician Hippocrates more than twenty-five hundred years ago[7]. Lavoisier's revolution was arguably as important as that of Copernicus[8], the man who showed that the Earth revolved around the sun and not vice versa, and the contribution of Darwin who argued that the origin of species[9], including man, arose by natural selection due to survival of the fittest of the offspring. The Oxygen Theory of Lavoisier falls in this same category. It was a revolution that reshaped science.

The experiments which started Lavoisier on his path toward the Oxygen Theory began in the late 1760s. His work on calorimetry was performed later, but it represents the initial studies of calorimetry and a key milestone in the battle of the bulge. I will begin with Lavoisier's early observations and then return to discuss his seminal contribution on calorimetry, which supported the hypothesis that metabolism is a form of slow combustion.

The period from 1770 to 1790 was one of great activity in the field of combustion chemistry. This era has excited the curiosity of many individuals and their viewpoints are aptly summarized in their various writings[5, 6, 10–13]. By 1772 Lavoisier appears to have reached the fundamental conclusions that served as the basis for his Oxygen Theory. When he began his studies on combustion, the phlogiston theory was the principal theory of combustion[5, 6, 14]. Phlogiston was hypothesized to be given off when an object burned. The demonstration that substances like sulfur and phosphorus gained weight rather than lost weight when they burned contradicted the phlogiston theory and perplexed Lavoisier. In Lavoisier's time, recognition that one had conceived an idea first could be gotten by depositing a letter with the Academy of Science indicating one's priority. Lavoisier did this. To quote from Lavoisier:

> This discovery which I have proved by experiments that I regard as decisive, has made me think that what was observed in the combustion of sulphur and phosphorous might take place in regard to all bodies which acquire weight in combustion or calcination, and I felt persuaded [*je me suis persuade*] that the increase in weight of the metallic calces was due to the same cause. My conjecture was completely confirmed by experiment. I reduced litharge (lead oxide) in closed vessels, with the apparatus of Hales [Lavoisier like Priestley goes back to Hales] and I observed that at the moment of the passage of calx (calcium oxide) into metal a considerable quantity of air was given off and that the volume of this air was at least a thousand times as great as that of the litharge used. As this discovery seemed to me one of the most interesting made since the work of Stahl [the man who proposed the phlo-

> giston theory[14]], I have thought it right to make certain that my claim to it by depositing the present note in the hands of the Secretary of the Academy [of Sciences] to remain secret till the moment when I publish my experiments. Paris 1, November 1772[11] (notes mine).

It was this discovery contained in a note deposited with the Academy of Sciences in 1772 which was elaborated in detail over the next fifteen years and published in detail in his *Elements of Chemistry* in 1789[15, 16]. This comprises his revolution in chemistry. The final step in the Oxygen Theory was made possible by a set of experiments performed by Henry Cavendish (1731–1810)[17]. Cavendish showed that when hydrogen gas was burned, a small moist vapor was left behind. Lavoisier proceeded to show that this vapor was water. Thus when oxygen and hydrogen burned, they produced water.

The Oxygen Theory was the death knell for the phlogiston theory, an idea which had served as the working hypothesis for Joseph Priestley (1733–1804) who discovered oxygen[18] (which he called eminently respirable gas), for Wilhelm Scheele (1742–1786) who also discovered oxygen, for Cavendish who showed that oxygen and hydrogen burned to give water[17] and for Crawford[4], who performed studies on calorimetry at the same time as Lavoisier. It was Lavoisier's genius that led him to realize that the Oxygen Theory provided a better way of viewing the chemical universe than was provided by the phlogiston theory. Joseph Priestley, the Quaker chemist who contributed so much to the isolation of gases and to the methodology needed for this purpose in the late eighteenth century, and who provided important information for Lavoisier, was never able to expel the old phlogiston theory of Stahl; neither was Crawford, who said:

> By some philosophers in the present age (referring to Lavoisier), the existence of the principle, which the chemists have termed phlogiston has been called in question. Mr. Lavoisier...is the principal opponent of the doctrine of phlogiston....[4]

With the concept of the Oxygen Theory clearly in mind, and phlogiston dismissed, Lavoisier began his collaboration with Laplace on the relation of respiration and heat production. The principle that Lavoisier used in his calorimeter came from the work of Joseph Black (1728–1799)[19], who showed that melting ice required heat. Lavoisier and Laplace used this principle to measure the amount of heat given off by a guinea pig in a measured interval of time. They also measured the amount of carbon dioxide (then called fixed air) given off by the guinea pig in this same interval. They found that a similar amount of ice was melted (i.e., heat produced) by a candle or a guinea pig when they produced the same amount of fixed air (carbon dioxide). From this, Lavoisier and Laplace concluded that respiration by an animal was similar to slow combustion. To quote from Lavoisier:

> Respiration is then a combustion, very slow, it is true, but otherwise perfectly analogous to the combustion of charcoal. It is made in the interior of the lungs without the disengagement of any appreciable amount of light, because the material of the fire on becoming free is immediately absorbed by the organic fluids. The heat developed in this combustion is communicated to the blood which passes through the lungs and is thence spread through the animal system. Thus, the air which we breathe serves two purposes equally necessary to our preservation: it carries off to the blood the "fixed air" (carbon dioxide) whose excess would be very harmful; and the heat which this combustion forms in the lungs repairs the continuous loss of heat which we give to the atmosphere and the surrounding bodies[10].

In 1962 Thomas Kuhn[20] published a seminal work titled *The Structure of Scientific Revolutions.* In reviewing the revolutions associated with the names of Copernicus, Newton, Lavoisier, and Einstein, Kuhn concluded that:

> Each of them necessitated the [scientific] community's rejection of one time-honored scientific theory in favor of another incompatible with it. Each produced a consequent shift in the problems available for scientific scrutiny and in the standards by which the profession determined what should count as an admissible problem or as a legitimate problem-solution. And each transformed the scientific imagination in ways that we shall ultimately need to describe as a transformation of the world within which scientific work was done. Such changes, together with the controversies that almost always accompany them, are the defining characteristics of scientific revolutions[20].

In Kuhn's view, a new theory, however special its range of application, is seldom or never just an increment to what is already known. Such a process is seldom completed by a single man and never occurs overnight. In terminology frequently used today, Kuhn's scientific revolution would be defined as a "paradigm shift." Kuhn goes on to discuss normal science, which is the science of textbooks and the science which most scientists participate in. This includes the "fact gatherers" and technological applications of existing theory. When a revolution or new paradigm arises that attracts most of the next generations of practitioners of science, an old field of science disappears. The chemical revolution is the first generally recognized major scientific revolution to have been called a revolution by its chief author, Antoine-Laurent Lavoisier. To quote from Foster's translation of Lavoisier:

> The importance of this subject has encouraged me to review all of the work which has seemed to me made to occasion a revolution in physics and chemistry; I have thought that I should regard only as indications all that has been performed before this time. I have proposed to repeat everything with fresh precautions in order to connect what we know about the air which is fixed or which sets itself free, with our other acquired knowledge and to form a new theory. The works of the different authors whom I have just mentioned, if they are considered from this point of view, present me with the separate portions of a chain, they are joined by links. But a great many experiments must be performed to make the sequence complete. An important point which most investigators have neglected is to put their attention on the origin of the air which is found in a great many bodies. They should have learned from Hales that one of the chief principles in the animal and vegetable economy is the fixation of air, (the combination of it with water, fire and earth to form all of the combinations with which we are familiar)... This method of looking at my object has made me feel the necessity of first repeating and then multiplying experiments on the absorption of air to the end that knowing the origin of these substances, I shall be able to trace their effects in all different combinations[10].

Acceptance of the chemical revolution fomented by Lavoisier began as early as 1778 in the work of Jean-Baptiste-Michel Bucquet. According to Guerlac[21], however, it was the work of Antoine François de Fourcroy[22] that was most responsible for the recognition of the scientific revolution in chemistry arising from Lavoisier's ideas. In his work titled *Leçons élémentaires d'histoire naturelle et de chimie,* published in 1782, Fourcroy notes the great revolution that was occurring in chemistry.

In his historical analysis of scientific revolutions, Bernard Cohen[23] has identified four stages in the process. The first stage he calls "the intellectual revolution or the revolution in itself." This occurs, he says, whenever a scientist or group of scientists devises a radical solution to some major problem or problems, finds a new method of using information, sets forth a new framework of knowledge, introduces a new set of concepts which changes the character of existing knowledge, or proposes a revolutionary theory. The second stage he labels "the write-up." The findings which lead to these new rules are recorded or written up first in an entry or diary book and subsequently in phase three published for wider dissemination. This third stage might be properly called the "revolution on paper." The fourth stage is broader acceptance of the revolution.

As Cohen says, even after publication, no revolution in science will occur until a sufficient number of other scientists become convinced of the theories or findings and begin to do their science in the revolutionary new way. The contribution of Lavoisier was rapidly taken up at the end of the eighteenth century and the early nineteenth century. The case of van't Hoff, a Dutch chemist of the late nineteenth century, shows that acceptance of revolutionary ideas can on occasion be delayed. He proposed in the 1870s that the carbon atom was asymmetrical, that is, that it had four attachment points and that different arrangements at these four attachments could produce mirror images. As Cohen notes, most chemists at that time were hostile to his ideas of asymmetry, and did not even give serious consideration to his proposed revolutionary revision of orthodox chemical theory. To quote Cohen:

> In part, the opposition to van't Hoff's ideas arose also from the fact that he had written of atoms and molecules as if they had physical reality, in direct opposition of the views of most organic chemists, who were willing to use the concept of atom and molecule but were skeptical as to their actuality. Today, van't Hoff's revolutionary ideas on the asymmetrical carbon are considered to be the foundation of stereo-chemistry[23].

To determine whether a scientific concept qualifies for a revolution, Cohen proposes four tests. First are the testimonies of witnesses, both scientists and non-scientists living at the time. His second criterion comes from examination of later documentary history of the subject, including, as an example, a study of treatises written before and after the period in which Copernicus published his ideas on the heliocentric structure of the planetary system. The third criterion that Cohen uses is the judgment of competent historians, and the final criterion is the opinion of scientists working in the field today. Using all of these criteria, it is evident that Lavoisier's chemical revolution would pass all of the criteria proposed both by Kuhn and by Cohen as a scientific revolution.

Some have attributed the beginning of modern chemistry to the work of Robert Boyle[24]. However, in his text *Chemistry in the Chemical Revolution*, Crossland[25] notes that Boyle effectively ended the period of alchemy with the publication of his book *The Skeptical Chemist* (1661) and states, "He launched some effective criticisms of traditional concepts, notably the Aristotelian theory of four elements and the Paracelsian theory of three principals, but he was not able to replace these theories with any more useful theories" (see reference 26 for more on Paracelsus). Indeed, up through most of the eighteenth century, the four Aristotelian elements of earth, air, fire, and water were the basis for many theories of life.

In his commentary about the contribution of Lavoisier, Popper, the twentieth century philosopher of science, suggested that although "Lavoisier's classical experiments which show that the volume of air decreases while a candle burns in a closed space... (they) do not establish the oxygen theory of combustion; yet they tend to refute the phlogiston theory"[27]. By negating, falsifying, or making implausible the phlogiston theory, Lavoisier went further with his new nomenclature, establishing the Oxygen Theory as the "new chemistry." As early as 1766, according to Gough, Lavoisier had planned to study, in turn, each of the four Aristotelian elements[28]. By 1772 his work on airs began his demolition of the four elements as a cosmology[15, 16].

With the Oxygen Theory of Lavoisier, the theory that the world is composed of the four elements reached its end. As Foucault has said of this transition period, "Modern medicine has fixed its own date of birth as being in the last years of the eighteenth century"[29], at the time that the Oxygen Theory revolutionized science and political revolutions convulsed France and the American colonies.

The concept of the four elements began with Thales, who attempted to identify a single element for all of nature. As different elements were "identified," the concept of air, water, earth, and fire as the four fundamental elements came to receive wide recognition in the ancient world. Its acceptance was such that it was the dominant idea for cosmology for much of the next two thousand years. It was a cosmology of simplicity. Empedocles and his Greek age constructed a theory of disease based in these four elements. It was adopted by Western medicine and by Buddhist and Tibetan medicine as well[30]. In 1785 Rigby[31] used these principles to account for the nutritional elements of food. To quote Rigby, "The principles into which the common articles of food, both animal and vegetable, are resolved by chemical analysis, are earth, water, air, phlogiston, and the matter of heat"[31]. It was not until the work of Priestley and Lavoisier, showing that there were many different kinds of air and that two airs (hydrogen and oxygen) could combine to form water, that this cosmology fundamentally died.

Lavoisier's Oxygen Theory necessitated a revolutionary change in theory. First, air, as we experience it, seems to be a single "element." During the eighteenth century, scientists gradually realized that air was composed of more than one substance. The first of these to be identified was fixed air (carbon dioxide). Priestley[18], using improved methods for collecting "airs" over mercury, was able to isolate oxygen (dephlogisticated air as he called it) or eminently respirable air (as Lavoisier called it). Thus the "air" of ancient times was not just "air" but a mixture of more than one type of air. The ordinary individual is unable to identify more than one component of air as part of their usual experience. It requires experimental manipulation to separate the air, as we breathe it, into its separate components. Doing so, however, makes "air" no longer a single element for the universe.

Second, Cavendish[17] showed that oxygen and hydrogen could be burned and Lavoisier showed unequivocally that the product was water. Thus, the "water" of the ancients was no longer a universal element. "Water" as we usually experience it is composed of two gases, oxygen and hydrogen. Thus, the Oxygen Theory of Lavoisier effectively destroyed the simple connection that existed between the perceived realities of everyday life in air and water and substituted a theory that moved beyond and behind the usual every day experience. Lavoisier had created a revolution in the framework in which people had to view the universe. From that point onward, the march of science involved ever more experimental manipulation and interpretation of information derived from instrumental interfaces with nature.

Biosketch

Antoine-Laurent Lavoisier (1743–1794) (Figure 10-2) was born in 1743, the son of well-to-do parents. He had all the advantages that education in the upper classes could provide[10]. He entered the College of Mazarin, where he received a law degree. His passion, however, was for science. He had received training in mathematics and astronomy and had studied botany, mineralogy, geology, and chemistry. In his scientific training he had come in contact with some of the most distinguished scientists in France, and by the age of twenty he began making barometric observations that he continued throughout his life. At the age of twenty-five, he became a junior member of the Academy of Sciences. He remained closely associated with the Academy until near the end of his life, when it was abolished. The events that led to his political persecution and death during the Revolution occurred when he became a member of the *Ferme Générale*, a semi-private corporation that collected tax revenues. Being involved with the *Ferme Générale* was an unpardonable sin to the leaders of the Reign of Terror, which ruled France from 1793. After a mockery of a trial, Lavoisier was guillotined on May 8, 1794. To end, I quote again from Lavoisier: "It is easy to see that from the year 1772, I had conceived the whole doctrine of combustion which I have since published"[11]. To slightly paraphrase Whitehead:

> The progress of science had reached a turning point. The stable foundations of physics have broken up...the old foundations of scientific thought all require reinterpretation.

This is what Lavoisier did.

References

1. Pais, A. *The Genius of Science: A Portrait Gallery of Twentieth Century Physicists.* Oxford: Oxford University Press, 2000.
2. Sarton, G. *Sarton on the History of Science.* Cambridge: Harvard University Press, 1962.
3. Lavoisier, A-L., P.S. Laplace. *Memoir on Heat.* Read to the Royal Academy of Sciences, 28 June 1783. Trans. H Guerlac. New York: Neale Watson Academic Publications, Inc., 1982.
4. Crawford, A. *Experiments and Observations on Animal Heat, and the Inflammation of Combustible Bodies; Being an Attempt to Resolve These Phenomena into a General Law of Nature.* 2nd ed. London: J. Johnson, 1788.
5. Mendelsohn, E. *Heat and Life: The Development of the Theory of Animal Heat.* Cambridge: Harvard University Press, 1964.
6. Goodfield, G.J. *The Growth of Scientific Physiology.* London: Hutchinson and Co., 1960.
7. Hippocrates. *Oeuvres complètes d'Hippocrate: traduction nouvelle avec le texte grec en regard, collationné sur les manuscrits et toutes les éditions; accompagnée d'une introduction, de commentaires medicaux, de variantes et de notes philologiques; suivie d'une table générale des matières par É. Littré.,* Paris: J.B. Baillière, 1839–1861.
7. Copernicus, N. *De revolutionibus orbium colestium.* Libri VI. Norimberg: Apud loh. Petreium, 1543.
8. Darwin, C. *On the Origin of Species by Means of Natural Selection or the Preservation of Favoured Races in the Struggle for Life.* London: John Murray, 1859.
10. Foster, M.L. *Life of Lavoisier.* Northampton, Mass.: Smith College, 1926.
11. Hartog, P.J. "The Newer Views of Priestley and Lavoisier." *Ann Sci.* 1941, 5:1–56.
12. Holmes, F.L. *Lavoisier and the Chemistry of Life: An Exploration of Scientific Creativity.* Madison: University of Wisconsin Press, 1985.
13. McKie, D. *Antoine Lavoisier.* London: Gollancz, 1935.
14. Stahl, G. *Theoria medica vera. Physiologiam and Pathologiam.* Halae: literis Ophanotrophei, 1708.
15. Lavoisier, A-L. *Traite élémentaire de chimie, présenté dans un ordre nouveau et d'après les découvertes modernes.* Paris: Chez Cuchet, 1789.
16. Lavoisier, A-L. *Elements of Chemistry, in a New Systematic Order, Containing all the Modern Discoveries.* 4th ed. Trans. R Kerr. Edinburgh: William Creech, 1799.
17. Cavendish, H. "Experiments on Air." *Phil Trans.* 74(1784): 119–153.
18. Priestley, J. *Experiments and Observations on Different Kinds of Air.* 3 vols. London: J. Johnson, 1774–1777.
19. Black, J. *Lectures on the Elements of Chemistry.* Ed. J Robinson.

Edinburgh, 1803.
20. Kuhn, T.S. *The Structure of Scientific Revolutions.* Chicago: University of Chicago Press, 1962.
21. Guerlac, H. "Chemistry as a Branch of Physics: Laplace's Collaboration with Lavoisier." *Historical Studies in the Physical Sciences.* 7(1976): 193–276.
22. Fourcroy, A.F. *Leçons élémentaires d'histoire naturelle et de chimie.* Paris, 1782.
23. Cohen, I.B. *Revolution in Science.* Cambridge: Belknap Press, 1985.
24. Boyle, R. *The Sceptical Chymist or Chymico-Physical Doubts Anti Paradoxes Touching the Spagyrist's Principles Commonly Called Hypostatical.* London: J.Caldwell for J. Crocke, 1661.
25. Crossland, N.I.P. *Chemistry and the Chemical Revolution.* Cambridge: Cambridge University Press, 1978.
26. Paracelsus. *Selected Writings, edited with an introduction by Jolande Jacobi, Translated by Norman Guterman.* Princeton, NJ: Princeton University Press, 1985.
27. *Popper Selections.* Ed. Miller D. Princeton: Princeton University Press, 1985.
28. Gough, J.B. "Lavoisier's Early Career in Science: An Examination of Some New Evidence." *Brit J His Sci.* 4(1968–1969): 52–57.
29. Foucault, M. *The Birth of the Clinic. An Archaeology of Medical Perception.* New York: Vintage Books, 1973.
30. Tibetan Medical Paintings. *Illustrations to the Blue Beryl Treatise of Sangye Guamtso (1653–1705).* Ed. Parfionovitch, Y., F. Meyer, G. Dorje. New York: Harry N. Abrams Inc., 1992.
31. Rigby, E. *An Essay on the Theory of the Production of Animal Heat, and on Its Application in the Treatment of Cutaneous Eruptions, Inflammation, and Some Other Diseases.* London: J. Johnson, 1785.

Chapter 11

Metabolic Rate–Are We Fat Because We Have Low Metabolism?

> *Far from being a sacrilege, the search and revelation of truth is a duty—it is not simply a scientific duty in a narrow sense, it is also a philanthropic duty and a religious one.*
>
> —Sarton

The French and American revolutions are seminal dates in human history. Each led to the founding of governments that were representative of the people. They were also important in the "battle of the bulge." This time period set the stage on which the idea that people could get fat without overeating would be played out. The initial setting on the stage was the calorimeter.

The development of calorimeters is usually identified with Antoine-Laurent Lavoisier (1743–1794) in Paris and with Adair Crawford[2] in England. Using these instruments at the end of the eighteenth century they each obtained similar results but reached different conclusions. Lavoisier saw his discovery as the demolition of the "phlogiston" theory that had permeated science during the eighteenth century. This theory argued that "combustion" produced the loss of something called "phlogiston." Lavoisier proved this wrong by showing that combustion increases weight rather than decreases it. Across the English Channel, Crawford obtained similar data as Lavoisier, but could never completely disown the phlogiston theory. Crawford concluded,

> ... the quantity of heat produced, when a given portion of pure air is altered by the respiration of an animal, is nearly equal to that which is produced when the same quantity of air is altered by the burning of wax or charcoal[2].

Crawford's important contributions have been summarized by Brownell:

1. Those animals which are furnished with lungs, and which continually respire fresh air in great quantities, have the power of keeping themselves at a temperature considerably higher than the surrounding atmosphere: but animals that are not furnished with respiratory organs are very nearly of the same temperature with the medium in which they live.
2. Among the hot-blooded animals, those are the warmest which have the largest respiratory organs and which consequently breathe the greatest quantity of air in proportion to their bulk.
3. In the same animal the degree of heat is in some measure proportionable to the quantity of air inspired in a given time; thus animal heat is increased by exercise and whatever accelerates respiration[3].

With the concept that "metabolism" was similar to "combustion" clearly established, the next great advance in the battle of the bulge came from two great German scientists, Robert Mayer and Hermann von Helmholtz (1821–1894), each of whom articulated the Law of Conservation of Energy[4, 5] at essentially the same time. The Law of Conservation of Energy describes the interconversion of different forms of energy but that mass and energy did not appear or disappear. Not until Einstein was this idea changed.

This central theory in the study of "animal heat" came from the German School of Laboratory Medicine. Both Robert Mayer[4], a ship's doctor, and Hermann von Helmholtz, a professor of physiology[5], independently described the Law of Conservation of Energy as applied to living systems. The second half of the nineteenth century was spent proving that this principle was also applicable to large animals and, more important, to human beings. It was calorimetry that made this possible[6, 7].

To test the applicability of the First Law of Thermodynamics to human beings required measuring the carbon and nitrogen in the urine and feces along with the quantity of oxygen taken up and the amount of carbon dioxide (CO_2) respired during the same time period. This is clearly easier in animals than in human beings. The development of a human calorimeter at the end of the nineteenth century was the second pillar for understanding metabolism following the Law of Conservation of Energy. The first human calorimeter was built in Germany by Pettenkofer and Voit[8] in 1865, but only a few studies were performed with it. The demonstration that the Law of Conservation of Energy applied to animals was performed using the calorimeter built in Marburg, Germany, by Max Rubner (1854–1932) in 1894[6]. The calorimeter used for human beings was built by Atwater and Rosa[7] at Wesleyan College in Connecticut in 1896.

Pettenkofer, in Voit's laboratory, built a small room that was large enough for a human subject. It was the first open-circuit calorimeter[8]. They used it to determine the amount of carbon dioxide that was produced by metabolism of carbon-containing molecules and the amount of nitrogen that was produced from the nitrogen-containing amino acids. From the carbon and nitrogen that were produced they could calculate the amount of oxygen that was required to oxidize the carbon and nitrogen.

The excitement of their discovery is apparent in Voit's obituary written for Pettenkofer[9]:

> Imagine our [Pettenkofer and Voit] sensations as the picture of the remarkable processes of the metabolism unrolled before our eyes, and a mass of new facts became known to us! We found that in starvation protein and fat alone were burned, that during work more fat was burned, and that less fat was consumed during rest, especially during sleep; that the carnivorous dog could maintain himself on an exclusively protein diet, and if to such a protein diet fat were added, the fat was almost entirely deposited in the body; that carbohydrates, on the contrary, were burned no matter how much was given, and that they, like the fat of the food, protected the body from fat loss, although more carbohydrates than fat had to be given to effect this purpose; that the metabolism in the body was not proportional to the combustibility of the substances outside the body, but that protein, which burns with difficulty outside, metabolizes with the greatest ease, then carbohydrates, while fat, which readily burns outside, is with the most difficulty combustible in the organism.

What was still needed, however, was the simultaneous measurement of carbon, nitrogen, and oxygen balance. Pettenkoffer and Voit had only "calculated" the amount of oxygen; they had not directly measured it, a measurement that was still missing. Both Rubner and Atwater had been in Voit's laboratory as these early studies by Pettenkoffer were being conducted. The race was on between Rubner and Atwater to be the first to measure nitrogen catabolism, oxygen uptake, and carbon dioxide production simultaneously. It took more than twenty-five years.

In 1892 Wilbur Atwater (1849–1907) began to develop a respiration calorimeter in collaboration with a physicist named Rosa on the faculty with him at Wesleyan College[7]. They initially used an open-circuit system[7] and later used a closed-circuit design[10,11], the difference being whether the carbon dioxide was trapped or not. Between 1892 and 1904 twenty-two experiments on five subjects were completed. The respiration calorimeter designed by Atwater and Rosa was a room-size chamber in which subjects could live for one or more days (Figure 11-1)[7]. It was equipped with an airtight door, ventilation system, electricity, phone, and pass-through devices for entry of food and passage of excretory products. The system measured oxygen consumption, carbon dioxide production, air flow rates, and heat production. The precision of their instrument is shown by the fact that the recovery of carbon dioxide was 99.6%, the recovery of water was 100.6%, and the recovery of heat was 99.9%.

Atwater and Rosa[7] say the following about their apparatus:

> The apparatus has been devised and the methods of experimenting have been elaborated for use in inquiries upon the transformation of matter and energy in the living organism. The ultimate purpose is the study of some of the fundamental laws of animal nutrition. The more immediate object, however, has been the study of the transformations of energy. This especial study is desirable for two purposes. One is the demonstration, if such be possible, that the law of conservation of energy holds in the living organism. The other is the practical application of this law in gaining more definite knowledge of the ways in which the body is nourished and the value and use of food.

As Webb notes, "[T]he final triumph was Atwater's. Energy in food came out as energy in heat and work, and the First Law of Thermodynamics, that energy is conserved, was established in the human animal"[12]. Webb observes:

> There were several reasons for beginning with men rather than with domestic animals. The study of human nutrition is very important. In the earlier development of the work, when many difficulties were to be overcome, it was very desirable to have inside the apparatus an intelligent person who could make and record important observations during the experiment, rather than an animal whose movements, even, could not be controlled. Indeed, the most advantageous way to develop methods and apparatus for experiments with animals is through such preliminary experience with men. The results of the experience thus far gained are now being utilized in planning apparatus and methods to

> be used not only with small animals, as rabbits, sheep, and dogs, but also with larger animals, as horses, oxen, and cows.
>
> For practical purposes we are therefore warranted in assuming that the law (of conservation of energy) obtains in general in the living organism as indeed there is every reason *a priori* to believe that it must.

With the demonstration that measuring oxygen uptake and carbohydrate production by the body produced quantitatively similar data to measurements of heat loss, measurements of gas exchange, i.e., oxygen uptake and carbohydrate production, have largely replaced direct calorimetry.

Construction and operation of the respiration calorimeter at Wesleyan College was "big science." It was made possible by what is now derogatorily called "pork-barrel science." To further expand this idea of an interaction of big science and society, I have chosen Atwater's application of the calorimeter to the study of alcohol metabolism. This illustrates the use of scientific instruments in a politically sensitive context.

Among nutritional scientists, Atwater is remembered for his confirmation that the First Law of Thermodynamics applied to human beings. He is also remembered for his development of tables of food composition and for the relative energy value of macronutrients oxidized in the body. He showed that carbohydrates contain 4 kcal/g, protein 4 kcal/g, and fat 9 kcal/g. He also showed that alcohol had 7 kcal/g[11].

In the late nineteenth and early twentieth century, the "drink problem" associated with alcohol played an important role in society and politics. The fervor and emotion associated with the "drink problem" have largely disappeared, and examination of this period can be done in a less passionate way. The confrontation between science and society illustrated by the "drink problem" in the late nineteenth and early twentieth century provides an instructive perspective on a number of current issues where science, society, and politics collide. Some of these contemporary issues are nuclear power, abortion, smoking, biotechnology applied to food, gene therapy, radiation of food, politically correct speech, human immunodeficiency virus, and evolution versus creationism.

Emotional issues with public overtones are often galvanized by pronouncements from activists or zealots. In the temperance movement of the late nineteenth century, a number of women played this activist role. Among them was Mary Hunt, who served as one of the powerful voices against "drink." She was born in 1830 and grew up in Connecticut. In 1852 she married Leander Hunt, a Boston businessman, and devoted the next twenty years to raising her family[13]. Her active involvement in what came to be called the Temperance and Science Movement developed in the mid-1870s. Like most members of the temperance movement, she believed that alcohol was a poison and that it had no nutritional value. Moreover, she believed that these concepts should be conveyed to school children prior to maturity. Beginning in 1878 she developed a model curriculum on "Temperance and Science" for the Boston schools. Her effectiveness as a lobbyist and spokesperson, along with her family wealth, made her a leading activist in the temperance crusade. Gradually, in the 1880s, an instructional curriculum based on the concepts of temperance morality became part of the schools in all states.

In contrast to the activist role of zealots like Hunt, the scientific community, represented by a growing number of American physiologists, mostly trained in Europe, remained largely aloof during the early development of temperance science. Men of science were concerned with issues other than alcohol and the "drink problem." Gradually, however, their reluctance to become involved in the scientific side of issues affecting society lessened and led a period of activism. This was formalized when the "Committee of Fifty for the Investigation of the Liquor Problem" was organized in 1893. The chairman of the committee was John Shaw Billings, surgeon general of the U.S. Army. He surrounded himself with a distinguished group of American physiologists and scholars.

The initial approach of the Committee of Fifty to the physiological and behavioral effects of alcohol was to review and survey the literature. These reports are contained in the final report of the Committee of Fifty published in 1902[14]. At the time of their first report in 1896, the respiration calorimeter developed by Professors Atwater and Rosa at Wesleyan offered an opportunity to investigate the effects of alcohol directly. The results of these studies by Atwater and his colleagues were published in the report of the Committee of Fifty[15] and as a memoir of the National Academy of Sciences[11].

The setting was now in place for a confrontation between Wesleyan University, a Methodist school that was on record as opposing alcohol, a professor of chemistry at Wesleyan University who was scientifically investigating alcohol and its nutritional effects, and the temperance movement. In June 1899 Atwater first publicized his work at an open meeting to the public in Middletown, Connecticut. In attendance at the meeting was a correspondent for the Associated Press who had used an advance summary of the talk to alert the press in New York City. The next morning the newspapers ran headlines such as "Alcohol Does Work of Starchy Foods." The Methodist denomination was up in arms. This notoriety began to shift the "drink problem" from a debate about the truth and weight of expert opinions to the drama of the conclusions from experimentation on alcohol itself.

From his studies, Atwater drew a number of conclusions about alcohol in the body. He found that more than 98 percent of the ingested alcohol was absorbed and oxidized in the body. The presence of alcohol in moderate amounts tended to increase very slightly the availability of other nutrients in the diet, especially proteins. He also found that alcohol was more completely absorbed than other nutrients in the ordinary mixed diet. The laws of conservation of energy applied to the metabolism of alcohol in the diet just as they did for other components of an ordinary diet. The potential energy of alcohol oxidized in the body was transformed completely into kinetic energy that appeared as heat, muscular work, or both. Finally, alcohol appeared to protect body fat by serving as a substrate for oxidation, but its effects in sparing body protein were somewhat more variable. The calories from alcohol may play a role in the bulge that we are battling.

The outpouring of hostility toward a Methodist university that was supporting a professor of chemistry who showed that alcohol behaved as a nutrient posed a major problem for the university and for Atwater. Beginning in 1900 Atwater began to defend his work vigorously to the public[16–18]. In his paper on temperance reform, Atwater noted that "the laws of nearly all our States require that the curricula of our public schools shall include the physiology with special reference to the action of alcoholic beverages." He goes on to quote from one of the commonly used school textbooks to point out its distortions: "If...you take into your stomach a little alcohol, it receives no welcome. Nature treats it as a poison. Every organ of elimination, all of the scavengers of the body...at once set to work to throw off the enemy." Yet this was contradicted by Atwater's own studies. Elimination of these erroneous ideas from educational materials was the goal of the Committee of Fifty. As Atwater notes, "These statements are misrepresentations. They belong to a kind of doctrine which pervades much of the...common temperance instruction," not only in the public schools, but also in the Sunday school and even in the pulpit. "The general character of the teaching is more or less opposed to scientific fact"[16–18].

With the direct focus on experimentation, one high-water mark for the temperance movement had been reached. In the ten years from 1889, when temperance science had appeared in all of the school textbooks, the physiologists had been galvanized to bring scientific fact to bear on an issue of public concern. In spite of these efforts by the physiologists, the momentum of the temperance movement continued and a Constitutional amendment forbidding the consumption of alcohol was passed in 1919. This dark day in American history was eventually undone, but the interval between the rise of the temperance movement and the amendment's repeal was nearly fifty years. However, the elimination of "temperance science" was an important step toward truth and was given a solid scientific impetus by the work of Atwater.

Biosketch

Hermann von Helmholtz (1821–1894) (Figure 11-2) was among the masters of medicine in the second half of the nineteenth century[19, 20]. He was preeminent in the physics related to optics and sound and is responsible for articulation of the Law of Conservation of Energy. von Helmholtz was born in Potsdam and educated as a surgeon for the Prussian army. While studying in Berlin, he came under the influence of Johannes Müller, M.D., professor of physiology, and the influence this man had on a whole generation of German physician-scientists. His inaugural dissertation dealt with the origin of nerve fibers from leeches and crabs that he had studied with a rudimentary compound microscope. While serving in the army he published in 1847 his first masterpiece on the conservation of energy *(Ueber die Erhaltung der Kraft)*. His academic appointments included professor of physiology and pathology at the University of Königsberg (1849–1855), professor of physiology and anatomy at the University of Bonn (1855–1858), professor of physiology at the University of Heidelberg (1858–1871), and professor of physics at the University of Berlin (1871–1894). Among his scientific contributions is the observation that muscle is the major source of animal heat (1848), the measurement of the velocity of the nervous impulse (1850–1852), and the invention of the ophthalmoscope (1851): His two other great works were his *Handbook of Physiological Optics* published in 1856–1867 and his acoustical masterpiece *Der Tonenfindungen* (1863). Although his contributions to physical medicine were extraordinary, he never forgot he was a physician. He once said, "Medicine was once the intellectual home in which I grew up; and even the emigrant best understands and is best understood by his native land"[21].

What matter titled? Helmholtz is a name
That challenges alone the award of fame!
When Emperors, Kings, Pretenders, shadows all,
Leave not a dust-trace on our swirling ball,
Thy work, oh grave-eyed searcher, shall endure,
Unmarred by faction, from low passion pure.

Biosketch

Max Josef von Pettenkofer (1818–1901) was intimately involved in the biomedical revolution in Germany in the mid-nineteenth century (Figure 11-3). He was born December 3, 1818, in Lichtenheim, about thirty miles north of Munich. He was the fifth of eight children in a farming family. At age eight, Pettenkofer moved to Munich where he lived with his uncle, who was court apothecary to Ludwig I of Bavaria. This is no doubt where the young Petterkofer developed his interest in medicine. He excelled at Greek and Latin in his high school *(Gymnasium)* and entered the University of Munich. He completed his training in medicine and in 1843 qualified with distinction in pharmacy, medicine and surgery. His professional career divides into three parts. The part dealing with metabolic studies was conducted with his student Carl Voit. The studies were initiated by a gift from the crown to build a human respiration chamber. His most significant studies were to show that protein breakdown did not increase with strenuous exercise. The second part of his career was marked by his interest in the design of buildings. Among other things he studied the ventilation of buildings. The final part of his career as professor of hygiene was devoted to studies on the epidemiology of cholera and typhoid fever[22].

Biosketch

Max Rubner (1854–1932) was one of the leading students of energy expenditure in the nineteenth century (Figure 11-4). One of Rubner's major intellectual accomplishments was the recognition that resting energy expenditure was proportional to the surface area of the body. In 1885 Rubner became professor of hygiene at Marburg University, where he constructed his own calorimeter in 1889. It was with this chamber that he demonstrated that the Law of Conservation of Energy or the First Law of Thermodynamics applied to experimental animals. In 1891 he followed Robert Koch as professor of hygiene in Berlin, where he subsequently became professor of physiology in 1909. In his eulogy in 1932 Graham Lusk said:

> Great men are very rare. They are worth knowing. They give impulse and stimulus to lesser men. They make the world more worthwhile for others to live in because of their presence in it. Max Rubner was the greatest man I ever knew[23].

Biosketch

Wilbur Olin Atwater (1849–1907) (Figure 11-5) was the son of a Methodist minister. He began his collegiate education at the University of Vermont but transferred to the Methodist-dominated Wesleyan University in Middletown, Connecticut, where he graduated in 1865. He earned his Ph.D. four years later from the Sheffield Scientific School at Yale University. Following two years of study at German universities in Leipzig and Berlin, Atwater returned to begin an academic career in the United States. After two initial appointments, he was recruited in 1873 to be professor of chemistry at his alma mater, Wesleyan University. He remained there until his death in 1907[24,25].

The first agricultural experiment station was established at Wesleyan College in 1875 as the result of two activities, effective lobbying by Atwater and Professor Johnson, his former instructor at Yale, and a contribution of one thousand dollars from Orange Judd, a wealthy philanthropist from

Hartford, Connecticut. Two years later, due to lobbying by Yale University, the scientific station was moved to Yale University under the direction of Professor Johnson. Following the lead of Connecticut, the federal government, through the Hatch Act of 1887, established the USDA Office of Experiment Stations. Funds for Connecticut were allocated between Yale University and a newly established Agricultural College at Storrs, Connecticut. Although forty miles from Wesleyan University, Atwater served as director of the program at Storrs while remaining professor of chemistry at Wesleyan. The studies on research with fertilizers and crops were gradually moved to the new agricultural experiment station, where Professor Atwater maintained research direction of this program over the next fourteen years. However, his interest shifted slowly from agricultural nutrition to human nutrition and energy expenditure.

Interest in energy expenditure had been reignited by a tour of Europe in 1882 and 1883. During the nineteenth century, Munich was a leading center for studies in nutritional science. Professor Justus von Liebig, one of the giants of nutrition and agriculture in the first half of the nineteenth century, eventually became a professor at the University of Munich. The University of Munich also counted Carl von Voit as professor of physiology and Max-Joseph Pettenkofer as professor of hygiene. As Kirkland says, "[F]or the devout nutritionist, Munich became a sort of Mecca"[26].

With his background in nutrition and his political skills in raising money, Atwater launched "big science" at Wesleyan College. At the physiological institute in Munich in 1882–83, Atwater had seen the respiration calorimeter invented by Professor Pettenkofer. With the availability of new funds from the state of Connecticut after 1887, Professor Atwater and E.B. Rosa, a new professor of physics, started to build a respiration calorimeter in 1892. The construction and operation costs were more than ten thousand dollars per year, a figure that exceeded the salary of a professor at Wesleyan by more than fivefold.

Following its construction, this singularly valuable instrument was put into operation by Atwater and Rosa. Its first subject was a twenty-nine-year-old Swede who was a laboratory janitor[7]. In 1893 support for these studies was provided by initial funding for human nutrition research from the U.S. Congress. In the hundred years since that time, human nutrition research centers supported by the Department of Agriculture have expanded greatly and are now located in Beltsville, Maryland; Boston; Houston; Grand Forks, North Dakota; Ames, Iowa; and San Francisco. The number of respiration calorimeters for the measurement of energy expenditure by respiratory gas exchange has mushroomed in the past twenty years[27–29].

References

1. Sarton G. *Sarton on the History of Science.* Cambridge: Harvard University Press; 1962.
2. Crawford A. *Experiments and observations on animal heat, and the inflammation of combustible bodies; being an attempt to resolve these phenomena into a general law of nature.* 2nd edition. London: J. Johnson; 1788.
3. Brownell P. *An inaugural dissertation on animal heat.* New York: I Riggs; 1814.
4. Mayer JR von. "Remarks on the forces of inorganic nature." *The London, Edinburgh, and Dublin Philosophical Magazine and Journal of Science.* 1862;24:371-377.
5. Helmholtz, HLF von. *Ueber die Erhaltung der Kraft, eine physikalische Abhandlung.* Berlin: G. Reimer; 1847.
6. Rubner M. "Die Quelle der Thierschen warme." Z *Biol.* 1894;30:73-142.
7. Atwater WO, Rosa EB. "Description of a new respiration calorimeter and experiments on the conservation of energy in the human body." US Department of Agriculture Office of Experimental Stations. 1899:63.
8. Pettenkofer M, Voit C. "Untersuchungen über den Stoffverbrauch des normalen Menschen." Z *Biol.* 1866;2:478-573.
9. Lusk G. "A respiration calorimeter for the study of disease." *Arch Intern Med.* 1915; 15:793-804.
10. Atwater WO, Benedict FG. *A respiration calorimeter with appliances for the direct determination of oxygen.* Washington, DC: Carnegie Institution of Washington; 1905. Publication No. 42.
11. Atwater WO, Benedict FG. An experimental inquiry regarding the nutritive value of alcohol. *Memoirs of the National Academy of Sciences.* 1902;8:235-272.
12. Webb P. *Human Calorimeter-Endocrinology and Metabolism Series.* No. 7. New York: Prager; 1985.
13. Pauly J. "The struggle for ignorance about alcohol: American physiologists, Wilber Olin Atwater and the Woman's Christian Temperance Union." *Bull Hist Med.* 1990;64:366-392.
14. Committee of Fifty. *Report of the Sub-Committee on the Physiological and Pathological Aspects of the Drink Problem.* 1903;2:11-13, 175-347
15. Billings JS, Atwater WO, Bowditch MP, Chittenden RH, Welch WH. "Report of the Sub-Committee on the Physiological and Pathological Aspects of the Drink Problem. Presented to the Committee of Fifty." 1903;I:xi-xxii.
16. Atwater WO. "Alcohol physiology and temperance reform." *Harper's* 1900;100:850-858.
17. Atwater WO. "False and true teaching in our schools concerning alcohol." *J Soc Sci.* 1909;37:107-116.

18. Atwater WO. "Alcohol physiology and superintendence." *Educ Rev.* 1900;20:1-29.
19. Helmholtz, H. von. *Über die Erhaltung der Kraft, ein physikalische Abhandlung, vorgetragen in der Sitzung der physicalischen Gesellschaft zu Berlin am 23sten Juli 1847.* Berlin: G. Reimer, 1847.
20. Helmholtz, H. von *Beschreibung eines Augen-spiegels zur Untersuchung der Netzhaut im lebenden Auge.* Berlin: A. Forstner'sche Verlagsbuchhandlung, 1851..
21. Helmholtz, H. von *Die Lehre von den Tonempfindungen als physiologische Grundlage fur die Theorie der Musik.* Braunschweig: Friedrich Vieweg und Sohn, 1863.
22. Trout DL. "Max Josef von Petternkofer (1818-1901). A biographical sketch." *J Nutr.* 1977;107:1569-1574.
23. Chambers WH. "Max Rubner." *J Nutr.* 1952;48:1-12.
24. Maynard LA, "Wilbur O. Atwater—A biographical sketch." *J Nutr.* 1962;78:3-952.
25. Potts DB. *Wesleyan University 1831-1910 Collegiate Enterprise in New England.* New Haven: Yale University Press; 1992.
26. Kirkland EC. "'Scientific eating': New Englanders prepare and promote a reform." *Proceedings of the Massachusetts Historical Society.* 1974;86:28-52.
27. Schutz Y, Jequier E. Resting energy expenditure, thermic effect of food, and total energy expenditure. *Handbook of Obesity: Etiology and Pathophysiology.* GA Bray and C Bouchard (eds). New York: Marcel Dekker, 1994.
28. McLean J.A. and G. Tobin. *Animal and Human Calorimetry.* Cambridge: Cambridge University Press, 1987.
29. DeLany J.P., G.A. Bray, D.W. Harsha and J. Volaufova. "Energy expenditure in preadolescent African American and white boys and girls: The Baton Rouge Children's Study." *Am J Clin Nutr.* 75:705-713, 2002.

Special thanks to the LSU Middleton Library and the Pennington Center Information Center for help in acquiring the Atwater selections.

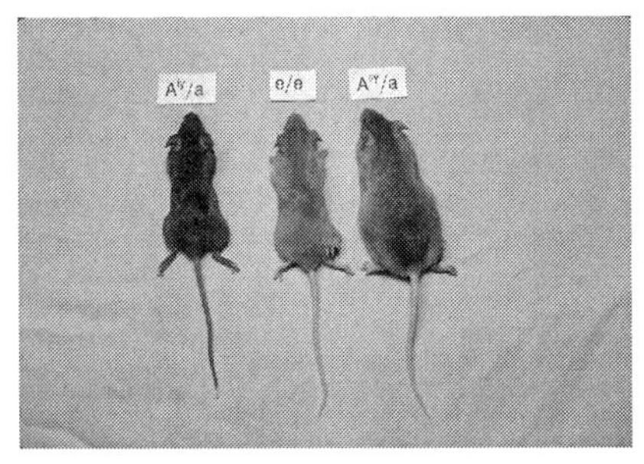

8-1

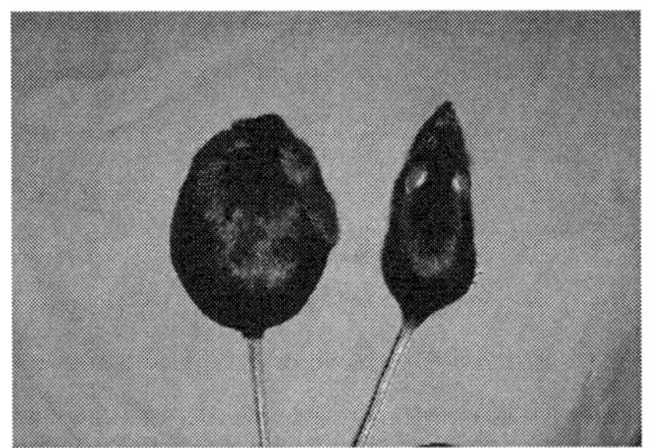

8-2

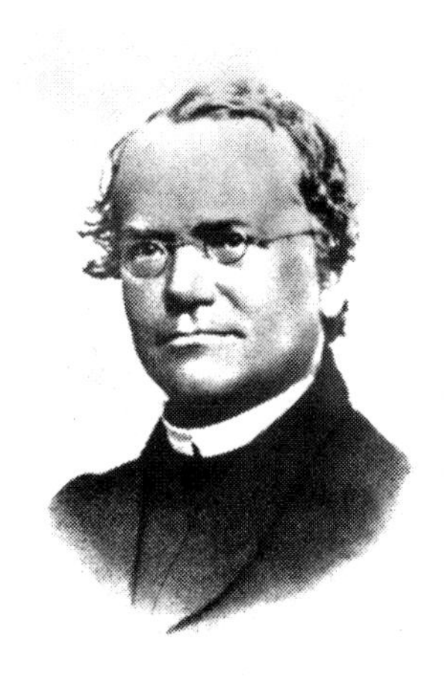

8-4

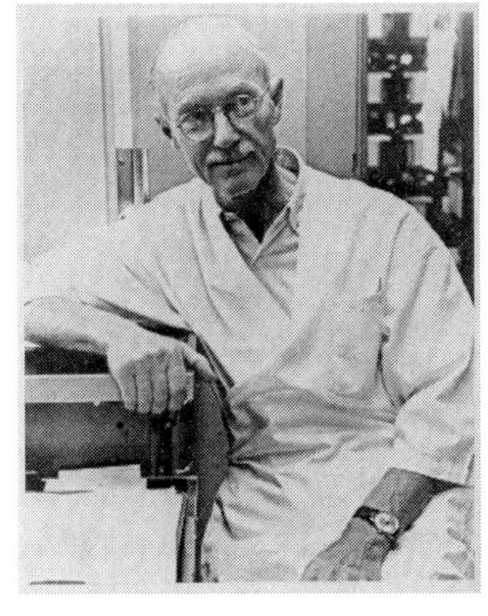

8-5

8-1 The Yellow Mouse is a dominantly inherited type of fat animal that is both large and fat. The genetic defect produces a yellow coat color and increased food intake. A^y/a indicates a yellow mouse; A/a indicates a black mouse; and Av^y/a indicates a fat yellow mouse. © George A. Bray, MD.

8-2 The obese (ob/ob) mouse is a recessively inherited type of fat animal. In contrast to the yellow mouse, the obese mouse is stunted in its growth in addition to being very fat and diabetic. This animal is deficient in leptin. When treated with leptin, food intake declines and the animal returns to normal proportions. © 2006 George A. Bray, MD.

8-4 Gregor Mendel (1822-1884). Courtesy of the National Library of Medicine.

8-5 George Davis Snell (1903-1996). Courtesy of the National Library of Medicine.

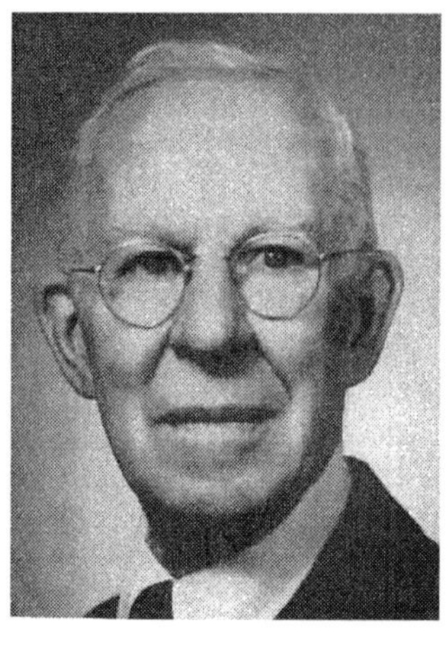

8-6

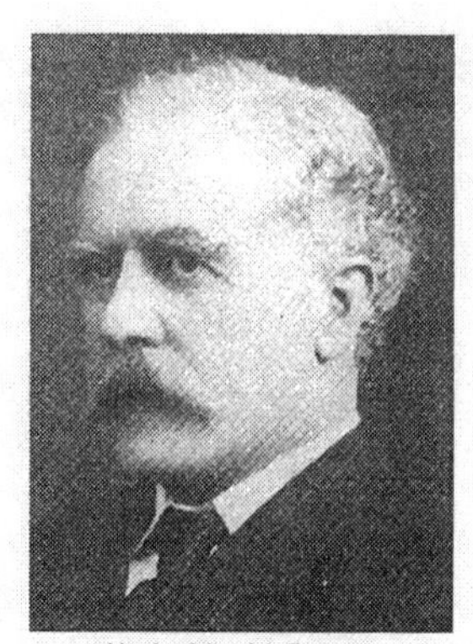

9-1

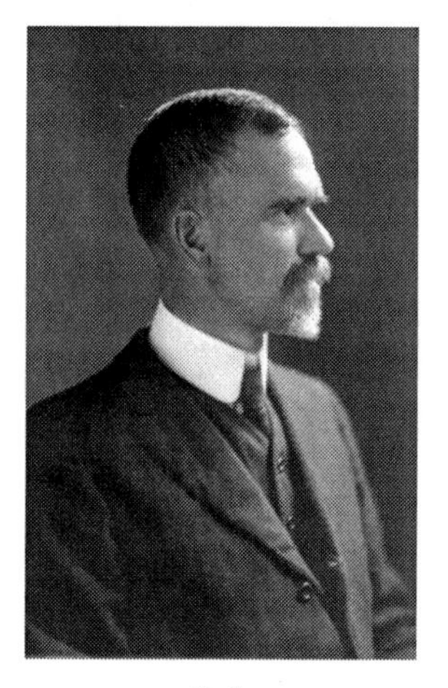

9-2

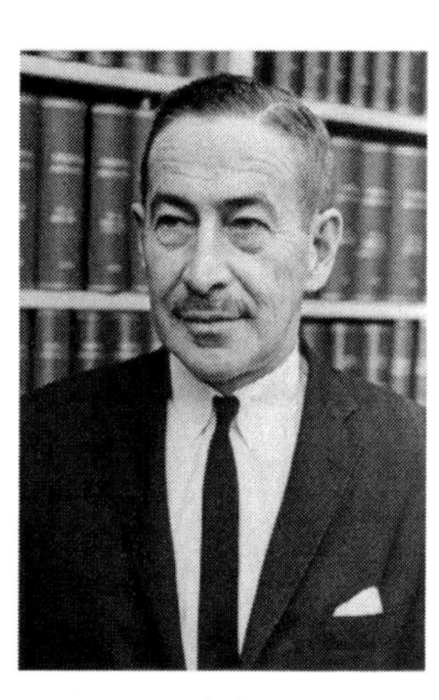

9-3

8-6 Charles Haskell Danforth (1883-1969). Courtesy of the National Library of Medicine.

9-1 Sir Archibald Edward Garrod (1857-1936). Reprinted with permission from Elsevier (*The Lancet*, April 4, 1936, p. 807).

9-2 Charles Benedict Davenport (1866-1944). Courtesy of the National Library of Medicine.

9-3 Edwin Bennett Astwood (1908-1976). Courtesy of the National Library of Medicine.

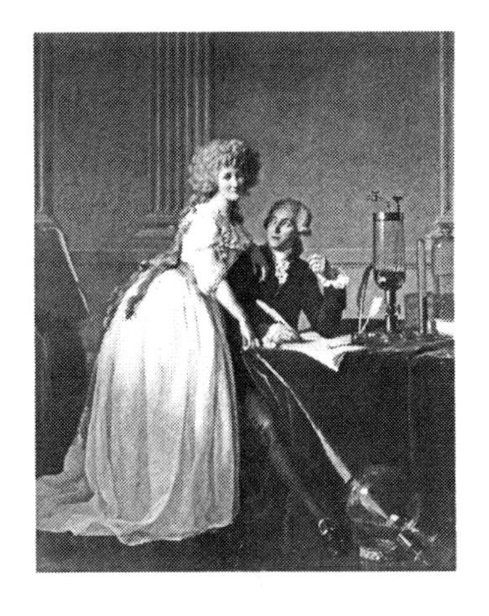

10-2

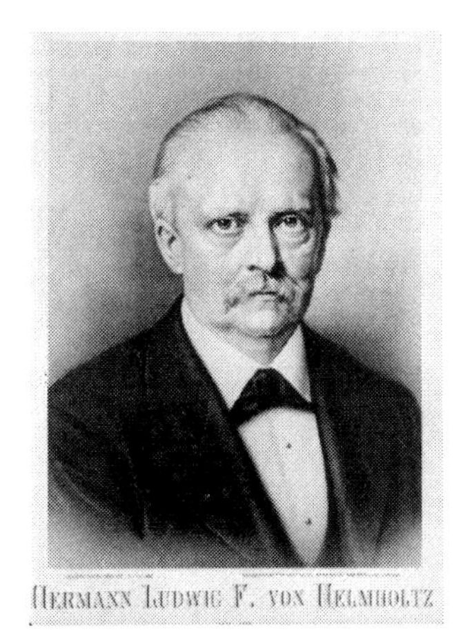

11-2

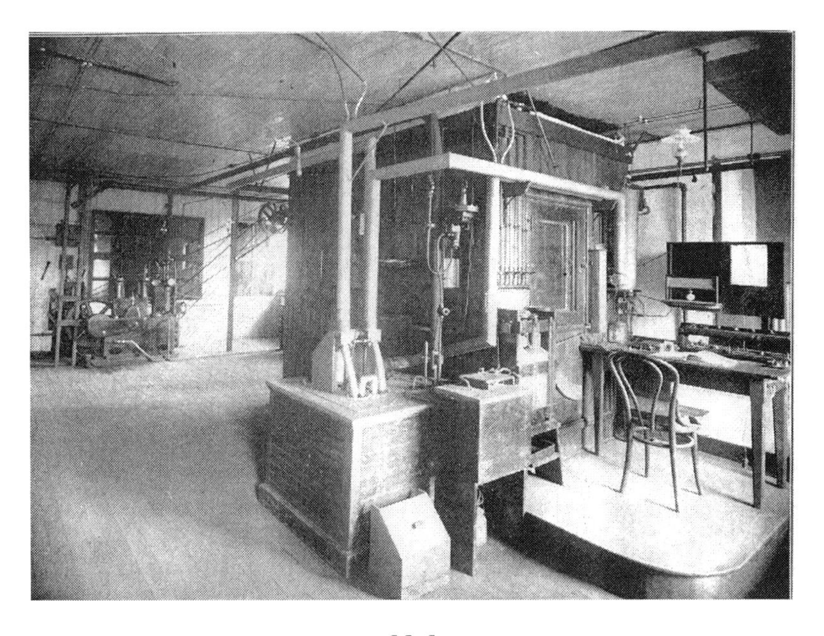

11-1

10-2 Antoine-Laurent Lavoisier (1743-1794). Courtesy of the National Library of Medicine.

11-1 Picture of the metabolic chamber developed by W.O. Atwater in which the energy expenditure of human beings could be measured. From the collection of the author.

11-2 Hermann von Helmholtz (1821-1894). Courtesy of the National Library of Medicine.

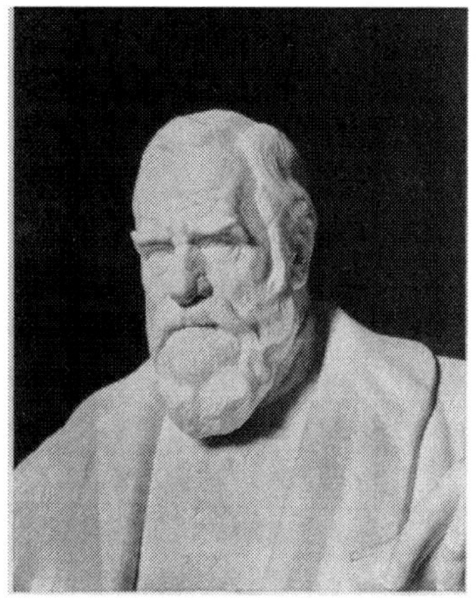

11-3

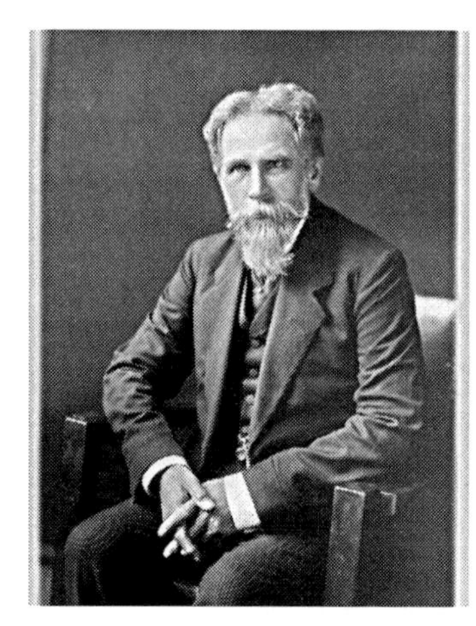

11-4

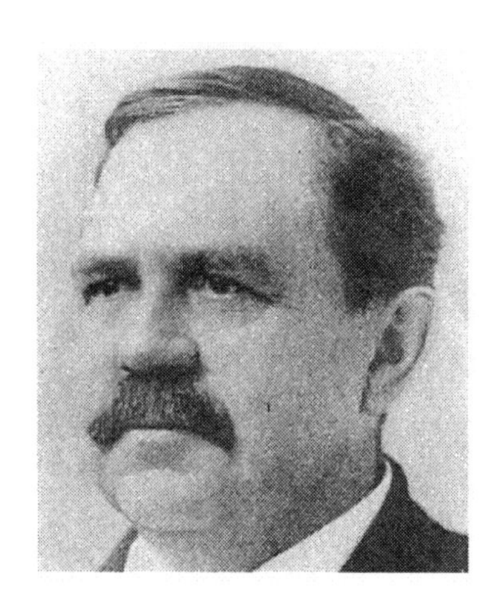

11-5

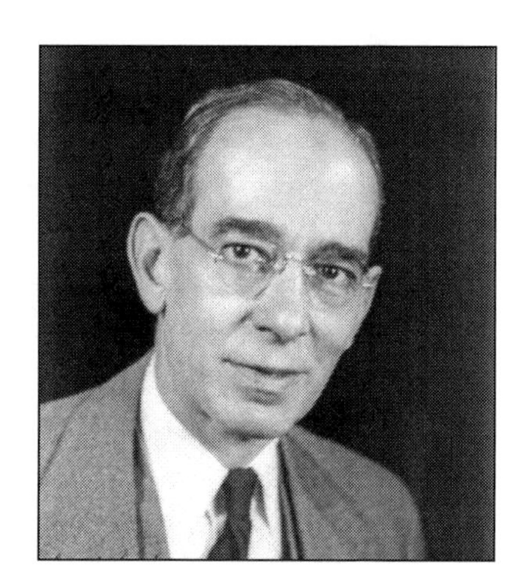

12-2

11-3 Max Josef Pettenkoffer (1818-1901). Courtesy of the National Library of Medicine.

11-4 Max Rubner (1854-1932). Courtesy of the National Library of Medicine.

11-5 Wilbur Olin Atwater (1849-1907). Courtesy of Special Collections, National Agricultural Library.

12-2 Louis Harry Newburgh (1883-1956). Courtesy of the National Library of Medicine.

Chapter 12

Can We Burn Off Unwanted Calories?

The important thing is to make the lesson of each case tell on your education. The value of experience is not in seeing much, but in seeing wisely.

—Sir William Osler[1]

Wouldn't it be wonderful if we could eat what we wanted and burn off what we didn't use rather than storing it as fat? This would turn the tide in the battle of the bulge more surely than anything else we have. This idea has surfaced periodically in scientific and popular publications. Each winter when people are looking forward to the summer, a new burst of enthusiasm for conquering the bulge reappears, and with it many ideas about ways to do this. Burning or getting rid of unwanted calories so we can eat all we want is always part of what we are offered. Is there any truth to this idea? Well, it has staying power—meaning it has reappeared from time to time over more than two hundred years. This is the story of three scientists who contributed to this study. It is also the story of how individual subjects can be used to help learn the truth. In two of these cases the subject was the scientist himself.

The German word *Luxuskonsumption* was coined early in the twentieth century to describe the idea that we could eat all we wanted and not get fat. With *luxuskonsumption* the body simply burns off the excess calories—a desire devoutly to be wished by anyone who is battling the bulge. However, this concept seems to fly in the face of the laws of conservation of mass and energy so painstakingly put together during the nineteenth century (see chapters 10 and 11). The work on the conservation of matter and energy in the middle of the nineteenth century by Mayer[2] and Helmholtz[3] had been well accepted. They showed that energy could be converted from one form (heat) to another, but that it did not vanish. The possibility that human beings might defy this law of nature by being more or less efficient was not so easily accepted. Indeed, it has been a recurring research theme during much of the twentieth century.

Three papers that are printed in the appendix deal with this important subject. The set includes two early papers, suggesting that there may be a form of *luxuskonsumption* (i.e., increased heat dissipation with increased food intake) and a third paper arguing that this does not exist. Each of the three papers is based on the study of a single case, yet the authors reach opposite conclusions. The question I am asking is, which author learned most wisely from his case?

Rudolf Otto Neumann was a careful scientist[4]. He was interested in the protein requirements of human beings because of the wide range of values that had been proposed as adequate for human nutrition. At one extreme were the recommendations that working men needed 118 g of protein per day. At the other extreme, Neumann noted data suggesting that as low as 30 g per day (g/d) was adequate, a finding that was supported by a number of other investigators who claimed 44.7 g/d, 41.7 g/d, 36.2 g/d, 34.7 g/d, or as low as 20.3 g/d. At the other end investigators reported the need for 64 g/d, or 79.8 g/d, or 83 g/d as adequate amounts of protein for the human body (see Reference 4 for details about the authors who made these claims).

What was the truth of protein needs? How much protein do we need?

Neumann set out to answer this question using himself as a subject. The use of oneself as a guinea pig for scientific experiments is well known in the field of human clinical investigation. To examine protein requirements and, interestingly, his weight stability, Neumann carried out three experiments on himself, in which his nitrogen intake was 15, 14.3, and 11.3 g per day (equivalent to 93.75 g, 89.38 g, and 70.625 g of protein per day). To put this into the context in the United States, recommended intakes of protein are about 50 g/d for women and 65 g/d for men. The ratio of fat to carbohydrate in these diets varied widely from a low of about one-third (36.7%) to a high of nearly two thirds (64.2%). These details aside, the changes in Neumann's weight are the central issue from our perspective in this history of the battle of the bulge. Could his weight stay constant with a wide range of energy and protein intakes? In the first two experiments his weight was stable at 67 kg (147.4 lb.) but rose to 70 kg (154 lb.) in the final experiment. Neumann concluded that the quantity of protein required for nitrogen equilibrium was substantially below what had been proposed and that weight stability can occur over a wide range of dietary intakes. It is this latter finding that led to the proposal of *luxuskonsumption*. Neumann had maintained a stable weight although his intake of protein and carbohydrate had changed widely. Grafe summarized Neumann's studies as follows:

> No differences in weight or well-being appeared regardless of whether he ate a daily diet of 1,760, 2,199 or 2,403

> calories. Neumann concludes from this that the human organism has the ability to get by on an insignificant intake of nutrients and that he can also set himself in balance with a more than sufficient diet because *luxuskonsumption* becomes apparent in the organism[5].

The idea of *luxuskonsumption* received a further boost from the next case study by Gulick[6]. Here again the investigator was the subject. He studied himself over several years of careful feeding and recording of his body weight. Two effects of food intake could be distinguished[7,8]. The first is the thermic effect of food, that is, the rise in oxygen consumption following ingestion of protein, carbohydrate, and to a lesser extent fat. This had been observed initially more than one hundred years earlier by Lavoisier in his pioneering studies. The second change is a stimulus to oxidation of food from the "plethora" of nitrogenous products in cell fluids[7]. To quote from Gulick, "To Rubner [a famous nineteenth century student of nutrition] this effect shows itself as a cumulative increase in the specific dynamic effect of heavy protein meals when they are administered on a series of days"[6]. To examine this question of change in the intake of protein in detail, Gulick carried out a set of careful feeding tests on himself in 1916 and 1917. Body composition was not measured nor was the energy content of his meals directly determined by precise methods such as bomb calorimetry. Fecal samples, however, were measured in one series of studies and showed that the dry weight was not affected by substantial changes in food intake. Gulick's energy intake during the periods of his studies varied from a low of 2725 calories per day to a high value of 3965 calories per day. Gulick concluded from his studies that "the prolonged diet has not raised the basal metabolic rate above the normal average." His highest period of caloric intake was 4115 calories per day and his lowest was 1874 calories per day, yet his body weight showed little change. He felt that the extravagance of calories at the high intake *(luxuskonsumption)* must be searched for elsewhere than in basal metabolism. This search for *luxuskonsumption* has occupied a greater deal of research time during the twentieth century.

Thirty years intervened between the study by Gulick and what was thought to be the "definitive" study. Methods for measuring human energy balance had continued to improve[9]. The observations of Gulick and those of Neumann seemed to violate the First Law of Thermodynamics[2, 3] that Atwater (see Chapter 11) found using room-size calorimeters in which human beings lived for several days[7, 10]. With the development of a new method for determining heat production over longer periods of time, the important question of *luxuskonsumption* was ripe for reexamination[9, 11]. The technique used here consisted of measuring heat production by determining insensible weight loss. With this technique, the loss of water through the lungs and skin is used to measure energy expenditure[10]. The energy cost of converting water to water vapor so it can evaporate was already known. It was this technique that Santorio pioneered at the beginning of the seventeenth century (see Chapter 4). By measuring the quantity of water lost in the expired air, the energy of insensible water loss could be calculated. When compared to energy expenditure in a calorimeter, insensible loss represented 24% of total energy expenditure. In a methodological study Newburgh fed eight normal individuals as nearly as possible a maintenance diet. The twenty-four-hour insensible weight loss was repeatedly measured and the average value for the insensible water calculated from it by subtracting the difference between the weights of the excreted carbon dioxide and absorbed oxygen. The heat removed by this water vapor was close to 24% of total heat production[11].

By the time Newburgh began his studies on *luxuskonsumption*, it was clearly established that prolonged starvation reduces basal metabolism and that a reduction in caloric intake short of starvation also produces a reduction in energy required to maintain weight in normal subjects. When men who habitually ate 3200 to 3600 kcal/day were reduced to eating a diet with 1400 kcal/d for three weeks their average body weight fell by 12% and their basal metabolism declined by 18%[12]. Of interest, these men were now able to maintain their new lower weight with an intake of only 1950 kcal/day. However, their basal metabolism remained low. This is similar to the more modern observations of Leibel and Hirsch on the reduced energy requirements for weight maintenance of previously obese subjects[13] and their data on systematic weight reduction of body weight in lean and obese subjects[14].

To study the question of whether *luxuskonsumption* exists, Wiley and Newburgh overfed a single subject who believed he remained lean because he oxidized all of the food taken into his body without regard to quantity. Using insensible water loss to measure energy expenditure, they found a slight increase in both basal and total metabolism on the overfeeding diet. This increase was entirely attributable to the increase in surface area plus the extra specific dynamic effect of the overfeeding diet. Moreover the subject gained the expected amount of weight when he took in food in excess of his habitual desire. Wiley and Newburgh thus concluded, "Clearly the body weight is affected on the one hand by the individual metabolic requirement and on the other hand by the total intake of energy. Evidently the mechanism, commonly called 'appetite,' functions to maintain a balance between the supply and demand"[9].

In spite of this clear and well-done study of a single subject, the issue of *luxuskonsumption* did not go away. It was revived in a particularly forceful manner by two studies: the first by Miller and colleagues[15, 16] and the second by Sims, et al.[17].

In spite of this definitive work in the first half of the twentieth century by Wiley and Newburgh[9], the issue of *luxuskonsumption* continued to raise its head in the second half of the twentieth century. Prior to the experiments of Miller and Mumford in 1963 and 1964, only three studies with humans had examined overfeeding, in contrast to the substantial literature on reduction in caloric intake[18]. As Miller and Mumford point out, "in animal husbandry it is recognized that animals fed isocaloric amounts of different diets do not necessarily gain equal weight"[15]. To examine whether this was true in human subjects the authors carried out the first experiment on themselves. They ate a diet with 2.8% of calories from protein with an additional 890 and 480 kcal/day respectively above their usual intake, followed by a second experiment on eight student volunteers who ate an additional 1330 kcal/day for four weeks and six subsequent students who volunteered to eat an additional 1530 kcal/day with diets containing either 2.8% or 14.9% of calories from protein. In the first experiment the overall weight gains were 1.3 and 1.2 kg, far short of the calculated 6.2 and 3.3 kg if all of the excess calories (37,300 and 20,100 kcal) had been converted to fat containing 66% triglyceride. Limitations in the measurements of body composition in the first experiment led to the additional two experiments. In the second experiment the excess caloric consumption was 35,000 kcal per person over the whole study. The low protein group gained only 0.9 kg compared to 3.7 kg in the high-protein diet. The calculated weight gains if the excess energy had been converted to adipose tissue with 66% triglyceride would be 5.9 kg per person. This led Miller and Mumford, his wife, to conclude that, "In our view, these results are direct evidence of *luxuskonsumption*"[15].

Miller and Mumford[15] suggest four possible explanations for their results: (1) increased activity, 2) reduced digestibility, (3) changes in body composition, or (4) increased heat production. Using pedometers to measure activity showed no change, but the authors did not examine the energy cost of carrying the extra weight. Other studies examined overeating and the efficiency of energy utilization coupled to external work. Whipp et al. showed that gaining weight following overeating did not alter the metabolic efficiency of muscular work[19]. However, more energy was needed to move the heavier body[20]. Measurements of the digestibility of food by Miller and Mumford[15] and by others[6] have shown no alterations with overfeeding. Changes in body composition measured as total body potassium, of nitrogen balance, and of urinary creatinine excretion do not appear to account for the difference in energy storage. The authors thus concluded that increased heat production (*luxuskonsumption*) must be the mechanism.

Their paper did not discuss the possibility that increased energy cost of nutrient storage could account for the changes. The traditional energy values assigned to fat, carbohydrate, and protein are 9 kcal/g, 4 kcal/g, and 4 kcal/g respectively. This is entirely fair when fat, carbohydrate, and protein are being metabolized by the body for "energy." In looking at the energy cost of weight gain, on the other hand, Donato and Hegsted[21] found that the energy cost for storing protein and carbohydrates was approximately 25%, and for fat approximately 10%. Thus corrected caloric values need to be used for estimating energy storage. In a subsequent paper, Miller et al.[16] concluded that "subjects who are overeating could convert their excessive caloric intake simply into heat and this paper provides evidence for the existence of this phenomenon." Within a few short years brown adipose tissue was suggested as one site for this process[22].

The next important contribution to the study of *luxuskonsumption* used a most unusual group of subjects. The Vermont study was organized and carried out by Ethan Sims and his colleagues. They were interested in the endocrine and metabolic effects that are produced when obesity is self-induced by overeating in men[17]. For subjects they needed individuals who would volunteer to gain 25% of their body weight and who were relatively confined. For inmates in the Vermont Penal system it was a win-win situation. They got good food and the investigators got good subjects. In this study, the authors noted that:

> there are marked differences in the ability of normal individuals to gain weight by taking calories in excess of those required for maintenance, that when weight is gained by (normal) subjects by increasing the intake of fat alone there is a higher proportion of weight gained to calories ingested and the weight gained may be maintained by an intake no greater than that required to maintain initial weight. Normal subjects fattened by eating a mixed diet required more calories in relation to their body surface for maintenance of the obese state than they require when at their natural weight and also more calories than the spontaneously obese generally require[17].

The studies of Miller et al. and of Sims and colleagues both cried out for a more precise measurements of energy expenditure and energy intake. Several such studies have now been done and some of them are summarized by Gilbert Forbes et al.[23]. The degree of weight gain and the extent of overfeeding shows a linear relationship for both males and females[24, 25]. The differences are accounted for by differences in the energy cost of storage, the increased energy cost for moving the body and by differences in the metabolic pathways through which ingested nutrients are metabolized. Supporting the conclusions of Forbes et al. are the studies of Claude Bouchard et al.[26] on identical twins in the last decade of the twentieth century. They showed a high degree of correlation in weight gain in total fat and in visceral fat within individual pairs of twins but a significant difference between pairs of twins. They attributed this to differences in metabolic channeling between subjects[26]. Such a change may well reflect the increased energy expenditure observed during overfeeding of lean and obese subjects by Leibel et al.[14], which might be accounted for by increased activity of the sympathetic nervous system that modulates, to variable degrees, the nutrient partitioning between carbohydrate storage and metabolism and protein storage and catabolism with fat storage being the pathway consuming the residual surplus energy.

The most recent study of *luxuskonsumption* used doubly labeled water to measure the energy expenditure of the volunteers that were overfed. As has often been the case before, they found a residual discrepancy in energy calculations that they attributed to non-exercise activity thermogenesis or NEAT[27]. We will await the next chapter in this ongoing saga of *luxuskonsumption*. But how do we make the three cases tell on our education, as Osler suggested they should? The answer is relatively simple: Analyze the data carefully. Neumann[4] and Gulick[6] concluded that the changes in calories did not produce the expected weight change. However, when Forbes replotted their data (Figure 12-1), both studies showed linear changes between calorie intake and weight change. As Forbes concluded, "The rather precise nature of the response...is a reminder of the central role of energy intake in weight homeostasis"[23]. To paraphrase Osler[1], Neumann and Gulick had seen much, but not wisely. Wiley and Newburgh, on the other hand, had seen wisely. Let us be among those who also see wisely.

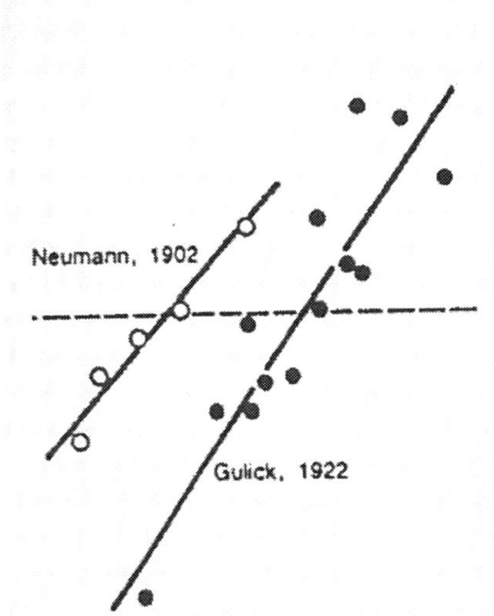

Figure 12-1: Relationship of food intake to changes in weight from two studies that claimed that individuals could maintain steady weight while "overeating." Note that in both cases there was a linear relationship between the small change in weight and the food intake indicating that if we overeat for an extended period the human body will store the extra energy as extra weight.

12-1 Plots weight change (g/day) against energy intake for Neumann's data (4) and for Gulick's data (6). Calculated regression line for the former is y = -230 + 0.109X, r = 0.969 and for the latter it is y = -430 + 0.140X, r = 0.902. [Reprinted from the American Society of Clinical Nutrition (23)].

Biosketch

Louis Harry Newburgh (1883–1956) was described by A. McGehee Harvey as "the compleat clinical investigator with a passion for measurement"[28]. Newburgh was born on June 17, 1883, in Cincinnati, Ohio (Figure 12-2). He received his A.B. degree from Harvard University in 1904 and his M.D. from Harvard Medical School in 1908. Upon completing a sixteen-month internship and a period of study at the Allgemeines Krankenhaus in Vienna, he returned to enter the private practice of medicine in Cincinnati. In a Harvard class report he wrote of his experience in private practice: "Cincinnati's medical ideas and ideals diverged so widely from the course which I'd laid out for myself that I became very unhappy and began to long for Boston, feeling that there I could work toward my goal in the way which I had so carefully planned"[28]. Newburgh did return to Boston in 1912, and under the tutelage of Dr. David Edsall, Jackson Professor of Clinical Medicine; James Howard Means, a subsequent Jackson Professor of Medicine; George Minot, a Nobel Prize winner; and William Townsend Porter, a professor of physiology, he honed his research skills until appointed in 1915 to an assistant professorship at the University of Michigan. He began this appointment at age thirty-three and within six years was professor of clinical investigation at the University of Michigan, where he remained for his academic career. He built a whole-body calorimeter and respirator in which subjects could reside for several days while having oxygen consumption and carbon dioxide production measured. His studies are summarized in a short monograph[29]. Newburgh follows in the long tradition of Sanctorius[30], Voit[8], Rubner[7] and Atwater and Benedict[10]. As A. McGehee Harvey observed,

> At a time when authorities denied that the first law of thermodynamics, the conservation of energy, applied to human metabolism, Newburgh proved irrefutably by meticulous determinations of calories in and calories out that this natural law applied to man as well as to inanimate matter[28].

Newburgh had made the lesson of his case tell on his education. With his experience, he had seen wisely and shown that *luxuskonsumption* was a myth.

Biosketch

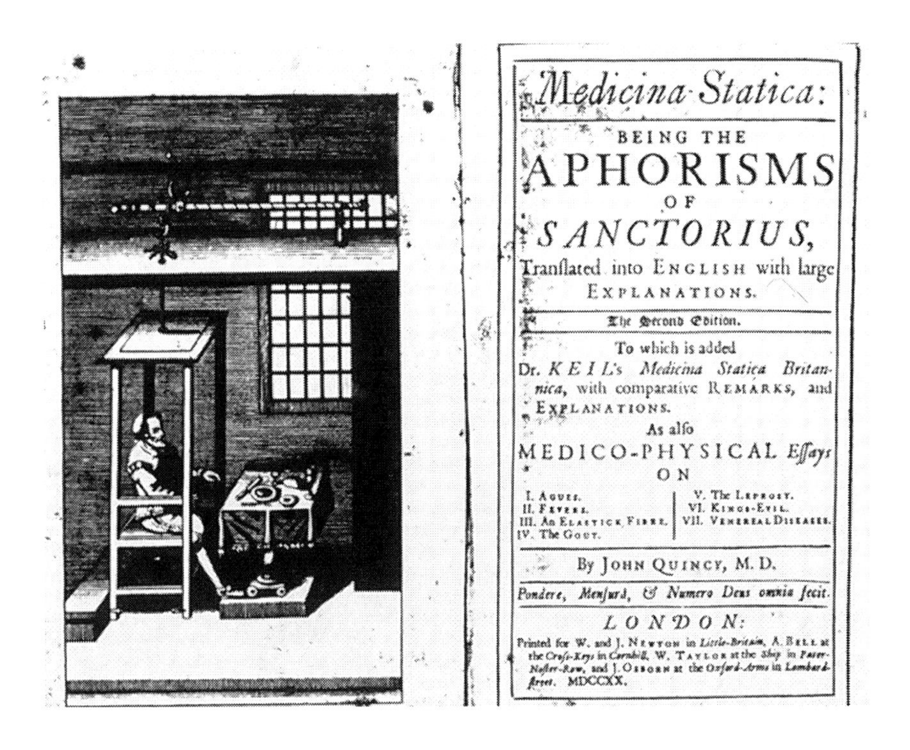

Medicina Statica:
BEING THE
APHORISMS
OF
SANCTORIUS,
Tranſlated into ENGLISH with large
EXPLANATIONS.
The Second Edition.
To which is added
Dr. *KEIL's Medicina Statica Britannica,* with comparative REMARKS, and
EXPLANATIONS.
As alſo
MEDICO-PHYSICAL *Eſſays*
ON

I. AGUES.
II. FEVERS.
III. An ELASTICK FIBRE.
IV. The GOUT.
V. The LEPROSY.
VI. KINGS-EVIL.
VII. VENEREAL DISEASES.

By JOHN QUINCY, M. D.

Pondere, Menſurâ, & Numero Deus omnia fecit.

LONDON:
Printed for W. and J. NEWTON in *Little-Britain*, A. BELL at the *Croſs-Keys* in *Cornhill*, W. TAYLOR at the *Ship* in *Pater-Noſter-Row*, and J. OSBORN at the *Oxford-Arms* in *Lombard-ſtreet*. MDCCXX.

4-1 Balance beam with Sanctorius sitting on it and cover from the 1720 edition of *Medicine Statica: Being the aphorisms of Sanctorius... (Transl. by John Quincy)*. From the collection of the author.

Ethan Allen Hitchcock Sims, M.D. (1916-XXXX) was born in Newport, Rhode Island on April 22, 1916, the youngest of five children where his father was president of the Naval War College. His interest in science began with the gift of a small 40-power microscope at age seven followed by a much better microscope a few years later. He completed Harvard College in 1938 and received his M.D. from the Columbia University College of Physicians and Surgeons in 1942. His career in endocrinology began at Yale-New Haven Medical Center where he was a younger faculty member working in the laboratory of John P. Peters. In 1950 he moved to the University of Vermont where he began and conducted an important series of experiments on the effects of voluntary weight gain of about 25 percent in healthy subjects who overate.

References

1. Osler, W. *Aequanimitas with Other Addresses to Medical Students, Nurses and Practitioners of Medicine.* 1st ed. Philadelphia: P. Blakiston's Son and Co., 1904.
2. Mayer, J.R. von. *"Bemerkungen über die Krafte der unbelebten Natur." Ann Chem Pharm (Lemgo).* 42(1842): 233–240.
3. von Helmholtz, H.L.F. *Ueber die Erhaltung der Kraft, eine physikalische Abhandlung.* Berlin: G. Reimer, 1847.
4. Neumann, R.O. "Experimentelle Beiträge zur Lehre von dem täglichen Nahrungsbedarf des Menschen unter besonderer Berücksichtigung der notwendigen Eiweissmenge." *Arch Hyg.* 45(1902): 1–87.
5. Grafe, E., D. Graham. "Ober die Anpassungsfabigkeit des tierischen Organismus an Uberreichliche Nahrungszufuhr." *Ztschr f. physiol. Chem.* (1911):lxxiii, 1:1–67.
6. Gulick, A. "A Study of Weight Regulation in the Adult Human Body During Overnutrition." *Am J Physiol.* 60(1922): 371–395.
7. Rubner, M. *Die Gesetze des Energieverbrauchs bei der Ernahrung.* Leipzig: Franz Deuticke, 1902.
8. Voit, C. von. "Untersuchungen über die Respiration." *Ann Chem Pharm (Heidelberg).* (1862–1863): suppl 2: 52–70.
9. Wiley, F.H., L.H. Newburgh. "The Doubtful Nature of 'Luxuskonsumption.'" *J Clin Invest.* 10(1931): 733–745.
10. Atwater, W.O., F.G. Benedict. *A Respiration Calorimeter with Appliances for the Direct Determination of Oxygen.* Washington, D.C.: Carnegie Institution of Washington, 1905. No. 42.
11. Newburgh, L.H., F.H. Wiley, F.H. Lashmet. "Method for determination of heat production over long periods of time." *J Clin Invest.* 10(1931): 703–721.
12. Benedict, F.G. *The Influence of Inanition on Metabolism.* Washington, D.C.: Carnegie Institution of Washington, 1907. Publication No. 77.
13. Leibel, R.L., J. Hirsch. "Diminished Energy Requirements in Reduced-Obese Patients." *Metabolism.* 33(1984): 164–170.
14. Leibel, R.L., M. Rosenbaum, J. Hirsch. "Changes in Energy Expenditure Resulting from Altered Body Weight." *N Engl J Med.* 1995:332:661–628.
15. Miller, D.S., P. Mumford. "Gluttony (1): An Experimental Study of Overeating Low- or High-Protein Diets" *Am J Clin Nutr.* 20(1967): 1212–1222.
16. Miller, D.S., P. Mumford, M.J. Stock. "Gluttony (2): Thermogenesis in Overeating Man." *Am J Clin Nutr.* 20(1967): 1223–1229.
17. Sims, E.A., E. Danforth, E.S. Horton, G.A. Bray, J.A. Glennon, B.

Salans. "Endocrine and Metabolic Effects of Experimental Obesity in Man." *Recent Prog Horm Res.* 29(1973): 457–487.

18. Lusk, G. *The Elements of Nutrition.* Philadelphia: W.B. Saunders, 1928.
19. Whipp, B.J., G.A. Bray, S.N. Koyal. "Exercise Energetics in Normal Man Following Acute Weight Gain." *Am J Clin Nutr.* 26(1973): 1284–1286.
20. Bray, G.A. "The Energetics of Obesity." *Med Sci Sports Exerc.* 15(1983): 32–40.
21. Donato, K., D.M. Hegsted. "Efficiency of Utilization of Various Sources of Energy for Growth." *Proc Natl Acad Sci USA.* 82(1985): 4866–4870.
22. Rothwell, N.J., M.J. Stock. "A Role for Brown Adipose Tissue in Diet-induced Thermogenesis." *Nature.* 281(1979): 31–35.
23. Forbes, G.B. "Energy Intake and Body Weight: A Reexamination of Two Classic Studies." *Am J Clin Nutr.* 39(1984): 349–350.
24. Forbes, G.B., M.R. Brown, S.L. Welle, B.A. Lipinski. "Deliberate Overfeeding in Women and Men: Energy Cost and Composition of the Weight Gain." *Br J Nutr.* 56(1986): 1–9.
25. Roberts, S.B., V.R. Young, P. Fuss, et. al. "Energy Expenditure and Subsequent Nutrient Intakes in Overfed Young Men." *Am J Physiol.* 259(1990): R461–R469.
26. Bouchard, C., A. Tremblay, J.P. Despres, et al. "The Response to Long-term Overfeeding in Identical Twins." *N Engl J Med.* 322(1990): 1522–1524.
27. Levine, J.A., N.L. Eberhardt, M.D. Jensen. "Role of Nonexercise Activity Thermogenesis in Resistance to Fat Gain in Humans." *Science.* No. 283 (1999): 212–214.
28. Harvey, A.M. "Louis Harry Newburgh: Compleat Clinical Investigator with a Passion for Measurement." *Am J Med.* 70(1981): 759–761.
29. Newburgh, L.H., M.W. Johnston. *The Exchange of Energy Between Man and the Environment.* Springfield, IL: Charles C. Thomas, 1930.
30. Sanctorius, S. *Medicina Statica: Or, Rules of Health, in Eight Sections of Aphorisms. English'd by J.D.* London: John Starkey, 1676.

Chapter 13

Unveiling of Objective Truth about Food Intake: People Don't Accurately Report What They Eat

Blessed is he who maketh due proofe.
With due proofe and with discreet assaye
Wise men may learn new things every day.
—Thomas Norton (G. 1493) in *Ordinall of Alkimy*[1]

Human beings as well as all other warm-blooded animals maintain a temperature that is higher than the environment. To do this requires us to produce heat everyday. We do this by burning food stuffs to make energy. If we eat more food than we need to keep warm, to move, and to satisfy the other needs of metabolism, we will store this extra energy in the form of fat. But do we know how much we eat? Our government spends large amounts of money on dietary surveys to find out. They store the data on computers and provide us with dietary guidelines based on this type of information. But how good is it? Understanding how much energy we need, and the processes by which foods are converted from the potential energy of food to our energy needs and/or stores in fat, has been an important part of biological science for over two hundred years, and is critically important if we are to know how to win the battle of the bulge.

The introduction of a method to measure energy expenditure with precision over several days rather than minutes to hours has revolutionized the study of energy expenditure and food intake. The original use of this technique called "doubly labeled water" to measure energy expenditure in animals was published fewer than fifty years ago. In the ensuing years it has been adapted to the study of energy expenditure in people with striking conclusions. We now know that our dietary records of food intake are woefully inadequate. Most people report eating less food than they would require to maintain their weight. This paper provided insights into the energy expenditure of free-living animals and human beings. Energy expenditure from the metabolism of ingested food or body nutrient stores is one-half of the equation for energy balance articulated by Hermann von Helmholtz (1821–1894) and Robert Mayer (1814–1878) in the nineteenth century as the First Law of Thermodynamics or the Law of Energy Conservation. However, this law did not pull back the veil of objective truth sufficiently for the work of Lifson et al.[2]. Their work required several additional unveilings of basic metabolism and isotope chemistry before their method could even be thought about. This new chemical understanding of the way the body functions was not possible until the mid-twentieth century.

New methods are one of the cornerstones for advances in science. The discovery of the microscope[3], the construction of calorimeters[4, 5] and the development of the radioimmunoassay to measure minute amounts of hormones in the blood[6] are but three in a long list. This section is about yet another method that was originally developed in animals and then applied to the study of energy expenditure in human beings with substantial new insights.

From the initial observations of Antoine Lavoisier (1743–1794)[4] that heat loss by animals could be measured by the rate of melting ice and the nearly simultaneous use of changing temperature of water to measure heat loss by Adair Crawford (1748–1795)[7] calorimetry had come a long way and contributed a lot to our understanding of the way human beings work by the time Lifson et al. began their important studies.

The importance of calorimeters in our study of the battle of the bulge is shown by the many types of calorimeters that have been produced over the last two hundred years and by the many scientists who have contributed by their use[4, 5, 9–38]. Table 13-1, adapted from McLean and Tobin[31] and from Webb[32], shows the calorimeters that have been developed over the past two centuries. The initial instruments were direct calorimeters which measured heat loss by the amount of ice that was melted or by the heating of water[4,7] The water bath used by Despretz[8] and by Dulong[9] in their work *On the Source of Animal Heat* was similar to the one used by Crawford. Their work won the prize offered by the Academie de Science in Paris in 1822 on energy expenditure. They confirmed the important hypothesis of Lavoisier, that metabolism was similar to burning of a candle.

Direct measurement of heat loss is essential to establish that animals and human beings obey the laws of nature. However, direct calorimeters are hard to use, and once it was clear that the utilization of oxygen and the production of carbon dioxide by the body gave the same answers as measuring heat loss directly, these "indirect" methods moved to the fore. The first closed-circuit calorimeter was developed by Regnault and Reiset in 1849[6] for the study of small animals. Because of poor temperature control in their chamber, they erroneously concluded that not all animal heat was caused by metabolism or oxidation within the body. The closed-circuit system absorbs the carbon dioxide produced by the animal or man and measures the oxygen that is utilized. Many subsequent respiration chambers have used the closed-circuit principle (Table 13-1). d'Arsonval[11] introduced the first heat-sink-direct calorimeter, the design adopted by Atwater and Rosa[5] for their first calorimeter. The isothermal or heat gradient calorimeter was the other design developed by Max Rubner[12] in his Marburg laboratory. Rubner also developed an open-circuit type of respiration calorimeter for animals. With this instrument, he provided "a triumphant demonstration of the law of conservation of energy." The amount of heat calculated by Rubner as the quantity that should have been derived from the metabolism of the dog during the day spent in the calorimeter was the amount actually given off by the dog to the calorimeter[12].

The first attempt at a human calorimeter came from the work of Max Pettenkofer and Carl Voit[21] in the middle of the nineteenth century. At that time, Voit's laboratory was a leading center for the study of human nutrition, particularly in energy metabolism. Pettenkofer, who developed the first human calorimeter; Rubner, another pioneer of energy expenditure; and Atwater, the American pioneer who built the first American calorimeters were all students in Carl Voit's laboratory during the 1860s the time of the American Civil War. By the end of the nineteenth century, both Rubner[12] and Atwater and Rosa[5] had succeeded in showing that the First Law of Thermodynamics applied to animals and to human beings. In addition Rubner[33] had enunciated the Law of Surface Area, which expressed the relation of the of energy expenditure in animals to their surface area.

During the twentieth century the techniques of calorimetry were applied to clinical medicine by Benedict, who inherited the mantle from W.O. Atwater. Parts of this work are enshrined in the famous Harris and Benedict equations published in 1919[39] that have received wide use in the estimation of basal energy needs of human beings. Lusk[19] built a human calorimeter in New York and trained many of the clinicians who used simple machines to measure basal metabolic rate used in the diagnosis of such diseases as hyperthyroidism. It was this same technique that led to the conclusion that basal metabolic rate was low in obesity. This had two consequences. First, it suggested that there was a metabolic basis for the "bulge" that accounted for the difficulty many people had in their battle against the bulge. And second, if metabolism was low then thyroid hormone, which increased metabolic rate, could be an appropriate treatment in our ongoing battle of the bulge. Other important contributors to measurement of resting and basal energy expenditure prior to World War II include DuBois[34], Newburgh[35], McCann [36], and King[37].

With the demonstration that measurements of gas exchange (oxygen uptake and carbon dioxide production) provided quantitatively similar data to measurements of heat loss, the measurement of gas exchange has largely

Table 13-1. Methods used to measure energy expenditure before 1950

I. Direct Calorimeters

Author	Year	Subject	Procedures
Crawford (7)	1778	Guinea Pig	Water Bath
Lavoisier (4)	1783	Guinea Pig	Ice Bath
Despretz (8)	1824	Rabbit	Water Bath; Respiration Calorimeter
Dulong (9)	1841	Rabbit	Water Bath; Respiration Calorimeter
Ott (10)	1889	Human	Water Bath
d'Arsonval (11)	1889	Rabbit	Adiabatic-(Heat Sink)-Isothermal
Rubner (12)	1894	Dog	Isothermal (heat gradient) Open Circuit; Air Bath-Water Bath.
Atwater and Rosa (5)	1899	Human	Heat Sink (Adiabatic). Open Circuit. Coined Respiration Calorimeter
Lefevre (13)	1896	Human	Bath Calorimeter.
Lefevre (14)	1911	Human	Convection air.
Hill and Hill (15)	1914	Sheep Dogs	Heat Sink (Adiabatic)

II. Respiration Chambers

A. Closed Circuit

Author	Year	Subject	Comments
Regnault & Reiset (16)	1849	Small animals and birds	Poor temperature control. CO_2 absorbed O_2 used. RQ varied with type of feed.
Laulanie (17)	1894	Guinea pigs, rabbits, dogs	Confinement Chamber
Atwater & Benedict (18)	1905	Human	5100 L volume
Lusk (19)	1915	Human	
Krogh (20)	1916	Human	Face Mask

B. Open Circuit

Author	Year	Subject	Procedures
Pettenkoffer/Voit (21)	1862/1866	Human	Carbon-Nitrogen Balance; O_2 calculated
Rubner (12)	1894	Dog	
Atwater & Benedict (22)	1903	Human	Heat Sink (Adiabatic)
Armsby (23)	1903	Cows and Oxen	Heat Sink (Adiabatic)
Zuntz (24)	1906	Human	Portable
Grafe (25)	1909	Human	First use of ventilated hood
Williams (26)	1912	Human	
Lusk (19)	1915	Human	

C. Total Collection

Author	Year	Subject	Procedures
Tissot (27)	1904	Human	Rigid spirometer for expired air.
Douglas bag	1911	Human	Canvas bag for expired air.

III. Other Indirect Methods

A. Insensible Losses

Author	Year	Subject	Procedures
Santorio (28)	1614		

B. Heart Rate and Activity Monitors and Records

Author	Year	Subject	Procedures
Zuntz (29)	1906	Human	Portable
Benedict and Collins (30)	1910		
Krogh (20)	1916		

Table 13-1 Methods used to measure energy expenditure before 1950. Adapted from Paul Webb, *Human Calorimeters*, 1985.[32]

replaced direct calorimetry[38]. However, room calorimeters cannot be used in field work and also restrict the level of activity of the participant. One of the early approaches to field work was to have subjects collect expired gas samples in a large backpack during various activities and then analyze these samples when brought back to the laboratory[24, 25, 29]. A second approach was to use the heart rate, which has a linear relationship with the energy expended in the activity itself at higher levels of activity[20, 29, 30]. Regrettably, heart rate is not a very good measure of resting metabolic rate. The development of doubly labeled water made a major advance in the measurement of energy expenditure over several days in animals and human beings.

One of the most common statements by many overweight people is that they eat very little. Indeed, there have been several studies designed to detect the metabolic differences between the "large eaters" and the "small eaters"[39, 40]. The possibility that such a phenomenon existed was supported by the dietary records that overweight patients ate no more than normal-weight ones. Yet measurements of energy expenditure using respiration chambers like those described in Table 13-1 had consistently shown an increasing energy need with increasing body size and weight[12]. More recently energy expenditure using metabolic chambers was shown to be related to fat-free mass[41]. Studies of energy expenditure had gone about as far as they could using the calorimeter.

Measuring energy expenditure with doubly labeled water solved this dilemma and provided a powerful new tool for measuring energy expenditure in free-living individuals. The new method developed by Lifson et al.[2] relied on the fact that the hydrogen and oxygen atoms in ingested water equilibrated with body water. Thus, measurement of the turnover (excretion) of water by the body and the production of carbon dioxide permitted them to estimate total carbon dioxide production and thus total metabolism. It allowed them to calculate oxygen uptake by the body by assuming or measuring the respiratory quotient (ratio of CO_2 production divided by oxygen uptake). As a preliminary to their work, they had to understand the steps by which metabolism through oxidation of foods produced useful energy for life. That is, they needed to understand the basics of intermediary metabolism or how foodstuffs were converted to energy within the body. An explosive growth in the study of intermediary metabolism began in the early twentieth century with the work of Otto Warburg (1883–1970)[42] and reached its peak in the late 1930s and 1940s with the work of Hans Adolph Krebs (1900–1981)[43, 44] and Fritz Lippman (1899–1986)[45] and many others. This background information served as a guide for the experiments of Lifson et al.[2].

The second prerequisite to the work of Lifson et al. was the availability of isotopes of oxygen and hydrogen. The steady growth in understanding of the atomic structure of chemical isotopes also began in the nineteenth century[46] and reached a peak during World War II[47]. By the time Lifson et al. were conducting their studies after World War II, the theoretical and methodological framework was in place.

In 1949 Lifson et al. used ^{18}O (oxygen-18) to identify the source of oxygen in respiratory carbon dioxide. This form of oxygen is rare compared to the common form of oxygen in air which is ^{16}O or oxygen-16. According to the concepts of intermediary metabolism known in 1949, labeled oxygen in water would be expected to equilibrate with body water and subsequently with the oxygen in CO_2[2]. The only study to examine this hypothesis prior to the work of Lifson et al.[48] had concluded that respiratory oxygen did not enter directly into carbon oxidation. Lifson et al. carried out two types of experiments. In the first one, respiratory oxygen, mainly ^{16}O, was enriched with ^{18}O. In the other, water was enriched with ^{18}O. The authors reached two conclusions: first, that the oxygen in respiratory CO_2 is in isotopic equilibrium with the oxygen in the body; second, that at least a large majority, and perhaps all, of the utilized oxygen is soon converted to body water[48]. Realizing that oxygen in CO_2 was in equilibrium with oxygen in water, the authors used the stable isotopic form of water ($D_2{}^{18}O$) to measure whole-body energy expenditure. To quote Lifson:

> This paper describes a method using $D_2{}^{18}O$ for measurement of total CO_2, production in the intact animal. The method was suggested by the finding that the oxygen of respiratory CO_2 and the oxygen of body water are in isotopic equilibrium with one another. It is unique in that it may permit determination of total CO_2 output (and hence an estimate of energy expenditure) over long periods merely by isotopic analysis of initial and final blood samples.

Mice were used in their studies because the isotopes were very expensive.

In the study of CO_2 output of species other than the mouse, the suitable time intervals will depend mainly on the absolute and relative magnitudes of the turnover rates of D_2 and ^{18}O, respectively. Optimum periods are those which produce decreases in S such that log (S_{inital}/S_{final}) can be measured accurately. In humans intervals of two to three weeks would correspond, in this respect, to those of two to three days in mice. Moreover, since any percentage error in (K_O–K_D) will reflect itself in a similar percentage error in the calculated CO_2 output, accuracy is favored by a high ratio of K_O–K_D.

In the mice K_O–K_D was approximately 1.6. Where this ratio is of the order of 1.4, as might be expected for the "typical" adult human, K_O and K_D will have to be determined with somewhat greater accuracy to make the method useful, even if uncertainty is introduced for no other reasons. Aside from theoretical considerations, the use of this approach in metabolic studies of larger animals, such as man, is at present limited because of the cost of $D_2{}^{18}O$.

This new method for measuring energy expenditure required support from several other scientific disciplines to allow Lifson et al.[2, 48] to propose it for general use. Figure 13-1 shows the method diagrammatically. After the water with the two different markers or isotopes is drunk it mixes with the rest of the water in the body which represents about 60–70% of normal weight, declining to 50–60% in people who are fighting the battle of the bulge. The hydrogen in water can only leave the body as water, but the oxygen can leave both as carbon dioxide and water. Thus the oxygen and hydrogen lines separate over time. Samples of body water obtained at the beginning and one to two weeks later are measured, and this separation between the loss of hydrogen and oxygen is used to calculate the amount of carbon dioxide that is produced and then used to calculate how much oxygen was used—a measure of overall metabolism.

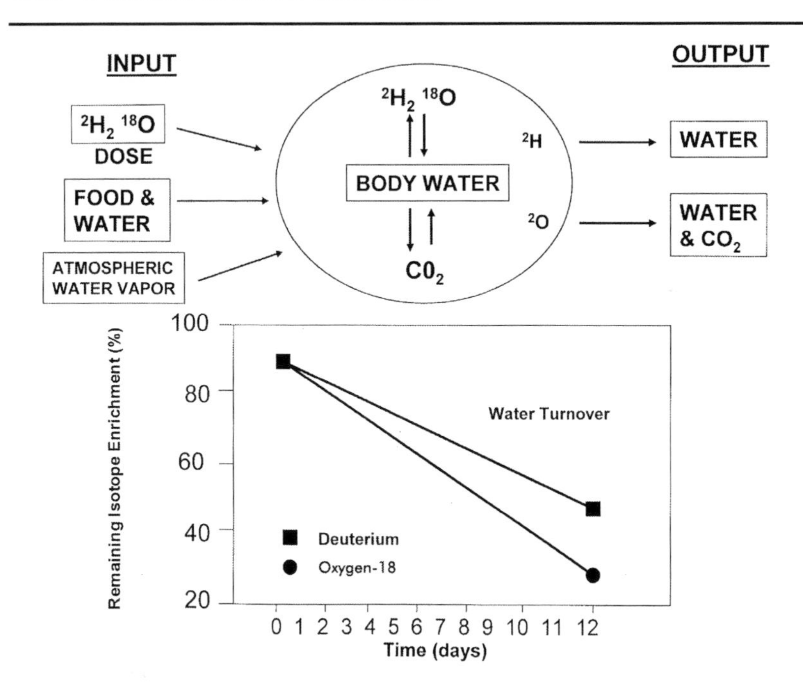

13-1 Routes of excretion for oxygen and hydrogen. When stable isotopes of each molecule are given the oxygen can appear in the urine as water and in the breath as carbon dioxide. The hydrogen can only appear as water in the urine. Thus the amount of each isotope remaining in the blood or other body fluid is a reflection of the overal metabolism.

In doing so they have fulfilled the words of Sarton cited below[49] and further unveiled the objective truth about nature. The following quotation summarizes the advance we have discussed above.

> The history of science may be defined as the story of the gradual unveiling of objective truth and the conquest of matter by mind; it describes the age-long and endless struggle for freedom of thought—freedom from violence, intolerance, error and superstition[49].

Biosketch

Carl von Voit (1831–1908) (Figure 13-2) is identified with the German Nutrition School of the mid-nineteenth century. He was born in Amberg, a Bavarian town in Germany, and spent most of his life there. After completing his medical training in 1854 he spent a year in Göttingen, Germany, with Wohler, the man who showed that inorganic materials could be used to synthesize urea, an organic molecule. Voit then returned to Munich where he rose to become professor of physiology in 1863. His seminal work was the measurement of metabolism in mammals and humans. He was the first to determine the amount of protein, carbohydrate, and fat broken down in the body. With Max von Pettenkofer he devised the first calorimeter large enough for human beings and proved the equality of total input and excretion of carbon, hydrogen, nitrogen, and oxygen, thus providing the first demonstration that the First Law of Thermodynamics applied to mammals[50].

References

1. Norton T. *Ordinall of Alkimy.*
2. Lifson, N., G.B. Gordon, M.B. Visscher, A.O. Nier. "The Fate of Utilized Molecular Oxygen and the Source of the Oxygen of Respiratory Carbon Dioxide Studied with the Aid of Heavy Oxygen." *J Biol Chem.* 180(1949): 803–811.
3. Leeuwenhoek, A. van. *The Selected Works of Antony van Leeuwenhoek Containing His Microscopical Discoveries in Many of the Works of Nature. Vol. 1, Parts 1 and 2.* Trans. S. Hoole. London: G. Sidney, 1800; Vol. 2, Part 3. London: Philanthropic Society, 1807.
4. Lavoisier, A-L, P.S. LaPlace, H. Guerlac. trans. *Memoir on Heat.* Read to the Royal Academy of Sciences, 28 June 1783. New York: Neale Watson Academic Publications, Inc., 1982.
5. Atwater, W.O., E.B. Rosa. "Description of a New Respiration Calorimeter and Experiments on the Conservation of Energy in the Human Body." U.S. Department of Agriculture Office of Experimental Stations. 1899: 63.
6. Berson, S.A., R.S. Yalow. "Quantitative Aspects of Reaction Between Insulin Serum." *J Clin Invest.* 38(1959): 2017–2025.
7. Crawford A. *Experiments and Observations on Animal Heat, and the Inflammation of Combustible Bodies; Being an Attempt to Resolve These Phenomena into a General Law of Nature.* 2nd ed. London: J. Johnson, 1788.
8. Despretz, C. "La cause de la chaleur animale." *J Physiol Exp Pathol.* 4(1824): 143–159.
9. Dulon, P.R. "Memoire sur la chaleur animale." *Anti Chilli Phys.* 3e serie. 1(1841): 440–455.
10. Ott, I. "Human Calorimetry." *NY Med J.* 49(1889): 342–345.
11. d'Arsonval, N.I.A. "Recherches de calorimetrie." *J Anat Physiol* (Paris). 22(1889): 113–161.
12. Rubner, M. "Die Quelle der thierschen Wärme." *Z Biol.* 30(1894): 73–142.
13. Lefevre, J. "Considerations generale sur la calorimetrie par les bains." *Arch Physiol (Paris).* 29(1896): 32–46.
14. Lefevre, J. *Chaleur animal et bioenergetique.* Paris: Masson et Cie, 1911.
15. Hill, A.V., A.M. Hill. "A Self-recording Calorimeter for Large Animals." *J. Physiol.* (Lond). 48(1914): 13–14.
16. Regnault, V., J. Reiset. "Recherches chimiques sur la respiration des animaux des diverses classes." *Ann Chim Phys. Ser Ill.* 26(1849): 299–519.
17. Laulanie, F. "De la marche des alterations de l'air dans l'asphyxie en vase clos." *Arch Physiol Norm Pathol.* 26(1894): 845–859.
18. Atwater, W.O., F.G. Benedict. "A Respiration Calorimeter with Appliances for the Direct Determination of Oxygen." Washington,

D.C.: Carnegie Institution of Washington, 1905. Publication No. 42.
19. Lusk, G. "A Respiration Calorimeter for the Study of Disease." *Arch Intern Med.* 15(1915): 793–804.
20. Krogh A. *The Respiratory Exchange of Animals and Man.* London: Lorigmans Green and Co., 1916.
21. Pettenkofer, M., C. Voit. "Untersuchungen über den Stoffverbrauch des normalen Menschen." *Z Biol.* 2(1866): 478–573.
22. Atwater, W.O., F.G. Benedict. "An Experimental Inquiry Regarding the Nutritive Value of Alcohol." *Mem Natl Acad Sci.*" 8(1902): 235–272.
23. Armsby, H.P. "The Respiration Calorimeter at the Pennsylvania Experiment Station." *Ann Rep Pennsylvania State College*, 1904.
24. Zuntz, N. "Ein nach dem Prinzip von Regnault and Reiset gebaulter Respirationapparat." *Arch Anat Physiol.* Suppl (1905): 431–435.
25. Grafe, E. "Einkopfrespiration apparat." *Deut Arch Klin Med.* 95(1909): 529–542)
26. Williams, H.B. "Animal Calorimetry. First Paper: A Small Respiration Calorimeter." *J Biol Chem.* 12(1912): 1317–1347.
27. Tissot, J. "Nouvelle méthode de mesure et d'inscription du debit et des mouvement respiratoire de l'homme et des animaux." *J Physiol Pathol Getz.* (Paris) 6(1904): 688–700.
28. Santorio, S. *Medicine statica.* 2nd ed. London: W. and J. Newton, A. Bell, W. Taylor, and J. Osborne, 1720.
29. Zuntz, N., A. Loewy, F. Muller, W. Caspar. *Hohenklima und bergwanderungen.* Berlin: Deutsches Verlagshaus Bong and Co., 1906.
30. Benedict, F.G., W.E Collins. "A Clinical Apparatus for Measuring Basal Metabolism." *Boston Med Surg J.* 183(1920): 449–458.
31. McLean, J.A., G. Tobin. *Animal and Human Calorimetry.* Cambridge: Cambridge University Press, 1987.
32. Webb, P. *Human Calorimeter-Endocrinology and Metabolism Series.* New York: Prager, 1985.
33. Rubner, M. *Die Gesetze des Energieverbrauches bei der Ernahrung.* Leipzig: Franz Deuticke, 1902.
34. Du Bois, E.F. *Basal Metabolism in Health and Disease.* Philadelphia: Lea and Febiger, 1924.
35. Newburgh, L.H., M.W. Johnston. *The Exchange of Energy Between Man and the Environment.* Springfield, IL: Charles C. Thomas, 1930.
36. McCann, S. *Calorimetry in Medicine.* Baltimore: Williams and Wilkins, 1924.
37. King, J.T., Jr. *Basal Metabolism Determination of the Metabolic Rate in the Practice of Medicine.* Baltimore: Williams and Wilkins Co., 1924.
38. Kleiber, M. *The Fire of Life.* New York: John Wiley, 1961.
39. George, V., A. Tremblay, J-P. Despres, C. Leblanc, L. Perusse, C. Bouchard. "Evidence for the Existence of Small Eaters and Large Eaters

of Similar Fat-free Mass and Activity Level." *Int J Obes.* 13(1989): 43–53.
40. Rose, G.A., R.T. William. "Metabolic Studies on Large and Small Eaters." *Br J Nutr.* 15(1961): 1–9.
41. Ravussin, E.., S. Lillioja, T.E. Anderson, et al. "Determination of 24-hour Energy Expenditure in Man. Methods and Results Using a Respiratory Chamber." *J Clin Invest.* 78(1986): 1568–1578.
42. Warburg, O. *Ueber die katalytische Wirkungen der legendigen Substanz.* Berlin: J Springer, 1928.
43. Krebs, H.A., W.A. Johnson. "Citric Acid in Intermediate Metabolism in Animal Tissues." *Enzymologia.* 4(1937): 148–156.
44. Holmes, F.L. *Hans Krebs. Architect of Intermediary Metabolism 1933–1937.* New York: Oxford University Press, 1993.
45. Lippmann, F.A., N.O. Kaplan. "A Common Factor in the Enzymatic Acetylation of Sulfanilamide and of Choline." *J Biol Chem.* 162(1946): 743–744.
46. Curie, M. *Traité de radioactivité.* Paris: Gauthier-Willars, 1910.
47. Hevesy, G. *Radioactive Indicatory Their Application in Biochemistry, Animal Physiology, and Pathology.* New York: Interscience Publishers, Inc., 1948.
48. Lifson, N., G.B. Gordon, R. McClintock. "Measurement of Total Carbon Dioxide Production by Means of $D_2{}^{18}O$." *J Appl Physiol.* 7(1955): 704–710.
49. Sarton, G. *Six Wings: Men of Science in the Renaissance.* Bloomington, IN: Indiana University Press,1952.
50. Holmes, F. "Carl von Voit." In *Dictionary of Scientific Biography.* New York: Charles Scribner's Sons.

CHAPTER 14

The Fat Cell Discovered: Units of Knowledge and the Illnesses from Overweight

> *In those days people often said to me, "Ah! The microscope is all very well as an amusement, but of what practical use is it in life?" These people little dreaming of the many and vastly important facts which in the future were to be brought to light by its instrumentality.*
>
> —Hassall[1]

Is obesity a disease? Is it just a "condition" that some people have but others don't? Are we battling a real enemy when we decide to reduce the bulge, or is it just a normal state of some people's bodies? These questions revolve around the issue of what we mean by "a disease" and how we measure it. In this section, I will introduce the topic of disease and how we define it and more particularly how it is related to obesity.

Disease and health are often viewed as opposites. When a disease is present, an individual is not healthy. The earliest explanations of disease were in terms of either loss of something needed for health or invasion of the body by some evil spirit. As the more systematic Western medicine developed in the seventeenth century, the idea of the "natural history of disease" gradually developed. Diseases start at some point, progress, and then either resolve or become chronic. The idea that obesity is a disease goes back nearly three hundred years. The argument then, and an argument that holds water today, is that when the proverbial bulge is sufficiently large it produces disability in walking, working, and living as well as other diseases, including sudden death. Several features are central to any disease. There must be a cause. There must be something that produces the suffering, in this case the excess amount of fat that damages joints that carry it around and that produces the agents that damage other tissues. The fat cell is thus a central player in the disease of obesity, and this is a story about how cells came to be considered basic units of biology and how the fat cell was identified.

The idea of the cell as a unit of biology and of enlarged fat cells as the basic problem in obesity has taken more than one hundred fifty years to develop. In the medical sense, the fat cell provides the basis for the pathology of obesity. Theodor Schwann (1810–1852)[2] identified the essential elements of cells in animals in 1839. His observations, coupled with the key insights of Max Schleiden[3] on the cellular structure of plants, led to the Cell Theory of Biology. Once the concept of a cell became clear, it was not long before Arthur Hassall[4] first described fat cells in an English-language publication.

Early microscopes appeared in the seventeenth century. Using these simple instruments, a Dutchman, Antony van Leeuwenhoek (1632–1723)[5], an Englishman, Robert Hooke (1635–1703)[6], and an Italian, Marcello Malpighi (1628–1694)[7] observed and described in considerable detail the particles and corpuscles of many plants and animals. To quote Leeuwenhoek,

> The blood is composed of exceeding small particles, named Globules, which in most animals are a red color, swimming in a liquor, called, by physicians, the serum: and by means of these Globules the motion of the blood becomes visible, which otherwise would not be discoverable by the sight. These particles or globules are so minute that 100 of them placed side by side would not equal the diameter of a common grain of sand; consequently a grain of sand is above a million times the size of one such Globule[5].

Leeuwenhoek, however, did not recognize the cellular nature of his "Globules."

Hooke[6] produced beautiful pictures of the external cellular structure of plants. The work of Hooke on cork is typical of the descriptions of plant structures, which were among the earliest carefully described histologic structures (Figure 14-1). Hooke says,

> These pores, or cells, were not very deep but consisted of a great many little boxes, separated out of one continuing long pore by certain diaphragms. I took a good clear piece of cork, and with a pen-knife sharpened as keen as a razor I cut a piece of it off, and thereby left the surface of it exceeding smooth, then examining it very diligently with a microscope, me thought I perceived it to appear a little porous; but I could not so plainly distinguish them, as to

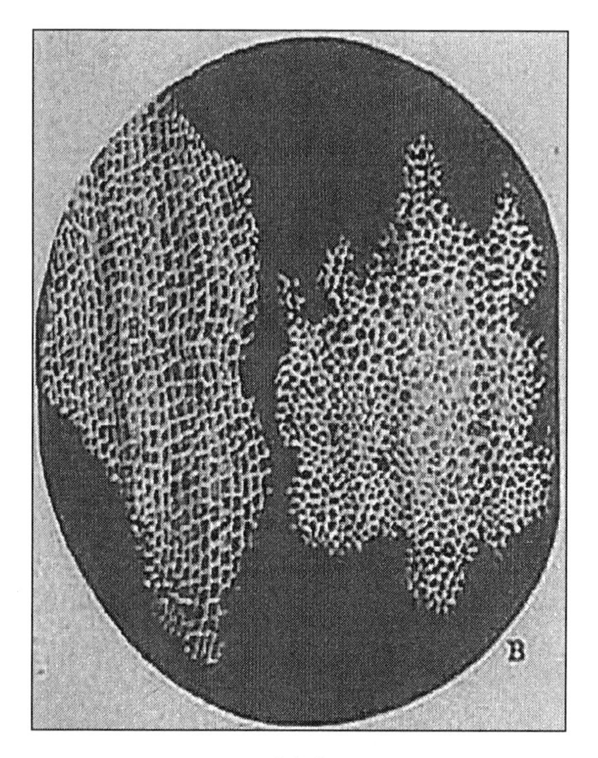

14-1

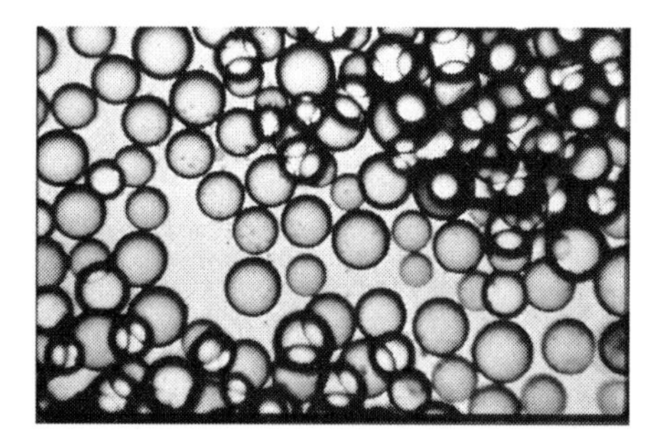

14-2

14-1 Micrograph of cork by Robert Hooke using an early type of microscope. From the collection of the author.

14-2 Picture of human fat cells which serve to store fat and to produce many important hormones that are secreted and circulate throughout the body. From the collection of the author.

> be sure they were pores, much less what figure they were of: but judging from the lightness and yielding quality of the cork that certainly the texture could not be so curious but that possibly, if I could use some further diligence I might find it to be discernible with a microscope, I with the same sharp pen-knife cut off from the former smooth surface an exceeding thin piece of it and placing it on a black object plate because it was itself a white body and crafting the light on it with a deep planoconvex glass I could exceedingly plainly perceive it to be perforated and porous, much like a honeycomb, but that the pores of it were not regular yet it was not unlike honeycomb in these particulars[6].

The simple microscopes available to Hooke and his contemporaries limited their ability to see the cell wall that circumscribed animal cells. Their microscopes also failed to detect the smaller structures that were inside cells. They failed for this or possibly other reasons to understand the concept of the cell as a unit of living matter. In addition to the problems with the level of magnification and resolution of their microscopes, there were also limitations of the tissue preparations with which they worked. Leeuwenhoek described the movements of the sperm and other objects in solutions, but he did not relate these observations to those he described in plants. The corpuscles that Malpighi saw also failed to set his mind to thinking about them as fundamental units of life.

Two things were essential for development of the Cell Theory: an intellectual framework and a microscope with greater resolution. A key factor for the development of the Cell Theory by Schwann[2] was the intellectual framework for discovery in nineteenth century Germany. With the dawn of the Renaissance and the development of printing as a tool for spreading ideas quickly, a tradition of descriptive knowledge in medicine began to develop. Among the pinnacles in this early development was the anatomical masterpiece titled *De humani corporis fabrica*, published in 1543 by Vesalius[8]. This monumental descriptive work on the organs, blood vessels, nerves, and bones of the human body was a major impetus to an anatomic understanding of the human body. As the organ basis for anatomy reached its pinnacle, an organ basis for pathology and disease emerged, epitomized by the powerful book titled *The Seats and Causes of Disease (De sedibus et causis morborum per anatomen indagatis Libriquinque)* by Giovanni Morgagni (1862–1771) published in 1761[9]. In this work we see the combination of an anatomist and a clinician applying his knowledge to understand the relationship between organs and the diseases they produced. This work was notable for both its size, the intelligence of his observations and the logical connections he made in analyzing his dissections.

The tissues composing the organs of the body were the next locus for explanations of disease. In his *Anatomie Générale*, the young Frenchman François Xavier Bichat[10], one of the great scientists during the French Revolution, proposed a tissue basis for pathology; however, neither he nor his French colleagues believed that the microscope could make an important contribution to furthering this area of study, and few important histologic works came from France in the early nineteenth century.

In contrast, the German school of the early nineteenth century readily took up the microscope as a basis for expanding knowledge about man and his environment. A number of explanations have been suggested for why the French failed to recognize the importance of the microscope while the Germans exploited it to exceptional value. Whatever the reason or reasons may be, it was the students of Johannes Müller, professor of physiology in Göttingen and then in Berlin in the early part of the nineteenth century, who revolutionized biology. Johannes Müller, a leading professor of Germany in the first half of the nineteenth century, was interested in both anatomic and histologic studies as well as physiologic and functional studies[11]. His two students Schwann and Schleiden followed the lead of the master to exceptional advantage.

A second factor in the development of the cell theory was the improvement of the microscope. About 1830 the optical system of the microscope was dramatically improved by the introduction of achromatic optics. This involves putting two lenses together to avoid the distortion that occurs near the edges of a single lens. This new type of lens was the most important advance in microscopy until the development of the electron microscope in the early twentieth century. It was the achromatic microscope that Schwann[2] and Schleiden[34] used for their epochal synthesis. As with many major advances, it was new or improved tools in the hand of creative scientists that led to progress.

Although observations on plant cell-like structures had been observed since the time of Hooke in 1665, the idea of a uniform "cell" took a stroke of imagination, since proving that all bodies of all organisms are composed solely of cells is no easy feat[12]. Indeed it is not possible to "prove" this; it is rather an idea or hypothesis that provides a basis for new experiments. Between the time the microscope was discovered in the early 1600s and the Cell Theory, more than two hundred years had elapsed. The work of Schwann, published in 1839, was done when he was twenty-nine years old. To quote from Schwann,

> Though the variety in the external structure of plants is great, their internal structure is very simple. This extraordinary

> range in external form is due only to a variation in the fitting together of elementary structures which, indeed, are subject to modification but are essentially identical—that is, they are cells. The entire class of cellular plants is composed solely of cells that can readily be recognized as such; some of them are composed merely of a series of similar or even only a single cell.

To quote further from Schwann:

> Animals being subject to a much greater range of variation in their external form than is found in plants also show (especially in the higher species) a much greater range of structure in their different tissues. A muscle differs from a nerve, the latter from a cellular tissue (which shares only its name with the cellular tissue of plant), or elastic tissue or horny tissue, etc.
>
> If, however, we go back to the development of these tissues, then it will appear that all of these many forms of tissues are constituted solely of cells that are quite analogous to plant cells...the purpose of the present treatise is to prove the forgoing by observations.
>
> The most frequent and important basis for recognizing the existence of a cell is the presence or absence of the nucleus. Its sharp outline and its dark color make it easily recognizable in most cells and its characteristic shape, especially if it contains nucleoli...identify the structure as a cell nucleus and make it analogous to the nucleus of the young cells contained in cartilage and plant cells...more than nine-tenths of the structures thought to be cells show such a nucleus and in many of these a distinct cell membrane can be made out and in most it is more or less distinct. Under these circumstances it is perhaps permissible to conclude that the spheres where no cell membranes be distinguished, but where a nucleus characteristic of its position and form is encountered, that a cell membrane is actually present but invisible[2].

The Cell Theory as described in this extract from Schwann's work arose out of the comparative study of tissue development. The first clear description of cells was probably around 1830. Von Baer, for example, described *Kugelchen* or *Komchen*, which were almost surely cells[13]. Other workers during the early 1830s also identified cells[13, 14]. From studies of animal cells,

Schwann[2] discovered that despite the numerous external differences from one tissue to another, there were several common features across all cells, which led him to conclude that they were the basic units of life. First was the nucleus. Although described earlier, it was Schwann and Schleiden who recognized the central place of the nucleus in the cell. The second was the cell membrane that separated the cell from the surrounding environment. Individual cells whether in single-celled organisms or as parts of larger tissue or organs were, according to Schwann and Schleiden, the basic units of life. They possessed the properties needed for multiplication and reproduction. They were the central units for metabolism and change of the environmental materials into the molecules needed by the cell. In his discussion in the growth of cells, Schwann contrasted them with crystals. Crystals grow, he noted, by adding similar materials that must be in the environment. Cells, on the other hand, grow in many environments by using elements from that environment to provide the things needed for the cell.

In his excellent historical review[13,14], Baker restated Schwann's hypotheses for the Cell Theory as follows:

1. Most organisms contain or consist of a large number of microscopical bodies called cells which in the less differentiated tissues, tend to be polyhedral or nearly spherical.
2. Cells have certain definable characters. These characters show that cells (A) are all of essentially the same nature and (B) are units of structure.
3. Cells always arise directly or indirectly from preexisting cells, usually by binary fission.
4. Cells sometimes become transformed into bodies no longer possessing all of the characters of cells.
5. Cells are to some extent individuals, and there are, therefore two grades of individuality in most organisms: that of the cells and that of the organism as a whole.
6. Each cell of a many-celled organism corresponds in certain respects to the whole body of a simple protist.
7. Many-celled plants and animals probably originated by the adherence of protist individuals after division.

The concept that the cell was the fundamental unit of life became the organizing principle for biology. From the idea of the cell as an organizing unit in life processes came the idea that disturbances in cells could produce "diseases," of which adiposity is one. Thus ideas about how to fight the battle of the bulging fat cell could now have a new focus and be dissected at the cellular level. As we now know, the cell membrane serves as a semi-crystalline structure composed of lipid bi-layers in which many protein molecules are situated and move. The cytoplasm consists of the many enzymes that carry out the metabolic functions of the cell. The mitochondria, primitive particles with their own genetic instructions, are the principle source for generation of energy by the cell. Mitochondria have an analogy with the chloroplast of plants. The mitochondrion takes the units of metabolism (acetyl-CoA) and converts this into metabolically useful energy for the cell by utilizing oxygen. The chloroplast in the plant cell uses energy from the sun to convert water and carbon dioxide into carbohydrate molecules with the release of oxygen. The reproductive capacity of the cell is located in the nucleus and the protein synthetic machinery in the reticulum and so-called Golgi apparatus.

Basic units are critical theoretical elements needed for progress in science. There are a number of such elements in various disciplines. In physics there are atomic and subatomic particles. In chemistry there are molecules and the atoms of which they are composed. At a more complicated level in biology there are genes, cells, and organs of animals or plants. The combination of elementary units into multi-unit organisms produces new properties which make the whole more than the sum of its parts. Understanding a process at one level may or may not contribute to understanding at other levels. The closer the units in functional terms, the more understanding one will contribute to the other. Thus knowledge of the mitochondrion sheds significant light on the function of the whole cell. However, knowing how cells work provides only one of many levels of knowledge needed to understand how whole animals or plants function and behave. Understanding the weak and strong atomic forces holds little likelihood of advancing our understanding of human beings and animals and their function in society or their ecological environment.

The discovery of globules in the blood was first made by Swammerdam[15] possibly in 1658. In 1665 Malpighi[7] also noted corpuscles in blood but regarded them as globules of fat. This description in 1665 by Malpighi was probably the first description of fat cells and appeared in his *Exercitatio de Omento* reprinted in his *Opera Omnia*[7]. He described them as *pinguedinis globul*, but Baker thinks there is little doubt that they were fat cells[13]. The second description of what is in retrospect probably fat cells was made by Monro in 1726 with cells he calls *partes adipose* in his description of the marrow from human bone[13].

Prior to the recognition of cells as the unit of biology, fat was thought to be stored in vesicles of which there was little further understanding[16]. Indeed even after publication of the epochal *Theory of the Cell*, fat in cells was perceived by some to be an epiphenomenon. Prior to Hassall, the fat cell was known to exist but had not been the subject of serious study. As Hassall noted, this was a "difficulty arising from the extreme tenuity of its cell wall and the opacity of its contents"[1]. In 1849 Hassall wrote the first

English-language histology book titled *The Microscopic Anatomy of the Human Body*[17]. In his subsequent work on the development of the fat cell or fat vesicle as he called it, he makes several points which are modern in their conclusions. He noted that "fat vesicles of children are not so large as those of the adult. This suggested that fat corpuscles grow slowly not attaining their full dimensions until near adult age"[4]. He went on to note, "[F]at was permanent in its character, enduring throughout life." He did not believe that fat cells divided, a conclusion that would fit with current observations. He also noted that "the development and growth of fat proceeds at different rates at different localities of the same body, it being more advanced in one situation than in another"[4]. He also noted that "[t]his superficial layer of fat is also generally thicker in children and in women than in men." He noted differences between families in their tendency to fatten. He also observed that "[i]n man, the fat usually undergoes augmentation after the meridian of life has passed. Castration peculiarly predisposes the system to the formation of fat"[4].

The work by Hassall quoted here was the first to deal with the concept of a fat cell as the unit that was related to obesity. It was nearly a century after the work of Schwann and of Hassall before the fat cell really came into its own. It was 1948 when Wertheimer and Shapiro[18] published their review pointing out that adipose tissue had major metabolic functions. During the next twenty years the functions of adipose tissue as a storage organ for fat and as a source of energy were the major areas of activity in this field[19]. Although Hassall the anatomist wrote about the size and number of fat cells, increased size of adipocytes in obesity was first clearly recognized by Bjurulf[20] and was extended to become the *Fat Cell Theory of Obesity* by Hirsch and Knittle[21] and by Bjorntorp and Sjostrom[22] in the 1970s.

Recently the fat cell has taken on a new role as a secretory or endocrine cell[23]. The work of Korn and Quigley in 1955[24] showed that the fat cell synthesizes and secretes an enzyme called lipoprotein lipase. This enzyme attaches to the surface of blood vessels and acts to split the triacylglycerols carried in blood lipids into the fatty acids and glycerol. The fatty acids can then enter fat cells to be stored in fat drops as triacylglycerol. The role of the fat cell was expanded further when it was found to secrete adipsin[25] in addition to lipoprotein lipase. The list of secretory products from the fat cell continues to grow. It produces leptin, an essential peptide in the regulation of body fat stores. It produces many small molecules called cytokines that are important for inflammation and for reactions of the cardiovascular system. For the fat cell, the twenty-first century looks to be most promising yet. In the century and a half since Schwann published his cell theory, the future for studies of the fat cell has never been brighter, now that the fat cell has become a member of the endocrine family[23].

With the discovery of the fat cell and its importance as a producer of messages that travel from one cell to the next, a new vista has been opened up in the battle of the bulge. We know that we bulge because fat cells become enlarged. One approach to winning this battle may well come from discoveries focusing on how to control the products that the fat cell makes.

Biosketch

Robert Hooke (1635–1703) was born on the Isle of Wight. In his childhood he demonstrated mechanical skills that were to become very important later in life. Following his father's death in 1648 when Hooke was thirteen, he moved to London and subsequently became a student at Oxford University, receiving his M.A. in 1663. During his Oxford years he worked with both Thomas Willis, the renowned physician, and Robert Boyle, the "Father of Chemistry." During much of his professional career he was associated with the Royal Society in London. His "Micrographia or Some Physiological Descriptions of Minute Bodies Made by Magnifying Glasses with Observations and Inquiries thereupon" was published in 1665 and stands as his most significant contribution to the body of scientific knowledge[26].

Biosketch

Theodor Schwann (1810–1882) was born near Düsseldorf in 1810 (Figure 14-3). His father was a jeweler and printer, and it is possible that Schwann's mechanical skill was learned at his father's side. Schwann began his advanced studies toward a degree in theology at the University of Bonn. It was there that he came under the influence of Johannes Müller, the professor of anatomy. This changed Schwann's life. He was granted an M.D. degree in 1834 from the University of Berlin. Schwann served as an assistant in experimental physiology for his first five post-doctoral years. Although his cell theory is his dominant legacy, he contributed three other important discoveries. He found that pepsin, an enzyme from the stomach, could convert albumen into peptones. He also described the organic nature of yeast and the production of alcohol by fermentation. And finally he showed that the particulate matter in air might be responsible for putrefaction since it could be destroyed by heat. All of these discoveries were completed by the age of twenty-nine. He was then appointed professor at the Catholic University of Louvain in Belgium and was awarded the Copley Medal of the Royal Society of London in 1845. In 1848, at the age of thirty-eight, he moved for the last time to become chair of anatomy at Liege in Belgium, where he remained until his death at age 72[27].

Biosketch

Arthur Hill Hassall (1817–1894) was born in Teddington, England[28] (Figure 14-4). He was the son of a general practitioner and is remembered for the unique thymic corpuscles that bear his name. Hassall received his medical training under Sir James Murray in Dublin, where he was indentured as an apprentice. Upon returning to England he developed a great interest in botany through his association with Sir William Hooker, who was then director of Kew Gardens. His work on a history of British freshwater algae is a classic. He received his fellowship in the Royal College of Surgeons in 1839 and obtained a diploma from the Apothecaries Hall in 1841. In 1851 he obtained membership in the Royal College of Physicians of London and later received an M.D. degree from the University of London. Based on his work in the post-mortem room at St. George's Hospital, where he studied the microscopic structure of tissues, he published the first complete book of histology in the English language in 1849 titled *The Microscopic Anatomy of the Human Body*[17]. Using his microscope, he next examined a large number of samples of foods. His seminal studies on food and its adulteration resulted in a book titled *Adulteration in Food and Medicine*, published in 1857[29]. This work was instrumental in establishing parliamentary legislation to control adulteration of food and drink. His next book dealt with urine in health and disease and was published in 1863. After he developed tuberculosis in 1866, he was instrumental in establishing the Ventnor Tuberculosis Hospital as a result of his experience with this disease. Under his portrait in the hospital are his words *"Non omnis moriar."* His life of great activity was summarized in his autobiography titled, *The Narrative of a Busy Life*. It begins:

> There are but few persons who have long passed the midday of their lives, who do not from time to time look back and recall the chief events and circumstances of their careers to determine there from how far these lives have been well or ill spent; what lessons are to be learned from the experience gained, what opportunities lost, what faults and sins committed; in fine, to judge whether they have been of any benefit to their fellow creatures, their country or the world[1].

The conclusion a century later is that Arthur Hill Hassall did indeed benefit his fellow creatures, his country, and the world.

References

1. Hassall, A. *The Narrative of a Busy Life; An Autobiography.* London: Longmans, Green, 1893.
2. Schwann, T.H. *Microsccopical Researches into the Accordance in the Structure and Growth of Animals and Plants.* Trans. H. Smith. London: Sydenham Society, 1847.
3. Schlieden, M.J. "Beiträge zur Phytogenesis." *Arch Anat Physiol Wiss Med.* (1838): 137–176.
4. Hassall, A. "Observations on the Development of the Fat Vesicle." *Lancet.* 1(1849): 63–64.
5. Leeuwenhoek van, A. *The Select Works of Antony van Leeuwenhoek, containing his microscopical discoveries in many of the works of nature, translated from the Dutch and Latin editions published by the author Samuel Hoole.* London: G. Sidney, 1800.
6. Hooke, R. *Micrographia, or some physiological descriptions of minute bodies made by magnifying glasses; with observations and inquiries thereupon.* London: J. Martyn & J. Allestry, 1665.
7. Malpighi, M. *Opera Omnia, figuris elegantissimis in aes incisis illustrata. Tomis duobus comprehensa. Quorum catalogum sequens pagina exhibet.* Londini: Apud Robert Scott & Georgium Wells, 1686.
8. Vesalius, A. *De humani corporis fabrica libri septem.* Basileae: ex. off. Ioannis Oporini, 1543.
9. Morgagni, G.B. *De sedibus, et causis morborum per anatomen indagatis libriquinque.* Venetiis, typog. Remordiniana, 1761.
10. Bichat, M.F.X. *Anatomie générale, appliqué à la physiologie et à la médicine.* Paris: Brosson, Gabon et Cie, 1802.
11. Muller, J. *De glandularum secemientium structura penitiori.* Lipsiae, sumpt L. Vossii, 1830.
12. Moore, J.A. *Science as a Way of Knowing the Foundations of Modern Biology.* Cambridge: Harvard University Press, 1993.
13. Baker, J.R. "The Cell-Theory: A Restatement, History, and Critique." *Quarterly Journal Microscopial Science,* no. 11 90(1949): 87–108.
14. Baker, J.R. "The Cell-Theory: A Restatement, History, and Critique." *Quarterly Journal Microscopial Science.* no 1. 89(1948): 103–125.
15. Swammerdam, J. *Biblia naturae; sive histgoria insectorum, in classes certas redacta, nec non exemplis, et anatomico variorum animalculorum examine, aeneisque tabulis illustrata.* Leyden: Isaacum Severinum, Balduinum Vander, Petrum Vander, 1737.
16. Bray, G.A. "Obesity: Historical Development of Scientific and Cultural Ideas." *Int J Obes.* 14(1990): 909–926
17. Hassall, A. *The Microscopic Anatomy of the Human Body, in Health and Disease.* London: Highly, 1849.

18. Wertheimer, E., B. Shapiro. "The Physiology of Adipose Tissue." *Physiol Rev.* 28(1948): 451–464.
19. *Handbook of Physiology: A Critical, Comprehensive Presentation of Physiological Knowledge and Concepts.* Ed. E. Renold and F. Cahill. Washington: American Physiological Society, 1959.
20. Bjurulf, P. "Atherosclerosis and Body Build with Special Reference to Size and Number of Subcutaneous Fat Cells." *Acta Med Scand* suppl 349 (1959): 7–99.
21. Hirsch, J., J.L. Knittle. "Cellularity of Obese and Nonobese Human Adipose Tissue." *Fed Proc.* 29(1970): 1516–1521.
22. Bjorntorp, P., L. Sjostrom. "Number and Size of Adipose Tissue Fat Cells in Relation to Metabolism in Human Obesity." *Metabolism.* 20(1971): 703–713.
23. Speigelman, B.M., J.S. Flier. "Adipogenesis and Obesity: Rounding Out the Big Picture." *Cell.* 87(1996): 377–389.
24. Korn, E.D., T.W. Quigley Jr. "Studies on Lipoprotein Lipase of Rat Heart and Adipose Tissue." *Biochim Biophys Acta.* 18(1955): 143–145.
25. Cook, K.S., H.Y. Min, D. Johnson, et al. "Adipsin: A Circulating Serine Protease Homolog Secreted by Adipose Tissue and Sciatic Nerve." *Science.* 237(1987): 402–405.
26. Clerke, A.M. "Robert Hooke (1635–1703)". In *The Dictionary of Scientific Biography.* Ed. L. Stephen and S. Lee. London: Vol. IX. Oxford University Press, 1937–38.
27. Talbott, J.H. *A Biographical History of Medicine: Excerpts and Essays on the Men and Their Work.* New York: Grune and Stratten, 1970.
28. Blau, G.N. "Hassall—Physician and Microscopist." *Brit Med J.* 3(1968): 617–619.
29. Hassall, A.H. *Food and Its Adulterations; Comprising the reports of the Analytical Sanitary Commission of "The Lancet" for the Years 1851 to 1854 Inclusive, Revised and Extended.* London: Longman, Brown, Green, and Longmans, 1855.

Chapter 15

The Science of Hunger: Gut-Brain Signals or the Wolf at the Door

Appetite, a universal wolf
So doubly seconded with will and power,
Must make perforce a universal prey,
And last eat up himself.
Troilus & Cressida, 1.iii.121

—William Shakespeare[1]

What is appetite? What is hunger? Understanding these two terms is important since an increased appetite or increased hunger may be the cause of the bulge that we are so often battling. The dictionary defines hunger as simply "a desire or need for food" and goes on to define it as "any appetite, strong desire or craving." *Appetite* is in turn defined as "a desire or longing to satisfy any conscious physical or mental need."

Appetite thus covers a broader range of desires than does hunger. Hunger may, in turn, be viewed as one kind of appetite. *Starvation* is used to refer to any lengthy and continuous deprivation of food. Hunger and appetite generally have none of the long-term connotations for deprivation and nutrient depletion that are associated with starvation. Hunger and appetite operate over the short term and signal mild levels of deprivation or depletion, as compared to that associated with starvation or malnutrition. Yet "hunger" is frequently used as a surrogate for "starvation." I will turn briefly to this latter context after discussing the scientific contributions of Drs. Cannon and Washburn[2] and of Dr. Carlson to our understanding of how the body recognizes hunger, which may give us clues in how to control it in our own battle of the bulge[3].

The two scientific papers reprinted in the appendix focus on gastrointestinal or gut signals for hunger. I have chosen these papers because they propose that hunger reflects gastric contractions. They were published at essentially the same time but used very different methods of approaching the problem. These authors were certainly not the first to ask questions about hunger, since this is a problem that has confronted humankind since the dawn of Homo sapiens one hundred thousand or more years ago. However, these papers provide a cohesive picture of how hunger might be produced and modulated. Moreover, the conclusions are based on experimental data used to support the theories.

Study of the role of the stomach in feeding was given impetus by the studies of military surgeon William Beaumont (1785-1853)[4]. Through an unfortunate but fortuitous accident, one of his patients suffered a gunshot wound to his stomach that healed with an opening to the outside. Through this opening Dr. Beaumont could examine the responses of the stomach lining to the ingestion of food and to external situations. This important clinical work carried out on the frontiers of the expanding United States was published in 1833 in a small book[4] and subsequently translated around the world.

Carlson provides a very nice review of the theories about hunger that had been put forward prior to 1916[5]. He divides them into three main groups: those theories in which the information about hunger comes from stimulation of peripheral nerves, those theories in which the message about hungers comes from a "hunger center" located in the brain, and a third group of theories labeled general sensation which involve both central and peripheral signals for hunger. The peripheral theories of hunger can be subdivided in two main categories: those related to stimulation of a strictly local group of sensory nerves, such as those in the stomach, and a second set of sensory nerves that receive signals from blood or from tissues and organs other than the stomach. Theories relating to the digestive tract include (1) hunger due to mechanical stimulation of sensory nerves caused by rubbing or pressure from the stomach; (2) hunger due to chemical stimulation of sensory nerves in the stomach wall; (3) stimulation of sensory nerves due to swelling of the gastric glands in the stomach; (4) effects on sensory nerves in the stomach resulting from changes in the blood flow due to food deprivation; (5) stimulation of sensory nerves due to the absence of contractions in the empty stomach; (6) and finally, hunger due to stimulation of sensory nerves in the wall of the stomach by contraction of the empty or partly empty stomach.

Carlson contends that the writings of Hippocrates and Galen do not contain specific theories concerning mechanisms for hunger or appetite. One of the earliest theories for the feelings of hunger is found in the eighteenth-century work of Albrecht von Haller (1708-1777)[6]. To quote from an English translation, Haller says, "The immediate cause of the sensation of hunger is the grinding or rubbing (tritus) of the delicate and vilous folds of the gastric mucosa against each other, through a motion or contraction inherent in the stomach, aided by the diaphragm and abdominal muscles"[5].

In contrast to Haller, Erasmus Darwin (1731-1802) and Johannes Müller (1801-1858) both thought that hunger was the absence of contractions in the stomach, which produced a variety of negative sensations. Yet another perspective was that of Weber and a number of other eminent nineteenth-century physiologists who perceived that hunger was "[s]udden and strong contractions of the empty stomach completely obliterating the gastric cavity, giving rise in part to the sensation we call hunger"[5]. Carlson believes that the turgescence theory of Beaumont[4] is untenable, since there is no accumulation of gastric juice in the crypts of the gastric glands in the empty stomach, which would stimulate gastric nerves by distention. The theory that hunger is merely a negative phenomenon due to the absence of a positive sensation accompanying the filled stomach has, in Carlson's view, not received much attention. The concept that hunger may be due to chemical stimulation of nerves in the gastric mucosa also dates back to the work of Albrecht von Haller[6].

The main arguments used by proponents of the theory that hunger is in the brain are that man and animals will eat after removal of the stomach or when the nerves to the stomach are cut, so that hunger may be present even when the stomach is partly filled with food and hunger may be appeased by feeding per rectum as well as by intravenous injections of nutrients.

In contrast to the peripheral theories, the great nineteenth-century French physiologist Francois Magendie (1783-1855)[7] thought that hunger was strictly of central origin, since the gastric sensations and general feelings of weakness that many associate with hunger have been observed to pass away without an individual partaking of food. The possibility that a hunger center in the brain could be stimulated by changes in the blood due to starvation is the theory held by many investigators[5]. In Carlson's view the main objection to this central theory is its failure to explain the reference of hunger sensations to the stomach, the fact that hunger may be temporarily abolished by eating of indigestible materials, and the periodicity of the sensations of hunger.

Theories of hunger originating in the brain assume that a hunger center in the brain is stimulated directly by changes in the composition of the blood resulting from nutrient deprivation as well as indirectly by afferent nervous impulses from many organs in the body. This theory according to Carlson[5] was accepted by a number of leading nineteenth-century scientists. The objections raised against this theory of hunger are that (1) hunger may set in before intestinal absorption is complete; (2) there may not be very marked chemical changes in the blood even in prolonged starvation; (3) hunger is abolished temporarily by eating indigestible matter; (4) that hunger is usually more or less periodic with sudden onsets; and (5) in very prolonged starvation hunger does not, at least in man, increase in intensity with the degree of depletion.

It was against this background that Cannon and Washburn in Boston and Carlson in Chicago conducted their studies. The study by Cannon and Washburn[2] was designed to answer the question of whether contractions in the stomach were associated with sensations of hunger. This was a clinical study, with Washburn, a medical student, acting as the subject. He is only one among many medical students who have contributed significant understanding to human biology during their years in medical training. A few others would include Charles Best (1899-1978), who worked with Frederick Banting (1891-1941) to isolate and inject the first insulin into a diabetic dog[8]; William Bowman (1816-1892), who described the structure of striated muscle as a medical student[9]; and Paul Lagerhans (1847-1888), who, during his early medical student years, identified the islet structure in the pancreas that produces insulin[10].

Washburn was the medical student who swallowed the intestinal balloons each experimental day. Based on the high level of congruence between his ratings of hunger and strong gastric contractions, Cannon and Washburn[2] concluded that gastric contractions were the cause of hunger sensations.

The experimental methods used by Carlson were different[3], but he reached the same conclusions as Cannon and Washburn. Carlson studied a patient with a gastric fistula, that is a hole from his skin into his stomach produced following closure of his esophagus from lye burns at an early age[5]. The use of subjects with gastric fistulas and other rare conditions has provided important opportunities for selected scientists to make outstanding contributions to medicine and particularly to the understanding of the battle of the bulge. Probably the most notable of these is William Beaumont's study of Alexis St. Martin[4], a frontiersman who suffered a gunshot wound to the stomach that healed with an opening through the skin. More recently Wolf and Wolff[11] used a similar unfortunate act of nature as the basis of their study of gastric function. The fistula present in the patient studied by Carlson allowed him to insert a tube with a balloon at the end from which recordings could be made. Like Cannon and Washburn, Carlson noted the high degree of relationship between strong contractions in the stomach and the reported feelings of hunger. Based on the work of these eminent scientists, the concept that gastric contractions produced hunger was widely accepted and became a standard explanation in textbooks.

The function of any good theory or hypothesis is to provide questions that lead to productive experiments and a framework for conceptualizing the results. One prediction would be that if you had no stomach, you might not have feelings of hunger. The demonstration by Grossman et al.[12] that animals with gastric denervation produced by vagotomy and sympathectomy could regulate food intake and the demonstration that removal of the entire stomach from human beings does not abolish their ability to detect sensations of hunger or to regulate food intake[12] challenged the hypothesis that gastric contractions are the primary mechanism for the sensation of hunger and led to the search for alternative explanations to help us understand why we bulge and how to battle it.

Another prediction for the gastric contraction theory of hunger is that if you become more sensitive to gastric contractions you might be better able to control hunger and eat when hunger was present and not otherwise. Neurotic obese subjects who originally could not distinguish gastric motility could be trained to do so. Almost every subject so trained could increase the ability to detect gastric contractions. The improved perception of gastric motility, however, had no effect on either hunger or the control of body weight in obese subjects[13].

Important information about the basic elements of hunger and satiety has come from elegant studies on insects[14] and experimental animals[15, 16]. Because of their greater simplicity, it is possible to isolate the elements of hunger in insects in great detail. Dethier[14] has shown that distention of the stomach in flies reduces feeding and that the absence of gastric contents is associated with feeding behavior in these same flies. It is now clear that the entire gastrointestinal tract has a neural innervation of its own with interconnections to the central autonomic nervous system. This rich gastrointestinal innervation involves monoamines as well as a variety of peptides in a complex neural network. There can be little doubt that distention or contraction of the stomach or intestines can provide us with information about how much food we have eaten, but there are other important mechanisms as well. Ghrelin, a peptide produced in the stomach, has provided a recent clue to the control of food intake. This substance is secreted into the blood. Its levels are high just before a meal and fall when we eat, only to rise again before the next meal. Moreover, people battling the bulge have lower levels of this substance in their blood than thinner people. Thus we have come full circle, from the contraction of the stomach to central controls and back to the stomach through release of an important hormone that may control feeding.

Hunger has more than one meaning. It is the internal recognition of food deprivation in a single individual. It is subjective and does not necessarily provide any information about how deprived of food we are (remember that the amount of food energy that we eat in a day is less than 2% of the amount of energy that is stored in our bulging fat stores.) Hunger does not tell us how much energy is stored in the body, but it does tell us about the absence of food in the stomach and upper intestines. One way some people battle the bulge is to consciously control these hunger signals — so-called retrained eaters. A restrained eater is an individual who makes conscious decisions when to eat and when not to eat. When this restrained control is lost, for whatever reason, there is often a tendency to overeat, with the expected consequences[17]. Indeed, among middle-aged, middle-class American women, there are only a small number who are not restraining their eating to some extent to avoid the consequences of the bulge.

The word *hunger* is often used in a much broader context related to shortages of food, malnutrition, and actual starvation. If I ask whether you are hungry and you answer yes, this does not necessarily tell either you or me anything about the true state of your body energy stores in fat.

Both people battling the bulge and normal people have sensations of hunger in relation to meals and intervals without food. However, the word *hunger* has taken on a political context in which it is often equated with malnutrition[18]. The two, however, differ in major ways. Hunger results from short-term and long-term deprivation. Malnutrition, on the other hand, results from deficiency of food and its nutrition that has occurred over a period of days, weeks, months, or even years.

A major impetus for the concern about world hunger and food supplies came from Malthus's book titled *An Essay on the Principle of Population*[19]. He pointed out that people multiplied geometrically but that the supply of food increased only arithmetically[19]. The implications are that as populations grow they will eventually run out of food and starvation will result. Two books on hunger[20, 21], along with periodic episodes of starvation around the globe, have served to highlight this problem. Malthus makes two important points. First he says:

> In taking a view of animated nature, we cannot fail to be struck with the prodigious power to increase in plants and animals...their natural tendency must be to increase in a geometrical ratio, that is, by multiplication...I think I may fairly make two postulates. First, that food is necessary to the existence of man. Secondly, that the passion between the sexes is necessary and will remain nearly in its present state.

He then goes on to conclude that the rate of population growth will eventually outstrip the ability of the land and agriculture to provide food for the growing number of people.

> I say, that the power of population is indefinitely greater than the power in the earth to produce subsistence for man...Population, when unchecked, increases in a geometrical ratio. Subsistence increases only in an arithmetical ratio...This implies a strong and constantly operating check on population from the difficulty of subsistence[19].

It is clear that over most of the millennia of human existence on Earth, indeed until the late nineteenth century, the rate of population growth had been relatively slow. "It is quite clear that a powerful check on the increase of population must be almost constantly in action," said Malthus. He goes on to define both preventive and positive checks on multiplication of the human species. Malthus viewed these checks largely as the supply of food. However, the presence of infectious diseases were an additional factor in controlling the size of the population. The twentieth-century has seen a remarkable control over these infectious diseases with a resulting explosion of the total population on earth in the last century.

Yet, in contrast to Malthus's dire predictions, the food supply has generally kept ahead of the growth of population. Since Malthus published his book in 1798, the world population has risen from nearly five hundred million to more than six billion people. Two important events could not be anticipated in Malthus's calculations. The first of these was the major impact of sanitation programs on the reduction in disease leading to a marked rise in population in the late nineteenth and early twentieth centuries, and the second was the improvement in agriculture. As Taylor notes, "Historically, a principal means of limiting population growth has been discrimination against the poor and against females. However, it is increasingly evident that a better balance between birth and death rates can be effectively achieved, providing special care to these groups"[21]. Taylor goes on to note that the synergism between nutrition and disease is highly related to socio-economic status and female gender. One major restraint on population growth until the late nineteenth and early twentieth centuries was early deaths due to infectious disease. This was often associated with low income levels, which decreased the food that these families could purchase and which in turn lowered their immunological resistance to bacterial diseases. This synergism between nutrition and infectious diseases has been an important event in the course of history.

The more than tenfold growth in world population between 1836 and 2000 has been more than matched by the chemical, green, and technological revolutions in food production, which have allowed smaller fractions of the population to produce substantially greater yields per acre of land and make adequate food available to the world population.

Clearly at some point in history, however, a balance will be restruck between the potential of all resources relating to population multiplication, including disease, availability of nutrients, and their interaction, which will lead to restabilization of the population. It is clear that Malthus's predictions of nearly two hundred years ago have yet to be fulfilled.

The word *hunger* in affluent countries often carries political connotations. Phrases such as "the war on hunger," "world hunger," and "hidden hunger" suggest deprivation and malnutrition in the midst of plenty. As

Rotberg and Rabb note, "For historians, part of the task of hunger studies is to encompass the complexity and variations of the phenomena of poverty and hunger, both socially loaded terms which refer, only indirectly, to the narrower nexus of individual human malnutrition and infection"[21]. Efforts to document this degree of deprivation and starvation have been difficult. At the time of the "war on poverty and hunger" in the United States, a survey of under-served groups was carried out. This showed pockets of poverty with malnutrition, but if malnutrition and starvation are criteria of hunger, it must be a rare event today in the absence of war or environmental catastrophe.

The major causes for malnutrition and starvation today are associated with civil war or internal strife. The recent events in Somalia, Ethiopia, Sudan, and North Korea are prime examples. Prior to the onset of centrally controlled governments with central planning, these countries had a surplus of food production. The disruption caused by civil war and the efforts to centrally plan the economies led to the current disastrous state of malnutrition and starvation. Nearly two hundred years ago, Malthus was aware of the limitations of central planning by governments in the provision of adequate food supplies. He said,

> There can be no well-founded hope of obtaining a large produce from the soil, but under a system of private property... it seems perfectly visionary to suppose that any stimulus short of that which is excited in man by the desire of providing for himself and his family, and of bettering his condition in life, should operate on the mass of society with sufficient force and constancy to overcome the natural indolence of mankind[19].

Overt hunger, noted above, differs from the concept of "hidden hunger." For example, as Newman[20] observed,

> [P]erinatal mortality was reduced most, when the diet of mothers was supplemented, particularly with iron and folic acid. Infection control had about half as much effect on perinatal mortality, mainly due to the reduction in neonatal tetanus by immunization of mothers and improved delivery practices of traditional birth attendance. Infant mortality was reduced most by infection control and less by improved nutrition. Mortality in children between the ages of 1 and 3 was reduced by both[21].

As Scrimshaw has pointed out, "The functional consequences of hidden hunger in the development of human society have probably been at least as important as those of hunger or famine"[21].

As I close this discussion we now see that hunger can be used in three contexts. In the first context, hunger is viewed as a reflection of individual experience of deprivation associated with gastric and/or intestinal contractions or events related to them which occur in the several hours following a meal. It is this sense of the word *hunger* that is most important to us in the battle of the bulge. In the second context, hunger was viewed as a surrogate for malnutrition and starvation which in present circumstances is seen primarily in conditions of civil war or international war. The third context and the one which may be most important in relation to population development is "hidden hunger," meaning the deficiency of selected components during essential parts of the developmental sequence that is life.

Biosketch

Walter Bradford Cannon (1871-1945) was an internationally known physiologist and chairman of the Department of Physiology at Harvard Medical School[22, 23]. He came from Prairie du Chien, a small town in Wisconsin, where he was born October 19, 1871. His mother died when he was ten. He received his early education in Milwaukee and St. Paul, from where he went to Harvard College on a scholarship, graduating *summa cum laude* 1896. (Figure 15-1)

He received his M.D. from Harvard Medical School in 1900 and joined the Department of Physiology as an instructor, only to be elevated to George Higginson Professor of Physiology in 1906, a position that he held until his retirement thirty-six years later in 1942. His early work was focused on the gastrointestinal tract, and his book titled *The Mechanical Factors of Digestion* is a classic in its field[24]. He was a skilled surgeon and used experimental animals frequently in his work. His devotion to animal welfare and to research led to his efforts throughout the pre-World War I period as an advocate of humane and proper care of experimental animals. His work on hunger, published in 1912, was followed three years later by one of his most popular books, *Bodily Changes in Pain, Hunger, Fear and Rage*[25]. His monograph *The Way of an Investigator* is a description of the life of a clinical investigator[26].

Biosketch

Anton Julius Carlson (1875-1956) was born in Sweden and immigrated to the United States alone in 1891 to join his brother in Chicago[27]. He worked for the next two years as a carpenter's helper while learning English. He enrolled in the Augustana College and Theological Seminary with the intention of becoming a Lutheran minister.

However, as biographer Visscher notes, "Within a year after beginning his ministerial post, he decided that he could not maintain his intellectual integrity while pretending adherence to dogma which he no longer believed." He therefore announced to his congregation that he was leaving the ministry to study neurophysiology, stating his reasons quite candidly[28]. He entered Stanford University, where he received his Ph.D. degree in 1902. A few years later he joined the University of Chicago as an associate in the Department of Physiology and rose to the rank of professor in 1914 and chairman in 1916. He retired from the University of Chicago in 1940. Carlson's first papers on the physiology of the stomach were published in 1912 and were followed by a long series in this field. Carlson's colorful personality made him a stimulating teacher and a sought-after lecturer. He was an ardent civil libertarian and was president of the American Association of University Professors[29]. (Figure 15-2)

References

1. Shakespeare, W. *Troilus and Cressida.* I.iii.121.
2. Cannon, W.B., A.L., Washburn. "An Explanation of Hunger." *Am J Physiol.* 29 (1912): 441-454.
3. Carlson, A.J. "Contributions to the Physiology of the Stomach. II. The Relation between the Concentrations of the Empty Stomach and the Sensation of Hunger." *Am J Physiol.* 31 (1912):175-192.
4. Beaumont, W. *Experiments and Observations on the Gastric Juices and the Physiology of Digestion.* Pittsburgh: F.P. Allen, 1833.
5. Carlson, A.J. *Control of Hunger in Health and Disease.* Chicago, IL: University of Chicago Press, 1916.
6. von Haller, A. *Elementa physiological corporis humani.* Lausanne: Marci-Michael Boursquet & Sociorurn, 1757:VI.
7. Magendie, F. *Precis elementaire de physiologie.* Paris: Mequignon-Marvis, 1816.
8. Banting, F.G., C.H. Best. "The Internal Secretion of the Pancreas." *J Lab Clin Med.* 7 (1921-1922): 251-256.
9. Bowman, W. "On the Minute Structure and Movements of Voluntary Muscle." *Phil Trans.* 130(1840): 457-501 and 131(1841): 69-72.
10. Langerhans, P. *Beiträge zur mikroskopischen Anatomie der Bauchspeicheldrilse. Inaugural Dissertation.* Berlin: Gustav Lange, 1869.
11. Wolf, S., H.G., Wolff. *Human Gastric Function: An Experimental Study of a Man and His Stomach.* New York: Oxford University Press, 1943.
12. Grossman, M.R., G.M. Cummins, A.C. Ivy. "The Effect of Insulin on Food Intake after Vagotomy and Sympathectomy." *Am J Physiol.* 149 (1947): 100-102.
13. Stunkard, A.J., S. Fox. "The Relationship of Motility and Hunger: A Summary of the Evidence." *Psychosomatic Medicine.* 33(1971): 123-134.
14. Dethier, V.G. *The Hungry Fly: A Physiological Study of the Behavior Associated with Feeding.* Cambridge: Harvard University Press, 1976.
15. Balagura, S. *Hunger: A Biopsychological Analysis.* New York: Basic Books Inc, 1973.
16. LeMagnen, J. *Hunger.* Cambridge: Cambridge University Press, 1985.
17. Williamson, D.A., O.J. Lawson, E.R. Brooks, P.J. Wozniak, D.H. Ryan, G.A. Bray. E.G. Duchman. "Association of Body-mass with Dietary Restraint and Disinhibition." *Appetite.* 25(1995): 31-41.
18. De Castro, J. *The Geography of Hunger.* Boston: Little, Brown and Co., 1952.
19. Malthus, T. *An Essay on the Principle of Population or, a view of its past and present effects on human happiness; with an inquiry into our prospects respecting the future removal or mitigation of the evils which it occasions.*

4th ed. London: J. Johnson, 1807.
20. Newman, L.F., ed. *Hunger in History: Food Shortage, Poverty, and Deprivation.* Cambridge, MA: Basil Blackwell Inc., 1990.
21. Rotberg, R.I., T.K. Rabb. *Hunger and History: The Impact of Changing Food Production and Consumption Patterns on Society.* Cambridge: Cambridge University Press, 1983.
22. Benison S., A.C. Barger, E.L. Wolfe W.B. Cannon. *The Life and Times of a Young Scientist.* Cambridge: Belknap Press, 1987.
23. Mayer, J. "Walter Bradford Cannon—A Biographical Sketch." *J Nutr.* 87(1965): 3-8.
24. Cannon, W.B. *The Mechanical Factors in Digestion.* London: E. Arnold, 1911.
25. Cannon, W.B. *Bodily Changes in Pain, Hunger, Fear, and Rage.* New York: D. Appleton & Co., 1915.
26. Cannon, W.B. *The Way of an Investigator.* New York: W.W., Norton & Co., 1945.
27. Talbott, J.H. *A Biographical History of Medicine: Excerpts and Essays on the Men and Their Work.* New York: Grune & Stratton, 1970.
28. Visscher, N.B. *Dictionary of Scientific Biography.* 3(1971): 68-70.
29. Kaufman, N.I., S. Galishoff, T.L. Savitt, eds. *Dictionary of American Medical Biography.* Westport, Conn.: Greenwood Press, 1984.

CHAPTER 16

The Science of Hunger: Revisiting Two Theories of Feeding

We must never make experiments to confirm our ideas, but simply to control them.

—Claude Bernard[1]

I. Background: The Science of Hunger

Breakfast is the time in the day when we break the fast of the previous night. Each morning we begin this meal and a short time later stop. What starts us eating? What stops us eating? What determines how long we eat? These questions have been the driving force in the search for the messages from the foods we eat. Knowing what these are will help us in the battle of the bulge. If we know what they are, then we have the potential for modifying them—for winning our fight against the bulge. If these signals work properly we maintain our weight. We are in homeostasis—that is, we are balancing our internal and external worlds to keep ourselves healthy. Two broad ideas surround this area. The first is that we respond to concentrations of things like glucose or blood sugar or to amino acids as messages about our nutritional status. These might be called "static" theories for the regulation of food intake and body weight. The other is that our brain and body respond not to the actual concentrations of glucose or amino acids but to the changes that occur after a meal or before a meal. These kinds of theories might be called "dynamic" theories. In this chapter we explore this approach to information about the battle of the bulge and how it might help us.

The three papers in the appendix relate to glucose and amino acids as peripheral signals for the control of food intake. The first paper is titled "Glucostatic Mechanism of Regulation of Food Intake" by Jean Mayer (1920-1993), which was published in 1953[2]. The second paper titled "A Fall in Blood Glucose Level Precedes Meal Onset in Free-Feeding Rats" by Jeanine Louis-Sylvestre and Jacques Le Magnen[3] recasts the glucostatic theory as a glucodynamic theory and opened the way to rethink other "static" theories in more dynamic terms. The third paper is titled "Relationship between Serum Amino Acid Concentration and Fluctuations in Appetite" and is by Sherman Mellinkoff and his associates, who articulated an "amino-static" theory for feeding in which protein or its amino acid components served as the signal to inhibit feeding[4].

From the early twentieth-century until World War II, theories about control of food intake were dominated by the work of Cannon and Washburn[5] and Carlson[6]. Their "peripheral" theories are described in Chapter 15 and were only gradually augmented or replaced by theories of central integration and by information about nutrients in the blood[7].

In 1940 Hetherington and Ranson at Northwestern University showed that tissue damage in the ventromedial hypothalamus of the brain would consistently produce an increase in food intake and began to change the framework of thought about control of food intake and body weight (See Chapter 24)[8]. This work was the definitive demonstration that the adiposo-genital syndrome (also called Frohlich's syndrome) was due to damage to hypothalamic structures at the base of the brain and not to damage to the pituitary—a conflict that had raged through the first quarter of the twentieth century[9]. It was the technical ability of Hetherington and Ranson to produce discrete anatomic destruction in the hypothalamus that provided the definitive experimental proof that it was the hypothalamus, not the pituitary, that was involved in controlling body fat. When they damaged the ventromedial hypothalamus on both sides, animals overate and became obese. Based on their work, a key role for the brain could no longer be denied. Brobeck and Anand, using similar precise techniques, showed that damaging hypothalamic lesions placed more laterally in the hypothalamus than the ones that produced obesity would produce loss of appetite and weight loss[10]. The pendulum was now swinging toward the brain for theories on the regulation of food intake. Using the experimental work of Hetherington and Ranson[8] and of Brobeck and his colleagues[11, 12], Eliot Stellar formulated the Dual Center hypothesis for regulation of food intake[13]. This theory postulated that the ventromedial hypothalamus located at the base of the brain functioned as a satiety center and centers located slightly lateral in the lateral hypothalamus served as a hunger center.

Close on the heels of the Dual Center hypothesis came several ideas about the nature of the signals to the brain that were called for by this theory[4]. Under the names of glucostatic[2], lipostatic[14], aminostatic[4], and thermostatic[12], several theories were proposed as a way of signaling to the brain about the need for food intake. An underlying assumption for all of these "static" proposals is that body weight and fat stores are stable. This apparent stability in the short term is associated with variations of food intake above and below the "stable" or preferred weight. Studies in both humans[15] and monkeys have shown that day-to-day food intake is a weak predictor of energy expenditure and body weight in the short term, suggesting that these day-to-day changes or oscillations in food intake provide error signals to the brain on which compensatory systems make corrections.

Although these theories all have the word *static* in them, they are in fact theories about how dynamic changes can be recognized by the body and appropriate adjustments made. Since they are dynamic rather than static, I have changed the terminology and will develop the concept of "dynamic" theories.

II. Glucodynamic (rather than glucostatic) Theory

In a very readable paper, Jean Mayer argued that body weight and fat stores are regulated, and he suggested that glucose concentration, or changes in glucose level was the primary, if not the only, signal needed to provide this regulation[16]. To support this concept, Mayer used the earlier work by Gasnier and Andre Mayer, his father [17-21]. With rabbits as their subjects, these scientists showed that there was only a very small short-term variation in body energy reserves about their preferred weight. There was also only a small variation in the day-to-day intake of food in rabbits that had access to food under uniform conditions. To show that the animals would adjust their intake to changing conditions, the animals were housed at several different environmental temperatures and food intake measured. Over the eighty days of the study, there was a spread of food intake and energy expenditure, indicating that day-to-day errors were detected and that changes of intake were made to compensate for these changes over time. Based on their studies, Gasnier and A. Mayer defined four parameters that described the day-to-day adjustments of energy or food intake in relation to energy expenditure. These parameters were the precision, reliability, sensitivity, and rapidity of response of the feeding system.

Precision is inversely proportional to the short-term difference between energy intake and expenditure and in the long term to the amplitude in body fat reserves for any given value of fat. Reliability refers to the temporal periodicity. Sensitivity, according to Gasnier and A. Mayer, is the distribution of values around the zero or privileged value of composition of fat or carbohydrate stores. Rapidity refers to the time constant or rate of oscillations.

From this analysis of the work by Gasnier and A. Mayer on rabbits, Jean Mayer concluded several things that might relate to human beings [16]. First, that there are upper and lower limits to food intake and energy expenditure, which are related to the biology of the stomach and other ingestive organs and the ability to use or conserve energy. Second, that there are day-to-day adjustments of energy intake to energy output. Third, that there is regulation of body fat reserves. Fourth, that the precision, reliability, sensitivity, and rapidity of response of the regulated system can be specified. Fifth, that a number of factors including cold and exercise can influence the regulation of this system. Sixth, that obese animals regulate intake, albeit with greater oscillations.

In looking for a short-term mechanism to explain the control of feeding, Jean Mayer set out several criteria [16]. First, the signal he was looking for must be integrated into the metabolism of the body. Second, it must have both an anatomic and physiologic basis. Third, it must account for the effects of variations in environmental conditions. Fourth, hormones such as insulin, growth hormone, and thyroxine must be integrated into the system. Finally, it must account for the state of hunger and satiety. Jean Mayer believed that the only mechanism that fulfilled all of these criteria was the availability of carbohydrates, primarily glucose. Glucose and carbohydrates have been a central theme in popular diet books. Some argue that glucose produced from carbohydrates stimulates insulin and that this is the reason that low carbohydrates are so useful in treating the battle of the bulge. We return to this theme later.

As he points out, glucose metabolism is pivotal for overall metabolic processes and is an essential fuel for the brain. In addition, there is anatomic evidence for glucose-responsive cells in the brain. When gold thioglucose is injected into animals, it enters the brain and destroys areas of the ventromedial hypothalamus with subsequent development of obesity[22]. Other data that are consistent with the idea of Mayer include the following: (1) that injections of insulin which lower blood glucose can stimulate feeding; (2) that 2-deoxy-D-glucose, an analogue of glucose that prevents glucose from being metabolized in cells, will stimulate feeding; and (3) that glucose injection[23] or mobilization of glycogen by glucagon[24] will reduce the differences in glucose between the arteries and veins and also reduce gastric contractions and abolish hunger.

Following the publication of Jean Mayer's hypothesis, Yutaka Oomura and his colleagues in Japan demonstrated the presence of neurons in the brain that were sensitive to the presence of glucose (glucosensitive neurons) or that responded to glucose (glucoresponsive neurons) in the ventromedial and lateral hypothalamus respectively[25]. Moreover, hormones such as insulin and growth hormone have important effects in the metabolism of glucose and on food intake. Finally, in the study of diabetics and normal subjects given injections of glucagon that will enhance the release of glucose, Mayer and his colleagues were able to show that it was the change in glucose utilization measured as the difference between the artery and vein that was the critical variable.

Albert Stunkard,[24] who was an initial contributor to work on the "glucostatic theory" for satiety, has given us a glimpse into the excitement that this theory brought to his early research career and to his eventual disillusion with this theory. In his very readable autobiographical work *The Pain of Obesity*, he summarized the status of the Glucostatic Theory in 1972 as follows:

> The more I thought about (the glucostatic) theory, the better it sounded. And it led directly into the next question. What went wrong in obesity...Two distinct possibilities suggested themselves. First, the glucostatic mechanism itself might break down. The second possibility was that the glucostatic mechanism itself might be intact, but for some reason the obese person might not have enough blood sugar available...There is a certain drama in any research, a drama that may hang on the simple behavior of a recording pen...After all the time spent in preparations, the actual experiments took only a few days...The experiments showed that the glucostatic mechanism seemed to work for both obese and non-obese people...In short, the results of all those years of work on sugar tolerance were negative. This long digression taught me a bitter lesson. Dogged persistence does not of itself bring rewards in the scientific enterprise...there is a law of diminishing returns in the pursuit of technical improvements...Where has all of this research brought the glucostatic theory, in the years since I left it?...Glucostatic mechanisms play a part in [the regulation of food intake]; but they cannot account fully for either short-term control, such as the ending of a meal, or for long-term control, such as the stability of body weight over months and years.[24].

The role of glucose in the modulation of feeding has not disappeared, but the focus has changed. The change was brought about by improved methodology, which often leads to improved theory[26, 27]. Jacques Le Magnen viewed the patterns of change in food intake as a response to alterations in the blood-borne signals from glucose and free fatty acids[28]. Early studies with measurements of glucose made at intervals of ten to thirty minutes had failed to find regular patterns of change in the concentration of glucose or blood sugar[29]. However, with an improved method for continuous measurement of blood glucose concentration, Jeanine Louis-Sylvestre and Jacques Le Magnen[3] observed a 6% to 8% decline in glucose concentration that occurred 5±0.3 minutes before the onset of most meals in both the light and dark parts of the day. L. Arthur Campfield et al. showed that if this decrease in glucose were delayed or prevented, initiation of a meal was delayed or did not occur. He has extended these findings to human beings[30] and shown that more than half of the meals occur following this small transient decrease in blood glucose—a biological response to a dynamic change in glucose, hence the glucodynamic theory.

The role of glucose in regulation of food intake has shifted from a satiety signal to an initiation signal. Moreover, its role has shifted from a static one aimed at maintaining constant levels to a dynamic one in which the brain or liver are responding to dynamic changes in glucose concentration to initiate food seeking. Thus, along with contractions of the stomach, a dip in glucose may be a signal that periodically initiates the search for food. Figure 16-1 shows schematically how these two signals may be put into a simple model for initiating the onset of food intake. The dip in glucose and request for a meal in human beings is shown in the accompanying figure.

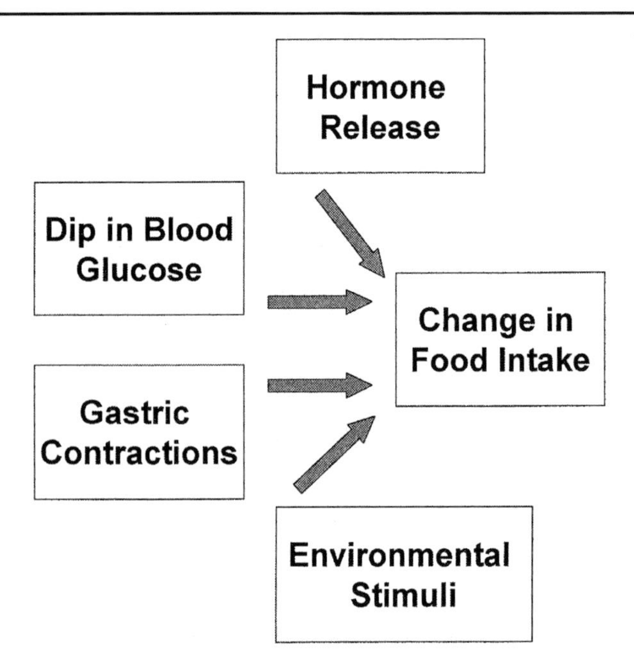

16-1 This figure shows three physiological ways in which the desire for food can be signaled. One is through contraction of the stomach that produces recognizable feelings in the abdomen. The second is a dip in blood glucose of 10-15% that precedes the initiation of eating in animals or the request for meals in human beings. The third is through a rise in blood levels of ghrelin, a hormone from the stomach that stimulates feeding. © George A. Bray, MD.

The use of the word *static* for the "glucostatic" theory is unfortunate, since it implies a static or unchanging system. Glucose oscillates in the plasma under normal circumstances and responds to a variety of external circumstances. The word ***dynamic*** would be more appropriate in light of the way in which food intake begins after the nadir in glucose, suggesting that it is the pattern of dynamic change in glucose that is sensed, rather than its level. It would thus be preferable to refer to this as the "glucodynamic theory" of food intake rather than the glucostatic theory.

III. Aminodynamic Theory

Changes in the levels of amino acids may provide another signaling system for feeding. When we eat protein, it is broken down in the intestine into amino acids that are absorbed into the blood. A high-protein diet may suppress feeding better than a low-protein diet and may stimulate energy expenditure more than a high-carbohydrate diet. This might suggest that the amino acids in these proteins could serve as messages to begin or to stop feeding.

The theory that amino acids might change food intake was tested by Sherman Mellinkoff and his colleagues[4]. For these studies they used normal, healthy volunteers who had no diseases that could affect their desire to eat. Each subject was asked to rate his hunger on a five-point scale that was then related to the level of amino acid nitrogen in the blood. At the time these studies were done, measurement of individual amino acids was not available, so they used total nitrogen in the blood as the index for changes in this dietary component. In the first experiment, blood was collected fasting and at four hourly intervals following breakfast. In the second and third experiments, each subject received an intravenous infusion of either a solution containing 5% amino acids and glucose or a 10% solution of amino acids obtained from digesting casein or milk protein enzymatically. In the final experiment, the subjects drank a 10% amino acid mixture. Appetite ratings and amino acid nitrogen levels showed reciprocal changes. That is, when the amino nitrogen was high hunger ratings were low, and when the nitrogen was low hunger ratings tended to be high. This suggested to them that amino acids may be involved in signaling hunger and satiety.

Protein-like materials have been measured for more than two centuries. Although the amino acids were isolated and synthesized in the nineteenth and early twentieth-centuries, reliable measurements of blood amino acids have come only in the past fifty years. The discovery of chromatography, a system that separates materials in blood or other solutions, made it possible to measure individual amino acids in biological fluids. In the 1940s, Martin and Synge[31] developed chromatography to separate individual chemical constituents from mixtures of these constituents. Moore and Stein[32] expanded this technique to the study of amino acids by developing a chromatographic system for separating and quantifying individual amino acids. All four men won the Nobel Prize for their work.

Tryptophan has been a particularly important amino acid in relation to feeding. In careful experimental studies, John Fernstrom and Richard

Wurtman showed that the levels of tryptophan in the brain reflected serum tryptophan levels[33]. The transport of tryptophan into the brain was also influenced by the concentration of other amino acids that are transported by the same transport system (phenylalanine, tyrosine, valine, leucine, and isoleucine). The importance of these observations on food intake is due to the fact that tryptophan is a precursor of serotonin, a neurotransmitter involved in modulating food intake.

But we are getting ahead of the story again. At the time of Hippocrates, more than two thousand years ago, many believed that there was a universal nutrient that was present in the food that entered the body[34]. The function of digestion was to extract this nutrient from the food. The fact that growth and development occurred on highly varied diets was certainly compatible with this idea. This concept of a single nutrient in food took a long time to be replaced and indeed persisted into the nineteenth century. A quote from a popular French textbook of physiology published in 1813 by A. Richerand titled *Elements of Physiology* gives the flavor of this idea:

> However various our aliments [food] may be, the action of our organs always separates from them the same nutritious principle; in fact, whether we live exclusively on animal or vegetable substances, the internal composition of our organs does not alter; an evident proof that the substance we obtain from aliments, to incorporate with our own, is always the same....[35]

The developments in chemistry in the eighteenth and early nineteenth-centuries abolished the one-nutrient hypothesis. In its place came the gradual recognition that there were three primary nutrients. William Prout (1785-1850)[36] proposed that all living bodies were composed of three great principles which he called saccharine (carbohydrate), oleosa (triglyceride), and albuminosa (protein). All of these are found in milk, the prototypical food. The essential nature of the nitrogenous or albuminous part of the diet was clearly demonstrated by Francois Magendie (1783-1855)[37], one of the great physiologists and nutrition scientists of the nineteenth-century. When dogs were given foods that contained no nitrogen, they began to fail and then died rapidly. The essential value of protein for life had been demonstrated; "protein was enthroned"[38].

However, not all proteins are equal, and the nineteenth-century gelatin crisis illustrates this clearly. Gelatin is a cheap source of protein made from tendons, hooves, bone, and skin[38, 39]. During the Napoleonic wars it was substituted in some hospitals for other forms of "protein" with the results we would now expect. However, it took the Gelatin Commission, which Magendie headed, to conclude that some proteins are better than others and that gelatin as the sole source of nitrogen was unable to sustain life[40].

The term *protein* was coined by G.J. Mulder (1802-1880) in 1839[41]. It symbolizes the broad importance now assigned to this component of animals and plants. Justus von Liebig (1803-1873)[42] was central among the individuals in giving protein its lofty status in the first part of the nineteenth century. Following the demonstration that nitrogen-containing substances were essential for life, Liebig formulated a concept of nutrition that put foodstuffs into two categories based on the role of protein in the formation of blood and its use in metabolism (a term not yet coined). Foods that were "proteinaceous" were in one group, and those that did not contain nitrogen were in the other. Because blood circulated and provided the tissues with the things that they needed to move and grow, Liebig argued that nutrients could be evaluated on their ability to provide substances to blood. In a step forward, yet still echoing some of the earlier concepts, Liebig said:

> The vegetable substances which serve for the production of blood, contain already the chief constituent of blood, ready formed, with all its elements. The nutritive power of vegetable food is directly proportional to the amount of these sanguingenous compounds in it....[43]

A nineteenth-century summary of Liebig's ideas was provided by an American, Austin Flint Jr. (1836-1915), in his book dealing with experiments on the effect of exercise on the excretion of urea. He said:

> Following the brilliant researches of Lavoisier upon the chemical phenomena of respiration and their relations to animal heat, the theories of Liebig, who divided the food into two classes, plastic (nitrogen containing) and calorific (without nitrogen), were almost universally adopted by physiologists. Liebig advanced the view that those articles of food composed of carbon, hydrogen and oxygen, were chiefly, if not entirely, useful in maintaining the animal temperature, by entering into combination with the oxygen of the inspirated air, producing carbonic acid, water and heat. He regarded that the elements of food composed of carbon, hydrogen, oxygen, and nitrogen, as concerned chiefly, if not entirely, in repairing the waste of the nitrogenized portions of the living body, particularly the muscular tissue. Applying these views to muscular action, Liebig assumed that exercise was always attended with an increased activity of the destructive metamorphosis of the nitrogenized substance of the muscular tissue; and that this could be measured by the amount of urea excreted[44].

It was only a few years later when Claude Bernard (1813-1878)[45] developed his concept of the internal milieu as a buffer against outside variations[46]. The concept of nutrition providing materials for blood may be viewed as a precursor to the concept of Bernard. The leading position of protein in nutrition was maintained throughout most of the nineteenth century and was only temporarily dethroned by the discovery of vitamins in the early twentieth-century[39, 47].

Between the discovery of cystine in 1810 and the discovery of the final amino acid, methionine, in 1922, a total of twenty-one amino acids had been identified[47]. When the study of protein and metabolism returned to center stage, amino acids occupied a larger portion of that stage. The classic studies of William C. Rose (1887-1985) and his colleagues[48] in the 1930s showed that amino acids could be divided into those that were "essential" and those that were "nonessential." The nine essential amino acids had to be provided to the body from animal or plant sources. The other eleven or so amino acids can be synthesized in the body—thus the amount in dietary proteins can be highly variable without affecting nutrition. Paralleling this was the demonstration that the adequacy of the amino acid composition of individual proteins varied substantially. This had been known since the days of the Gelatin Commission, but with newer technologies it was possible to show that the adequacy of proteins for growth depended on the similarity of their amino acid composition to that of animal proteins. Proteins where one or more amino acids were in low concentration relative to animal proteins were less effective in supporting growth in young animals[37].

As has so often been the case in science, the introduction of new methods has revolutionized our concepts. Following the discovery of radioactivity, additional nonradioactive isotopes were discovered. Using nonradioactive isotopic forms of nitrogen and carbon, Rudolf Schoenheimer (1898-1941)[49] and his associates drastically changed the concept of protein metabolism. Using nitrogen-15-labeled amino acids, Schoenheimer showed that the body proteins were in a constant state of flux. This dynamic state of protein and other body constituents opened new vistas for research. If the body proteins were being continually destroyed, they must be continually remade, and for this to happen there must be a regular supply of the amino acid building blocks.

Turning from whole proteins to amino acids has greatly expanded our scientific horizon as the veil of truth has been steadily pulled back using the technique of amino acid chromatography. Corpulent human beings were found to have elevated circulating levels of several amino acids including alanine, cystine, methionine, threonine, tyrosine, phenylalanine, leucine, valine, and arginine[50]. Other amino acids were normal. The removal of individual amino acids from the diet was found to reduce food intake[51, 52]. The center for this sensitivity to diets deficient in one amino acid was in the pyriform cortex where alpha-1 adrenergic receptors play a key role[51].

The level of brain tryptophan and the level of serotonin were found to relate to the blood level of tryptophan relative to the other large neutral amino acids (phenylalanine, leucine, isoleucine, and valine) that are transported across the blood brain barrier by the same transport system[33]. The tryptophan entry system thus provided a direct mechanism for the brain to monitor circulating levels of an amino acid.

Tryptophan and its metabolite 5-hydroxytryptophan can both reduce food intake; the most likely explanation for this is the rise in brain tryptophan and the corresponding rise in 5-hydroxy-tryptamine or serotonin, an important neurotransmitter that suppresses feeding. On first glance, one might expect tryptophan and serotonin to be involved indirectly in modulating protein intake. As Rene Dubos has said, "Logic is an unreliable instrument for the discovery of the truth"[53]. Serotonin and drugs that act like serotonin specifically reduce fat intake and do not affect carbohydrate or protein[54-57].The saga of amino acids as regulators of food intake has taken another turn. Not only can they affect food intake but they also can selectively affect the intake of a single macronutrient: fat.

In the dynamic sense, then, it may be the rate of change in a nutrient (glucose, amino acids, or fatty acid), one compartment relative to another, that provides the more important signal for regulating nutrient stores. This can be true of amino acids and protein as the dynamic changes in glucose signal readiness to eat[30]. Dynamic changes in amino acids, particularly when one is deficient, may also fit this concept[51]. A final set of observations which may fit this concept are related to growth and fat storage.

During childhood and the adolescent growth spurt, protein intake is channeled to "linear growth"[58]. One of the hormones involved in this process is growth hormone. In human beings, both children and adults, growth hormone will increase body protein and decrease body fat. In the adult, this is most evident when acromegalics that produce excess quantities of growth hormone are treated in ways that reduce the levels of growth hormone[59]. A fall in levels of growth hormone lowers body protein and increases body fat, particularly visceral fat.

Similarly, the changes in testosterone relative to estrogen at puberty play a major role in the differential changes in fat and protein as boys and girls mature into men and women. However, as Bacon said, "Excess of nourishment is hurtful; for it maketh the child corpulent," an observation that was documented in overfeeding studies by Bouchard and his colleagues[60]. When protein formation or turnover is stimulated in the presence of adequate amounts of all of the amino acids from the diet, body fat may be reduced. A shift toward protein accretion and away from fat synthesis has already been noted for growth hormone and for testosterone. Some drugs and natural hormones (norepinephrine and epinephrine) that stimulate the ß2 and ß3 adrenergic receptors also stimulate protein formation and reduce body fat. Enhanced protein synthesis and turnover may thus be a signal to reduce body fat.

The effects suggested by Mellinkoff et al. in their "aminostatic" or, more appropriately, aminodynamic hypothesis[3] may be most appropriately viewed in the context of protein synthesis and breakdown. When a single amino acid is deficient, complete proteins cannot be made. This will reduce food intake. When amino acids are adequate, their concentrations are controlled by rates of protein synthesis and breakdown. Insulin plays a central role in this process by regulating amino acid use for cycling to the liver and for production of amino acid carbons for oxidation and amino acid nitrogen for acid/base balance in the kidney.

The changes in amino acid levels after meals noted by Mellinkoff et al.[3] may reflect the changes in insulin, which rises with food ingestion and then falls. The pattern of amino acid change, like the pattern of glucose change, may be a dynamic signal for initiating or terminating feeding.

In closing, one recent concept may be worth noting. The loss of protein during fasting is related to the amount of body fat that is stored. The larger the amount of fat, the smaller the amount of protein that is lost with partial or complete fasting. When refeeding is begun, the storage of protein, like the breakdown during fasting, is specific to an individual. This may relate to the higher insulin levels in obese individuals. In their studies with overfeeding, Bouchard et al.[60] noted that a compartment which they labeled "nutrient partitioning" was needed to match the differences in rates of nutrient storage and oxidation among these subjects. A number of adrenergic drugs that have been tested have shown the ability to increase protein accretion relative to fat. This mechanism for shifting or channeling the intake of amino acids to protein rather than to oxidation and fat storage may be an important link in the role of protein in the development of obesity.

In this discussion of protein and amino acids, I have traced some of the changing views over the past two centuries. A more detailed review of this subject can be found in the monograph of Kenneth Carpenter[38]. One conclusion about the general view of nutrition is summarized by Hopkins[61]:

> In connection with his own nutrition, Man's experience has been—needless to say—coterminous with his whole existence. Science may explain that experience, but is unlikely it might seem, to improve upon experience as a guide. It may supply theory, but where experience has been so great and so continuous it seems unlikely that it could do much to guide practice. This consideration, consciously or subconsciously accounts, I think, for the widespread feeling that the teachings of science about our food are of academic interest only.[61]

Biosketch

Justus von Liebig (1803-1873) was born in Darmstedt. After receiving his doctoral degree in 1822, he went to Paris to continue his work in chemistry with Gay-Lussac, one of the leading chemists of the day (Figure 16-2). He returned to Germany and had become professor with four years—a clear example of his intellectual prowess. So was his founding in 1832 of a scientific journal called *Liebigs Annalen*, a journal that survived till 1874.

Liebig began as a chemist, but his interests shifted to the chemistry of plants and animals. His analytical techniques facilitated his studies of body tissues and fluids. He emphasized the importance of protein in human nutrition.

He contributed both to human nutrition and to the development of agriculture. He introduced the use of fertilizers that helped increase agricultural output.

He discovered the amino acid tyrosine, and he also isolated hippuric acid and chloroform.

He studied uric acid, so important in gout, and developed a method to measure urea[62, 66].

Biosketch

Claude Bernard (1813-1878) stands along with Helmholtz and Ludwig as the leading scientific figures of physiology in the nineteenth-century (Figure 16-3). He was born into a vintner's family at St. Julien in the Beaujolais region of France on July 12, 1813.

Because of financial difficulties, he became a pharmacist's assistant in Lyons, France. The young Bernard at first turned his attention to writing plays, one of which, a vaudeville comedy, met with some success. Armed with two plays, one of which had been performed, he went to Paris, where the critic Girardin advised him that medicine was a better choice to make a living. Bernard completed his seven-year medical curriculum in 1841 at the age of twenty-eight. Under the tutelage of Magendie, the leading French physiologist of the time, Bernard matured to be a better scientist than his master. Bernard was a genius at the experimental method and founded experimental medicine by which disease states were induced by chemical or physical manipulation. His discovery that the liver released glucose into the circulation revolutionized the concept of metabolism. His idea of the "internal milieu" as a buffer against the outside world is still an important concept. His mastery of the entire range of physiology is shown in the series of lectures that were published between 1855 and 1879. In February 1878 he died a lonely death from acute nephritis as his wife and two daughters lived away from him because they felt distaste for his life's work[62]. His genius, however, was recognized by the pomp and circumstance of the public funeral held at State expense[63-64].

Biosketch

Rudolf Schoenheimer (1898-1941) was born and educated in Berlin. With the rise of the Nazis in Germany, Schoenheimer fled, settling in New York and working at Columbia University. His central scientific contribution was to show that the body fat and protein were in dynamic state by using stable isotopes attached in fatty acids and proteins. His findings were set out in a small monograph called *The Dynamic State of Bodily Constituents.* With the onset of World War II, he committed suicide.

Biosketch

Jean Mayer (1920-1993) was born in Paris on February 19, 1920. He received his undergraduate education in Paris before World War II, and he was active in the Resistance during the war. When peace arrived in 1945, Mayer began his work for the Ph.D., which was awarded in 1948 by Yale University, followed by a Sc.D. from the Sorbonne in 1950. (Figure 16-4)

During the 1950s, Mayer was an active scholar in obesity and nutrition working at the Harvard School of Public Health. In 1969 President Nixon named him to chair the White House Conference on Food, Nutrition and Health. This conference developed many of the models for nutrition policy for the next twenty-five years. In 1976, he became the tenth president of Tufts University. In this role he established the only school of veterinary medicine in New England and founded the USDA Human Nutrition Research Institute on Aging. He died of a heart attack at age seventy-two in 1993[65].

References

1. Bernard, C. *Introduction a l'étude de la médecine expérimentale.* Paris: J.B. Bailliere et Fils, 1865.
2. Mayer, J. "Glucostatic Mechanism of Regulation of Food Intake." *N Engl J Med.* 249(1953): 13-16.
3. Louis-Sylvestre, J., J. LeMagnen. "A Fall in Blood Glucose Level Precedes Meal Onset in Free-Feeding Rats." *Neurosci Biobehav Rev.* 4(1989): 13-15.
4. Mellinkoff, S.M, M. Frankland, D. Boyle, M. Greipel. "Relationship between Serum Amino Acid Concentration and Fluctuations in Appetite." *J Appl Physiol.* 8(1956): 535-538.
5. Cannon, W.B., A.L. Washburn. "An Explanation of Hunger." *Am J Physiol.* 29(1912): 441-454.
6. Carlson, A.J. *The Control of Hunger in Health and Disease.* Chicago: University of Chicago Press, 1916.
7. Bouchard, C., G.A. Bray. "Introduction." In. Bouchard, C., G.A. Bray, eds. *Regulation of Body Weight: Biological and Behavioral Mechanisms.* Chichester: John Wiley & Sons Ltd., 1996.
8. Hetherington, A.W., S.W. Ranson. "Hypothalamic Lesions and Adiposity in Rat." *Anal Rec.* 78 (1940): 149-172.
9. Bray, G.A., T.F. Gallagher Jr. "Manifestations of Hypothalamic Obesity in Man: A Comprehensive Investigation of Eight Patients and a Review of the Literature." *Medicine.* 54(1975): 301-330.
10. Anand, B.K., J.R. Brobeck. "Localization of "Feeding Center" in Hypothalamus of Rat." *Proc Soc Exper Biol Med.* 77(1951): 323.
11. Brobeck, J.R., J. Tepperman, C.N.H. Long. "The Effect of Experimental Obesity upon Carbohydrate Metabolism." *Yale J Biol Med.* 15 (1942): 893-904.
12. Brobeck, J.R. "Food and Temperature." *Rec Prog Hormone Res.* 16(1960): 439-459.
13. Stellar, E. "The Physiology of Motivation." *Psychol Rev.* (1954): 5-22.
14. Kennedy, G.C. "The Role of Depot Fat in the Hypothalamic Control of Food Intake in the Rat." *Proc Royal Soc.* 140(1953): 578-592.
15. Edholm, O.G., J.M. Adam, M.J.R. Healy, H.S. Wolff, R. Goldsmith, T.W. Best. "Food Intake and Energy Expenditure of Army Recruits." *Br J Nutr.* 24(1970): 1091-1107.
16. Mayer, J. "Regulation of Energy Intake and the Body Weight: The Glucostatic Theory and the Lipostatic Hypothesis." *Ann N Y Acad Sci.* 63(1955): 15-43.
17. Gasnier, A., A. Mayer. "Recherches sur la régulation de la nutrition, I. Qualités et cotes des mécanismes régulateurs." *Ann Physiol Physiocochim Biol.* 15(1939): 145-156.

18. Gasnier, A., A. Mayer. "Recherches sur la régulation de la nutrition, II. Les mécanismes régulateurs de la nutrition chez le lapin domestique." *Ann Physiol Physicochim Biol.* 15 (1939): 157-185.
19. Gasnier A., A. Mayer. "Recherches sur la régulation de la nutrition, III. Mecanismes régulateurs de la nutrition et intensité du métabolisme." *Ann Physiol Physicochim Biol.* 15(1939): 186-194.
20. Gasnier, A., A. Mayer. "Recherches sur la régulation de la nutrition, IV. Différences entre deux races de lapins domestiques." *Ann Physiol Physicochim Biol.* 15(1939): 195-209.
21. Gasnier, A., A. Mayer. "Recherches sur la régulation de la nutrition, V. Caractères individuels." *Ann Physiol Physicochim Biol.* 15(1939): 210-214.
22. Debons, A.F., I. Krimsky, A. From, R.J. Cloutier. "Site of Action of Gold Thioglucose in the Hypothalamic Satiety Center." *Am J Physiol.* 219(1970): 1397 1402.
23. Van Itallie, T.B. "Peripheral Assimilation of Fructose in Man." *Proc Soc Exp Biol Med.* 84(1953): 713-715.
24. Stunkard, A.J. *The Pain of Obesity.* Palo Alto: Bull Publishing Co, 1976.
25. Oomura, Y. "Glucose and Osmosensitive Neurones of the Rat Hypothalamus." *Nature.* 222(1969): 282-294.
26. Bray, G.A., L.A. Campfield. "Metabolic Factors in the Control of Energy Stores." *Metabolism.* 24(1975): 99-117.
27. FIatt, J.P. "Assessment of Daily and Cumulative Carbohydrate and Fat Balances in Mice." *J Nutr Biochem.* 2(1991): 193-202.
28. LeMagnen, J. *Hunger.* Cambridge: Cambridge University Press, 1985.
29. Strubbe, J.H., A.B. Steffens, L. De Ruiter. "Plasma Insulin and the Time Pattern of Feeding in the Rat." *Physiol Behav.* 18(1977): 81-86.
30. Campfield, L.A., P. Brandon, F.J. Smith. "On-line Continuous Measurement of Blood Glucose and Meal Pattern in Free-Feeding Rats: The Role of Glucose in Meal Initiation." *Brain Res Bull.* 14(1985): 605-616.
31. Martin, A.J.P., R.L.M. Synge. "Analytical Chemical of the Proteins." *Adv Protein Chem.* 2(1945): 1-83.
32. Moore, S., W.H. Stein. "Chemical Structures of Pancreatic Ribonuclease and Deoxyribonuclease." *Science.* 180(1973): 458-464.
33. Fernstrorrm, J.D., R.J. Wurtman. "Brain Serotonin Content: Physiological Dependence on Plasma Tryptophan Levels." *Science.* 173(1971): 149-152.
34. Mendel, L.B. *Nutrition: The Chemistry of Life.* New Haven: Yale University Press, 1923.
35. Richerand, A. *Elements of Physiology.* Transl. G.J.M. De Lys. Philadelphia: Thomas Dobson, 1813.
36. Prout, W. *Chemistry, Meteorology and the Function of Digestion.* London: Churchill, 1845.
37. Magendie, F. "Sur les propriétés nutritives des substances qui ne conti-

ennent pas d'azote." *Ann Client (Ser2).* 3(1816): 66-77, 408-410.
38. Carpenter, K.J. *Protein and Energy: A Study of Changing Ideas in Nutrition.* Cambridge: Cambridge University Press, 1994.
39. McCollum, E.V. *A History of Nutrition.* Boston: Houghton Mifflin, 1957.
40. Magendie, F. "Rapport fait a l'Académie des Sciences au nom de la Commission dite de la gelatine." *C R Acad Sci (Paris).* (1841): 237-283.
41. Mulder, G.J. "Über die Zusammensetzung einiger thierischen Substanzen." *J Prakt Chem.* 16 (1839): 129-152.
42. von Liebig, J. *Animal Chemistry, or Organic Chemistry in its Application to Physiology and Pathology.* Transl. W. Gregory. London: Taylor and Walton, 1842.
43. von Liebig, J. *Familiar Letter on Chemistry.* London: Taylor & Walton, 1851.
44. FIint, A. Jr. *On the Physiological Effects of Severe and Protracted Muscular Exercise, with Special Reference to its Influence upon the Excretion of Nitrogen.* New York: D. Appleton & Co., 1981.
45. Bernard, C. "Sur le mécanisme de la formation du sucre dans le foie." *C R Acad Sci* 41 (1855): 461-469.
46. Cannon, W.B. *The Wisdom of the Body.* New York: Norton & Co., 1932.
47. McCay, C.M. *Notes on the History of Nutrition Research.* Ed. F. Verzer. Berne: Huber Publisher, 1972.
48. Rose, W.C. "Amino Acid Requirements of Man." Fed Proc. 8(1949): 546-552.
49. Schoenheimer, R. *The Dynamic State of Body Constituents.* Cambridge: Harvard University Press, 1941.
50. Felig, P. "The Glucose-Alanine Cycle." *Metabolism.* 2(1973): 179.
51. Gietzen, D.W. "Neural Mechanisms in the Responses to Amino Acid Deficiency." *J Nutr.* 123(1993): 610-625.
52. Harper, A.E. "Effects of Disproportionate Amounts of Amino Acids." In Harper, A.E. and D.M. Hegsted, eds. *Improvement of Protein Nutrition.* Washington, DC: National Academy of Science, 1988.
53. Dubos, R.J. *Louis Pasteur, Free Lance of Science.* Boston: Little, Brown & Co., 1950.
54. Lawton, C.L., J.K. Wales, A.J. Hill, J.E. Blundell. "Serotinergic Manipulation, Meal-Induced Satiety and Eating Pattern: Effect of Fluoxetine in Obese Female Subjects." *Obes Res.* 3(1995): 345-356.
55. Kanarek, R.B., H. Dushkin. "Serotonin Administration Selectively Reduces Fat Intake in Rats." *Pharmacol Biochem Behav.* 31(1988): 113-122.
56. Goodall, E.M., P.J. Cowen, M. Frankon, T. Silverstone. "Ritanserin Attenuates Anorectic, Endocrine and Thermic Responses to D-Fenfluramine in Human Volunteers." *Psychopharmacology.* 112(1993): 461-466.

57. Smith, B.K., D.A. York, G.A. Bray. "Chronic D-Fenfluramine Treatment Reduces Fat Intake Independent of Macronutrient Preference." *Pharmacol Biochem Behav.* 60(1983): 105-114.
58. Tanner, J.M. *A History of the Study of Human Growth.* Cambridge: Cambridge University Press, 1981.
59. Bengtsson, B.A., R.J.M. Brummer, S. Eden, T. Rosen, L. Sjostrom. "Effects of Growth Hormone on Fat Mass and Fat Distribution." *Acta Paediatr Suppl.* 383(1992): 62-65.
60. Bouchard, C., A. Tremblay, J.P. Despres, et al. "The Response to Long-Term Overfeeding in Identical Twins." *N Engl J Med.* 322(1990): 1477-1482.
61. Hopkins, F.G. *Physiology and National Needs.* Ed. W.D. Hall. London: Constable and Co.; 1919.
62. Garrison, F.H. *Introduction to Medicine.* Philadelphia: W.B. Saunders, 1929.
63. Mayer, J. Claude Bernard. *J Nutr.* 45(1951): 3-19.
64. Holmes, F.L. *Claude Bernard and Animal Chemistry: The Emergence of a Scientist.* Cambridge: Harvard University Press, 1974.
65. Jean Mayer biography.
66. Mettler, C.C., F.A. Mettler. *History of Medicine.* Philadelphia: Blakiston, 1947, p 162.
67. Guggenheim, K.Y. "Rudolf Schoenheimer and the concept of the dynamic state of body constituents." *J NUtr.* 1991; 121:1701-4.

Chapter 17

The Science of Hunger: From a Physiologic to a Molecular Basis for Hunger

> *It is often difficult to identify the "who, when, and where" of advances in medicine and surgery because it's a rare advance indeed (such as the use of digitalis by William Withering) that can be clearly related to the astuteness of one person at one time and place.*
>
> —Comroe[1]

The cell is a basic unit of life. This truth was first recognized more than one hundred fifty years ago, and has stimulated advances in understanding human and animal behavior. For psychology and the brain, the nineteenth and twentieth centuries have seen enormous advances. We have recognized the reflex arc[5]. We have learned that the brain is constructed with a series of cell clusters, called ganglia, that underlie much of its structure and function[4]. The idea that many brain functions have a specific location in one part of the brain or another is one outgrowth of these newer ideas. Finally, we have learned about the chemical or rather the neurochemical transmission of information between one cell and another in the brain[7,8]. This chapter is about the transition from the functional to the neurochemical understanding of food intake as it relates to obesity. These neurochemicals form the basis for "behavior" and thus for the decisions we make about eating, exercising, and other activities related to our weight. The more we know about these neurochemicals, the more effectively we will be able to prepare for our battle against the bulge.

Reports on the neurochemical basis for the control of food intake have exploded in the last quarter century. As Ackerknecht and Vallois, two of the leading historians of medicine have put it,

> Modern psychology (physiological, experimental psychology) is faced by the same problems as all other scientific

> disciplines. In order not to go astray, in order to find new, safer and more direct paths, she must continuously re-examine her premises. In such re-examinations, it is not sufficient to analyze some recent work; one must go back to the real sources because they are the ones to reveal most clearly the virtues and the vices of a method.[2]

Thus, the history of research in psychology and the understanding of brain function and its neurochemical basis should be viewed as a development away from philosophy and toward general biology[3].

Because several minds nearly converged simultaneously on the idea of chemical neurotransmission as the basis for feeding behavior, I will discuss several of them. The first paper showed that localized injection of the neurotransmitter norepinephrine into the region of the brain called the hypothalamus increased food intake in animals[9]. The second paper showed that a peptide from the gastro-intestinal track called cholecystokinin (CCK) may act as a signal for satiety when released from the gut[10]. The final paper extended the field of gut-brain communication by showing that neuropeptide-Y which is found in both was one of the strongest stimulants of feeding yet described[11].

To understand the historical significance of our modern views of the brain and its control of food intake, we need to take a brief trip through the history of ideas about the brain. The concepts about the functions of the brain developed in Greece and more particularly by Galen in Roman times dominated thinking until the nineteenth century[12]. Galen viewed the brain as presiding over bodily functions through the spinal marrow and nerves. He thought that the innate powers and faculties resided in the ventricles of the brain. Sensation and imagination were assigned to the anterior ventricular chamber, reason to the middle chamber, and memory to the posterior ventricular chamber. The spinal cord was viewed as a prolongation of the cerebral mass. With the spinal cord as a large nerve, the brain was perceived as the source of all nervous power and as the seat of life[3].

With the development of physical sciences from the time of Galileo and Newton in the seventeenth-century until the beginning of the nineteenth century, the mind tended to be isolated outside of this physical environment in part to avoid problems with religious institutions. As Young puts it, "The fragmentation of the world into primary and secondary qualities, outer and inner, body and mind, and the exclusions of final causes from science have plagued the study of mind and behavior at least since Descartes in the sixteenth-century.[3]" Replacement of this Cartesian dualism, that is that mind and the body are separate[13], has been slow because the veil of ignorance has only been pulled back slowly to reveal scientific truth. The events of the nineteenth century went a long way toward the goal of bridging the gap between the mind and the body.

The major impetus for a change from the Galenic concept of the organization of the central nervous system to the modern neuroanatomic basis came from German scientists in the mid-nineteenth century. Romanticism is the name given to the philosophy of nature which was central to German thought at this time. A fundamental axiom of this philosophy was the unity of nature. Such a concept put human beings in the same system as other animals. Thus, the same laws that worked in animals and plants were at work in human beings. This idea of unity made the conceptualization of the cell as the unit of biology a possibility for the German scientists Schwann[14] and Schleiden[15]. Similarly this concept of unity provided a powerful impetus for embryological studies and for the idea that fetal development recapitulates the steps of phylogenetic development from conception to birth. That is, "ontogeny recapitulates phylogeny." Nature does not progress by inventing new structures and chemicals, so much as it adapts the existing structures and chemicals to its changing needs.

In the early nineteenth-century the concept of the brain as a branch of biology was given significant support by the comparative anatomists and embryologists. The concept was stated by Grainger in 1842 as follows: "We are enabled by a judicious selection of those classes of animals which exhibit the simplest structure, to seize the essential typical form of organs, which, in many, although fashioned in the same model, are obscured by their amazing intricacy"[16]. In the early nineteenth-century, largely through comparative anatomical studies, the spinal cord was recognized to be a series of ganglia, or collections of neural cells, rather than merely an extension of the brain as Galen had proposed. This ganglionic structure of neural tissues was first evident in the vegetative or autonomic nervous system which controls our breathing, heart rate, and other automatic functions. This structure also applied to the spinal cord as a whole. Moreover, functions involving the spinal cord persisted even when separated from the brain. Thus, the concept of the spinal cord as an extension from the brain was no longer tenable.

The idea that specific functions had specific locations within the brain gave an impetus to reunification of the "mind and brain." One of the first to advance this idea was Gall, whose landmark work (1822-1826) extended the idea of ganglionic structure to the brain itself[4]. Franz Joseph Gall (1758-1828) and his contemporary Johann Caspar Spurzheim (1776 - 1832) were leaders in demonstrating the specific localization of function within the cranium. When they carried this idea to the concept that one could identify features of the individual from the shape of the skull, an art called phrenology, they partially delayed the acceptance of their views. In retrospect, Gall made three major contributions to the study of the mind-brain problem[3]. First, he documented the many functions that man and animals have in common. Of the twenty-seven fundamental faculties that he identified, nineteen are shared between man and animals. Second, he rejected the speculative concepts of imagination, reason, and memory, which had been the center of Greek concepts, as inadequate for the explanation of the differences among species in nature and individual men and animals within their respective societies. Finally, he believed that he had identified a way to establish functions in definable regions of the brain. Although this idea developed into the pseudo-science of phrenology, it does not detract from the fundamental advances which Gall and Spurzheim's work made in the field of localizing brain function. As the author R.M. Young noted, "In his vision of Psychology as a branch of Biology, subject therefore to all biological laws, and to be pursued by biological methods, he [Gall] may be said to have given the science [of psychology] its basis"[3].

The next major advance that applied specific functions to regions of the brain came nearly forty years later, just after the middle of the nineteenth-century. Paul Broca (1824-1880), after whom Broca's area of the brain is named, described a localized region in the brain that was associated with one form of loss of speech (aphasia). Destruction of a small region in the third convolution of the brain produced this problem in two of his patients. Of interest is that the lesion was only on the left side. Broca's area is thus known as the speech area.

It was shortly after this that the work of Ivan Pavlov (1849-1936) on conditioned reflexes came to the fore and dominated the field of feeding behavior for the next fifty years[17,18]. Even though the work of Joseph Babinski (1857-1932)[19] and Alfred Frohlich (1871-1953)[20] at the turn of the twentieth-century demonstrated the ganglionic nature of damage to the hypothalamus that produced obesity, the central concepts about feeding continued to focus on the role of the gastrointestinal tract and peripheral signals[21]. In his historical review of this period, Eliot Stellar (1919-1993)[22] says, "it is hard to imagine, but in the late thirties [1930s]...our concepts of hunger, appetite and food intake were primarily peripheralist and environmentalist. Thinking in physiology was dominated by Cannon's gastric contraction concept. In psychology, classic behaviorism was still the dominant force...." What was lacking in the thinking about food intake was an anatomic basis for integrating central and peripheralist views. It was the work of Hetherington and Ranson[23] and of Anand and Brobeck[24] that provided a ganglionic location for feeding. Their identification of the ventromedial hypothalamus[23] and lateral hypothalamus[24] as key sites for the integration of feeding would be consistent with the "ganglionic" organization of the brain pioneered in the nineteenth-century.

In his classic review, Eliot Stellar (1919-1993)[25] also put learning, behavior, and anatomy into a new context. It was this context which provided the framework for the neurochemical discoveries about feeding that occurred in the four succeeding decades. In the early part of the twentieth-century, Cannon and his associates[26] had been leaders in studying the biology of the sympathetic nervous system. By World War II, they had divided the activities of the sympathetic nervous system into excitatory (sympathin E) and inhibitory (sympathin I) effects[27]. This is where the problem rested until after World War II when Ulf von Euler (1905-1983) showed that norepinephrine was the noradrenergic neurotransmitter[28]. von Euler was one of the leading Swedish scholars of the middle part of the twentieth-century. He took up the problem of the sympathetic nervous system and demonstrated that there were two neurotransmitters called adrenaline and noradrenaline that are also called epinephrine and norepinephrine. For these key advances he shared the Nobel prize in medicine and physiology.

With the gradual recognition that hormones and drugs interacted with a lock-and-key mechanism at the cell surface, the way was open to study the biology of neural function in more detail. To account for the different patterns of response to norepinephrine and epinephrine in different tissues, Ahlquist[29] proposed that there were two receptors involved in their action. He called the receptors alpha (α) and beta (ß). This hypothesis opened the door to understanding the role of norepinephrine and epinephrine in feeding. Grossman[9] injected norepineprine directly into the brain and showed that it stimulated food intake when applied directly to the ventromedial hypothalamus. In contrast to the feeding response to norepinephrine, another neurotransmitter, acetylcholine, had no effect on food intake but did alter water intake. Shortly after the work of Grossman, Sarah Leibowitz[39] showed that norepinephrine had both stimulatory and inhibitory effects on food intake, depending on the area of the brain into which it was injected. The ventromedial hypothalamic area was called the "satiety center" by Stellar[5], since it responded with an increase in food intake when norepinephrine was injected. This effect of norepinephrine could be blocked by injection of α-adrenergic antagonists into the ventromedial area. More laterally in the perifornical area, injection of norepinephrine reduced food intake through adrenergic receptors that were blocked by ß-adrenergic antagonists. Following the recognition that there were two α receptors, it was shown that stimulation of the α-1 adrenergic receptor reduced food intake[31] whereas stimulation of the α-2 receptor increased food intake[32].

As the biology of α and ß receptors in the control of feeding was being explored, more receptors were being identified. Both ß-1 and ß-2 receptors as well as α-1 and α-2 receptors were recognized. In addition to showing that α and ß receptors were involved in food intake, Leibowitz and her colleagues showed that stimulation of the α-2 receptors in the paraventricular nucleus increased carbohydrate intake, but not fat intake[32]. These experiments opened up the idea that selection of specific macronutrients could be modulated by different neurotransmitters[33].

In addition to the monoamines, norepinephrine and epinephrine, that we have just been discussing, there are a number of peptides that also control food intake. The first peptide to attract attention was cholecystokinin or CCK, a small peptide found in the gastrointestinal tract. CCK was originally identified in 1928 by its ability to produce contractions of the gall bladder. Its role in food intake was not recognized for many years, until James Gibbs and his colleagues[10] carried out the critical experiments. They showed that when nutrients are injected into the intestines they would reduce food intake of sham-feeding animals (an animal that is eating a liquid diet that will drain out of an opening in the stomach. These animals have a drain surgically placed in their stomachs. It can be opened or closed by removing a cap over the drainage tube). These scientists tested the idea that CCK might duplicate the reduction of food intake that occurred when food was put in the duodenum. They were elated to find that the more of CCK that they injected, the greater the decrease in food that was eaten. That is, CCK produced a dose-related reduction in feeding. Since CCK is released by eating a meal, these seminal studies suggested that this peptide might be important in reducing food intake as a way of preventing the bulge we are battling. The reduction of food intake by injecting CCK has been repeated many times, and efforts have been made to find drugs that act like CCK that might be used in the battle of the bulge, but as yet no clinically useful ones have been found.

As the sophistication of the peptide chemists has increased, a number of new peptides were isolated from the intestine and various other tissue that were subsequently synthesized[34]. The skin of amphibia, particularly a toad known as *Bombina bombina*, and the gastrointestinal tract were major sources for these peptides. Of these peptides, one called neuropeptide Y[34] proved to be one of the most potent stimulators of food intake. Neuropeptide Y is so named because it has the amino acid tyrosine, which is abbreviated "Y" by biochemists, at one end of the molecule. NPY is found in the gut and the brain. The fact these peptides are found in both the gut and the brain may stem from the fact that both tissues originate during fetal life from the same set of ectodermal/endodermal cells that line the gut and skin. The discovery of peptides as important micromodulators of feeding has also destroyed another long-held belief. Monoamines, like norepinephrine, epinephrine, and serotonin, are stored in granules or little packets that are found in neurons and other cells. It had been scientific dogma that a single neuron held only a single type of neurotransmitter in these granules. The development of sophisticated techniques for identifying these peptides by their reaction with antibodies (immunocytochemistry) has shown that a single neuron can co-secrete more than one neurotransmitter. And so another theory is cast into the dust-bin of history.

Shortly after the discovery of neuropeptide Y, Clark and his colleagues[11] showed that it would stimulate feeding and reduce reproductive function.

Stanley and associates[35] showed that repeated injections of this peptide would produce obesity. Thus, a new type of obesity was born, one that depended entirely on overeating or hyperphagia. In addition, NPY was shown to increase the preference for carbohydrates[36]. Gradually, the concept that the intake of fat, carbohydrate, and protein, might be controlled individually was born, stimulated in part by the discovery of a small molecule that specifically inhibits the intake of dietary fat[33,37].

In the past three hundred years, we have come a long way from the mind-brain dualism of Descartes[13] toward a biological basis of behavior. It is clear that the veil of mystery has gradually been lifted from the chemical basis of behavior but that much more will be added to the story in the new millennium. We are continuing to identify new peptides that are involved in the battle of the bulge and to understand how they work. With this new information, the outlook for effective treatments in the battle of the bulge steadily improves.

Biosketch

Paul Broca (1824-1880) was born in southwest France to a Protestant Calvinist family (Figure 17-1). After completing his early education he headed toward mathematics, but changed directions to medicine after the death of his older sister. He was a multi-talented man as professor and surgeon, founder of the Society of Anthropology (France), neurologist, and political activist. Following the death of Professor Claude Bernard, Broca became a senator in France, representing the medical interests in the French legislature. It was, however, his work in neurology that has brought his name down to us.

Biosketch

Ulf Svante von Euler (1905-1983) made three major contributions during his scientific career at the Karolinska Institute in Stockholm. He discovered and characterized norepinephrine. Second, with Henry Dale he discovered Substance P, an important peptide involved in sensations of pain. And third, he isolated the prostaglandins from the human prostate. von Euler was the second son of five siblings, born in Stockholm and raised in a family where his father received the Nobel Prize for chemistry in 1929. (Figure 17-2)

von Euler entered medical school in 1922 and completed his thesis in 1930. This was followed by a year of travel and research with Henry Dale in London where he isolated Substance P from the intestine. He then returned to his research work at the Karolinska, where over the years he discovered prostanglandins in 1935, piperidine in 1942, and norepinephrine in 1946 and rose from lecturer in physiology in 1933 to professor in 1939[38].

Biosketch

Eliot Stellar (1919-1993) (Figure 17-3) was born and educated in Boston, Massachusetts, and received an undergraduate education at Harvard where he published his first paper in psychology. His graduate work was done at Brown University where he began his lifelong work on motivation. After service in World War II, Eliot joined the faculty at Johns Hopkins where he worked with Morgan to prepare the second edition of *Physiological Psychology*, a leading text in the field. A classic paper on "The Physiology of Motivation" in 1954 was to dominate the field for the next thirty years. In 1954 Stellar moved to the University of Pennsylvania where he spent the rest of his professional career in the Institute of Neurological Sciences, Department of Anatomy, and as Provost of the University[39].

References

1. Comroe, J. *Retrospectroscope: Insights into Medical Discovery.* Menlo Park, CA: Von Gehr Press, 1977.
2. Ackerknecht, E.H., H.V. Vallois. "Contributions of Gall and the Phrenologists to Knowledge of Brain Function." In Poynter, F.N.L. (ed). *The Brain and Its Functions.* Oxford: Blackwell, 1958.
3. Young, R.M. *Mind, Brain and Adaptation in the Nineteenth Century.* Oxford: Clarendon Press, 1970.
4. Gall, F.J. *Sur les Fonctions du Cerveau et sur Celles de Chacune de ses Parties.* Paris: l'Auteur, 1822-1825
5. Sherington, C.S. *The Integrative Action of the Nervous System.* New York: Charles Scribner's Sons, 1906.
6. Ferrier, D. *The Functions of the Brain.* London: Smith, Elder & Co., 1876.
7. Dale, H.H. "The Action of Certain Esters and Ethers of Choline, and Their Relation to Muscarine." *J Pharmacol.* 6(1914): 147-190.
8. Loewi, O. "Ueber humorale Uebertragbarkeit der Herznerven wirkung." *Pflug Arch Ges Physiol.* 189(1921): 239-242.
9. Grossman, S.P. "Eating or Drinking Elicited by Direct Adrenergic or Cholinergic Stimulation of Hypothalamus." *Science.* 132(1960): 301-302.
10. Gibbs, J., R.C. Young, G.P. Smith. "Cholecystokinin Decreases Food Intake in Rats." *J Comp Physiol Psychol.* 84(1973): 488-495.
11. Clark, J.T., P.S. Kalra, S.P. Kalra. "Neuropeptide Y Stimulates Feeding but Inhibits Sexual Behavior in Rats." *Endocrinology.* No. 6. 117(1985): 2435-2442.
12. Galen, C. *Pergameni Opera, iarn Recens ver sa; Quorum Cataloguin Proxima Indicabit Pagina.* Basileae ex aedivus, 1531.
13. Descartes, R. *De Homine Figures et Latinitate Donatus a Florentio Schuyl.* Lugduni Batavorum, apud F Moyardum, P Leffen, 1662.
14. Schwann, T. *Mikroscopische Untersuchungen über die Übereinstimmung in der Struktur und dem Wachstum der Thiere and Pflanzen.* Berlin: Sander, 1839.
15. Schleiden, M.J. "Beiträge zur Phytogenesis." *Arch Anat Physiol wiss Med.* (1838): 137-176.
16. Clarke, E., L.S. Jacyna. "Nineteenth-century Origins of Neuroscientific Concepts." *Med Hist.* 32(1988): 42, 211-213.
17. Bray, G.A. "Commentary on Classics of Obesity. Eat slowly—From Laboratory to Clinic: Behavioral Control of Eating." *Obes Res.* 4(1996): 397-400.
18. Pavlov, I.P. *Dvadtsstiletniy opyt ob' yektwnogo izucheniya Akromegalee. Vysshey nervnoy deyatelnosti (Povedeniya) zhivotaykh 883-886 (Twenty*

years of experiments in the objective study of higher nervous activity (behavior) of animals). Moscow & Leningrad: State Publishing House, 1923.

19. Babinski, J.F.F. "Tumeur de corps pituitaire sans acromégalie et avec arrêt de développement des organes génitaux." *Rev Neurosci.* 8(1900): 531-533.
20. Frohlich, A. "Ein Fall von Tumor der Hypophysis cerebri ohne Akromegalie." *Wiener Klinisch Rundschau.* 15(1901): 883-886
21. Bray, G.A. "Commentary on Classics of Obesity 6. Science and Politics of Hunger." *Obes Res.* 1(1993): 489·493.
22. Stellar, E. "The CNS and Appetite: Historical Introduction." *Proc Dahlem Workshop on Appetite and Feeding.* May(1997): 15-20.
23. Hetherington, A.W., S.W. Ranson. "Hypothalamic Lesions and Adiposity in the Rat." *Anat Rec.* 78(1946): 149-172.
24. Anand, B.K., J.R. Brobeck. "Localization of a "Feeding Center" in the Hypothalamus of Rat." *Proc Soc Exp Biol Med.* 77(1951): 323-324.
25. Stellar, E. "Physiology and Motivation." *Psychol Rev.* 61(1954): 5-22.
26. Cannon, W.B., A.L. Washburn. "An Explanation of Hunger." *Am J Physiol.* 29(1912): 441-454.
27. Cannon, W.B., A. Rosenbleuth. *Autonomic Neuro-effector Systems.* New York: Macmillan, 1937.
28. Euler, U.S. von. "A Specific Sympathetornimetic Ergone in Adrenergic Nerve Fiber (Sympathin) and its Relations to Adrenaline and Noradrenaline." *Acta Physiol Scand.* 12(1946): 73-97.
29. Ahlquist, R.P. "A Study of the Adrenotropic Receptors." *Am J Physiol.* 153(1948): 586-600.
30. Leibowitz, S.F. "Role of Alpha and Beta Receptors in Mediating Effects of Hypothalamic Adrenergic Stimulation." *Physiol Behav.* 14(1975): 743.
31. Wellman, P.J., B.T. Davies. "Suppression of Feeding Induced by Phenylephrine Microinjections within the Paraventricular Hypothalamus in Rats." *Appetite.* 17(1991): 121-128.
32. Leibowitz, S.F. "Hypothalamic Paraventricular Nucleus: Interaction between the Noradrenergic System and Circulating Hormones and Nutrients in Relation to Energy Balance." *Neurosci Biobehav Rev.* 12(1988): 11-109.
33. Bray, G.A. "The Effect of Peptides on Nutrient Intake and the Sympathetic Nervous System." In Bray, G.A., D.H. Ryan (eds). *The Science of Food Regulation: Food Intake, Taste, Nutrient Partitioning, and Energy Expenditure.* Baton Rouge: Louisiana State University Press, 2(1992): 257-276.
34. Tatemoto, K., M. Carlquist, V. Mutt. "Neuropeptide Y: A Novel Brain Peptide with Structural Similarities to Peptide YY and Pancreatic

Polypeptide." *Nature.* 296(1982): 659-662.

35. Stanley, B.G., K.C. Anderson, M.H. Grayson, S.F. Leibowitz. "Repeat Hypothalamic Stimulation with Neuropeptide Y Increases Daily Carbohydrate and Fat Intake and Body Weight Gain in Female Rats." *Physiol Behav.* 46(1989): 173-177.
36. Stanley, B.G., D.R. Daniel S. Chin, S.F. Leibowitz. "Paraventricular Nucleus Injections of Neuropeptide Y Preferentially Enhance Carbohydrate Ingestion." *Peptides.* 6(1985): 1205-1211.
37. Okada, S., D.A. York, G.A. Bray., C. Erlanson-Albertsson. "Enterostatin (Val-Pro-Asp-Pro-Arg), the activation peptide of procolipase, selectively reduces fat intake." *Physiol Behav.* 49(1991): 1185-1189.
38. Blashko, H.K.F. "Ulf Svante von Euler." In *Proceedings of the Royal Society.* (1984): 145-170.
39. Schulkin, J. Eliot Stellar November 1, 1919-October 12, 1993. *Biogr Mem Natl Acad Sci.* 1996; 69:315-322.

Chapter 18

Overweight in a Social Setting: Psychoanalysis and Anorexia

> *To tell us that every Species of Things is endow'd with an occult specifick Quality by which it acts and produces manifest effects is to tell us nothing: But to derive two or three general Principles of Motion from Phenomena, and afterwards to tell us how the Properties and Actions of all corporeal Things follow from those manifest Principles, would be a very great step in Philosophy, though the Causes of these Principles were not yet discover'd.*
>
> —Newton (cited by Dingle[1])

A. Introduction

Recognizing who is overweight is easy. You just have to look. You can tell it in yourself by looking in a mirror; in others by looking for the bulges. It differs from elevated cholesterol or high blood pressure, which require special tests for their detection. For corpulence, it only takes a pair of eyes. Because it is a problem for the bearer and for society, it is important to put the battle of the bulge into a social context.

The Victorian era of the nineteenth century was a period of great change. In their fascinating book on fasting and anorexia, Vandereycken and van Deth[2] described four revolutionary themes that characterized the period from the Napoleonic era at the beginning of the nineteenth century through the Victorian era one century later. The first was the Industrial Revolution, reflected by the harnessing of steam to do man's work; the second was the urbanization of the population, a trend that still goes on; the third was the beginning of the women's revolution; and the fourth was the economic revolution. The appearance of anorexia in the late nineteenth century and bulimia in the twentieth century may be an outgrowth of the effect of these revolutionary forces on women as they battle the bulge.

The status of women has been changing steadily and often rapidly for nearly two centuries. Efforts to obtain the right to vote began in the mid-nineteenth century, with New Zealand becoming the first country to grant that right in 1894. Gradually, however, the right was acquired in all countries. The struggle for economic equity was accelerated by World War II, and almost all job categories are now open to women.

The reproductive revolution also began in the nineteenth-century. Birth control clinics began sporadically early in the twentieth century[3], and the entire movement received a great impetus from the discovery and marketing of birth control pills in the 1960s[4]. These elements made it possible for women to choose whether and when to become pregnant. It is against this background of revolutionary changes in society and the changing roles of women that anorexia nervosa and the much more common problem of bulimia nervosa can best be viewed. Kim Chernin has summarized this from the perspective of a twentieth century feminist:

> During the 19th century woman's experience entered the realm of written and spoken debate. Marriage, domestic labor, child raising, and prostitution, which had not seemed worthy of intellectual consideration, now became serious topics as women began to philosophize about their own condition. In our own time, the female experience of rape, the sexual abuse of female children, the existence of pornography, and domestic violence, come increasingly to be examined for the larger meaning in our culture's treatment of women.[5]

A fear of fat has been attributed as a trigger for a second disease called bulimia nervosa. This disease is characterized by uncontrolled bingeing and then purging[6-10]; weight loss may or may not occur. Again, this syndrome seems to be most common in the upper social and economic groups where there is a high level of concern about obesity.

The four papers from scholarly journals printed in the appendix were chosen to put obesity and underweight into a psychological and socio-economic context of the nineteenth and twentieth century. The context for these papers was the transition from the social and cultural features of the Victorian era in the nineteenth century to the modern scientific era interspersed by two World Wars and a variety of other conflicts. Both anorexia nervosa and the psychoanalytic theories of Freud were the products of the Victorian era. As the context of obesity has expanded over the ensuing century, the psychoanalytic approach has been replaced by a socio-economic and bio-medical context for viewing the problem.

The clinical descriptions of anorexia nervosa were published almost simultaneously by Ernest Charles Lasegue (1816-1883) in 1873[11] and by William Withey Gull (1816-1890) in 1874[12]; a psychoanalytic perspective on anorexia nervosa was published by Hilda Bruch (1904-1984)[13] seventy years later. The social context of obesity as a problem of lower socio-economic groups occurred only in the latter half of the twentieth century[14].

B. Anorexia Nervosa

Several features characterize anorexia nervosa [2, 6-12]. It occurs almost entirely in young women at or just after the onset of menses and includes emaciation, decreased food intake, constipation, and absence of menstruation. It is largely restricted to upper-class women who display a lack of concern or *"belle indifference"* about their emaciated look. These young women tend to be physically very active and respond poorly to most treatments. When the disease was first recognized in the last quarter of the nineteenth-century during the Victorian era, it was difficult to determine whether it was a new disease arising from the social-cultural context of the time or an ancient disease that appeared in new trappings. Sir William Withey Gull is usually given credit as the first person to describe the disease in the English language[12]. His publication in 1874 begins as follows:

> In an address on medicine delivered at Oxford in the autumn of 1868, I referred to a peculiar form of disease occurring mostly in young women, and characterized by extreme emaciation, and often referred to latent tubercle, and mesenteric disease. I remarked that at present our diagnosis of this affection is negative, so far as determining any positive cause from which it springs; that it is mostly one of inference from our clinical knowledge of the liability of the pulmonary or abdominal organs to particular lesions, and by proving the absence of these lesions in the cases in question. The subjects of this affection are mostly of the female sex, and chiefly between the ages of 16 and 23. I have occasionally seen it in males at the same age.[12]

However, nearly one year earlier, Lasegue in Paris had provided a nearly identical description. In English translation, Lasegue says:

> The object of this memoir is to make known one of the forms of hysteria of the gastric centre which is of sufficient frequency for its description not to be, as too readily happens, the artificial generalization of a particular case, and constant enough in its symptoms to allow physicians who

> have met with it controlling the accuracy of the description, and to prevent those who have yet to meet with it in their practice being taken unawares. The term "anorexia" might have been replaced by "hysterical inanition," which would better represent the most characteristic of the accidents; but I have preferred the former term, without otherwise defending it, precisely because it refers to a phenomenology which is less superficial, more delicate, and also more medical.[11]

Was Gull aware of the work by his French contemporary? The evidence on this question is unclear. Although English translations of French papers were quite common, it may have been either the rumor or the actual knowledge of Lasegue's work that prompted Gull to publish his own paper. On the other hand, it may have been two eminent clinicians arriving at the same syndrome simultaneously, which has certainly happened on other occasions. As the number of clinical scholars increased in the nineteenth century, the probability of reaching the same conclusion increased. In the review of literature on fasting by Vandereycken and van Deth[2], they conclude that priority probably belongs to neither Gull nor Lasegue but rather to Richard Morton (1637-1698)[15].

In 1689 Richard Morton described two patients who in retrospect would appear to have symptoms similar to anorexia nervosa. Morton's depiction of atrophia or phthisis nervosa in 1689 is the first detailed medical description of the syndrome we call anorexia nervosa, and for many the history of this syndrome begins with Morton's treatise[15]. However, as Vandereycken and van Deth note, "it was not until 1900 that the famous Sir William Osler in a lecture on Morton's Phthisiologia[16] stated almost in passing: 'Under what he [Morton] terms nervous consumption, I think we may recognize Gull's anorexia nervosa, particularly in the history of the two cases which he narrates'"[16]. However, it is appropriate to credit both Gull[12] and Lasegue[11] with the independent identification of this syndrome, because their two reports marked a watershed in the study of anorexia nervosa.

C. The Archeology of Mind

Obesity is at the other extreme of body weight from anorexia nervosa but, like anorexia nervosa, has been a major research subject for psychiatrists. Sigmund Freud (1856-1938) was a major intellectual force in psychiatry in the twentieth century[17], bringing psychoanalysis to life almost single-handedly. However, Freud's training was during the waning years of the Victorian era, and he carried this framework with him during his life. Freud made us aware of the power of the subconscious mind and developed a theory of personality. His archeological approach of delving into the recesses of the subconscious mind has, however, proven to be highly controversial. It is this controversy that makes the introductory quote by Newton so poignant. Freud's early work dealt with cocaine, and with neurology and hypnotism. The year 1895 was a pivotal one for Freud. It saw the publication of *Studies of Hysteria* with Josef Breuer[18], which set forth the idea that hysterical patients were suffering from repression into the subconscious mind of traumatic events that could not be faced without distressing emotional consequences[18]. Freud and Breuer also proposed that the secret to caring for these hysterical symptoms was to unblock the pent-up emotions through free expression.

Freud later introduced the method of free association as a way to probe the unconscious mind. The approach might also be called the "archeology of the mind." An archeologist digs through the remains of ancient civilizations and pieces them together through the items he finds. The psychoanalyst, a term Freud first used in 1896, helps the patient dig through his unconscious mind to bring out buried, emotionally charged memories. An underlying assumption of this approach is that the memory traces that are unearthed by the psychoanalyst are representations of earlier events. Freud's development of psychoanalysis was paralleled by a personal interest in archeology. Many archeological artifacts that he collected are on display at his former homes in Vienna and London[19].

From 1920 until his death in 1939, Freud's work centered on systematic inquires into the human personality and the structure of society. As the historian Gaarder says in his discussion of the development of a theory of personality structures, "It is no exaggeration to say that Freud discovered human drives"[20]. These human drives are the non-rational elements of which human sexual drive is a prime example. Freud identified a pleasure principle that he called the id. Society will not generally allow free expression of the pleasure principle. Rather, it must be controlled by a reality principle which Freud called the ego. The third element in personality is the superego that embodies our conscience. Along with this structure of personality, the psychoanalysts defined several stages of development beginning with the stage of oral and anal gratification and moving on to more advanced stages.

With this theoretical framework for personality structure and an archeological approach to unearthing repressed memories, psychoanalysis rose to a dominant position in psychiatry by the time of World War II. Albert Stunkard, a leading psychiatrist with a lifelong interest in obesity described the relation of psychoanalysis to medicine and to obesity in these words:

> Psychoanalysis was just reaching its position of preeminence in American psychiatry when I began my career (1945). It had already become the dominant theoretical system in the field, and for good reason. A new and fundamental understanding of the human condition seemed at

> hand, not just the relief of symptoms, but the very transformation of human nature itself. At a time when most medical research was leading away from the patient and into the laboratory, psychoanalysis held forth the promise of the most basic kind of clinical investigation into the human condition in the context of deep and meaningful personal relationships.[21]

Thus, it is not surprising that psychoanalytic thought should impact thinking about obesity. In 1939-1940, Hilda Bruch (1904-1984) published five studies reporting on her psychoanalytic experience with a group of corpulent children who were fighting the battle of the bulge [13, 22-26]. A number of features were common in these overweight children with adiposity, including immaturity, over-dependence, and lack of aggressiveness. She says, "[O]vereating is the weapon with which he (the obese child) meets traumatic experiences, failure and disappointment"[24]. She goes on to say, "In his insecure and unstable relation to his surroundings, physical size gives him a certain feeling of safety and strength. The heavy layer of fat acts like a wall behind which the child seeks protection against a threatening outside world"[24].

Many psychoanalytically oriented physicians have explained overweight and overeating as a fixation of the personality at the early oral stage of psychosexual development. In discussing one of his cases, the psychiatrist Bychowski elaborates as follows: "In surrounding herself with a cushion of fat, she was unconsciously attempting to avoid her mother's wrath since she was eliminating herself as a rival (Oedipus) and her father's anger at her potential relations with other men"[27].

In her classic book, *The Importance of Overweight*[28], Bruch classifies children with obesity into three groups. The first group are overweight children whose obesity is not related to emotional problems. The second group she calls "reactive obesity." These are children who overeat in times of stress or psychological deprivation. The third type is "developmental obesity." These are the individuals who have been fighting the battle of the bulge their entire life. They have surrendered to overfeeding and overprotection early in life. Bruch says "...concern with size and weight, and inability to tolerate frustration or delay in gratification seems to be the center, the very core, of their whole development." In two 1961 papers[29,30], Bruch began with a critical re-evaluation of the psychoanalytic principles cited by her as a reminder that in spite of our acceptance of scientific principles, psychoanalysis had not completely avoided the error of attributing names to "occult phenomena and then using these descriptive terms as if they were explanations"[30]. Bruch notes that

> psychoanalysts on the other hand have been slow and reluctant, even hostile, to the idea of critical reappraisal of their concepts...[O]ne implicit error was related to psychoanalysts' exclusive preoccupation with motivations underlying patients' communication and actions[30].

Bruch continues, "Along with [a] change in technique, a re-evaluation of the theoretical considerations was necessary." In the traditional psychoanalytic approach to abnormal food intake, food and eating are interpreted as a substitute activity in conflict situations. Bruch had to admit that she was responsible for having started some of these by now widely popularized notions. The trouble with such interpretations is not that they are wrong. On the contrary, many additional illustrations could easily be given. The trouble is that they do not really say anything. To go back to the introductory quotation by Newton, "they tell us nothing"[1].

Bruch continues with her critique of the deficiency of the psychoanalytic method as a way of dealing with the obese child:

> A large part of the theoretical structure of the psychoanalytic edifice is built on the theory of "drives"...Failure of appropriate response to signs and signals originating in the child has been singled out as the outstanding deficiency in the transmission of information that is essential for learning to identify body states correctly[30].
>
> Psychoanalytic concepts helped to clarify the psychodynamics of disturbed eating behavior and the symbolic significance of food and body size, they were not effective in therapeutic applications.[29]

One limitation of the free association techniques of psychoanalysis is that they deal with one patient at a time. Thus, the usual kind of randomized controlled clinical trial that is so essential to establishing that a technique is effective cannot be used with psychoanalytic approaches—they are too "personal." The randomized clinical trial has proven to be a powerful technique for evaluating treatments, including those for battling the bulge. They include, at a minimum, the use of two different groups of subjects with a defined set of trial conditions. One group receives the standard treatment, and the other an experimental treatment. The individuals are assigned to standard treatment or experimental treatment in a random way in order to avoid biases. During the treatment period, ideally, neither those giving the treatment nor those receiving it know which group they are in.

Randomized controlled trials don't exist in psychoanalysis, since the treatment is individual. Thus, to try and evaluate whether weight loss might occur as a result of the psychoanalytic process, Rand and Stunkard[31] sent questionnaires to 572 fellows of the American Academy of Psychoanalysis. Of these, 55% responded and 104 indicated that they had at least one overweight patient in individual treatment. Based on two separate questionnaires comparing results of the 84 overweight patients and 63 matched controls, Rand and Stunkard found that the weight loss in the patients with obesity in psychoanalytic treatment was similar to that of standard methods of weight loss. A large part of the weight loss had been at a rate of 0.1 kg/week. The unexpectedly large weight losses compared favorably to losses produced by behavior therapy. In the second questionnaire, the rate of weight loss had risen to 0.9 kg/week. It is unusual, however, to have the rate of weight gain increase later in treatment. As Rand and Stunkard noted, the increased rate of weight loss may reflect a different level of "attention" to the patient's weight status in the free-association sessions. A number of differences between the corpulent and control subjects were observed. Disturbances in body image of the patients with adiposity were substantial and decreased with weight loss. All data in this study were subjective. When the authors approached some of the analysts about the possibility of validating their reports of weight loss, the analysts stated that

> weighing their patients could constitute undue intrusion of research into the analytic process....This problem of validation will continue to affect studies of outcome research in psychoanalysis, including studies that use less objective measures than weight loss. It clearly constitutes an impediment to such research.[31]

This inability to use objective evaluation in psychoanalytic studies has led to a decrease in the influence of psychoanalysis during the last third of the twentieth-century. As research has increased the demand for verification of its findings, the shortcomings of psychoanalytic procedures with respect to verification has become ever more apparent. This delusion has been nicely summarized by Dr. Albert Stunkard in his autobiographical book titled *The Pain of Obesity*. He concluded:

> [P]sychoanalysis proved ultimately disillusioning. The generalizations which had stirred such enthusiasm in a generation of psychiatrists did not generate a systematic program of research. And worse, they diverted attention from the real work that had to be done on a lower and much more laborious level, to build a solid structure of knowledge.[25]
>
> It would be difficult to overestimate the impact that the psychoanalytic movement had upon American psychiatry.[25]

> World War II accelerated a number of technological developments. We are still assimilating some of these developments. One of these was a growing understanding of the chemistry of the brain. The introduction of chemical agents that can be used for treating schizophrenia and depression based on a theory of neurotransmitter derangements as the cause of these illnesses has been very fruitful. Coupled with the difficulties of "validation" of the psychoanalytic process, there has been a gradual shift in the focus of research on mental illness.
>
> That psychoanalysis, as a mode of treatment, has been experiencing a long institutional decline is no longer in serious dispute. Nor is the reason: though some patients claim to have acquired profound self-insight and even alterations of personality, in the aggregate psychoanalysis has proved to be an indifferently successful and vastly inefficient method of removing neurotic systems.[2,1]

The archeology of the mind, the process of digging for lost memories buried in the past of an individual is central to the psychoanalytic approach. Recovered memory is one name for this process. Recovered memory has been used frequently in court. In the field of child abuse, some think that the idea of recovered memory has done irreparable harm. To quote from Crews, who is a serious critic of recovered memory:

> Freud had launched a pseudoscience, that is, a nominally scientific enterprise which is so faulty at the core that it cannot afford to submit its hypotheses for unsparing peer review by the wider community, but must instead resort to provisos that forestall any possibility of refutation.[2]

In his book *Wittgenstein's Freud*, Cioffi cryptically paraphrases the problem that Newton had identified three centuries earlier: "What a psychoanalytic explanation tells us is itself"[33]. "As I write," Crews says, "a number of parents and child-care providers are serving long prison terms, and others are awaiting trial, on the basis of therapeutically induced 'memories' of child sexual abuse that never in fact occurred"[32]. This is an example of distorted archeology similar to the hoax of the Piltdown man, a skeleton that was identified amid great fanfare and subsequently shown to be a recent skeleton buried to make it appear to be from an earlier era.

The limits of psychoanalysis are aptly stated by the great historian of science, Dr. Karl Popper: "Those clinical observations which analysts naively believe confirm their theory cannot do this any more than the daily confirmations which astrologers find in their practice....Belief in repression has the same standing as belief in God. The idea may be true, but it is consistent with too many eventualities to be falsifiable that is amenable to scientific assessment"[34].

D. Obesity and Socioeconomic Status

The scene now shifts from the decline of psychoanalytic influence on obesity to the more modern views of obesity in a socio-economic context. In the early post-war period there were reconstruction projects in many American cities that displaced people from their homes while new buildings were being built. As part of this process, the Mid-Manhattan Survey was set up to examine the health and behavioral consequences of this dislocation. Using the data collected from this study in the 1960s, Moore, Stunkard, and Srole[14] asked whether there was any relation between body weight and social class. They assessed social class on the basis of an individual's occupation and education and combined it with economic status to provide twelve categories. The prevalence of overweight in the lowest of these twelve groups—the lowest socio-economic group with the least education and lowest income—was seven times higher than among those in the most educated individuals and those with the highest income. The gradient of economic and occupational status on weight was more evident in women and much less evident in men. Since this initial report by Moore et al.[14], the inverse relationship between social class and overweight in women has been widely reported by many other scientific authors. In their discussion of their findings the authors of this seminal paper weigh in on the role of nature and nurture in the development of obesity and point to what a strong influence the social environment can have:

> One of the most interesting findings of this study is the high correlation between obesity and social class. Clinical investigations had previously suggested such a relationship, but this is the first controlled study, as far as we know, that has demonstrated it. The fact that obesity is 7 times more frequent in lower-class than in upper-class women has profound implications for theory and for therapy. For it means that whatever its genetic and biochemical determinants, obesity in man is susceptible to an extraordinary degree of control by social factors[14].

One explanation for the inverse relationship in women of weight and social class is that women in the upper social class consciously reduce their overall food intake. Restraint of food intake was first identified by Herman and Polivy[35] and is common in many, if not most, middle-aged women[36]. A breakdown in this restraint mechanism may provide an explanation for the rising prevalence of overweight in the United States[37]. However, the fact that overweight has risen to a comparable degree in both men and women of all social classes makes this an unlikely explanation.

In this social context, fat can be viewed as a feminist issue[5,38]. It is more prevalent in women where the social pressures toward thinness are greatest. This changing social context over the past century[39] may provide a way of linking the appearance of anorexia nervosa, bulimia nervosa, and restrained eating with the inverse relation of weight and social class. Orbach has put this case most strongly:

> Fat is a social disease, and fat is a feminist issue. Fat is *not* about lack of self-control or lack of will power. Fat *is* about protection, sex, nurturance, strength, boundaries, nothing, substance, assertion, and rage.
>
> In this way, fat expresses a rebellion against the powerlessness of the woman, against the pressure to look and act in a certain way and against being evaluated on her ability to create an image of herself.
>
> In this context, just as many women first become fat in an attempt to avoid being made into sexual objects at the beginning of their adult lives, so many women remain fat as a way of neutralizing their sexual identity in the eyes of others who are important to them as their life progresses.[38]

Some of these ideas are reminiscent of those put forward by Dr. Hilda Bruch[6] nearly fifty years ago and subsequently modified by her. Gordon[9] has described this change as follows:

> In her last paper, Bruch suggested that within her own lifetime she witnessed the transformation of anorexia nervosa from an individual into a social disease. Even as recently as the 1960s, she suggested, cases of anorexia nervosa occurred in individuals who had never heard about the disorder; it was as if each created the symptoms anew out of the crucible of their own individual experience. But more recently, she suggested, as the disease has become more common and increasingly known, the clinical picture has undergone a subtle transformation...Bruch even goes so far as to suggest that the numerous programs for the treatment of eating disorders may have contributed to the socialization of the disease.[9]

The impact of the social environment on behavioral disease seems evident.

What is missing in this formulation is the impact of drugs on bulimia. According to Gordon:

> During the 1980s a further treatment approach has emerged, one based on the idea that bulimia is mediated by biological depression...[A] certain number of normal-weight bulimics respond favorably to antidepressant medications, such as the tricyclic antidepressants and the MAO inhibitors.[9]

These dramatic findings led Pope and Hudson to argue that bulimia is grounded in an endogenous depression or primary affective disorder."[9]

This suggests that the biological changes which are reflected in the behavior associated with bulimia may involve a serotonergic neurotransmitter system that is directed in a certain way by the culture in which it is expressed. Until a treatment modality is found for anorexia nervosa, it will not be possible to know whether a similar explanation may apply. Simmonds's Syndrome or pituitary cachexia[40]and the effects of lateral hypothalamic damage to reduce food intake and body weight suggest that a neuroanatomic basis for anorexia nervosa may lie behind the veil of truth, waiting for the veil to be pulled back.

This survey of behavioral and social correlates of obesity and its opposite, anorexia, is important because it gives us a perspective on the battle of the bulge. As weight is lost it affects both the one losing weight and people in the same environment. Depending on the social and cultural factors the reactions to success in battling the bulge can be either positive or negative. When positive they can reinforce success. When negative they can undermine it. It is thus important to have a picture of the environment as one begins a battle of the bulge.

Biosketch

Richard Morton (1637-1698) is described by the *Dictionary of National Biography* as an "ejected minister and physician"[41]. His initial education led him to Oxford, where he received a M.A. in 1659 when he was serving as chaplain to the family of Philip Foley of Prestwood. With the Reformation, he was unable to comply with the requirement of the "Act of Uniformity" and was ejected from his livelihood as a minister in 1662.

He then turned his attention to medicine and received an M.D. in 1670 on nomination of the Prince of Orange. He subsequently moved to London and became a member and then fellow of the Royal College of Physicians in 1679 (Figure 18-1). His most important work for us is his *Phthisiologia: seu Exercitationes de Phthisi*, published in 1689. This work follows the principles of clinical observation espoused by Thomas

Sydenham. His book describes all of the conditions of "wasting" that he personally saw. It was Sir William Osler who noted that one of Morton's cases was probably "Anorexia nervosa"[16].

Biosketch

Sir William Withey Gull (1816-1890) (Figure 18-2) was born in Colchester, near London. His father, a barge owner, died when he was ten, and his early education was mostly home schooling. In 1836 he entered Guy's Hospital and received his M.B. in 1841 and his M.D. in 1846.

He gradually rose through the ranks at Guy's Hospital becoming a full physician in 1856. He resigned in 1865 due to his growing private practice but continued an active role in administrative and clinical medicine. He was elected a Fellow of the Royal Society in 1869. His baronetcy came in 1872 for treatment of the Prince of Wales for typhoid fever. Gull was an eminent clinical teacher and clinician. He is probably best known for his classical description of myxedema. His lecture describing anorexia nervosa is the basis for his inclusion here[42,43].

Biosketch

Ernest Charles Lasegue (1816-1883) ranks as one of the great French psychiatrists in the mid-nineteenth century. He was born in 1816, the same year as Gull, but across the English Channel. They were thus contemporaries.

However, Lasegue's career "developed more slowly." Only in 1867 did he become professor of general pathology and in 1869 he became chair of clinical medicine at La Pitie Hospital. (Figure 18-3)[2].

Biosketch

Sigmund Freud (1856-1938) (Figure 18-4) changed the world with his ideas about the subconscious, about the role of repressed experience in behavioral patterns that could be understood through psychoanalysis, a kind of archeology of the mind. Freud was born in Freiberg in 1856. His parents moved to Vienna when he was four. He received his medical degree in 1881, and his initial medical studies dealt with physiology, but he quickly turned to neurology and neuropathology.

During these years he conducted his "cocaine" studies, hoping it would be a substitute for morphine. His first work on the subconscious mind was published with Breuer in 1895. The publication of *The Interpretation of Dreams* in 1900 is Freud's most important contribution[44]. It was the cornerstone for the psychoanalytic approach to the unconscious. Development of this method occupied Freud from 1895 to 1920. Among the landmarks in this period were *The Psychopathology of Everyday Life* in 1901[45], *Three Essays on Sexuality*[46] in 1905 and *Introductory Lectures in Psychoanalysis*[47] in 1916-1917. Freud became a magnet for the training of the psychoanalysts of the twentieth-century. After the rise of the Nazis and their occupation of Austria, Freud fled to London where he lived out the final years of his life[48].

Biosketch

Hilda Bruch (1904-1984) (Figure 18-5) is noted for her contributions to the study of childhood obesity and to anorexia nervosa. Dr. Bruch grew up in a Jewish family with six siblings in Dulken, Germany. For practical reasons, she did not pursue mathematics or her interest in dress design but graduated with a medical degree from the University of Freiburg in 1929. As the climate for tolerance deteriorated in Germany with the rise of Hitler, she emigrated first to London, where she spent one year, and then to Houston.

Her initial work in pediatrics shifted into psychiatry as the Second World War began. In 1943 she became a professor of psychiatry at Columbia University, College of Physicians and Surgeons. Her early contribution showing that most childhood obesity was not due to Frohlich's Syndrome or hypothalamic obesity was a landmark. As an older single woman, she finally decided to leave New York and accepted a position at the Baylor College of Medicine as professor of psychiatry. During these years she made significant contributions to understanding the psychiatric aspects of childhood obesity[49,50].

References

1. Dingle, H. "Cosmology and Science." *Sci Am.* X(1956): 224-236.
2. Vandereycken, W., R. Van Deth. *From Fasting Saints to Anorexic Girls: The History of Self Starvation.* London: Athlone Press, 1994.
3. Stopes, M.C.C. *Contraception.* London: John Bale Reproductions 1923.
4. Rock, J., C.M. Garcia, G. Pincus. "Synthetic Progestins in the Normal Human Menstrual Cycle." *Recent Prog Horm Res.* 13(1957): 323-339.
5. Chernin, K. *The Obsession: Reflections on the Tyranny of Slenderness.* New York: Harper & Row, 1981.
6. Bruch, H. *The Golden Cage: The Enigma of Anorexia Nervosa.* Cambridge: Harvard University Press, 1978.
7. Crisp, A.H. *Anorexia Nervosa. Let Me Be.* London: Academic Press, 1980.
8. Daily, P., J. Gornez. *Anorexia and Obesity: A Sense of Proportion.* London: Faber and Faber, Ltd., 1990.
9. Gordon, R.A. *Anorexia and Bulimia: Anatomy of a Social Epidemic.* Cambridge, MA: Basil Blackwell, Inc., 1990.
10. Lui, A. *Solitaire.* New York: Harper and Row, 1979.
11. Lasègue, E.C. "De l'anorexie hystérique." *Archives générales de médecine.* 21(1873): 385-403.
12. Gull, M. "Anorexia Nervosa (apepsia hysterica, anorexia hysterica)." *Trans Clin Soc London.* 7(1874): 22-28.
13. Bruch, H. "Obesity in Childhood. III. Physiologic and Psychologic Aspects of the Food Intake of Obese Children." *Am J Dis Child* 58(1940): 738-781.
14. Moore, M.E., A. Stunkard, L. Srole. "Obesity, Social Class, and Mental Illness." *JAMA.* 181(1962): 962-6.
15. Morton, R. *Phthisiologia, or, a treatise of consumptions. Wherein the difference, nature, causes, signs, and cure of all sorts of consumptions are explained.* London: Samuel Smith and Benjamin Walfoni, 1694.
16. Osler, W. "The 'Phthisologia' of Richard Morton, M.D." *Med Lib Hist J.* (1904).
17. Alexander, F.G., S.T. Selesnicki. *The History of Psychiatry: An Evaluation of Psychiatry Thought and Practice from Prehistoric Times to the Present.* New York: Harper and Row Publishers, 1966.
18. Breuer, J., S. Freud. *Studien über hysterie.* Lepzig & Wien: F Deuticke, 1895. *Studies on hysteria.* Translated from German and edited by J. Strachey in collaboration with Anna Freud. New York: Basic Books, Inc., 1957.
19. *Sigmund Freud and Art: His Personal Collection of Antiquities.* G. Gamwell and R. Wells, eds. Syracuse: State University of New York,

1990.
20. Gaarder, J. *Sophie's World: A Novel about the History of Philosophy.* Transl. P. Moller. London: Phoenix House, 1955.
21. Stunkard, A.J. *The Pain of Obesity.* Palo Alto, CA: Bull Publishing Co., 1976.
22. Bruch, H. "The Frohlich Syndrome: Report of the Original Case." *Am J Dis Child.* 58(1939): 1282.
23. Bruch, H. "Obesity in Childhood: II. Basal Metabolism and Serum Cholesterol of Obese Children." *Am J Dis Child.* 58(1939): 1001-1022.
24. Bruch, H. "Obesity in Childhood and Personality Development." *Am J Orthopsychiatry.* ii(1941): 467-74.
25. Bruch, H. "Studies in Obesity in Childhood: 1. Physical Growth and Development of Obese Children." *Am J Dis Child.* 58(1939): 457.
26. Bruch, H., G. Touraine. "Obesity in Childhood: V. The Family Frame of Obese Children." *Psychosom Med.* 2(1940): 141-206.
27. Bychowski, G. "On Neurotic Obesity." *Am J Psychoanal.* 37(1950): 301-319.
28. Bruch, H. *The Importance of Overweight.* New York: W.W. Norton and Co, Inc., 1957.
29. Bruch, H. "Conceptual Confusion in Eating Disorders." *J Nerv Ment Dis.* 133(1961): 46-54.
30. Bruch, H. "Transformation of Oral Impulses in Eating Disorders: A Conceptual Approach." *Psychiatr Q* 35(1961): 458-481.
31. Crews, F. "The Memory Wars: Freud's Legacy in Dispute." New York: New York Review, 1995.
32. Cioffi, F. "Wittgenstein's Freud." In *Studies in the Philosophy of Wittgenstein.* P. Winch, ed. London: Routledge, 1969.
33. Popper, K.R. *Conjectures and Refutations: The Growth of Scientific Knowledge.* New York: Basic Books, 1965.
34. Herman, C.P., J. Polivy. "Anxiety, Restraint and Eating Behavior." *J Abnorm Psychol.* 84(1975): 666-672.
35. Lawson, O.J., D.A. Williamson, C.M. Champagne, et al. "The Association of Body Weight, Dietary Intake, and Energy Expenditure with Dietary Restraint and Disinhibition." *Obes Res.* 3(1995): 153-161.
36. Kuczmarski, R.J., K.M., Flegal, S.M., Campbell, C.L. Johnson. "Increasing Prevalence of Overweight Among U.S. Adults." *JAMA.* 272(1994): 205-211.
37. Orbach, S. *Fat Is a Feminist Issue: The Anti-diet Guide to Permanent Weight Loss.* New York & London: Paddington Press Ltd., 1978.
38. Schwartz, H. *Never Satisfied: A Cultural History of Diets, Fantasies and Fat.* NewYork: Free Press, 1986
39. Simmonds, M. "Über Hypophysisschwund mit tödlichem Ausgang."

Deutsche medizinische Wochenschrift. 40(1914): 322 323.
40. Porter, B. "Richard Morton (1637-1698)." In *The Dictionary of National Biography.* L. Stephens and S. Lee, eds. London: Oxford University Press, Vol XIII, 1937-1938.
41. Bettany, G.T. "Sir William Withey Gull (1816-1890)." In *The Dictionary of National Biography.* L. Stephens and S. Lee, eds. London: Oxford University Press, Vol VIII, 1937-1938.
42. Medvei, V.C. *A History of Endocrinology.* Lancaster: MTP Press, 1982.
43. Freud, S. *Die Traumdeutung. [The Interpretation of Dreams.]* Wein: F. Deuticke, 1900.
44. Freud, S. *Zur Psychopathologie des Alltagslebens. [Psychopathology of Everyday Life]* Berlin: S. Karger, 1901.
45. Freud, S. *Drei Abhandlungen zur Sexual Theorie. [Three Essays on Sexuality.]* Vienna: F. Deuticke, 1905.
46. Freud, S. *Vorlesungen zur Einfuhrung in die Psychoanalyse. [Introductory Lectures in Psychoanalysis.]* Vienna: F. Deuticke, 1916-1917.
47. Major, R. *A History of Medicine.* Springfield, IL: Charles C. Thomas, 1954.
48. Gallo, S. "Short Biographies of Mabel Giddings Wilkin, M.D., and Hilda Bruch, M.D." *Texas Med.* 10(1994): 60-70.
49. Garfinkel, P.E. "Hilda Bruch, M.D.: A Seeker of Truth." In *Women Physicians in Leadership Roles.* Arlington, VA: American Psychiatric Press, 1986.

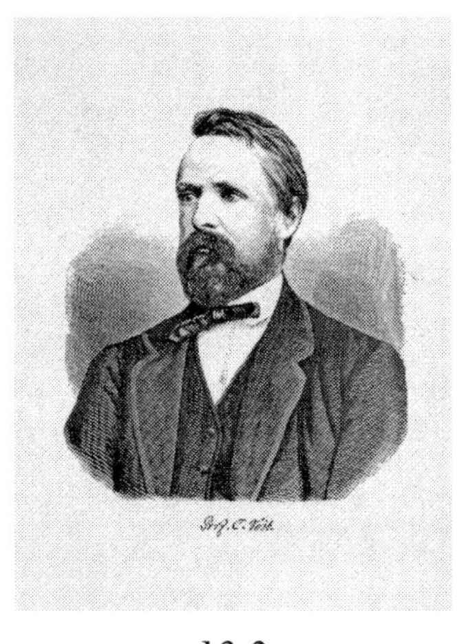

13-2

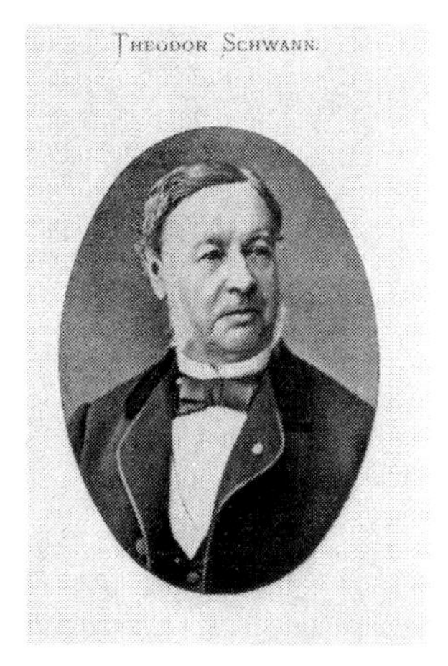

14-3

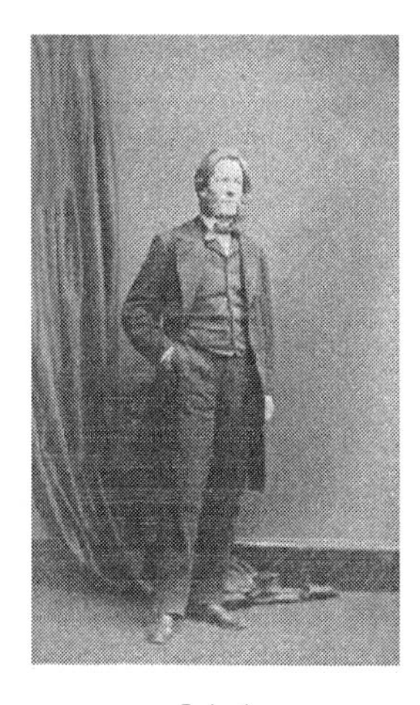

14-4

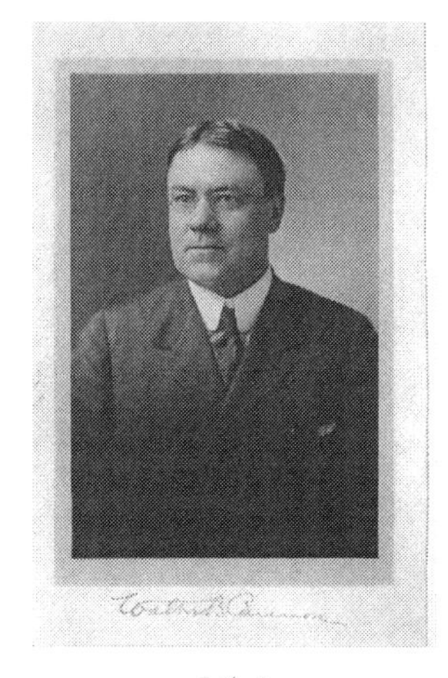

15-1

13-2 Carl von Voit (1831-1908). Courtesy of the National Library of Medicine.

14-3 Theodor Schwann (1810-1882). Courtesy of the National Library of Medicine.

14-4 Arthur Hill Hassall (1817-1894). Courtesy of Charles C. Thomas Publisher Ltd.

15-1 Walter Bradford Cannon (1871-1945). Courtesy of the Francis A. Countway Library of Medicine.

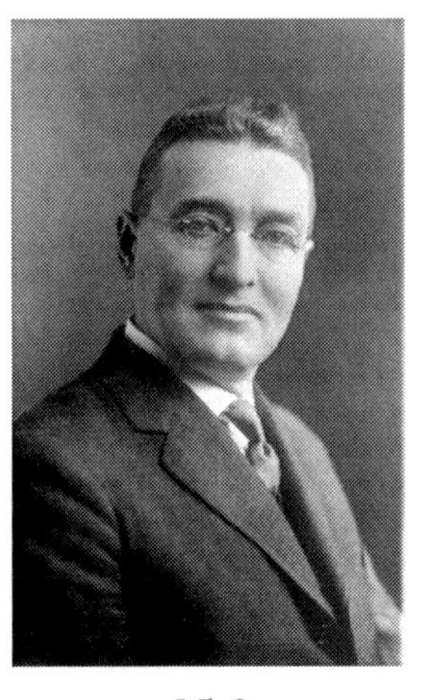

15-2

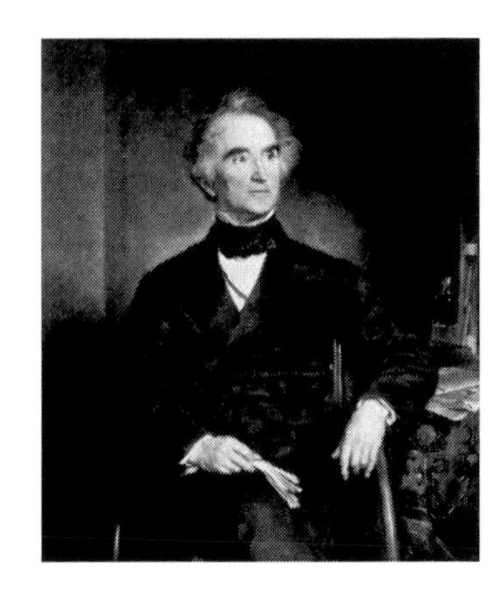

16-2

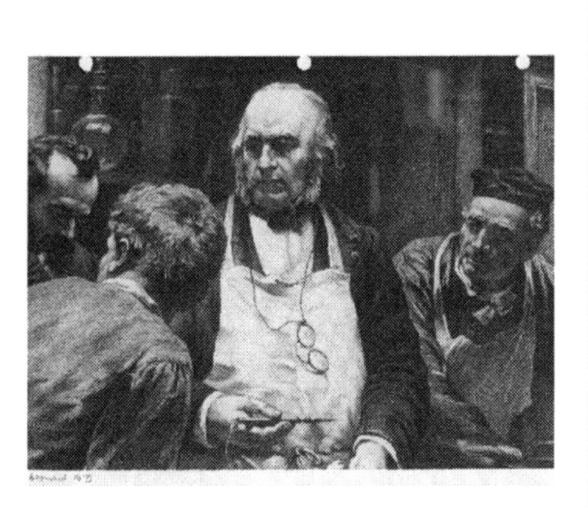

16-3

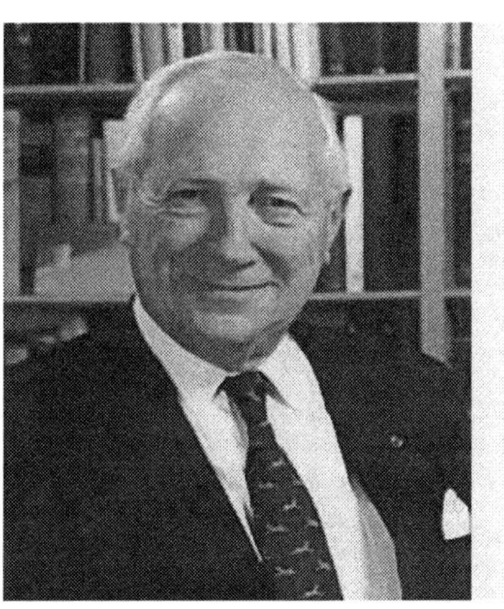

16-4

15-2 Anton Julius Carlson (1875-1956). Courtesy of the National Library of Medicine.

16-2 Justus von Liebig (1803-1873). Courtesy of the National Library of Medicine.

16-3 Claude Bernard (1813-1878) From the collection of the author.

16-4 Jean Mayer (1920-1993). Courtesy of Tufts University Archives.

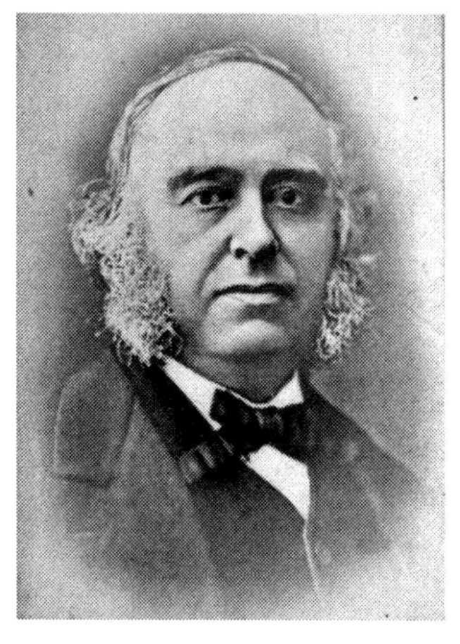

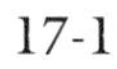

17-1

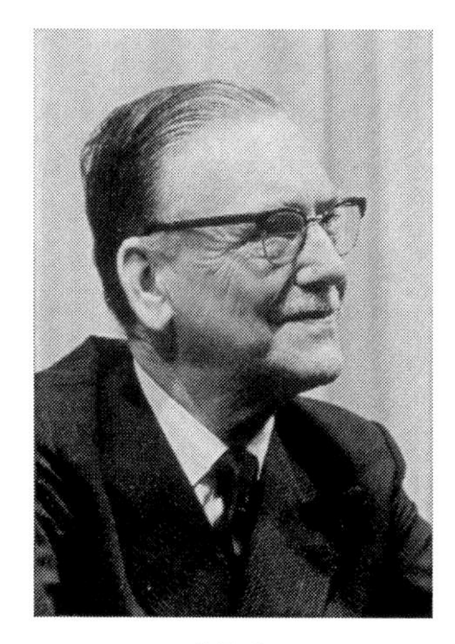

17-2

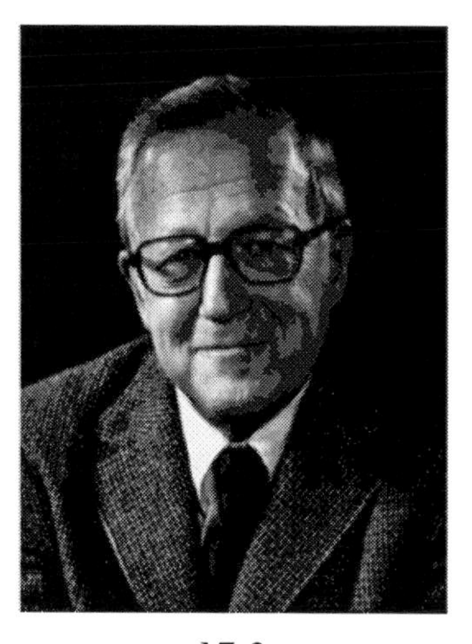

17-3

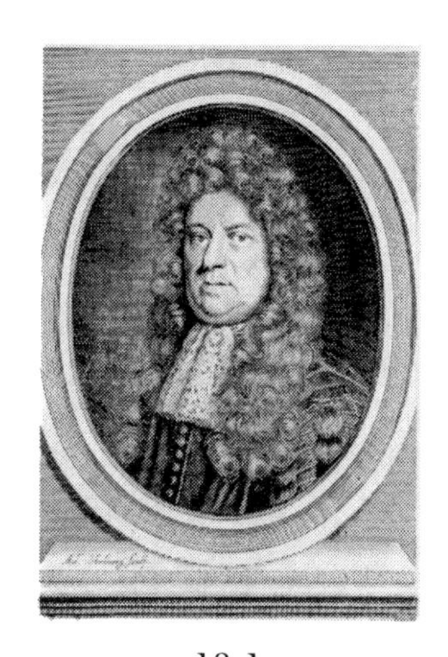

18-1

17-1 Paul Broca (1924-1980). Courtesy of the National Library of Medicine.

17-2 Ulf Svante von Euler (1905-1983). Courtesy of the National Library of Medicine.

17-3 Eliot Stellar (1919-1993). http://www.psych.upenn.edu/history/bushtext.htm

18-1 Richard Morton (1637-1698). Courtesy of the National Library of Medicine.

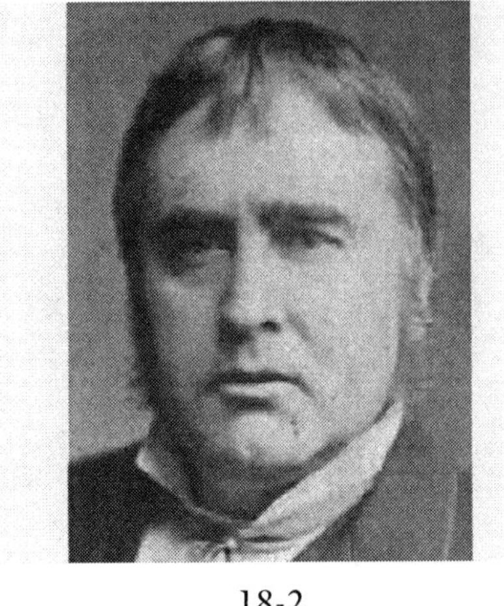

18-2

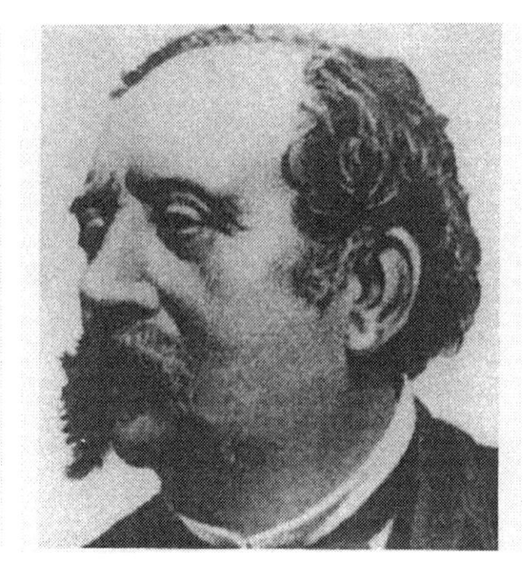

18-3

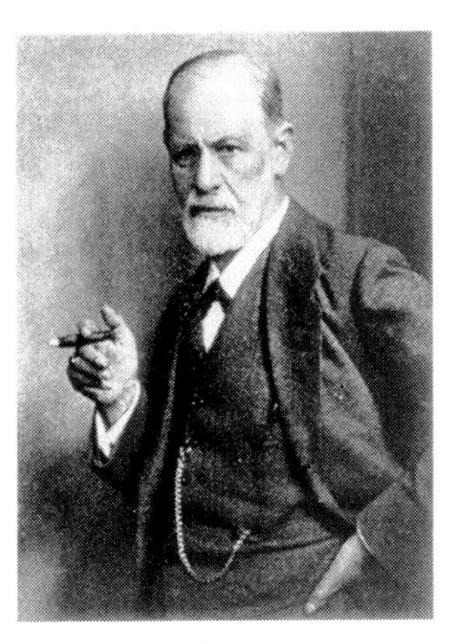

18-4

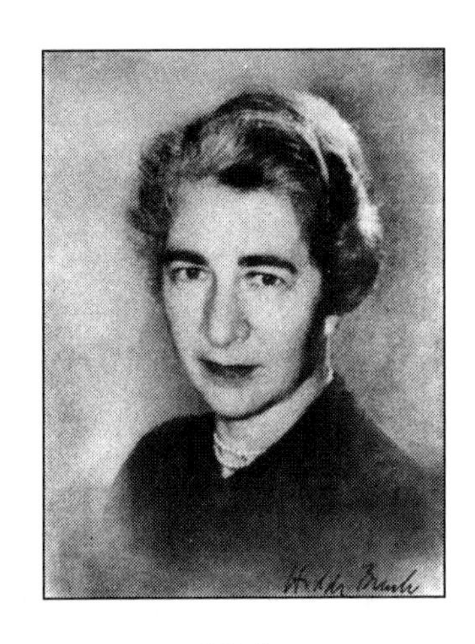

18-5

18-2 William Withey Gull (1816-1890). Courtesy of the National Library of Medicine.

18-3 Ernest Charles Lasegue (1816-1883). Courtesy of Charles C. Thomas Publisher Ltd.

18-4 Sigmund Freud (1856-1938). Courtesy of the National Library of Medicine.

18-5 Hilda Bruch (1904-1994). Courtesy of the National Library of Medicine.

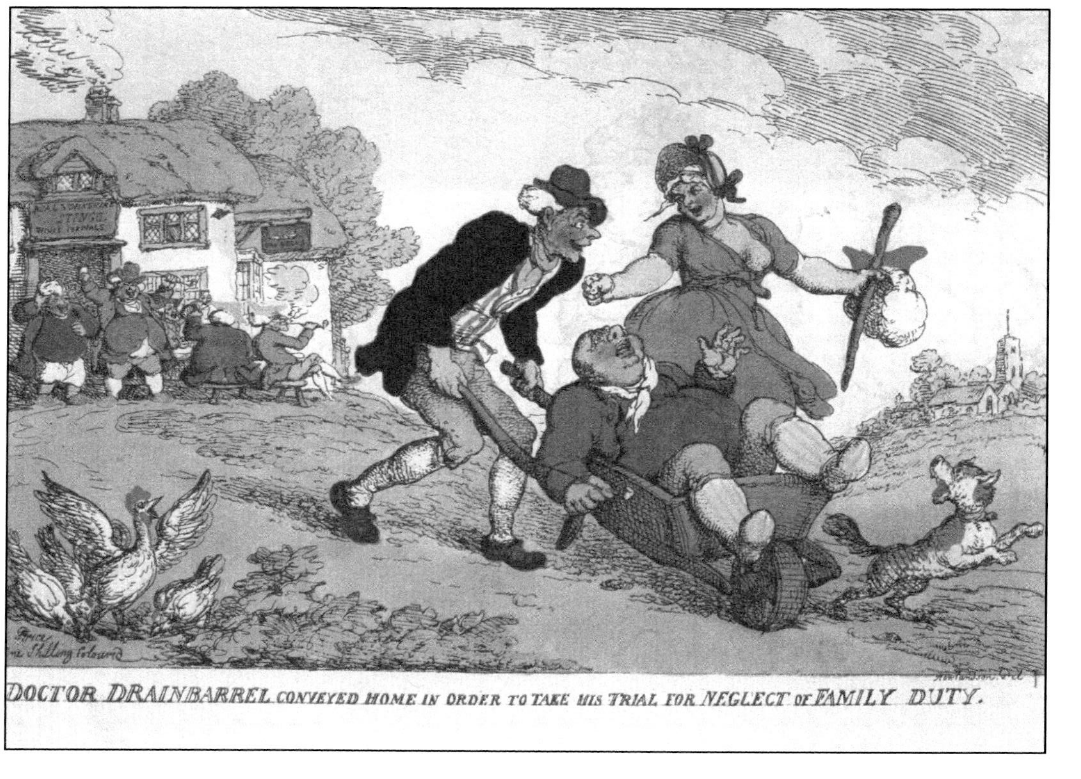

19-1 Rowlandson cartoon. From the collection of the author.

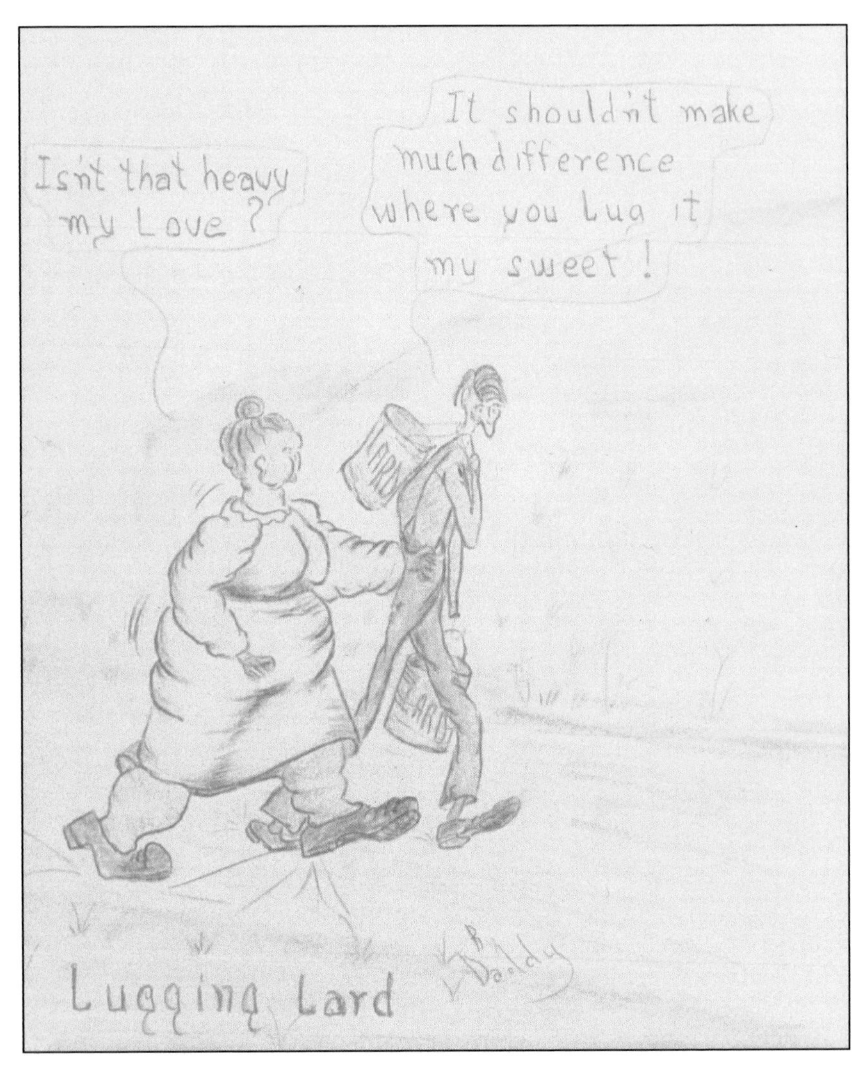

19-2 "Lugging Lard," Carl O. Rice. From the collection of the author.

Chapter 19

The Pain of Overweight

> *It's amazing how insensitive people can be to fat people. You wouldn't walk up to a cripple in the street and say, 'How did you lose the use of your legs?' So I don't know why people think it's all right to say these things to us.*
>
> —Interview with Laura Campbell[1]

Overweight Americans are continually subjected to all sorts of prejudice[2]. These negative reactions come in many forms. Individuals who are overweight can be the subject of ridicule, negative comments, and insensitive behaviors that combine to make overweight an even less bearable condition. In one sense overweight is a "disability" just as injuries and amputations are disabilities.

> One of the powerful things I remember about weight from my childhood is that my older sister (who is three years older than I) was quite overweight—she was about 25 pounds overweight in high school. My mother would ridicule and torment her, and call her Fatty or Fatso, under the guise of trying to help her lose weight. I remember once in the guise of "helping" her my mother grabbed my sister's dress and pulled it up and grabbed her thigh and said, "Look at this ham."[1]

These reactions of normal-weight people to people who are overweight produce some of the pain of obesity. As the scientific background to this section, I have selected a classic paper that is reprinted in the appendix to show that prejudice toward those battling the bulge begins in early childhood[3,4].

The pain or stigma associated with obesity drives many people to extreme means to lose weight, particularly women. Scientific documentation of this prejudice is poignantly illustrated by the two papers I have selected. They tell us that prejudice toward obesity is already present in childhood. The project was designed to examine the way children view disabilities in other children. For this purpose a series of picture cards were prepared showing six different disabilities in boys or in girls. Included among these six pictures of disabilities was a picture card showing a fat boy or a fat girl. The children who participated in this initial study were fifth graders in schools around the United States. There were wealthy and poorer children, children from rural and urban schools, and children from both the North and South. In each case the boys were shown the six cards with pictures of boys and the girls the cards with girls. The children were asked to look at the cards and pick the child that it would be easiest to play with. When the first card was selected, the process was repeated with the remaining cards until all of the six cards had been chosen. The remarkable finding was that the fat child was almost always the child that would be hardest to play with—they were the least preferred as a playmate by both the boys and girls everywhere. When the children were asked why this was so, most of them indicated that the children with amputations, blindness, scars, etc., could not help themselves. They were not responsible for their disability. However, the fat children were perceived as responsible for their fatness and were therefore less likeable.

The authors were surprised by their findings and decided to expand their work. They conducted an additional study in preschool children, reasoning that it might be the exposure to the prejudices of other children in school that had already occurred during the first few years in school that led to the prejudices toward fat fifth grade children. Again they studied children from around the United States, and again they found that the fat child was the least popular child to have as a playmate. Other replicates of this approach revealed that the negative attitudes toward fatness are widespread through adults from all walks of life in American society.

Prejudice against the obese has some fascinating historical examples. The story of King Sancho I, also called Sancho the Fat, from tenth-century Spain is most intriguing[5]. After his brother King Ordono III died, Sancho I became king of León in Spain in A.D. 958. His reign was short because his fatness became an impediment to his rule. "The nobility of León began to think of him as weak-willed because of his obesity"[5], and he was deposed. The physicians in León were unsuccessful in helping Sancho lose weight. Tota, Sancho's grandmother, who had once ruled the kingdom, was determined to help Sancho regain the throne. Although she loathed the Muslims who occupied the southern part of Spain in the tenth-century, Tota and Sancho sought the help of the brilliant and learned Jewish physician Hisdai ibn Shaprut, physician to the caliph in the southern Spanish city of Cordoba. In the tenth-century, Cordoba was one of the leading cultural cities of the world. It was also renowned as one of the great medical centers of the late Middle Ages.

In a day when house calls were still in fashion, Shaprut went to Pamplona to evaluate Sancho. Shaprut agreed to take Sancho as a patient but advised him that it would be a long treatment requiring him to relocate to Cordoba. Because of the seriousness of the problem, Sancho and his grandmother Tota moved from the Christian section in the north of Spain to the Muslim southern part of the Iberian Peninsula to receive treatment for obesity. The medicine that Shaprut prescribed was "Theriaca," a mixture that probably contained opiates and that was often taken with wine and oils. Over time Sancho gradually lost weight. When he returned to León as a lean man, his throne was restored. From this story it is clear that even kings are not immune from the prejudice associated with obesity. "Apparently a King may be cruel, but not fat"[5]. Moreover, this shows that more than one thousand years ago, obesity of mammoth proportions could be treated effectively.

A second story from Constantinople in the fourteenth-century, four hundred years after Sancho[6], illustrates the prejudice engendered by obesity. Although overweight, John Gavalas was a distinguished military commander and foreign minister in Byzantium during the transition of power in 1354. Apocaucus, the new governor to Constantinople, promised his daughter's hand in marriage to Gavalas as part of a deal to enlist Gavalas's aid. This promise was to be honored and the marriage consummated, even if Gavalas became ill with the sacred disease (leprosy) or developed epilepsy or mental illness (melancholy). However, the bride and her mother thought that Gavalas was too fat. Apocaucus had studied medicine and advised Gavalas to lose weight so "his belly would go down and he would appear slimmer and worthy to love because as he was he appeared disgusting with the asymmetry of his flesh"[6]. Gavalos was treated by an Italian physician who used baths, drugs, emetics, purgatives, and a strict diet. In spite of the treatments, Gavalos lost only a little weight. Contrast this with the successful long-term weight loss produced by the Muslim physicians in Spain. Clearly some treatments and some physicians are more successful at helping overweight people than others.

Prejudice against the overweight isn't just in ancient times or just about kings[7-10]. Prejudice is clearly illustrated in a story about the selection of the person to play Ronald McDonald, the mascot of McDonald's food chain. It is told by Eric Schlosser in his book *Fast Food Nation:*

> The McDonald's Corporation's first mascot was Speedee, a winking little chef with a hamburger for a head. The character was later renamed Archie McDonald. Speedee was the name of Alka-Seltzer's mascot, and it seemed unwise to imply any connection between the two brands. In 1960,

> Oscar Goldstein, a McDonald's franchisee in Washington D.C. decided to sponsor *Bozo's Circus*, a local children's television show. Bozo's appearance at a McDonald's restaurant drew large crowds. When the local NBC station canceled *Bozo's Circus* in 1963, Goldstein hired its star—Willard Scott, later the weatherman on NBC's *Today Show*—to invent a new clown who could make restaurant appearances. An ad agency designed the outfit, Scott came up with the name Ronald McDonald, and a star was born. Two years later the McDonald's Corporation introduced Ronald McDonald to the rest of the United States through a major ad campaign. But Willard Scott no longer played the part. He was deemed too overweight; McDonald's wanted someone thinner to sell its burgers, shakes, and fries.[7]

A movie that screened in 2001 also illustrates this prejudice toward obese women. *Shallow Hal* is about a man who is hypnotized to recognize only the inner beauty of a woman. He then meets Rosemary, who is an obese woman, but he can only see the thin woman and he falls in love with her. The lead actress, Gwyneth Paltrow, became fat by wearing a fat suit that made her appear two hundred pounds heavier. When interviewed, she described the response when she sat in the lobby of a New York hotel wearing her fat suit. No one was willing to help her when she asked questions. According to a newspaper story[8], Ms. Paltrow expressed her sympathy for the obscene discrimination against fat people and "the despair of being morbidly obese." This movie has touched off considerable discussion, pro and con, about the pain of obesity as experienced by fat people in everyday life and whether there are ways to help them.

A sympathetic view of the problems confronting the afflicted overweight is presented in *Such a Pretty Face* by Marcia Millman[1]. Her interviews with overweight people all associated with various organizations concerned with the overweight provide telling insights into their lives. Included in the list of organizations were the National Association to Aid Fat Acceptance, which is working to reduce prejudice toward the overweight; the self-help group Overeaters Anonymous, which patterns its sessions after those of Alcoholic Anonymous; and a summer camp for adolescents. The pain of being overweight is easily detected in these interviews. In another part of the interview with Laura Campbell, who was quoted at the beginning of this chapter, she says:

> People are always making loud remarks about me in the street, like, "Look at that woman. She should be in a circus," or, "Look at that fat elephant."

> One day I was in the supermarket and a four-year-old kid was marching around and around me in circles, screaming at the top of his lungs, *"You are fat. You are fat. You are fat"*—over and over again. I wanted to choke the kid, or say to his mother, "You should teach your child some manners." But it's complicated. Sometimes children are only stating a fact, and by saying they shouldn't say it, it's like agreeing that being fat is bad.[1]

At an Overeaters Anonymous meeting, Millman recorded this comment from Laura R.:

> My daughter was going to spend Christmas with her grandmother and she baked some cookies to bring along. I'm jealous of my daughter because she's a beautiful nine-year-old who has her whole life ahead of her. While she was at school I ate all of the cookies she baked for her grandmother.
>
> There was no way I could replace them for her. They were love. She and my husband couldn't believe that I ate those cookies. My husband asked me how I could do it.[1]

The title of another book, *Fat—A Fate Worse Than Death?*[11] captures the essence of the pain of being overweight. The question mark in the title indicates that the answer to the question may depend. In the book *Such a Pretty Face*[1], one of the respondents says, "I feel so terrible about the way I look that I cut off connection with my body. I operate from the neck up. I do not look in mirrors." It is a common observation that very overweight women tend to avoid looking at themselves in mirrors. One of my patients finally came to seek help when she got stuck in the turnstile of a grocery store because she was unaware that she was too large to get through it. The turnstile had to be taken apart to free her. This woman's humiliation while waiting for that to happen was unforgettably painful.

The pain of overweight as a disability are again captured in a repeat of the survey in children described at the beginning of this chapter and in a survey of adults seeking surgical treatment in their battle of the bulge. In 2003 Latner and Stunkard[10] repeated the study done in 1961-63[3,4]. This modern repeat of the earlier seminal studies was done in New Jersey and included fifth and sixth graders who were from upper-middle and lower-middle income households. The 485 children were more than half white children, but there were non-white, African-American and Asian-American children, too. A total of six drawings of the same sex were shown to each child with the question of which one would they like to have as a playmate. The drawings included a "healthy" child, four children with various disabilities, and an overweight child. Children in this study, like those in 1961, liked the overweight child least. More disturbing was that the overweight child was liked even less well than in the earlier study. It is an unhappy experience to be an overweight child, compared to their normal-weight peers.

The depth of the disability from being overweight and the reaction to the slings and arrows it brings is brought to light by a survey of people who were seeking surgery to conquer the battle of the bulge[11]. This study looked at the response of 47 people who had kept off one hundred pounds or more for three years following surgical treatment in their battle of the bulge. These individuals said that they would prefer to be of normal weight with a major handicap (deaf, dyslexic, diabetic, legally blind, very bad acne, heart disease, or one leg amputated) than return to their original weight. Clearly the stigma of being overweight is a strong one.

Prejudicial attitudes toward those battling the bulge can also be seen in many cartoons. "[Their] intention is often merely to amuse, to deflate the pretentious or expose a plump backside for a coarse laugh. [Caricature] is also a blunt instrument for the expression of national prejudices"[12]. However, obese individuals often the bear the brunt of the joke in cartoons and prints, adding to their stigmatized roles.

> Mockery of the individual was but one function of caricatures...The theme of the caricaturists was the progress of folly, of greed and lechery, often embodied in the corruption of such professions as the Army, the Church, the Law and Medicine. Added to this was humour of the simplest kind: hen-pecked husbands and *stout* (italics mine) wives.[12]

William Hogarth's work (1697-1764) dominated the caricaturists during the first half of the eighteenth-century. Most of his works were caricatures of the human condition with such titles as *The Harlot's Progress, The Rake's Progress,* or *Election Entertainment.*

> Hogarth visited France in 1748 and on his return from Paris was arrested while sketching the English Gate at Calais. He took his revenge in this classic exercise in English xenophobia, which determined an English image of the lean and beggarly French. Hogarth said of Calais that the "farcical pomp of war, parade of religion and bustle with very little business—in short poverty, slavery and insolence, with an affectation of politeness give you even here the first specimen of the whole country." On the right is "a poor highlander fled thither on account of the

> Rebellion the year before brozing on scanty French fare in sight of a sirloin of beef, a present from England...my own figure in the corner with the soldier's hand upon my shoulder is said to be tolerably like." (original in the Tate Gallery, London; Yale University)[12]

James Gillray (1756-1815) is principally remembered for his satires of George III and the Revolutionary War period in the United States—a contrast between England and France. In a cartoon titled "French Liberty-British Slavery" there is:

> The Juxtaposition of a starving Frenchman and a plump (obese) Englishman feasting on roast beef had been a common place of English satires since Hogarth. The events of the French Revolution inspired Gillray to give it definitive form in a print that was copied in France and Germany. Such images gave foreigners an idea of the English physical type that could lead to disappointment. Louis Simond arrived in London from New York in 1809 and noted that "Prepossessed with a high opinion of English corpulency, I expected everywhere to see the original of Jacques Roast-Beef. No such thing; the human race is here rather of mean stature—less so, perhaps than the true Parisian race; but there is really no difference."[12]

Thomas Rowlandson (1756-1827) along with Gillray represent the supreme English caricaturists[12]. As an example of the work of Rowlandson, I have selected one that depicts an overweight individual being treated in *Dr. Graham's Earth Bathing Establishment.* This print caricatures the lengths that overweight people will go to get "treated" and the quackery that some of these treatments involve. (Figure 19-1)

> James Graham (1745-1794), "Emperor of the Quacks," began his medical career in Edinburgh and Philadelphia as an ear-and-throat specialist and pedlar of miraculous nostrums. From the mid 1770s he operated in London a number of health spas, with such features as magnetic thrones, electrical baths, "celestial" beds for relief from sterility, and immersions. Mocked as a charlatan, he nevertheless believed in his methods, and his establishment provided first-rate entertainment for the beau-monde. He publicly demonstrated his belief in earth-bathing by having himself buried to the chin, his powdered, bewigged

> head protruding from the slime and resembling, as one wit observed, a head of cauliflower.[12]

Rowlandson depicts Graham's earth-bathing establishment in Fleet Street. This treatment was advertised for virtually every ailment, including leprosy, gout, and corpulency. As an example of his nutritional naiveté, he published a pamphlet in 1793 on "How to live for many weeks, months, years [sic] without eating anything whatever"[12].

Honore Daumier (1808-1879) began his satirical lithographs in 1830 and continued for nearly twenty years. During this time he lampooned the royalty, as well as doctors, lawyers, bureaucrats, and the overweight. Finally, I present one of a series of cartoons by a well-known surgeon to show that some of the attitudes toward overweight individuals are also prevalent in the medical profession[13]. (Figure 19-2)

The stigma carried by overweight Americans who are fighting the battle of the bulge is oppressive. This is obviously one reason why the battle rages. The illustrations in this chapter show that this stigma has a long history. I start with the assumption that no one wants to be overweight and that the stigma associated with this problem serves as one motive for change. Compassion for those fighting the battle of the bulge from those who aren't could help ease the pain of obesity.

References

1. Millman, M. *Such a Pretty Face: Being Fat in America.* New York: Horton, 1980.
2. Stunkard, A.J. *The Pain of Obesity.* Palo Alto: Bull, 1976.
3. Richardson, S.A., A.H. Hastorf, N. Goodman, S.M. Dornbusch. "Cultural Uniformity in Reaction to Physical Disabilities." *Am Sociol Res.* 26(1961): 241-247.
4. Goodman, N., S.A. Richardson, S.M. Dornbusch, A.H. Hastorf. "Variant Reactions to Physical Disabilities." *Am Sociol Res.* 28(1963): 429 435.
5. Hopkins, K.D., E.D. Lehmann. "Successful Medical Treatment of Obesity in 10th Century Spain." *Lancet.* (1995): 316.
6. Lascaratos, J. "Medical Management of Obesity in 14th Century Byzantium." *Lancet.* 346(1995): 54-5.
7. Schlosser, E. *Fast Food Nation: The Dark Side of the All-American Meal.* New York: Houghton Mifflin, 2000.
8. Kuczynski, A. "Movie Is 'Shallow' Indeed, Critics Say." *San Francisco Chronicle.* Nov. 25, 2001, A18.
9. Thone, R.R. *Fat—A Fate Worse Than Death?* New York: Haworth, 1997.
10. Latner, J.C., A.J. Stunkard. "Getting worse: The stigmatization of Obese Children." *Obes Res.* 11(2003): 452-456.
11. Rand, C.S., A.M. Macgregor. "Successful Weight Loss Following Obesity Surgery and the Perceived Liability of Morbid Obesity." *Int J Obes Relat Metab Disord.* 15(1991): 577-579.
12. *English Caricature 1620 to the Present.* London: Victoria and Albert Museum, 1984. Museum catalogue.
13. Rice, C.O. *Musings of a Surgeon: An autobiography.* Unpublished manuscript.

PART 4.

The Pathology and Clinical Causes of the Bulge

Chapter 20

William Wadd and Obesity as a Disease

Anatomy is to physiology, as geography to history; it describes the theater of events.

—Jean Fernel[1]

Dissect in anatomy, experiment in physiology, follow the disease and make the necropsy in medicine; this is the three-fold path, without which, there can be no anatomist, no physiologist, no physician.

—F.X. Bichat[2]

Science advances, but the advances are not always linear. One step forward does not necessarily lead to the next forward step. There are often deviations, missteps, or steps backwards. If it were otherwise, the discovery of new knowledge through scientific research would be far more predictable[3]. It is this lack of predictability of the results of the next experiment that makes the research endeavor so expensive. If it were easy to read the crystal ball and our guesses were always right, or right even a modest amount of the time, we would already have won the battle of the bulge. The fact that you and I are facing an epidemic of obesity means that we still have many more steps to take before we will be able to declare victory in this battle.

Fat in excess is a visible sign of disease. Signs such as the bulging fat deposits or "beer belly" in an individual reflect the underlying pathology of the illness or disease. *Pathology* is a word derived from the Greek *pathos* for "suffering" and *logos* for "study." I will use the word *pathology* to develop ideas about the "study of suffering." The argument that obesity or corpulence is a disease was made by William Wadd[4] and even earlier by Malcolm Flemyng[5] and will be echoed here. The words of Flemyng written in 1760 clearly state the idea that obesity is a disease:

> Corpulency, when in an extraordinary degree, may be reckoned a disease, as it in some measure obstructs the free exercise of the animal functions; and has a tendency to shorten life, by paving the way to dangerous distempers.[5]

Two examples of 'corpulence in an extraordinary degree' are shown in Figures 20-1 and 20-2. Both men died at relatively young ages. The short book by William Wadd (1776-1829) written in 1810[4] titled *Cursory Remarks on Corpulence; or Obesity Considered as a Disease* gives an interesting account of this disease and its "cure" in the early nineteenth-century. This book was written anonymously by a surgeon, believe it or not. We usually think of surgeons as doing gastric operations, but Wadd worked at a time before germs were known to cause disease and before there was anesthesia or antisepsis to help the patient, to say nothing of antibiotics and blood transfusions. Wadd's book is the first English-language monograph on obesity in the nineteenth-century. This small book was written at the time when the leading teaching hospitals in clinical medicine were shifting from Edinburgh, which reached its zenith at the end of the eighteenth-century, to Paris, which dominated teaching and research in clinical medicine during the first half of the nineteenth-century[6,7]. But before I return to the book by Wadd[4,8-12], I want to trace the growth of ideas about illness, pathology, and disease to the beginning of the nineteenth-century[13].

Patients come to doctors and other healers because they are ill. Their illness consists of its outward manifestations, the things the doctor can see or identify, and the internal feelings and changes that the patient describes. Disease is an abstract construct as opposed to the illness that an individual patient has. As human understanding of the world has advanced, so has our understanding of disease and pathology. The generalized complaint "I feel bad" has gradually been resolved into many different ways of looking at the signs, that is, those things the doctor sees, like too much fat, and the symptoms the patient has of "feeling bad"—in the case of obesity, one of these would be running out of breath or shortness of breath. From simple roundness or *embonpoint*, as obesity was called in France in the eighteenth-century, the idea of obesity has gradually become more refined and differentiated.

Pathology as the study of suffering can provide several important needs, as noted by Duffin[13]. It can provide an explanation of the illness to the health care provider, to the individual who has the illness, and to society in general. It can also define the ailment and in so doing provide a separation between health and illness. From an understanding of the illness comes the diagnosis and prognosis for its future course. Finally, the disease framework that an illness falls into provides a basis for treatment.

From a Western perspective, the beginnings of pathology can be traced to Greco-Roman times, when disease was perceived as an imbalance in the natural order[13,14]. These Hippocratic writings were done several centuries before the time of Christ[15]. Their influence survived until the eighteenth century, in part through the writings of Galen who lived and practiced in Rome after the death of Christ but before Christianity was accepted[16]. The relationship of the four humors can be viewed as the corners of a rectangle (Figure 20-3). At one corner is fire and its equivalent, yellow bile, which is associated with the liver.

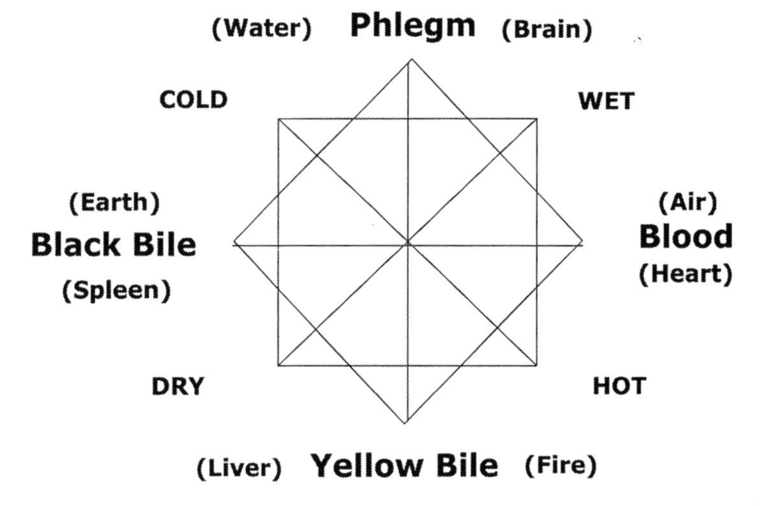

20-3 Properties and relationships of the four humors model, a key element of Greek science and medicine.

At the opposite corner is water, with phlegm and the brain as the humor and organ. On the corner between fire and water is earth and black bile, which are associated with the spleen. Opposite to earth and black bile is air and blood, which comes from the heart. This system of viewing the humoral balances held sway for nearly two thousand years. As an example of this concept of pathology, medical historian Jaclyn Duffin uses epilepsy. After an accurate description of the clinical course of what was referred to as the "Sacred Disease" by some, the authors of the Hippocratic corpus went on to explain that epilepsy resulted from an obstruction of phlegm in the brain[13].

With the advent of the seventeenth century, however, disease began to take on new forms based on patterns of suffering. Pathology became a grouping of symptoms into patterns of suffering and illness. By observing patients, astute physicians were able to separate "diseases" one from another. In his twenty-volume series, the Muslim physician Rhazes in the tenth century accurately distinguished measles and smallpox, two diseases that manifested their clinical state with a rash[17].

With the advent of the seventeenth century, the clinical observation of symptoms produced by sick patients led to attempts to classify disease. With the introduction of the binary system for classifying plants by Linnaeus[18] in Sweden, in which a plant was given a genus and species name, the idea of a binary system spread to classifying diseases. People who classify diseases are called "nosologists." A little more than two centuries ago, these nosologists used a tree-like structure of "class," "order," "genus," and "species" to sort out their concepts about disease. At its peak, some of these classifications recognized several thousand "entities" that medical students were expected to know[19,21]. The futility of this approach at the end of the eighteenth-century opened the field for viewing disease as "altered anatomy."

Following the publication of the first modern anatomy book by Andreas Vesalius (1514-1564) in 1543[22], the next step from a clinical perspective was the application of this anatomical knowledge to the interpretation of disease. Pathologic anatomy is a direct outgrowth of the gross anatomy that was advancing so rapidly following the work of Vesalius. Vesalius was the professor of anatomy at the University of Padua and was elected to this chair by age twenty-seven. As Esmond Long (1890-1973) remarked in his *History of Pathology*, "On the whole...the balance of power, at the end of the sixteenth-century remained with Galen, in spite of Vesalius and the anatomical pathologists"[14]. Prior to the time when dissection became widespread, an anatomical basis for pathology was not possible. As anatomical study expanded in the sixteenth-century, anatomists began to codify the observations of "abnormal" organs that they dissected. The first such collection was that of Antonio Benvieni (1440-1502)[23], whose 111 autopsies were published posthumously in 1507. In spite of this contribution, the sixteenth century contributed little to the advancement of pathology in general and nothing to obesity.

The story in the seventeenth century is very different. This was the century in which William Harvey (1578-1657) discovered the circulation of the blood, where Robert Boyle (1627-1691), John Mayow (1643-1679), Richard Lower (1631-1691), and Thomas Willis (1621-1675) of the Oxford University school of physiology did the first transfusion of blood. It also saw the publication of the first great book dealing with anatomical pathology. This book by Theophile Bonet (1620-1689) titled *Sepulchretum, sive anatomia practica*[24] is a weighty tome running to more than one thousand seven hundred pages. Sadly, it lacks organization. It is rather one man's compilation of his experiences with autopsies. In part the lack of organization may have been a deficiency of the author, but in part it was the limitations of the concepts of disease at this time. This was the time of mechanical explanations for bodily function. Microscopy was just beginning and the modern microscope as we know it was nearly two hundred years away. Thus, the idea of an anatomic pathology evolved slowly.

The seventeenth-century work of Bonet, however, has been viewed as a direct predecessor to the eighteenth-century work of Giovanni Morgagni (1682-1771), who is justifiably called the "Father of Pathology." The Latin name of Morgagni's book was *De Sedibus and Causis Morborum per Anatomen Indagitis (On the Sites and Causes of Diseases Discovered by the Anatomist)*[25]. As the first great anatomical pathology textbook, it is fitting that its author was a professor at the University of Padua where Vesalius, Galileo, and Santorio had labored nearly two centuries earlier. Written long after the intellectual impact of the University of Padua had peaked, the book was published in 1761 when Morgagni was seventy-nine years old and remains a classic in the field. Anatomical descriptions of obese individuals were published in this book and in an eighteenth-book by Albrecht von Haller (1708-1777)[26].

However, it was not until the late eighteenth century and early nineteenth century that the post-mortem pathological examination became an essential element in the diagnosis of disease. The first steps were the gradual development of an organ-based pathology. Standing at the opening of the nineteenth-century is a young Frenchman named François-Xavier Bichat (1771-1802)[2] who moved the pathological explanations of disease from an organ-based approach to a tissue-based approach. During his short thirty years of life, he reframed the concept of pathology. His moment in the sun followed the end of the French Revolution, which also brought a revolution to the teaching of medicine[7]. Before the Revolution, the medical and surgical faculties in France and elsewhere had been separated. Following the Revolution, they combined for the first time, and the hospital, not the lecture hall, became the site for teaching medicine. These developments, along with the clinical technique of percussion discovered by Leopold Auenbrugger (1722-1809) and popularized by Jean-Nicholas Corvisart (1755-1821)[27] and the discovery of the stethoscope by René-Théophile-Hyacinthe Laennec (1781-1826)[28], opened a new frontier in medicine and an exciting three decades that medical historian Erwin Ackerknecht[7] has referred to as "The Paris Hospital."

Emblematic of early nineteenth-century medicine was the tissue pathology of Bichat[2]. If disease arose from organs and tissues, a new approach to disease was possible. As Charcot[29] said, "Symptoms, then, are in reality nothing but the cry from suffering organs." To take another view, Logan Clendenning[30] said, "Surgery does the ideal thing—it separates the patient from the disease. It puts the patient back to bed and the disease in a bottle." The early part of the nineteenth century saw the continuing delineation of disease using anatomic findings as its basis. In England four diseases were defined this way and carried their author's names to fame. Thomas Addison (1793-1860)[31] described the clinical condition of weight loss, emaciation, and brownish pigmentation to the skin associated with loss of functional adrenal glands. Richard Bright (1789-1858)[32] described the withered kidneys associated with renal failure. Thomas Hodgkin (1798-1866)[33] described the malignant lymphomatous disease that carries his name. Finally, Robert Graves (1797-1853)[34] described hyperthyroidism, a disease of overactivity of the thyroid gland. These disease entities encompassed illnesses that were associated with internal changes in organs.

The next step after an organ based pathology was one located in the cell. With the newer microscopes after 1840 Virchow (1821-1902) provided such a new cellular pathology.[30]

In spite of the advances in developing an organ-based pathology of disease, treatment for illnesses in the early part of the nineteenth-century was still rooted in the balance of the four humors. Bleeding was still widely practiced, although declining somewhat from its peak at the end of the eighteenth century. To quote from Williams[35], "let out the blood, let out the disease" was the rallying cry for bleeding that had long been a mainstay of medical intervention. A variety of techniques were developed, including leeches, scarificators, and opening of a vein. The difficulty of identifying veins in corpulent people was recognized as early as 1669 when Cinton D'Amato published a practical book on bleeding. In it he said, "When confronted with a corpulent patient, the ligature around the arm should be tied very tightly, as opposed to thin persons on whom the ligature was to be placed should not be too tight"[37].

The delightful book by William Wadd Esq.[5], who was surgeon to the king of England, was published during the time that the Paris School of Medicine flowered and the clinical descriptions of disease were published in England. In the introduction, Wadd[4] begins by telling a story of a patient:

> A Gentleman with whom I was early in the habit of conversing on professional subjects, had often introduced his tendency to corpulence, expressing his fears, less his pursuits, which were sedentary, should increase, what he already felt a growing inconvenience. At length he addressed a letter, earnestly requesting my reference, as to which authors as might satisfy his curiosity, or give him information, on a subject which so much engrossed his thoughts. At the same time stating, some circumstances of his life illustrative of his complaints; particularly his observations of the effect a vegetable diet had on them.
>
> He had approached his thirtieth year before he experienced any great inconvenience from his increase of bulk. From this period his mind was deeply impressed with the

> apprehension of corpulency. Indeed inactivity, somnolency, depression of spirits, and an inaptitude for study, were symptoms sufficient to produce anxiety. By an abstemious mode of living, and a vegetable diet, he became lighter, more capable of mental exertion, and in every respect improved in health—but whenever he resumed his former habits, his complaints returned in full force.

Wadd uses this case as an introduction. He then goes on to describe the relation of national wealth to the problems in English society:

> If the increase of wealth and refinement of modern times have tended to banish plague and pestilence from our cities, they have probably introduced the whole train of nervous disorders, and increased the frequency of corpulence (p. 3).
>
> It has been conjectured by some, that for one fat person in France or Spain, there are an hundred in England. I shall leave others to determine the fairness of such a calculation (p. 5).

Next Wadd turns to a discussion of the omentum and of the nature of fat.

> Fat is, of all the humours or substances forming part of the human body, the most diffused; a certain proportion of it is indicative of health, and denotes being in good condition—nay, is even conducive to beauty; but when in excess—amounting to what may be termed OBESITY—it is not only in itself a disease, but may be the cause of many fatal effects, particularly in acute disorders (5 pp. 29-30).
>
> Boerhaave mentions a case of a man whose belly grew so large that he was obliged to have it supported by a sash; and had a piece of the table cut out to enable him to reach it with his hands. After death his omentum weighed thirty pounds (p. 13).

On the formation of fat Wadd[4] notes that

> Boerhaave and Van Swieten were of opinion, that fat is deposited from the blood by its slower circulation in the extreme vessels. Malpighi and other anatomists have thought that there was a glandular apparatus superadded to the cellular membrane, to assist in the formation of fat. But this, though consistent with the general system of the

> economy, has never been discovered... But when excessive, [fat] is not only burthensome, but becomes a disease, disposes to other diseases, and to sudden death (p. 15).

According to Wadd[4] "...a predisposition (to corpulency) is often hereditary..." (p. 16). Exciting factors include "...a free indulgence of the table...." Wadd quotes Arbuthnot: "Spare diet and labour will keep constitutions, where this disposition (to corpulency) is strongest, from being fat. You may see an army of forty thousand foot soldiers without a fat man; and I dare affirm, that by plenty, and rest, twenty of the forty shall grow fat" (p. 17). On inactivity: "Thus we find persons who have been long confined to their rooms, from any accident, not interfering with the digestive powers, usually grow corpulent."

Finally, Wadd reviews treatments for obesity by discussing the earlier literature—literature, that is prior to 1810.

> Coelius Aurelianus, to whose diligence in collecting the opinions of preceding writers, we are much indebted, divided the mode of cure into two parts; first, taking food that has little nutrition in it; secondly, by observing certain rules of exercise (p. 19).
>
> Borelli advised chewing tobacco; a practice objected to by Etmuller, as he thinks it may lead to consumption [tuberculosis].
>
> Few things have been more generally administered in the cure of corpulency, than acids of various kinds. The emaciating properties of acid liquors, particularly vinegar, are very well known. It is said, that the famous Spanish General, Chiapin Vitellis, well known in the time he lived for his enormous size, reduced himself, solely by drinking of vinegar, to such a degree, that he could fold his skin around his body (p. 20).
>
> Castile soap is strongly recommended by Dr. Flemyng (p. 21). Over a 2 year period, his patient lost 2 stones (28 pounds) with this treatment (p. 22).
>
> Dr. Cullen is, however, of opinion, "that the inducing a saline and acrid state of the blood," (which are supposed to be the effect of vinegar and soap) may have worse consequences than the corpulency it was intended to correct, and that no person should hazard those, while he may have recourse to the more safe and certain means of abstinence and exercise (p. 26). The diet, he adds, must be sparing, for rather, what is more admissible, it must be such as affords little nutritious matter; it must therefore be chiefly or almost

> only of vegetable matter, and at the very utmost, milk (p. 26).
>
> According to Dr. Fothergill: "A strict vegetable diet reduces exuberant fat more certainly than any other means I know" (p. 27).

Dr. Beddoes, a famous early nineteenth-century physician, believed corpulency was due to deficiency of oxygen. His cure was to diffuse more oxygen into the system. When referring to Dr. Beddoes, Wadd notes, "But Dr. B remained so inconveniently fat during his life, that a lady of Clifton used to denominate him the walking feather-bed."

> Mr. Wood, Miller of Billericay, in the *Med Trans Royal College of Phys* by using animal food, sparingly, and leaving off malt liquor, and by degrees, he brought himself to do without any liquor whatever, except what he took in the form of medicine; and latterly the whole of his diet consisted of a pudding made of sea biscuit; by this plan, it is supposed he reduced himself ten or eleven stone weight [140-154 pounds] (p. 37).
>
> By far the greater part of the medical tribe (physicians) are satisfied with attending only to actual disease, as being the only source of profit, while the preventive part, though far the most important, but as furnishing no emolument, is generally disregarded (p. 41).
>
> I have always found it difficult to get corpulent persons to give up those habits which lead to obesity (p. 50).
>
> A sudden palpitation excited in the heart of a fat man has often proved as fatal as a bullet through the thorax (p. 66).
>
> Asked the Patient: "Now what do you recommend me to do?
>
> Doctor: "Keep your eyes open and your mouth shut."
>
> Patient: "Poh...that won't do for me—give me something to take—have you no pills?"

This delightful book by Wadd argues that obesity is a disease. I would also argue that obesity is a disease. It has a cause—eating too much and exercising too little, or as we have learned, a positive energy balance. It has its own pathology—enlargement of the fat cells. Some overweight people may also have more fat cells than normal, but all overweight people have large fat cells. These large fat cells produce more and more hormones and other unneeded chemicals that act throughout the body to produce other disease. The inability to relate needed intake to expenditure led me to call obesity a chronic, relapsing, neurochemical disease. It is chronic in the sense that there are no cures, and once fat, people tend to stay that way. It is relapsing because most people regain weight once they lose it, unless they have serious illnesses. Finally, it is neurochemical because it is the monoamines and peptides in the brain that control food intake and the balance between food and activity that lead to obesity.

Biosketch

Giovanni Battista Morgagni (1682-1771) was born in Forli, Italy, in 1682. He was a precocious youth and at the age of nineteen received his degree in medicine and philosophy from the University of Bologna in 1701 (Figure 20-4). His anatomical interests, born in part of his association with Marcello Malpighi the great microscopist, focused on dissections of large fishes and on human cadavers.

He practiced medicine from 1709 to 1711. In 1711 he was appointed professor of practical medicine at the University of Padua and, four years later as professor of anatomy, positions he held until his death in 1771 at the age of 89[36,37].

Biosketch

William Wadd (1776-1829), surgeon, the eldest son of Solomon Wadd, a surgeon, who lived and practiced for more than half a century in Basinghall Street, London, was born on June 21, 1776, and was entered at Merchant Taylors' school late in 1784. He was apprenticed to Sir James Earle in 1797 and thus became one of the privileged class of surgeon's pupils at St. Bartholomew's Hospital. He was admitted a member of the Royal College of Surgeons on December 18, 1801, and in 1816 he contested the post of assistant-surgeon to St. Bartholomew's Hospital, when John Painter Vincent was elected. Wadd was chosen a member of the council of the College of Surgeons in 1824 and was appointed a member of the court of examiners in succession to John Abernethy on August 3, 1829. He was appointed one of the surgeons extraordinary to the Prince Regent on August 19, 1817, and surgeon extraordinary to George IV on March 30, 1821. A life-size half-length in oils painted by John Jackson is in the secretary's office at the Royal College of Surgeons in Lincoln's Inn Fields, London (Figure 20-5).

Dr. Wadd was killed instantaneously on August 29, 1829, by jumping off a runaway railway car on the road from Killarney to Mitchelstown while he was making a holiday tour in Ireland. At the time of his death he was a fellow of the Linnean Society and an associate of the Société de Médecine of Paris. A man of high talents, Wadd had a rich fund of anecdote. He was an excellent draughtsman and learned etching to such good effect that the illustrations in his works are all the products of his own needle. (Figure 20-6) He married, on July 8, 1806, Caroline Mackenzie, who survived him, and by her had two children, a son who was drowned at Mauritius and a daughter[38].

Biosketch

Rudolf Virchow (1821-1902), the father of modern pathology, was born in Schievelbein. He received his medical education at Berlin, and after graduation in 1843 he became the prosector for Froriep in 1845. It was only two years later, in 1847, that he founded the *Archiv für pathologische Anatomie*, which was known until after World War II as Virchow's Archive. His early views landed him in trouble with the government just before the revolutions of 1848. He moved to Wurzberg, but because of his eminence, he was appointed professor and head of the Pathological Institute in Berlin in 1856. It was only a year later that one of his most influential books, *Die Cellularpathologie*, was published, proclaiming to the world that pathological changes were at the cellular level (Figure 20-7). His work was the obvious outgrowth of Morgagni's organ pathology, Bichat's tissue pathology, and the cell theory of Schwann, published just as Virchow was in medical school.

Of interest is that he opposed the Darwinian theory and the theories of Koch and Behring dealing with toxins and anti-toxins. He was active not only in medicine and science but in politics, where he served in the Reichstag from 1880 to 1893. During the Franco-Prussian War of 1870-71, he organized the German ambulance corps. He received many awards recognizing his contributions to medicine and society prior to his death in 1902[36].

References

1. Fernel, J. *On the Natural Part of Medicine*, 1542. Cited by Sherrington, *The Endeavor of John Fernel*, Cambridge: Cambridge University Press. 1946.
2. Bichat, F.X. *Traité d'anatomie descriptive.* Transl. E.R. Long, 1802.
3. Wilson, E.O. *Concilience: A Unity of Knowledge.* New York: Alfred A. Knopf, 1998.
4. [Wadd, W.] *Cursory Remarks on Corpulence: By a Member of the Royal College of Surgeons.* London: J Callow, 1810.
5. Flemyng, M. *A Discourse on the Nature, Causes and Cure of Corpulency. Illustrated by a remarkable case.* 1760.
6. Garrison, F.H. *Introduction of the History of Medicine.* Philadelphia: W.B. Saunders, 1929.
7. Ackerknecht, E.H. *Medicine at the Paris Hospital.* Baltimore: Johns Hopkins University Press, 1967.
8. [Wadd, W.] *Cursory Remarks on Corpulence: By a Member of the Royal College of Surgeons.* London: J. Calow, 1813.
9. Wadd, W. *On Corpulence; Or Obesity Considered as a Disease. With a Critical Examination of Ancient and Modern Opinions, Relative to Its Causes and Cure. Third Edition, Containing a reference to the most remarkable cases that have occurred in this country.* London: J. Callow, 1816.
10. Wadd, W. Esq, F.R.S. *Cursory Remarks on Corpulence; or Obesity Considered as a Disease: With a Critical Examination of Ancient and Modern Opinions Relative to its Cause and Cure. 3rd ed. Containing a reference to the most remarkable cases that have occurred in this country.* London: J. Callow, 1822.
11. Wadd, W. Esq., F.L.S. *Surgeon Extraordinary to the King etc. etc. etc. Comments on Corpulence Lineaments of Leanness Mems on Diet and Dietetics.* London: John Ebers &Co., 1829.
12. Wadd, W. *L'Embonpoint consideré comme maladie, avec un examen critique des opinions anciennes et moderne relative à ce sujet; ses cause, ses guérison.* Transl. Dr. Leon. Paris: Chez le docteur Leon, 1838.
13. Duffin, J. *History of Medicine: A Scandalously Short Introduction.* Toronto: University of Toronto Press, 1999.
14. Long, R. *A History of Pathology.* Baltimore: Williams and Wilkins Co., 1928.
15. Hippocrates. *Oeuvres complétes d'Hippocrate : traduction nouvelle avec le texte grec en regard, collationné sur les manuscrits et toutes les éditions; accompagnée d'une introduction,...suivie d'une table générale des matières /par E. Littre.* Paris: J.B. Balliere, 1839.
16. Green, R.M. *A Translation of Galen's Hygiene (De Sanitate Tuenda).*

Springfield, IL: Charles C. Thomas, 1951.
17. Rhazes. *A Treatise on the Small-Pox and Measles (transl. from the original Arabic by W.A. Greenhill, M.D.)*. London: Sydenham Society, 1848. Reprinted by the Classics of Medicine Library, 1987.
18. Linnaeus, C.V. *Species Plantarum*. Stockholm: Salvius, 1753.
19. Sauvages, F.B. *Nosologia methodica sistens morborum classes juxta Sydenhami menten and botanicorum ordinem*. Amstelodami: Fratrum de Tournes, 1768, 2 vols.
20. Cullen, W. *First Lines of the Practice of Physic, by William Cullen, M.D. late professor of the practice of physic in the University of Edinburgh, and including the definitions of the nosology; with supplementary notes chiefly selected from recent authors, who have contributed to the improvement of medicine by Peter Reid, M.D.* Edinburgh: Abernethy and Walker, 1810, 2 vols.
21. Pinel, P. *A Treatise on Insanity, in Which Are Contained the Principles of a New and More Practical Nosology of Maniacal Disorders*. Sheffield: W. Todd, 1806. Reprinted by Classics of Medicine Library, 1983.
22. Vesalius, A. *De humani corporis fabrica*. Basileae: ex off. Joannis Oporini, 1543.
23. Benvieni, A. *De abditis nonnulis ac mirandis morborum et sanationum causis*. 1507.
24. Bonetus, T. *Sepulchretum, sive anatomia practica, ex cadaveribus morbo denatis, proponens historias omnium humani corporis affectum*. Genevae: Sumptibus Cramer & Perachon, 1700.
25. Morgagni, G.B. *De sedibus, et causis morborum per anatomen indagatis libriquinque*. Venetiis: typog. Remordiniana, 1761.
26. von Haller, A. "Corpulence Ill Cured; Large Cryptae of the Stomach (etc)." *Path Observ.* (1756): 44-49.
27. Auenbrugger, L. *Nouvelle méthode pour reconnaître las maladies internes de la poitrine par la percussion de cette cavité (Traduire par J.N. Corvisart)*. Paris: Mignert, 1808.
28. Laennec, R.T.H. *De l'Auscultation Médiate, ou Traité du Diagnostic des Maladies des Poumons et du Coeur.* Paris: J-A Brosson et J-S Chaude, 1819.
29. Charcot. In: Duffin, J. *History of Medicine: A Scandalously Short Introduction*. Toronto: University of Toronto Press, 1999.
30. Virchow, R. *Die Cellular pathologie in ihrer Begründung auf physiologische und pathologische Gewebelehre*. Berlin: August Hirschwald, 1858.
31. Addison, T. *On the Constitutional and Local Effects of Disease of the Suprarenal Capsules*. London: Samuel Highley, 1855.
32. Bright, R. *Reports of Medical Cases, Selected with a View of Illustrating Symptoms and Cure of Diseases by a Reference to Morbid Anatomy.* London: Longmans, 1827-431.

33. Hodgkin, T. "On Some Morbid Appearances of the Absorbent Glands and Spleen." *Med Chir.* 17(1832): 68-114.
34. Graves, R.J. "Palpitation of the Heart with Enlargement of the Thyroid Gland". *Lond Med Surg J (Renshaw).* 7(1845): 516-517.
35. Williams, G. *The Age of Agony: The Art of Healing 1700-1800.* Chicago: Academy Chicago Publishers, 1986.
36. Medvei, V.C. *A History of Endocrinology.* Lancaster: MTP Press, 1982.
37. Garrison, F. *Introduction to the History of Medicine.* Philadelphia: W.B. Saunders, 1910.
38. Power, D.A. "William Wadd (1776-1829)." In *The Dictionary of National Biography.* Ed. L. Stephen and S. Lee. London: Oxford University Press, 1937-1938. Vol. XX.

Chapter 21

Is Overweight Risking Fate? Light from the Beginning of the Twentieth-Century

Knowledge comes, but wisdom lingers.

—Tennyson[1]

Nothing is certain but death and taxes. All of us try to avoid taxes, but avoiding death is impossible. Since we can't predict when we will die, we buy life insurance to protect our families in the event that we should have an early and untimely death. As a result, the insurance companies have a vast store of information about the average duration of life and the causes of death. To them, knowing how to gauge life expectancy for the lives they insure means the difference between making and losing money—of being profitable or going bankrupt. One of the earliest observations that the life insurance industry made was that their clients who were overweight were more likely to die earlier than their normal-weight insured participants. This message that "overweight is hazardous to your health" has been broadcast often during the twentieth century but often fell on deaf ears or was ignored. This is the story of when that message was recognized within the insurance industry and the difficulties of transferring it to the broader public. This story is important because it tells how we came to recognize the hazards of the bulge and why winning the battle of the bulge is so important for our long-term health and well being. To reach this goal we must also deal with those who contend that "overweight" is a myth or trumped up[2,3].

The importance of life insurance data to our understanding of the epidemic of obesity is emphasized by an extract from the *Report of the Joint Committee on the Medico-Actuarial Mortality Investigation* published in 1913, at a time when most people were more concerned about undernutrition than obesity[4]. In this publication, the life insurance industry threw down the gauntlet and stated that being overweight is hazardous to our health. Thus, winning the battle of the bulge became important to the life insurance industry because it increased profits. As the twentieth-century moved toward its end, this message became important to all of us as obesity became epidemic in this country[5,6].

One of the champions for the life insurance case that "overweight was risking fate" was Dr. Louis Dublin, (1882-1964), a leading actuary for the life insurance industry. In a lecture in 1926, Dublin said, "The conviction that body build affects longevity has been general for a long time"[7], although not many people paid much attention to it. When, then, was this concept that overweight is hazardous to your health first identified, and how long did it take to impact public perceptions about the hazards of obesity?

The idea that obesity carried extra risk was clearly enunciated as early as 1913 in the material published by the Association of Life Insurance Medical Directors and the Actuarial Society of America[4]. Indeed it was recognized much earlier than this in published medical writings[8,11]. To show this, I have made a graph of the 1913 data to compare with the more recent data to show their similarity (Figure 21-1). As weight rises the increase in risk of dying rises, as this figure clearly shows. In contrast there is little, if any, effect of having a lower-than-average weight.

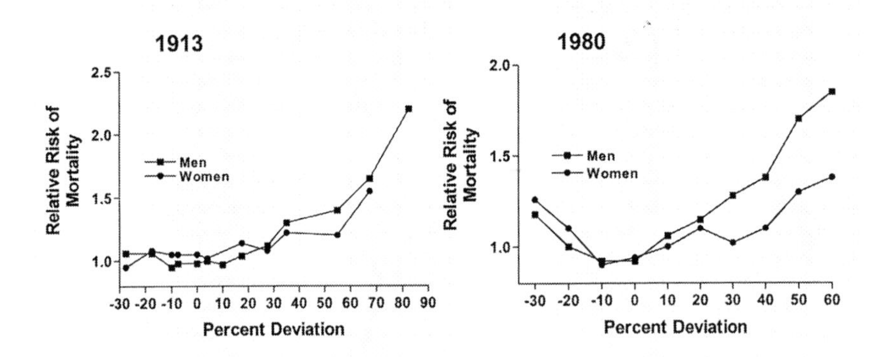

21-1 Relation of relative mortality to body weight in life insurance data from 1913 and 1983. Note that for each time period there was a significant increase in mortality for the overweight compared to people within the normal weight range. Adapted with permission of the Society of Actuaries and the American Academy of Insurance Medicine.

Following the important publication in 1913 titled *Mortality Statistics of Insured Wage-Earners and Their Families,* the insurance industry didn't reemphasize the effect of weight in their next major publication in 1919[12]. In fact the 1919 report made no mention at all of overweight as a health risk. There was a very thorough review of deaths from many causes and a discussion of tuberculosis and heart diseases in great detail. However, nowhere in the discussion of the organic heart diseases is there any mention of the importance of excess body weight or overweight to the development of heart disease.

It now seems clear that this 1919 report was an aberration, since the problem of overweight and health risks resurfaced in the 1922 *Statistical Bulletin of the Metropolitan Life Insurance Company* and continued to receive emphasis from that time forward. The 1922 report said:

> It is generally recognized that weight of the human body in relation to its height plays a part in determining the health and longevity of the individual. It is only recently, however, that the long experience of the insurance companies has made possible the crystallization of this impression into a series of definite propositions. We know now, for example, that overweight is a serious impairment among insured lives, the gravity increasing with the excess in weight over the average for the height and age. But, even this statement has its exceptions because, at younger ages, a limited amount of overweight is apparently an advantage. Such persons have uniformly lower death rates from tuberculosis. It is after age 35 that overweight, even in relatively small amounts, begins to be dangerous. The seriousness increases with advancing age and with the amount of overweight[13].

As a final conclusion the report notes, "The important lesson taught by these propositions is that there is an optimum build with reference to mortality. The average build is not the best build. Those who weigh between 10 and 20 per cent below the average show the optimum condition of longevity at most of the ages after early adult life"[13]. The 1922 report also emphasizes the importance of age. Overweight begins to make its impact at ages over thirty-five.

With the recognition that obesity increased the health risks for the life insurance industry and for the public, it became clear that the relation of these events might provide important opportunities for investigation[14]. The life insurance report noted that:

> A promising field of investigation is opened up for the physiologist to determine why the body mechanisms function

> better in those who are of lighter build than in heavier set persons. Common observation confirms these statistical findings. We can all recall from our personal observation that a large majority of our friends who have reached a ripe old age are of slight build. Large persons more often succumb at an earlier age to the diseases of the heart or kidneys, to pneumonia and to disorders which affect the worn-out machinery of the body. To discover the reason for this is the problem of the physiologist[14].

One of the issues that has plagued the study of obesity during the last half of the twentieth-century was the relationship between the average weight of a group of people and the optimal weight for that same group of individuals. What we obviously want to provide is guidance for weight goals—healthy or optimal weight, if you like. These concepts gradually arose from the writings of the life insurance industry[13].

It appears to have taken nearly a decade from 1913 to 1922 for the life insurance industry to recognize the full impact of overweight on reducing health and increasing risk for disease. From this time through World War II, Dublin and the Metropolitan Life Insurance Company repeatedly warned the public about the dangers of being overweight. Their message was that overweight was a risk to health[7,12-18]. Indeed it was probably this repeated hammering home of this message that helped stimulate prospective studies to determine whether this relationship was real.

To help Americans decide an appropriate weight for themselves, the life insurance industry has issued tables of called "desirable" weight or "ideal" weight tables. The first of these was during World War II, but the more influential ones were issued in 1959 and 1983. These tables served as a guide to weights for Americans. They also provided reference points for the early post-World War II epidemiological studies. The Framingham Study defined a "Metropolitan Relative Weight" as the basis for describing the weight status of the men and women who volunteered for this study. The table used for this purpose was the one issued in 1959. This table defined three frame sizes—a small, medium, and large frame. However, there were never any criteria about how to use frame size. Of course, everyone who was a little overweight had a "large" frame. When the 1983 tables were issued, there was an uproar. People had gotten used to the 1959 tables. The newer tables raised the upper and lower weights for large and small frame sizes. The basis for deriving these newer standards, or even the 1959 table, were never identified. How did the insurance industry divide people into frame sizes when the data they had was height and weight? The best guess is that they used the middle half of the population (±1 standard deviation) for the medium frame size and the upper and lower quarters (±1-2 SD) as the small and large frame size. Because of this uncertainty, a meeting at the National Institutes of Health in 1973 defined a new table based on the "middle" weight and provided an upper and lower limit that were the upper and lower weights for the large and small frame size respectively[19].

One problem with life insurance company data was that it came from the people they insured. The insured population is not representative of the population as a whole. People who buy life insurance tend to be better educated, to have a higher income and to be predominantly white, compared to the general population. Thus the question of whether life insurance data could be extrapolated to the entire population was a most important question and needed to be answered. With the end of World War II, money and effort were available to focus on this important question.

One of the key figures tackling this important question was Ancel Keys (1904-2004) from the University of Minnesota. During World War II he had conducted a series of landmark studies on the response to underfeeding and refeeding that provided the strategy for refeeding prisoners of war as they were liberated from concentration camps[20]. K-rations, the food used by so many soldiers during World War II, were named for Dr. Keys.

When the war finished, he launched a collaborative study with colleagues in several countries. In his book titled the *Seven Countries Study*[21], which recounts the development of this study and its results, Keys said:

> Before coronary heart disease was credited as being a major cause of death, American Insurance Companies, led by the Metropolitan Life Insurance Company, were pointing to overweight as a serious impairment associated with undue probability of premature death....[F]rom the mortality experience of policyholders, it was concluded to be justifiable to charge extra premiums to insurance applicants who are grossly overweight according to the standard tables. With recognition that coronary heart disease was the leading killer in the United States, it was assumed that overweight promotes the disease, though the insurance actuaries did not provide any convincing data in confirmation. Still, relative weight was the first variable proposed for control in efforts to prevent heart attacks.

The study that Keys and his international team conducted played an important role in supporting the importance of overweight in the development of heart disease. By today's standards it was a small study involving fewer than ten thousand people. Contrast this with the five million people available for the insurance company analyses. These differences in sizes of populations will be important when we consider the proposition that "obesity" is a myth.

A second major study that has provided additional support to the relation of body weight to the development of heart disease was begun in Framingham, Massachusetts, in 1948. The well known *Framingham Study*, like the *Seven Countries Study* described earlier, showed the detrimental effects of overweight on heart disease and overall mortality, just as the life insurance industry had predicted. However, it took many years of observation before obesity was recognized as an independent predictor of heart disease and mortality in the Framingham Study [22]. In his book describing the Framingham Study, Dr. Dawber said:

> A century ago the risk of death from infectious disease and other severely debilitating disorders was sufficiently high that a moderate degree of excess weight was considered medically desirable. Nutritionists advocated intake of high-calorie food by the young. The effect of this apparently "good" nutrition was to create a population in the Western countries that was over nourished and better able to withstand the infectious killer diseases of that era. The concept of desirable overnutrition has not been easy to overcome, even though the major risks of death are now those of atherosclerosis and cancer. Unfortunately, the development and progression of atherosclerotic disease is aided and abetted by the same rich diet that was so helpful in combating disease hazards 100 years ago. Life insurance data have long suggested that excess weight limits life expectancy. Epidemiologic studies have shown that over nutrition is a definite risk factor for certain manifestations of atherosclerotic disease. Today's physician constantly cautions against weight gain and endeavors to keep his patients well below the supposedly ideal weight of a generation or more ago.[23].

The Framingham Study has taught us many important lessons about body weight and the battle of the bulge. One of the most important is the value of long-term studies. After the first six years of this study, it actually appeared that mortality was lower in the overweight citizens of Framingham than in those who were normal or underweight[24]. Several other studies also questioned the importance of overweight in relation to mortality,[21,25] and this has been a recurring theme[3]. As time passed, the impact of excess weight on longevity in the Framingham population became clear. Indeed, when the residents of this New England community had been studied for twenty-six years, overweight was found to be an independent predictor of early death and heart disease[22].

Why did it take so long to document this relationship? It is interesting to compare the mortality curve from the 1913 life insurance data[2] with data from the Build Study of 1980 in Figure 21-1[26]. They are almost identical. In his recent careful analysis of the long interval between the 1913 publication by the life insurance industry and its eventual acceptance, Lars Sjostrom[27] noted two important reasons for the difficulty in showing the relation of overweight to increased risks of health in some studies. The first problem is the small number of people who were included in the study. The second problem is the relatively short length of time that people were followed as part of the study. The Framingham Study[23], *The Seven Countries Study*[21], and many other early studies only included a few thousand people in comparison to the life insurance pool of several million people. With small sample sizes, a much longer follow-up is needed to show the relationship between overweight and risk to health. This became particularly clear in the Framingham Study. After eighteen and twenty-four years of follow-up, but not after six or twelve years, it was clear that excess weight increased the risk of dying prematurely[24]. In contrast, a large population, such as the insured clients of a life insurance company, allows the impact of excess weight on longevity to become clear in a shorter period of time.

Several large studies are now underway that have profited from these lessons. One of these is the American Cancer Society study, where more than one million people were enrolled for a long-term follow-up. A second study is the Nurses Health Study that enrolled more than one hundred thousand healthy nurses and then noted the time it took for various diseases to develop and the relationship of these diseases to the nutritional and body weight status of these nurses[18]. Like the life insurance data, the American Cancer Society study and the Nurses Health Study have all documented the increased risk associated with higher body weight.

The knowledge that overweight is hazardous to your health took more than half a century to become widely recognized. The wisdom associated with this knowledge has enlightened the way we design and conduct studies of how our behavior impacts on our health. Knowledge comes, but wisdom lingers.

However, it was not that simple. The idea that some people could be overweight without risks to their health received support from a book titled *Obesity Myth*, an article published in the prestigious *Journal of the American Medical Association* that suggested that it might be better to be slightly overweight than normal weight, and a commentary on this issue in the highly regarded *Scientific American* in June 2005. The basic information used for all of these articles was the representative sample of the American population collected by the National Center for Health Statistics. This agency of the U.S. Government conducts periodic surveys of samples of the American population to obtain information related to health and nutrition. The first of these surveys was done under a slightly different name (Health Examination Survey) in 1960-1962. Following up, examinations under the name National Health and Nutrition Examination (NHANES) have been conducted from 1970-74 (NHANES I), 1976-1980 (NHANES II), from 1988-1994 (NHANES III), and NHANES 1999-2002. It was the analysis of the first three of these surveys in 1994 that showed the sudden increase in number of overweight Americans between 1980 and 1992[5]. The increased number of overweight Americans has been confirmed in each subsequent survey. Each of these surveys contains between eight thousand and fourteen thousand people.

An analysis of deaths among these samples and the changes in risk factors for heart disease have raised some interesting issues and thrown fuel on the fire of whether it is worth fighting the battle of the bulge. Maybe being overweight is not bad for you; it may be good for you[28,29]. One analysis showed that over the time interval from 1970 to 1994 there had been improvements in blood pressure and blood lipids that would tend to reduce the likelihood of early death from heart disease. In another analysis of these same surveys the authors found that the risk of dying was less in those in the overweight category than those in the "normal weight" category. Can this be true? Are all of our previous data wrong? I think not.

The problem with interpreting these data is the same one raised earlier—size of sample and duration of follow-up. There is a third issue for this study, and that is the basis for comparison. Earlier we defined the body mass index and suggested that it was a useful measurement to compare populations. When this unit was adopted for evaluating population data by the National Heart, Lung and Blood Institute (NHLBI) and the World Health Organization (WHO), they selected 18.5 to 25 as the normal range for body weight. This lower limit is of concern. Using the life insurance tables discussed earlier the body mass index for the lowest weight at each height in the small frame category and the highest weight for each height in the large frame category can be calculated. These numbers are approximately 20 to 25 for both men and women. They are slightly higher in the 1983 life insurance table than in the 1959 life insurance table. The lower limit in the WHO/NHLBI recommendations of 18.5 includes a number of people who are quite thin relative to American standards.

Are thinner people at higher risk? The answer is yes, if they are thin enough. Population surveys have repeatedly found that low BMI is associated with increased risk. The relation of body mass index and age for the two million Norwegians living outside of the capital, Oslo[30], allows us to make several conclusions. First there is a "J" shaped relationship for each age group and for men and women. At low levels of BMI and at higher levels of BMI there is increased risk of death. Second, there is a relatively flat area between a BMI of 20 and 26 where there is little extra risk from overweight.

Third, the entire curve flattens in older decades of life, indicating that the major effects of excess weight are among the young and middle-aged people. The value of the American Cancer Society study described earlier, and the life insurance data is that they are very large, in excess of one million people. As Sjostrom[27] showed years ago, these large studies allow conclusions about health risks to be reached in a short period of time. In contrast, smaller studies take longer because there is more uncertainty in their data.

Let's take the life insurance data and the NHANES data. According to the NHANES data about one third of Americans have a BMI between 18.5 and 25, another third between a BMI of 25 and 30, and the other third have a BMI above 30. If we divide the life insurance data with about 4.5 million people into thirds this would give us about 1.5 million people in each category or something less than three hundred thousand for each BMI unit. If we divide the NHANES approximately fifteen thousand people into thirds we have about five thousand people in each category or about one thousand for each BMI unit. It is obvious that we have much less certainty from the NHANES data because of its much smaller size. If we pool or lump all of the people with a BMI of 18.5 to 25, we will be including people at the lower end who are at higher risk. This will make the risk associated with the beginning of the upper end (25 and up) appear better than if the people in the BMI group 18.5 to 20 had been excluded. Since the lowest risk appears to be for people with a BMI between 22 and 23, BMI values that are higher or lower will be a high, albeit only slightly higher, risk. The farther we move on each side of the 22-23 mark the greater the risk.

Biosketch

Louis Dublin (1882-1969) was the vice president and statistician to the Metropolitan Life Insurance Company that provided "weight tables" during much of the twentieth-century (Figure 21-2). He was educated in biology and statistics at City College of New York and Columbia University.

His entire professional career was spent at the Metropolitan Life Insurance Company, from which he became a champion of public health issues that were pointed out in the analyses of life insurance data[31].

Biosketch

Ancel Keys (1904-2004) (Figure 21-3) was born January 26, 1904. He received a bachelor's degree from the University of California in Berkeley, which was followed by a Ph.D. in oceanography and biology in 1930. A second Ph.D. was awarded from Cambridge University in 1938. Keys is noted for several important things. During World War II he was responsible for the design of military field rations known as K-rations.

His two-volume classic study *The Biology of Human Starvation* was conducted during World War II to assess the effects of semi-starvation on function and behavior of human beings. He showed that the body mass index (BMI) had a better relation to body fat than other anthropometric formulas. Following these important contributions he turned his attention to the relation of diet and heart diseases, specifically cholesterol. With colleagues Francisco Grande and Joseph Anderson he developed the equations for predicting the changes in cholesterol when dietary fats are modified. The genesis of the *Seven Countries Study* was the hypothesis that diet was related to heart disease. These important epidemiological findings were the result of Keys's work[32].

References

1. Tennyson, A. "Locksley Hall." Line 141.
2. Campos, P. *The Obesity Myth: Why America's Obsession with Weight Is Hazardous to Your Health.* New York: Gotham Books, 2004.
3. Gibbs, W.W. "Obesity: An Overblown Epidemic?" *Scientific American.* No. 292 (2005)6: 70-77.
4. The Association of Life Insurance Medical Directors and The Actuarial Society of America. *Medico Actuarial Mortality Investigation.* New York: The Association of Life Insurance Medical Directors and The Actuarial Society of America, 1913.
5. Kuczmarski, R.J., K.M. Flegal, S.M. Campbell, C.L. Johnson. "Increasing Prevalence of Overweight Among U.S. Adults." The National Health and Nutrition Examination Surveys, 1960 to 1991. *JAMA.* No. 272 3(1994): 205-211.
6. Hedley, A., G.L. Ogden, C.L. Johnson, M.D. Carroll, L.R. Curtin, K.M. Flegal. "Prevalence of Overweight and Obesity among U.S. Children, Adolescents, and Adults. 1999-2002." *JAMA.* No. 291 23(2004): 2847-2850.
7. Dublin, L.L. "Body Build and Longevity: The Johns Hopkins University De Lamar Lectures, 1925-1926." Baltimore: Williams and Wilkens, 1927.
8. Hippocrates. *Oeuvres complètes d'Hippocrate: traduction nouvelle avec le texte grec en regard, collationné sur les manuscrits et toutes les éditions; accompagnée d'une introduction, de commentaires médicaux, de variantes et de notes philologiques; suivie d'une table générale des matières / par E. Littre.* Paris: J.B. Bailliere, 1839-1861.
9. Flemyng, M. *A Discourse on the Nature, Causes, and Cure of Corpulency. Illustrated by a Remarkable Case. Read before the Royal Society November 1757.* London: L. Davis and C. Reymers, 1760.
10. [Wadd, W.] *Cursory Remarks on Corpulence: By a Member of the Royal College of Surgeons.* London: J. Callow, 1810.
11. Chambers, T.K. "The Gulstonian Lectures On Corpulence." *Lancet.* 2(1850): 11-19, 342-350, 437-445.
12. Dublin, L.I, E.W. Kopf, G.H. Van Buren. *Mortality Statistics of Insured Wage-Earners and Their Families.* New York: Metropolitan Life Insurance Company, 1919.
13. Metropolitan Life Insurance Company. "Body Weight and Longevity." *Stat Bull Met Life Ins.* 3(1922): 3-4.
14. Association of Life Insurance Medical Directors. Actuarial Society of America, 1918.
15. "Further Facts on Body-weight and Longevity." *Stat Bull Met Life Ins.* 4(1923): 2-4.

16. Dublin, L.I., H.H. Marks. *The Build of Women According to Build-Experience on Substandard Issues.* New York: Press of Recording & Statistical Corp, 1939.
17. "Ideal Weights for Men." *Stat Bull Met Life Ins.* 24(1943): 6-8.
18. "Ideal Weights for Women." *Stat Bull Met Life Ins.* 23(1942):6-8
19. Bray, G.A. Fogarty Center conference proceedings. 1973.
20. Keys, A. *The Biology of Human Starvation.* Minneapolis, MN: University of Minnesota, 1950.
21. Keys, A. *Seven Countries: A Multivariate Analysis of Death and Coronary Heart Disease.* Cambridge: Harvard University Press, 1980.
22. Hubert, H.B., M. Feinleib, P.M. McNamara, W..P Castelli. "Obesity as an Independent Risk Factor for Cardiovascular Disease: A 26-year Follow-up of Participants in the Framingham Heart Study." *Circulation.* 67(1983): 986977.
23. Dawber, T.R. *The Framingham Study: The Epidemiology of Atherosclerotic Disease.* Cambridge: Harvard University Press, 1980.
24. Feinleib, M. "Epidemiology of Obesity in Relation to Health Hazards." *Ann Intern Med.* 103(1985): 1019 1024.
25. Man, G.V. "The Influence of Obesity on Health." *N Engl J Med.* 291(1974): 178-185, 226-232.
26. Society of Actuaries and Association of Life Insurance Medical Directors of America. *Build Study 1979.* Schaumburg, IL: Society of Actuaries and Association of Life Insurance Medical Directors of America, 1980
27. Sjostrom, L. "Mortality of Severely Obese Subjects." *Am J Clin Nutr.* 55(1992): 516S-523S.
28. Manson, J.E., G.A. Colditz, M.J. Stampfer, et al. "A Prospective Study of Obesity and Risk of Coronary Heart Disease in Women." *N Engl J Med.* 322(1990): 882-889.
29. Gregg. E.N., Y.J. Cheng, B.L. Cadwell, et al. "Secular Trends in Cardiovascular Disease Risk Factors According to Body Mass Index in U.S. Adults." *JAMA.* no. 293 15(2005): 1868-1874.
30. Waaler, H.T. "Height, Weight and Mortality: The Norwegian Experience." *Acta Med Scand Suppl.* 79(1984): 1-56.
31. Dublin, Louis I.: Editorial. November 1, 1882-March 7, 1969. *Am J Public Health.* 59(1969): 1083-5.
32. *Morbidity and Mortality Weekly Report.* 48(1999): 651.

Chapter 22

Body Fat Distribution and the Distribution of Scientific Knowledge

Next to nature there is nothing more
wonderful than man's gradual understanding of it.

—Sarton[1]

Science advances one step at a time. Moving ideas and inventions from the laboratory to the clinic and then to the population at large takes time. Sometimes this transition is fast, sometimes painstakingly slow. This is a story about the relatively long time needed to accept the idea that fat distribution was very important to health. During the last decade of the twentieth century, newspapers and magazines began to refer to people as "pear-shaped" or "apple-shaped." Pear-shaped people are those with fat located from the waist downward; apple-shaped people are the ones with the "beer belly" or "barrel-chested" shape. People with apple-shaped distribution of their body fat are the ones at highest risks for health problems. Yet it took nearly one hundred years for this idea to move from conception to a wide public recognition as a key element of the battle of the bulge. This is the story of that discovery.

Four original papers in the appendix provide the basis for understanding the idea that where your body fat is located is important to your health. The first two are short excerpts from the transactions of the Actuarial Society of America published in 1901-1903 and 1904[2-4]. The other two papers are the first publications of Professor Jean Vague (1911-2002)[5,6] on regional fat distribution that were published nearly fifty years after the life insurance observations. Vague's initial scientific publication in May 1947 was in French and appeared in *La Presse Médicale*, a journal that is not widely read outside of France. Professor Vague has kindly translated it into English[5] for this book. His second paper was published in the *American Journal of Clinical Nutrition* in 1956, which made his work widely available to English-speaking scientists[6].

The life insurance industry was at the forefront in recognizing the extra risk to health associated with the "apple-shaped" person. They made this observation early in the twentieth century. It was nearly fifty years later in France right after World War II that Professor Jean Vague made the next big step by recognizing that relation of body fat distribution in diabetes, and it was a full thirty years longer before the health writers for our newspapers picked up this story. Overall it took eighty years after the work by the Society of Actuaries for fat distribution to become recognized as an important cause of disease for those battling the bulge.

In the first part of the twentieth century, obesity was divided into two types, endogenous and exogenous[7]. This idea was championed by one of the leading German physicians, Carl H. von Noorden (1858-1944). Endogenous obesity occurred in people with "glandular" diseases or metabolic diseases that were the cause of their obesity. In contrast, exogenous obesity resulted from eating too much or exercising too little. This same classification of obesity was used in the United States. In a leading American textbook from the 1920s titled *Endocrinology and Metabolism*, compiled by physicians at John Hopkins[8], Tileston classified obesity as "endogeneous" or "exogenous." Neither von Noorden nor Tileston included any mention of how body fat was distributed or that being apple-shaped might be bad for your health.

This then was the setting for classifying obesity as World War II broke out in 1939. Shortly after the end of the World War II, the issue initially identified by the life insurance industry resurfaced. In 1947, two years after the end of World War II, a young French physician named Jean Vague published his first paper on the subject of regional fat distribution. In this paper Vague says, "The classical divisions into endogenous and exogenous obesity, those of endocrine origin and those due to overfeeding and insufficient movement, do not provide a key to the problem." He goes on to suggest that "sexual differentiation could throw some light on the mechanisms of obesity"[5].

With the concept of sexual differences in mind, Vague concluded that it was essential to examine the total biotype of an individual. He included in this concept the anatomic or morphological components, the functional or physiological components, and the behavioral or psychological aspects needed for a thorough understanding of the problem of obesity. To provide a measure of fat distribution he developed an index called the 'adipomuscular ratio.' His idea of trying to relate the amount of muscle and fat to one another in both men and women was very incisive, but as we will see, the method was cumbersome.

To calculate the adipomuscular ratio you need two measurements of the arm and two measurements of the leg. Two of the four measurements are skinfolds and the other two are circumferences. The skinfold thicknesses are measured at the upper part of the upper arm and the upper part of the leg.

The circumference of the upper arm and leg are obtained at the same place that the skinfolds were measured. Each of these skinfolds is divided by the circumference of the arm or thigh at the same point. This ratio is the femoral adipomuscular ratio (FAMR) when the measures are done on the leg and the brachial adipomuscular ratio (BAMR) when done on the arm. For a normal-weight male, the BAMR was approximately 0.21 and the FAMR approximately 0.19. To give an overall index, Vague divided these ratios by each other. That is, he divided the BAMR by the FAMR to give a brachio/femoral AMR. For men this was about 1.10. In women it was about 0.77. These differences reflect the differences in the amount of fat in the thigh and arm relative to circumferences. The individual ratios in females are a BAMR of 0.48, indicating a relatively thicker fat fold on the arm in women than in men and a FAMR of 0.63, showing that the thighs of women were relatively fatter than the arms in women. The brachio/femoral ratio, or AMR, in women aged twenty-five to thirty was 0.77, which is considerably lower than in men. Vague went one step further and included two other skinfold measures in his fat distribution index (FDI). For the FDI Vague adds a term related to skinfold thickness at the nape of the neck (N) and the sacral skinfold (F), both squared. Thus,

$$FDI = B/F\ AMR + (N)^2 + (F)^2$$

This index is very different between men and women. This is shown in Table 22-1, taken from the 1947 paper[5]. It should be obvious by now that Vague was on the right path but that the method he had developed for his purpose was difficult to apply and as a result was not widely used.

Table 22-1. Classifying adult obesity using the mean value of the Fat Distribution Index (FDI)

	Classification				
	Hyperandroid	Android	Mixed (Fat Distribution Index)	Gynoid	Hypergynoid
Men	> 3	2 to 3	1 to 2	0.70 to 1	< 0.70
Women	> 1	0.81 to 1	0.61 to 0.80	0.40 to 0.60	<0.40

From Vague (5,6,9).

In spite of the difficulty of this method, Vague was able to show the increased risk for diabetes and high blood pressure associated with increased central fat, i.e., increased brachio/femoral ratios. Vague's first paper in English on this subject appeared in 1956 in the *American Journal of Clinical Nutrition*[6] and contained an extension of his original observations. Over the next thirty-five years, Vague and his colleagues[9] continued to pursue and probe this problem before his work was finally taken up by others. For the excellence of his research, Vague eventually received the Willendorf Award, the highest award for clinical research in obesity.

In spite of the importance of Vague's concept it took another method for measuring the distribution of fat before the idea finally came into the mainstream a quarter of a century later[10]. Although one other author had picked up on Vague's original idea[11], it was not until 1982 and the work of Dr. Ahmed Kissebah and his colleagues in the United States[12] and the work of the late Professor Per Bjorntorp and his colleagues in Sweden[13-15] that this concept became widely accepted.

The idea that an increased amount of fat on the abdomen, the so-called apple shape, is more hazardous to health than fat on the hips and thighs, the so-called pear shape, is now taken for granted and has become a key element in a newly recognized group of findings called the "metabolic syndrome." The metabolic syndrome is a collection of findings that often go together and includes central adiposity or the apple shape, abnormal blood lipids, high blood pressure, and abnormal glucose metabolism. Using widely accepted criteria for making the diagnosis of the metabolic syndrome, we find that nearly one-quarter of adult Americans have this problem as part of their battle of the bulge. Central adiposity is part of this syndrome. These apple-shaped individuals are at risk for heart disease, diabetes, high blood pressure, gall bladder disease, and some forms of cancer[17].

Why the delay in recognizing the hazards associated with the "apple-shaped" distribution of fat when it had been pointed out as early as 1904? Rogers provides some insight into this delay in recognition of new ideas when he said:

> Many technologists think that advantageous innovations will sell themselves, that the obvious benefits of a new idea will be widely realized by potential adopters, and that the innovation will therefore diffuse rapidly. Unfortunately, this is very seldom the case. Most innovations, in fact, diffuse at a surprisingly slow rate[18].

What was the setting that led to a thirty-year delay between the initial paper by Vague and the acceptance of this idea? Several reasons may be suggested. These include the complexity of the index he used, the state of the field when the concept was first put forward, the relative inaccessibility of the original paper, and the diffusion time required for new ideas which lead to a shift in the paradigm of scientific thought.

The adipomuscular ratio proposed by Vague[6] was cumbersome. It required four separate measurements (circumference of the arm and leg and skinfold measurements at the same two sites). Vague's fat distribution index (FDI) was even more difficult, requiring six measurements. In addition to the number of different measurements that had to be made was the problem of precision. If the same measurement is made several times, there is always a variation in the values. For skinfolds these measures by a single person are often large, but when more than one person makes the measurements the differences are even larger. Thus, unless the measurements were done by a single person, they could be quite unreliable.

In contrast to the difficulty of using the system developed by Vague is the simplicity of the waist circumference divided by the hip circumference (WHR) which requires only two measurements, one at the circumference of the waist and the other the circumference of the hips. In addition, the variability in measuring the circumference is less than in measuring a skinfold. It was the use of the WHR by Professor Ahmid Kissebah et al.[12], by Professor Per Bjorntorp (1931-2003)[14-16] and his colleagues in the set of papers in 1982 that put this concept of apple-shaped body fatness on the map. The subscapular skinfold which was used by Donahue et al.[19] and by Stokes et al.[20] to reach the same conclusions was an even simpler but equally powerful measurement. The waist circumference alone has supplanted all of these simple methods since it is as good as these others in estimating the apple shape and pear shape.

Some concepts are picked up and rapidly translated from laboratory to patients; others suffer long delays. The initial publication on the stethoscope by René T.H. Laennec (1781-1826) in 1819[21] was met with almost immediate and widespread acceptance. Laennec's work was translated into English within two years[22]. An overweight woman played a key role in the discovery of the stethoscope. In the early nineteenth-century, it was the "custom...to apply the ear directly to the heart or chest (direct auscultation)" to listen for heart sounds or diseases in the chest[23]. Many physicians objected to this technique for two reasons. First, codes of modesty often made it difficult to get patients to remove enough clothing to hear well. Second, lice were common on many of the patients in public hospitals. This deterred many physicians from putting their ear to a lice-infested chest. In addition, the rush of blood to the head as it was lowered to the chest would sometimes cause confusing noises. However, it was obesity and not these other problems that led Laennec to his discovery. An obese girl at the Necker Hospital in Paris where he worked was suffering from a heart condition, and because of her obesity, direct auscultation by placing his ear to her chest was not possible. From watching a group of children listening to sounds through rolled up papers, Laennec got the idea for rolling up paper and applying it directly to the chest of the obese girl. His original discovery was called a "*cornet de papier*" (paper cornet) but was rapidly translated into the single wooden tube stethoscope that became so popular[23]. His initial wooden stethoscope that could be carried under the hat was an immediate success. Its introduction into clinical medicine marked one of the earliest instruments that would help physicians diagnose diseases of the chest. Publication of his discovery in French was part of the swift recognition of this method. Laennec was an active physician practicing medicine at the height of the dominance of the French Clinical School[24] in the early years of the nineteenth-century. This made his technique something that would be readily distributed to other physicians and students from many countries who were in Paris to learn medicine.

Percussion, a second clinical technique for evaluating chest diseases, fared less well. Thumping on a barrel had long been used as a way to determine the quantity of wine or other liquid in a barrel. Leopold Auenbrugger (1722-1809)[25] recognized this principle and applied it to the clinical problem of detecting fluid or air in the chest. He published his work in 1761, but it largely fell on "deaf ears." One problem with its acceptance was that it was published in Latin, at a time when medicine was switching to the vernacular languages, such as German, French, or English. It was printed in the latter half of the eighteenth-century, a half century marked by the American Revolution and the French Revolution. Moreover, the method was not accepted by the leaders of the Austrian school where Auenbrugger taught. All of these events conspired to delay the acceptance of this important clinical technique.

How then was it finally recognized? It was the translation of his work into French in 1808 by Jean Corvisart (1755-1821)[26] that popularized this valuable clinical tool. Like the stethoscope, the rapid acceptance of percussion after its translation in 1808 may be related to the dominance of the French Clinical School during these years and Corvisart's leadership role in that school.

Vague's paper was published in French at the end of World War II. During the 1940s the Second World War had taken a major toll on the European countries. In the late 1940s, the Marshall Plan was providing vast amounts of financial aid to help rebuild Europe. American medicine was in the ascendancy[27], and research in Europe was at a low ebb. This important work by Vague, published in French in the early years after World War II, may have suffered from its limited availability in a manner similar to the work of Auenbrugger on percussion.

X-rays, like the stethoscope, were rapidly adopted for diagnostic use in medicine. The original paper by Wilhelm Roentgen (1845-1923)[28], showing the ability of x-rays to penetrate the skin and show the underlying bones, was published in a relatively obscure German journal on December 28, 1895, but by early January of 1896, one month later, his discovery was being commented on in the scientific and popular press[29]. At the time of his discovery, the German Laboratory School was the dominant school for medicine. It was only a few months after Roentgen's original publication that the first paper on x-rays was published in English[30]. For his work Roentgen was awarded the Nobel Prize in 1901, just six years after the publication of his findings. Thus there was almost no delay between publication by Roentgen and the adaptation of x-rays to experimental research and clinical investigation.

Ideas that require a paradigm shift may take longer to be accepted[18,31]. Two examples will be used to illustrate this point. The first is the discovery by James Lind (1716-1794)[32] that oranges and limes would prevent scurvy in British sailors. The observation that citrus fruits were beneficial for people with scurvy was made in 1601 by the English sea captain James Lancaster. Lind was aware of Lancaster's work when he conducted his experiments more than one hundred fifty years later[33]. At the time of Lind's work, scurvy was a major cause of death and disability for British seamen. Lind conducted what may be the first controlled clinical study. It was done on board the *H.M.S. Salisbury* where small groups of two to three sailors each with scurvy were given different treatments that had been proposed to "cure" scurvy. The ones who received the mixture of lemon and orange juice recovered rapidly. The ones who received other treatments, such as vinegar, got worse. Lind published these results in his treatise of 1754[32,33]. Lind went on to prepare a potion that he believed would cure scurvy, but he did not do any further clinical trials. It was more than forty-five years after Lind's publication before the Royal Navy adopted the eating of limes as a way to prevent scurvy among British sailors.

Acceptance of the work of Gregor Johann Mendel (1822-1884) on heredity is another example of a long delay between the original publication and its acceptance. As Bateson notes, "To appreciate what Mendel did the reader should refer to the original paper which is a model of lucidity and expository skill. His success is due to the clearness with which he thought out the problem"[34]. Yet, it was over forty years before Bateson picked up this original paper and widely disseminated it.

Bateson described his views about why the work of Mendel was so long in being recognized:

> The fact that the Brunn journal [where Mendel published] is rather scarce does not in itself explain why the work was not noticed...The cause is unquestionably to be found in that neglect of the experimental study of the problem of Species which supervened with the general acceptance of

> the Darwinian doctrines. The problem of Species...attracted thenceforth no workers. The question it was imagined had been answered and the debate ended. No one felt much interest in the matter[34].

During the twentieth-century, the importance of the concept of unitary inheritance described by Mendel became obvious. It was highlighted by the work of Watson and Crick in 1957[35] when they described the helical structure of the deoxyribonucleic acid (DNA) that forms the chemical basis for the Mendelian traits. Their seminal paper set in motion the revolution in molecular biology that ended with the publication of the human genome along with the genome structures of several other species by the end of the` twentieth-century—a truly phenomenal growth in our understanding of the basic biology of human beings.

Understanding that the bulge we battle is divided into more than one part provided important new ideas for our fight. We now know, after a long delay in dissemination of the idea, that centrally located fat or the "apple shape" is associated with increased health risks. Reducing these central bulges would be a good target in the battle of the bulge using diet, exercise, lifestyle, and other treatments that are discussed later.

Biosketch

Leopold Auenbrugger (1722-1809) was born in Austria and introduced the art of physical diagnosis into clinical medicine with his publication on the use of percussion (Figure 22-1). Percussion is a technique for determining the amount of wine in a wine barrel and had been in long use for this purpose.

It was Auenbrugger who recognized that this same technique could be used to evaluate the presence of fluid in the human chest. His small monograph, published in 1761, drew scant attention[25]. It was not until the translation of his work into French in 1808 by Corvisart that it achieved its current status as a diagnostic technique[26]. It was at the Hospital of the Holy Trinity in Vienna where he was physician-in-chief and where he did the work on percussion that is the basis for his fame[36].

Biosketch

René-Théophile-Hyacinthe Laennec (1781-1826) is noted for his discovery of the stethoscope[23]. He was born in Quimper, a small town in the Bretonne region of northwest France. His father was a lawyer and a mediocre writer of verse. After his mother's death when he was age six, Laennec was raised by his uncle who was a physician in nearby Nantes. He began his studies in medicine with his uncle, but these were interrupted by the French Revolution. In 1801 he went to Paris and enrolled at the Charité Hôpital, where he became a pupil of Corvisart, the man who translated

Auenbrugger's technique of percussion into French. After receiving his doctoral degree in 1804, he worked in pathological anatomy. He was appointed to the Necker Hospital in 1814, where he discovered the principle of the stethoscope in 1816[37]. (Figure 22-2)

Biosketch

James Lind (1716-1794) (Figure 22-3) was born in Edinburgh. By age fifteen he had become apprenticed to a surgeon. In 1739 at the age of twenty-three he entered the navy where he served as a surgeon in many regions of the world, including the Mediterranean, off the Guinea coast and in the West Indies. He developed an interest in tropical diseases and became interested in naval hygiene. He left the Royal Navy in 1848 after nine years and proceeded to earn his M.D. degree from the University of Edinburgh and then to set up a practice of medicine in the city. After ten years he left for Haslar Hospital, a naval hospital near the southern English city of Portsmouth where he remained for the next twenty-five years. His famous book on his experiments at sea was published in 1757, but it was more than forty years before his findings came into use leading to British sailors being called "limeys" for the limes they ate to prevent scurvy.

Biosketch

Professor Jean Vague (1911-2002) (Figure 22-4) was born in 1911 and received his undergraduate education in Aix-en-Provence and his medical education at the University of Marseilles. Following an internship at the Hôtel Dieu Conception in Marseilles, he began his practice and research in endocrinology and rose through the ranks at the university to become professor in 1957.

He served in the French army and was decorated with the Legion of Honor. Among many other distinctions, he was a member of the French Academy of Medicine[38].

Biosketch

Per Bjorntorp, M.D. (1931-2003) was born in Linkoping, Sweden in 1931 and received his medical education from the University of Gothenburg. Following completion of his MD degree, he did a fellowship at the Oklahoma Research Foundation in Oklahoma City, where he began his work on the metabolism of adipose tissue. Upon returning to Gothenburg, where he spent most of his career, Dr. Bjorntorp set up a laboratory for the study of obesity at a time when the subject was not very popular. He continued to lead the work in obesity and adipose tissue while serving as chair of medicine at Gothenburg from 1977 until his retirement in 1996. Over the years, his outgoing personality attracted a number of young men and women to work with him who in turn have established highly regarded programs of their own. Bjorntorp was noted for his work on the metabolic syndrome and was one of the pioneers in its recognition. He was chairman of the third International Congress on Obesity in Rome in 1980 and editor of the *International Journal of Obesity* from 1983-1989. In addition to being an eminent physician scholar who was honored in a number of awards, Bjorntorp was a skilled cellist and played regularly in the local orchestras. He was also an avid sailor[39].

References

1. Sarton, G. *The History of Science and the New Humanism.* New York: Henry Holt and Co., 1931.
2. Actuarial Society of America. *Transactions.* 7(1901-1903): 492-497.
3. Weeks, R.W. "An Experiment with the Specialized Investigation." Actuarial Society of America. *Transactions.* 8(1904): 17-23.
4. Kahn, H.S., D.F. Williamson. "Abdominal Obesity and Mortality Risk among Men in Nineteenth-Century North America." *Int J Obes.* No. 18 10(1994): 686-691.
5. Vague, J. *"La differenciation sexuelle facteur determinant des formes de l'obésité."* Transl. J. Vague. *Presse Médicale.* 55(1947): 339-340.
6. Vague, J. "The Degree of Masculine Differentiation of Obesities: A Factor Determining Predisposition to Diabetes, Atherosclerosis, Gout, and Uric Calculous Disease." *Am J Clin Nutr.* 4(1956): 20-34.
7. von Noorden, C. "Obesity." In von Noorden, C., ed. *Metabolism and Practical Medicine.* Chicago: W.T. Keener & Company, 1907.
8. Tileston, W. "Obesity." In Barker, L.F., ed. *Endocrinology and Metabolism.* New York: D. Appleton and Co., 1922.
9. Vague, J. *Obesities.* London: John Libbey & Company, Ltd., 1991.
10. Bray, G.A. "Topography of Body Fat." *Adv Endocrinol Metab.* 5(1994): 297-322.
11. Feldman, R., A.J. Sender, A.B. Sieglaub. "Differences in Diabetic and Non-diabetic Fat Distribution Patterned by Skin-fold Measurements." *Diabetes.* 18(1969): 478-486.
12. Kissebah, A.H. "Relation of Body Fat Distribution to Metabolic Complications of Obesity." *J Clin Endocrinol Metab.* 54(1982): 254-260.
13. Bjorntorp, P. "Visceral Obesity: A 'Civilization Syndrome.'" *Obes Res.* 1(1993): 206-222.
14. Lapidus, L., C. Bengtsson, B. Larsson, K. Pennert, E. Rybo, L. Sjostrom. "Distribution of Adipose Tissue and Risk of Cardiovascular Disease and Death: A 12 Year Follow-up of Participants in the Population Study of 1462 Women in Gothenberg, Sweden." *Br Med J.* 289(1984): 1257-1261.
15. Larsson, B., K. Svardsudd, L. Welin, L. Wilhelmsen, P. Bjorntorp, G. Tibblin. "Abdominal Adipose Tissue Distribution, Obesity and Risk of Cardiovascular Disease and Death: 13 Year Follow-up of Participants in the Study of 792 Men Born in 1913." *Br Med J.* 288(1984): 1401.1404.
16. Krotkiewskl, M., T. Bjorntorp, L. Sjostrom U. Smith. "Impact of Obesity on Metabolism in Men and Women: Importance of Regional Adipose Tissue Distribution." *J Clin Invest.* 72(1983): 1150-1162.

17. National Cholesterol Education Program. "Executive Summary of the Third Report of the National Cholesterol Education Program (NCEP) Expert Panel on Detection, Evaluation, and Treatment of High Blood Cholesterol in Adults (Adult Treatment Panel III)." *JAMA.* 285(1002): 2486-2497.
18. Rogers, E.M. *Diffusion of Innovations.* 3rd ed. New York: Free Press, 1983.
19. Donahue, R.P., R.D. Abbott, E. Blood, D.J. Reed, K. Yano. "Central Obesity and Coronary Heart Disease in Men." *Lancet.* 1(1987): 821-824.
20. Stokes, J. III, R.J. Garrison, W.B. Kannel. "The Independent Contribution of Various Indices of Obesity to the 22-year Incidence of Coronary Heart Disease: The Framingham Heart Study." In Vague, J., P. Bjorntorp, B. Guy-grand, M. Rebuffe-Scrive, M. Vague, P.H., eds. *Metabolic Complications of Human Obesity.* Amsterdam: Excerpta Medics, (1985): 49-57.
21. Laennec, R.T.H. *De l'auscultation médiate, ou traité du diagnostic des maladies des poumons et du coeur.* Paris: J-A Brosson et J-S Chaude, 1819.
22. Laennec, R.T.H. *A Treatise on the Diseases of the Chest, in Which They are Described According to their Anatomical Characters, and their Diagnosis Established on a New Principle by Means of Acoustic Instruments.* Transl. J Forbes. London: T. and G. Underwood, 1821.
23. Webb, G.B. *René Théophile Hyacinthe Laennec: A Memoir.* New York: Paul B. Hoeber, 1928.
24. Ackerknecht, E.H. *Medicine at the Paris Hospital.* Baltimore: Johns Hopkins University Press, 1967.
25. Auenbrugger, L. *Inventum novum ex percussione thoracis humani ut signo abstrusos.* 1st ed. Vindobonae: J.T. Trattnerr, 1761.
26. Auenbrugger, L. *Nouvelle Méthode pour reconnaître les Maladies Internes de la Poitrine par la Percussion de cette Cavité* (*Par J.N. Corvisart*). Paris: Migneret, 1808.
27. Bray, G.A. "The Tide Shifts Again: The Ebb and Flow of History." *Obes Res.* 3(1995): 605-608.
28. Roentgen, W.C. "Ueber eine neue Art von Strahlen." *S.B. Phys-med Ges Wurzburg.* (1895): 132-141.
29. Glasser, O. *Wilhelm Conrad Roentgen and the Early History of the Roentgen Rays.* Springfield, IL: Charles C. Thomas, 1934.
30. Jones, R., O. Lodge. "The Discovery of a Bullet Lost in the Wrist by Means of the Roentgen Rays." *Lancet.* 1(1896): 476-477.
31. Kuhn, T.S. *The Structure of Scientific Revolutions.* Chicago: University of Chicago Press, 1962.
32. Lind, J. A. *Treatise on the Scurvy in Three Parts Containing an Inquiry*

into the Nature, Causes and Cure of that Disease Together with a Critical and Chronological View of what has been Published on the Subject. 2nd ed. London: A. Millar, 1757.

33. Carpenter, K.J. *The History of Scurvy and Vitamin C.* Cambridge: Cambridge University Press, 1986.
34. Bateson, W. *Mendel's Principles of Heredity.* Cambridge: Cambridge University Press, 1909.
35. Watson, J.B., F.H.C. Crick. "Molecular Structure of Nucleic Acids: A Structure for Deoxyribose Nucleic Acid." *Nature (Lond).* 171(1953): 737-738.
36. Garrison, F.H. *An Introduction to the History of Medicine.* Philadelphia: W.B. Saunders, 1914.
37. Major, R.H. *A History of Medicine.* Springfield, IL: Charles C. Thomas, 1954.
38. Jaffiol, C. "de Jean Vague." *Bulletin Academie Nationale de Médecine.* 188 (2004): 895.
39. Sjostrom, L. "Obituary: Per Bjorntorp." Int J Obes Relat Metab Disord 2004;28:351.

Chapter 23

What's in a Name?
Mr. Dickens's "Pickwickian" Fat Boy Syndrome

What's in a name? That which we call a rose
By any other name would smell as sweet.
Romeo and Juliet[1] *II.ii.43-44*

—William Shakespeare

Corpulency, when in an extraordinary degree, may be reckoned a disease, as it in some measure obstructs the free exercise of the animal functions; and has a tendency to shorten life, by paving the way to dangerous distempers.

—Malcolm Flemyng[2]

There is an epidemic of obesity galloping through the world. Why does this concern us? In part because we believe that obesity is hazardous to our health. The information from many sources says obesity increases the odds that you will get diabetes, heart disease, high blood pressure, joint troubles, and certain forms of cancer. For this reason the life insurance industry has been exhorting us throughout the twentieth-century to weigh less. If we weigh less we will be at lower risk for these unwanted outcomes. If we are successful in the battle of the bulge, we will also have defeated a number of other enemies of health.

This chapter is the story of one of the conditions that is associated with corpulence. It is an interesting story with a long historical record. It is also an interesting story because of its association with the literary world. The charming Mr. Pickwick was the leading character in Charles Dickens's *The Posthumous Papers of the Pickwick Club*, and the man who created him was a keen observer of the human condition. In *The Pickwick Papers* there is a fat boy named Joe who readily falls asleep. The medical condition in this chapter is the one that Joe has—a form of breathing problem. Its historical roots date back to antiquity. But there is also the question raised by this disease of whether it is appropriate to name diseases after people. In this case, the lung condition has been called The Pickwickian Syndrome.

Four papers are included in the discussion of The Pickwickian Syndrome. The first is a case by Russell[3] published in 1866. It is one of the earliest descriptions that I have identified in English of a Pickwickian-like syndrome, describing the association between obesity and daytime somnolence. The second paper by Bramwell[4] and the third paper by Morrison[5] are cases of the same syndrome published in 1889, more than twenty years later. They contain the first reference to the fat boy in *The Pickwick Papers.* The fourth paper is by Burwell and colleagues[6], and is the one which firmly implanted the term "The Pickwickian Syndrome" in the medical literature.

Although Joe (Figure 23-1), the fat boy in Charles Dickens's *The Posthumous Papers of the Pickwick Club*[7] had no other name, he was modeled after James Budden, a real-life fat boy[8]. Joe is referred to at various places in Dickens's novel as "a fat and red-faced boy in a state of somnolency," a "Young Dropsy," a "Young Opium-Eater," and "Young Boa Constrictor."

Joe was a servant to Mr. Wardle. The following passage describes his sleepiness and obesity:

> A most violent and startling knocking was heard at the door; it was not an ordinary double knock, but a constant and uninterrupted succession of the loudest single raps, as if the knocker were endowed with the perpetual motion, or the person outside had forgotten to leave off.
>
> Mr. Lowton hurried to the door...The object that presented itself to the eyes of the astonished clerk was a boy—a wonderfully fat boy—standing upright on the mat, with his eyes closed as if in sleep. He had never seen such a fat boy, in or out of a traveling caravan; and this, coupled with the utter calmness and repose of his appearance, so very different from what was reasonably to have been expected of the inflicter of such knocks, smote him with wonder.
>
> "What's the matter?" inquired the clerk.
>
> The extraordinary boy replied not a word; but he nodded once, and seemed, to the clerk's imagination, to snore feebly.
>
> "Where do you come from?" inquired the clerk.
>
> The boy made no sign. He breathed heavily, but in all other respects was motionless.
>
> The clerk repeated the question thrice, and receiving no answer, prepared to shut the door, when the boy suddenly

> opened his eyes, winked several times, sneezed once, and raised his hand as if to repeat the knocking. Finding the door open, he stared about him with astonishment, and at length fixed his eyes on Mr. Lowton's face.
>
> "What the devil do you knock in that way for?" inquired the clerk, angrily.
>
> "Which way?" said the boy, in a slow, sleepy voice.
>
> "Why, like forty hackney-coachmen," replied the clerk.
>
> "Because master said I wasn't to leave off knocking till they opened the door, for fear I should go to sleep," said the boy[7].

Introduction into medical circles of the name Pickwick and its association with the syndrome of obesity and daytime somnolence can be traced back to a remark by Christopher Heath in 1889[9]. It occurred during the discussion of a patient that had been presented to the Clinical Society, a society of clinicians, by Dr. Richard Caton (1842-1926)[9]. Dr. Heath, the president of the Clinical Society, alluded to the classical case of Joe, the fat boy in *The Pickwick Papers*[7]. More than twenty years later, Sir Byron Bramwell (1847-1931) published another case of a seventeen-year-old fat boy and said, "He (the patient) presents in a minor degree a condition similar to the Fat Boy in *Pickwick*—whenever he sits down he seems to go to sleep"[4].

Whether the term "Pickwickian Syndrome" should be applied to the clinical features ascribed to Joe by Charles Dickens has generated considerable literary and medical controversy[9-17]. Julius Comroe (1911-1984), a noted heart specialist, for example, points out that the term "Pickwickian" has been applied inappropriately to describe the clinical syndrome of obesity, daytime somnolence, and hypoventilation[10]. In the concluding remarks in his paper, Comroe says, "Someone once wrote: 'Scientists who introduce new terminology should, by law, be required to post a $1,000 bond, to be forfeited if the terminology is both misleading and used.'" To quote Comroe again[10], "Scientists who are painfully wounded by scientific errors that find their way into medical journals, actually seem to be amused—even delighted—by literary errors that happily accept and perpetuate them."

The use of the "Pickwickian" term is described by Keelan as "errored terminology of scientific expression...compounded by errors both literary and scientific"[11]. James and associates[18] call the Pickwickian Syndrome a "charming sobriquet more justified by poetic license than by literary history," but then go right ahead and title their paper, "Pickwickian Syndrome." Says Comroe, "I believe that dubbing 'the fat boy' a Pickwickian, is much like calling the transformation of Lot's wife into a pillar of salt the 'biblical syndrome' because she was a minor character who appeared in a well-known book called 'The Bible.'"

Fashions in terminology for describing diseases and indeed the meaning of diseases themselves have changed over time. Efforts at classification can be traced back at least as far as Aristotle in the fourth-century B.C.[19]. Following his successful development of the binomial genus and species classification of plants and animals[20], Carl von Linne (1707-1778) who was also a physician, developed a classification system for "disease" which divided them into classes[21]. One major problem for this brilliant eighteenth-century innovator was the difficulty of separating symptoms of a disease from the disease itself. This difficulty reached its extreme in the system of Sauvages, who enumerated 2,400 different kinds of diseases[22]. He started with 10 classes, a number similar to Linne but then expanded to 40 orders and 78 genera for the final division into 2,400 species of "disease"[22]. William Cullen (1710-1790)[23], professor of medicine in Edinburgh during the late eighteenth-century when the medical school and university were among the most prestigious in the world, produced significant improvement in a less extensive classification using only four classes.

The term *polysarka* used by Russell in his paper to describe obesity is also the term used by Sauvages[22] and by Cullen[23] for obesity[24]. *Polysarka* was replaced by *corpulence* or *obesity* during the first half of the nineteenth century. With the increase in post-mortem examination of patients[25] and improved diagnostic techniques in the nineteenth century, classification of diseases changed to introduce more descriptive terms. It also helped make the distinction between symptoms that the patient has and the disease that is causing them clearer. Eponyms associating an individual's name with clinical symptoms of disease have been common in the nineteenth and twentieth-centuries. These eponyms often reflected astute clinical observations, as in Addison's disease, a disease of the adrenal glands, or Frohlich's syndrome, the syndrome of obesity associated with damage to the hypothalamic portion of the brain.

Charles Dickens, although not a physician, was an astute observer of diseased individuals and accurately described at least two other clinical conditions. His description of the association of somnolence, obesity, snoring, and a ruddy face also accurately reflected many features of the obesity-sleep apnea syndrome. Referring to this syndrome as the "Dickens' Pickwickian fat boy syndrome" would, in my view, be entirely appropriate, and in this respect I agree with Eugene Robin, a lung specialist from Stanford University who suggested this name[26].

In his review of historical accounts of the sleep apnea syndrome, Lavie[13] attributes the first description of what we call today "mixed sleep apnea" to Broadbent in 1877[27]. A second early clinical report from 1889 by Caton[9] described a thirty-seven-year-old poulterer who complained of intense drowsiness, appearing at the time of weight gain. A third report in 1889 by Morison[5] reported on a sixty-three-year-old obese man who had suffered from drowsiness that became increasingly more severe. The earlier case by Russell[3] and the one described by Wadd[28] antedate all of these. The patient in Russell's report was a forty-five-year-old woman who for two years had been exceedingly drowsy. Quoting Russell, "To such an extent had this been the case, that she had been afraid to sit near the fire; and, whilst, attending as an outpatient, she requested to be dismissed speedily, lest she should fall asleep in the hall"[3]. In addition to being a very corpulent woman, her face was described as

> injected with dark blood, and she stated that the lividity was often intense; the jugulars were not distended. Her urine was loaded with albumen and presented a large number of hyaline and waxy casts, small and of full size. She continued to attend as an out-patient for some weeks, and then was admitted into the hospital. At this time she was very dull and torpid; her face was completely livid. There was oedema but not copious anasarca of the trunk and lower extremities. Yet, she was able to lie down easily and presented no important symptoms of chest disturbance.[3]

The case reported by Wadd in his 1810 and 1816 editions may antedate even the one by Russell:

> A country tradesman, aged about thirty, of a short stature, and naturally of a fresh sanguine complexion, and very fat, applied to me for assistance. He complained of perpetual drowsiness and inactivity; his countenance was almost livid, and such a degree of somnolency attended him, that he could scarce keep awake whilst he described his situation. In other respects he was well[28].
>
> Elizabeth Stuart who died at Cambridge on the 28th of March 1807, aged 44, weighed twenty-three stone (146 kg or 322 lb). She was inclined to be corpulent from her infancy; lived a regular inactive and indolent life. A few years before her death she had a severe illness, occasioned by an inflammation in her limbs, of which she afterwards perfectly recovered. She was of a cheerful disposition, but so little inclined to move, that the only mode by which she could be induced to get from bed, was by drawing her and the feather bed on to the floor, and then it required the aid of three strong men to place her in a chair, in which she was wheeled to the fire place. An attempt was three times made to bleed her on account of a drowsiness, but each time it

> was found impossible to open a vein, from the quantity of fat surrounding it. Her diet was chiefly vegetables and pastry; but she was constantly drinking milk and water, consuming above a gallon in the course of each night, which she voided almost as soon as drank, never sleeping more than three quarters of an hour from this distressing interruption. Her death was sudden. The sleeves of her gown measured three feet in circumference[29].

There is no notation of snoring in the case report by Russell, nor in the ones from Wadd. Figure 23-2 is an etching of one of Wadd's somnulent patients.

The fourth report is that of extreme obesity associated with alveolar hypoventilation, a case of the Dickens's Pickwickian Fat Boy Syndrome. Although the term Pickwickian had been used by Osler long before Burwell[6], it was the paper of Burwell and his colleagues that tied the description of the fat boy Joe in The Pickwick Papers to the syndrome of obesity and hypoventilation. Clinically, there appear to be two syndromes of hypoventilation and obesity. The first is the syndrome of sleep apnea with airway obstruction, which appears to be worsened by the presence of obesity[30]. For these individuals, obstructive sleep apnea at night leads to many interruptions of sleep, with somnolence appearing during the day as a way to trying to make up for the lost sleep[31]. A second syndrome of hypoventilation does not appear to involve obstructive sleep apnea but is rather hypoventilation without obstruction which is not improved by weight loss.

The relationship of obesity to somnolence has a long history which is nicely described by Kryger[12,32] in two reviews. Dionysius, the tyrant of Heracleia of Pontus who reigned about 360 B.C., is one of the first historical figures afflicted with obesity and somnolence. This enormously fat man frequently fell asleep. As a way of awakening him, servants used long needles which were inserted through his skin and fat to awaken him when he fell asleep. Kryger cites a second case of Magas, King of Cyrene, who died in 258 B.C. He was a man "weighted down with monstrous masses of flesh in his last days; in fact he choked himself to death." Each of these individuals might be entitled to the eponym associated with obesity hypoventilation and sonmolence.

For me, Dickens's Pickwickian Fat Boy Syndrome is as appropriate as any, and I will continue to use it.

Biosketch

James Russell, M.D., (1818-1885) was the son of a Birmingham surgeon who received his medical training at King's College, London.

He was a physician at the Birmingham General Hospital from 1859 to 1884, and he was largely responsible for amalgamation of the Queen's College with Sydenham College. He was elected chairman of the local medical societies and president of the Birmingham Medical Institute. He was described as a liberal and a nonconformist[33].

Biosketch

Richard Caton, M.D, (1842-1926) was educated at Edinburgh University where his interests in neurology and brain function developed under the tutelage of Sir David Ferrier.

He moved from Edinburgh to Liverpool where he began his studies on the electrical properties of nerve and brain. Using rabbits and monkeys as subjects, he made recordings with new nonpolarizable electrodes and showed the presence of feeble electrical potentials which varied with the degree of alertness and were abolished by anesthesia. His work was initially presented at a meeting of the British Medical Association in 1874 in Edinburgh and subsequently at the Ninth International Medical Congress held in Washington, D.C., in 1887. This was the beginning of electroencephalography, but its beginnings were largely ignored. No work on the EEG appeared in the United States until after the first quarter of the twentieth-century[34]. In 1891 Caton resigned his professorship of physiology in Liverpool and subsequently became Lord Mayor of Liverpool in 1907. He is one of a number of famous scientists including Newton and Virchow who have taken up important political positions later in life. Caton died in 1926 before the first publication about EEGs had even appeared in the United States[35].

Biosketch

Sir Byron Bramwell (1847-1931) (Figure 23-3) was the son of a physician. Following his education at Edinburgh University, he became the house surgeon to the professor of surgery who is alleged to have "advised him to write as much as he could in order to become known."

This advice has often been repeated and is aptly summarized by the phrase "publish or perish." Bramwell published. Following an interval in medical practice with his father, Bramwell returned to Edinburgh as lecturer in the Extramural School of the Royal College of Physicians and Surgeons. His published work dealt largely with neurology. In 1882 Bramwell was appointed pathologist at the Edinburgh Royal Infirmary, and in 1897 he became a full physician. His clinical skills "in harvesting facts and reaching clinicopathological correlations" is demonstrated in the paper reported here. He died in 1931[36].

Biosketch

Charles Sidney Burwell (1893-1967) (Figure 23-4) was a graduate of the Harvard Medical School class of 1919. Following completion of his house staff training at the Massachusetts General Hospital, he was instructor at Johns Hopkins Medical School from 1921-1922 and an associate in medicine until

1924 when he moved to Vanderbilt University. In 1935 Burwell was appointed dean of the Harvard School of Medicine, and after relinquishing this position following World War II, he returned to head the pulmonary group at the Peter Bent Brigham Hospital where the work on Dickens's Pickwickian Fat Boy Syndrome was published[37,38].

References

1. Shakespeare, W. *Romeo and Juliet.* II.ii.43-44.
2. Flemyng, M. *A Discourse on the Nature, Causes and Cure of Corpulency. Illustrated by a Remarkable Case, Read before the Royal Society, November 1757 and Now First Published.* London: L. Davis and C. Reymers, 1760.
3. Russell, J. "A Case of Polysarka, in Which Death Resulted from Deficient Arterialisation of the Blood." *Br Med J.* (1866): 220-221.
4. Bramwell, B. "Case XXII Excessive Sleepiness." *Clinical Studies: A Quarterly Journal of Clinical Medicine.* Edinburgh: R&R Clark-Ltd, 1910.
5. Morison, A. "Somnolence with Cyanosis Cured by Massage." *Practitioner.* 442(1889): 277-281.
6. Burwell, C.S., E.D. Robin, R.D. Whaley, A.G. Bickelmann. "Extreme Obesity Associated with Alveolar Hypoventilation—a Pickwickian Syndrome." *Am J Med.* 21(1956): 811-818.
7. Dickens, C. *The Posthumous Papers of the Pickwick Club.* London: Chapman and Halt, 1837.
8. Waugh, A. "The Fat Boy." In *A Pickwick Portrait Gallery.* New York: Charles Scribner's Sons, 1936.
9. Caton, R. Clinical Society of London. "Narcolepsy." *Br Med J.* (1889): 358-359.
10. Comroe, J.H. Jr. "Frankenstein, Pickwick, and Ondine." *Am Rev Respir Dis.* 111(1975): 689-692.
11. Keelan, P. "Of Pickwick and Ondine." *Irish Med J.* 74(1991): 339-340.
12. Kryger, M.H. "Fat, Sleep and Charles Dickens: Literacy and Medical Contributions to the Understanding of Sleep Apnea." *Clin Chest Med.* 6(1985): 555-562.
13. Lavie, P. "Nothing New Under the Moon: Historical Accounts of Sleep Apnea Syndrome." *Arch Intern Med.* 144(1984): 2025-2028.
14. Markel, H. "Charles Dickens and the Art of Medicine." *Ann Intern Med.* 101(1984): 408-411.
15. Millman, R.P. "Did the Fat Boy Snore? Editorial." *Chest.* 89(1986): 621-622.
16. Phillipson, E.A. "Pickwickian, Obesity-Hypoventilation, or Fee-Fi-Fo-Fum Syndrome? Editorial." *Am Rev Resp Dis.* 121(1980): 781-782.
17. Vaisrub, S. "Pickwickian Syndrome? The Dickens!" *JAMA.* 239(1978): 645.
18. Jame, T.N., B. Frame, E.O. Coates. "*De subitaneis mortibus.* 3. Pickwickian syndrome." *Circulation.* No. 48 6(1973): 1311-1320.
19. King, L.S. *The Medical World of the Eighteenth Century.* Huntington, NY: Robert E. Krieger Publishing Co., Inc, 1971.

20. Linne, C.V. *Systema naturae.* Lugduni Batavorurn. apud Theodorum Haak, 1735.
21. Linne, C.V. *Genera Morborum sistens morborum classes, genera et species.* Amstelodami: Fratrum de Tourmesr, 1763.
22. Sauvages, F.B. *Nosologia methodica sistens morborum classes juxta Sydenhami menten and botanicorum ordinem.* Amstelodami: Fratrum de Tournes, 1768.
23. Cullen, W. *The Works of William Cullen.* Edinburgh, 1827.
24. Bray, G.A. "Obesity: Historical Development of Scientific and Cultural Ideas." *Int J Obes.* 14(1990): 909-926.
25. Long, E.R. *A History of Pathology.* Baltimore: Williams and Wilkins, 1928.
26. Robin, E.D. "Of Sleep and Seals and Many Things: Pickwickians—1978." *West J Med.* No.129 5(1978): 419-421.
27. Broadbent, W.H. "Cheyne-Stokes' Respiration in Cerebral Haemorhage." *Lancet.* (1977): 307-309.
28. Wadd, W. *Cursory Remarks on Corpulence: By a Member of the Royal College of Surgeons.* London: 1810.
29. Wadd, W. *On Corpulence; Or Obesity Considered as a Disease. With a Critical Examination of Ancient and Modern Opinions, Relative to Its Causes and Cure. Third Edition, Containing a reference to the most remarkable cases that have occurred in this country.* London: J. Callow, 1816.
30. Auchincloss, J.H., E. Cook, A.D. Renzetti. "Clinical and Physiological Aspects of a Case of Obesity, Polycythemia and Hypoventilation." *J. Clin Invest.* 34(1995): 1537-1545.
31. Gastart, H, C. A. Tassarini, B. Duron. "Polygraphic Study of the Episodic Diurnal and Nocturnal Manifestations of the Pickwick Syndrome." *Brain Res.* 2(1966): 167-186.
32. Kryger, M.H. "Sleep Apnea: From the Needles of Dionysius to Continuous Positive Airway Pressure." *Arch Intern Med.* 143(1983): 2301-2303.
33. Brown, G.H. *Munk's Rolls: Lives of the Fellows of the Royal College of Physicians of London.* 1826-1925. London: The College, 1955.
34. Brazier, M.A.B. *A History, of Neurophysiology in the 19th Century.* New York: Raven Press, 1987.
35. Schoenberg, B.S. "Richard Caton and the Electrical Activity of the Brain." *Mayo Clinic Proc.* 49(1974): 474-481.
36. Ashworth, B. "The Bramwells and Neurology in Edinburgh." *Scott Med J.* 26(1981): 364-370.
37. Eppinger, E.C. "Memorial. Charles Sidney Burwell, M.D." *Trans of the Clin Climatol Assoc.* 79(1968): 1-11.
38. Harvard Editorial Department. "A New Dean at Harvard." *N Engl J Med.* 212(1935): 451.

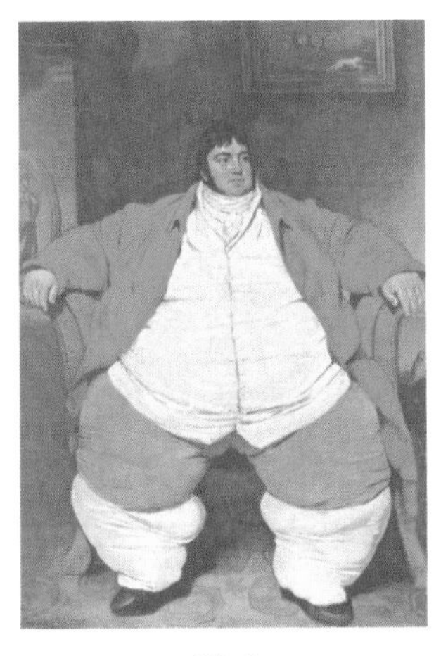

20-1

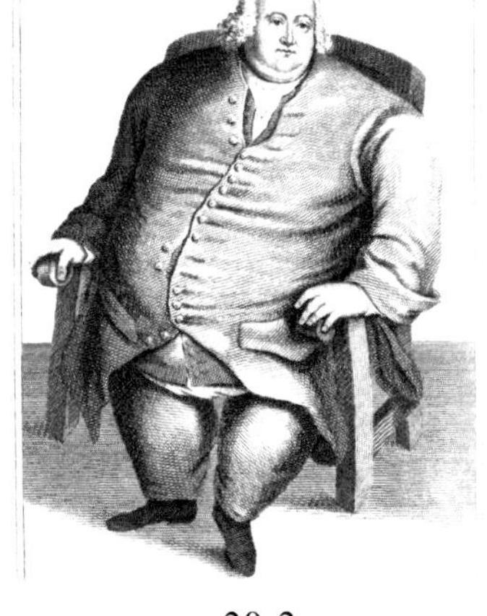

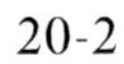

20-2

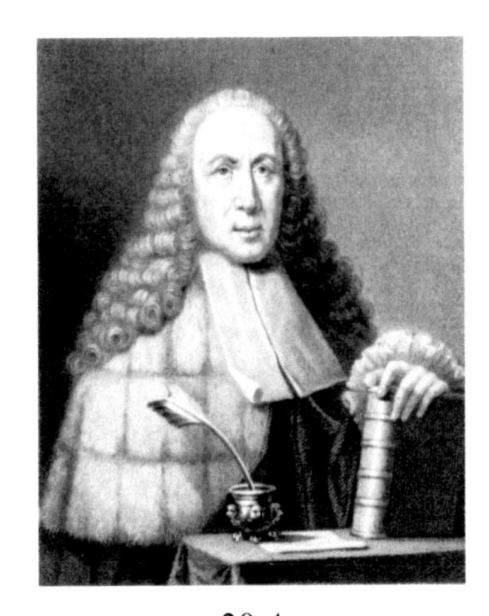

20-4

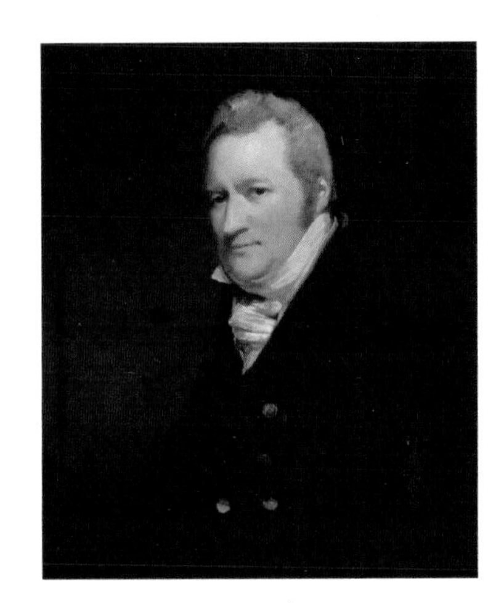

20-5

20-1 Daniel Lambert the Great, who died in 1839 weighing 739 lbs. From the collection of the author.

20-2 Edward Bright of Malden in Essex. From the collection of the author.

20-4 Giovanni Battista Morgagni (1682-1771). Courtesy of the National Library of Medicine.

20-5 William Wadd. From the Royal College of Surgeons.

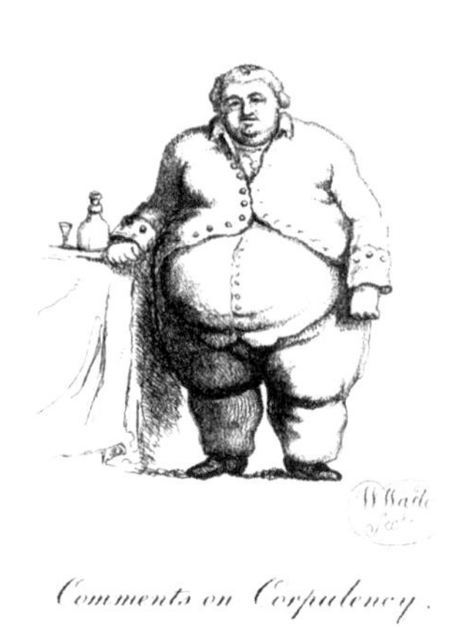

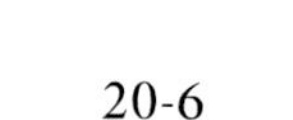

20-6

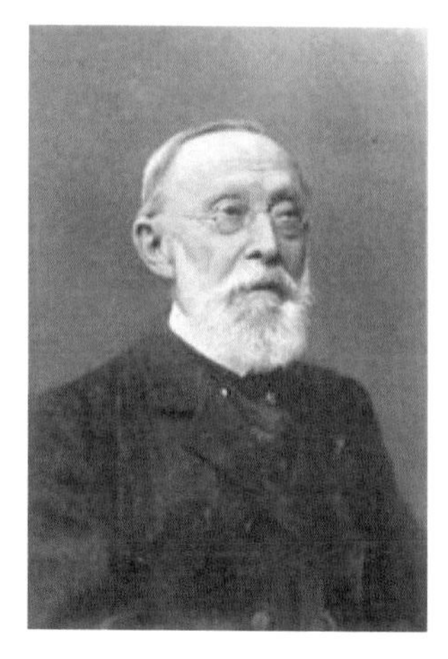

20-7

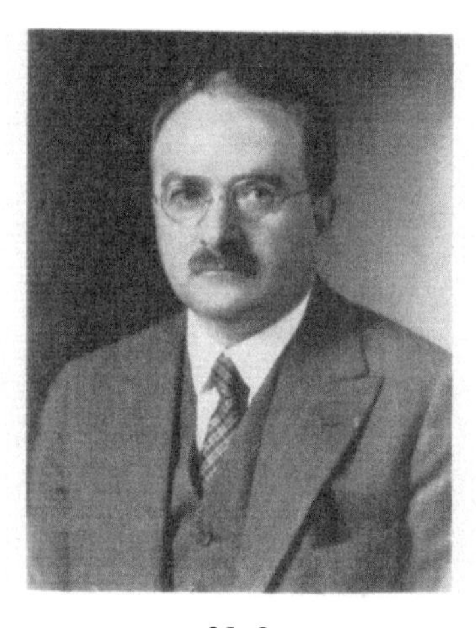

21-2

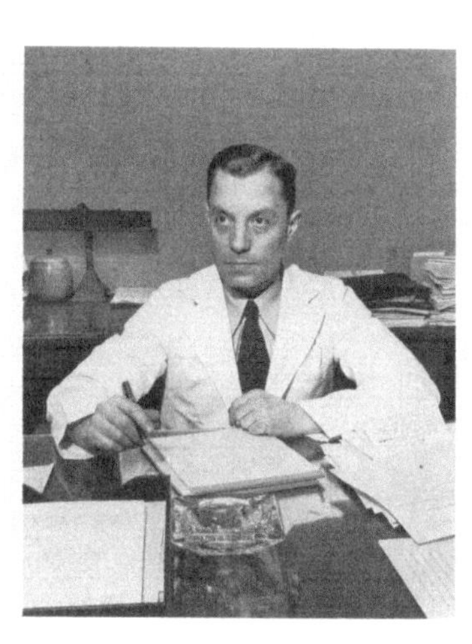

21-3

20-6 An etching from Dr. Wadd's monograph. From the collection of the author.

20-7 Rudolf Virchow (1821-1902). Courtesy of the National Library of Medicine.

21-2 Louis Dublin (1882-1969). Courtesy of MetLife Archives.

21-3 Ancel Keys (1904-2004). Courtesy of the Ancel Keys Collection of the University of Minnesota.

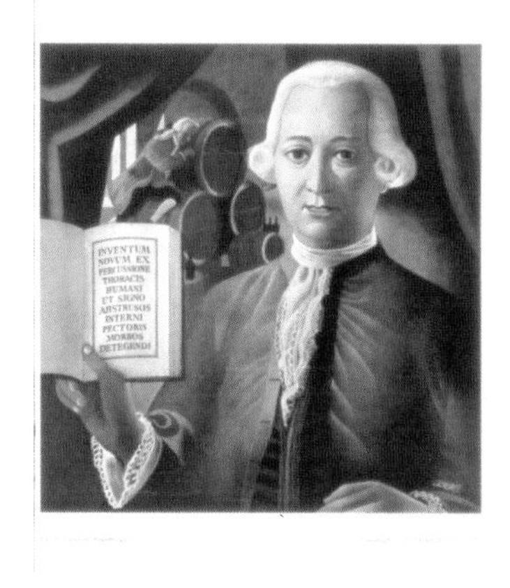

22-1

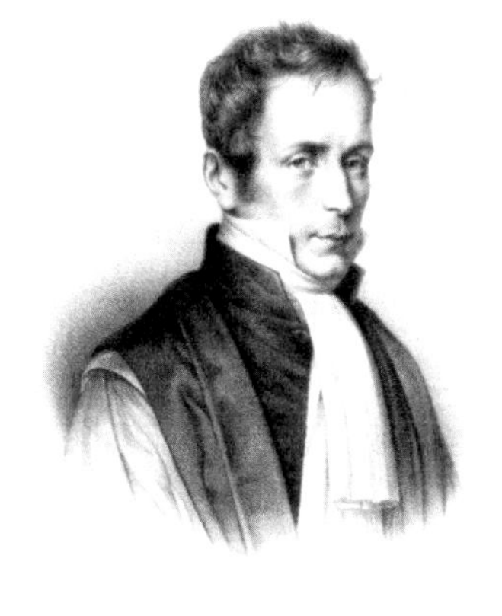

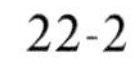

22-2

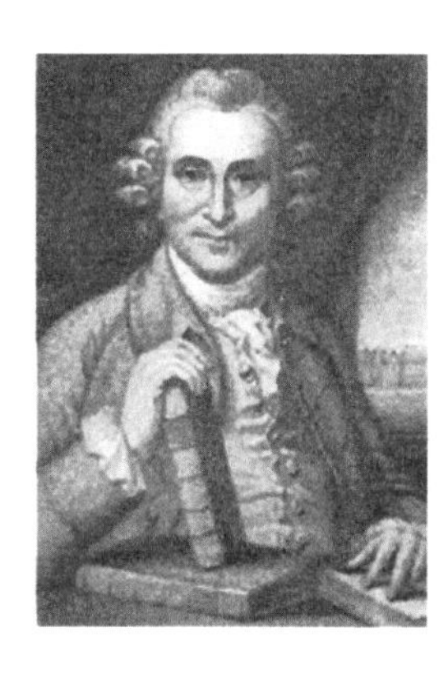

22-3

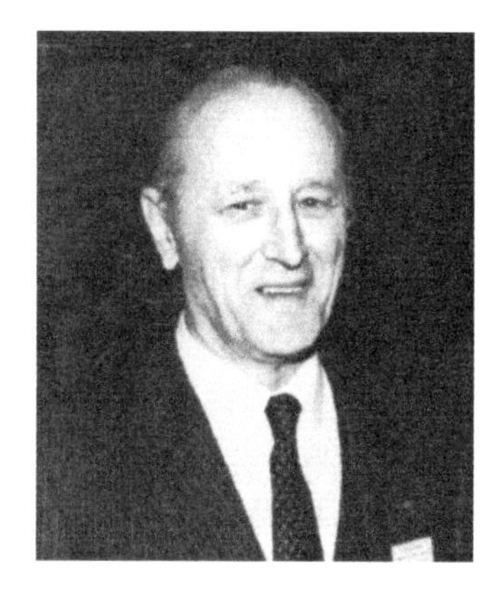

22-4

22-1 Leopold Auenbrugger (1722-1809). Courtesy of the National Library of Medicine.

22-2 René-Théophile-Hyacinthe Laennec (1781-1826). Courtesy of the National Library of Medicine.

22-3 James Lind (1716-1794). Courtesy of The Journal of the Royal Naval Medical Service—Vol. XIII (1927).

22-4 Jean Vague (1911-2002). From the collection of the author.

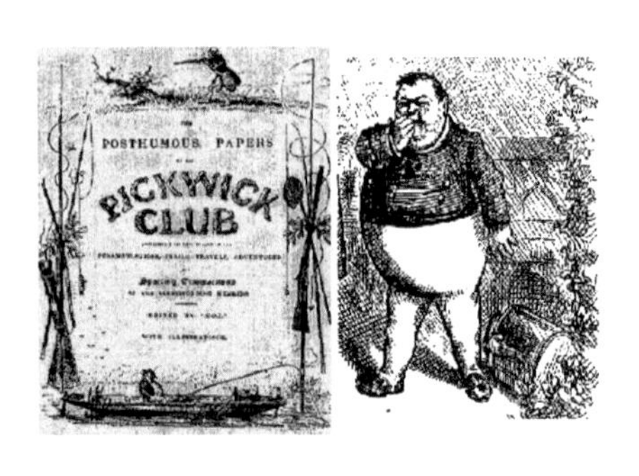

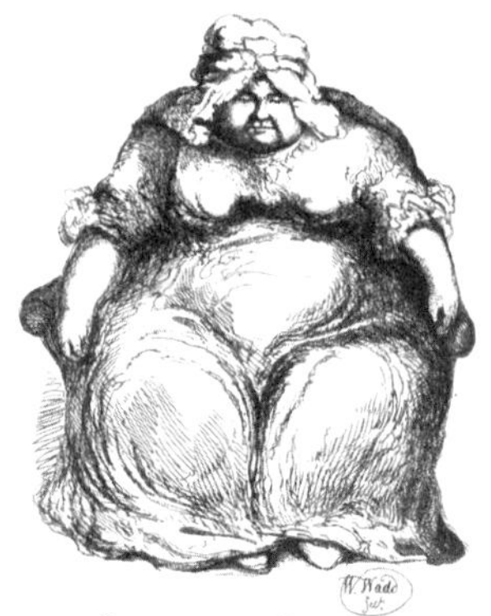

23-1

23-2

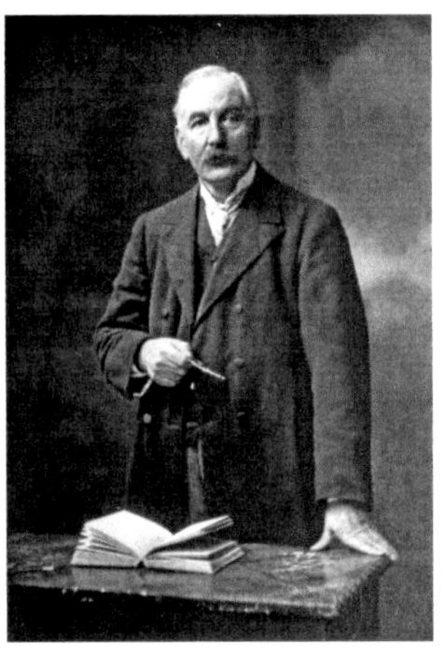

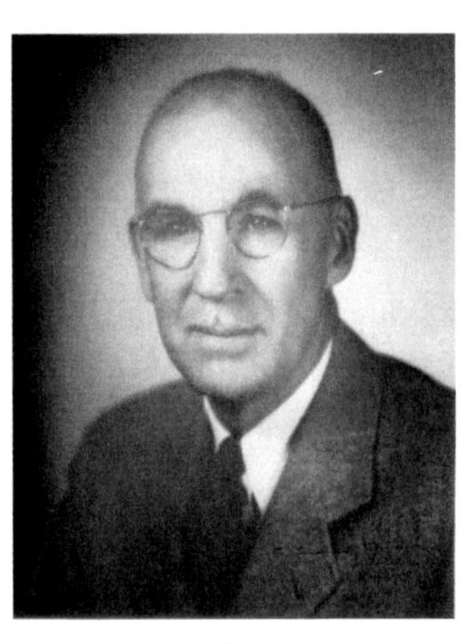

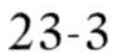

23-3

23-4

23-1 "... and on the box sat a fat and red-faced boy, in a state of somnolency...the fat boy rose, opened his eyes, swallowed a huge piece of pie he had been in the act of masticating when he fell asleep..." *The posthumous paper of the Pickwick Club, Charles Dickens 1836*

23-2 Snoring subject from "Comments on Corpulency. Lineaments of Leanness Mems on Diet and Dietetics" by William Wadd (1829). From the collection of the author.

23-3 Sir Byron Bramwell (1847-1931). Courtesy of the National Library of Medicine.

23-4 Charles Sidney Burwell (1893-1967). Courtesy of the National Library of Medicine.

Chapter 24

Reflections on a Syndrome: Laurence, Moon, Bardet, and Biedl

Dans les champs de l'observation
Le hasard favorise que les ésprit preparée
[In the field of observation
Chance favors the prepared mind]

—Pasteur[1]

Experiments of nature often lead to new truths. For medicine, these come in the form of unusual clinical diseases or syndromes that may provide important insights into the way the body works. This has been demonstrated over and over again. Several such experiments of nature have provided new ideas about the battle of the bulge. Understanding these experiments of nature can be facilitated by new techniques. In this chapter, I will describe an experiment of nature whose description became possible with a new medical instrument—the ophthalmoscope that allows the doctor to see the back of the eye clearly. The new disease involves obesity, short stature, and an eye disease called *retinitis pigmentosa* which is detected as blackening of the usually red retinal color. This disease is a leading cause of human blindness. This syndrome was initially described by two doctors, John Zachariah Laurence (1829-1870) and Robert Moon (1844-1914). Dr. Laurence was a leading ophthalmologist in the last half of the nineteenth-century; the other author was a young physician. Laurence and Moon reported on four cases of *retinitis pigmentosa* that occurred in the same family and was accompanied by what they called "general imperfections" in development[2]. This paper reports on four out of eight siblings who had a rare type of kidney disease and who were short for their age. The three males showed significant delay in sexual development, called hypogenitalism. None of the children had extra fingers (polydactyly) and there was no apparent intermarriage or consanguinity in the family. However, since it appeared that four of the eight children were affected, it was suggestive that each parent must have had one defect or allele for the gene that produces this syndrome. Since they were the first to describe the collection of findings, the syndrome was called the Laurence-Moon syndrome.

At the time this paper was published, Laurence was in the prime of his professional career and Moon was a young physician. The description of the changes in the eye (retina) in the publication by Laurence and Moon was made possible by using the ophthalmoscope. This instrument was one of the many "brain children" of Hermann von Helmholtz (see Biosketch in Chapter 11) (1821-1894). He published his description of this instrument in 1851[3] and with it went on to develop a solid theory of vision that he published as a book in 1867 on physiological optics[4,5]. In describing his discovery many years later, Helmholtz said:

> A teacher in a university is subject to excellent discipline, in that he is obliged each year not only to give at least an outline of the whole of his science, but also to convince and satisfy the clear heads among his hearers, some of whom will be the great men of the next generation. This necessity was most beneficial to myself. In preparing my lectures, I was led to devise the method of measuring the velocity of the nervous impulse, and also to the conception of the ophthalmoscope...I was endeavoring to explain to my pupils the emission of reflected light from the eye...I turned the problem over and over to ascertain the simplest way in which I could demonstrate the phenomenon to my students. The first model was constructed of paste-board, eye lenses and cover glasses used in the microscopic work. It was at first so difficult to use, that I doubt if I should have persevered, unless I had felt that it must succeed; but in eight days I had the great joy of being the first who saw before him a living human retina[6].

It was with this instrument that Laurence and Moon described the eye changes of *retinitis pigmentosa* that characterized this hereditary syndrome. The reflections of light from the eye were the stimulus for the discovery by Helmholtz who in turn provided the instrument, allowing these reflections to be examined in detail. This development by Helmholtz and the rapid progress in understanding vision and ways of treating it led to ophthalmology becoming one of the first subspecialty areas of medicine.

The observations of Laurence and Moon were "rediscovered" more than half a century later when two other papers reawakened the field. In his doctoral thesis, the young French physician Bardet[7] begins with a general discussion of obesity and its features. He then presents the details of his patient, Ms. Odette P., an eleven-year-old girl who is an example of infantile obesity associated with too many toes or hexadactyly of the right foot and *retinitis pigmentosa* in the eyes of this child who was obese from birth.

Following the detailed presentation of the syndrome, Bardet then collected eight other cases published in medical journals that were similar to his. He also discussed the much larger literature on hypothalamic obesity and pointed out the differences.

Bardet had the "prepared mind" to which Louis Pasteur (1822-1895)[1], the great French scientist and developer of the germ theory, alluded in the quote at the beginning of this chapter. Bardet was confronted with clinical findings. He was astute enough to recognize that there were features in this case such as too many toes (hexadactyly) and a peculiar eye disease called *retinitis pigmentosa* that did not fit with the other cases of hypothalamic obesity, such as those described by Joseph F.F. Babinski (1857-1932)[8] and by Frohlich (1871-1953)[9]. In this sense he was like the great neurosurgeon Harvey Cushing (1869-1939)[10,11], who unraveled the role of the basophilic adenoma of the pituitary gland as the cause of the symptom complex of obesity that now bears his name. (See Chapter 26)

Although Bardet[7] recognized the triad (obesity, polydactyly, and *retinitis pigmentosa*) that forms the basis of this syndrome, he explained it by reference to the pituitary. The normal size of the pituitary gland that was observed using x-rays of the skull of his patient did not dissuade him from arguing that this syndrome was due to a lesion in the posterior part of the pituitary gland. Pituitary obesity of the adiposo-genital type described by Babinski[8] and Frolich[9] was well recognized and much over diagnosed. At the time Bardet published his paper, the fact that "pituitary obesity" was not actually due to damage to the pituitary but to injury in the hypothalamic region of the brain had not yet been demonstrated conclusively. Cushing had published his classic monograph on the pituitary at the time that Bardet was in his impressionable years of training. He thus made the best argument he could that the posterior pituitary gland was involved as a cause of the syndrome in his patient. All of us are creatures of our times, and, although Bardet did recognize the unique features of his patient, the interpretation was in the "traditional" framework.

The short scientific paper by Arthur Biedl (1869-1933)[12] reported two children who were siblings and both of whom had congenital deformations, eye disease described as *retinitis pigmentosa*, an extra finger (called polydactyly), and an intellectual slowness or torpidity. There were no signs by x-ray of alteration in the pituitary gland or brain nor were there any characteristic signs of an obstruction of development of the brain. In spite of this, Biedl argued that the pathogenesis of this syndrome would lie in a disturbance somewhere between the brain and the pituitary. These cases in siblings were thought to be an unusual variety of adiposo-genital syndrome, although there was no evidence of pressure at the base of the brain (hypothalamus) or other symptoms.

Neither the thesis by Bardet[7] nor the brief case report by Biedl[12], one of the foremost endocrinologists of the early twentieth-century[13], referred to the earlier case report by Laurence and Moon[2], which had come from the ophthalmological literature in a journal that had ceased publication after its third year, a not uncommon problem[14].

With the stature of Biedl behind it, the syndrome gradually came to be recognized. Rony[15], in the first American book devoted solely to obesity, referred to it as the Laurence-Biedl syndrome and gave a rather complete review of the literature on this syndrome:

> The complete syndrome consists of obesity, retinal degeneration, mental retardation, polydactyly, stunted growth and hypogenitalism. In incomplete or atypical forms any or all of the last named four signs may be missing. In some cases other skeletal anomalies than polydactyly are present; retinal degeneration may appear in the form of typical retinitis pigmentosa. In most cases the obesity shows no special types of fat distribution. It is a rare disease; Reilly and Lisser found altogether 73 cases reported in the literature. According to Cockayne, Krestin and Sorsby, the syndrome is inherited as a recessive mutation of a single gene causing the skeletal defects as well as the retinal and diencephalic change. J. Bauer believed that polydactyly is transmitted as a dominant factor, independently from the retino-diencephalic process which is recessive. The histological character of the pathological process supposed to be located in the hypothalamus or hypophysis is not known as no case has come to autopsy[15].

The small book on obesity authored by Rynearson and Gastineau[16] and published shortly after World War II is one of the very nice books about obesity. In their book, the syndrome we are discussing was called the Laurence-Moon-Biedl Syndrome, even though the two clinical pictures are somewhat different. This is also the name used by several other authors over the next two decades[17,18]. Rynearson and Gastineau described the Laurence-Moon-Biedl syndrome thus:

> This [syndrome] consists of (1) mental deficiency, (2) retinitis pigmentosa, (3) hypogenitalism, (4) obesity and (5) polydactyly. It appears to be inherited in a recessive

> manner. This syndrome was first described by Laurence and Moon in 1866 and interest in it was reawakened by reports of several cases by Bardet in 1920 and by Biedl in 1922. Biedl suggested that the syndrome could be described as a dystrophia adiposogenitalis of cerebral origin. He considered that the pituitary played no part in the manifestations of the condition, but more recently a somewhat tenuous and complicated theory, which involves the concept that hypopituitarism is followed by hyperpituitarism, and has been proposed by Jason and Curbelo...An important observation by these workers is that the obesity does not appear until after one month of age...In summary, it can be said that the Laurence-Moon-Biedl syndrome does not appear to be endocrine in origin, that it is an ill-defined and poorly understood entity and that no proof has been advanced that the obesity results from any factor other than a large appetite and decreased activity. What may cause the increased intake of food is not known[16].

By the time I wrote my book titled *The Obese Patient* in 1976[19], all four authors were lumped into the same syndrome as the Laurence-Moon-Bardet-Biedl Syndrome. By this time a large number of families, each with many affected children, had been described and the unity of the syndrome began to splinter. In 1934 Biemond described four generations in which there was a syndrome of unusual eye findings (coloboma), and increased number of fingers or toes on the hand or foot (polydactyly), mental retardation, a female or gynoid type of obesity, and sexual immaturity due to gonadal hypotrophy[19,20]. In 1954 Alstrom described another syndrome with eye problems (retinal degeneration), a female or gynoid type of obesity, diabetes mellitus, deafness due to nerve problems, and sexual immaturity (hypogonadotrophic hypogonadism)[21].

The Laurence-Moon-Bardet-Biedl Syndrome includes five central features: a specific eye problem called retinal degeneration, obesity, mental deficiency, extra fingers or toes (polydactyly), and sexual immaturity called hypogenitalism. In 1866 Laurence and Moon[2] described four patients with this syndrome. Bardet noted the polydactyly[7] in 1920 and Biedl[12] demonstrated the familial occurrence in 1922. In addition to these major features, clinical findings of congenital heart disease, rapid eye movements (strabismus), and kidney disease may be detected.

In a review of this syndrome in 1958, Bell[22] collected 368 families or pedigrees from the literature and found parental intermarriage or consanguinity in 23.4%. Among 26 pedigrees (38 sibsips) in Switzerland, Klein and Ammann[23] found consanguinity in 52.6%. In Israel consanguinity was present in 50%. Decreased visual acuity at school age is frequently the first sign of this disease, but it may be preceded by night blindness. The eye disease (pigmentary retinopathy) is typical in only 18.7% of the Swiss cases. Whether typical or atypical, vision steadily deteriorated and most patients were blind by age thirty.

Sexual immaturity with inadequately developed sexual organs or hypogenitalism is more common in men than in women. There are reports of women with LMBB Syndrome having children but no reports of men being fathers. Small testes, feminine hair distribution, and occasionally formation of breast tissue (gynecomastia) have been described in the males. Increased numbers of fingers or toes, called polydactylism, is usually manifested as an extra digit on the hypothenar (cubital) side. It may occur on any extremity and all four were involved in 26.3%. Syndactyly, or fusion between pairs of fingers or toes, is less frequent. The fifth cardinal feature is mental retardation, which is present in over 70%; it is generally a mild feeble-mindedness. The obesity usually appears in childhood and is progressive. It is present in 88.8% of the men and 93.8% of the women reviewed by Bell[22]. In well over half of the patients, body weight was more than three standard deviations above normal, and in one patient body weight was over 200 kg (440 lbs.).

Although the Laurence-Moon and Bardet-Biedl syndromes are often considered together, they are probably distinctly different diseases. The four patients reported by Laurence and Moon had eye disease (retinal degeneration), mental retardation, hypogenitalism, and a neurologic defect characterized as difficulty moving the legs (spastic paraplegia), but without obesity or extra fingers or toes.

The case of Bardet and the two cases of Biedl described a syndrome consisting of eye disease (*retinitis pigmentosa*), obesity, extra fingers or toes (polydactyly), sexually immature reproductive organs (genital hypoplasia), mental retardation, and anal atresia. There subsequently have been more than five hundred cases that fit into this group of findings. Although both syndromes are inherited, they have a number of important differences. Both are inherited as autosomal recessive traits, meaning both parents have one copy of the defective gene. The eye disease (pigmentary retinopathy) is present in the Laurence-Moon syndrome, but a different type of eye disease (tapetoretinal degeneration) occurs in the Bardet-Biedl Syndrome. Obesity, which is an almost uniform feature of the Bardet-Biedl syndrome, is uncommon in the Laurence-Moon syndrome. In addition the Bardet-Biedl syndrome may be associated with congenital heart disease and kidney disease, which has been reported to be as high as 71% in one autopsy series.

The original identification of the Laurence-Moon syndrome depended on the invention of the ophthalmoscope by Helmholtz. Further advances in subdivision of this syndrome have relied mainly on clinical acumen, such as that displayed in the papers by Bardet and Biedl. As is so often the case in science, new advances come from new techniques[24]. The heterogeneity in the clinical presentation of the Laurence-Moon and the Bardet-Biedl syndromes which led to their subdivision into the Laurence-Moon and Bardet-Biedl syndromes again shows itself using these newer techniques. As we look back at this syndrome which causes one form of bulging, we note the importance of experiments of nature and new methods for making clinical diagnoses. As we develop even newer methods and a progressively better understanding of the types of obesity, we will be better able to win the battle of the bulge.

Several human chromosomes have been implicated in the Bardet-Biedl syndrome. A detailed study of Canadians in the Maritime Provinces with Bardet-Biedl Syndrome has shown its genetic relationship to another genetic syndrome called the McKusick-Kaplan Syndrome[25]. The genetic studies suggested that the gene chaperonin may produce a defective protein that leads to the clinical features[26].

Above the door of his Montreal office, the famous Canadian endocrinologist Hans Selye is reported to have the following saying by Medvei:

> *Neither the prestige of your theme*
> *Nor the power of your tools*
> *The breadth of your knowledge*
> *The care of your planning*
> *will ever take the place of the originality of your thought, and*
> *the acuity of your power of observations*[27].

Acuity of observation fits the contribution of all of the physician-scientists whose work forms the basis for the identification of the Bardet-Biedl Syndrome.

Biosketch

John Zachariah Laurence (1826-1870) received his M.B. degree and established the South London Ophthalmic Hospital, which became the Royal Eye Hospital in 1857 (Figure 24-1). He was one of the leading ophthalmologists of his period and founded and edited the *Ophthalmic Review*, in which he and Moon published their paper.

Biosketch

Robert Charles Moon (1844-1914) was born in 1844 and received his medical training at Jefferson Medical College[28]. He was the son of Dr. William Moon, who invented the raised type used by the blind. He died in Lansdowne, Pennsylvania, in 1914 at the age of sixty-eight[29].

Biosketch

Arthur Biedl (1869-1933) was born in Osztern, a part of Hungary, in 1869. He received his medical training in Vienna. He rose rapidly through the ranks from 1893 to 1899, when he was given the title of professor. In 1914 he became professor and chair of general and experimental pathology at the University in Prague. His interest in endocrinology dates from 1895, when he began his studies on the physiology of the adrenal glands. (Figure 24-2)

He published a short monograph on internal secretions entitled *Internal Secretion* in 1903, which was eventually expanded into the large two-volume work in 1910. With Aschner he founded the journal *Endokrinologie*, and in 1922 he published a monograph on the pituitary, the same year in which he made presentations of his patients with mental deficiency, reduced metabolic rate, a disturbance of digestion, and polydactyly[27].

References

1. Pasteur, L. *Études sur la bière, ses maladies, causes qui les provoquent, procédé pour la rendre inaltérable, avec une théorie nouvelle de la fermentation.* Paris: Gauthier-Villars, 1876.
2. Laurence, J.Z., R.C. Moon. "Four Cases of 'Retinitis Pigmentosa,' Occurring in the Same Family, and Accompanied by General Imperfections of Development." *Opthalmol Rev.* 2(1866): 32-41.
3. von Helmholtz, H. *Beschreibung eines Augen-spiegels zur Untersuchung der Netzhaut im lebenden Auge.* Berlin: A. Forstner'sche Verlagsbuchhandlung, 1851.
4. von Helmholtz, H. *Handbuch der Physiologischen Optik I vol.* Leipzig: L. Voss, 1867.
5. Koenigsberger, L. *Hermann von Helmholtz.* Welby, F.A., trans. Oxford: Clarendon Press, 1906.
6. McKendrick, J.G. *Hermann Ludwig Ferdinand von Helmholtz.* London: T. Fisher Unwin, 1899.
7. Bardet, G. *Sur un Syndrome d'Obésité Congénitale avec Polydactylie et Retinite Pigmentaire (Contribution a étude des formes clinique de l'Obésité hypophysaire).* Paris: 1920. Thesis.
8. Babinski, J.F.F. "Tumeur du corps pituitaire sans acromegalie et avec arrêt de développement des organes génitaux." *Rev Neurol (Paris).* 8(1900): 531-533.
9. Frohlich, A. "Ein Fall von Tumor der Hypophysis cerebri ohne Akromegalie." *Wien klin Rdsch.* 15(1901): 883-886, 906 -908.
10. Cushing, H. *The Pituitary Body and Its Disorders: Clinical States Produced by Disorders of the Hypophysis Cerebri.* Philadelphia: J.B. Lippincott & Co., 1912.
11 Cushing, H. "The Basophil Adenomas of the Pituitary Body and their Clinical Manifestations: Pituitary Basophilism." *Bull Johns Hopkins Hospital.* L(1932): 137-195.
12. Biedl, A. "Geschwisterpaar mit adiposo-genitaler Dystrophie." *Deutsche Med Wochen.* 48(1922): 1630.
13. Biedl, A. *The Internal Secretory Organs: Their Physiology and Pathology.* New York: William Wood and Co., 1913.
14. Bray, G.A. "Obesity Research and Medical Journalism." *Obes Res.* 3(1995): 65-7 1.
15. Rony, H.R. *Obesity and Leanness.* Philadelphia: Lea and Febiger, 1940.
16. Rynearson, E.H., C.F. Gastineau. *Obesity.* Springfield, IL: Charles C. Thomas, 1949.
17. Gries, F.A., P. Berchtold, M. Berger. *Adipositas: Pathophysiologie, Klinik and Therapie.* Berlin: SpringerVerlag, 1976.
18. Jung, I.T. *A Colour Atlas of Obesity.* London: Wolfe Medical

Publications, 1990.
19. Bray, G.A. *The Obese Patient.* Philadelphia: W.B. Saunders, 1976.
20. Vague, J. *Obesities.* London: J. Libbey & Co., 1991.
21. Alstrom, C.H., B. Hallgren, L.B. Nilsson, H. Asander. "Retinal Degeneration Combined with Obesity, Diabetes Mellitus and Neurogenous Deafness." *Acta Psychiatr Scand.* 34(1959) (Suppl 129): 1-35.
22. Bell, J. "The Laurence-Moon Syndrome." In *The Treasure of Human Inheritance.* Ed. L.S. Penrose. London: Cambridge University Press: 1958. Vol 5, Part 3.
23. Klein, O., F. Ammann. "The Syndrome of Laurence-Moon-Bardet-Biedl and Allied Diseases in Switzerland." *J Neurol Sci.* 9(1969): 479-513.
24. Watson, J.D., F.H.C. Crick. "Molecular Structure of Nucleic Acids: A Structure for Deoxyribose Nucleic Acid." *Nature (Lond).* 171(1953): 737-738.
25. McKuslick, V.A. *Mendelian Inheritance in Man: Catalogs of Autosomal Dominant, Autosomal Recessive, and X-Linked Phenotypes.* 10th ed. Baltimore: Johns Hopkins University Press, 1992.
26. Sheffield, V.C., R. Carml, A. Kwitek-Black, et al. "Identification of a Bardet-Biedl Syndrome Locus on Chromosome 3 and Evaluation of an Efficient Approach to Homozygosity Mapping." *Hum Molec Genet.* 3(1994): 1133-1135.
27. Medvei, V.C. *A History of Endocrinology.* Lancaster: MTP Press, 1982.
28. Drews, R.C. "Ophthalmology 100 Years Ago." *Ann Ophthalmol.* 3(1971): 322-324.
29. Robert Charles Moon. *JAMA* 62(1819): 712.

Chapter 25

Brain Injury and Overweight

Life is short, the art long, opportunity fleeting, experience treacherous, judgment difficult.

—Hippocrates[1]

Once again experiments of nature rise to help us in our battle of the bulge. The recognition that there were many different types of obesity came slowly. It was facilitated by the gradual acceptance by the public that post-mortem examination of the bodies of people who died could help the family understand the reason for death and could contribute to the advancement of knowledge about disease. With the advent of frequent autopsy examination at the beginning of the nineteenth century, many reports began to appear of diseases involving the pituitary gland and hypothalamus located at the base of the brain[2]. The autopsy findings related to diseases of the pituitary gland and the adjacent hypothalamic regions of the brain can be grouped into several disease categories[3], including inflammatory disease, brain damage caused by bleeding into the brain, cysts containing fluid, and a variety of tumors or cancerous growths.

The first recognition that a disorder of the pituitary gland could produce a disease with generalized systematic symptoms became clear when Dr. Pierre Marie (1853-1940)[4] described a case of acromegaly in 1886. Acromegaly is a disease that results from excess secretion of growth hormone from the pituitary gland. Growth hormone is essential during the growing years in children, but in adults it produces gigantism and enlargement of many organs, including heart, liver, and kidneys, along with thickening of the skin. The report of acromegaly by Dr. Marie aroused considerable clinical interest and was translated into English in 1891. An earlier description of acromegaly by Nicholas Saucerotte (1741-1821) in 1772[5] was only subsequently recognized as a case of acromegaly.

The three papers that form the basis for this chapter deal with our understanding of the process by which obesity results from damage to the hypothalamus or pituitary. The published versions are translations of a paper by Bernard Mohr[6] (1809-1848) titled "Hypertrophy of the Hypophysis Cerebri and Its Pressure on the Ventral Brain Surface, particularly on the Optic Tract and Chiasm of the Left Hemisphere;" a paper by Joseph Francois Felix Babinski[7] (1857-1932) titled, "Tumor of the Pituitary Body without Acromegaly and with the Arrest of the Genital Organ;" and a translation by Hilda Bruch[8] of the paper by Alfred Fröhlich[9] (1871-1953) titled "A Case of Tumor of the Hypophysis without Acromegaly."

The earliest record of a patient with obesity and brain disease was described by Bernard Mohr (1809-1848)[6] in 1840. This report is sometimes credited as the initial description of the association of a pituitary tumor as the possible cause of obesity. Although his paper showed an association of a pituitary tumor in an overweight individual, a cause-and-effect relationship was not suggested by the author nor was there any evidence of a temporal relationship between the pituitary disease and the patient's weight gain. A second paper published in French at almost the same time[10] has also been identified as a paper relating pituitary tumors and obesity. On reading this paper, there is no report of obesity among the cases with pituitary tumors. It is thus more appropriate to accord recognition for the association between a pituitary tumor and obesity to the two papers published at the beginning of the twentieth century by Fröhlich[9] and Babinski[7].

The description by Fröhlich of the relation of a pituitary tumor and obesity attracted much attention. He described the syndrome as the adiposogenital syndrome, but his name was subsequently given to it by Bartels[11]. The name Fröhlich's Syndrome was used more widely as a general label for obese children with delayed sexual development, whether or not there was a hypothalamic tumor. It is instructive to examine the original patient described by Fröhlich and the changes this patient experienced over the ensuing years.

The patient (Figure 25-1) described by Fröhlich was a twelve-year-old boy complaining of severe headaches[8,9]. These headaches were associated with vomiting but no other complaints. In 1901, two years following the first evaluation, the boy, now age fifteen, returned to the clinic with a number of serious complaints. The patient, who originally had been slim, had been gaining weight rapidly. Beginning in January 1901 his sight in the left eye began to diminish. Six months later the headaches recurred and increased in severity. The boy became tired very easily and vomited repeatedly, most commonly after meals. His vision declined steadily until he was blind in the left eye. He was short, standing 1.45 meters (4 ft. 9 in.) tall, and he was overweight, weighing 54 kg (119 lb.), giving him a body mass index of 25.7 kg/m^2, well above the normal limits for a boy of fifteen years. The largest accumulation of fat was in the tissues of the trunk, particularly on the abdomen and in the neighborhood of the genitals. The testes were small and axillary hair was absent. Based on these findings, Fröhlich made the diagnosis of a tumor (neoplasm) of the pituitary gland. The patient continued to be followed in the clinic. In 1907 an x-ray of the skull showed destruction of part of the bones surrounding the pituitary called the *dorsum sellae*, with preservation of other parts of this structure, the anterior clinoid process, which are bony spurs that normally hold the pituitary gland in place[11]. Parenthetically, it was only in 1895 that Wilhelm Roentgen (1845-1923) had originally reported the discovery of x-rays, which were used in diagnosing this boy. Examination of the eyes showed atrophy of the optic disc. He had gained more weight and now weighed 65.2 kg (147 lb.), which is quite fat for an immature boy of average height. In 1907 an operation was performed on his brain (craniotomy). The surgeon removed fluid from a hazelnut-sized cyst containing several spoonfuls of fluid resembling old blood[12]. Microscopic examination revealed an abnormality of the pituitary with a precancerous tumor. Following surgery the patient improved and showed development of his sexual function. The last report on this patient is in 1913[13] and showed that improvement had persisted but the patient maintained his infantile appearance.

In reaching his diagnosis of a brain tumor, Fröhlich[9] used several findings from this boy. First, the boy had headaches and vomiting which slowly progressed. This suggested a slowly expanding tumor located at the base of the skull. Because of the decreased vision, Fröhlich reasoned that the lesion was in the region where the optic nerves cross (chiasm) on their way to the brain. Since the left eye was involved more than the right, he assumed there was a neoplasm in the region of the pituitary. In reviewing the older literature, Fröhlich noted that several authors had commented on the presence of adiposity with an effeminate appearance as a coexisting symptom. None of these earlier authors, however, had recognized the diagnostic importance of these associated symptoms nor their potential causal relationship. Only with the syndrome of acromegaly described in 1886 by Marie[4] had the connection been made between pituitary enlargement and the development of disease.

In contrast with the patient of Fröhlich[9], the case published by Babinski[7] is shorter in length and there is little discussion of other scientific reports. The patient was a seventeen-year-old girl who had been observed for ten years and was the basis for a doctoral thesis by Onanoff[14]. The 17-year-old female patient of Babinski, like the patient of Fröhlich, had complained for several years of headaches that increased in intensity. Her vision was diminished. On examination Babinski was struck by the excess adipose tissue on her body and the infantile nature of her sexual organs. Babinski's paper contained the autopsy examination showing a tumor of the bony regions where the pituitary sits (*sella turcica*) that was adhering to the pituitary gland and engulfing the surrounding tissues (the *tuber cinereum*). As Babinski noted, this case was interesting from two perspectives. The first was the absence of gigantism (acromegaly) in the presence of a large pituitary tumor. The second was the coexistence of the pituitary lesion and infantilism with an arrest in the development of the sexual organs. As Babinski noted, "the idea of a cause and effect relationship between the tumor of the pituitary and infantilism is very acceptable." Because Babinski's patient was obese and his focus was on the impaired sexual development, this would lead me to believe that Frohlich deserves the primary credit for recognizing the relationship between a tumor of the pituitary gland and obesity.

Immediately after recognition by Fröhlich of the relation of a tumor at the base of the brain and obesity, the question of whether it was a tumor of the pituitary or a tumor outside the pituitary became the subject of a raging debate. In 1904 Erdheim, a leading German pathologist of the time[15], wrote a long and detailed scientific paper that took issue with Fröhlich's conclusion that his patient had a pituitary tumor. Erdheim offered an alternative conclusion suggesting that a tumor in the hypothalamus just above the pituitary was more likely the cause of obesity than a tumor within the pituitary. By reviewing a series of post-mortem exams, Erdheim demonstrated that only tumors of the pituitary which grow beyond the bony cup (*sella turcica*) in which this gland sits are associated with obesity. Moreover, he noted that tumors limited to the pituitary gland did not produce adiposity. Finally, tumors of the pituitary stalk, which connects the pituitary to the brain and which originates in or near the pituitary but without the involvement of the pituitary, could also produce obesity. On the basis of this evidence Erdheim argued that the syndrome of adiposity was caused by tumors outside the pituitary impinging on the base of the brain.

In 1938 Dr. Hilda Bruch (1904-1984), a psychiatrist interested in childhood obesity, provided a translation of the patient reported by Fröhlich and a gave a detailed discussion of the role of tumors of the pituitary versus the hypothalamus as causes of this syndrome. She said, "For a long time it seemed that the conflicting theories (pituitary versus hypothalamus) could be reconciled by the assumption that an intimate anatomic and physiologic connection existed between the pituitary (hypophysis) and the surrounding nerve centers"[8]. Recent anatomic investigations, she said, "have shown this concept to be false. There are no veins of any consequence passing from the [base of the brain] infundibular stem to the hypothalamic region or vice versa"[16]. Bruch was wrong. Unfortunately the studies that she relied on to reach this conclusion were inaccurate[16]. The existence of a blood supply from the brain to the pituitary, called the hypothalamic pituitary-portal system, was proven in 1955 by Geoffrey Harris (1913-1972)[17] just longer than fifty years after the original reports by Fröhlich and Babinski.

The syndrome of obesity and delayed development of the reproductive organs was reproduced experimentally by Samuel Crowe et al. (1883-1955) in 1910[18]. In their review, two leading neurologists, Dr. John F. Fulton (1899-1960) and Percival Bailey (1892-1935) suggested that "it is doubtful whether the pituitary (hypophysis) plays an essential role in the production of sleepiness (hypersomnia), adiposity and genital dystrophy"[19]. A clear-cut experimental demonstration that the infantilism of this syndrome was a result of pituitary damage was furnished by the experiments of Herbert Evans (1882-1971) and C.N.H. Long in 1921[20] and by Philip Smith (1884-1970) in 1927[21]. After it became clear by 1927 that the destruction of the pituitary produced shrinkage in size (atrophy) of the thyroid gland, the adrenal gland, and the gonads, but not obesity, Hetherington and Ranson[22] showed that discrete damage to the ventromedial hypothalamus uniformly produced obesity but did not lead to loss of function of the thyroid, adrenal, or gonads. Damage to the hypothalamus a small distance to either side of the central hypothalamus was shown to produce anorexia and weight loss[23]. The presence of regions in the brain that could produce weight gain or weight loss when damaged led to the dual center hypothesis as an explanation of hunger and satiety[24].

More recently it has been shown that a lesion in either the ventromedial hypothalamus or paraventricular nucleus, a region just above the ventromedial hypothalamus, will produce obesity. The effects of damage to these two regions of the hypothalamus with obesity differ in a number of respects. Damage to the paraventricular nucleus produces increased feeding or hyperphagia, which is essential for development of the syndrome. When food intake in such animals is restricted to normal levels following a lesion in the paraventricular nucleus, obesity does not occur. In contrast, a lesion in the ventromedial nucleus produces an imbalance between the sympathetic and parasympathetic limbs of the autonomic nervous system. The autonomic nervous system consists of two principal parts. The parasympathetic part of this system controls emptying of the stomach, slows the heart rate, and controls bladder and colon function. The sympathetic part of the autonomic nervous system controls constriction of the blood vessels and can increase energy expenditure. The disruption to the autonomic nervous system after damage to the ventromedial hypothalamus results in increased levels of insulin and decreased heat production (thermogenesis) by the sympathetic nervous system. There is also a reduction in growth hormone secretion with stunting of body growth (the opposite of the acromegalic syndrome reported by Dr. Marie). Thus, current work nearly a century after the classic description by Fröhlich[9] and Babinski[7] suggests that there are two distinctive syndromes in hypothalamic obesity: (1) a hyperphagic syndrome due to increased food intake and (2) a metabolic syndrome with altered balance between the sympathetic and parasympathetic components of the autonomic nervous system.

The discovery of leptin, a peptide produced by adipose tissue, has provided an important link between fat and the brain—and specifically to the hypothalamic brain structures involved in regulation of food intake. Leptin acts on cells located in the areas of the hypothalamus that we have been describing. Diseases of the hypothalamus, including tumors, infectious diseases, and congenital malformaltions, destroy the cells that can respond to leptin. In the absence of leptin, or with loss of cells that respond to it, obesity results. Thus the reports early in the twentieth-century that hypothalamic injury produces obesity have shown us where the brain cells are that respond to leptin. As we continue to understand better how the signals from fat tissue influence the function of the hypothalamic part of the brain, we will gain new tools needed in our battle of the bulge.

Biosketch

Alfred Fröhlich (1871-1953) (Figure 25-2) was born in Vienna, where he received his M.D. degree in 1895.

Following graduation, he joined the department of medicine under the direction of Dr. Nothnagel and worked in experimental pathology and in the neurology clinic. It was during his stay in Sherrington's laboratory in Liverpool, England, that Fröhlich met Harvey Cushing. Frohlich's first academic appointment with tenure was in the department of pharmacology and toxicology in Vienna. He was subsequently appointed a full professor and served in that position from 1919-1939. He came to the U.S. in 1939, a victim of the German-Austrian *Anschluss.* He continued his pharmacologic studies as a member of the May Institute of Medical Research at the Jewish Hospital in Cincinnati, Ohio. Fröhlich's work touched almost all areas of vertebrate and invertebrate pathology[25].

Biosketch

Joseph François Felix Babinski (1857-1932) (Figure 25-3) was born in Paris of Polish parents.

Under the influence of the famous Charcot, he became a neurologist and was appointed to the Hôpital de la Pitie in 1890, where he became a senior neurologist in 1914. He is best known for his description of the turning up of the big toe when the sole of the foot is stroked, the so-called plantar reflex, which bears his name. Babinski was a prolific writer, publishing in areas of physiology, neurosurgery, medical endocrinology, psychiatry, and medical editing. His first scientific contribution in 1882 concerned typhoid fever. His graduate thesis, published in 1885, was on multiple sclerosis. At age thirty, he became chief assistant to Professor Charcot at Hôpital Salpétrière and shortly after became Médecin aux Hôpitaux. He was an editor of the *Revue Neurologique* and a founder of the Société de Neurologie de Paris[26].

References:

1. Hippocrates. *Aphorisms* I. 1.
2. Michel, M. "Pathology of the Pituitary Body." *Charleston Med J Rev.* 15(1860): 145-175.
3. Boyce, R.W., C.F. Beadles. "A Further Contribution to the Study of the Pathology of the Hypophysis Cerebri." *J Path Bacteriol.* 1(1893): 359-383.
4. Marie, P. "Sur deux cas d'acromegalie. Hypertrophie singuliere non congénitale des extrémités superieures, inférieures et céphalique." *Rev Med.* 6(1886): 297-333.
5. Sauccrotte, N. "Accriossement singulier en grosseur des os d'un homme âge de 39 ans." *Melanges de chirurgie.* (1801): 407-411.
6. Mohr, B. "Hypertrophie der Hypophysis cerebri und durch bedingter Druck auf die Hirngrundfläche, ins besondere auf die Sehnerven, das Chiasma derselben und den linkseitigen Hirnschenkel." *Wschr ges Heilk.* 6(1840): 565-571.
7. Babinski, A.F.F. "Tumeur du corps pituitaire sans acromégalie et avec arrêt de développement des organes génitaux." *Rev Neurol.* 8(1900): 531-533.
8. Bruch, H. "The Frohlich Syndrome: Report of the Original Case." *Am J Dis Child.* 58(1939): 1281-1289.
9. Frohlich, A. "Ein Fall von Tumor der Hypophysis cerebri ohne Akromegalie." *Wien kiln Rundschau.* 15(1901): 883-886, 906-908.
10. Rayer, P.F.O. "Observations sur les maladies de l'appendice sus-sphenoidal (glande pituitaire) du cerveau." *Arch Gen Med.* 3(1823): 350-367.
11. Bartels, M. "Ueber Plattenepithelgeschwulste der Hypophysengegend (des Infundubulums)." *Ztschr auf Augenh.* 16(1906): 407-438, 530-560.
12. von Eiselsberg, A., L. von Frankl-Hochwart. "Ein neuer Fall von Hypophysisoperation bei Degeneratio adiposo-genitalis." *Wien klin Wchnschr.* 21(1908): 1115.
13. Biedl, A. *Innere Sekretion: Ihre physologischen Grundlagen und ihre Bedeutung fur die Pathologie.* 2nd ed. Berlin: Urban & Schwarzenberg, 1913.
14. Onanoff. *Sur un cas d'epithelioma.* These de Paris, 1892.
15. Erdheim, J. "Ueber Hypophysengangsgeschwulste und Hirncholesteatome." *Sitzungsb d k Akad d Wissensch Math-naturw CI, Wien.* 113(1904): 537-726.
16. Wislocki, G.B., L.S. King. "The Permeability of the Hypophysis and Hypothalamus to Vital Dyes, with a Study of the Hypophyseal Vascular Supply." *Am J Anat.* 58(1936): 421-472.

17. Harris, G.W. *Neural Control of the Pituitary Gland.* London: Edward Arnold Ltd., 1955.
18. Crowd, S.J., H. Cushing, J. Homans. "Experimental Hypophysectomy." *Johns Hopk Hosp Bull.* 21(1910): 127-169.
19. Fulton, J.F., P. Bailey. "Tumors in the Region of the Third Ventricle: The Diagnosis and Relation to Pathological Sleep." *J Nerv Ment Dis.* 69(1929): 1-125, 145-164, 261-277.
20. Evans, H.M., J.A. Long. "The Effect of the Anterior Lobe Administered Intraperitoneally upon Growth, Maturity and Oestrus Cycles of the Rat." *Anat Rec.* 21(1921): 62-63.
21. Smith, P.E. "The Disabilities Caused by Hypophysectomy and Their Repair: The Tuberal (Hypothalamic) Syndrome in the Rat." *JAMA.* 88(1927): 159-161
22. Hetherington, A.W., S.W. Ranson. "Hypothalamic Lesions and Adiposity in the Rat." *Anat Rec.* 78(1940): 149-172.
23. Anand, B.K., J.R. Brobeck. "Hypothalamic Control of Food Intake in Rats and Cats." *Yale J Biol Med.* 24(1951): 123-146.
24. Stellar, E. "The Physiology of Motivation." *Psychol Rev.* (1954): 5-22.
25. Editorial on Alfred Frohlich. *JAMA* 207(1969): 2275-2276.
26. Talbott, J.H. *A Biographical History of Medicine: Excerpts and Essays on the Men and Their Work.* New York: Grune & Strattory, 1970.

Chapter 26

Glandular Imbalance Can Produce Overweight: Harvey Cushing

All disease entities are abstract concepts created by the human mind.

—Faber[1]

Is one person's battle of the bulge the same as another's? Are we able to tailor the strategies we use to the needs of the individual? If so, we need to know how to tell one overweight person from another. One way to do this is by their names, Social Security number, driver's license number, gender, age, race, place of residence, or other similar identifiers. This tells us something about the person, but it doesn't address the question of whether one type of person's battle of the bulge is like the next person's. Understanding the causes of why we are bulging has been one of the major results of research on overweight during the twentieth century. In this chapter, I will tell the story of a brilliant neurosurgeon who separated one cause of obesity from other causes by careful clinical observations.

Dr. Harvey Williams Cushing (1869-1939) was one of the leading medical figures in the first half of the twentieth century. He was a faculty member of Johns Hopkins Hospital in Baltimore during his early years and was the first chief of surgery at the Peter Bent Brigham Hospital of the Harvard Medical School in Boston from 1912 to 1932. He was a founder of the subspecialty of neurosurgery. He had the unusual ability to couple an active surgical career with exceptional scientific productivity. In addition, he was a noted lover of books, a collector of books by the famous anatomist Andreas Vesalius[2] and a Pulitzer Prize-winning biographer to boot[3].

In a scientific paper published in 1932, Cushing described the details of a group of patients for whom obesity was an important symptom. They also had high blood pressure, a truncal or central location for their fat, and unusual purplish marks on the abdomen. This report, in 1932, had been preceded by an earlier description of the syndrome in a book he wrote in 1912[4]. This "monograph on the pituitary stands as a milestone in American medicine, and more particularly in the history of endocrinology"[5]. It is detailed and profusely illustrated and brought together Cushing's thinking about acromegaly and hypopituitarism into a single volume. In this book he described his first case of what is now known as Cushing's Syndrome. This monograph has the distinction of being the first full-length book in American medicine, and it is a classic in the study of glandular diseases, or endocrinology as this field of study is now called. Cushing's careful medical reasoning integrated the symptoms of his patient with those of other patients to develop the features of a new syndrome. He showed how the concept of a disease entity including obesity evolved over twenty years. The importance of Cushing's work has been elegantly summarized by one of his biographers, Dr. John Fulton (1899-1960), who said:

> For those who believe that the originality of most men reaches its peak before the age of forty and that it would be a good thing if most of us were chloroformed at sixty[7], it is a fact of some significance that one of Cushing's most original single contributions to clinical medicine was made in his sixty-third year as he was about to retire. He had done many other things that exhibited originality and scientific imagination, but his primary achievements had come by dint of hard work. However, the recognition of an entirely new disease entity and the establishment of its pathogenesis must be regarded in the same category as the recognition of other eponymic syndromes, such as Addison's disease [tuberculosis of the adrenal glands], Graves' disease [hyperthyroidism], and Bright's disease [end-stage renal disease.[6]]. (items in brackets added.)

In his book Cushing described this first case of the disease that would bear his name as follows (Figure 26-1):

> Case XLV. (Surgical No. 27140) A syndrome of painful obesity, hypertrichosis and amenorrhea, with over-development of secondary sexual characteristics accompanying a low grade of hydrocephalus and increased cerebral tension. Pituitary, adrenal, pineal or ovary? Subtemporal exploration and decompression[4].

Cushing went on to say:

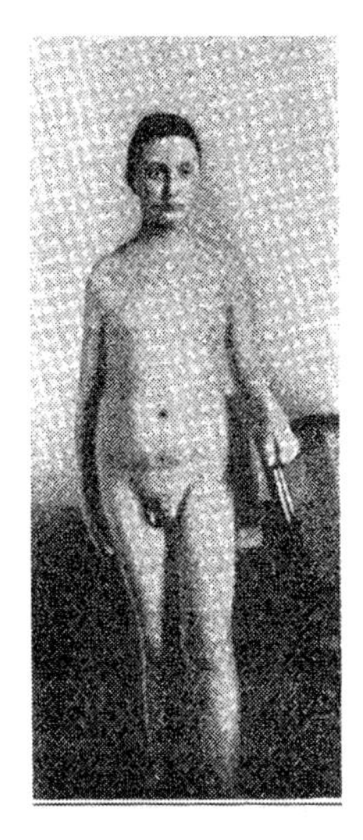

Figure 1

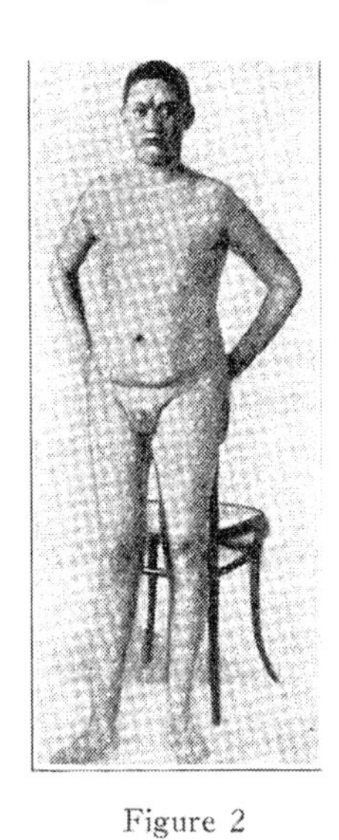

Figure 2

25-1

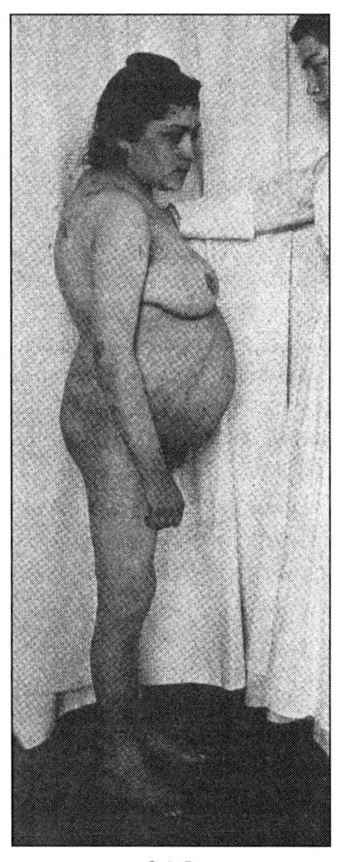

26-1

25-1 Classics in Obesity, "The Fröhlich Syndrome Report of the original case.

26-1 Patient LVI from Cushing. From the collection of the author.

> The case is an instance of the combination of intracranial pressure symptoms with amenorrhea, adiposity and low physical stature—a syndrome which might well be due to hypophyseal [pituitary gland] deficiency. But here, however, the similarity to the cases of hypopituitarism [low function of the pituitary], which have been heretofore discussed, ends, and instead of the sexual infantilism of reversive type with which we have become familiar, the patient shows the secondary sexual development, mammary and genitalia of a nullipara with unusual and recently acquired hirsuties [excess body hair].
>
> Other cases with precisely the same syndrome have been recorded in the past...In all of them adenomatous or hyperplastic adrenal tumors have been found and in some instances the constitutional transformation of the afflicted individual into an adipose and hirsute creature has been extraordinary. It will thus be seen that we may perchance be, on the way toward the recognition of the consequences of *hyperadrenalism*. Heretofore the only recognizable clinical state associated with primary adrenal disease has been the syndrome of Addison [failure of the adrenal glands], and the grouping of these cases may possibly add one more to the series of clinical conditions related to primary maladies of the ductless glands[4]. (Items in brackets added.)

In 1932 Cushing described twelve similar clinical cases that he pulled together from his own experience and from other published scientific reports. It shows Cushing's genius at abstracting clinical symptoms and findings into an integrated disease entity with a pathologic basis. Two of the cases were from Cushing's series and the other ten cases were reported by other physicians. The first case, that of Minnie G., is described in the earlier quote as Case XLV. After this patient's initial admission in 1910, follow-up admissions to the hospital occurred in 1913, 1922, and 1932. Between 1910 and 1932 a series of six other patients with the same or a highly similar disorder were carefully studied at the Peter Bent Brigham Hospital in Boston. In reviewing the records of these patients and others published in medical reports, Cushing found that a "basophilic adenoma of the pituitary gland" was present in three cases, an undifferentiated adenoma of the pituitary in two cases, and that an adenomatous-like structure was described in an additional case. Cushing reasoned as follows:

> The usual method of progression has been somewhat as follows. A peculiar clinical syndrome has first been described by someone with a clarity sufficient to make it easily recognizable to others. This syndrome, in course of time, has been found to be associated either with a destructive lesion or with a tumefaction primarily involving one or another of the organs in question. These tumefactions have proved in most cases to be of an adenomatous character and it was finally recognized (first in the case of the thyroid) that adenomata of this kind were functionally active structures that produced hypersecretory effects. It then gradually came to be realized that the tumor need not necessarily be bulky, but quite to the contrary, striking clinical effects might be produced by minute, symptomatically predictable adenomas. So it is the degree of secretory activity of an adenoma, which may be out of all proportion to its dimensions, that evokes the recognizable symptom-complex in all hypersecretory states.[8].

Continuing, he wrote:

> It was at this stage of the story that the case was first reported (1912). Its most striking feature was the rapidly acquired adiposity of peculiar distribution in an amenorrheic young woman. At the time, Dercum's adiposis dororosa (usually a menopausal disorder), Bartel's and Frohlich's adiposogenital dystrophy (commonly associated with hypophysial-duct tumors) and the adipositas cerebralis of Asheim and Erdheim (due to hypothalamic lesions) were but vague terms; and the possible relation of the basophilic elements in the anterior pituitary to the reproductive functions was not even suspected...In commenting on the case at the time, it was pointed out...that the source of the trouble in all probability lay in the adrenal gland[8].

In reviewing these twelve patients, Cushing found several features that were commonly present. All of the patients were comparatively young women who had more or less abrupt cessation of their menstrual periods (amenorrhea) and had become obese quite rapidly with a peculiar tense and more or less painful adiposity chiefly affecting the head, neck, and trunk. The average age at onset of the malady was approximately eighteen years. The female patients were short. Cushing described the clinical characteristics succinctly as follows:

> (1) A rapidly acquired, peculiarly disposed and usually painful adiposity confined to the face, neck and trunk, the extremities being spared; (2) A tendency to become round shouldered (kyphotic) even to the point of measurable loss of height associated with lumbo-spinal pains; (3) A sexual dystrophy shown by early *amenorrhoea* in the females and ultimate functional impotence in the males; (4) An alteration in normal hirsuties, shown by a tendency to *hypertrichosis* [excess hair] of the face and trunk in all the females as well as the preadolescent males and possibly reversed in the adult males; (5) A dusky or plethoric [reddish] appearance of the skin with *purplish lineae atrophicae* [purplish stretch marks on the abdomen]; (6) *Vascular hypertension* present in all except three cases where no mention was made of blood pressure; (7) A tendency to *erythremia*...; (8) Variable *backaches, abdominal pains, fatigability*, and ultimate extreme weakness[7]. (Italics added.)

This paper by Cushing identified a specific cause for obesity and added to the list of definable types of adiposity[9]. Cushing's interest in basophilic adenomas was aroused by a report by Dr. Raab from Professor Biedl's clinic in 1924[10]. This was a report of a patient with a basophilic tumor identified at autopsy whose clinical features resembled a patient that Cushing was following. Report of another patient published by Teel in 1931[11] stimulated Cushing's interest further and the deductions from his clinical experience were presented and published in 1932[7]. It was not until 1935, however, that Minnie G., his first patient, died and the presence of a basophilic adenoma was proven at post-mortem examination of the pituitary[9]. Even without the post-mortem data, however, Cushing reached the following conclusion:

> An excess or deficiency of anterior-pituitary hormones... secondarily affects the function of the adrenal cortex with established certainty, whereas nothing comparable to this occurs in the reverse direction. Hence, if further study should prove that adrenal tumors in the absence of any demonstrable change in the pituitary body may cause a polyglandular syndrome in many respects similar to that under discussion, it may well enough be assumed that when the same features characterize the syndrome of a basophilic adenoma, they in all probability are secondarily ascribable to a hypersecretory influence of the adrenal cortex even in the absence of any histologically appreciable abnormality[8].

Cushing identified and described with great accuracy the features of the syndrome that bears his name. They include a centrally located type of obesity, the purplish stretch marks on the abdomen, and increased blood pressure. Although he concluded that this syndrome was due to a small tumor or adenoma in the pituitary gland composed of basophilic cells (determined by the color the cells stain when looked at microscopically), definitive documentation that these tumors caused the disease awaited measurements of the hormones secreted by the pituitary gland. The radioimmunoassay to measure adrenocorticotropic hormone (ACTH) accurately had to await the work of Solomon Berson and Rosalind Yalow. Definitive proof that these tumors caused the syndrome was obtained by surgically removing the adenoma from the pituitary with remission of the disease. This didn't occur until almost forty years after Cushing's description.

It is interesting to examine the reason for the delay between the clear-cut demonstration that a basophilic adenoma of the pituitary gland could produce this entire syndrome and the routine use of partial pituitary removal (hypophysectomy) as opposed to total adrenalectomy for its treatment. First, the tumors in the pituitary are very small, and improvements in x-ray techniques were needed before they could be routinely identified. Second, it required laboratory measurements to separate the obesity of Cushing's Syndrome from other types of obesity in some cases. Finally, the radioimmunoassay was only developed in 1967, and it was this technique that allowed a definitive measurement of the pituitary hormone that was secreted in excess and that produced this syndrome.

During Cushing's active years at the Peter Bent Brigham Hospital in Boston from 1912 to 1932, endocrinology, the study of glandular function in the body, made great strides. The physiological effects of experimental removal of the adrenal glands (adrenalectomy) or removal of the pituitary gland (hypophysectomy) became well recognized. When the adrenal glands are removed or destroyed by disease, the body loses sodium in the urine, and patients are unable to metabolize foods properly and lose weight. When the pituitary is removed, the control over the thyroid gland, adrenal glands, and testis or ovary are lost. Deficiency of thyroid hormone and loss of menstrual cycles in women and impotence in men are seen. However, no commercially available form of adrenal steroids was available until the late 1930s and early 1940s. Indeed, it was at the Peter Bent Brigham Hospital, following Cushing's retirement, that the first use of adrenal steroids was undertaken for treatment of insufficiency of the adrenal glands[12]. When these steroids became available, treatment of Cushing's Syndrome by removal of the adrenal glands and replacement of normal amounts of steroid became possible. Only when the laboratory methods were developed to measure the cortisol that is produced by the adrenal gland and the ACTH that is produced by the pituitary gland did it become possible to identify reliably patients with

Cushing's Syndrome. It is interesting to note that the radioimmunoassay for ACTH was developed by Berson and Yalow, the same two scientists who developed the radioimmunoassay for insulin.

Identification of a new disease of the pituitary gland has depended on the introduction of sophisticated techniques. The first of these techniques was the x-ray, discovered by Wilhelm C. Roentgen (1845-1923) in 1895[13]. Most patients with Cushing's syndrome have pituitary tumors that are so small that there would be no evidence of enlargement of the pituitary when the patient was alive. Since these tumors are usually small in size, they are not detected with standard x-ray techniques. After the discovery of x-rays by Roentgen in 1895, diagnosis of pituitary diseases took a big leap forward. Using x-rays it was possible to see enlargement of the pituitary gland, providing the increase in size was sufficiently great. Most small tumors, however, like the basophilic adenomas that produce Cushing's Syndrome, do not enlarge the pituitary enough to be seen with ordinary x-ray techniques. The larger tumors or tumors that destroy the bony socket in which the pituitary sits (the *sella turcica*) were detectable with standard x-rays. Just as x-rays provided a big advance in diagnosis of pituitary disease, the use of contrast techniques such as putting air or some substance that x-rays cannot penetrate into the brain area advanced diagnostic power of x-rays. The biggest advance, however, was the introduction of computed tomography by Hounsfield in the 1960s[14]. With CT scans of the head it became possible to identify the presence of pituitary microadenomas with great precision. Once the presence of a small tumor could be precisely located, surgical removal was possible without having to remove the entire pituitary and induce pituitary insufficiency.

In this story of Cushing's discovery of a new syndrome of obesity, we can begin to understand how techniques to treat this type of obesity can produce a success in battling the bulge. In many patients whose pituitary is successfully removed, weight loss follows. Body weight may not return to normal, but here we have a clear success in the battle of the bulge by preventing further weight gain and usually inducing a cure with long-term weight loss.

Biosketch

Harvey Williams Cushing (1869-1939) came from a family with a long medical tradition[5]. He could trace his ancestry back to the Massachusetts Bay Colony in 1638. Both his father and his grandfather were physicians in Cleveland, Ohio. Harvey Cushing was the youngest child in a family of ten. He received his collegiate education at Yale University, where he graduated in 1891. After Yale he entered Harvard Medical School, where he was a classmate of the famous diabetologist, Elliott Joslin, whose clinic in Boston still carries Joslin's name. Drawings from Harvey Cushing's notebooks in medical school[6,15] gave evidence of his skills as a minute and careful observer. Following one year of post-graduate education at the Massachusetts General Hospital in Boston, Massachusetts, Cushing began his work as an assistant surgical resident with the famous William Halsted (1852-1922) of the Johns Hopkins Hospital. Following two years of training at major European clinics, he returned to Johns Hopkins in 1901, where he remained until 1912 when he became the professor of surgery at the newly opened Peter Bent Brigham Hospital in Boston across the street from the Harvard Medical School. (Figure 26-2)

Cushing's friendship with Sir William Osler during his years at Johns Hopkins made a significant imprint on the young Cushing's interest in the history of medicine. Cushing's collection of books, now residing in the Yale library, and his collection of works by and about the famous anatomist Vesalius, are evidence of his historical perspective.

Cushing's bio-bibliography of Andreas Vesalius, published posthumously, is a classic in the field of historical bibliography[2].

In addition to his work on the syndrome that bears his name, Cushing, along with Sir Victor Horsley (1857-1916) in England, pioneered microsurgery. Cushing studied many neurosurgical diseases including acromegaly, meningiomas, gliomas, and intracranial physiology. He published twelve books. The first of these on the pituitary gland appeared in 1912[4], the year in which Cushing moved from Johns Hopkins Hospital to become professor of surgery and surgeon-in-chief at the Peter Bent Brigham Hospital in Boston. His work in Boston was interrupted by the first World War. The surgical unit at Base Hospital #5 in France was organized by Cushing, and his wartime experiences were subsequently published in an account of this surgical unit[16]. Cushing's most notable literary contribution, however, was his two-volume work titled *The Life of Sir William Osler*, written between 1921 and 1924[7]. It earned him the Pulitzer Prize for biography in 1925. In 1932, at the age of sixty-three, Cushing retired from the Harvard Medical School through an agreement Cushing made with Dr. Henry Christian, professor of medicine, upon his arrival in Boston in 1912. In spite of his long attachments to the Harvard Medical School, Cushing moved his book collection to Yale University, from which he had received his undergraduate degree, and bequeathed his library to Yale upon his death in 1938. The words used by Cushing in 1927 at the centenary of the birth of Lord Lister, the surgeon who introduced antisepsis into surgery, can equally be applied to Harvey Williams Cushing:

> Rarely is it safe to prophesy any durability of recognition whatsoever the accomplishment. Fame that is contemporary, fame that for a time endures, and fame that actually

> accumulates, differ in quality as differ the flash of a meteor, the glow of a comet and the permanence of a fixed star. Only when the contemplation of both the man and his achievement truly inspires and ennobles us will they remain indivisible to be, praised by the people for time everlasting[17].

With the passage of time, Harvey Cushing's place as a medical pioneer in the twentieth-century seems "everlasting."

References

1. Faber, K. *Nosography in Modern Internal Medicine.* New York: Paul B. Hoeber, Inc., 1923.
2. Cushing, H. *A Bio-bibliography of Andreas Vesalius.* New York: Schuman's, 1943.
3. Cushing, H. *The Life of Sir William Osler.* Oxford: Clarendon Press, 1925.
4. Cushing, H. *The Pituitary Body and Its Disorders.* Philadelphia: J.B. Lippincott, 1912.
5. Loriaux, D.L. "Harvey Williams Cushing 1869-1939." *Endocrinologist.* No. 2 1(1992): 2-5.
6. Fulton, J. *Harvey Cushing: A Biography.* Springfield, IL: Charles C. Thomas, 1946.
7. Osler, W. "The Fixed Period." In *Aequinimatis.* Philadelphia: Blakiston and Sons, 1932.
8. Cushing, H. "The Basophil Adenomas of the Pituitary Body and Their Clinical Manifestations: Pituitary Basophilism." *Bull Johns Hopkins Hospital.* L(1932): 137-195.
9. Bray, G.A. "Commentary on Classics of Obesity. 4. Hypothalamic Obesity." *Obes Res.* 1(1993): 325-328.
10. Raab, W. "Klinische und röntgenologische Beiträge zur hypophysären zerebralen. Fettsucht und Genitalatrophie. (Case 2)." *Wien Archif inn Med.* 7(1924): 443-530.
11. Teel, F.N. "Basophilic Adenoma of the Hypophysis with Associated Pluriglandular Syndrome." *Arch Neurol Psychiat.* 26(1931): 593-599.
12. Thorn, G.W., L.L. Engel, H. Eisenberg. "Treatment of Adrenal Insufficiency by Means of Subcutaneous Implants of Pellets of Desoxycorticosterone Acetate (A Synthetic Adrenal Cortical Hormone)." *Bull Johns Hopkins Hosp.* 64(1939): 155-166.
13. Roentgen, W. "Ueber eine neue Art von Strahlen. (Vorlaufige Mittheilung.)" *Sitzber. phys. med. Ges. Wurzburg.* 132(1895): 132-141.
14. Hounsfield, G.N. "Computerized Transverse Axial Scanning (Tomography)." *Br J Radiol.* 46(1973): 1016-1022.
15. Thomson, E.H. *Harvey Cushing. Surgeon, Author, Artist.* New York: Schuman, 1950.
16. Cushing, H. *From a Surgeon's Journal, 1915-1918.* Boston: Little, Brown and Co., 1936.
17. Cushing, H. "The Emancipator." In *Consecratio Medici and Other Papers.* Boston: Little, Brown, and Co., 1928.

Chapter 27

The First Diet Book: "A Letter on Corpulence Addressed to the Public"

In practice therefore there was only one test of effective treatment. Did it work.

—Poynter & Keele[1]

Diet books storm on to bookstore shelves every January, promising miracle cures and advice for people who are battling the bulge—some of this advice is good and some not. The successful books among each new crop have a few characteristics. There is always some "theory" that will help melt fat away. There are the reports of overweight individuals who have successfully used the ideas propounded by the author to successfully win their personal battle of the bulge. The author is usually a doctor, sometimes a physician, but not always. When doctors or celebrities write these books they carry an additional aura of authenticity. Rarely have the results from using the method in the book been put before other scientists for critical examination. Freedom of the press allows publication of books that may be scientifically dubious if not downright ludicrous.

Each crop of new books suggests that they have a "magic" cure that previous ones did not have. However, the history of books for treating obesity goes back more than one hundred fifty years, and there are many recurrent themes, including low-carbohydrate diets for quick and permanent weight loss, low-fat diets to lose weight and improve your health, or combinations of food that are guaranteed to relieve your hunger. If any of these diets had been successful in curing the battle of the bulge, there would be no room for next year's crop. It is as certain that new diet books claiming the final cure for obesity will appear with the melting of the snow as it is that birds will migrate north.

In this chapter, I will tell the story of diet books, beginning with the pamphlet that is arguably the first diet book. It was published in 1863 by

Mr. William Banting (1796-1878). It is a pamphlet of twenty-one pages and can appropriately be called the first popular diet book published by a layman. It is, however, only the first in a long series of low-carbohydrate, high-protein diets that have been published under many names for one hundred fifty years. Mr. Banting's *Letter on Corpulence Addressed to the Public*, as it was titled, is a short twenty-one pages in length, written by a businessman and undertaker[2]. It was originally published privately in 1863 but went through many editions and was translated into many languages. In it Banting related his successful weight loss using a diet provided by his physician Dr. William Harvey (1806-1876), who was no relation to the William Harvey who discovered the circulation of the blood more than two hundred years earlier.

In the final edition of this pamphlet, published in 1902, Mr. Broadley, the editor, said the following:

> William Banting in the early 1860s and Captain Boycott in the early 1880s achieved, in turn, the notable feat of adding a new verb to the English language. Although well nye 40 years have rolled by since Mr. Banting published his modest "Letter on Corpulence, Addressed to the Public", he still remains the undisputed pioneer of all modern crusades against corpulence and the term Banting-System has even become part and parcel of the various languages into which the famous pamphlet of 1863 was promptly translated.[3]

The relationship of the name Banting to diet and obesity has dimmed in the twentieth century, but the importance of this first diet book has not.

The one thousand copies of the first edition, published in May 1863[2], were given away and are hard to find in libraries. A second edition was published in December of 1863 by Harrison & Sons[4]. The one thousand five hundred copies of this second edition describe Mr. Banting's continued weight loss and give some additional details about the diet. The version selected for reproduction here is the third edition, of which sixty-three thousand copies were printed in three different versions. The first version contains a concluding addendum[5], the second version adds an appendix[6], and the final version includes a letter from Dr. William Harvey, an ear surgeon[7]. It was the former Dr. Harvey who had originally prescribed the diet to Mr. Banting. The version reprinted here is from the more extensive edition published in 1869 along with numerous testimonials to the benefit of this diet sent to Mr. Banting[8]. This third London edition also contains the translation of a paper by Professor Niemeyer of Halle, Germany[9]. In addition to the pamphlet by Mr. Banting, we are republishing three letters from Mr. Banting to the owner of the 1869 edition[12] (see appendix.)

The importance of Mr. Banting's pamphlet lies in two directions. First, it was enormously popular—people wanted to lose weight, even in 1863, and here was a diet that worked, and Banting showed from his own experience just how well it worked. Before beginning his diet, Mr. Banting, who was in his sixties, was having trouble hearing and found it difficult to go down stairs. To keep from falling, he went down stairs backwards. For help with the decrease in his hearing, he consulted Dr. William Harvey, who prescribed the successful diet. The second impact of the pamphlet was the subsequent medical response to its popularity. In medical circles it was roundly condemned, a situation which is reminiscent of many recent professional responses to other popular diet books.

The rationale for this diet is described in a letter from Dr. Harvey to Mr. Banting that was part of the third edition of the *Letter on Corpulence Addressed to the Public*[7,20]. When Dr. Harvey was in Paris in 1856, he learned about the discoveries by the famous French physiologist Claude Bernard (1813-1878) on the role of the liver in the control of blood sugar. The series of lectures delivered by Bernard in 1855 and 1856 included, among other things, his discoveries of the way that the liver stored and broke down glycogen to produce blood sugar. Dr. Harvey knew that a purely animal diet was of great value in checking the secretion of diabetic urine and it seemed to follow, "[a]s a matter of course, that the total abstinence from saccharine and farinaceous matter [carbohydrates and starch], must drain the liver of this excessive amount of glucose and thus arrest in a similar proportion the diabetic tendency." With this idea in mind, he reasoned that a diet low in carbohydrate, or as he termed it, "saccharine and farinaceous matter," might be beneficial in the treatment of diabetes. If a purely animal diet was useful in treating diabetes, he reasoned that such a diet might also be useful in treating obesity.

The first patient to use Dr. Harvey's low-carbohydrate animal protein diet in his battle of the bulge was an enormously corpulent man who consulted Dr. Harvey for deafness. In addition to the non-farinaceous, non-saccharine diet (i.e., a low-carbohydrate, high-protein diet), he used a volatile alkali described in the second edition of Mr. Banting's pamphlet[4]. The diet was eminently successful and within seven months, the first patient had returned to almost normal proportions and his hearing problems were completely cured. With this success, Dr. Harvey recommended his diet to William Banting who had consulted him for a similar problem of decreased hearing.

The diet that Mr. Banting used is shown in Table 27-1, along with an analysis of its food composition.

Table 27-1: Mr. Banting's Average Daily Diet
Total Estimated Daily kilocalorie intake: 1714

Protein intake, grams	115 (27% of kilocalories)
Fat intake, grams	42 (22% of kilocalorie)
Carbohydrate intake, grams	119 (28% of kilocalories)
Alcohol, grams	56 (23% of kilocalories)

Kilocalories allocated to each meal were as follows:

Breakfast	319
Dinner	835
Tea	240
Supper	320

* Data Analysis done by Dr. Catherine Champagne using Moore's Extended Nutrient Data Base at the Pennington Biomedical Research Center, Baton Rouge, LA

The diet contained approximately 1700 calories. It would be described as a low-carbohydrate, high-protein, high-fat diet, with a moderate amount of alcohol as shown by the table. Mr. Banting's weight loss is plotted from the numbers he provided in the third edition of his pamphlet (Figure 27-1). His weight declined from 202 pounds to 156 pounds, a loss of nearly 50 pounds (23 kg) in one year.

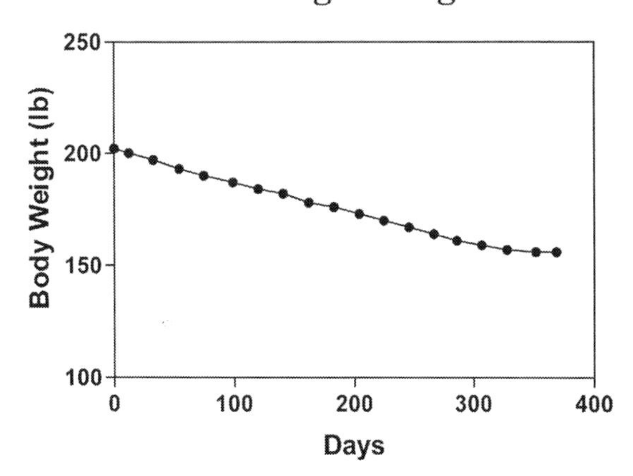

27-1 Weight loss curve for Mr. William Banting during the first year that he used the diet prescribed for him by Dr. William Harvey. © 2006 George A. Bray, MD.

Table 27-2: William Banting's Paper on Corpulence:
Editions Available in National Library of Medicine

Year	Publisher	Initial Leaves	Pp.	Addenda: Addenda I	Addenda: Concl. Add. II	Append	Mr. Harvey's Letter	Other	Edition	Comments
May 1863	Harrison & Sons, London	–	1-21	–	–	–	–	8°	1st edition	1000 copies given away; Hard tan cover
Dec. 1863	Harrison & Sons, London	–	1-16	17-22	–	–	–	8°	2nd edition	1000 copies–free; 500 sold
Apr. 1864	Harrison, London	iii-iv	5-25	27-34	35-45	–	–	8°	3rd edition preface dated	63,000 copies sold
1864	Mohun Ebbs & Hough, NY	–	5-16	17-22	–	–	–	–	3rd edition with addenda	Rebound–hard cover. No original cover
1865	Mohun & Ebbs, NY	–	1-16	17-22	23-30	31-33	34-36	–	4th edition with addenda	Gray cover– 58,000 copies sold in England at top of page (1865 on cover 1864 on title page)
1865	Mohun & Ebbs, NY	–	5-13	14-18	19-25	26-28	29-31	–	5th edition with addenda	
1865	A Roman & Co., San Francisco	–	1-14	15-19	21-27	–	–	Blackwood's on Corpulence Harper's Weekly 29-53	Reprinted from 3rd edition	pp 29-53, Banting On Corpulence, Review from Blackwood Magazine; pp55-64, On Corpulence and Leaness, from Harper's Weekly
1868	J.B. Lippincott & Co., Philadelphia	Pref 3-4	7-26	27-34	35-46	47-51	–	12°	6th edition	
May 1869	Harrison, London	Preface iii-xvi	1-22	–	–	–	–	8° Correspondence 23-99	4th edition	*See below
1902	Harrison & Sons, London	i-ix	1-22	23-48	–	49	–	8° omits correspondence & Dr. Harvey's Letter	re-edited by A. Barnister	

* Following Correspondence in 1869 ed. in NLM: 1.The treatment of corpulence by the so-called Banting System. A popular and scientific lecture, delivered in the Hall of Konigsbau at Stuttgart on the 23rd Dec. 1865 by Professor Niemeyer M.D. consulting physician extradordinary to his Majesty the King of Wurtenberg. Published by August Hirschwald 68, Unterden Linden. Berlin 1866 pp101-116, pp117-118. 2.William Banting to the Public. 3.Prospector for the purpose of funding and endowing a new institution in the service of humanity to be called The Middlesex Country Convalescent Hospital pp119-127.

The *Letter on Corpulence Addressed to the Public* was an immediate success. By 1865 more than fifty-eight thousand copies had been sold in England and subsequent editions followed[4,7,8]. It was published in India[25] and translated into Polish[26], German[9,7], French[28], and recently into Swedish[29]. International conferences were held on Bantingism, the term introduced into the English language to describe his diet.

Success often breeds contempt, and this was certainly true in this case. In an article from *The Albion*, published in New York on October 15, 1864, there is a brief comment on the discussion of the Banting System at a meeting of the British Association for the Advancement of Science at Bath, England, in 1864. One speaker concluded that "it would be an evil to the nation (England), both bodily and mentally, if the Banting system of reduction were to become at all general, and that, regarding the whole population there was more need to add to than to lessen the weight of the body." An article from the *Providence Press* (Rhode Island) dated Friday, November 11, 1864, goes on to say, "Mr. Banting's plan, which was good enough for himself, has been tried by others and caused great injury and suffering. Probably the surest way to grow lean in this country is to immigrate to the nation originated by Jefferson Davis, and live on food procured at famine prices."

In an article appearing in the January 25, 1865, issue of *Commercial Advertiser*, the moral issues of obesity and the focus on dieting were clearly stated.

> Good Heavens! The ill of the world is not repletion [obesity], it is emptiness and all the other fat men are running about in their own puffery and breathless manner asking: What about malt? How is it as to chocolate? Are anchovies bad for me? Must I cut off my Stilton? To these I say: Let me be your doctor. Retrench your all-absorbing self-interest. Turn your thoughts from your duodenum to the famishing creatures who peer down through the railings of your areas at the blazing fire in your kitchen grate. Give up this filthy selfishness that takes for its worship all that is least worthy in humanity. Walk, ride, bathe, swim, fast if you must but take your thoughts off this detestable theme and try to remember that the subject you want to popularize is in its details of the coarsest that can be made matter for conversation.

Further in the article the writer said, "[F]rom Falstaff [In Shakespeare] downward, I have ever liked fat men; they are all nothing but the pleasantist fellows that walk the earth. They are genial by force of temperament; and there is neither ungenerous sarcasm in their jowlery nor malicious malice in their wit." Clearly Mr. Banting's diet had stirred up a hornet's nest of concerns by health professionals and health non-professionals alike.

In the preface to the fourth edition of 1869[8] Mr. Banting took on his accusers, saying:

> I believe I have subdued my discourteous assailants...and can now look with pity, not unmixed with sorrow, upon the men of eminence who had the rashness and folly to denigrate the dietary system as humbug and to hold up to scorn the men who put it forth... I heartily thank the public press for the general fairness of the criticisms and feel deeply indebted to the *Morning Advertiser* for its able article of 3 October 1865 when I was so sadly and unjustly attacked by certain prominent members of the British Association, whose feelings now that the subject has been more widely and intelligently examined and discussed, I do not envy...Two or three unfavorable results having been reported in the public press, I instantly set out work to trace them, and prove them to have no better foundation than the frequent reports of my death.

Following publication of his pamphlet, Mr. Banting said, "I have been told again and again, that the system was as old as the hills. I will not deny it...but I can say for myself that it was quite new to me"[8]. Several authors had indeed previously suggested the use of a low-carbohydrate diets, but these had not been widely disseminated.

Jean Anthelme Brillat-Savarin (1755-1825) who wrote *Physiologie du Goût*[21], may have been the first to recommend a low-carbohydrate diet. "From all that I have discussed," Brillat-Savarin said,

> it is plain that if obesity is not actually a disease, it is at least a most unpleasant state of ill health, and one into which we almost always fall because of our own fault...Obesity is a distressing influence on the two sexes in that it destroys both strength and beauty...It also predisposes its victims to various illnesses, such as apoplexy, dropsy, and ulcers on the legs, and makes all other afflictions more difficult to cure[21].

As to the causes of obesity, Brillat-Savarin noted that "[t]he first [cause] is the natural temperament of the individual. It follows therefore that some people [are]...destined to be obese"[21]. Beyond natural temperament, Brillat-Savarin observes that "the second principal cause of obesity lies in the starches and flours which man uses as the base of his daily nourishment. As we have already stated, all animals who live on farinaceous foods grow fat whether they will or no; man follows the common rule." Additionally he notes that "[a] double cause of obesity results from too much sleep combined with too little exercise"[21]. With the causes of obesity duly outlined, Brillat-Savarin offers a plan to intercede in the course of obesity that, without help, awaits the hapless patient. According to Brillat-Savarin, "Any cure of obesity must begin with the three following and absolute precepts: discretion in eating, moderation in sleeping, and exercise on foot or on horseback"[21]. But after uttering them, Brillat-Savarin says he places little credence in these guidelines and for the following reasons:

> Now in the first place it needs great strength of character for a man to get up from the table while he is still hungry... As for the second prohibition, it is a painful insult to fat people to tell them to get up early in the morning... Exercise on foot...is horribly tiring, and the perspiration it rings out places one in grave danger of false pleurisy...therefore, while it is admitted that anyone who wishes to reduce his weight should eat moderately, sleep but little, and exercise as much as possible, another method must be sought to attain the same end.[21].

Brillat-Savarin then goes on to recommend an anti-fat diet that involves a "more or less rigid abstinence from everything that is starchy or floury...Any anti-fat diet should be accompanied by a precaution which I had forgotten, and which I should have mentioned at the very beginning: it consists of wearing day and night a belt which supports the belly at the same time that it moderately confines it"[21].

The concept of a low-carbohydrate diet was expanded in two books by Dancel[22,23]. Dancel's rationale for his diet was that fat contains hydrocarbons. Thus corpulent individuals must eliminate those foods and focus on the nitrogen-containing foods. His method recommended roasted meat, game, and poultry, with fish in moderation, accompanied by dried toast or firm cheese. To be avoided were *pate de fois gras*, brain, feet, lobsters, and crab, as well as most vegetables, including artichokes, lettuce, carrots, rice, peas, beans, potatoes, beets, and cabbages. Taking a cue from the success of William Banting's pamphlet and the one by Dancel, Dr. John Harvey—no relation to Dr. William Harvey, Mr. Banting's doctor—published a pamphlet in 1864 titled *Corpulence: Its Diminution and Cure without Injury to Health*[24]. Dr. John Harvey adapted the Dancel-System and claimed to have done so prior to Banting's pamphlet, although his work was not published until afterwards. In the fourth edition of his pamphlet in 1869, William Banting[8] noted, "As I find, there are more Mr. Harveys than one concerned in the question of the cure of corpulence and as I have been much troubled by the correspondence on the subject, I am glad to repeat that the medical advisor to whom I am so much indebted is Dr. William Harvey, F.R.C.S. of #2 Soho Square, London, W."

The saga of diet books didn't end here—it just began. The high-protein, low-carbohydrate diet recommended by Mr. Banting is a regular on the diet book circuit. It is accompanied by other themes, too. The low-fat diet, the balanced deficit diet, and the special food diet are also recurring themes. I guess the public just needs a periodic rest from one theme before it is ready to be enticed into trying the same type of medicine wrapped in a different package. As of this writing, neither diets nor any other form of treatment short of surgery are "cures" in the battle of the bulge.

Biosketch

Jean Anthelme Brillat-Savarin (1755-1826) (Figure 27-2) came from a family of lawyers and was neither an academic nor a cook. Born in the town of Belley, his studies took him into the family profession of the law. At one point prior to his appointment in 1802 as a judge in the Supreme Court of Appeals in Paris he had been mayor of Belley. He survived the French Revolution, but barely. In 1789 he was the representative of Belley to the Third Estate. He narrowly escaped the guillotine in 1793 and fled to Switzerland and then to America, where he spent three years before returning to France. Compiling his masterpiece took thirty years[21].

Biosketch

William Banting (1797-1878) was born in 1797 and worked as an undertaker (Figure 27-3). He was 65 inches tall and as he grew older, suffered great personal inconvenience from his increasing stoutness. Before sixty years of age, he found himself unable to stoop to tie his shoes or to attend to the little offices which humanity requires, without considerable pain and difficulty.

He was compelled to go down stairs slowly backwards to avoid the jar of increased weight on the ankle joints and with every exertion huffed and puffed in a way that was unseemly and disagreeable. His efforts to obtain help from the medical profession were generally unsuccessful. His encounter with Dr. William Harvey in the early 1860s turned out to be eminently successful, and it was on this basis and his experiences with this low carbohydrate, non-farinaceous, non-saccharin diet that his dietary plan was based[30].

References

1. Poynter, F.N.L., K.D. Keele. *A Short History of Medicine*. London: Mills and Boon, 1961.
2. Banting, W. *Letter on Corpulence Addressed to the Public*. London: Harrison and Sons, 1863. 1-21.
3. Banting, W. *The Rational Cure of Obesity, Being a Letter on Corpulence Addressed to the Public. Re-edited with notes, addenda and a preface by A. Barrister*. [Broadley] London: Harrison and Sons, 1902. 1-49.
4. Banting, W. *Letter on Corpulence Addressed to the Public. 2nd edition*. London: Harrison and Sons, 1863. 1-22.
5. Banting, W. *Letter on Corpulence Addressed to the Public: 3rd edition with addenda*. London: Harrison and Sons, 1864. v, 7-45.
6. Banting, W. *Letter on Corpulence Addressed to the Public. 3rd edition with addenda and appendix*. London: Harrison and Sons, 1864. v, 7-50.
7. Banting, W.
8. Banting, W. *Letter on Corpulence, Addressed to the Public. 4th edition with prefatory remarks by the author, copious information from correspondents, and confirmatory evidence of the benefit of the dietary system which he recommended to public notice*. London: Harrison and Sons, 1869. 1-127.
9. Niemeyer, F. *Die Behandlung der Korpulenz nachdem sogenannten Bantingsystem. Ein popularwissenschaftliger Vortrag gehalten zu Stuttgart*. Berlin: A. Hirschwald, 1866. 1-37.
10. Banting, W. *Letter on Corpulence Addressed to the Public: 4th Edition with addenda*. New York: Mohun, Ebbs and Hough Booksellers and Importers, 1864.
11. Banting, W. *Letter on Corpulence Addressed to the Public. 4th edition with addenda, appendix, and remarks by Mr. Harvey*. New York: Mohun, Ebbs and Hough Booksellers and Importers, 1865. 1-36.
12. Banting, W. *Letter on Corpulence Addressed to the Public. 5th edition with addendas and remarks by Mr. Harvey*. New York: Mohun and Ebbs, 1865. 5-131.
13. Banting, W. *Letter on Corpulence Addressed to the Public: Reprinted from the 3rd London edition with a review of the work from Blackwood's Magazine and an article on Corpulency and Leanness from Harper's Weekly*. San Francisco: A. Roman & Company Booksellers, Importers & Publishers, 1865. 5-64.
14. Banting, W. *Letter on Corpulence, Addressed to the Public. By William Banting 3rd edition*. Philadelphia: 1866. 50.
15. Banting, W. Letter on corpulence addressed to the public. 6th Edition. Philadelphia: Lippincott, 1868.
16. Banting, W. *Letter on Corpulence Addressed to the Public. 8th Edition*. Philadelphia: Lippincott, 1873. 51.

17. Banting, W. *Letter on Corpulence Addressed to the Public. 10th Edition.* Philadelphia: Lippincott, 1875. 51.
18. Banting, W. *Letter on Corpulence Addressed to the Public by William Banting. 12th Edition.* Philadelphia: Lippincott, 1877. 51.
19. Banting, W. *Letter on Corpulence Addressed to the Public. 4th Edition, reprinted.* London: Harrison, 1885. 116.
20. Harvey, W. *On Corpulence in Relation to Disease: With Some Remarks on Diet.* London: Henry Renshaw, 1872.
21. Brillat-Savarin, A. *Physiologie du goût, ou méditations de gastronomie transcendant, ouvrage théorique, historique, et à l'ordre du jour, dedié aux gastronomes parisiens, par un professeur.* Bruxelles: A. Wahlen & Co., 1839.
22. Dancel, R. *Preceptes fondes sur la chimie organique pour diminuer l'embonpoint sans alterer la santé.* 2nd edition. Paris: LeBlanc 1850. 1-213.
23. Dancel, J.F. *Traité théorique et pratique de l'obésité (trop grand embonpoint). Avec plusiers observations de guérison de maladies occasionées ou entretenues par cet état anormal.* Paris: J.B. Bailliere et fils, 1861. 1-357.
24. Harvey, J. *Corpulence, Its Diminution and Cure Without Injury to Health. 3rd edition.* London: Smith, 1864. 1-37.
25. Duke, J. *How to Get Thin; or, Banting in India. 2nd edition.* Calcutta: Thacker, Spink, 1878. 1-37.
26. Mokricki, T. "Mleko jako srodek przeciwko otylosci." *Pam towarz Lek Warszaw.* 69(1873): 328-342.
27. Vogel, J. *Korpulenz ihre Ursachen, Verhütung und Heilung durch einfache diatetische mittel, mit Benutzung der Erfahrugen von William Banting.* Leipzig: L. Denicke. 6(1864): 1-59.
28. Vacher, L. *De l'obésité et de son traitement.* Paris: Savy, 1873. 1-39. With: Niemeyer, *Du Traitement de l'obésité part la methode Banting.* Conference. 41-67.
29. Banting, W. *Bantings kur Mot Fetma.* Transl. and ed. J. Torgerson & K. Stenlof from the Mohun & Ebbs edition, New York, 1865, based on the London 1864 edition. Goteborg, Sweden: Aros, 1999.
30. Harrison, R. "William Banting (1797-1878)." In *The Dictionary of National Biography.* Ed. L. Stephen and S. Lee. Vol. I. London: Oxford University Press, 1937-1938.

Chapter 28

Very-Low-Energy Diets and Fasting: Are They Good for You?

We must never make experiments to confirm our ideas, but simply to control them.

—Claude Bernard[1]

Concern for man himself and his fate must always form the chief interest of all technical endeavors.

—Albert Einstein[2]

For most of human history famine and food shortages have been the plight of man. During the long epochs of human evolution, food shortages were certainly more common than excesses. The human being adapted to periods of famine by using the energy that was stored in fat. This put a premium on the efficiency with which fat could be stored during times of plenty. In this setting human genes adapted to become "thrifty" in using energy and efficient in its storage. Our human genes are thus ill adapted to dealing with our current surfeit of food and abundant food choices. For this reason, many people steadily gain weight in the face of readily available food supplies. The hazards to health produced by this accumulation of fat and the social stigma that is attached to it lead to the continuing search for effective strategies in the battle of the bulge. One of these has been short-term starvation or near-starvation levels of energy intake. This chapter traces some of the developments in the use of these very-low-energy approaches in treating our current epidemic of obesity.

In 1928 Evans and Strang[4] published a new approach to the treatment of obesity. The title of their paper, "A Departure from the Usual Methods in Treating Obesity," identifies the fact that they thought it was "new." Their paper was the forerunner of the very-low-calorie diet craze that became a major treatment for obesity in the 1980s[5], some fifty years after their seminal paper was published. The paper by Evans and Strang provides a scientific rationale for the use of very-low-calorie diets with obese patients, but they lacked the commercial marketing know-how to capitalize on it as the entrepreneurs did fifty years later.

First let me define what I mean by a very-low-calorie diet. A very-low-calorie diet (VLCD), also called a very-low-energy diet (VLED), covers the range of energy intakes between 200 and 800 kcal/d. I will call a fasting diet one with less than 200 kcal/d of energy.

Although Evans and his colleagues had published earlier[6] as well as later[7-9] summaries of this diet, the paper reprinted below is his definitive use of a diet in the range of 400 kcal/d. (See appendix)

The authors begin their paper by noting, as did Hippocrates two thousand five hundred years earlier, that obesity is a hazard to continued good health. They go on to discuss the apparent paradox that some people appear to get fat while others do not on equivalent diets. They dismiss as insignificant the number of people who have a low metabolic rate as the cause of their obesity. By 1929 there was already a substantial number of scientific publications showing that "when calculated by the usual methods, [metabolic rate] is within normal limits" in obese people. They also discuss and dismiss the idea or hypothesis that the specific dynamic action of food (now called thermic effect of food or TEF) related to metabolism of protein may be abnormally low among the obese. When a meal is eaten, there is a rise in energy expenditure that may be 10% of the energy or caloric value of that meal. This increase is called the thermic effect of the meal. Except in the rare cases where a glandular disease is the cause of obesity (Cushing's disease, discussed in Chapter 25), Evans and Strang go on to say, "The treatment should be dietary, and dietary alone." They add, "No special article of food has any merit with regard to losing weight. Total calories must be reduced." They then go on to the dietary approach which they claim is based on new metabolic insight. They asked the following question: Instead of cautiously reducing the diets of the obese to 14 or 15 kcal/kg of body weight per day [1200 to 1600 kcal for people weighing 80 to 120 kg (175 to 265 pounds)] with a resulting weight loss of 6 to 8 lbs. (2.7 to 3.6 kg) a month, would it not be safe in some cases to give them half as many calories, say, 6 to 8 kcal/kg, and get a more rapid reduction? They tried it and it worked very well.

The diet, which they then describe, consists of 1 g of protein per kg of desirable body weight. This would provide approximately 60 g of protein for an individual whose desirable body weight is 60 kg. This is similar to the lower limits of normal using the current Dietary Reference Intakes. In their initial diets they used 45 g of carbohydrate with as much fat omitted from the diet as possible when using whole foods. They gave the following example: For a woman weighing 80 kg (176 pounds), the diet consisted of 60 g of protein, 45 g of carbohydrate, and 29 g of fat for a total of 681 kcal, or 8.5 kcal/kg. This diet was maintained for ten weeks, during which time she lost 42 lbs. (19 kg).

This is the menu and list of rules that Evans and Strang provided for use of their dietary approach:

1. If bread is eaten as toast, it must be weighed before toasting.
2. Eggs may be taken boiled, poached, or raw.
3. Meat may be boiled, broiled, or roasted.
4. No fried foods may be eaten.
5. No lard or butter may be used in cooking.
6. Vegetables must be prepared without milk, oil, or egg dressing.
7. Water may be taken as desired.
8. Salt, pepper, and vinegar (not lemon juice) may be used as desired.
9. It is just as important that all this be eaten as that nothing not on the list be taken.
10. Take a level teaspoon full of soda and a half glass of water twice a day.

No special vitamin or salt supplements were used with this diet, since the authors considered the diets as satisfactory sources of vitamins and salts for the limited periods of dieting required. Of the 98 patients who completed the diet, the average time on the diet was 8.75 weeks, with a weight loss of 12 kg (26.4 lbs.) or an average weight loss of 1.37 kg/wk (3.02 lbs./wk). This is at the upper end for the range of weight losses produced by most diets. In 33 of the 111 patients with systolic blood pressure elevated above 150 mmHg (Stage I hypertension), all but one showed a reduction in blood pressure during treatment with this diet. Thus began the use of very-low-energy diets, defined as those below 800 kcal/d, as a treatment in the battle of the bulge. The uses of these diets continued until the beginning of World War II[7]. Rationing during World War II and the focus of medical research on needs of the military terminated these studies on treatment of obesity.

Almost twenty years elapsed from the beginning of World War II in 1939 before there was any new therapeutic progress in the use of very-low-energy diets. The next step came with the introduction by Bloom and Duncan in 1959[11,12] of short-term fasting as a treatment for obesity. Starvation of obese patients, however, may be dated much earlier in the century. Folin and Denis[13] noted that the two obese women whom they studied during short fasts lost less nitrogen than leaner subjects under similar conditions, indicating that they were more effective in conserving protein. The most comprehensive studies of fasting and inanition, however, were published by Benedict[14,15]. For these studies he used a "professional faster," an individual who went off and on fasts. Benedict[14] confined this individual for twenty-eight days to the metabolic chambers designed by Atwater and Rosa (Chapter 11). During this stay, Benedict measured the carbohydrate, protein, and fat that was metabolized by this individual to maintain body temperature and to sustain life. He found that glycogen stores in liver and muscle were quickly exhausted, usually within thirty-six hours. Thereafter the fuel for daily energy needs came from the stores of fat in the body.

The excretion of nitrogen in the urine fell gradually as the fasting individual conserved his protein stores. The respiratory quotient (RQ), an indicator of how much fat is being oxidized, fell to 0.7, indicating that fat was the principal metabolic fuel. Metabolic rate also declined slightly. This decline in metabolic rate during starvation, and with very-low-calorie diets in obese subjects[16,17], as well as lean ones[3,4] is now well recognized. When metabolic rate falls, less energy is needed, thus slowing the rate of weight loss. In a study on semi-starvation of conscientious objectors during World War II, Keys et al.[3] restricted calorie intake by 50%. Mobilization of fat was the predominant source of energy for these healthy men. As they withdrew fuel from body fat stores, they lost weight. When they were given food again to mimic refeeding of concentration camp prisoners that was anticipated at the end of the war, there was an initial overshoot in the percent body fat which gradually returned to its usual level. That is, these men were fatter after refeeding than they had been when the semi-starvation began. The brain also adapts to starvation. As glycogen stores are depleted, glucose is produced from muscle and the brain gradually adapts to metabolize ketone bodies that are transported into the brain to provide for fuel to replace the glucose that is not available to the brain.

In 1959 Bloom[11] reported on nine very overweight patients who had fasted for a short period in the hospital with rapid weight loss and no ill effects. The weight loss during short periods of fasting is predictable and ranges from 3.2 to 5.9 kg/wk (7 to 13 lbs./wk) after the first ten days in patients weighing in excess of 120 kg (264 lbs.). A series of fasts lasting more than two hundred days were reported between 1966 and 1970. Many overweight individuals have energy stores that can support them for more than a year without food. In contrast, for normal weight people, death usually occurs after a fast of thirty to forty days. Among the overweight patients prolonged fasts of more than one year have been reported, but there have also been several deaths[18].

Although fat was the primary tissue consumed during starvation, the continuing loss of nitrogen from amino acids in muscle tissue provided the carbon skeletons for formation of glucose in the liver and kidney (hepatic and renal gluconeogenesis) and suggested the possibility, as Evans had originally proposed, that adding protein during the individual's fast might prevent nitrogen loss[6].

Apfelbaum and his colleagues in Paris[19] and Bollinger et al. in Kansas[20] were the first to demonstrate the protein-sparing effect of providing protein as the sole source of nutrition during starvation. Subsequently, several other groups showed that the loss of nitrogen from the body could be reduced significantly by giving protein-containing foods[21-23]. Application of these principles led to the marketing of several different dietary protein formulations and began a major boom in the health industry known as the protein-sparing or very-low-calorie diets[14,22,24]. One of these diets was popularized in a book called the *Last Chance Diet*[25] Alas, it was indeed the last diet for some people. This diet used protein from collagen. The collagen produced from gelatin in horse hooves and connective tissues is inadequate for human survival[26,27]. Because collagen is a cheap source of protein, it had first been tried as the sole source of protein during the Napoleonic wars in the early 1800s, but with disastrous results. Even when "essential" amino acids were added to the gelatin-based diets similar to the one described in the Last Chance Diet, there were reports to the FDA of more than fifty deaths[28]. Other very-low-calorie diets, including the Balanced Deficit Diet, the Optifast Diet, and the Cambridge Diet, used high-quality protein from milk or egg in their diets and avoided the calamity of the Last Chance Diet[25]. These commercial programs were launched on the heels of the initial scientific publications in the early 1970s and by the late 1970s and early 1980s were major products for the dietary treatment of obesity. Like so many diets, however, the public interest and consumption exploded and then imploded. One of the first widely sold formula diets collapsed after sales peaked at over $125 million. This was followed a few years later by the Cambridge Diet that was alleged to have sales of more than a billion dollars. Hospital-based programs, such as Optifast and Medifast, grew more slowly and imploded only after the Congressional hearings in the early 1990s threw an unfavorable light on this industry.

A recent study brings this story full circle. It compares the rates of weight loss with diets containing either 425 or 800 calories[29]. The rate of weight loss was not significantly different. This suggests that the extra reduction in calories with the very-low-energy diets were compensated for by either a decrease in metabolic rate or a decrease in energy expenditure or a combination of both. Thus, the original diet of 700 to 900 kcal/d proposed by Evans and Strang[6] more than fifty years ago still represents an effective approach to treating obesity, but more restrictive diets do not seem to add any value in terms of additional weight loss.

Biosketch

Francis Gano Benedict (1870-1957) (Figure 28-1) was a giant in the field of metabolism who contributed classic studies to the literature on starvation. He was born in Milwaukee and lived in both Florida and Boston during his youth. After a year at the Massachusetts College of Pharmacy, he received his A.B. and M.A. degrees from Harvard and a Ph.D. from Heidelberg in 1895. As fortune would have it, he began his academic career at Wesleyan University in 1895 as Atwater was completing his calorimeter. He began his work with Atwater, and when Atwater died, Benedict was appointed director. Shortly after that, the Nutrition Laboratory was moved to Boston to be nearer clinical facilities. From 1897 to 1937 when he retired, more than five hundred experiments were carried out which were presented in some four hundred publications. His work on human starvation was conducted in 1915 and is a classic in the field[30].

Biosketch

Frank Alexander Evans (1889-1956) (Figure 28-2) was born in Pittsburgh in 1889. He graduated from Washington and Jefferson College in 1910 and attended Johns Hopkins Medical School where he received his M.D. in 1914.

Following an internship at the Johns Hopkins Hospital, he received training in pathology at Presbyterian Hospital in New York City before returning to Johns Hopkins. Following service in World War I he again returned to Johns Hopkins until 1922, when he joined Western Pennsylvania Hospital in Pittsburgh and rose from attending physician to physician-in-chief in 1931. In addition to his contributions to metabolism reviewed here, Evans wrote a book on pernicious anemia, which had the unfortunate timing to appear in the same year that George Minot reported his Nobel Prize-winning discovery that liver therapy prevented pernicious anemia, a discovery that did not appear in Evans's monograph[31].

References

1. Bernard, C. *Introduction a l'étude de la médicine expérimentale.* Paris: J.B. Bailliere et fils, 1865.
2. Einstein, A. In Duffin, J. *History of Medicine.* Toronto: University of Toronto Press, 1999.
3. Keys, A., J. Brozek, A. Henschel, O.Mickelsen, H.L. Taylor. *The Biology of Human Starvation, Vols. 1, 2.* Minneapolis: University of Minnesota Press, 1950.
4. Evans, F.A., J.M. Strang. "A Departure from the Usual Methods in Treating Obesity." *Am J Med Sci.* 177(1929): 339-348.
5. Blackburn, G.L., G.A. Bray. *Management of Obesity by Severe Caloric Restriction.* Littleton, MA: PSO Publishing Co. Inc., 1985.
6. Evans, F.A. "A Radical Cure of Simple Obesity by Dietary Measures Alone." *Atlantic Med J.* (1926): 240-241.
7. Evans, F.A. "Treatment of Obesity with Low-Calorie Diets: Report of 121 Additional Cases." *International Clinics.* 2(1938): 19-23.
8. Evans, F.A., J.M. Strang. "The Treatment of Obesity With Low-Calorie Diets." *JAMA.* 97(1931): 1063-1068.
9. Strang, J.M., H.B. McClugage, F.A. Evans. "The Nitrogen Balance During Dietary Correction of Obesity." *Am J Med Sci.* 181(1931): 336-349.
10. *Dietary Reference Intakes for Energy Carbohydrate, Fiber, Fat, Fatty Acids, Cholesterol, Protein and Amino Acids (Macronutrients).* Washington, DC: National Academies Press, 2002.
11. Bloom, W.L. "Fasting as an Introduction to the Treatment of Obesity." *Metabolism.* 8(1959): 214-220.
12. Duncan, G.G., W.K. Jenson, R.I. Fraser, F.C. Cristofori. "Correction and Control of Intractable Obesity: Practicable Applications of Intermittent Periods of Total Fasting." *JAMA* 181(1962): 309-312.
13. Folln, O., W. Denis. "On Starvation and Obesity, with Special Reference to Acidosis." *J Biol Chem.* 21 (1915): 183-192.
14. Benedict, F.G. "A Study of Prolonged Fasting." Pub. No. 203. Washington: Carnegie Institution of Washington, 1915.
15. Benedict, F.G., W.R. Miles, P. Roth, H.M. Smith. "Human Vitality and Efficiency Under Prolonged Restricted Diet." Carnegie Institute of Washington, Pub. No. 280. Washington: Carnegie Institution of Washington, 1919.
16. Bray, G.A. "Effect of Caloric Restriction on Energy Expenditure in Obese Patients." *Lancet.* 2(1969): 397-398.
17. Drenick, E.J., M.E. Swendseld, W.H. Bland, et al. "Prolonged Starvation as Treatment for Severe Obesity." *JAMA* 187(1964): 100-105.

18. Bray, G.A. *The Obese Patient. Major Problems in Internal Medicine.* Philadelphia: W.B. Saunders, 1976.
19. Apfelbaum, M., J. Bostsarron, L. Brigant et al. "La composition du poids perdu au cours de la diète hydrigue." *Gastroenterol Biol Med.* 108(1967): 121-134.
20. Bollinger, R.E., B.P. Lukert, R.V. Brown, et al. "Metabolic Balance of Obese Subjects During Fasting." *Arch Intern Med.* 18(1966): 3-8.
21. Blackburn, G.L. J.P. Flatt, G.H.A. Cloves, et al. "Protein Sparing Therapy during Periods of Starvation with Sepsis of Trauma." *Ann Surg.* 177(1973): 588-593.
22. Genuth, S.M., J.H. Castro, V. Vertes. "Weight Reduction in Obesity by Outpatient Semistarvation." *JAMA* 230(1974): 987-991.
23. McLean-Baird, I.M., R.L. Parsons, A.N. Howard. "Clinical and Metabolic Studies of Chemically Defined Diets in the Study of Obesity." *Metabolism.* 23(1974): 645-657.
24. Howard, A.N., A. Grant, O. Edwards, et al. "The Treatment of Obesity with a Very-Low-Calorie Liquid Formula Diet: An Inpatient/ Outpatient Comparison Using Skimmed-Milk Protein as the Chief Protein Source." *Int J Obes.* 2(1978): 321-332
25. Linn, R., S.L. Stuart. *The Last Chance Diet.* Secaucus, NJ: Lyie Stuart, 1976.
26. McCollum, E.V. *A History of Nutrition.* Boston: Houghton-Mifflin, 1957.
27. Carpenter, K.J. *Protein and Energy: A Study of Changing Ideas in Nutrition.* Cambridge: Cambridge University Press, 1994.
28. Sours, H.E, V.P. Frattali, C.D. Brand et al. "Sudden Death Associated with Very Low Calorie Weight Regimes." *Am J Clin Nutr.* 34(1981): 453-461.
29. Hoerr, R.A., H.W. Kohl, M.Z. Nichaman, R.S. McPherson, A. Bunker, S.N. Blair. "Differences in Weight Loss Between Two Levels of Energy Intake During a 26 Week Very Low Calorie Weight Loss Program." *Obes Res.* (suppl)19(1993): 21S.
30. Maynard, L.A. "Francis Gano Benedict—A Biographical Sketch." *J Nutr.* 98(1969): 1-8.
31. Minot, G.R., and W.P. Murphy. "Treatmnet of pernicious anemia by a special diet." *JAMA* 87(1926):470-476.

Chapter 29

Behavioral Control of Eating

Eat slowly: Only men in rags
And gluttons old in sin
Mistake themselves for carpet bags
And shovel victuals in.

—Sir Walter Raleigh[1]

Battling the bulge is a form of behavior. It is a decision—a decision that you or I must make to behave in a different way, a way that can prevent us from getting fatter or from staying fat if we are already there. Although eating is a "behavior," the idea of adapting psychological theories about behavior to changing this behavior is a relatively recent idea. This chapter describes how this came about and how it was used to further successful efforts in the battle of the bulge.

The quote from Sir Walter Raleigh captures two perceptions about obesity and behavior: First, it says that the obese are behaving as hyperphagic (overstuffing) gluttons, a concept that goes back at least to early Christendom. Second, it implies that changing behavior by using techniques of behavioral therapy may be useful in correcting the problem.

There is a substantial stigma or social disapproval to obesity[2-4] (see also Chapter 19). Prejudice against overweight people is present in all age groups, in both men and women, and at all levels of income and education. Some progress in changing these negative and prejudicial attitudes was made by the discovery of leptin in 1994[5]. Leptin is a protein that is made in fat cells and then secreted into the bloodstream where it tells the brain about how much fat we have. Profound obesity occurs in the rare individuals and animals that lack leptin. This "molecular" discovery has breathed new respectability into the study of obesity. As public views about obesity change, the use of behavioral treatment may become more effective.

The concept of transferring behavioral research from the laboratory into the clinic for the treatment of obesity occurred in two steps. A seminal paper in 1964 titled "The Control of Eating" provided the theoretical background for applying behavioral therapy to the treatment of obesity[6]. This paper outlines a four-step process of analyzing and developing self-control over human eating behaviors which are the essential ingredients for the program. These steps include:

1. Determining the variables that influence eating
2. Determining how these variables can be manipulated
3. Identifying the unwanted effects of overeating
4. Arranging a method of developing required self-control.[6].

Step 2 was the application of this theory to real patients who were battling the bulge. Only a few years after the first study, Richard Stuart applied these principles with amazing success and published the results in an important scientific paper titled "Behavioral Control of Overeating"[7]. This was in 1967, three years after the theoretical paper noted above. Stuart's paper turned these theoretical ideas[6] into practice. This seminal work by Stuart was followed by a surge of other behavioral studies that resulted in behavioral therapy becoming a cornerstone in the treatment of obesity[8-10].

The framework for understanding human behavior has evolved steadily. Advancements in this field have occurred as the scientific understanding of human nature has increased. Following Johannes Kepler's (1571-1630) discovery of the laws of celestial motion and Isaac Newton's (1642-1727) publication on the laws of mechanics in the seventeenth-century, human behavior was formulated in mechanical terms. Man was viewed as a machine. Indeed one author, Denis Diderot (1713-1784) in the eighteenth-century, published a book called *Man as Machine*[11]. This analogy used pistons as the basis for a hydraulic system that accounted for some kinds of human behavior, particularly movements. However, other parts of behavior, such as that belonging to the "soul," were reserved for the spiritual sphere of control[12].

The next step forward in formulating concepts of behavior also occurred in the eighteenth century with the demonstration that nerves were irritable[13]. That is, stimulation or irritation of a nerve could elicit muscular contraction. This was the beginning of the expansion of knowledge about the reflex arc, where a stimulus to the skin or a nerve leads to a predictable response. The so-called reflex arc came to be closely identified with the nineteenth-century neurologists and most notably Charles Sherrington (1857-1952)[14]. For all its attractiveness, explanations in terms of reflexes like those using mechanical analogies were limited. As B.F. Skinner (1904-1990)[15], a famous Harvard psychologist, noted, "In spite of the importance [of the reflex] it is still true that if we were to assemble all of the behavior which falls into the pattern of a simple reflex, we should have only a very small fraction of the total behavior of the organism"[15].

In the late nineteenth century and certainly by the beginning of the twentieth century it had become clear that our conscious activity and behavior were controlled largely by the brain. Two experimental approaches were developed to study the way the brain controlled behavior. They became the scientific underpinnings for the development of behavior therapy for obesity. One line of work was initiated by Ivan P. Pavlov (1849-1936)[16,17], on conditioned reflexes. The other line of work began with Thorndike[18] and more recently Skinner[19] on behavior and operant conditioning.

Pavlov was a Russian physiologist through and through. He transferred to the study of the brain his know-how in general from studies on the physiology of digestion[16]. He substituted physiological mechanisms for psychic mechanisms. He identified and explored with great vigor the concept of the conditioned reflex. As Babkin notes, "Pavlov argues that if [unconditioned] reflex actions can be studied successfully by physiological methods...there can be no reason to doubt the validity of the physiological method for the study of the conditioned reflexes"[21].

Pavlov's great contribution lay in bringing to fruition a method by which cortical or higher brain activity could be studied effectively. Conditioning is a process of stimulus substitution by giving food and the sound of the bell together. When this is done on repeated occasions he could get his dogs to salivate in response to the ring of a bell. To use Skinner's words, "Pavlov's achievement was the discovery, not of neural processes, but of important quantitative relations which permit us, regardless of neurological hypotheses, to give a direct account of behavior in the field of the conditioned reflex"[15]. Pavlov's work was highly meritorious and he received the Nobel Prize in 1904.

The second approach to the study of the consequences of behavior was made by Thorndike[18] and by Skinner[19]. Thorndike evaluated the learning curves from repeated exposure to experimental settings that initiated spontaneous inborn (innate) behavior. Operant conditioning as pioneered by Thorndike, and developed more fully by Skinner, consists of increasing the probability that a given consequence will follow upon a given environmental stimulus. This means rewarding good behavior to increase the likelihood that it will be repeated, rather than punishing bad behavior.

According to Skinner, "In operant conditioning we 'strengthen' an operant in the sense of making a response more probable or, in actual fact, more frequent"[15]. As with conditioned reflexes, operant conditioning can also be extinguished. In his book titled *Contingencies of Reinforcement*[19], Skinner outlines the features that are the basis for much of what Stuart[7] applied to his obese patients when he says, "An adequate formulation of the interaction between an organism and its environment must always specify three things: 1) the occasion upon which a response occurs, 2) the response itself, and 3) the reinforcing consequences. This list is similar to the steps taken by Stuart[7] in applying operant conditioning to behavior therapy for battling the bulge.

Both the principles of extinction of "conditioned reflexes" based on Pavlov's ideas and the principles of operant conditioning based on Skinner's work have been applied to treatment of obesity. Aversive methods have proven effective in treating smoking but do not work very well in treating obesity. Operant conditioning, on the other hand, has become the hallmark for most modern behavioral treatment programs for obesity. A theoretical framework can be a major stimulus to research. Productive and fruitful hypotheses are among the most important elements in scientific thought, as Hans Popper, the twentieth-century philosopher of science, has said so well[22]. Among the most fruitful hypotheses have been Newton's Laws of Motion[23], Darwin's ideas on the origin of species[24], and Einstein's theory of relativity[25]. In the context of the present discussion the theoretical framework of Ferster et al.[6] was the behavioral therapy to the treatment of obesity by Stuart[7].

In his paper Stuart[7] outlines the four steps he used to achieve weight losses that averaged 17.1 kg (37.75 lb.) or 19.1% of the initial weight of 89.2 kg (196.25 lb.) in eight women. These four steps in self-control include:

1. An analysis of the response to be controlled along with its antecedents and consequences;

2. The identification of the behavior which facilitates eating the right amount of food;

3. The identification of the positive and negative reinforcers that control eating; and

4. Using reinforcement to alter the probability of the pre-related response[7].

These are very similar to Ferster's ideas that I listed above.

To carry out these steps, Stuart used several procedures[7,26]. Paper forms were used to allow his overweight subjects to record the time, nature, quantity, and circumstances for all eating events, related to both food or drink. Next he kept a running record of fluctuations in body weight. He obtained a list of behavior patterns with a high likelihood of occurring in his patients such as reading, watching television, etc. Stuart also gathered information on the patients' fears that were most weight related. These might be social, sexual, or health related. During the first session he introduced the behavioral curriculum in which he emphasized action as a means of attaining the desired goal. One piece of advice noted in our first quote was to "eat slowly." Conscious interruption of eating, such as getting a glass of water during a meal, was another such example. The second step in the behavioral curriculum was to instruct the client or patient to remove food from all places in the house except the kitchen. Only one serving of food was to be prepared at a time. Complementing this was the third step, which focused on eating and how to make it a more circumscribed event. With none of his patients did Stuart consciously limit the intake of food.

Step four was introduced at the beginning of the second week. The patient was instructed to place a small amount of food in his mouth and then put the utensils down until the food was thoroughly chewed and swallowed. The patient was only trained to control eating under conditions of high arousal, such as when they were hungry. At step five the patient was instructed in substituting one of their preferred activities for eating. The sixth and final step combines thinking about eating and then an aversive situation. It is interesting that Stuart in his first paper produced better results than almost any paper that has been published since[27]. (See p. 797)

Stuart's work was based on the theories of Ferster et al.[6], but there are several differences. First, Ferster's treatment was purely operant on the model of Skinner. In contrast, Stuart combined operant and respondent techniques[7]. Second, Ferster treated his patients in groups, whereas Stuart treated them individually. Finally, Ferster emphasized the aversive consequences of obesity while Stuart made little use of aversion.

Following the publication of Stuart's paper, a veritable avalanche of studies appeared along with many popular books using behavior therapy[10,26]. In addition, a large amount of scientific work was begun to understand and refine the experimental basis of behavioral therapy for obesity. From these studies a number of working manuals have become available[27,28].

A summary of the current results is shown in Table 29-1. In the nearly thirty years since behavior therapy was introduced, several trends are obvious.

The length of treatment has risen steadily from an average of 8.4 weeks to 27 weeks. This longer treatment period has more than doubled the weight loss from 3.8 to 9.4 kg. The rate of weight loss, however, has remained the same. The low initial attrition rates have increased somewhat, as has the weight of the individual seeking to battle the bulge. The disappointing aspect of these studies is that the weight loss was never as great as reported by Stuart, and weight loss at follow-up has not improved.

Table 29-1 Table of Results with Behavioral Therapy

Variable	1970's	1980-89	1989-1995	1995-
Number of Studies	15	15	5	13
Sample Size	51.3	71.3	21.2	34.0
Initial Weight (kg)	73.4	87	91.9	92.2
Length of Treatment (wk)	8.4	13.2	21.3	27.0
Weight Loss (kg)	3.8	6.9	8.5	9.4
Loss per week (kg)	0.5	0.5	0.4	0.4
Attrition (%)	11.4	10.6	21.8	18.0
Length of follow-up (wk)	15.3	58.4	53.0	39.0
Weight loss at follow-up	4.0	4.4	5.6	5.4

Biosketch

Sir Charles Scott Sherrington (1857-1952) was the oldest of three boys (Figure 29-1). Following his preparatory education, he entered Gonville and Caius College of Cambridge University in England. Here he came under the tutelage of Sir Michael Foster, the leading nineteenth-century physiologist. His first paper was presented in 1884 while he was still a student. After completing his clinical work at St. Thomas's Hospital in London, he received his M.B. from Cambridge in 1885 and his M.D. in 1892. His work was greatly influenced by a visit from Ramón y Cajal, the Spanish neuroanatomist who held that the neuron was the central cell of the nervous system. In 1895 he moved to Liverpool as professor of physiology and spent the next sixteen years developing the reflex as a basic connective structure of the neurons within the nervous system. In 1904 he gave the Silliman Lecture at Yale, which was subsequently published under the title "The Integrative Action of the Nervous System."

He received the Nobel Prize in 1932. In 1913 he accepted the Waynflete Chair of Physiology at Oxford, where he remained until 1935[29].

Biosketch

Ivan Petrovich Pavlov (1849-1936) was the world-famous physiologist who was awarded the Nobel Prize in 1904 with the citation "In recognition of his work on the physiology of digestion, in essential respects, he has transformed and enlarged our knowledge of this subject." He was born in the city of Ryazan and received his early education in the theological seminary. His interest in science led him to St. Petersburg University, where he studied chemistry and physiology. He received his medical degree in 1883 from the Military Medical Academy. Post-doctoral research training in Leipzig with Ludwig and in Breslau with Heidenhain taught him techniques that would serve him well for his entire life (Figure 29-2). His chair in physiology, awarded in 1895, was the one he held until he retired in 1924[32].

His most famous work is on the conditioned reflexes[21,30,31].

Biosketch

Burrhus Frederic Skinner (1904-1990) was born in Pennsylvania (Figure 29-3). His father was a lawyer, but Skinner was an independent soul. He attended Hamilton College in upstate New York and was an atheist in a school that required attendance in chapel. Although he tried his hand at writing, he didn't make the grade and in 1928 began his graduate studies at Harvard University where he received a master's in 1931 and a Ph.D. in 1932 in psychology. He remained there doing research until 1936 when he moved to the University of Minnesota where he remained until he became chairman of psychology at the University of Indiana in 1945. He moved to Harvard in 1948, where he remained for the rest of his life. During his career he guided many young men and women to become psychologists, and, according to his biographer Boeree, he may "perhaps be the most celebrated psychologist since Sigmund Freud."

References

1. Quote (Sir Walter Raleigh).
2. Allon, N. "The Stigma of Overweight in Everyday Life." In Bray, G.A. *Obesity in Perspective.* DHEW publication no. (NIH) 5-708.197;83-102.
3. Goodman, N., S.A. Richardson, S.M. Dornbusch, A.H. Hastorf. "Variant Reactions to Physical Disabilities." *Am Sociolog Rev.* 28(1963): 429-435.
4. Gortmaker, S.L., A. Must, J.M. Peru, A.M. Sobol, W.H. Dietz. "Social Consequences of Overweight in Adolescence and Young Adulthood." *N Engl J Med.* 329(1993): 1008-1012.
5. Zhang, Y.Y., R. Proenca, M. Maffei, M. Barone, L. Leopold, J.M. Friedman. "Positional Cloning of the Mouse Obese Gene and Its Human Homolog." *Nature.* 372(1994): 425-432.
6. Ferster, C.B., J.I. Nurenberger, E.B. Levitt. "The Control of Eating." *J Math.* 1(1964):87-109.
7. Stuart, R.B. "Behavioral Control of Overeating." *Behav Res Ther.* 5(1967): 357-365.
8. Stunkard, A.J. "New Therapies for the Eating Disorders: Behavior Modification of Obesity and Anorexia Nervosa." *Arch Gen Psychiat.* 26(1972): 391-398
9. Fore, J.P., G.K. Goodrick. "Evidence for Success of Behavior Modification in Weight Loss and Control." *Ann Intern Med.* 119(1993): 698-701.
10. Perri, M.G., A.M. Nezu, B.J. Viegener. *Improving the Long-term Management of Obesity: Theory, Research and Clinical Guidelines.* New York: John Wiley & Sons, 1992.
11. de la Mettrie, J.O. *L'homme machine.* Leyde: E. Luzac, fils, 1748.
12. Descartes, R. *Treatise of Man.* Trans. T.S. Hall. Cambridge, MA, 1972.
13. von Haller, A. "A Dissertation on the Sensible and Irritable Parts of Animals." Trans. M. Tissot. *Bull Hist Med.* 4(1937): 651-699.
14. Sherrington, C.S. "On the Proprioceptive System, Especially in Its Reflex Aspect." *Brain.* 29(1906): 467-482.
15. Skinner, B.F. *Science and Human Behavior.* New York: Macmillan, 1953.
16. Pavlov, I.P. *The Work of the Digestive Glands.* Trans. Thompson, W.H. London: Charles Griffin and Co., 1910.
17. Pavlov, I.P. *Conditioned Reflexes: An Investigation of the Physiological Activity of the Cerebral Cortex.* Trans. Anrep, G.V. London: Oxford University Press, 1928.
18. Thorndike, E.L. *Animal Intelligence: An Experimental Study of the Associative Processes in Animals.* New York: Columbia University, 1898. Thesis.

19. Skinner, B.F. *Contingencies of Reinforcement: A Theoretical Analysis.* New York: Meredith Corp., 1969.
20. Konorski, J., I.P. Pavlov. *Br Med J.* (1949): 949-950.
21. Babkin, B.P. *Pavlov: A Biography.* Chicago: University of Chicago Press, 1949.
22. Popper, H. *Conjectures and Refutations: The Growth of Scientific Knowledge.* New York: Basic Books, 1962.
23. Newton, I. *Mathematical Principles on Natural Philosophy and his System of the World.* Original translations by A. Motte, revised translations by F. Cajori. Berkeley: University of California Press, 1934.
24. Darwin, C. *The Origin of Species by Means of Natural Selection of the Preservation of Favoured Races in the Struggle for Life.* 6th ed. London: John Murray, 1885.
25. Einstein, A. *The Collected Papers of Albert Einstein: Volume 1. The Early Years 1879 to 1902.* Ed. J. Stachel. Princeton: Princeton University Press, 1987.
26. Stuart, R.B., B. Davis. *Slim Chance in a Fat World.* Champaign, IL: Research Press Co., 1972.
27. Wing, R.R. "Behavioral Treatment of Obesity: Its Application to Type 2 Diabetes." *Diabetes Care.* 16(1993): 193-199.
28. Brownell, K.W. *The LEARN Program for Weight Control.* Philadelphia: University of Pennsylvania Press, 1985.
29. Ferguson, J.M. *Habits, Not Diets: The Real Way to Weight Control.* Palo Alto, CA: Bull Publishing, 1976.
30. Penfield, W. "Sir Charles Scott Sherrington (1857-1952)." In *The Dictionary of National Biography 1951-1960.* Ed. E.T. Williams and H.M. Palmer. London: Oxford University Press, 1971.
31. Stevenson, L.G. *Nobel Prize Winners in Medicine & Physiology 1901-1950.* New York: Henry Schuman, 1953.
32. Mitchell, H.S. "Ivan Petrovich Pavlov—A Biographical Sketch." *J Nutr.* 88(1966): 3-8.

Chapter 30

Amphetamine: The Janus of Treatment for Overweight

A desire to take medicine is, perhaps, the great feature which distinguishes man from other animals.

—Sir William Osler[1]

Janus was the Roman god with two faces—one face smiling, one scowling[2,3]. Amphetamine, the first drug with a clinical trial showing effectiveness in the battle of the bulge, also has two faces. One face is suppression of appetite; the other face is addiction. It is this latter frowning face that has cast a cloud of doubt and concern over pharmacological agents developed to help in the battle of the bulge. This is the story.

The report by Lesses and Myerson[4] on the use of amphetamines in the treatment of corpulence was published in the prestigious *New England Journal of Medicine* in 1938. It stands as a landmark in the field of drug development for battling the bulge, because it was the first clinical trial of a potential weight-loss drug. It provided important lessons on the consequences of use and abuse of drugs for treatment of corpulence and was selected for that reason. Amphetamine and drug addiction are a good example of the "law of unintended consequences." Appetite suppression and weight loss were the intended consequences, drug dependency the unintended consequence. I will trace the development and disappointments of using drugs as a strategy for battling the bulge over the past one hundred years, since it was just longer than one hundred years ago that drugs were first used in treating overweight.

The introduction of drugs in the battle of the bulge can be dated to at least 1893. The first bona fide drug to be used was thyroid extract[5]. In the years before 1890, a clinical condition called myxedema had been clearly identified[6] to result from failure of the thyroid gland. Patients with myxedema have a puffy type of weight gain, slowing of their thought processes, slow speech, and if severe, a drop in body temperature and coma. When patients with myxedema were treated with thyroid extract, all of these symptoms improved. They became less sluggish, they slept less, and most important for us, they lost weight. Removal of the thyroid gland will produce a myxedema-like picture in animals and humans, and thyroid replacement corrects it, indicating a cause-and-effect relationship for thyroid deficiency and myxedema. Patients with myxedema are often overweight. The treatment of overweight patients with thyroid extract was empirically supported by the fact that thyroid extract produced weight loss in patients with myxedema. These observations prompted Baron (see Putnam[5]) to use thyroid extract to treat overweight non-myxedematous patients.

Thyroid extract is rich in iodine. These molecules of iodine are attached to thyroxine, triiodothyronine, and iodo-tyrosine that are part of a large protein, thyroglobulin, stored in the thyroid gland. When this large molecule is broken down, these iodine-containing hormones are released into the blood. Thyroxine was one of the first hormones to be isolated and then synthesized by organic chemists[7,8]. The thyroxine in thyroid extract can be converted to the active hormone triiodothyronine[9] by chemical changes called deiodination that can occur in several tissues in the body.

Following the invention of a room-sized calorimeter to study human metabolism by Atwater and Rosa in 1895[10], smaller instruments to measure "basal metabolism" came into wide clinical use in many hospitals and clinics across America. Thyroid hormone increases basal metabolism, and a high or low basal metabolism was widely used in the first half of the twentieth century to diagnose the overactivity or underactivity of the thyroid gland that produced hyperthyroidism or hypothyroidism[11]. Measurement of basal metabolism in overweight people was often reported as low[11], although the total amount of oxygen used by overweight patients in this test was higher than normal. The reason tests were often reported as low, when in fact they were not low, is that this test is expressed in relation to body weight. When expressed in relation to body weight, the metabolism of people who were battling the bulge was low. This led to the erroneous concept that obesity might be due to "low metabolism," and it provided a rationale for treatment of corpulent patients with thyroid hormone. With improved methods measuring metabolic rate that were developed after World War II (1939-1945), we have learned that total energy expenditure in overweight individuals is actually increased[12]; they almost never have low metabolism.

Thyroid extract and the thyroxine and triiodothyronine that it contains have all been used to treat obesity[5,13-16]. A major consequence of treatment with thyroid hormone is an increased metabolic rate. When the metabolic rate is increased, we burn up or metabolize fat. We also burn up some of the lean tissue, including muscle and bone that are essential for life[13]. Since obesity is not due to low basal metabolism or low thyroid hormone levels, treatment with thyroid hormone is not indicated unless the patient is also hypothyroid and suffering from insufficiency of the thyroid gland.

The rapid growth of the chemical industry in Germany in the nineteenth and early twentieth-centuries produced many compounds for dyeing cloth. One major impact of this commercial development was the introduction of dyes to stain histological samples for study of tissue structure. Another outgrowth was a supply of chemicals to the synthetic organic chemist to use for making "new molecules." One of the medical pioneers whose work was dependent on these dyes was Paul Ehrlich (1854-1915), the father of drug therapy. Among his many contributions to biomedical science was his concept of the "magic bullet"—the molecule that would act as the key to a lock and provide a way to target chemicals to disease. One of the fruits of his labor was salvarsan, also called "707," a drug that saw wide use in the treatment of syphilis before penicillin became available. The number "707" was the number of different molecules he had to test before finding the "magic bullet"[17].

Another product of this industry that had a direct impact on obesity was dinitrophenol. Factory workers preparing this chemical were noted to lose weight. This finding led doctors to use dinitrophenol in the battle of the bulge without adequate clinical testing. The results were unhappy—the unhappy side of Janus[18]. Use of dinitrophenol was discontinued after the development of skin rash, cataracts, and neuropathy, but this was only after considerable damage had been done[19].

Just after dinitrophenol disappeared as a strategy in the battle of the bulge in the early 1930s, Lesses and Myerson[4] published their paper on the use of amphetamine. Amphetamine was first synthesized by Edeleano in 1887, but it was not until 1927 that Alles described its psychopharmacologic effects. Its two major effects are an increase in alertness and a decrease in food intake[20]. Trials of this drug as a treatment for narcolepsy, or sleepiness, were initiated in the 1930s, and as a pseudo-serendipitous part of these trials it was observed that patients treated with amphetamine lost weight. Following this observation, Lesses and Myerson[4] conducted a clinical trial and demonstrated that amphetamine (Benzedrine®) was effective in producing weight loss. This observation has stimulated controversy and comment ever since.

Amphetamine produces weight loss by reducing food intake[21]. When ten human subjects were maintained on a constant food intake and treated with amphetamine for fifty-six days, there was some weight loss in the first four to eight days in seven of the subjects, which was attributed to a slight increase in energy metabolism[21]. Other than that, weight remained stable. When dogs were treated with 5 to 10 mg of amphetamine just prior to presentation of their daily allotment of food, the drug caused complete abolition of the desire to eat food for a period of ten to twenty-one days in some of these animals. Based on these studies, it was concluded that amphetamine significantly reduced food intake and thus reduced body weight. Following the demonstration that amphetamine suppressed appetite, it was soon realized that the drug was addictive[20]. Appetite suppression and drug abuse are two sides of the same compound—its Janus faces.

After World War II, amphetamine became a street drug that was widely abused and had significant potential for harm. Amphetamine was also widely used in the 1950s by college students to stay awake while studying for examinations and by truck drivers to stay awake when driving long hours. "Benzedrine® inhalers" with amphetamine turned into delivery systems for abusive drugs. In the 1960s restrictive measures curtailed this public health problem, but amphetamine is still an abused drug.

Amphetamine [Benzedrine® chemically identified by the structure alpha-methyl-beta-phenethylamine = amphetamine] is a compound of the ß-phenethylamine chemical series. In this way it resembles norepinephrine, an important neurotransmitter in the brain and autonomic nervous system. Amphetamine also resembles ephedrine, another drug that has been used to treat both asthma and the bulge. To learn about the actions of these drugs, Barger and Dale[22] evaluated a series of similar drugs to find out what they did and what parts of the molecule were important for this effect. They found that a number of these chemical compounds could mimic the effects on the body of the sympathetic nervous system, hence they are called "sympathomimetic" amines. This work was largely forgotten until more than a decade later, when ephedrine was "rediscovered" to produce sympathomimetic effects, including dilatation or enlargement of the pupils, constriction of the bronchi in the lungs with wheezing, constriction of blood vessels with a rise in blood pressure, and stimulation of the heart rate[20].

Because amphetamine stimulates wakefulness, several studies in the mid-1930s examined the effect on narcolepsy, a state of increased sleepiness. In a study of nine cases of narcolepsy treated with amphetamine, Prinzmetal and Bloomberg[23] did not report any effects on body weight. Similarly, Myerson[24] in his first report on the treatment of fatness using Benzedrine® in normal and neurotic persons did not note any weight loss. However in 1937 Nathanson[25] reported a study of forty patients and noted that ten of them had a marked loss of appetite with a definite reduction in body weight. Losses of weight varied between 3.2 to 9 kg (7 and 20 lbs.). The loss of weight appeared to be explained by the lessened appetite and increased physical activity. Davidoff and Reifenstein[26] concluded from their studies with amphetamine that "it may be of use in reducing weight"—an aid in the battle of the bulge. Ulrich[27] in his report on the treatment of narcolepsy with Benzedrine® sulfate also noted that seven obese patients lost weight. It is against this background that the clinical study of Lesses and Myerson[4] was conducted. They studied seventeen overweight patients from their private medical practice. Each individual was given a 1400 kcal/d diet and provided with enough medication to last until their next visit two weeks later. During the observation period, which lasted from six to twenty-five weeks, patients lost an average of 0.66 kg/wk (1.45 lb./wk). A promising beginning, but for the Janus properties of amphetamine.

It was not long before the abuse potential was recognized and the drug's use for obesity came under a cloud of disapproval. This Janus side of the problem stimulated pharmaceutical chemists to synthesize other drugs that would reduce hunger but not have the potential that amphetamine had. A variety of new drugs were made, tested, and marketed, but with the drug abuse epidemic of the 1960s, all of the derivatives of amphetamine have been tarred with the same brush. As amphetamine fell from grace, a similar pall fell over the entire class of compounds for better or for worse, and whether deserved or not. As we will see, one of these "derivatives" had no abuse potential at all, yet was regulated by the U.S. Government as though it did.

To their credit, the pharmaceutical chemists developed compounds that reduced or eliminated the risk of habituation, yet retained appetite-suppressing properties. One of these provides a particularly important lesson in the semantic pitfalls of tarring all compounds that look alike structurally with the same mechanism of action. It is now known, through the work of Leibowitz and Rossakis[28], that direct hypothalamic injections of amphetamine will significantly reduce food intake. This effect involves the release of two neurotransmitters, norepinephrine and dopamine, that act on adjacent cells to activate signals that tell animals they are not hungry. In all likelihood, it is the response to dopamine that is associated with the risk of habituation. Three different groups of chemical compounds were developed as the result of this work by the organic chemists.

The first group of compounds was similar to amphetamine, but had lower or very much lower abuse potential, yet retained the appetite-suppressing effects so needed in the battle of the bulge. For this group of compounds, the mechanism of action appeared to be the release of the neurotransmitter norepinephrine, but not dopamine, from nerve endings in the brain. More recent data sugests that the higher extraneuronal level of norepinephrine may be due to blockade of re-entry into the neuron rather than simply being metabolized.

A second group of compounds in this group, typified by mazindol, arose from the observation that a tricyclic inhibitor of norepinephrine reuptake could reduce food intake. Tricyclic drugs provide an important group of drugs for treatment of depression. Indeed, the weight loss produced by mazindol was detected during its tests as a potential anti-depressant drug. This relationship between drugs that affect depressed mood and weight loss has been observed several times. Two widely used anti-depressants, fluoxetine (Prozac®) and sertraline (Zoloft®), produce weight loss.

Venlafaxine (Effexor®) is an antidepressant that is very similar chemically to a weight-loss drug, sibutramine, that was also identified during trials for an anti-depressant. The third compound has structural similarities to amphetamine but acts by a totally different mechanism. This molecule, d,l-fenfluramine, works by releasing serotonin and partially blocking its re-uptake into nerve endings. On paper, d,l-fenfluramine is similar to amphetamine, but it differs in a major way from other derivatives of amphetamine. Whereas treatment of animals with most of the derivatives of amphetamine reduces brain norepinephrine, treatment with fenfluramine does not. Rather, d,l-fenfluramine reduces brain serotonin, whereas other amphetamine derivatives do not. Its mechanism of action is through serotonergic receptors, not norepinephrine receptors. Thus, it is very different in the way it works and is without addictive potential.

This discovery opened a whole new area of research into serotonergic agents as drugs for use in the battle of the bulge. Serotonin is also involved in depression. This was a problem for some patients taking d,l-fenfluramine. When the drug was stopped abruptly, many patients experienced a mild depression. To avoid this, the drug is usually discontinued over several days.

Most of the chemical modifications of the amphetamine molecule mimic the effects of activation of the sympathetic nervous system but have little or no risk of habituation or abuse since they do not affect the dopaminergic neurotransmitters that are so often associated with drugs of abuse.

Serendipity is an important ingredient in human progress. Serendipity refers to making discoveries that aren't directly related to your major efforts. There are two kinds of serendipity[29]. The first is true serendipity, in which the discovery has no relationship to the usual activity of the individual. Three such examples would be the discovery of the Rosetta Stone by Napoleon's army engineers in Egypt, the discovery of the Dead Sea Scrolls by boys playing in caves in Israel, and the discovery of the Lascaux Caves in France by young boys playing in the mountainous areas of Southern France. In each case, the individual making the discovery had not been trained in scientific disciplines or for "discovery."

Pseudo-serendipity is a second sort of serendipity. It occurs to individuals who are highly trained in their field but who make accidental but often momentous discoveries. The discovery of the explosive dynamite by Alfred Nobel and the discovery of x-rays by Wilhelm Roentgen are two good examples of accidental discoveries by trained minds but in areas that were unrelated to their primary search. The observation by Lesses and Myerson that opened up the field of appetite suppressants in the treatment of obesity extended the pseudo-serendipitous observation that a drug being tested for narcolepsy could reduce appetite and body weight.

The report of cardiac disease (valvular insufficiency)[30] associated with the use of the fenfluramine drugs is an example of the "law of unintended consequences" which has plagued the treatment of obesity. This disaster also adds to the concern and doubt that surround the use of drugs as aids in the battle of the bulge. The story began in the 1980s with a scientific hypothesis. By that time it was well known that fenfluramine acted on the serotonin system to reduce food intake and that the other appetite suppressants acted on the norepinephrine (noradrenergic) system. It was a logical question to ask whether combining drugs acting on each of these two different receptor systems would produce greater weight loss or have fewer side effects than a single drug alone. This was initially tested in a pilot study and then in a drug trial sponsored for four years by the National Institutes of Health[31]. In this study the outcome supported the initial idea. Corpulent participants treated with both drugs lost more weight than in trials with single agents alone, and in many cases were able to keep this weight off for more than three years during this study of the battle of the bulge.

When the dramatic weight-loss results of combining fenfluramine and phentermine became known, the use of "Fen/Phen," as it was widely called, exploded across the country. Patients and doctors alike were thrilled with the results of using Fen/Phen. For the first time it appeared that corpulent Americans were winning the battle of the bulge as they had rarely done before. Offices dispensing Fen/Phen opened up all over the country. Then came the surprise—or rather the calamity. In July 1997 the first cases of valvular heart disease in patients taking Fen/Phen were reported[30]. Urgent meetings by the U.S. Food and Drug Administration assembled enough information to convince them that up to 30% of the patients treated with Fen/Phen might develop valvular heart disease. On September 15, 1997, fenfluramine and dexfenfluramine were pulled from the market worldwide. The Fen/Phen success had been shattered by the "law of unintended consequences" and added another sad ending to a therapy that offered such promise in the battle of the bulge.

This is not the first disaster to befall overweight patients treated for their obesity. Table 30-1 provides several more examples. We can see that even with thyroid hormone, first used more than one hundred years ago, there were unwanted and potentially hazardous problems. This litany of difficulties associated with many treatments should give us pause when new ones are developed. Careful testing is most important to keep the smiling Janus face looking down on us.

Biosketch

Paul Ehrlich (1854-1915) was born in Strehlen, a small town in Silesia. After completing his basic education at Breslau he moved to Strasbourg, where he received his medical education. His initial interest in aniline dyes formed the basis for his work in histology. He was forced to give up his work for a year and a half after contracting tuberculosis in 1886. (Figure 30-1)

In 1896 he was appointed director of the newly opened Serum Institute at Steglitz. From there he moved in 1899 to become director of the Royal Institute for Experimental Therapy in Frankfurt am Main, a position he held until his death in 1915. In addition to his early work on the application of aniline dyes as stains to the study of tissues, he also contributed pioneering studies to immunology, for which he won the Nobel Prize in 1908. His legacy is most famously associated with his work on chemotherapeutics. His concept of the "magic bullet" as a concept for the drug targeted for a specific disease is an important part of his legacy[32,33].

Biosketch

William Henry Dale (1875-1968) was the third son and third of seven children. His education began in London and required competitive receipt of fellowships and scholarships. He entered the Leys School in Cambridge for three years on scholarship and then went to Trinity College on a minor scholarship. His medical education at St. Bartholomew's in London was interrupted for financial reasons. Among his mentorships were positions with J.N. Langley at Cambridge, with E.H. Starling at University College in London, and with Paul Ehrlich in Frankfurt. From 1904-1914 he was researcher and subsequently director of research for the Wellcome Company. In 1914 he was appointed director of the Department of Biochemistry and Pharmacology of the projected Institute for Medical Researches, which became the National Institute for Medical Research at Hampstead. From 1923 to 1942 he was director of this institute. Upon Sir Henry Wellcome's death in 1936, Dr. Dale became director of the Wellcome Institute and was its chairman from 1938 to 1960 and thereafter a scientific adviser. His research focused around adrenergic amines, histamine, and acetyl choline[34].

Biosketch

Abraham Myerson (1881-1948) was a neuropsychiatrist born in Yanova, Lithuania. He moved to the United States in 1892 at age eleven. In Myerson's early years he demonstrated his phenomenal memory and unusual skills at speed reading. During his years at English High School in Boston, he developed a strong interest in biology. After an interval of six years while he worked to save money, he entered the Columbia University College of Physicians and Surgeons in New York but transferred to Tufts Medical School where he received his M.D. in 1908. His major teaching activities were at Tufts University, where he rose from an assistant professor in 1918 to professor in 1921 and professor emeritus in 1940. (Figure 30-2)

His major work was in neurology, which is noted by the eponym Myerson's Sign, referring to the glabellar reflex. He also developed a procedure for obtaining carotid artery and internal jugular vein samples for study of brain metabolism. Myerson's interest in psychiatry was at the physiological level, and he was a strong anti-Freudian during most of his life. It was in his role as a neuropsychiatrist that his studies with amphetamine to relieve narcolepsy were conducted. He was a talented speaker and a man of great zest and enthusiasm. He chaired the research committee for the American Psychiatric Association from 1939 until 1947 and during World War II was on the National Research Council representing the American Psychiatric Association[35].

References

1. Osler, W. "Recent Advances in Medicine." *Science.* 17(1891): 170-171.
2. Temkin, O. "The Double Face of Janus." In *The Double Face of Janus and Other Essays in the History of Medicine.* Baltimore: Johns Hopkins University Press, 1977.
3. Koestler, A. *Janus: A Summing Up.* New York: Random House, 1978.
4. Lesses, M.F., A. Myerson. "Human Autonomic Pharmacology XVI: Benzedrine Sulfate as an Aid in the Treatment of Obesity." *N Engl J Med.* 218(1938): 119-124.
5. Putnam, J.J. "Cases of Myxoedema and Acromegalia Treated with Benefit by Sheep's Thyroids: Recent Observations Respecting the Pathology of the Cachexias Following Disease of the Thyroid; Clinical Relationships of Graves's Disease and Acromegalia." *Am J Med Sci.* 106(1893): 125-148.
6. Gull, W.W. "On a Cretinoid State Supervening in Adult Life in Women." *Trans Clin Soc Lond.* 7(1873-74): 180-185
7. Kendall, E.C. "The Isolation in Crystalline Form of the Compound Containing Iodine, Which Occurs in the Thyroid; Its Chemical Nature and Physiologic Activity." *JAMA.* 54(1915): 2042-2043.
8. Harington, C.R. "Chemistry of Thyroxine I." *Biochem J.* 20(1926): 293-313.
9. Gross, J., R.V. Pitt-Rivers. "3:5:3'-Triiodothyronine. I. Isolation from Thyroid Gland and Synthesis." *Biochem J.* 53(1953): 645-650.
10. Atwater, W.O., E.B. Rosa. "Description of a New Respiration Calorimeter and Experiments on the Conservation of Energy in the Human Body." U.S. Department of Agriculture Office of Experimental Stations, 1899.
11. DuBois, E.F. *Basal Metabolism in Health and Disease.* Philadelphia: Lea & Febiger, 1924.
12. Ravussin, E., S. Lillioja, T.E. Anderson, L. Christin, C. Bogardus. "Determinants of 24-Hour Energy Expenditure in Man: Methods and Results Using a Respiratory Chamber." *J Clin Invest.* 78(1986): 1568-1578.
13. Bray, G.A., K.E.W. Melvin, I.J. Chopra. "Effect of Triiodothyronine on some Metabolic Responses of Obese Patients." *Am J Clin Nutr.* 26(1973): 715-721.
14. Edward, D.A.W., G.I.M. Sawyer. "The Comparative Values of Dextroamphetamine Sulphate, Dried Thyroid Gland and a Placebo in the Treatment of Obesity." *Clin Sci.* no. 9 2(1950): 115-126.
15. Gelvin, E.P., T.H. McGavack. "Dexedrine and Weight Reduction." *NY State J Med.* 49(194): 279-282.
16. Lyon, D.M., D.M. Dunlop. "The Treatment of Obesity: A Comparison

of the Effects of Diet and of Thyroid Extract." *Quart J Med.* 1(1932): 331-352.

17. Ehrlich, P. and S. Mata. *Die experimentelle chemotherapie der Spirillosen.* Berlin: Julius Springer, 1910.
18. Bray, G.A. *The Obese Patient: Major Problems in Internal Medicine.* Philadelphia: W.B. Saunders, 1976.
19. Simkins, S. "Dinitrophenol and Desiccated Thyroid in the Treatment of Obesity: A Comprehensive Clinical and Laboratory Study." *JAMA* 108(1937): 2110-2193.
20. Leake, C.D. *The Amphetamines: Their Actions and Uses.* Springfield, IL: Charles C. Thomas, 1958.
21. Harris, S.C., A.C. Ivy, L.M. Searle. "The Mechanism of Amphetamine-induced Loss of Weight: A Correlation of the Theory of Hunger and Appetite." *JAMA* 134(1947): 1468-1474
22. Barger, G., H.H. Dale. "Chemical Structure and Sympathomimetic Action of Amines." *J Physiol.* 41(1910): 19-59.
23. Prinzmetal, M., W. Bloomberg. "The Use of Benzedrine for the Treatment of Narcolepsy." *JAMA.* 105(1935): 2051-2053.
24. Myerson, A. "Effect of Benzedrine Sulfate on Mood and Fatigue in Normal and in Neurotic Persons." *Arch Neurol Psych.* 36(1936): 816-822.
25. Nathanson, M.H. "The Central Action of Beta-aminopropylbenzene (Benzedrine)." *JAMA.* 108(1937): 528-531.
26. Davidoff, E., E.C. Reifenstein Jr. "The Stimulating Action of Benzedrine Sulfate: A Comparative Study of the Responses of Normal Persons and of Depressed Patients." *JAMA* 108(1937): 1770-1776.
27. Ulrich, H. "Narcolepsy and Its Treatment with Benzedrine Sulfate." *N Engl J Med.* 217(1937): 696-701.
28. Leibowitz, S.F., C. Rossakis. "Analysis of Feeding Suppression Produced by Perifornical Hypothalamic Injection of Catecholamines, Amphetamines and Mazindol." *Eur Pharm.* 53(1978): 69-81.
29. Roberts, R.M. *Serendipity: Accidental Discoveries in Science.* New York: John Wiley & Sons, Inc., 1989.
30. Connolly, H.M., M.D. McGoon, D.D. Hensrud, B.S. Edwards, W.D. Edwards, et al. "Valvular Heart Disease Associated with Fenfluramine-Phentermine." *N Engl J Med.* 337(1997): 581-588.
31. Weintraub, M., P.M. Sundarensan, M. Madan, et al. "Long-term Weight Control (Parts 1-7), the National Heart, Lung and Blood Institute Funded Multimodal Intervention Study." *Clin Pharmacol Ther.* No. 51 5(1992): 581-646.
32. Stevenson, L.G. *Nobel Prize Winners in Medicine & Physiology 1901-1950.* New York: Henry Schuman, 1953.
33. Garrison, H. *An Introduction to the History of Medicine with Medical*

Chronology Bibliographic Data and Test Questions. Philadelphia: W.B. Saunders, 1914.

34. Feldberg, W. "Sir Henry Hallett Dale (1875-1968)." In *The Dictionary of National Biography 1961-1970.* London: Oxford University Press, 1981.
35. Walter, R.D. "Abraham Myerson." *Dictionary of American Biography.* 24(1974): 617-618.

Chapter 31

Surgery for Overweight Individuals

Tradition has always been a restraining barrier to innovation.

—Wangensteen & Wangensteen[1]

Any fool can cut off a leg. It takes a surgeon to save one.

—George Ross of Montreal[2]

Would you consider surgery in the battle of the bulge? You wouldn't need to remember to stick with your diet, to exercise, or to take medications. For some "a consummation devoutly to be wished." However, you would be trading one kind of problem for another. The surgical scars and reworking of your stomach and intestine would replace your diets and exercise with physical constraints on food intake that produce some of the most dramatic results in the battle of the bulge, but which also have their problems. This chapter will explore the developments in surgery that have made this drastic but effective approach grow in popularity as the final treatment for many desperate overweight people

Surgical treatment for disease has a long history[1,3-5]. Trephination, or the drilling of holes into the skull, was one of the earliest surgical techniques developed by early human cultures. These procedures date from Neolithic times more than five thousand years ago up to the twentieth-century. Prior to the discovery of anesthesia, they were done without any good procedures to relieve pain. Some skulls show evidence of more than one operation, and long survival after trephination is well known.

Military surgeons have treated wounded soldiers since armies formed. Galen (ca A.D. 130-200) is thought to have learned much of his human anatomy from repairing wounds to gladiators and Roman soldiers. Ambroise Paré (1509-1590)[6], the great sixteenth-century French surgeon, and Jean-Dominque Larrey (1766-1842)[7], Napoleon's surgeon, are two of the best known. In spite of the important role in treating injuries, the training of surgeons was separate from the education of physicians until after the French Revolution[8]. Indeed, surgeons were part of the Guild of Barber-Surgeons until the early nineteenth century when these guilds separated.

Many of the early surgeons were anatomists. John Hunter (1728-1793), for example, was an inveterate collector of pathological specimens, many of which are now on display at the Royal College of Surgeons in London[9]. He founded the Windmill School of Anatomy in London.

A major turn of events in medical/surgical education dates from the French Revolution, when the training of surgeons and physicians was finally put under the same faculty[8] and teaching of medicine and surgery were consolidated in hospitals.

Four themes have moved surgeons from the anatomist technician to the forefront of medical practice: (1) The discovery of anesthesia[10,11]; (2) the germ theory of disease, which resulted in the practice of washing hands before entering the delivery room[12] and in the development of antisepsis[13], antibiotics[14], and immunology[15]; (3) blood transfusion, fluid replacement, and nutritional support therapy[17], and (4) development of plastics and technical devices[18].

Prior to the discovery of anesthesia in the 1840s, surgery inflicted much pain[11]. Amputations and other procedures were done as rapidly as possible. Scenes of operations prior to discovery of anesthesia showed patients being forcibly restrained[4,5]. With the introduction of ether[10], nitrous oxide[19], and chloroform[20] between 1842 and 1850, the acute pain of surgery was alleviated, but the problem of infection remained. The original use of ether anesthesia is attributed to Crawford Long (1815-1878). Dr. Long was a general physician practicing in rural Georgia. He noticed that ether inhalation at social events often produced "anesthesia" for injuries that occurred while under its influence. He decided to try the use of ether for a local surgical removal. The operation was a success, but he did not publish the results until a number of years later. It was, however, William T.G. Morton (1819-1868) who demonstrated ether anesthesia at the Massachusetts General Hospital in 1846, who brought the value of the technique to public awareness.

The next fifty years saw enormous progress in surgery, improving both the tools of the surgeon and the safety of his patients. Shortly after the discovery of anesthesia, Ignaz Semmelweis (1818-1865) in Vienna recognized the relation of childbed fever in women who had just delivered their babies and the failure of physicians to wash hands when going from the autopsy room to the delivery room. In 1847 he introduced hand washing, which dramatically reduced the transmission of disease.

Antiseptic procedures were introduced into the operating room by Lord Joseph Lister (1827-1912)[13] in 1865. This was followed by the introduction of latex gloves in about 1895[21], to reduce the transmission of germs from the hands to the open wounds of surgically treated patients. The discovery of antibiotics[15] and sulfa drugs[22] in the period just before World War II made surgery safer from all perspectives. Blood transfusion and fluid replacement were also important preconditions for modern surgery. Replacement parts, prostheses, and the introduction of sophisticated instruments like heart pumps[18] were important post-conditions.

Blood transfusion took somewhat longer to move from conception to practice. Richard Lower (1631-1691) first transfused dogs in 1665[23], and the first human transfusions were done shortly after in France. However, it required the understanding of blood groups[15] and immunology to make blood transfusions safe. The impact of the development of anesthesia, antisepsis, and blood transfusions can be seen most dramatically by the reduction of deaths in military forces. It was not until the twentieth-century that deaths in battle exceeded deaths due to disease and injury (Table 31-1).

Table 31-1. Impact of Medical Developments on Military Mortality

War	Years	Deaths due to combat	Deaths due non-combat diseases*
Peninsular War	1808-1824	8,889	24,930
Crimean War	1854-1856	7,000	14,000
Boer War	1899-1902	7,500	14,500
World War I	1914-1918	52,967	31,304

* Disease includes typhoid, typhus, cholera and dysentery (figures for World War I include 1917 only). Source: Wellcome Collection, Science Museum, London

Surgical treatment prior to the introduction of anesthesia to relieve the pain of operation in 1846 was only conducted under dire circumstances. Over the past one hundred fifty years as surgical techniques and the pre-operative and post-operative support have improved, surgeons have tackled more and more difficult problems, including the battle of the bulge.

Surgical approaches for battling the bulge were developed over the last quarter of the twentieth-century.

The two papers in the appendix illustrate the use of two surgical innovations for treating obesity. The first is the paper by Payne et al.[24] describing jejunocolic anastomosis, and the second is the paper by Mason and Ito[25] describing the first series of gastric reduction operations to treat obesity.

In 1963 Payne and DeWind published their results with an operation that they soon abandoned. The operation involved cutting the small intestine and attaching it to the colon. In this way the contents of the small intestine were drained into the colon before digestion was complete. This operation produced malabsorption of partially digested food. This operation produced major weight loss along with diarrhea. In summarizing the results with this jejuno-colic bypass procedure, Payne and DeWind said:

> In accord with the plan adopted before our first study was undertaken in 1956, intestinal continuity was re-established when the desired weight was reached or when electrolyte disturbance required it. Weight gain to pre-shunt levels occurred promptly in all subjects whose intestinal continuity was restored to normal. For these reasons, this approach, jejunocolic shunt, was abandoned[24].

The fact that their patients regained weight was disturbing to the authors, who believed that if these patients could achieve normal weight they would be able to maintain that weight. An alternative view is that weight regain is to be expected when treatments for obesity are terminated because obesity is a chronic disease that was not cured but only treated[26]. The jejuno-colic bypass had been abandoned for some years by the community of academic surgeons, yet it was abandoned much more slowly by other surgeons. This is illustrated by a comment of Farris at a surgical meeting:

> It is amazing to me that although the jejuno-colic fistula really has no place in the treatment of obesity...it is still being used in a great number of centers. It is obvious that the dissemination of medical information is slow since many are still performing an operation which has been obsolete on the West Coast for several years.[27].

Similar delays of a number of years in the dissemination of scientific findings have been noted on many occasions[28].

The failure of the jejuno-colic operation was followed by the introduction of a modified intestinal operation. The two principal forms were the end-to-end or end-to-side jejuno-ileal anastomosis[29,33].

As with the jejuno-colic procedure, Payne and DeWind were among its early pioneers[30], although Kremen et al.[29] reported the first case. Soon there were a number of surgical groups performing this operation. Figure 31-1 shows the end-to-side jejuno-ileal operation that was so popular during the 1970s. Numerous complications followed this operation, and the operation was gradually replaced by the gastric operations that were pioneered by Mason and Ito. A number of gastric restriction operations have been developed (Figure 31-1) that slowed the flow of food from the upper stomach to the lower one.

At the same time a gastric bypass was developed that short-circuited food from a small upper gastric pouch into the intestine. This operation produced greater weight loss than the gastric restriction operations (Figure 31-1). A final operation, a joint gastric-intestinal and intestinal-intestine bypass, called the Scopinaro procedure after its pioneer, was also introduced. This operation is sometimes associated with malnutrition.

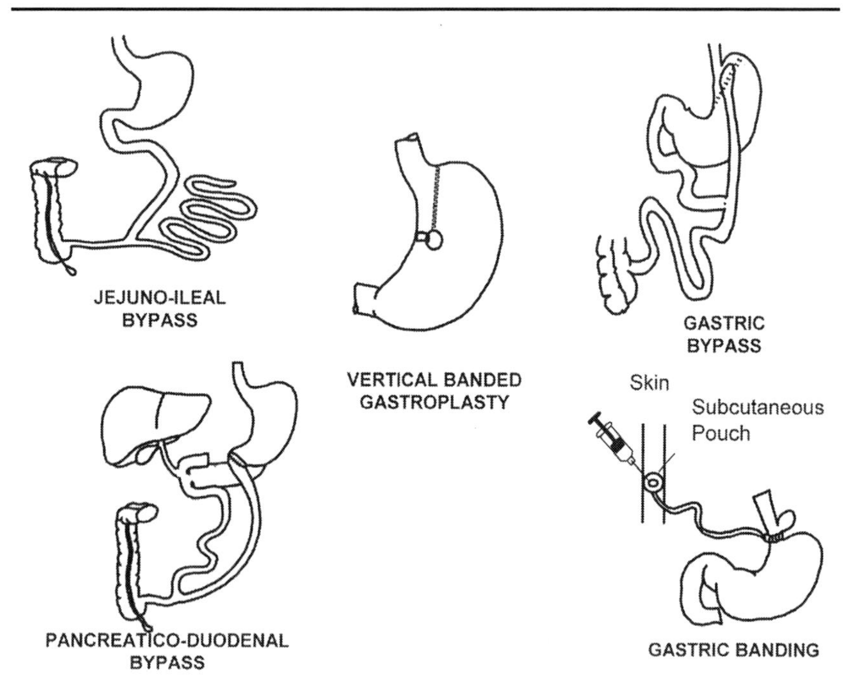

31-1 Diagram of bariatric operations developed for obesity since 1950. © 2006 George A. Bray, MD.

In the broad sense, at least two types of surgical procedures can be identified. The first are operations that repair traumatic damage—the type that occurs in automobile accidents, military encounters, or other acute injuries. Many orthopedic surgical operations fall into this group, as well as surgery for gunshot wounds. Also conditions like appendicitis, where inflammation produces much of the disease process and where surgery eliminates or corrects the disease, would fall in this group.

A second broad group of surgical operations treat chronic diseases. Repair of a dilated aorta or coronary vascular occlusion are two such examples. The operation of sympathectomy for hypertension[34] is an example of a surgical procedure that has been replaced by effective pharmacological intervention for treating hypertension. The operative procedures for peptic ulcer disease would also be in this group[35]. The gastric operations for obesity, like sympathectomy for hypertension, are surgical approaches that will probably be abandoned when better prevention and pharmacological treatment becomes available for the battle of the bulge. However that day is not here yet, and surgery clearly offers some hope for treatment of obesity.

The jejuno-ileal bypass has been used to lower cholesterol[31] as well as to treat obesity. As a surgical treatment for hypercholesterolemia it met with a measure of success. As a treatment for obesity, jejuno-ileal by-pass had serious problems. It led to long-term weight loss, reduced food intake, and improvement in social functioning[33]. However, a new disease was often produced consisting of fluid and electrolyte problems due to diarrhea and a series of problems, including arthritis and liver disease due to changes in the bacteria growing in the intestine. Surgical efforts to reduce these complications included attaching the unused portion of the jejunum to the gall bladder. In spite of these efforts, the problems associated with jejuno-ileal bypass were sufficiently troublesome that it has been abandoned.

Mason and Ito[25] introduced a new procedure based on the work of Theodor Billroth (1829-1894) who pioneered the surgical treatment of gastric and peptic ulcers[35]. The surgical history of gastric operations dates to the nineteenth-century. The work of William Beaumont (1785-1853)[37], who directly observed the human gastric mucosa in a patient with an accidental gastric fistula, was but the first in a long line of studies that directly observed the stomach[34]. The work of Ivan P. Pavlov (1849-1936)[38], who pioneered the cerebral control of conditioned reflexes, and of Walter Cannon (1871-1945)[39], who led the way in using x-rays to study gastric function, set the stage for advances in gastric surgery. Billroth, the famous Viennese surgeon, tackled the problem of peptic ulcer disease surgically. The operations for antral exclusion and gastric resection that Billroth pioneered were the cornerstones for the gastric operations for obesity. He developed two procedures that were widely used to treat this problem[35] before the discovery of drugs that block histamine H-2 receptors to treat the disease and the role of *Helicobacter pyloris* in causing it[41].

Mason and Ito[25] began their studies of surgery for obesity by using dogs and then proceeding to human beings. The initial procedure diverted food from a small upper pouch into the jejunum through an anastomosis between stomach and intestine after closing the lower stomach off. Several versions were tested. The initial procedures used surgical techniques developed in the earlier part of the century, including traditional sutures. With the introduction of stapling instruments and new synthetic fibers, new innovative approaches became possible.

Since gastric restriction was successful in reducing weight, it was a small step to reducing gastric filling by preventing the jaws from opening. Mandibular fixation, as it is called, was shown to reduce food intake. It had little long-term use, however, because patients uniformly regained weight when the wires were removed and the mouth could open. This finding, and the regaining after reversal of jejuno-colic and jejuno-ileal operations, reinforces our views of the chronicity of obesity and the fact that treatments don't work when they are discontinued.

Biosketch

John Hunter (1728-1793) led surgery from its barber-surgeon days into the broader daylight of a physiologically based discipline (Figure 31-2)[42]. As Garrison says, "Hunter came up to London in 1748 (from Scotland) a raw, uncouth Scotch lad, fonder of taverns and theater galleries than of book-learning"[42].

Under the wing of his older brother William, who became known for his classic monograph and work in obstetrics, Hunter became an anatomist and in his life dissected more than five hundred different species. Once he had found himself in anatomy he began surgical work with Cheselden and Pott. His experience in gunshot wounds was obtained on an expedition to Belleisle in 1761; the remainder of his career was spent in London. He was an inveterate collector and left some thirteen thousand specimens to the Royal College of Surgeons[9] where those that survived the bombing during World War II can still be seen in the Hunter Museum. Many famous students worked with him, including William Jenner who introduced vaccination, Parkinson of Parkinson's disease, and Physick, the American physician from Philadelphia. To quote Garrison, "His permanent position in science is based upon the fact that he was the founder of experimental and surgical pathology as well as a pioneer in comparative physiology and experimental morphology"[3].

Biosketch

Theodor Billroth (1829-1894) was a pioneer of gastrointestinal surgery in the nineteenth century, as those who pioneered gastrointestinal surgery for obesity were in the twentieth century (Figure 31-3).

He was born on the island of Rügen and graduated with a medical degree from Berlin in 1852. He learned his early surgery at the time that anesthesia and the antiseptic methods were being introduced. After training with Langenbeck he became professor of surgery at Zurich from 1860 to 1887 (the time of the American Civil War) and the professor of surgery at Vienna from 1867 to 1894. He was the first to resect the esophagus and to resect the pylorus for cancer. Billroth was a musician and a poet as well as having a charming and genial personality[3].

References

1. Wangensteen, O.H., S.D. Wangensteen. *The Rise of Surgery: From Empiric Craft to Scientific Discipline.* Minneapolis: University of Minnesota Press, 1978.
2. Duffin, J. *History of Medicine: A Scandalously Short Introduction.* Toronto: University of Toronto Press, 1999.
3. Garrison, F. *An Introduction to the History of Medicine.* Philadelphia: W.B. Saunders and Co., 1914.
4. Haeger, K. *An Illustrated History of Surgery.* New York: Bell Publishing Co., 1988.
5. Rutkow, I.M. *Surgery: An Illustrated History.* St Louis: Mosby-Year Book, 1993.
6. Paré, A. *Les oeuvres de M. Ambroise Paré.* Paris: G. Buon, 1575.
7. Larrey, D.J. *Memoires de chirurgie militaire.* Paris: J. Smith, 1812.
8. Ackerknecht, E.H. *Medicine at the Paris Hospital.* Baltimore: Johns Hopkins University Press, 1967.
9. Descriptive catalogue of the Pathological Series in the Hunterian Museum of the Royal College of Surgeons of London. Edinburgh: E&S Livingstone Ltd., 1966.
10. Bigelow, N.J. "Insensibility during Surgical Operations Produced by Inhalation." *Boston Med Surg J.* 35(1846): 309-317.
11. Fulop-Muller, R. *Triumph over Pain.* New York: Literary Guild, 1938.
12. Semmelweis, I.O. *Die Aetiologie der Begriff und die Prophylaxis des Kinderbettfiebers.* Pes, Vienna & Leipzig: C.A. Hartleben's Verlags-Expedition, 1861.
13. Lister, J. *Observations on Ligature of Arteries in the Antiseptic System.* Edinburgh: Edmonston & Douglas, 1869.
14. Fleming, A. "On the Antibacterial Action of Cultures of a Penicillium, with Special Reference to Their Use in the Isolation of B. Influenza." *Brit J Exp Pathol.* 10(1929): 226-236.
15. Landsteiner, K. "Zur Kenntnis der antifermentativen, lytischen, und agglutinierenden Wirkungen des Blutes und der Lymphe." *Zbl Bakt.* 27(1900): 357-362.
16. Hunter, J. "A Case of Paralysis of the Muscles of Deglutition, Cured by an Artificial Mode of Conveying Food and Medicines into the Stomach." *Trans Soc Improvement Med Chir Knowledge.* 1(1793): 182-188.
17. Dudrick, S.J., D.W. Wilmore, H.M. Vars, J.E. Rhoads. "Long-Term Parenteral Nutrition with Growth and Development and Positive Nitrogen Balance." *Surgery.* 64(1968): 134-142.

18 Gibbon, J.H. "Application of a Mechanical Heart and Lung Apparatus to Cardiac Surgery." *Minn Med.* 37(1954): 171-180.

19. Wells, H. *Horrace Wells, Dentist, Father of Surgical Anesthesia: Proceedings of Centenary Commemorations of Wells' Discovery in 1844 of Lists of Wells' Memorabilia, Including Bibliographies, Memorials and Testimonials.* Hartford: Case, Lockwood and Brainard, 1948.
20. Simpson, J.Y. *Remarks on the Superinduction of Anesthesia in Natural and Morbid Parturition: With Cases Illustrative of the Use and Effects of Chloroform in Obstetric Practice.* Boston: William B. Little & Co., 1848.
21. Halsted, W.S. *Johns Hopk Hosp Rep.* 4(1894): Plate XII.
22. Domagk, G. "Ein Beitrag zur Chemotherapie der bakteriellen Infektionen." *Dtsch Med Wschr.* 61(1935): 250-253.
23. Lower, R. *Tractatus de Corde.* Londini: J Allestry, 1669
24. Payne, J.H., L.T. DeWind, R.R. Commons. "Metabolic Observations in Patients with Jejunocolic Shunts." *Am J Surg.* 106(1963): 173-189.
25. Mason, E.E., C. Ito. "Gastric Bypass in Obesity." *Surg Clin North Am.* 47(1967): 1345-1351.
26. Bray, G.A. "Barriers to Treatment of Obesity." *Ann Intern Med.* 115(1991): 152-153.
27. Farris, J.M. "Discussion of Payne and DeWind." *Am J Surg.* 118(1969): 147.
28. Rogers, E.M. *Diffusion of Innovations.* 3rd ed. New York: Free Press, 1983.
29. Kremen, A.J., J.H. Linner, C.H. Nelson. "An Experimental Evaluation of the Nutritional Importance of Proximal and Distal Small Intestine." *Ann Surg.* 140(1954): 439-448.
30. Payne, J.H., and L.T. DeWind. "Surgical Treatment of Obesity." *Am J Surg.* 118(1969): 141-147.
31. Buchwald, H., R.L. Varco. "Partial Ileal Bypass for Hypercholesterolemia and Atherosclerosis." *Surg Gynecol Obstet.* 124(1967): 1231-1238.
32. Scott, H.W., D.H. Law. "Clinical Appraisal of Jejunoileal Shunt in Patients with Morbid Obesity." *Am J Surg.* 117(1969): 246-253.
33. Bray, G.A., F.L. Greenway, R.E. Barry. "Surgical Treatment of Obesity: A Review of Our Experience and an Analysis of Published Reports." *Int J Obes.* 1(1977): 331-367
34. Smithwick, R.H. "A Technique for Splanchnic Resection for Hypertension: Preliminary Report." *Surgery.* 7(1940): 1-8.
35. Billroth, T. *General Surgical Pathology and Therapeutics in Fifty Lectures: A Textbook for Students and Physicians.* Birmingham: Classics of Medicine, 1987.
36. Beaumont, W. *Experiments and Observations on the Gastric Juice and the Physiology of Digestion.* Plattsburgh: F.P. Allen, 1833.
37. Wolf, S., H.G. Wolff. *Human Gastric Function: An Experimental Study of a Man and His Stomach.* London: Oxford University Press, 1943.

38. Pavlov, I.P. Transl. W.H. Thompson. *The Work of the Digestive Glands.* 2nd edition. London: Charles Griffin and Co., 1910.
39. Cannon, W.B. *The Mechanical Factors of Digestion.* London: Edward Arnold, 1911.
40. Black, J.W., W.A.M. Duncan, C.J. Durant, C.R. Ganellin, E.M. Parsons. "Definition and Antagonism of Histamine H2 Receptors." *Nature.* 236(1972): 385-390.
41. Bettany, G.T. "John Hunter (1728-1793)." In *The Dictionary of National Biography.* Ed. L. Stephen and S. Lee. London: Oxford University Press, 1937-1938. Vol X. pp. 287-293.

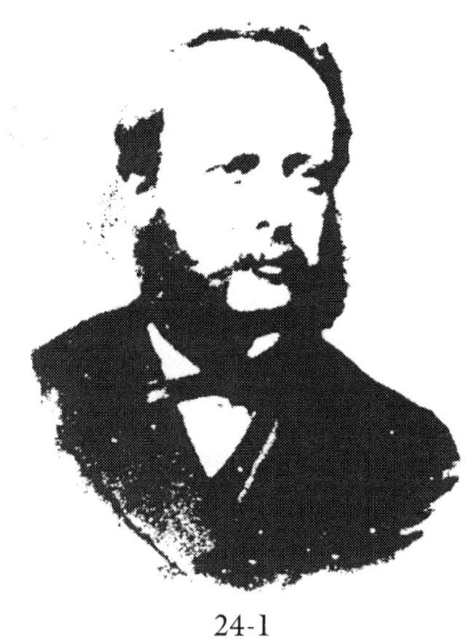

24-1

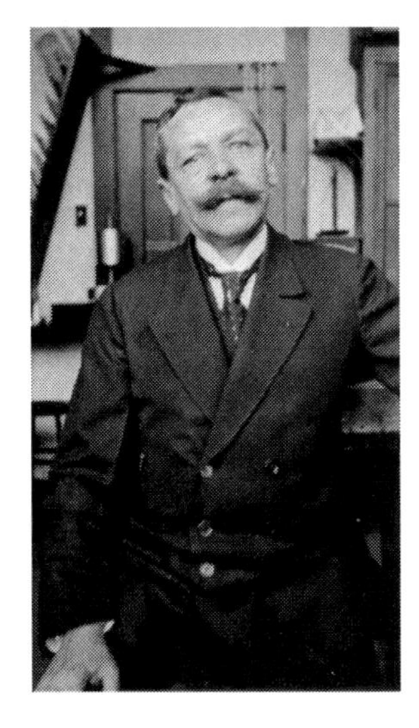

24-2

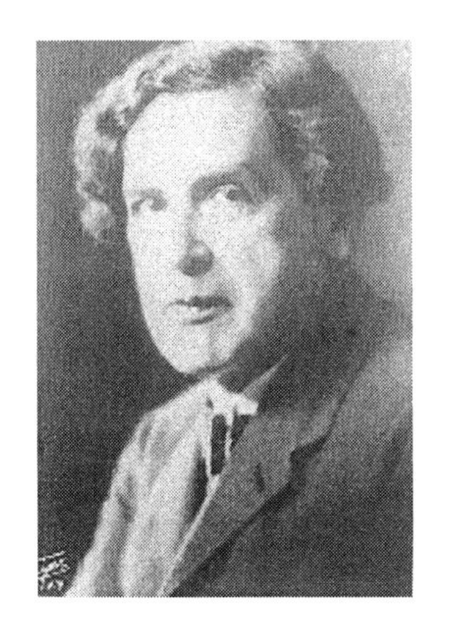

25-2

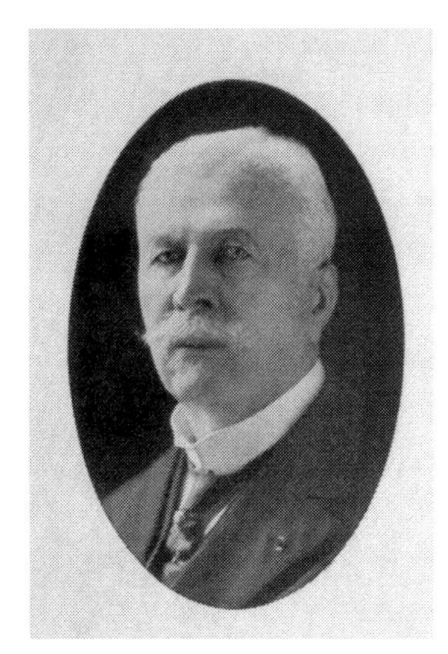

25-3

24-1 John Zachariah Laurence (1826-1870). http://www.isgrd.umds.ac.uk/laurence/

24-2 Arthur Biedl (1844-1914). Courtesy of the National Library of Medicine.

25-2 Alfred Frohlich (1871-1953). http://www.uic.edu/depts/mcne/founders/page 0037.html

25-3 Joseph Francois Felix Babinski (1857-1932). Courtesy of the National Library of Medicine.

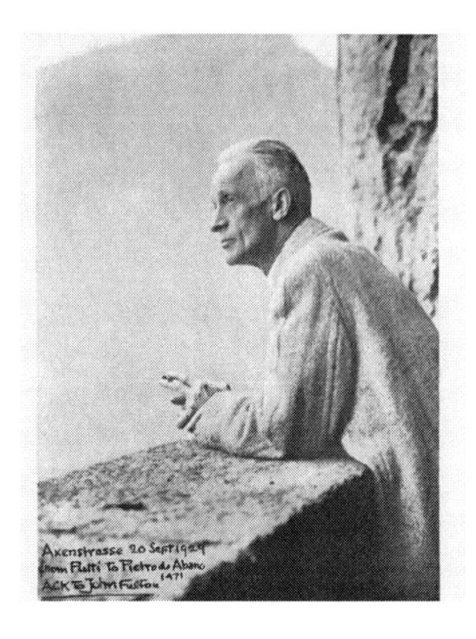

26-2

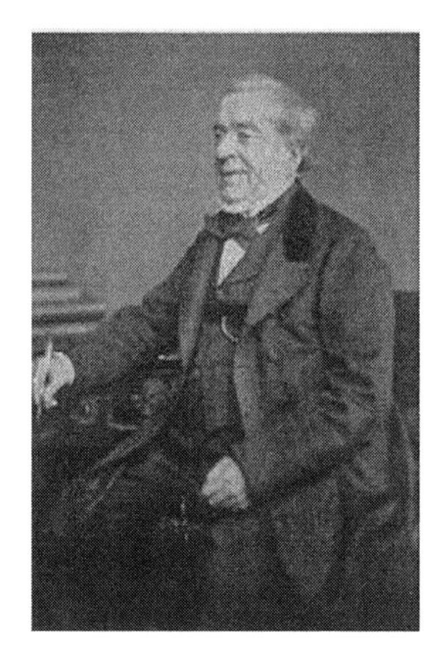

27-2

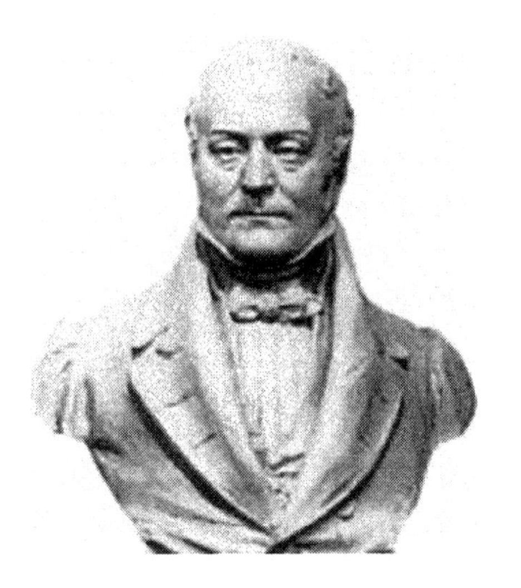

27-3

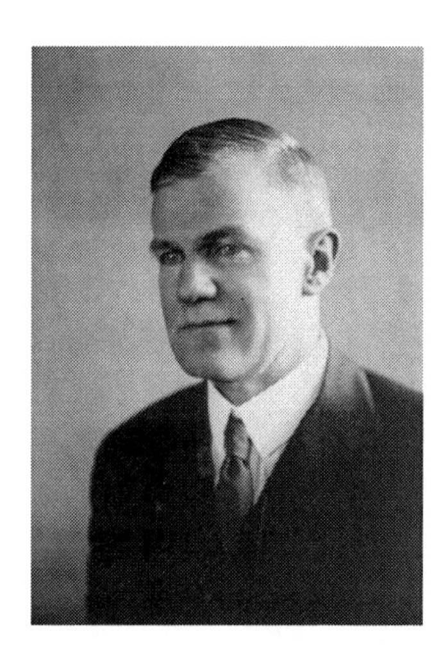

28-1

26-2 Harvey Williams Cushing (1869-1939). From the collection of the author.

27-2 William Banting (1797-1878)
http://www.mercola.com/2002/oct/16/banting.htm

27-3 Jean-Anthelme Brillat-Savarin (1755-1826)
http://www.chm.bris.ac.uk/motm/dimethylsulphide/dmsh.htm

28-1 Francis Gano Benedict (1870-1857). Courtesy of the National Library of Medicine.

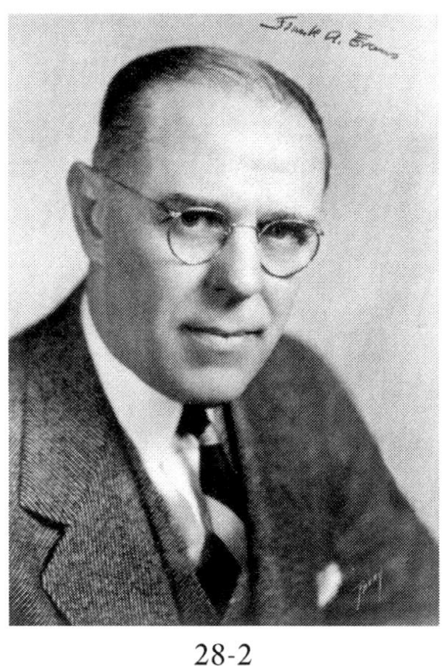

28-2

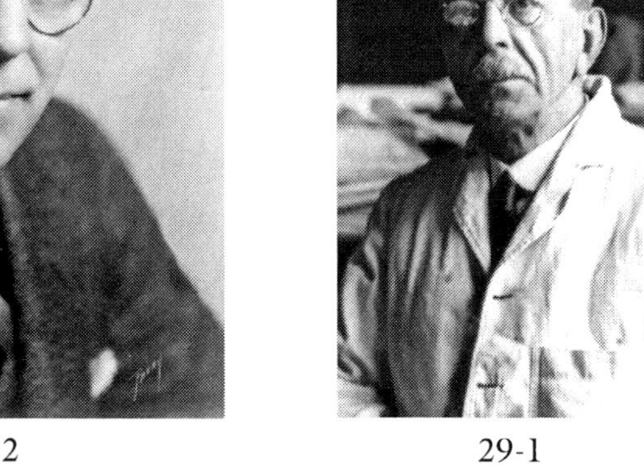

29-1

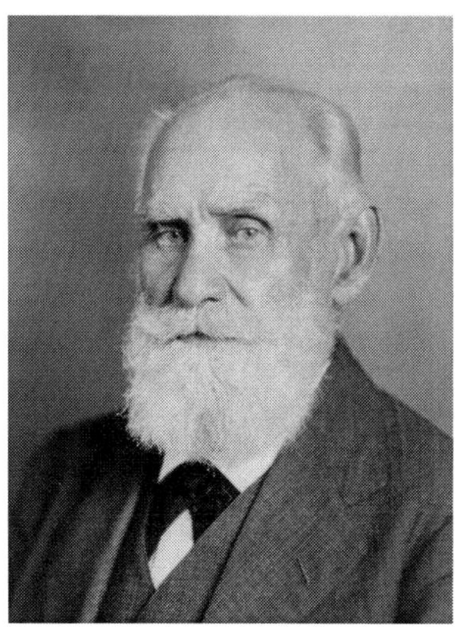

29-2

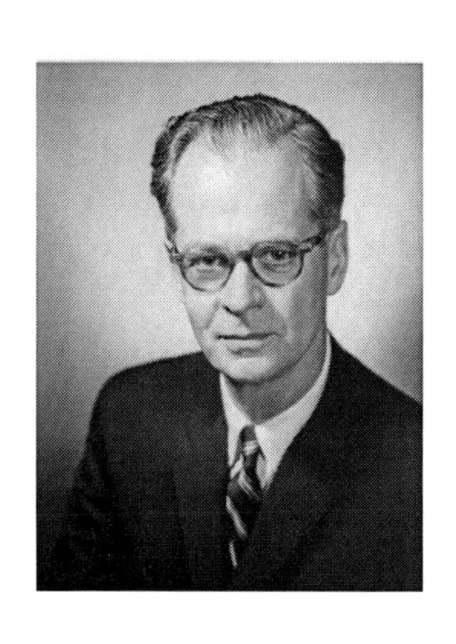

29-3

28-2 Frank Evans (1889-1956). Courtesy of the National Library of Medicine.

29-1 Sir Charles Scott Sherrington (1857-1952). Courtesy of the National Library of Medicine.

29-2 Ivan Petrovich Pavlov (1849-1952). Courtesy of the National Library of Medicine.

29-3 Burrhus Frederic Skinner (1904-1990). Courtesy of the National Library of Medicine.

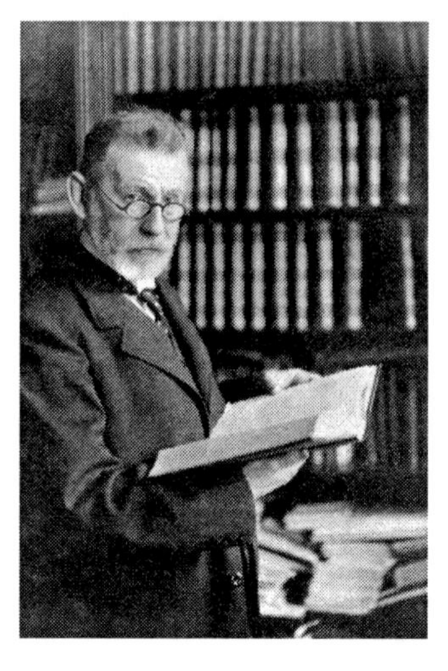

30-1

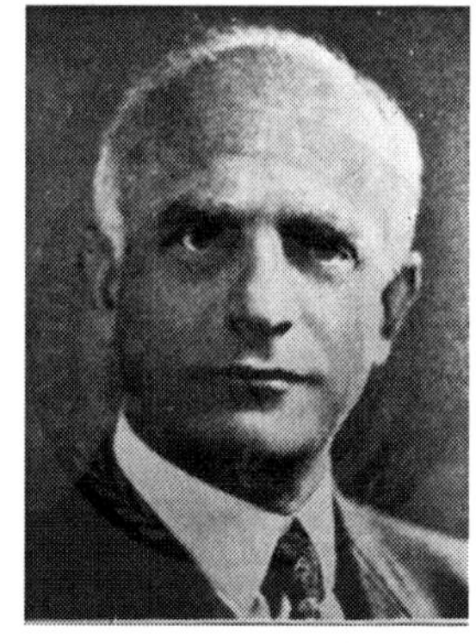

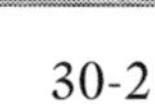

30-2

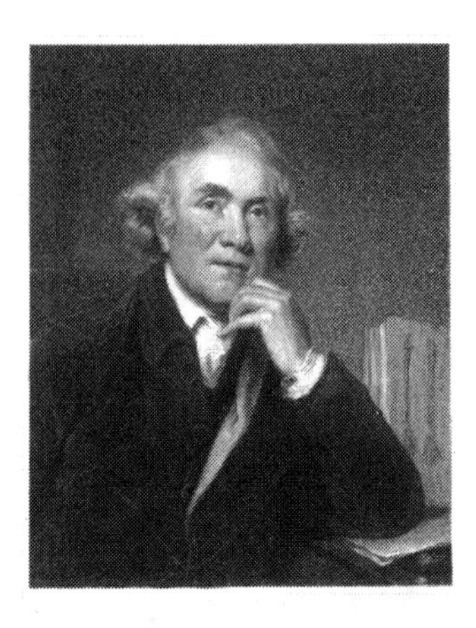

31-2

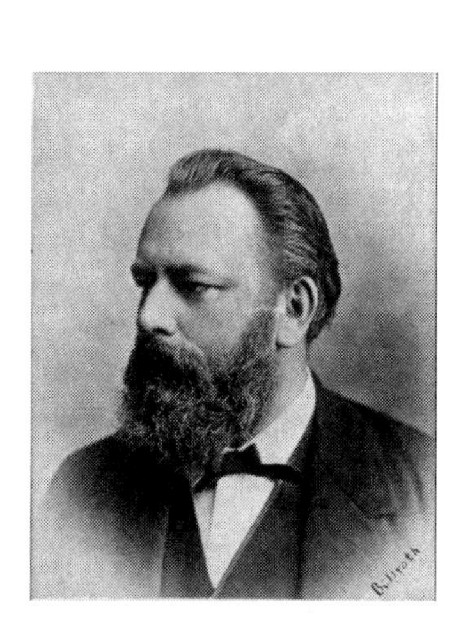

31-3

30-1 Paul Ehrlich (1854-1915) Courtesy of the National Library of Medicine.

30-2 Abraham Myerson (1881-1948). Courtesy of the National Library of Medicine.

31-2 John Hunter (1728-1793). Courtesy of the National Library of Medicine.

31-3 Theodor Billroth (1829-1894). Courtesy of the National Library of Medicine.

Appendices

Classic Papers

A Treatise on Man and the Development of His Faculties

Lambert-Adolf-Jacques Quetelet

BOOK SECOND.

DEVELOPMENT OF STATURE, WEIGHT, STRENGTH, &C.

APPARENTLY but little interest is attached to the determination of the stature and weight of man, or to his physical development at different ages; nor, until the present time, has any one particularly attended to this subject. Man has only been studied in his most conspicuous relations; the correlative study of his qualities, and the numerical determination of the modifications which are consequent upon age, have been neglected. This state of things leaves immense voids in science, and the result is that we generally want the necessary means for solving a great number of interesting questions, especially relating to the natural history of man. For example, we are almost totally ignorant of the ratios which may exist between the laws of development of his different faculties, and what are the elements which predominate at such or such an age: hence the critical periods of life can only be determined in a very indefinite manner.

The researches which have been made to measure the height and weight of man, especially relate either to the period of birth or to the period of complete development; but the intermediate ages have scarcely been attended to. Physiologists have connected the first of these determinations with a question in legal medicine; they have even anticipated the period of birth, and sought to value the size and weight of the fœtus. Natural philosophers, who studied man as a mechanical agent, have rather been occupied with the determination of his weight when he has acquired complete development. La Hire has made some very remarkable researches of this kind, which prove that the subject now occupying us has a much deeper interest than that resulting from mere curiosity.

Quetelet LAJ. A Treatise on Man and the Development of his Faculties. Edinburgh: William and Robert Chambers; 1842. In: Comparative statistics in the 19th century. Farnborough: Gregg International Publishers; 1973.
Reprinted with permission from Gregg Publishing, 60 High Street, Godstone, Surrey RH9 8LW.

To show how little advanced is the state of the study of the progressive development of man, let us suppose that we want to establish the age of an individual, from the aggregate of his physical qualities: we may be allowed to say, that we shall not find in science any assistance for the determination of this question–we shall be reduced to mere empirical conjecture. However, legal medicine presents numerous examples where such determinations become necessary. We may ask, no doubt, if it will ever be possible to obtain them, especially for advanced ages? This fear, well founded as it may appear, ought not, however, to lead us to reject such researches: that would not be very philosophic. If to the data furnished by the habit of observation, and the *tact* resulting therefrom, we can join physical qualities susceptible of measurement, prudence bids us not neglect them. When a physician is called to examine the body of an infant found lifeless, and when, in a legal inquiry, he, from simple inspection, establishes the presumed age of this child, it is evident that he cannot but impose his judgment on those who read the inquiry, however erroneous it may otherwise be, since there are no elements existing for the verification of it. If, on the contrary, to the assistance of the estimate which has been made of the age, is joined the height and weight of the child, and some other physical qualities susceptible of computation; and if, moreover, there were exact tables which might enable one to ascertain, at different ages, the values of these physical qualities, and the limits within which they are found connected in individuals regularly formed, the judgment given of the age would be capable of verification–it would even become useless, if the elements of verification admitted of great accuracy. Such appreciations, then, ought not to be neglected by legal medicine, since they tend to substitute precise characters and exact data for conjectural estimates, which are always vague and often faulty.

Thus, apart from the interest which is presented by the determination of man at different ages, and in researches relating to the average man, it may present another important element, as we shall see more perfectly farther on, for the solution of the following problem of legal medicine: *To determine the age of an individual after death, from the aggregate of his physical qualities.* In this sense, weight would be one of the elements which it would be necessary to connect with the distinguishing of individuals; and this physical character naturally takes a place near that of the stature.

Researrches on the height of man, and on his development, may have another useful end, that of enlightening governments on many points; as, for example, as regards the fixing of the age of recruits.

There is another element, the determination of which is equally important, and which, also, is but little known, namely, the strength. I do not flatter myself that I have filled up the voids which science presented on this subject, but I shall think myself happy if my researches may induce other persons to attempt it.

CHAPTER I.

OF THE DEVELOPMENT OF THE HEIGHT.

I DO not think that, before Buffon, any inquiries had been made to determine the rate of human growth successively from birth to maturity; and even this celebrated naturalist cites only a single particular example; neither has he examined the modifying influences which age exerts on height. The only researches at all precise which science possesses, refer to the length of the child before birth, and to that of the fully developed man.*

Chaussier, who invented the *mecometre*, an instrument adapted to measure the length of children, thought that we might view as regular the increase in length of the child for six months before its birth; and he estimated this increase at two inches per month. In the *Dictionnaire des Sciences Medicales,* the length of the fœtus is estimated by the following numbers:–

	Metres.
At birth,	0•487 to 0•541
On month before birth,	0•433 to 0•487
Two months	0•379 to 0•433
Three months	0•300 to 0•379
Four months	0•216 to 0•300
Five months	0•162 to 0•216

The medium length of the child at birth would then be 0•514 metres: this estimate differs but slightly from that obtained at the Foundling Hospital in Brussels, by means, also, of Chaussier's *mecomtre*. On measuring the length of fifty male and as many female children immediately at birth, the following numbers were obtained:‡–

Length.	Boys.	Girls.	Total.
From 16 to 17 inches French,	2	4	6
" 17 to 18 "	8	19	27
" 18 to 19 "	28	18	46
" 19 to 20 "	12	8	20
" 20 to 21 "	"	1	1
	50	50	100

With regard to the mediums or averages and the limits, they have given the following values for the two sexes:–

Value.	Boys.	Girls.
Minimum,	16 inches 2 lines.§	16 inches 2 lines.
Medium,	18 " 6 " nearly	18 " 1.5 " nearly
Maximum,	19 " 8 "	20 " 6 "

From these results it follows, that, from the period of birth, the height or length of one sex is superior to the other; being, for boys, 0•4999; for girls, 0•4896; giving thus in favour of boys a trifle less than half an inch.

By uniting these numbers to those which have been obtained in the junior schools of Brussels, the Orphan Hospital, boarding-houses, and in public life, in respect to young persons of different classes, I have been able to construct the following table, comprising the rate of growth from birth to 20 years: the height of the shoe is not included:–

Table showing the rate of Growth in the two Sexes.

Ages.	Boys.	Girls.	Difference
	metres.	metres.	metres.
Birth,	0•500	0•490	0•010
1 year,	0•608	..	..
2 years,	0•796	0•780	0•016
3 years,	0•867	0•853	0•014
4 years,	0•930	0•913	0•017
5 years,	0•986	0•978	0•008
6 years,	1•045	1•035	0•010
7 years,	..	1•091	..
8 years,	1•160	1•134	0•003
9 years,	1•221	1•205	0•016
10 years,	1•280	1•256	0•024
11 years,	1•334	1•286	0•048
12 years,	1•431	1•340	0•044
13 years,	1•489	1•417	0•014
14 years,	1•549	1•475	0•014
15 years,	1•600	1•496	0•053
16 years,	1•640	1•518	0•082
17 years,	..	1•553	0•087
18 years,	1•665	1•564	..
19 years,	..	1•570	0•095
20 years,	1•684	1•574	..
Growth terminated,	..	1•579	0•105

*See on this latter subject an excellent memoir of M. Villermé, inserted in the first volume of the *Annales d'Hygiene*. †[The French metre is equal to 3 feet English and •2808 of a decimal; or 3 feet and 2*10ths.] ‡I have been greatly aided in numberous researches into the height, weight, strength, and other physical qualities of man, by Messrs Guiette and Van Esschen, Professors in the School of Medicine at Brussels, as well as by M. Plataw. Without their assistance, it would have been impossible for me to have obtained all the measurements in the various charities, hospitals, public schools, Prison of Vilvorde, &c.

§ [The French line is equal to 12th part of an inch.

We observe by this table that, towards the age of 16 to 17, the growth of girls is already, *relatively*, almost as much advanced as that of boys from 18 to 19.‡ Moreover, the annual growth for boys is about 56 millimetres [somewhat more than two inches] between 5 and 15 years of age; whilst for girls it is only about 52 millimetres [or rather less than two inches.] In the *Dictionnaire des Sciences Medicales*, in the article *Giants*, M. Virey attributes the lower stature of woman to the circumstance of her arriving sooner at the age of puberty, or having reached perfection, and also to her having less vital energy. We may add, that her annual growth, up to the age of puberty, is also less rapid than that of man.

After having spoken of what relates to the sexes, it must be interesting to consider the influence of a town or a country residence upon human growth. Already Dr. Villermé, in the second part of the *Annales of Hygiene*, had proved, contrary to the generally received notion, that the inhabitants of towns are taller than those of the country. I have arrived at the same conclusion in respect to the inhabitants of Brabant. Extracts from the government militia that registers, which I communicated at time to Dr. Villermé, were published in the fifth number of the *Annales of Hygiene;* they gave the following numbers: –

Arrondissements.	1823.	1824.	1825.	1826.	1827.	Average.
	metres.	metres.	metres.	metres.	metres.	metres.
1. Brussels,	1•6719	1•6640	1•6631	1•6647	1•6528	1•6633
Rural Communes,	1•6325	1•6317	1•6343	1•6353	1•6296	1•6325
2. Louvain,	1•6424	1•6349	1•6399	1•6460	1•6335	1•6393
Rural Communes,	1•6296	1•6229	1•6090	1•6145	1•6127	1•6177
3. Nivelles,	1•6398	1•6446	1•6581	1•6384	1•6330	1•6428
Rural Communes,	1•6264	1•6260	1•6409	1•6431	1•6053	1•6323
Annual {Cities,	1•6514	1•6478	1•6537	1•6497	1•6398	1•6485
Averages {Rural Communes,	1•6295	1•6269	1•6280	1•6309	1•6225	1•6275
General Average,						1•6380

The averages of each year were taken from 400 individuals for Brussels, and from 150 for Louvain and Nivelles. Those of the rural parishes were deduced from 400 individuals for each district. Thus, the general average for the whole province was drawn from 3500 individuals living in towns, and from 6000 living in the country.

By these numbers, we see that the inhabitant of towns is taller than the inhabitant of the country; and in arranging the cities and rural districts according to the respective height which man attains in them *in his nineteenth year*, the order would be as follows:–Brussels, Nivelles, Louvain; and the same order for the rural districts around these towns. In spite of the differences we have thus remarked as taking place at the age of 19, it might still happen that the inhabitant of the country might attain a greater height than the inhabitant of the town previous to the completion of his full growth, in such a way that the growth of man in cities might be at first more rapid up to a certain point than in the country, and might even be nearly terminated in cities, whilst in the country the growth would be very far from having attained its complete development. And these remarks coincide pretty nearly with the deductions of Dr. Villermé, in respect to the height of man in France. The doctor remarks, that "human height becomes greater, and the growth takes place more rapidly, other circumstances being equal, in proportion as the country is richer, the comfort more general, houses, clothes, and nourishment better, and labour, fatigue, and privations during infancy and youth less; or, in other words, the circumstances accompanying misery put off the period of the complete development of the body, and stint human stature."

It becomes, then, important to determine the epoch at which human growth terminates; and the government registers for Brussels, being examined with this view, gave the following results. These registers refer to a great levy made about eighteen years ago; I have divided them into three series, each comprising 300 individuals:–

	19 Years.	25 Years.	30 Years.
	1•6630 metre.	1•6822 metre.	1•6834 metre.
	1•6695 metre.	1•6735 metre.	1•6873 metre.
	1•6620 metre.	1•6692 metre.	1•6817 metre.
Medium,	1•6648 metre.	1•6750 metre.	1•6841 metre.

Thus we see that human growth,* as regards height, does not terminate at 19, or even invariably at 25. I have

‡The proposition may be easier understood by stating it in this way: A girl is relatively as tall at 16 as a boy is at 18, the sex and full growth of each being taken into account.

*[The translator had observed some years ago, that the male human height had exidently not attained its maximum previous to at least 30 years of age, and probably not even then. This he was led to remark by observing large numbers of students, who, leaving college at the age of 20, 21, or 22, have returned seven or eight years afterwards. Examination proved that these persons had grown very considerably, not only in breadth but also in height.]

to regret exceedingly that the state of the government registers does not allow of my making similar researches in regard to the inhabitants of the country; we might then have known if the growth in towns terminates more rapidly than in the country, and also if man, when fully developed, is tallest in the country.

When we class the 900 individuals of whom I have spoken above, in order of their height, we come to the following results:–

Heights	Number of Individuals		
	of 19 Years.	of 25 Years.	of 30 Years.
From 15 to 16 decimetres....	32	17	15
" 16 to 17, "	173	174	163
" 17 to 18, "	92	103	109
" 18 to 19, "	3	5	12
" 19 to 20, "	..	1	1
	300	300	300*

Thus, at 19, 3 individuals only were more than 18 decimetres [above 5 feet 10 inches] high; at the age of 25, there were 6; and at the age of 30 there were 13.† It seems to me that we are entitled to conclude, from the whole of these results, that human growth, in respect to height, does not terminate in Brussels even at the age of 25, which is very much opposed to the generally received opinion.

According to M. Hargenvilliers, ‡ the average height of conscripts of 20 years, taken for all France, is 1•615 metre [4 feet 10 inches nearly]; and of 100,000 there were as follows:–

Under 1•570 metres,..	28,620
1•570 to 1•598 "..	11,590
1•598 to 1•624 "..	13,990
1•624 to 1•651 "..	14,410
1•651 to 1•678 "..	11,410
1•678 to 1•705 "..	8,780
1•705 to 1•732 "..	5,530
1•732 to 1•759 "..	3,190
Above 1•759 "..	2,490

*[The value of the decimetre in English measures is 3 inches and •937 decimal parts, or nearly 4 English inches.] †In the preceding numbers were comprised the men who were rejected, or had leave to withdraw from the corps, as of under size. ‡*Inquiries and Considerations on the Formation and Recruitment of the French Army:* 1817. M. Villermé, in his Memoir on the Height of Man in France, quotes the opinion of Tenon and also some facts, which show that, during the time of the Empire, continual wars had lowered the human stature. [A question naturally arises here, whether the stature was actually lowered, or the yound conscripts merely called on before their time of full development; but the remark of Dr. Villermé suggests other considerations, well worthy the attention of statisticians–such, for example, as the effects produced in Prussia, by the maintaining of a standing army of somewhat more than 200,000 men in time of peace, it being admitted that these are the finest and best proportioned men in the kingdom. For we have first the withdrawal of the very choices: of the male population from the exercise of the arts and the cultivation of science, at precisely that period of life when they are best fitted for such pursuits; and, secondly, the effects upon the population in respect to the restraints upon marriage, and the preference given by the soldier to a debauched and irregular life. The same remarks, modified, apply to all other European nations, none of them being without standing armies of greater or less magnitude.]

We might consider the inhabitants of the ancient department of Bouches-de-la-Meuse, which was partly formed of Holland, and of which the Hague was the chief place, as affording the limits of the statures observed in France from the time of the Empire. The average height of conscripts for the years 1808, 1809, and 1810, raised before the age of 260, was 1•677 metre.* On the other hand, in the ancient department of the Appennines, of which Chiavari was the chief place, the country mountainous, without industrious occupations, extremely poor, and where the men toil from a very early age and are ill fed, the average stature of the conscripts for the same three years, was 1•560 metre. "The difference of these results," says M. Villermé, "is striking. In the former place, where the stature is highest, there were but few excused or rejected even for diseases; on the contrary, in the latter place, where the stature is very low, there are many excused even for this latter cause; so that all the advantages are in favour of men of high stature."†

It is remarkable that the inequality of statures is not merely observed between the inhabitants of town and country, but is also felt in the interior of towns between individuals of different professions, and having different degrees of affluence, as M. Villermé has shown for the different arrondissements of Paris, where the stature of men seems to be, all other things being equal, in proportion to the good fortune, or at least in inverse proportion to the difficulties, toils, and privations experienced in infancy and youth.‡ Of 41 young persons between 17 and 20 years of age, measured at the Athenæum of Brussels, 13 were found between 16 and 17 decimetres, 26 between 17 and 18 decimetres, and 2 between 18 and 19 decimetres; so that the young persons between 17 and 18 were double the number of those between 16 and 17 decimetres; whilst, in the interior of the town, the number of the former is not equal to the latter, even at the age of 30 years.

The young girls measured in the Female Orphan Hospital of Brussels, and who, during their infancy, have been brought up in the country, are generally smaller than girls of the same age, in easy circumstances, who have been measured in town.

In the Prison (*Maison de Détention*) of Vilvorde, by forming three groups, each of 23 individuals for each

*Sur la Taille, &c. †[The translator is firmly persuaded that Dr. Villermé and M. Quetelet, have failed to detect the real cause of difference of stature in those two departments: it is a question purely of *race*, and not of feeding or locality. The taller conscripts were Saxons, drawn from the departments of Holland and the Mouths of the Meuse; the shorter conscripts, found in the Apennines and around Chiavari, were the decendants of the ancient Celtic population of that country. The difference in stature, then, depends, in this instance, in a great measure on the difference in blood, or on the race of men: it has existed for thousands of years, and will continue so, altogether independent of locality, feeding, or government. ‡Annales d'Hygiène, No. 2, p. 370.

sex, the average results have been–

	For men.	For Women.
	1•657 met.	1•572 met.
	1•664 met.	1•581 met.
	1•670 met	1•585 met.
General average,..................	1•664 met.	1•579 met.

Classing them according to size, we find–

Sizes.	Men.	Women.
From 14 to 15 decimetres,.............	1	3
From 15 to 16 decimetres,.............	6	36
From 16 to 17 decimetres,.............	42	27
From 17 to 18 decimetres,.............	19	3
From 18 to 19 decimetres,.............	1	..
	60	69

These results show that the prisoners were generally shorter than fully developed individuals measured in Brussels; their average stature being nearly equal to that of young persons of 19 years of age, and it may correspond with the average stature of the inhabitants of the province.

With the view of appreciating the modifications which painful toil in manufactories may produce on the development of children, Mr. J.W. Cowell has made different observations at Manchester and Stockport he has inserted the details in the first volume of *Factory Reports*, and has kindly assisted me in obtaining the results, which I have reduced to the métrical measure. The girls and boys have been measured with their shoes on; no deduction has been made for this circumstance: but, as the observations were made on the Sunday, the thickness of the soles for boys would probably be from one-half to one-third of an inch (English), and for girls from one-eighth to one-sixth of an inch. This being laid down, the following are the values obtained:*–

Average Stature of Children of the Lower Orders, at Manchester and Stockport.†

Ages.	Boys		Girls	
	Working in Factories.	not Working in Factories.	Working in Factories.	not Working in Factories.
	metres.	metres.	metres.	metres.
9 years,	1•222	1•233	1•218	1•236
10 years,	1•270	1•286	1•260	1•254
11 years,	1•302	1•296	1•299	1•323
12 years,	1•355	1•345	1•364	1•363
13 years,	1•383	1•396	1•413	1•399
14 years,	1•437	1•440	1•467	1•479
15 years,	1•515	1•474	1•486	1•502
16 years,	1•563	1•605	1•521	1•475
17 years,	1•592	1•627	1•531	1•542
18 years,	1•608	1•775	1•593	1•645

It appears, from these numbers, that the statures of male and female children do not differ much in Belgium and England: we also see that, until the age of puberty, there is no great difference in size of the children of the lower orders, whether they work in factories or not. But for the latter years of the table, there is a very sensible difference. Will it be found that the growth in factories, after puberty, is diminished, or only retarded? or, which seems more probable, does not the amelioration remarked for the lower ages proceed from the useful changes which have already been made, from the apprehension of parliamentary inquiries?‡

When, in England, we chose the terms of comparison from rather higher classes of society, we find the stature of men higher than in France or the Low Countries, at least for young persons between 18 and 23 years of age. The following are the results of 80 measurements made on students of the University of Cambridge, in groups of 10 each:§–

Ten individuals................................	58 feet 3 1/2 inches.
"	58 " 6 1/2 "
"	58 " 9 "
"	57 " 7 1/2 "
"	56 " 9 1/2 "
"	57 " 9 1/2 "
"	58 " 3 "
"	58 " .. "
Average,..	58
Height of one person,........................	5 feet 9 3-5th inches.

I have enumerated different causes which influence the growth of man in town, but their number increases when the researches embrace a large extent of territory; thus, the complete development stature stops more suddenly in very hot or very cold countries than in those of a moderate temperature; more suddenly in low plains than on mountainous heights, where the climate is severe. The kind of food and drink farther influence growth; and individuals have been known to grow considerably by changing their mode of life, and making use of moist food calculated to distend and increase their organisation. Some diseases, and particularly fevers, may also excite rapid and extraordinary growth.

*[It has been suggested to the translator, by a gentleman well acquainted with the manufacturing districts of Yorkshire and Lancashire, that wooden clogs, and not shoes, seemed almost universally worn by the manufacturing propulation of these countries, more especially of Lancashire. Now, the soles and heels of these clogs are of great thickness: a question then arises with respect to Mr. Cowell's measurements. If this class of the population wear clogs on Sundays, this circumstance may partially affect the value of Mr. Cowell's statements.] †The number of children measured was–factory boys, 410; others, 227: female factory children, 652; others, 201. Very few non-factory children, of the ages of 16, 17, and 18, have been measured. ‡It has been found, by this inquiry, that in some districts the children were forced to work standing upright, with the legs fastened in tin pipes. §It is a custom at Cambridge to measure and weigh the young persons coming to the university with great accuracy, at a merchant's warehouse, where a book is kept for the purpose of entering the data. It is from this book that, through the kindness of Mr. Whewell, the accompanying numbers have been taken.

The case of a young girl is related, who, becoming unwell (*pendant ses menstrues*) by an attack of fever which she had, acquired a gigantic stature.* Lastly, it has also been remarked that lying in bed is favourable to growth, and that a man in the morning is somewhat taller than in the evening; during the day, he undergoes a degree of depression.†

I shall now pass to a more particular examination of the law of growth of man, from birth to complete development. The numbers on which my results are based, have been collected at Brussels, and as much as possible from individuals of different classes: by the side of the observed values, I have written down the calculated ones, according to an empirical formula, which I shall explain subsequently.

Table of the Growth of Man.

Ages.	Stature Observed.	Stature from Calculation.	Difference.
	metres.	metres.	metres.
Birth,........................	0•500	0•500	0•000
1 year,......................	0•608	0•698	0•000
2 "	0•796	0•791	+0•005
3 "	0•867	0•864	+0•003
4 "	0•930	0•928	+0•002
5 "	0•986	0•988	-0•002
6 "	1•045	1•047	-0•002
7 "	..	1•105	..
8 "	1•160	1•162	-0•002
9 "	1•221	1•219	+0•002
10 "	1•280	1•275	+0•005
11 "	1•334	1•330	+0•004
12 "	1•384	1•385	-0•001
13 "	1•431	1•439	-0•008
14 "	1•489	1•493	-0•004
15 "	1•549	1•546	+0•003
16 "	1•600	1•594	+0•006
17 "	1•640	1•634	+0•006
18 "	..	1•658	..
19 "	1•665	1•669	-0•004
25 "	1•675	1•680	-0•005
30 "	1•684	1•684	0•000

I have endeavoured to render the preceding results *sensible* by the construction of a line, which indicates the growth at different ages, but in one-tenth of the real proportions.

Thus, supposing that the new-born infant sets out from the point *o*, and proceeds along the axis *o*A, reaching in succession the points I., II., III., IV., &c., at the age of 1, 2, 3, 4, &c., years, his head will always be at the height of the curve *o*B, at the different points 1, 2, 3, 4, &c. We see that–

1. The most rapid growth takes place immediately after birth: the child in the course of one year grows 2 decimetres [7 8-10th inches] nearly.

2. The growth of a child diminishes as its age increases, until towards the age of four or five years, the period at which it reaches the maximum of probable life. Thus, during the second year after birth, the growth is only one-half of what it was during the first; and during the third year, only about one-third.

3. Proceeding from the fourth or fifth year, the increase of stature becomes almost exactly regular until about the sixteenth year, that is to say, until the age of puberty, and the annual increase is 56 millimetres [2 2-10th inches] nearly.

4. After the age of puberty, the stature still continues to increase, but only inconsiderably: from the sixteenth to the seventeenth year, it increases 4 centimetres [1 5-10th inches]; in the two succeeding years, it only increases 2 1/2 centimetres [or a little less than 1 inch; in exact numbers, 0•984].

5. The full growth of man does not appear to be attained at his twenty-fifth year.

In what has just been said, I have only spoken of absolute growth: if we compare the annual growth with the stature already acquired, we shall find that the child increases in size two-fifths from birth to the end of the first year; during the second year, one-seventh; during the third, one-eleventh; during the fourth year, one-fourteenth; during the fifth year, one-fifteenth; during the sixth year, one-eighteenth, &c.; so that the relative growth is continually decreasing from the time of birth.

The curve representing the growth of females, would be a little under that of males, and would be nearly equidistant from it, until the age of eleven or twelve years, when it tends more rapidly to become parallel to the axis *o*A.

It remains for me to speak of the formula by which I have calculated the numbers shown in the table given above. Letting the co-ordinates y and z represent the stature and the age corresponding to it, we have the following equation:–

*See *Dictionnaire de Medicine*, article*Geant*, by Virey. †[M. Quetelet has unaccountably omitted, in the above paragraph, the great cause productive of differences in stature of men and animals–to wit, difference in race or blood. The diminutive Bosjeman of Southern Africa, the athletic Caffre, reaching the full European stature, and the gigantic Boor, the descendant of the Saxon race, are as nearly alike in respect to food and climate as may be; the extraordinary differences, therefore, which these men present, are ascribable to one cause alone–a difference of blood or origin; and the historic evidence derived from ancient Rome, and from the equally authentic figures depicted in the tombs of Egyptian Thebes, prove that these differences caused by blood or race are now neither greater nor less than they were at least 4000 years ago, thus, as it were, setting at defiance all minor causes, such as food, climate, localities, &c. Whether the Hun resides in the fertile plains of Hungary, the shores of the Caspian, or the frozen regions of Scandinavia or of Lapland, the general stature of the race remains perfectly unaltered. In respect to what M. Quetelet observes regarding the influence of rest and horizontal position on the stature, it is a fact well established that, by such a position, in bed for example, the elastic fibro-cartilages connecting the spinal bones together, seem to recover their full depth, and the stature may gain an inch or more thereby. Recruits for the army and deserters avail themselves of a knowledge of this fact, and occasionally succeed in making their identity difficult to be established.]

$$y+\frac{y}{1000(T-y)}=ax+\frac{t+x}{1+\frac{4}{3}x};$$

t and T are two constants which indicate the stature of the child at birth, and that of the fully developed individual: their value for Brussels are 0•500 and 1•684 metre. The coefficient a of the first term in the second number, will be calculated according to the different localities, from the regular growth which annually takes place between the fourth and fifth, to the fifteenth or sixteenth year: for Brussels, its value has been made equal to 0•0545 metre. I think that in giving these three constants, we may use this formula with considerable advantage for other localities.

If we make t=0.49 metre, T=1•579 metre, a=0•052 metre, agreeably to the observations above quoted for calculating the law of the growth of women for Brussels, we shall have–

$$y+\frac{y}{1000(1\cdot 579-y)}=0\cdot 0521x+\frac{0\cdot 49+x}{1+\frac{4}{3}}.$$

By using this formula, I have calculated the numbers which appear in the third column of the following table:–

Law of the Growth of Woman.

Ages.	Stature Observed.	Stature Calculated.	Difference
	metres.	metres.	metres.
Birth,........................	0•490	0•490	0•000
1 year,......................	..	0•690	..
2 "	0•730	0•781	-0•001
3 "	0•853	0•852	+0•001
4 "	0•913	0•915	-0•002
5 "	0•978	0•974	+0•004
6 "	1•035	1•031	+0•004
7 "	1•091	1•086	+0•005
8 "	1•154	1•141	+0•013
9 "	1•205	1•195	+0•010
10 "	1•256	1•248	+0•008
11 "	1•286	1•299	-0•013
12 "	1•340	1•353	-0•013
13 "	1•417	1•403	+0•014
14 "	1•475	1•453	+0•022
15 "	1•496	1•499	-0•003
16 "	1•518	1•535	-0•017
17 "	1•553	1•555	-0•002
18 "	1•564	1•564	0•000
19 "	1•570	1•569	+0•001
20 "	1•574	1•572	+0•002
Growth terminated.	1•579	1•579	0•000

The differences between the observed numbers and the calculated ones, are greater than in the table (already given) of the growth of man. It may be owing to the circumstance, that the observations have been less numerous, and made on fewer of the different classes of society, for the one sex than for the other. What appears to give additional support to my conjecture is, the manner in which the positive and negative signs succeed each other in the differences of the observed and calculated numbers. Moreover, it is remarkable that the formula may be entirely determined, when we have been enabled to give the statures of an individual corresponding to three different ages, sufficiently distant from each other.

Although the equation of which I have availed myself in the calculations, is of the third order, it resolves itself, like those of the second, into an unknown one, when we give the successive values of the other. Considered as belonging to a curve, it points out to us that there still exists another branch than the one we are occupied with; for to each value of the abscissa x, there are two values of y.

The curve of growths oB has an asymptote parallel to the axes of the abscissæ, situate at a distance from this axis equal to T, which is the height of man fully developed; moreover, this curve, proceeding from the point o, which corresponds to birth, towards the thirteenth or fourteenth years, is sensibly confounded with an hyperbola; for in these limits, the second term of the first order is so small as to be considered nothing, so that we shall have–

$$y=ax+\frac{t+x}{1+\frac{4}{3}x}.$$

The curve oB does not merely indicate the growth of man from birth to complete maturity, but also those of the other side of the axis Oo; that is to say, for the months which precede birth, the results which it presents are conformable to those observed with regard to the fœtus. This concordance is not always manifested until towards the fifth or sixth month before birth, which is the age at which the embryo becomes a fœtus. It is, moreover, true, that before this period the child is in a state which hardly yet appears to belong to human nature. The curve singularly represents this state, if we give any significance to it; for between five and six months before birth, it suddenly passes under the axis oA, and the values of statures, positive as they were, become negative: the curve in the negative region is lost in infinity, approaching an asymptote which corresponds to a value of x=-3/4; or, in other words, at nine months before birth, the period of conception. Without occupying ourselves with the stature of the infant while it is still an embryo, or altogether unformed, if we confine our calculations to the growth of the fœtus about five months before birth, we shall find the following results, by the side of which are written the results of measurements given in the *Dictionnaire des Sciences Medicales*:–

Age of the Infant.	Stature Calculated.	Stature Observed.
	metres.	metres.
Birth,............................	0•500	From 0•487 to 0•541
1 month before birth.....	0•464	" 0•433 to 0•487
2 " " "	0•419	" 0•379 to 0•433
3 " " "	0•361	" 0•300 to 0•379
4 " " "	0•281	" 0•216 to 0•300
5 " " "	0•165	" 0•162 to 0•216

The calculated values fall, for each month, between the limits of the results of the observations. Moreover, it is well to observe that these results do not carry the same degree of exactness as those obtained after birth, because of the uncertainty of the period of conception, as well as the varying duration of pregnancy. What is most important for us to observe here, in my opinion, is the law of continuity which exists for the growth of the child immediately before and after birth. Admitting the approximative calculations of M. Chaussier, it will be found that *the fœtus increases almost as much in length in one month, as a child between six and sixteen years does in one year.*

In what has preceded, I have endeavoured to point out how the development of the stature of man and woman takes place: it now remains for me to say some words on the diminution which this element undergoes by age. From a great number of observations, of which we shall make greater use of when speaking of the corresponding diminution of weight, it appears that it is chiefly towards the fiftieth year that the decrease becomes most apparent, and towards the end of life it amounts to about 6 or 7 centimetres [2 3-10th inches, or 2 6-10th inches]. From the number of individuals who have been measured, those have been carefully excluded who were much roundshouldered, or who could not make themselves straight during the observation.

Ages.	Stature of Men.	Stature of Women.
40 years................	1•684 metre.	1•579 metre.
50 ".....................	1•674 "	1•536 "
60 ".....................	1•639 "	1•516 "
70 ".....................	1•623 "	1•514 "
80 ".....................	1•613 "	1•506 "
90 ".....................	1•613 "	1•505 "

It may be asked if the diminution of stature towards the end of life is not rather apparent than real, and if it be not owing to the circumstance that longevity is generally shorter for individuals of great stature. At least, it would be interesting to examine if the size of man has any influence on the duration of his life.

I shall endeavour, in a few words, to present such of the results of my researches as appear to me most interesting: it is almost unnecessary to observe that these results only apply to Brussels and the province of Brabant.

1. The limits of growth in the two sexes are unequal: first, because woman is born smaller than man; second, because she sooner finishes her complete development; third, because the annual increase which she receives is smaller than that of man.

2. The stature of the inhabitant of towns, at the age of 19, is greater than that of the country person by 2 to 3 centimetres [7-10ths to 1 inch nearly].

3. It does not appear that the growth of man is entirely completed at 25 years of age.

4. Individuals who live in affluence generally exceed the average height: misery and hard labour, on the contrary, appear to be obstacles to growth.

5. The growth of the child, even from several months before birth until complete development, follows such a law of continuity, that the increase diminishes successively with age.

6. Between the 5th and 16th years nearly, the annual growth is pretty regular, and it is one-twelfth of the growth of the fœtus during the months before birth.

7. Subsequently to the 50th year, man and woman undergo a diminution of stature which becomes more and more marked, and may amount to from 6 to 7 centimetres [2 3-10ths or 2 0-10th inches] nearly, about the age of 80 years.

CHAPTER II.

OF THE DEVELOPMENT OF THE WEIGHT, AND OF ITS RELATIONS TO THE DEVELOPMENT OF THE HEIGHT OF THE BODY.

1. Weight and Height at Different Ages

Researches on the height and weight of new-born infants have been made at the Foundling Hospital of Brussels. To ascertain the weight, the ordinary balance has been used; but in the different observations, the weight of the swaddling clothes has been taken. The average values obtained for 63 male and 56 female children, are as follows:–

	Weight.	Height.
Male children,................	3•20 kilogrammes.	0•496 metre.*
Female children,............	2•91 "	0•483 " †

*Here those children only have been measured whose weight had been ascertained. The number of observations is greater than I could avail myself of in my former researches. †[The kilogramme is, as nearly as possible, 2 1-5ths lbs. English.]

Thus, *from the time of birth, there is an inequality in the weight and height of children of the two sexes, and this inequality is in favour of males.* The height corresponds nearly with what I have found from other observations.

By classing the infants who furnished the preceding average values according to their total weight, we find–

Infants Weighing	Boys.	Girls.	Total.
From 1•0 to 1•5 kilog..........	..	1	1
" 1•5 to 2•0 "	..	1	1
" 2•0 to 2•5 "	3	7	10
" 2•5 to 3•0 "	13	14	27
" 3•0 to 3•5 "	28	23	51
" 3•5 to 4•0 "	14	7	21
" 4•0 to 4•5 "	5	3	8
	63	56	119

The extremes were as follows:–

	Boys.	Girls.
Minimum............................	2•34 kilog.	1•12 kilog.
Maximum...........................	4•50 kilog.	4•25 kilog.

Professor Richter has made researches similar to the preceding at the Foundling Hospital of Moscow;* and, according to his observations, of 44 new-born children, the sexes of whom are not stated, the average value was 9 1-15th pounds in weight, and 18 1/2 inches (Paris) in length. I regret that I do not know the value of the weight which he employed. The height, which is 0•501 metres, new measure, is almost precisely the same as we have found for boys. The extremes obtained by M. Richter were as follows:–

	Weight.	Height.
Minimum,............................	5 pounds	15 inches.
Maximum,...........................	11 "	21 "

Thus, the weight of boys varies as 1 to 2, as I have found at Brussels. The extremes of length do not differ so much, and present values which differ very little from those which we have obtained.

Moreover, the extremes, at least of weight, may differ as much as the averages. We read in the *Dictionnaire des Sciences Medicales*, article *Fœtus*–"The researches made at the Foundling Hospital, on more than 20,000 infants, prove that one infant, born at the full period and well-formed, generally weighs 6 1/4 pounds. Only a very small number of infants have been seen at this hospital weighing 10 1/2 pounds, or others weighting only 3 pounds, or 2 pounds and some ounces." This value of 6 1/4 pounds, or 3•059 kilogrammes, obtained from so great a number of observations, agrees very nearly with the value–3•055 kilogrammes–obtained for Brussels, leaving out of consideration the distinction of the sexes: the extreme values likewise present very little difference.

It is remarkable that learned men who have made observations on the weight and height of new-born infants, should have attended so little to the distinction of the sexes. Although our results are not deduced from so large a number of observations as could be desired, yet we think we may conclude, with sufficient probability, that the average values of the weight and height of children of the two sexes present a very sensible difference.

From all the researches which have been made on the relations existing between the weight and the age of the fœtus, it appears that the ratios present so much uncertainty, that we can scarcely make any use of them.

It is M. Chaussier, if I am not mistaken, who has made the remark, that an infant diminishes a little in weight immediately after birth. This curious remark deserves to be carefully verified: unfortunately, I have only been able to procure seven series of observations, which do not extend beyond the seventh day after birth. The average calculations for each day present the following values:–

	Weight of the Infant.
After birth,..	3•126 kilog.
On the 2d day,..	3•057 kilog.
" 3d "	3•017 "
" 4th "	3•035 "
" 5th "	3•030 "
" 6th "	3•035 "
" 7th "	3•060 "

It really appears, then, from these numbers, that *the weight of the child diminishes a little immediately after birth,* and that it does not begin to increase in a sensible manner until after the first week.

Thus we see that, from birth, there is an inequality in the weight of children of the two sexes: however, we shall examine if this inequality is produced again at different ages, and examine the modifications which it undergoes. I have already stated the analogous results for height; nevertheless, I thought it would be useful to state again the new numbers which have been obtained from the individuals of both sexes, on whom observations were made to determine the weight. It was interesting to place these two elements during their progressive development in the same individual, opposite each other.

In estimating the weight, I have generally used the balance of Sanctorius. Since this balance is not so sensible when slightly charged, and also since great care is required in placing the bodies to be weighed by it, chil-

*Synops, Praxis Medico-Obstetriciae: 1810.

dren of tender age have been almost constantly weighed in the arms of persons whose weight had previously been taken.

The observations on children from 4 to 12 years of age, have for the most part been made in the schools of Brussels and at the Orphan Hospital. The weights of young persons have been taken more especially in the colleges and at the Medical School of Brussels. For more advanced ages, individuals of different classes have been taken, though those of the lower orders have been least numerous.

For old men, the weights have chiefly been taken in the large and magnificent hospital recently erected at Brussels. The two following tables point out the results, such as they are, for men and women.

The first column gives the ages; the second and third point out the average values of the height and weight which correspond to these different ages. The values of the height are almost the same as those previously given, except for individuals who are more than 16 or 17 years of age; which no doubt arises from individuals of the lower class having been less numerous in these than in the former observations. Indeed, I have already shown that young persons who apply themselves to study, and persons in the affluent classes generally, are taller than others. In the third column, the ratios of weight and size for different ages are calculated, their values being considered as abstract numbers. These ratios are not deduced immediately from the numbers contained in the two preceding columns, but are the average of the ratios calculated for each individual. In the last place, the four last columns point out the maximum and minimum of height and weight at each age, for individuals who are well-formed.

Table of the Size and Weight of Man at Different Ages.

Ages.	Size.	Weight.	Ratio of Weight to Size.	Size Observed. Max.	Size Observed. Min.	Weight Observed. Max.	Weight Observed. Min.
	met.	kilog.		met.	met.	kilog.	kilog.
Birth	0•496	3•20	6•19	0•532	0•438	4•30	2•34
1 year	0•696	10•00	14•20	0•750	0•682	11•00	9•00
2 "	0•797	12•00	15•00	0•824	0•730	13•50	10•50
3 "	0•860	13•21	15•36	0•875	0•840	13•60	12•10
4 "	0•932	15•07	16•32	0•963	0•840	18•20	12•50
5 "	0•990	16•70	16•98	1•080	0•915	28•50	14•00
6 "	1•046	18•04	17•44	1•115	0•960	20•40	15•80
7 "	1•112	20•16	18•31	1•162	1•109	24•50	17•20
8 "	1•170	22•26	18•92	1•260	1•120	28•50	19•00
9 "	1•227	24•09	19•68	1•325	1•150	29•00	22•20
10 "	1•282	26•12	20•37	1•325*	1•163	32•00	22•70
11 "	1•327	27•85	21•58	1•405	1•215	33•80	25•00
12 "	1•359	31•00	22•80	1•450	1•270	36•30	25•00
13 "	1•403	35•32	25•30	1•490	1•300	39•50	34•60
14 "	1•487	40•50	27•49	1•630	1•330	45•00	37•00
15 "	1•559	46•41	29•88	1•658	1•380	61•50	37•00
16 "	1•610	53•39	33•00	1•730	1•430	61•50	40•00
17 "	1•670	57•40	34•25	1•790	1•467	65•50	45•00
18 "	1•700	61•26	35•67	1•790	..	67•00	45•00
19 "	1•706	63•32	37•00	1•800	..	70•00	48•20
20 "	1•711	65•00	37•99	1•838	..	72•70	..
25 "	1•722	68•29	39•66	1•890	..	98•50	..
30 "	1•722	68•90	40•02	..	..	..	..
40 "	1•713	68•81	40•03	..	..	..	..
50 "	1•674	67•45	40•14	..	..	..	..
60 "	1•639	65•50	40•01	..	..	..	..
70 "	1•623	63•03	38•83	..	..	..	49•1
80 "	1•613	61•22	37•96	1•820	1•467	83•00	49•7

Table of the Size and Weight of Woman at Different Ages.

Ages.	Size.	Weight.	Ratio of Weight to Size.	Size Observed. Max.	Size Observed. Min.	Weight Observed. Max.	Weight Observed. Min.
	met.	kilog.		met.	met.	kilog.	kilog.
Birth	0•483	2•91	6•15	0•555	0•438	4•25	1•12
1 year	0•690	9•30	13•50	0•704	0•660	10•5	8•3
2 "	0•780	11•40	14•50	0•798	0•720	12•0	8•3
3 "	0•850	12•45	14•70	0•895	0•795	15•8	10•5
4 "	0•910	14•18	15•10	0•950	0•810	15•8	11•5
5 "	0•974	15•50	15•70	1•085	0•876	17•5	13•3
6 "	1•032	16•74	16•24	1•085	0•956	20•3	13•3
7 "	1•096	18•45	16•85	1•177	1•050	23•4	16•0
8 "	1•139	19•82	17•45	1•380	1•050	23•4	16•0
9 "	1•200	22•44	18•65	1•380	1•110	25•7	18•3
10 "	1•248	24•24	19•45	1•380	1•160	28•3	20•3
11 "	1•275	26•25	20•60	1•385	1•160	39•8	21•6
12 "	1•327	30•54	23•00	1•476	1•160	42•8	21•6
13 "	1•386	34•65	24•50	1•580	1•160	42•8	21•6
14 "	1•447	38•10	25•35	1•580	1•160	51•0	32•0
15 "	1•475	41•30	28•10	1•638	1•160	55•2	32•0
16 "	1•500	44•44	29•62	1•638	1•160	57•6	32•0
17 "	1•544	49•08	31•75	1•688	1•284	61•6	..
18 "	1•562	53•10	34•05	1•740	..	79•9	..
20 "	1•570	54•46	34•70	..	..	..	..
25 "	1•577	55•08	35•26	..	..	..	..
30 "	1•579	55•14	35•90	..	..	..	..
40 "	1•555	56•65	36•50	..	..	..	..
50 "	1•536	58•45	38•15	..	1•444	90•5	39•8
60 "	1•516	56•73	37•28	..	1•436	..	..
70 "	1•514	53•72	35•49	..	1•431	93•8	..
80 "	1•506	51•52	34•21	1•701	1•408	72•5	33•0

The numbers in the preceding tables are such as have been obtained from direct observation; but they must be subjected to two corrections–in the first place, because the persons have always been weighed in their dresses; and, secondly, because observations have not been made on all classes of society.

The first cause of error which has been pointed out, may be removed, or at least diminished to some extent. The average weight of the clothes at different ages may be determined very precisely, and then it is only necessary to subtract its value from each of the corresponding numbers of the table of weights. From different experiments, I think we may admit, as near the truth, that the average weight of the clothes at different ages is one-eighteenth of the total weight of the male body, and a twenty-fourth part of the total weight of the

*When a number is repeated, it is because the maximum of this year was less than that of the preceding. The inverse takes place in the cloumn of the minima.

female. With this value, I have corrected the numbers of the preceding table, except for new-born infants, because the numbers had already undergone this correction, from direct experiment, immediately after weighing them [the infants].

The second cause of error may also be removed: indeed, we shall soon see, that of individuals of the same age, the weight may be considered as having a pretty constant relation to the size of the body. It will be sufficient, then, to know the ratios inserted in the fourth column of the preceding tables, and to have a good general table of the growths, to deduce the corresponding table of the weight. It is in making use of the *table of growths* given above, and constructed with elements collected from all classes of society, that I have calculated the following table, in which I have also made the necessary corrections for clothing:–

Table of the Development of the Height and Weight.

Ages.	Men.		Women.	
	Height.	Weight.	Height.	Weight.
	metres.	kilog.	metres.	kilog.
Birth	0•500	3•20	0•490	2•91
1 year	0•698	9•45	0•690	8•79
2 "	0•791	11•34	0•781	10•67
3 "	0•864	12•47	0•852	11•79
4 "	0•928	14•23	0•915	13•00
5 "	0•988	15•77	0•974	14•36
6 "	1•047	17•24	1•031	16•00
7 "	1•105	19•10	1•086	17•54
8 "	1•162	20•76	1•141	19•08
9 "	1•219	22•65	1•195	21•36
10 "	1•275	24•52	1•248	23•52
11 "	1•330	27•10	1•299	25•65
12 "	1•385	29•82	1•353	29•82
13 "	1•439	34•38	1•403	32•94
14 "	1•493	38•76	1•453	36•70
15 "	1•546	43•02	1•499	40•37
16 "	1•594	49•67	1•535	43•57
17 "	1•634	52•85	1•555	47•31
18 "	1•658	57•85	1•564	51•03
20 "	1•674	60•06	1•572	52•28
25 "	1•680	62•93	1•577	53•28
30 "	1•684	63•65	1•579	54•33
40 "	1•684	63•67	1•579	55•23
50 "	1•674	63•46	1•536	56•16
60 "	1•639	61•94	1•516	54•30
70 "	1•623	59•52	1•514	51•51
80 "	1•613	57•83	1•506	49•37
	1•613	57•83	1•505	49•31

To render the preceding results more apparent, I have constructed two lines, which represent the increase of weight which men and women undergo at different ages: these lines have, for abscissæ, the ages, and for ordinates, the corresponding weights. We perceive, at the first glance, that, *at equal ages, man is generally heavier than woman; about the age of twelve years only are individuals of both sexes nearly of the same weight.* This circumstance is owing to the development of the weight being inconsiderable in both sexes, until the time of puberty, when, on the contrary, it becomes very apparent. Now, since puberty takes place sooner in woman, this acceleration causes a temporary disappearance of the inequality of weight which existed between children of both sexes, and which is, for children between one and eleven years of age, from one kilogramme to one and a half. The difference of weight of the sexes is more considerable in adult persons; it is about five kilogrammes between the sixteenth and twentieth years, and more than seven after this period.

Man reaches his maximum of weight about the age of 40, *and he begins to waste in a sensible manner about the age of* 60: *at the age of* 80 *he has lost about six kilogrammes* [16 lbs. troy]. *His height has also diminished, and this diminution is about seven centimetres* [2 7-10ths inches].

The same observation applies to women: in old age, they generally lose from six to seven kilogrammes in weight, and seven centimetres in stature. I have taken care not to include ricketty individuals in these valuations, or badly formed persons, or even those who were round-shouldered, and unable to stand upright for many minutes.

Woman attains her maximum of weight later than man; she weighs the most about the age of 50 *years:* setting out from about the age of 19, the development of her weight is nearly stationary, until the period of procreation is passed.

The extreme limits of the weight of well-formed individuals have been 49•1 and 98•5 kilogrammes for men; and for women 39•8 and 93•8 kilogrammes.

The limits of height have been 1•467 and 1•890 metres for men; and 1•444 and 1•740 metres for women.

The average weight at 19 years, is nearly that of old persons of the two sexes.

When man and woman have attained their complete development, they weigh nearly exactly twenty times as much as at birth; whilst the height is only about three and one-fourth times what it was at the same period.

One year after birth, children of both sexes have tripled their weight; boys weight 9•45 kilogrammes, and girls 8•79 kilogrammes. At 6 years, they have doubled this latter weight, and at 13, they have quadrupled it.

Immediately before puberty, man and woman have one-half the weight which they have after their complete development.

I am indebted to the kindness of M. Villermé for the communication of the unpublished researches of Tenon on the weight of man, which appear to have been made in 1783. They were made in a village in the environs of Paris–the village of Massy–where Tenon had his country house. These researches, which comprise observations on 60 men between 25 and 40 years of age, and as many women of the same ages, give the following results:–

	Maximum. kilog.	Minimum. kilog.	Average. kilog.
Weight of man.....	83•307	51•398	62•071
" woman.....	74•038	36•805	54•916

In all these observations, the weight of the clothes has been subtracted, and care has been taken not to include any female who was pregnant.

If we now compare these numbers with those I obtained at Cambridge, made on men from 18 to 23 years of age, weighed with clothes, we shall find, dividing into series of tens the 80 individuals whose weights were obtained–

	Stones.	Pounds.
1st series,	108	9
2d "	111	2 3/4
3d "	114	6 3/4
4th "	101	0 1/4
5th "	102	5
6th "	107	12 1/2
7th "	103	6 1/4
8th "	112	2 1/4
Average,	107	10 27/32

Which gives, for the weight of one individual, about 151 pounds, or 68•465 kilogrammes, which is nearly the weight of a man of 30 in Brabant, when weighed with his clothes on.

If, on the other hand, we compare the weight of children of the lower classes in England, we shall find the following results, which have been communicated to me by Mr. J.W. Cowell, taken on 420 boys working in the factories, and 223 not working in factories; and 651 girls working in factories, and 201 not working in those places.

Average Weight of Children of the Lower Orders.

Ages.	Boys		Girls	
	Working in Factories.	not Working in Factories.	Working in Factories.	not Working in Factories.
	kilog.	kilog.	kilog.	kilog.
9 years,	23•47	24•15	23•18	22•87
10 "	25•84	27•33	24•85	24•68
11 "	28•04	26•46	27•06	27•72
12 "	29•91	30•49	29•96	29•96
13 "	32•69	34•17	33•21	32•97
14 "	34•95	35•67	37•82	37•83
15 "	40•06	39•37	39•84	42•44
16 "	44•43	50•01	43•62	41•33
17 "	47•36	53•41	45•44	46•45
18 "	48•12	57•27	48•22	55•32

These numbers were collected at Manchester and Stockport: the children were weighed in summer, and consequently were lightly clothed, and they had nothing in their pockets. We see here again, as in the height, that it is only after puberty that, at equal ages, we observe a difference in weight. The comparison of weights seems to be rather in favour of Belgic children; it is true that those of England were taken from the lower orders.

2. Relations between the Weight and Height

If man increased equally in all his dimensions, his weight at different ages would be as the cube of his height. Now, this is not what we really observe. The increase of weight is slower, except during the first year after birth; then the proportion which we have just pointed out is pretty regularly observed. But after this period, and until near the age of puberty, the weight increases nearly as the square of the height. The development of the weight again becomes very rapid at the time of puberty, and almost stops at the twenty-fifth year. In general, we do not err much when we assume that, *during development, the squares of the weight at different ages are as the fifth powers of the height;* which naturally leads to this conclusion, in supposing the specific gravity constant, that the transverse growth of man is less than the vertical.

However, if we compare two individuals who are fully developed and well-formed with each other, to ascertain the relations existing between the weight and stature, we shall find that *the weight of developed persons, of different heights, is nearly as the square of the stature.* Whence it naturally follows, that a *transverse section, giving both the breadth and thickness, is just proportioned to the height of the individual.* We furthermore conclude that, proportion still being attended width predominates in individuals of small stature.

Taking twelve of the smallest individuals of both sexes, and twelve of the largest, of those who have been submitted to our observations, we have obtained the following values as the average of stature, and the ratio of weight to the stature:–

Men.	Stature.	Ratio of Weight to Stature.
The smallest,	1•511 metre.	36•7 kilog.
The largest,	1•822 "	41•4 "
Women.		
The smallest,	1•456 metre.	35•6 kilog.
The largest,	1•672 "	38•0 "

Thus, the stature of men and women, fully developed and well-formed, varied in the proportion of five to six nearly: it is almost the same with the ratios of the weight to the stature of the two sexes: whence it naturally follows, as we have already said above, that the weight is in proportion to the square of the stature.*

Now, let us suppose that we have the individuals grouped, not according to age, but to stature, and that we have taken the average of the weight of each group, for example, and that we proceed by ten centimetres at a time: we shall have groups of children at first, then groups of children with whom some adult persons are classed, which will be the case with men commencing at 1•47 metres nearly, and women at 1•41 metres. If we afterwards reduce these numbers to a tabular form, we shall arrive at the following results, the weight of the clothes having been subtracted:–

Relation of Stature to Weight.

Stature.	Men.		Women.	
	Weight.	Ratio.	Weight.	Ratio.
At Birth,.........	3•20	6•19	2•91	6•03
0•60 metre,......	6•20	10•33	..	..
0•70 "	9•30	13•27	9•06	12•94
0•80 "	11•36	14•20	11•21	14•01
0•90 "	13•50	15•00	13•42	14•91
1•00 "	15•90	15•90	15•82	15•82
1•10 "	18•50	16•82	18•30	16•64
1•20 "	21•72	18•10	21•51	17•82
1•30 "	26•63	20•04	26•83	20•64
1•40 "	34•48	24•63	37•28	26•63
1•50 "	46•29	30•86	48•00	32•00
1•60 "	57•15	35•72	56•73	35•45
1•70 "	63•28	37•22	65•20	38•35
1•80 "	70•61	39•23	..	..
1•90 "	75•56	39•77	..	..

We see that, statures being equal, woman weighs a little less than man until she attains the height of 1 metre 3 decimetres, which nearly corresponds to the period of puberty, and that she weighs a little more for higher statures. This difference, for the most part, proceeds from aged females being mingled with groups of a moderate stature sooner than males are; and, at equal statures, as we have already stated, aged persons weigh more than young ones.

To apply the preceding to determine the age of a *non-adult* person, from a knowledge of the weight and stature only, let us suppose the height of the person to be 1•23 metre, and the weight 24 kilogrammes, he being, moreover, of the male sex. We shall immediately see, from the preceding table, that he is heavy in proportion to his stature; the table before informs us that, by taking the height alone, he ought to be a little more than nine years of age, and considering the weight alone, he should be under ten; so that we may pronounce, with great probability of truth, that the individual in question must be between nine and ten.

*Calling *t* and T the statures, and *p* and P the corresponding weights of the smallest and the largest individuals, we have, in fact, almost exactly, t:T::5:6, by the numbers of the first column, belonging to men, and *p/t*: P/T::5:6 for those of the second; from which we find that *t*:T::*p/* :P/T, or, in other words, t^2:T^2::*p*:P. It is the same with the numbers belonging to females.

3. Weight of a Population–Weight of the Human Skeleton

The following table may serve to determine the weight of a population composed of men, women, and children, or of a population composed of individuals of certain limited ages: it has been formed by taking the numbers belonging to each age from a population table, and multiplying them by the weight of individuals of this age.*

Table of the Weight of a Population of 10,000 Souls.

Ages.	Men.	Women.	Total.
	kilog.	kilog.	kilog.
0 to 1 year,......................	0•894	0•903	1•697
1 to 2 "	1•462	1•324	2•786
2 to 3 "	1•504	1•372	2•876
3 to 4 "	1•676	1•485	3•161
4 to 5 "	1•864	1•658	3•522
5 to 6 "	2•017	1•765	3•782
6 to 8 "	4•251	3•796	8•037
8 to 10 "	4•768	4•318	9•086
10 to 12 "	5•263	4•827	10•090
12 to 14 "	6•332	5•977	12•309
14 to 16 "	8•805	7•801	16•606
16 to 20 "	18•902	17•700	36•602
20 to 25 "	25•292	23•308	48•600
25 to 30 "	25•603	22•770	48•373
30 to 40 "	39•396	39•548	78•944
40 to 50 "	28•720	31•470	60•190
50 to 60 "	24•122	24•634	48•756
60 to 70 "	23•620	16•458	40•118
70 to 80 "	9•620	7•908	17•428
80 and upwards	2•320	1•998	4•318
Total.................................	236•471	220•810	457•281

Thus, taking at once a population of 10,000 souls, without distinction of age or sex, the weight will be 457,000 kilogrammes nearly, 236,000 being that of the male portion. Thus we see that *the average weight of an individual, without reference to age or sex, is* 45•7 *kilo-*

*The population table made use of in these calculations is one which will be found above, taken from the *Recherches sur la Mortalité et la Reproduction. Bruxelles:* 1839.

grammes nearly; and, considering the sexes, 47 *kilogrammes for a man* [125 9-10ths lbs. troy], *and* 42 1/2 *kilogrammes for a woman* [74 lbs. troy]. The whole population of Brussels, which amounts to 100,000, would weigh 4,572,810 kilogrammes; or nearly four and a half times as much as a cube of water 10 metres square: and the whole human race, computed at 737,000,000, would not weigh as much as 33 cubes of water 100 metres square: a value which at first sight appears small, since such a volume of water might be contained in a basin having a surface of less than one-third of an acre [*hectare*], and a depth of 100 metres.

To the preceding data, I shall add some measurements of the human skeleton, which have been communicated to me by MM. Van Esschen and Guiette. They will throw additional light on our present subject.

Dimensions.	Number of Skeletons.				
	No. 1*	No. 2†	No. 3‡	No. 4§	No. 5∞
	kilog.	kilog.	kilog.	kilog.	kilog.
Weights................	4•2	4•4	5•7	5•2	3•0
	met.	met.	met.	met.	met.
Statures,................	1•685	1•640	1•667	1•755	1•500
Height of head,....	0•138	0•134	0•136	0•135	0•135
" of spinal column	0•590	0•560	0•563	0•550	0•470
" of pelvis,...........	0•210	0•186	0•182	0•225	0•152
Length of the upper extremities,.......	0•779	0•735	0•754	0•790	0•662
Length of the lower extremities,...........	0•917	0•870	0•885	0•970	0•800

The two last skeletons, belonging to females, did not present any essential difference from the three first, which were males.

We see, from the preceding table, that the weight of a skeleton prepared some years, scarcely exceeds the weight of a child at birth.

From the foregoing, we deduce the following conclusions:–

1. From birth there is an inequality, both in weight and stature, between children of the two sexes; the average weight of a boy being 3•20 kilogrammes [8 5-10ths lbs. troy], that of a girl 2•91 kilogrammes [7 7-10ths lbs. troy]; the stature of a boy is 0•496 metres, and that of a girl 0•483 metres.

2. The weight of a child diminishes a little towards the third day after birth, and does not begin to increase sensibly until after the first week.

* No.1. Natural skeleton of a man of about thirty-five years of age, prepared seven years. † No. 2. Skeleton of a man about twenty-five years of age, prepared six years. ‡ No. 3. Skeleton of a man. Age and date of the preparation unknown. § No. 4. Skeleton of a woman. Age and date of the preparation unknown. ∞ No. 5. Skeleton of a woman aged fifteen years, prepared one year.

3. At equal ages, man is generally heavier than woman: about the age of 12 years only are the individuals of both sexes of about the same weight. Between 1 and 11 years, the difference in weight is from one kilogramme to one and a half: between 16 and 20, it is six kilogrammes nearly; and after this period eight to nine kilogrammes.

4. When man and woman have attained their full development, they weigh almost exactly twenty times as much as at birth; and their stature is about three and one-fourth times greater than it was at the same period.

5. In old age, man and woman lose about six or seven kilogrammes in weight, and seven centimetres in stature.

6. During the development of individuals of both sexes, we may consider the square of the weight, at different ages, as proportioned to the fifth power of their stature.

7. After the full development of individuals of both sexes, the weight is almost as the square of the stature.

From the two preceding relations, we infer, that increase in height is greater than the transverse increase, including breadth and thickness.

8. Man attains the maximum of his weight at about 40, and begins to waste in a sensible degree about the 60th year.

9. Woman attains the maximum of her weight about the age of 50. During the period of reproduction, namely, from the 18th to the 40th year, her weight scarcely increases in a perceptible degree.

10. The weight of individuals who have been measured, and who were fully developed and well-formed, varies within extremes which are nearly as 1 to 2; whilst the stature only varies within limits which, at the most, are as 1 to 1 1/3. This is inferred from the following values, furnished by observation:–

	Maximum.	Minimum.	Average.
Weight of man,	98•5 kilog.	49•1 kilog.	63•7 kilog.
" woman,	93•8 "	39•8 "	55•2 "
Stature of man,	1•890 met.	1•467 met.	1•684 met.
" woman,	1•740 "	1•408 "	1•579 "

11. At equal statures, woman weighs a little less than man before reaching the height of 1•3 metres, which almost corresponds to the period of puberty; and she weighs a little more for higher statures.

12. The average weight of an individual, without reference to age or sex, is 45•7 kilogrammes; and, taking sex into account, 47 kilogrammes for man, and 42•5 kilogrammes for woman.

CLASSICS IN OBESITY

THE SPECIFIC GRAVITY OF HEALTHY MEN

BODY WEIGHT ÷ VOLUME AS AN INDEX OF OBESITY

A. R. Behnke, Jr., M.D.
Lieutenant Commander, M. C., U.S. Navy

B. G. Feen, M.D.
Lieutenant, M.C., U.S. Navy

AND

W. C. Welham, M.D.
Lieutenant, M.C., U.S. Navy

The fundamental biologic determination of corporeal specific gravity, essentially a relationship between weight and unit volume, has been neglected in the modern classification of healthy persons. Stern (1) and Spivak (2) emphasized the value of the measurement of corporeal density, but their experimental data are not conclusive. Of especial interest is the relationship between gravity and the fat content of the body.

The presence of an indeterminate amount of excess adipose tissue renders difficult any precise computation, for example, of metabolic rate or dosage of drugs in terms of total body weight. The important consideration should be the weight of the lean body representing the active mass of protoplasm.

In this paper the data support the concept that the comparatively low specific gravity of fat makes the measurement of the specific gravity of the body mass valid for the estimation of fat content.

The comprehensive, statistical analysis of Boyd (3), however, covering seven hundred and eighty-seven values reported since 1906 does not permit a classification of individuals with respect to obesity. The analyzed results (3), moreover, obtained by different investigators elude comparison by reason of the unknown quantity of air present in the lungs when the measurements were made.

In the present investigation the values of specific gravity obtained on ninety-nine healthy naval men in the 20 to 40 year age group were corrected by determining the residual air volume. The results obtained permit the classification of individuals as to degree of obesity and serve as a single index of physical fitness to supplement the standard age-height-weight tables which frequently lead to a designation of overweight for well developed men in contrast with a designation of normal weight for more obese individuals who fall into a lower weight group.

METHOD OF PROCEDURE

The essential measurement is that of body volume, which, based on Archimedes' principle, can be conve-

Behnke AR, Feen BG, Welham WC. The specific gravity of healthy men. *JAMA*. 1942;118:495-498.

Special thanks to Judy Roberts of the Pennington Information Center for help in acquiring this and reference documents.

The material in this article should be construed only as the personal opinion of the writers and not as representing the opinion of the writers and not as representing the opinion of the Navy Department officially.

1. Stern, H.: Investigations on Corporeal Specific Gravity and on the Value of This Factor in Physical Diagnosis, M. Rec. 59: 204-207, 1901.

2. Spivak, C. D.: The Specific Gravity of the Human Body, Arch. Int. Med. 15: 628-642 (April) 1915.

3. Boyd, Edith: The Specific Gravity of the Human Body, Human Biology 5: 646-672 (Dec.) 1933.

TABLE 1.–*Example Illustrating the Method of Computing Specific Gravity*

		Pounds	Kilograms
Weight of the body in air		183.00	83.20
Weight in water, full inspiration		14.20	6.45
Weight in water, complete expiration		23.20	10.55
Vital capacity computed from the volume of water displaced	4,090 cc.		
Vital capacity by spirometric measurements	4,150 cc.		
Volume of residual air	1,200 cc.		
Weight of abdominal belt		13.75	6.25
Corrections			
Gross weight in water		23.20	10.55
Weight of belt		13.75	6.25
Weight in water, not corrected for residual air		9.45	4.30
Correction for residual air (1,200/453)		2.65	1.20
Net weight in water		12.10	5.50

$$\text{Specific gravity} = \frac{\text{Weight}}{\text{Volume}} = \frac{183}{170.9} = 1.071$$

niently determined by the method of hydrostatic weighing, i.e. equivalent volume = weight in air – weight in water. The weight in water is determined by suspending a subject below the surface of the water on a line leading up to a spring scale graduated in ounces. A weighted lead belt maintains negative buoyancy for all types of persons.

Two weighings in water serve to check the accuracy of the procedure: one at the completion of maximum inspiration and the other at the end of maximum expiration.

The difference in weight obtained record hydrostatic displacement, which serves as a measure of vital capacity. This determination of vital capacity when corrected for the effect of the mean hydrostatic pressure on thoracic volume gives values comparable to those obtained by the standard method employing spirometry.

In the determination of residual air, the inhalation of a helium-oxygen mixture for a period of three minutes following maximal expiration brought about a removal of the residual nitrogen. The subsequent washing out during normal respiration of the previously inhaled helium with 50 liters of air or oxygen permitted an accurate computation of residual pulmonary volume comparable to unpublished results obtained by Willmon and Behnke using the nitrogen dilution method. Duplicate determinations usually gave values which dif-

TABLE 2.–*Residual Air and Vital Capacity Values*

Specific Gravity	Number of Men	Average Residual Air, Liters	Residual Air, Range	Average Vital Capacity, Liters	Vital Capacity, Range
1.020-1.029	2	1.315	1.312-1.317	4.350	4.100-4.600
1.030-1.039	2	1.357	1.200-1.513	4.125	4.100-4.150
1.040-1.049	4	1.131	0.850-1.486	4.575	3.700-5.000
1.050-1.059	20	1.525	1.060-2.398	4.888	3.575-6.000
1.060-1.069	23	1.179	0.707-1.643	4.757	3.975-6.095
1.070-1.079	27	1.504	0.858-2.650	4.820	3.875-6.200
1.080-1.089	14	1.379	0.706-2.126	5.003	4.400-5.750
1.090-1.099	7	1.730	1.098-2.204	5.085	4.250-5.970

TABLE 3.–*Individual Loss of Weight in Relation to Specific Gravity*

		Weight				Circumference			
		In Air		In Water (Net)		Chest		Abdomen	
Date	Gravity	Pounds	Kg.	Pounds	Kg.	Inches	Cm.	Inches	Cm.
3/12	1.056	202.5	92.0	10.8	4.9	38.5	97.8	35.2	89.4
7/ 1	1.060	194.5	88.4	11.0	5.0	...	...	...	...
8/13	1.066	187.0	85.0	11.6	5.3	38.7	98.3	33.0	83.8
10/9	1.071	183.0	83.2	12.1	5.5	39.1	99.3	31.4	79.7

fered by not more than 150 cc.

CIRCUMFERENTIAL MEASUREMENTS OF CHEST AND ABDOMEN

The circumferential measurements of the chest and the abdomen are subject to considerable variation unless special care is exercised. The values recorded were obtained usually in the midmorning, during quiet respiration and with the arms of the subject extended vertically. Under these circumstances errors arising from altered muscular tonus or voluntary retraction of the abdomen were minimized. The chest measurement was made at the level of the nipples, the abdominal measurement at the level of the umbilicus.

SOURCES OF ERROR

The greatest error arises from the determination of residual lung volume. If the variation in this measurement is of the order of 200 cc., values for specific gravity will be subject to an error of $\pm$ 0.003.

Repeated determinations on the same individual permitting the use of a constant volume for residual air give values that agree to within 0.003.

A second error may arise from the presence of gas in the abdominal viscera. In an attempt to minimize this error, determinations were made in the morning on the fasting individual.

RESULTS OBTAINED

In table 4 are listed values obtained on ninety-nine healthy men in military service. From analysis of the data, two facts are apparent: 1. Specific gravity increases inversely in relation to weight. 2. The difference between abdominal and thoracic girth can be correlated with specific gravity.

In table 2 the values for residual air indicate that any error in the determinations will not appreciably alter the relative classification of the subjects with respect to specific gravity. It is apparent that the range of values for residual air is large so that any individual measurement of specific gravity must be accompanied by an actual determination of residual air. For groups of twenty or more men, however, when average values are compared, an arbitrary figure of 1,450 cc. for residual

TABLE 4.–*Specific Gravity in Relation to Weight, Age, Height and Measurements of Thoracic and Abdominal Circumference*

		Average Weight				Average Height		Average Circumference					
								Chest		Abdomen			
Specific Gravity	Number of Men	Pounds	Kg.	Range, Pounds	Average Age	Inches	Cm.	Inches	Cm.	Inches	Cm.	Average Difference Inches	Difference Range
1.020-1.029	2	233	105.9	221-245	34	68.9	175.0	41.5	105.4	41.6	105.7	–0.1	–0.75-0.50
1.030-1.039	2	187	85.0	174-200	48	71.0	180.3	36.7	93.2	35.9	91.2	0.9	0.75-1.00
1.040-1.049	4	166	75.4	145-184	31	66.9	169.9	38.0	96.5	33.7	85.6	4.2	3.00-5.25
1.050-1.059	20	171	77.7	126-208	33	69.3	176.0	37.2	94.5	33.0	83.8	4.2	1.00-7.25
1.060-1.069	23	158	71.8	131-202	24	68.1	173.0	35.6	90.4	30.3	77.0	5.2	3.25-7.00
1.070-1.079	27	153	69.5	131-199	26	69.4	176.3	35.7	90.7	30.0	76.2	5.6	2.50-8.50
1.080-1.089	14	148	67.3	130-164	24	69.4	176.3	35.7	90.7	29.7	75.4	6.1	275.-7.75
1.090-1.099	7	140	63.5	125-163	23	69.9	177.5	35.5	90.2	28.6	72.6	6.9	5.25-8.25

TABLE 5.–*High, Intermediate and Low Specific Gravity Group Values in Relation to Weight and Circumferential Measurements*

Number of Men	Average Specific Gravity	Range	Average Weight		Average Circumference					Average Height	
					Chest		Abdomen				
			Pounds	Kg.	Inches	Cm.	Inches	Cm.	Difference, Inches	Inches	Cm.
38	1.081	1.075-1.097	148.7	67.6	35.3	89.7	29.6	75.2	5.7	69.7	177.0
33	1.066	1.060-1.074	156.6	71.2	35.8	90.9	30.4	77.2	5.4	68.3	173.5
28	1.056	1.021-1.059	176.0	80.0	37.6	95.5	33.9	86.1	3.7	69.0	175.3

pulmonary volume will not introduce an error greater than ±0.003 in the computation of specific gravity.

In table 5 the ninety-nine subjects are divided into three groups on the basis of high low and middle range values for specific gravity. In the low group are listed all values below 1.060, and in the high group are values above 1.074.

Table 3 indicates how the loss of 19.5 pounds of adipose tissue in one subject results in a change in specific gravity. The values for the weight in water have been corrected for a residual air volume of 1,200 cc. One notes that a decrease in abdominal girth is followed by an increase in specific gravity.

COMMENT

Difference in Thoracic and Abdominal Girth as an Index of Corpulence.– Although variation in individual values except for the most obese subjects is considerable, the group values in relation to specific gravity show a definite trend according to table 4. The lean subjects on inspection possess the greater circumferential difference between chest and abdomen in comparison with the corresponding difference in fat men.

Body Weight and Specific Gravity.– The relationship between body weight and specific gravity (table 4) is not absolute but relative in the sense that for any selected group of homogeneous persons the heaviest men tend to have specific gravity values in the low range of the scale. The rather uniform decrease in average weight in relation to specific gravity is to be regarded as coincidental. Lean men, for example, weighing 200 pounds will have high specific gravity values in contrast with the measurements on fat men of the same weight.

The average weight, for example, of thirty-eight men in the high specific gravity group (table 5) was 148.7 pounds. In a separate series of determinations on exceptional athletes, presented in the second paper, a similar high value for specific gravity was associated with an average weight of 200 pounds. These facts suggest a fundamental relationship between adiposity and specific gravity.

Specific Gravity and Obesity.– Corporeal density serves as an index of the amount of excess adipose tissue. In table 5 the average weight in water of the low specific gravity group was 9.4 pounds, corresponding to a specific gravity value of 1.056. The corresponding values for the high specific gravity group were 11.1 and 1.081. The difference in weight in air between the two groups is 27.3 pounds.

On the assumption that a loss of 27.3 pounds of body weight in air is associated with a gain of weight in water of 1.7 pounds (11.1 - 9.4), the specific gravity of the low group following this loss of weight will be raised from an initial value of 1.056 to 1.081.

Thus, for every pound of weight lost the weight of the body in water is increased 0.062 pound (1.7 ÷ 27.3). The specific gravity of the reduced tissues is therefore 0.94 (1 ÷ 1.062), or a value in accord with the specific gravity of adipose tissue.

The average difference in thoracic and abdominal measurements of 5.8 and 3.7 inches for the high and low groups respectively suggests that excess adipose tissue accounts essentially for the difference in values for specific gravity of the two groups.

Individual Loss in Weight (table 3).– A man placed on a restricted diet and engaging in systematic exercise lost 19.5 pounds over a period of seven months. The net weight in water increased from 10.8 pounds to 12.1 pounds, although the corresponding weight in air decreased from 202.5 pounds to 183.0 pounds. Thus, for every pound of weight lost in air the weight in water increased 0.067 pound (1.3 ÷ 19.5). The specific gravity of the reduced tissue is therefor 0.937 (1.000 ÷ 1.067), or a value again in accord with the specific gravity of neutral fat.

The reduction in abdominal girth further suggests that the eliminated tissue was chiefly fat.

Specific Gravity and Composition of the Body.– Of all the constituents of the tissues of the body, fat and

TABLE 6.–*Body Composition, Showing the Effect of Variations in the Percentage of Bone and of Fat on Specific Gravity*

		Percentage of Bone (10)			Percentage of Bone (14)			Variation in Fat Content		
	Specific Gravity	Percentage	Weight, Pounds	Volume	Percentage	Weight, Pounds	Volume	Percentage	Weight, Pounds	Volume
Bone salts*...............	3.0	5	10	3.3	7	14	4.66	5	7.0	2.3
Essential lipoids........	0.94	10	20	21.2	10	20	21.20	10	14.0	14.9
Tissue........................	1.06	85	170	160.4	83	166	156.60	85	119.0	112.2
Totals..			200	184.9		200	182.46	Lean Man	140.0†	129.4
									60.0‡	63.8
								Fat Man	200.0§	193.2
Specific gravity of the body as a whole.........		1.082				1.095		† 1.082; § 1.035		

*$Ca_2(PO_4)_3$ and $Ca\ (CO_3)_2$, approximately one half the weight of marrow free bone. ‡Excess adipose tissue.

bone appear to be the chief determinants of the ultimate values for specific gravity. In the comparison of the three groups (table 5) the difference between the average of the high and low values could best be attributed to a variation in adipose tissue. On the other hand, it is expected that the relative amount of bone may alter individual values within a limited range.

In table 6 hypothetic examples are presented to clarify the relationship between specific gravity and the composition of the body especially with respect to variation in the percentage of bone and fat.

For the purpose of our analysis the body may be viewed as comprising calcium salts representing 50 per cent of the weight of bone, essential or irreducible lipoid substance, excess adipose tissue, and all other tissues of the body embracing chiefly muscle, organs, brain, skin and blood.

The specific gravity of the mineral substance of bone is of the order of 3.0, adipose tissue 0.94, and all other tissue 1.060. This last figure is an approximation based on the specific gravity of blood and various other tissues according to Vierordt (4) and Nadeshdin (5).

With reference to the specific gravity of blood, eighty-one determinations made according to the method of Barbour and Hamilton on eighteen of the ninety-nine subjects reported on in this paper gave an average in agreement with the data of Stern (1) of 1.060, standard deviation 0.002.

The percentage of skeletal weight in relation to the body as a whole exclusive of excess adipose tissue may not be expected to vary more than 4 units. Corresponding to this variation of 4 units in the percent-

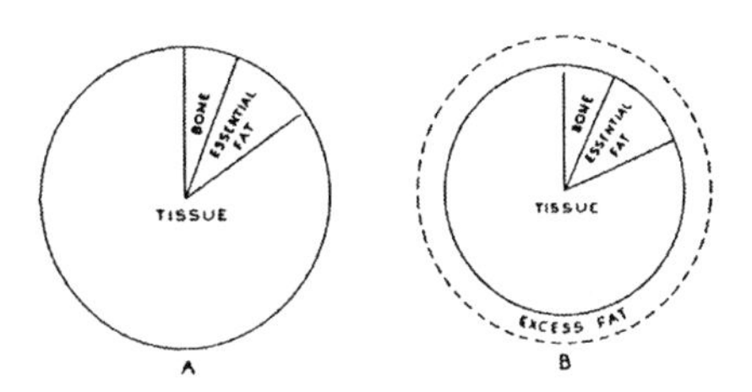

A represents the volume percentages of the three major specific gravity determinants of the body for a 200 pound, 90.9 Kg., lean man. The calculations were based on the following data: bone 10 per cent of body weight, specific gravity 1.60; essential fat 10 per cent, specific gravity 0.94; tissue 80 per cent, specific gravity 1.06. The volume percentages are therefore bone 6.8 per cent, essential fat 11.5 per cent, tissue volume 81.7 per cent. The specific gravity of this man would be 1.082. The solid inner circle in B represents the volume percentages for a 140 pound, 63.6 Kg., lean man. The volume percentages and specific gravity are the same as for the 200 pound (90.9 Kg.) lean man. The dotted outer circle represents the addition of 60 pounds of excess fat to the 140 pound lean man. The bone volume percentage is lowered to 4.5 per cent, the fat volume percentage is increased to 40.8 per cent and the tissue volume is reduced to 54.7 per cent in this man. Thus the specific gravity of the body is reduced to 1.035.

4. Vierordt, H.: Anatomische, physiologische und physikalische Daten und Tabellen, 3d rev. ed., Jena, Gustav Fischer, 1906.

5. Nadeshdin, W. A.: Zur Untersuchung der Minderwertigkeit der Organe an Leichen, Deutsche Ztsch. f. d. ges. gerichtl. Med. 18: 426-431, 1932.

age of body weight attributed to bone is a fluctuation of specific gravity of 13 units (table 6).

In contrast with bone, the amount of excess fat is subject to wide variations and a value of 30 per cent of the total body weight is not unreasonable for obese persons. If a lean man weighing 140 pounds, for example, accumulates 60 pounds of adipose tissue, the corporeal specific gravity will be lowered from 1.082 to 1.035, representing a difference of 46 units.

Since the density of the mass of tissue exclusive of bone and fat is probably constant for healthy men, the amount of fat appears to be the main factor affecting the specific gravity of a person.

Our concepts with regard to the composition of the body can be summarized by the accompanying diagrams. A, for example, the volume of a lean body mass weighing 200 pounds (90.9 Kg.), specific gravity 1.082. is divided into its components 1, 2 and 3.

In B the inner circle encompasses a mass similar to weight by 60 pounds (27.3 Kg.). The outer circle circumscribes an accumulation of 60 pounds (27.3 Kg.) of adipose tissue. The specific gravity of this 200 pound mass can be computed as 1.035, in contrast with the value of 1.082 for the mass represented by the inner circle.

The fundamental problem of the amount of variation of constituents 1 and 2 within the lean body mass remains to be determined. For the present the assumption is made that the percentage variation of these constituents based on body weight is small for lean men.

Excess fat therefore is viewed as the prime factor governing the level of specific gravity.

Precise measurements, however, of this excess fat will necessarily await a knowledge of the relative percentage variation of the weight of the skeleton in lean persons.

Of the anthropometric measurements, the chest diameters and height are expected to modify the values for specific gravity in persons possessing the same degree of obesity.

CONCLUSIONS

1. The fundamental biologic characteristic of corporeal density can be accurately measured usually within 0.004 unit by the method of hydrostatic weighing, provided a correction is made for the air in the lungs.
2. Values of specific gravity for healthy men ranging in age between 20 and 40 fall between 1.021 and 1.097.
3. Low values for specific gravity indicate obesity and, conversely, high values denote leanness.
4. Individual loss in weight through exercise and a restricted diet is associated with an increase in specific gravity.
5. Difference in the circumferential measurements of chest and abdomen serve as a criterion of obesity and can be correlated with specific gravity.
6. Variation in the percentage of bone in relation to body weight, excluding excess fat, is not expected to produce deviation of more than 0.013 units in comparable values.

CLASSICS IN OBESITY

IMMUNOASSAY OF ENDOGENOUS PLASMA INSULIN IN MAN

BY ROSALYN S. YALOW AND SOLOMON A. BERSON
(From the Radioisotope Service, Veterans Administration Hospital, New York, N.Y.)

(submitted for publication March 7, 1960; accepted March 22, 1960)

For years investigators have sought an assay for insulin which would combine virtually absolute specificity with a high degree of sensitivity, sufficiently exquisite for measurement of the minute insulin concentrations usually present in the circulation. Methods in use recently depend on the ability of insulin to exert an effect on the metabolism of glucose *in vivo* or in excised muscle or adipose tissue. Thus, the insulin concentration in plasma has been estimated: a) from the degree of hypoglycemia produced in hypophysectomized, adrenalectomized, alloxan-diabetic rats (1); b) from the augmentation of glucose uptake by isolated rat hemidiaphragm (2); or c) from the increased oxidation of glucose-1-C^{14} by the rat epididymal fat pad (3). Since there have been reports indicating the presence, in plasma, of inhibitors of insulin action (4) and of noninsulin substances capable of inducing an insulin-like effect (5,6), these procedures, while yielding interesting information regarding the effects of various plasmas on glucose metabolism in tissues, are of doubtful specificity for the measurement of insulin per se (5).

Recently it has been shown (7,8) that insulins from various species (pork, beef, horse and sheep) show quantitative differences in reaction and cross reaction with antisera obtained from human subjects treated with commercial insulin preparations (beef, pork insulin mixtures). An immunoassay method for beef insulin has been reported in which the insulin content is determined from the degree of competitive inhibition which the insulin offers to the binding of beef insulin-I^{131} by human antisera (9-12). Although human insulin reacts with human antibeef, pork insulin antiserum and displaces beef insulin-I^{131} by competitive inhibition (7,8,10), the reaction is too weak to permit measurement of the low insulin concentrations present in human plasma (7,8,11-13). In preliminary communications we have reported that the competitive inhibition by human insulin of binding of crystalline beef insulin-I^{131} to guinea pig antibeef insulin antibodies is sufficiently marked to permit measurement of plasma insulin in man (11,12,14), and to be capable of detecting as little as a fraction of a microunit of human insulin (12,14). Preliminary data on insulin concentrations in man before and after glucose loading have been reported (12,14,15). The present communication describes in detail the methods employed in the immunoassay of endogenous insulin in the plasma of man, and reports plasma insulin concentrations during glucose tolerance tests in nondiabetic and in early diabetic subjects and plasma insulin concentrations in subjects with functioning islet cell tumors or leucine-sensitive hypoglycemia.

RS Yalow, SA Berson. Immunoassay of endogenous plasma insulin in man. J Clin Invest. 1960;39:1157-1175.

METHODS

Immunization of guinea pigs. Guinea pigs were injected subcutaneously at 1 to 4 week intervals with 5 to 10 units of either protamine zinc beef insulin (Squibb) or commercial regular beef insulin (Squibb) emulsified with mannide mono-oleate. Insulin-binding antibodies were detected in all animals after 2 to 3 injections. The antiserum employed in the present study (GP 49, serum 6-25-59) was obtained from a guinea pig immunized with protamine zinc beef insulin without adjuvant and was selected for its relatively high antibody concentration and other suitable characteristics described below.

Preparation of insulin-I^{131}. Because of the desirability of keeping the concentration of added insulin-I^{131} as low as possible and yet assuring an adequate counting rate, it is necessary to prepare the insulin-I^{131} with a high specific activity. The lots of insulin-I^{131} employed in this study had specific activities of 75 to 300 mc per mg at the time of use. The preparation of such highly labeled preparations entails difficulties not encountered when the specific activity is very much lower. The Newerly modification (16) of the Pressman-Eisen method (17) was used for labeling with several further modifications designed to increase specific activity and to minimize damage to the insulin from irradiation and other causes. To approximately 0.3 ml chloroform in a 50 ml separatory funnel are added in turn, 0.2 ml of 2.5 N HCl, 20 µl of 10^{-3} M KI, 30 to 80 mc I^{131} (as iodide) and 1 drop of 1 M $NaNO_2$. Immediately after addition of the last reagent, the funnel is stoppered to prevent loss I^{131} of into

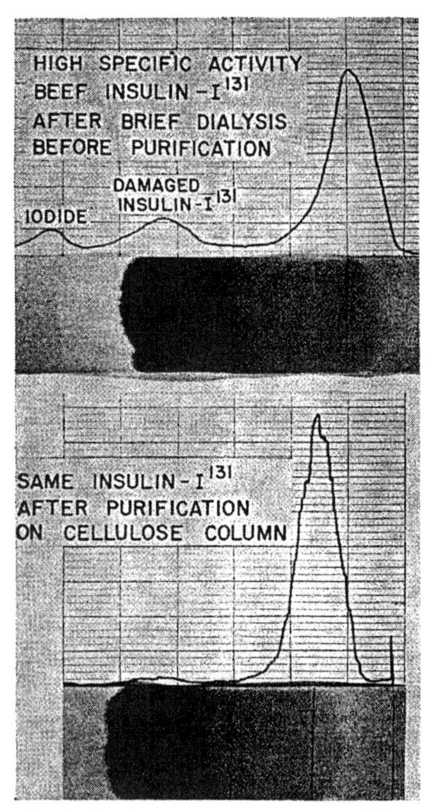

FIG. 1. PURIFICATION OF DAMAGED INSULIN-I^{131} BY CELLULOSE COLUMN ADSORPTION. *Top:* Chromato-electrophoretograms of beef insulin-I^{131}, with specific activity about 300 mc per mg, after 30 minutes' dialysis. *Bottom:* Same preparation after elution from cellulose column with control (nonimmune) plasma. At significantly lower specific activities the preparations appear as in the bottom figure *without* purification.

the atmosphere and is shaken vigorously for 2 to 3 minutes. The chloroform layer (bottom) is then drawn into a test tube beneath a layer of a few drops of water (to prevent loss of I^{131} into the air) and assayed for radioactivity in any low-sensitivity counting device. If much less than one-half of the starting radioactivity has been extracted, a second extraction with 0.2 to 0.3 ml chloroform is performed. The total amount of chloroform should be kept as small as possible to facilitate the subsequent extraction of iodine into the aqueous protein solution. The volume of the aqueous phase in the separatory funnel also should be kept small to favor the initial extraction of iodine into the chloroform. The chloroform-iodine mixture is added to 0.5 ml of 0.2 M borate buffer, pH 8, containing 20 μg of crystalline beef insulin in a 50 ml centrifuge tube, which provides for a broad interface between the two phases. The tube is shaken briskly but not violently for not more than 2 to 3 minutes following which an additional 1.0 ml borate buffer is mixed into the contents. A barely visible flocculate appears occasionally and should be allowed to settle, whereupon the top 0.5 ml (one-third of total) of the water phase is quickly removed and dialyzed against 2 L of distilled water[1]. Owing to the high concentration of radioactivity and low concentration of protein, the insulin is very susceptible to radiation damage (18,19); therefore, exposure to I^{131} at this stage should be as brief as possible, not more than 5 to 10 minutes elapsing between addition of I^{131} to the insulin and the start of dialysis. Of the total radioactivity in the dialysis bag, approximately 65 to 80 per cent represents unbound I^{131} which is reduced to less than 1 per cent of the I^{131} bound to insulin after 2 hours of dialysis. Between 20 and 60 per cent of the insulin-I^{131} is adsorbed to the dialysis membrane during this time so that the procedure yields approximately 3 to 5 μg insulin labeled with about 1.0 to 2.0 mc I^{131}. Considerable sacrifices in total yield are made to expedite the procuring of a highly labeled preparation which usually contains no more than 4 to 6 per cent damaged components. We have the impression that the addition of 10^{-2} M KI or phenol (as radical scavengers) to the dialyzing solution may help to minimize radiation damage, but this has been difficult to establish since other factors are also responsible for damage to the protein during the procedure. Distilled water is used in the last dialysis following which 1 drop of human serum albumin (250 mg per ml) is added to the insulin-I^{131} solution to prevent losses of labeled insulin by adsorption to glassware (20,21) and to minimize any further irradiation damage (18,19). Solutions are kept frozen when not in use.

If the insulin-I^{131} solution is surveyed for radioactivity at completion of dialysis, the specific activity of the insulin-I^{131} may be estimated approximately. If the yield of labeled insulin has been sufficient to produce a specific activity in excess of 150 mc per mg, it can be anticipated that damage will be significantly in excess of 4 to 6 per cent, and at 300 mc per mg may be as great as 15 to 18 per cent. It is then necessary to effect partial purification of the insulin-I^{131}. Since the damaged components do not adsorb to paper but are observed to migrate with serum proteins on paper strip chromatography or electrophoresis (22), it is possible to use a cellulose column for the purification procedure as follows: The dialyzed insulin-I^{131} solution is added to 0.1 ml control (nonimmune) serum and the mixture is then passed through a column packed with a cellu-

[1] Removal of unbound iodide^{131} by anionic exchange resins is usually unsatisfactory because much of the insulin-I^{131} at this low concentration is lost by adsorption to the resin.

lose powder[2] about 1 ml in volume following which the column is washed 3 or 4 times with 1 ml of veronal buffer, 0.1 ionic strength. Most of the damaged components pass through the column with the serum while the undamaged insulin remains adsorbed to the cellulose in the column and can now be eluted slowly with undiluted control serum or plasma. Usually 3 to 4 eluates (each 0.5 ml of plasma) are collected and diluted immediately 1:20 to 1:100 with veronal buffer containing 0.025 per cent serum albumin to prevent further damage to the insulin by the concentrated plasma. Although the elution of insulin-I^{131} from the column is far from complete, adequate amounts are obtained for almost any number of insulin assays. Most of the damaged fraction is removed by this procedure (Figure 1).

Principles of immunoassay. The basis of the technique resides in the ability of human insulin to react strongly with the insulin-binding antibodies present in guinea pig antibeef insulin serum (11,12,14), and by so doing, to inhibit competitively the binding of crystalline beef insulin-I^{131} to antibody. The assay of human insulin in unknown solutions is accomplished by comparison with known concentrations of human insulin. The use of I^{131} -labeled animal insulin as a tracer is necessitated by the lack of a crystalline preparation of human insulin.

The determination of antibody-bound insulin-I^{131} and free insulin-I^{131} by paper chromato-electrophoresis has been described previously (22). Briefly, the separation of antibody-bound insulin from unbound insulin in plasma results from the adsorption of all free insulin (when present in amounts less that 1 to 5 µg) to the paper at the site of application ("origin"), while the antibody-bound insulin migrates toward the anode with the inter-β-γ-globulins. Thus, in the presence of insulin-I^{131} there appear two separate peaks of radioactivity; measurement of the areas beneath the two peaks (by planimetry) yields the relative proportion of bound insulin-I^{131} (migrating with serum globulins) and free insulin-I^{131} (remaining at origin). The ratio of bound insulin-I^{131} to free insulin-I^{131} (B/F) is a function of the concentration of insulin-binding antibodies, of both insulin concentrations, and of the characteristic kinetic and thermodynamic constants for the reactions between the insulins and the particular antiserum (23). Selection of an antiserum for purposes of this assay is determined primarily by the desirability of obtaining a relatively marked decrease in B/F ratio with small increments in the concentration of human insulin. Although the antibody concentration is of only secondary importance, it should be high enough to permit at least 1:100 dilution of the antiserum (preferably 1:1,000 or greater). On the basis of preliminary tests the antiserum is diluted appropriately to yield an initial B/F ratio between 2 and 4 for tracer beef insulin-I^{131} alone, in the absence of added human insulin. Provided that the amount of the beef insulin -I^{131} used is truly a tracer quantity, the initial B/F ratio is inversely proportional to the dilution factor (23). In the presence of human insulin, the B/F ratio decreases progressively with increase in insulin concentration; with sensitive antisera the B/F ratio is reduced by about 50 per cent in the presence of 15 µU per ml human insulin.

Standard curves. Two preparations of human insulin were employed as standards. The first ("Tietze human insulin")[3] is reported (24) to have a potency of 1.8 U per mg crude preparation; the second ("Fisher human insulin")[3], was assayed at 6.8 U per mg in 1956 (25), but it was believed that the activity of the latter preparation might have decreased slightly since its initial preparation (25). A tentative value of 6 U per mg for the Fisher insulin was assigned. However, since a value as low as 22 U per mg could be placed on a crystalline sample of the latter preparation (25), whereas the Tietze insulin was assayed relative to a standard of 27 to 29 U per mg, we have regarded the Tietze crude insulin preparation as 1.8/28 x 100 = 6.45 per cent pure insulin by weight, and the Fisher insulin powder preparation as 6/22 x 100=28.2 per cent pure insulin by weight. When compared on this basis, no consistent differences in potencies of the two preparations were observed in the immunoassay procedure and the value of 6 U per mg for the Fisher preparation was accepted as the correct value. Since the Fisher preparation is the more highly purified, it was employed as standard in most of the studies.

All dilutions of insulin and antiserum are prepared in 0.1 ionic strength veronal buffer containing 0.25 per cent human serum albumin to prevent adsorption of reactants to glassware. (There is no detectable insulin in commercial supplies of human serum albumin.) Standard solutions each contain identical concentrations of tracer beef insulin-I^{131} (about 0.05 to 0.15 mµg per ml but differing in different runs) and antiserum, but varying concentrations of human insulin ranging from 0.05 to 5.0 mµg per ml (calculated as "pure" human insulin). The antiserum is added last in all cases. Mixtures are refrigerated at 4 degrees C for 4 days. These conditions provide sufficient time to reach equilibrium between bound and free insulin. The mixtures are then subjected to chromato-electrophoresis (22) in a cold room at 4 degrees C (Whatman 3 MM paper, veronal buffer, 0.1 ionic strength, pH 8.6, constant voltage 20 to 25 v per cm, cover of apparatus open), which produces a satisfactory separation of the peaks of bound and free insulin-I^{131} in about 1 to 1.5 hours. Earlier immunoassays (10) were performed after prolonged incubation at 37 degrees C. However, it has since been shown (23) that the standard free energy change of the reaction in the direction of antigen-antibody complex formation is increased considerably at 4 degrees C, which results in an approximately twofold

[2] Genuine Whatman Cellulose Powder, W & R Balston Ltd., England.

[3] We are greatly indebted to Dr. F. Tietze of the National Institutes of Health and Dr. A. M. Fisher of the Connaught Laboratories, Toronto, Canada, for these preparations.

greater slope in the B/F versus insulin concentration curves at low insulin concentrations. Just prior to chromato-electrophoresis, control (nonimmune) guinea pig plasma is added to the mixtures to prevent trailing of antibody-bound insulin on the paper strips, since the very low concentrations of serum proteins in these mixtures are insufficient in themselves to prevent adsorption of the serum proteins (including antibody) to the paper.

The chromato-electrophoretograms are developed until the albumin band has moved about 2.5 to 3 inches from the origin, which, under the conditions employed here, usually takes about an hour. The peak of antibody-bound insulin-I^{131} moves about 2.25 inches under these conditions. The use of several large boxes, each with a capacity for 16 strips, makes it possible to run 250 to 300 strips a day. After drying, the strips are assayed for radioactivity in an automatic strip counter (Figure 2A). A "standard curve" is obtained by plotting the B/F ratio as a function of the concentration of added human insulin (Figure 2B) after correction for damaged components of insulin-I^{131}. From 3 to 6 per cent of the insulin-I^{131} was damaged after final preparation of the lots employed in this study. These damaged components migrate nonspecifically with the serum proteins, primarily with the α-globulins (22), and are demonstrably not available for binding by antibody. The short run chromato-electrophoresis does not resolve the serum proteins well enough to distinguish between antibody-bound insulin-I^{131} and damaged insulin-I^{131} so that the damaged fraction is determined by using either control (nonimmune) plasma, or antiserum whose binding capacity for undamaged insulin-I^{131} is completely saturated with beef insulin. Since the antiserum used here has a maximal beef insulin-binding capacity of about 1 mμg per ml at the dilutions employed, it has been general practice to include one or more samples made up with 1 to 4 μg per ml beef insulin for the purpose of determining the damaged fraction.

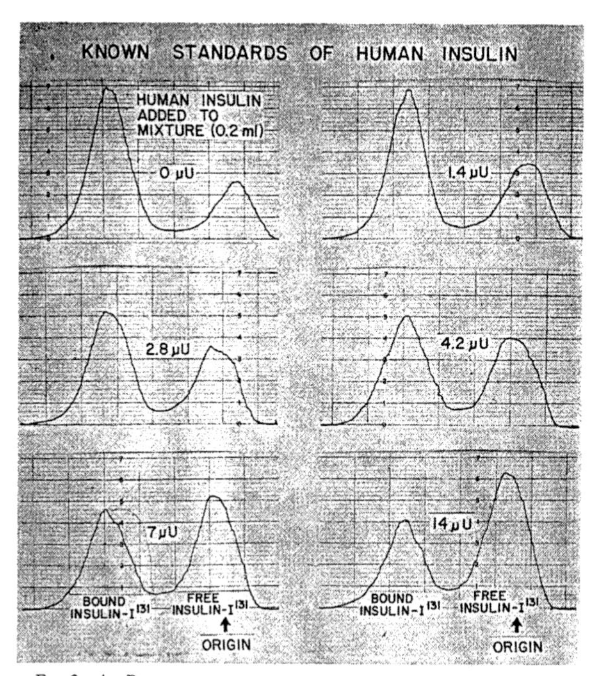

FIG. 2. A: RADIOCHROMATO-ELECTROPHORETOGRAMS OF ANTISERUM, INSULIN MIXTURES. Mixtures contained the same concentrations of guinea pig antibeef insulin serum and beef insulin-I^{131} but varying concentrations of human insulin as indicated.

Damaged insulin-I^{131} migrating with serum proteins is corrected for by subtracting the fraction damaged from the total area in the chromato-electrophoretogram. The area under the free insulin peak is then divided by the corrected total area to yield the fraction of free insulin. The fraction "bound insulin" is then 1.00 minus the fraction "free insulin."

It is evident that variation in the volumes of solution applied to the paper strips is of no consequence. Generally 100 to 200 µl is applied, the larger volume permitting use of a smaller quantity of tracer beef insulin-I^{131} for the same counting rate.

Assay of insulin in plasma. Mixtures containing unknown samples are prepared at the same time and in the same way as are standard solutions except that the unknown sample is substituted for the human insulin. Plasma insulin is best determined in a 1:10 final dilution unless the insulin concentration is unusually high; then a 1:20 or 1:40 dilution may be used. Mixtures may be made up to any desired volume. However, since only 100 to 200 µl is applied to the paper strips, it is convenient to prepare all mixtures in 0.2 or 0.5 ml volumes containing 20 or 50 µl of plasma, respectively.

Since insulin may be damaged by plasma during incubation (22), an effect which is more marked in concentrated plasma than in diluted plasma, and at 37 degrees rather than at 4 degrees C[4], it is advisable to run a control mixture with unknown plasma but without antiserum to correct for "incubation damage." However, at 1:10 dilution of plasma after 4 days at 4 degrees C, incubation damage amounts only to 0 to 3 per cent, an observation which contributed to the selection of these conditions. Therefore, only a negligible additional correction for damage is required in the plasma samples.

The insulin concentration in each plasma sample is determined from the standard curve by referring to the insulin concentration which corresponds to the corrected B/F ratio observed in the plasma sample (10-12,14,15).

Subjects for glucose tolerance tests. Subjects were chosen at random from patients sent to the general laboratory for glucose tolerance tests and from known diabetic and apparently nondiabetic patients on the wards of the Veterans Administration Hospital, Bronx, N.Y. Patients who had *ever* been treated with insulin were excluded from this study in order to obviate effects of antibodies in their own serum (22). Other than the exception noted below, subjects were classified as diabetic or nondiabetic on the basis of the following criteria applied to the 2-hour blood sugar curve following oral ingestion of 100 g of glucose: *diabetic* --a peak blood sugar concentration of 180 mg per

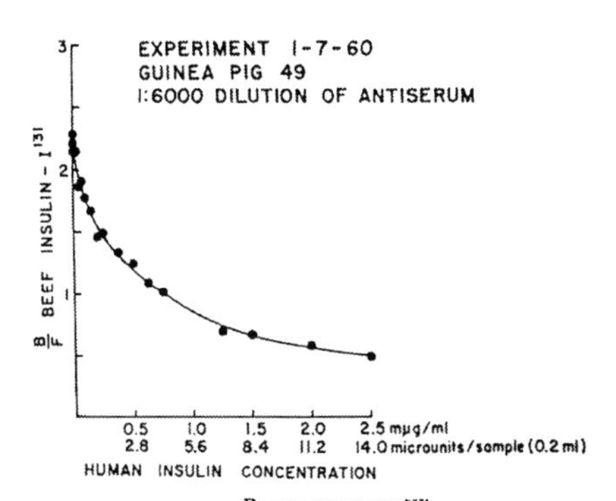

FIG. 2. B: RATIO, $\frac{\text{BOUND INSULIN-I}^{131}}{\text{FREE INSULIN-I}^{131}}$, AS A FUNCTION OF THE CONCENTRATION OF ADDED HUMAN INSULIN. The ratios were obtained from the complete series of radio-chromato-electrophoretograms, a few of which are shown in Figure 2A.

100 ml or greater; and a 2-hour blood sugar concentration of 120mg per 100 ml or greater; nondiabetic --a peak blood sugar concentration not exceeding 160 mg per 100 ml, and 2-hour level no more than 120 mg per 100 ml. One subject with marginal ulcer and a dumping syndrome, with a blood sugar concentration of 286 mg per 100 ml at 0.5 hour falling to 134 mg per 100 ml at 1 hour and 44 mg per 100 ml at 2 hours, is included in this group. Because of the exclusion of insulin-treated patients, only mild or early maturity-onset diabetes is represented in the diabetic group. Subjects who did not qualify by these criteria for either group are considered in an "*undetermined status.*" The criteria employed are modified from those suggested by Fajans and Conn (26) and are designed to eliminate questionable cases from diabetic and nondiabetic categories.

All subjects were to have fasted for 14 hours prior to the glucose tolerance test, but from the fasting blood sugar concentration in one subject (Ri) it is suspected that this restriction was not observed in his case. All subjects were to have consumed a diet containing at least 300 g carbohydrate per day for 3 days preceding the glucose tolerance test, but there is no assurance that this regimen was followed in all cases. Blood samples were obtained in the fasting state immediately before, and 0.5 hour, 1 hour and 2 hours following glucose feeding. In a small group of cases an additional 50 g glucose was administered at 1.5, 2 and 2.5 hours, and blood collections were continued to 3 hours.

Blood sugar determinations were determined according to the method of Somogyi (27).

RESULTS

Standard curves. Several representative standard curves are shown in Figure 3. The amount of insulin-I^{131}

[4] For this reason plasma is separated in a refrigerated centrifuge immediately after withdrawal of blood and is used immediately or kept frozen until used in order to minimize loss of the endogenous insulin present.

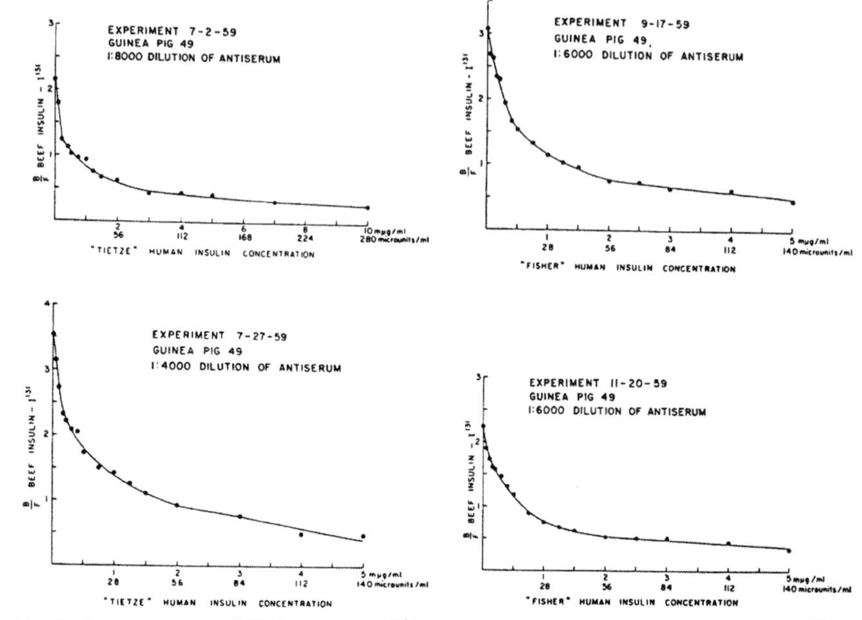

FIG. 3. STANDARD CURVES: B/F (BEEF INSULIN-I^{131}) RATIO AS A FUNCTION OF THE CONCENTRATION OF TIETZE OR FISHER HUMAN INSULIN.

employed as tracer varied somewhat from experiment to experiment. In the experiments shown in Figure 4, the effects of Tietze and Fisher insulins are compared with each other and with the effect of crystalline beef insulin. As in other experiments no significant differences between the two human insulin preparations were observed. Since 100 to 200 μl of solution was assayed, less than 1 μU of human insulin was readily detectable with this antiserum. At low insulin concentrations, random variations in B/F produce only small errors in the absolute quantity of insulin but the percentage error is high; conversely, at high insulin concentrations the absolute error is likely to be higher but the percentage error lower. By increasing the dilution of the antiserum, the entire concentration range is easily scaled down by a factor of 2 or 3 and the limit of sensitivity increased to about 0.1 to 0.2 μU of insulin. However, the conditions employed are suitable for determination over the 50- to 100-fold range of insulin concentrations ordinarily encountered in man.

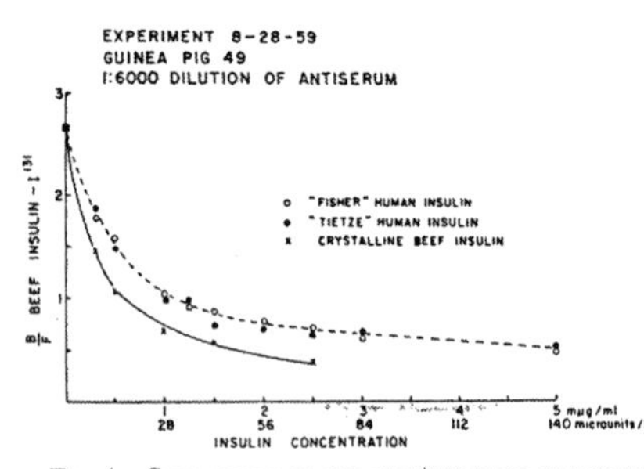

FIG. 4. COMPARISON OF THE EFFECTIVENESS OF VARIOUS CONCENTRATIONS OF TIETZE AND FISHER HUMAN INSULINS AND CRYSTALLINE BEEF INSULIN IN REDUCING THE B/F RATIO FOR BEEF INSULIN-I^{131}.

It is evident that beef insulin reacts about two to four times more strongly (depending on the insulin concentration employed) with the guinea pig antibeef insulin serum than does human insulin (Figure 4). Other guinea pig antisera to beef insulin have shown even greater differences in reaction of beef insulin and human insulin. On this account *beef insulin cannot be used as a standard for the assay of human insulin in the guinea pig antibeef insulin system.* Because of the differences in reactivity of human and beef insulin, differences in the specific activity of the beef insulin-I^{131} preparations result in different initial B/F values and somewhat differently shaped curves even at the same dilution of

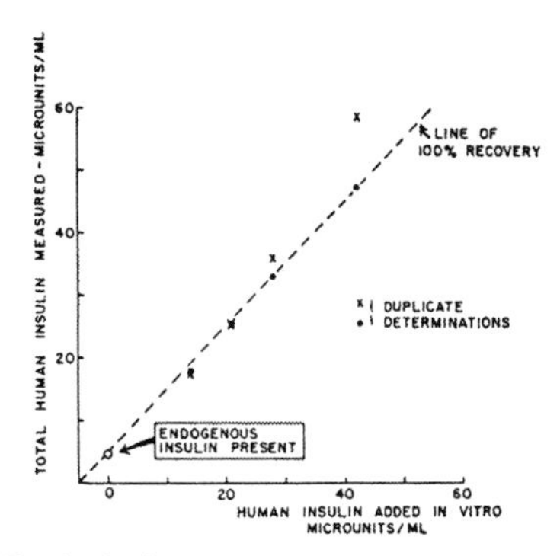

FIG. 5. A: RECOVERY OF HUMAN INSULIN ADDED *IN VITRO* TO A FASTING PLASMA SAMPLE. Endogenous insulin concentration in undiluted plasma was 48 μU per ml. All assays were performed in 1:10 dilution of plasma.

TABLE I

*Effect of cysteine on endogenous plasma insulin**

Subj.	Plasma sample	Original plasma before incubation and dialysis	Control sample incubated and dialyzed without cysteine	Sample incubated with cysteine and dialyzed
		μU/ml	μU/ml	μU/ml
Yo.	1 hr	324	238	14
Un.	1 hr	337	216	0

(Insulin concentration spans the last three columns.)

* See text for conditions of experiments.

antiserum if approximately the same radioactivity (and therefore different amounts of beef insulin) is used. These differences could be abolished if each lot of beef insulin-I[131] were assayed for its beef insulin concentration and if the same amount of beef insulin were employed, independent of its content of radioactivity. However, it is more expedient to include a standard curve with human insulin for each run of unknowns. When 250 or more unknown samples have been run in a single experiment, an added set of 15 to 16 standard solutions is a negligible addition.

Recovery of added human insulin and effect of plasma dilution. The virtually quantitative recovery of human insulin added to plasma *in vitro* (Figure 5A) indicates that the plasma has neither an inhibitory nor an augmentative effect and this conclusion is confirmed by the proportionate decrease in measured insulin concentration when the plasma is diluted over a large range (Figure 5B).

Effect of cysteine and cellulose on endogenous plasma insulin. Since insulin is destroyed by incubation with cysteine at alkaline pH and is adsorbed by powdered cellulose, the effects of these agents on endogenous insulin were tested. Plasmas of relatively high insulin concentration were incubated at 37 degrees C with 0.02 M cysteine at pH 8 for 1.5 hours and then dialyzed against normal saline for 3 hours to remove the cysteine. Aliquots of the same serum samples were treated similarly except that cysteine was omitted. Although incubation and dialysis alone led to a 26 to 36 per cent loss in endogenous insulin concentration in the control samples, cysteine was almost completely effective in destroying the endogenous insulin (Table I). In simultaneous experiments insulin-I[131] was found to be virtually completely destroyed under these conditions as determined by paper chromato-electrophoresis.

To evaluate cellulose adsorption of endogenous insulin, a minute amount of tracer beef insulin-I[131], negligible compared to the amounts used in the immunoassay, was added to 0.1 or 0.2 ml plasma which was then passed

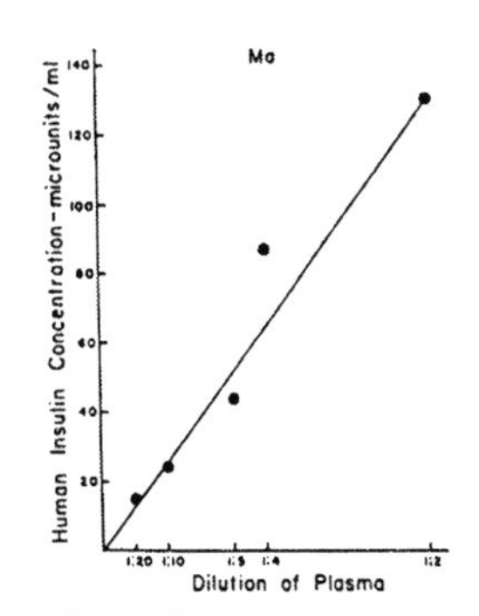

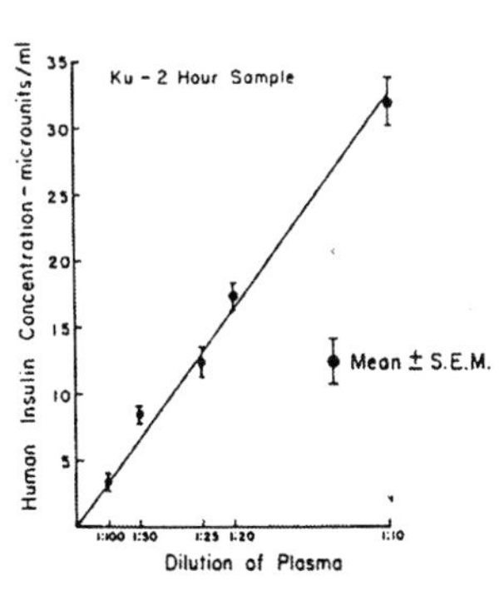

FIG. 5. B: EFFECT OF DILUTION OF PLASMA ON MEASURED CONCENTRATION OF ENDOGENOUS PLASMA INSULIN. Four replicate determinations were made for each point in the experiment on the right.

TABLE II

Cellulose adsorption of beef insulin-I^{131} and endogenous human plasma insulin

Subj.	Plasma	Per cent adsorbed by cellulose column: Beef insulin-I^{131}	Endogenous human insulin
	ml		
Y.	0.1	69	64
	0.2	49	44
U.	0.1	71	88
E.	0.1	81	84

though a packed powdered cellulose column (about 0.5 ml in volume) and eluted, by suction, with veronal buffer to recover all the plasma. Assay of the radioactivity remaining on the column and that eluted from the column, and immunoassay of endogenous insulin eluted from the column revealed that approximately the same fractions of endogenous insulin and added beef insulin-I^{131} were adsorbed by the cellulose (Table II). The larger the amount of plasma per unit volume of cellulose the less the fraction of insulin that was adsorbed. With significantly smaller amounts of plasma virtually all insulin-I^{131} and endogenous insulin are adsorbed, but the insulin concentrations then become unmeasurable. Only negligible fractions of albumin-I^{131} and γ–globulin-I^{131} are adsorbed by cellulose under these conditions.

Insulin concentration in early maturity-onset diabetic and control subjects. The average fasting insulin concentrations tended to be only slightly higher in the diabetic (mean, 27 μU per ml) than in the nondiabetic (mean, 21 μU per ml) subjects, although 34 per cent of the diabetics exceeded 40 μU per ml in contrast to only 10 per cent of the nondiabetics. In none of the 68 patients in both of these groups did the fasting level exceed 70 μU per ml (Table III, A and B, Figure 6). These values are in good agreement with those reported earlier in a smaller series of subjects (15). The responses to orally administered glucose in diabetic and nondiabetic patients differed more markedly than did the fasting insulin concentrations. Nondiabetic subjects were about equally divided in showing the peak insulin concentration at 0.5 hour or 1 hour (Table IIIA), whereas with few definite exceptions diabetic patients showed the maximal insulin concentration at 2 hours (Table IIIB). The average insulin concentration at 0.5 hour was lower in diabetic (mean, 97 μU per ml) than in nondiabetic (mean, 143 μU per ml) subjects, but the diabetics appeared to form two groups at this point (Figure 6). A delayed insulin response is suggestive in the lower of these two groups.

Although there is a large scatter of individual values, the mean curves for the two groups illustrate these differ-

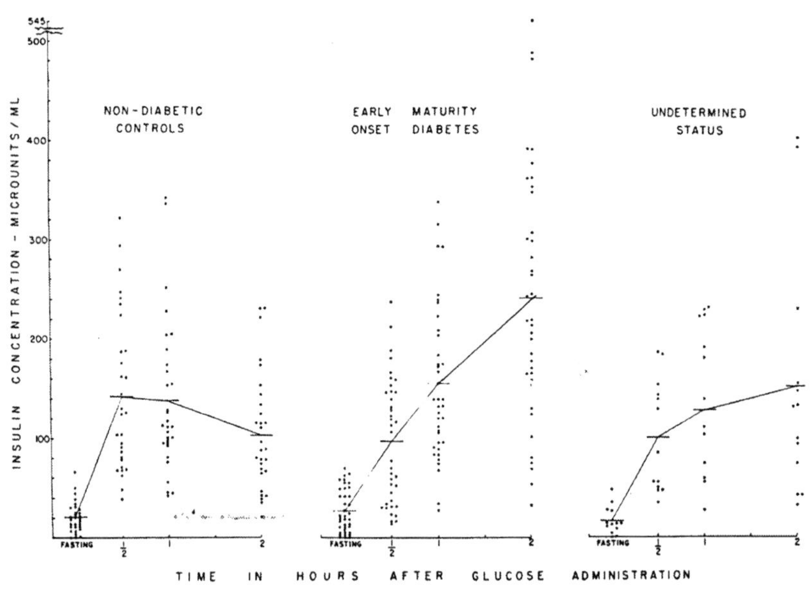

FIG. 6. PLASMA INSULIN CONCENTRATIONS DURING STANDARD 100 G (P.O.) GLUCOSE TOLERANCE TEST IN VARIOUS GROUPS OF SUBJECTS.

TABLE III

Blood sugar and plasma insulin concentrations during a standard 100 g oral glucose tolerance test

Subj.	Blood sugars						Plasma insulin concentrations					
	F	0.5 hr	1 hr	2 hrs	3 hrs	4 hrs	F	0.5 hr	1 hr	2 hrs	3 hrs	4 hrs
	mg/100 ml						*μU/ml*					
A. *Nondiabetic controls*												
La.	87	122	78	91			31	162	112	89		
Pa.	73	109	68	77			25	270	154	155		
Hu. J.	85	120	113	113			7	103	95	116		
Wh.	78	110	85	88			66	294	168	174		
Don.	88	108	135	115			45	67	98	39		
St.	89	120	104	93			13	95	46	43		
Kan.	83	113	103	83			28	62	229	117		
Ra.	91	131	135	90			20	176	128	112		
Jo.	92	113	113	80			25	124	118	21		
Wa.	98	128	147	118			20	68	93	75		
Dor.	90	140	148	118			31	81	126	90		
Ei.	83	100	70	95			50	235	101	79		
Cor.	110	133	133	115			21	130	155	145		
Cal.	91	117	147	119			7	39	76	47		
Te.	83	143	155	73			17	78	190	126		
Ru.	83	103	113	98			3	145	204	222		
Dam.	90	118	120	110			18	187	205	180		
Kas.	98	150	135	108			11	48	112	65		
Kr.	98	115	125	120			2	71	95	117		
Him.	93	140	120	108			22	322	252	232		
Hu. J. J.	95	128	110	105			9	126	56			
Dan.	83	115	73	100			0	224	18	98		
Sc.	83	158	140	113			22	91	114	135		
Un.	88	133	153	115			0	247	337	233		
Ke.	103	138	128	112			34	163	174	67		
Hig.	100	148	88	120			14	241	42	70		
Con.	90	133	135	115			11	104	45	36		
Pop.	93	148	143	95			39	67	101	79		
Ry.	90	143	150	110			11	84	107	81		
Al.	96	296	134	44			14	188	342	42		
						Mean	21	143	139	106		
B. *Early maturity-onset diabetes*												
Ri.	245	346	436	472			51	123	173	179		
Wa. D.	96	178	218	150			6	32	97	166		
Mor.	93	110	180	218			3	77	158	300		
Moh.	95	145	193	135			59	162	339	355		
Ko.	93	240	360	120			3	14	294	364		
Fl.	138	173	248	266			56	70	190	270		
Fel.	100	152	190	141			19	107	121	102		
Fr.	113	238	310	195			35	113	316	378		
Sh.	118	232	300	190			13	38	175	76		
Go.	100	146	218	173			22	54	156	216		
Bl.	114	168	236	223			19	59	108	221		
Ma.	163	240	256	320			51	46	35	54		
We.	96	178	218	150			6	32	97	166		
Qu.	93	155	180	178			56	120	121	283		
Ok.	143	202	244	204			11	24	79	160		
Ha.	110	155	193	200			50	154	185	482		
Cr.	92	200	245	225			0	31	75	70		
Mi.	105	180	211	170			25	117	112	187		
Ro.	113	177	233	240			0	182	224	266		
Wo.	100	163	170	180			42	160	168	207		
Poi.	103	188	243	190			5	17	83	173		
Fo. F.	152	244	266	380			11	22	28	23		
No.	105	195	215	185	91	83	59	190	238	392	159	59
Ny.	93	158	193	138	60		11	53	90	154	17	
Moo.	113	153	205	268			63	148	91	131		
Fo. J.	90	169	193	185	83		34	238	249	490	173	
Br.	90	167	198	163	86	67	20	62	133	201	79	29
Pl.	100	183	193	160	63		42	168	241	308	191	
Mu.	130	233	326	374			3	17	68	126		
Fla.	93	140	170	178			22	140	126	220		

TABLE III—*Continued*

Subj.	Blood sugars F	0.5 hr	1 hr	2 hrs	3 hrs	4 hrs	Plasma insulin concentrations F	0.5 hr	1 hr	2 hrs	3 hrs	4 hrs
	mg/100 ml						*μU/ml*					
B. *Early maturity-onset diabetes*—Continued												
Car.	108	165	238	183	90		42	34	106	247	106	
How.	125	198	223	250			14	132	140	245		
Coo.	95	145	163	178	128		28	213	205	350	233	
Fele.	100	193	266	235			0	31	84	81		
Le.	90	173	250	193			65	65	294	392		
Ga.	105	148	178	135			70	148	210	302		
Hor.	95	165	147	195	211		8	148	140	364	386	
Eh.	91	156	211	309	246		17	129	176	545	531	
						Mean	27	97	156	243		
C. *Undetermined status*												
Wa. D.	85	100	150	148			0	35	56	42		
Wr.	98	123	158	138			27	86	75	75		
Ric.	100	138	158	143			13	140	226	100		
Ba.	88	140	150	129			14	144	230	405		
Har.	88	148	178	140			36	187	232	134		
Hew.	83	145	163	105			4	56	64	94		
Jos.	95	147	171	136			49	130	192	157		
Leh.	100	152	162	145			14	186	224	395		
Wis.	103	150	158	128			0	155	182	148		
Doh.	70	110	155	128			8	48	28	33		
Lut.	100	118	160	130			28	51	112	132		
Sa.	100	170	143	110			11	48	140	42		
Wi.	90	123	164	118			14	56	104	233		
						Mean	17	101	128	153		
D. *Decompensated cirrhosis*												
Man.	96	164	146	136			54	240	356	486		
Mar.	92	168	150	100			8	140	226	143		
Cara.	95	143	140	93			14	40	57	30		
Cro.	85	143	118	85			2	16	14	8		
Di.	78	100	82	65			25	33	19	5		
Fo.	80	135	100	80			5	36	22	8		
E. *Pituitary tumors*												
Sil.*	92	122	147	134			32	350	570	175		
Sin.†	90	135	140	117			5	177	192	180		
Led. (Acromegaly)	93	163	174	103			8	156	203	109		
F. *Thyrotoxicosis*												
El.	103	215	240	210			38	275	230	240		
Yo.	93	170	184	103			65	247	324	81		
G. *Others*												
Ku. (Hemochromatosis)	73	135	175	160			48	121	321	330		
Cra. (Acute pancreatitis)	100	120	138	125			5	20	100	135		
Bl.‡	48	108	148	135			28	90	56	67		
Coh.§	36	52	78	76			118	190	199	98		

* Chromophobe adenoma.
† Eosinophilic and chromophobe adenoma with acromegaly.
‡ Hypoglycemia, cause undetermined, after partial pancreatectomy.
§ Proven islet cell adenoma (courtesy of Dr. H. Epstein).

ences clearly (Figure 6). The average integrated insulin concentration during the 2 hour glucose tolerance test was 26 per cent higher for the diabetic (147 μU per ml) than for the nondiabetic (117 μU per ml) group. The "undetermined" group (Table IIIC) probably represents a mixture of early diabetic and nondiabetic subjects and nothing can be concluded definitely about the variable insulin response to glucose loading.

Insulin concentrations in four diabetic and five nondiabetic subjects given an additional 50 g of glucose at half hour intervals from 1.5 to 2.5 hours are shown in Figure 7 and Table IV. Insulin concentrations rose to higher levels in both groups but more marked increases were observed in the diabetic subjects.

It should be emphasized that insulin-I[131] when administered intravenously exhibits a rapid fall in concentration due to a marked and continuous increase in its apparent volume of distribution for a period of about 30 to 60 minutes and to a metabolic turnover rate with a half-time of about 35 minutes (22). It may be reasonably expected that endogenously secreted insulin behaves similarly[5], and therefore that any particular peak concentration depends on the precise moment of sampling. A very rapid and pronounced fall from the peak concentration would be anticipated in the case of a single secretory spurt. Conversely, a sustained elevation or continued rise in insulin concentration implies a continued secretion during the time interval under observation.

Insulin concentrations in patients with islet cell tumors or leucine-induced hypoglycemia. Insulin concentrations in fasting plasmas from five of seven patients[6] with proven islet cell tumors were elevated above normal levels (Figure 8), but the response to glucose was normal in the one patient studied during a glucose tolerance test (Coh., Table IIIG).

Four of six subjects[7] with leucine-induced hypoglycemia showed increased insulin concentrations following administration of L-leucine (75 to 150 mg per kg) in six of nine experiments (Figure 9), although fasting insulin concentrations were elevated in only a single patient (Figure 8), the only adult in the series and the one patient suspected on clinical grounds to have an islet cell tumor[8]. The peaks of insulin concentration, when observed, were in good time correspondence with the induced hypoglycemia.

Plasma insulin in cirrhosis, acromegaly and hyperthyroidism. Six patients with decompensated cirrhosis were

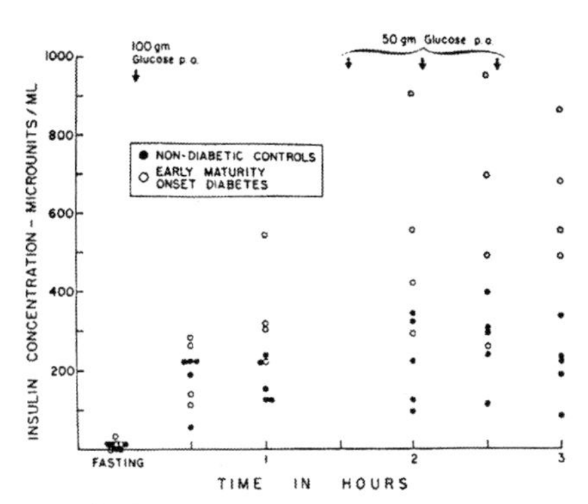

FIG. 7. PLASMA INSULIN CONCENTRATIONS DURING HEAVY GLUCOSE LOADING EXPERIMENTS IN DIABETIC AND NONDIABETIC SUBJECTS.

studied (Table IIID). In two cases the glucose curves were high, but not within the diabetic range, and were associated with relatively high insulin concentrations. In three cases insulin concentrations were very low throughout the 2 hour glucose tolerance test, and in two of these the glucose concentration curves were quite flat. Intravenous glucose tolerance tests are necessary before it can be decided whether the observed association in the latter cases is to be attributed to poor glucose absorption or to heightened insulin sensitivity.

In three patients with pituitary tumors, two of whom had clinical acromegaly, and in two thyrotoxic subjects, insulin concentrations during the glucose tolerance test were

[5] Endogenously secreted insulin is, in addition, subject to removal by the liver before it reaches the peripheral circulation (28, 29).

TABLE IV

Effect of heavy glucose loading on blood sugars and plasma insulin levels*

Subj.	Blood sugars F	0.5 hr	1 hr	2 hrs	2.5 hrs	3 hrs	Plasma insulin concentrations F	0.5 hr	1 hr	2 hrs	2.5 hrs	3 hrs
	mg/100 ml						µU/ml					
Nondiabetic controls												
Hea.	84	136	106	130	108	110	3	190	129	345	308	190
Gas.	78	118	86	108	104	98	14	224	129	322	300	341
Rei.	90	127	129	105	103	101	15	224	224	125	400	225
Keh.	94	158	142	98	90	86	0	224	238	224	241	235
McC.	100	144	150	104	102	90	17	56	151	98	118	84
Maturity-onset diabetes												
Cri.	100	188	214	208	188	162	17	265	548	910	960	685
All.	86	140	152	166	126	122	12	284	223	560	496	496
Ab.	90	143	170	167	177	155	31	112	309	420	700	870
Ti.	86	170	181	155	149	145	3	140	313	294	255	578

* Glucose 100 g p.o., immediately after fasting specimen; glucose, 50 g p. o., at 1.5, 2 and 2.5 hours.

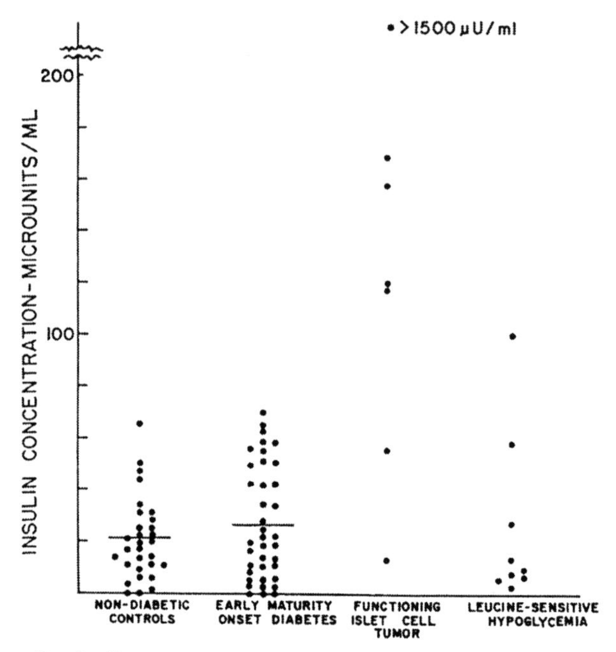

FIG. 8. FASTING PLASMA INSULIN CONCENTRATIONS IN VARIOUS GROUPS OF SUBJECTS. The subject with plasma insulin concentration greater than 1,500 μU per ml had an islet cell adenocarcinoma with widespread metastases (patient of Dr. J. Field).

in the high normal range (Table III, E and F).

Results in a few individual cases that do not fall into the other categories are also included in Table IIIG.

In the absence of glucose loading, plasma insulin concentrations did not change significantly in two control subjects (Fra. and Gre., Table V).

In seven cases, sera were refrozen and repeat determinations were performed one or more months later with a different lot of insulin-I^{131}. The reproducibility of determinations performed under these conditions is shown in Figure 10.

DISCUSSION

The demonstration that unlabeled insulin could displace insulin-I^{131} from complexes with insulin-binding antibody (22) and that the fraction of insulin-I^{131} bound to antibody decreases progressively with increase in insulin concentration (22) laid the foundation for the immunoassay of insulin employing isotopically labeled insulin. In initial reports describing results with the present method for immunoassay of beef insulin (9,10) it was emphasized that species differences in the reaction of insulin with insulin antisera exist and that human antibeef, pork insulin serum is useful for microassay of animal insulins (10). However, the human antisera react too weakly with human insulin (7,8,11) to serve as a basis for assay of the latter hormone in plasma. Fortunately, however, the serum of guinea pigs immunized with beef insulin was reported to react sufficiently strongly with human insulin for purposes of assay (11,14) and this finding has recently been confirmed by Grodsky and Forsham (30). The latter workers have employed a salt fractionation technique that produces a partial separation of antibody-bound insulin-I^{131} from free insulin-I^{131} and have measured insulin concentrations in extracts of plasma. However, since, in the assays of Grodsky and Forsham, human insulin was assumed to react

[6] We are indebted to Doctors H. Epstein, J. Field, E. D. Furth, E. Gordon, A. Renold, and J. Steinke for these sera.

[7] We are indebted to Doctors A. DiGeroge, M. Goldner, M. Grumbach, I Rosenthal and S. Weisenfeld for these sera.

[8] Courtesy of Doctors S. Weisenfeld and M. Goldner.

quantitatively like beef insulin, which is not valid for guinea pig antibeef insulin serum, their absolute values for human plasma insulin concentrations are questionable. Furthermore, since the *relative* degree to which human insulin and beef insulin react at different insulin concentrations varies several-fold, even relative values obtained with beef insulin as a standard are subject to large errors. Grodsky and Forsham (30) were unable to detect insulin in most fasting plasmas and reported mean values of 31 μU per ml after glucose loading in five patients. These values are very much smaller than those reported earlier by us (14) or those of the much larger series presented here. However, a significant underestimate of human insulin concentration is precisely the anticipated consequence of the invalid assumption of equal reactivity of beef and human insulins in the guinea pig antibeef insulin system.

TABLE V

*Blood sugar and plasma insulin concentrations in the absence of glucose loading**

Nondiabetic controls	Time	Blood sugar	Plasma insulin concentrations
	min	*mg/100 ml*	*μU/ml*
Gre.	0	93	17
	20	90	19
	40	90	18
	60	88	18
	120	78	25
Fra.	0	85	3
	20	85	5
	40	80	5
	60	85	3
	120	88	3

* Subjects were fasted overnight and throughout the period of blood sampling.

To our knowledge there have been only two other immunologic methods employed for the assay of insulin. Arquilla and Stavitsky (31) developed an assay for insulin based on the inhibition of hemolysis of insulin-sensitized red blood cells; however, the lower limit of detectability by this technique was approximately 0.1 μg (2.8 mU) making it unsuitable for determination of plasma insulin. Loveless (32) has used certain normal human subjects, in whom the skin can be locally sensitized to insulin (by the intracutaneous injection of human anti-insulin serum) to assay insulin by the whealing response obtained. Aside from the inconvenience associated with this method, the lower limit of detectability was 200 μU beef insulin per ml and human plasma insulin was not detectable, a result attributed in part to the lesser reactivity of human insulin (32).

Reported estimates of plasma insulin concentrations, derived from the various biological assay procedures, have varied widely. Thus, the *in vitro* diaphragm assay has

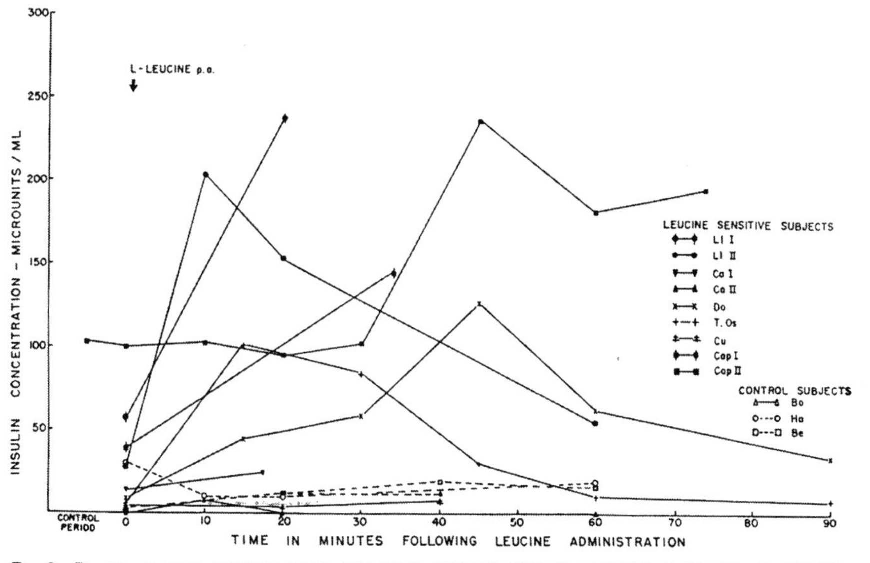

FIG. 9. PLASMA INSULIN CONCENTRATIONS FOLLOWING ADMINISTRATION OF L-LEUCINE TO CONTROL AND LEUCINE-SENSITIVE HYPOGLYCEMIC SUBJECTS.

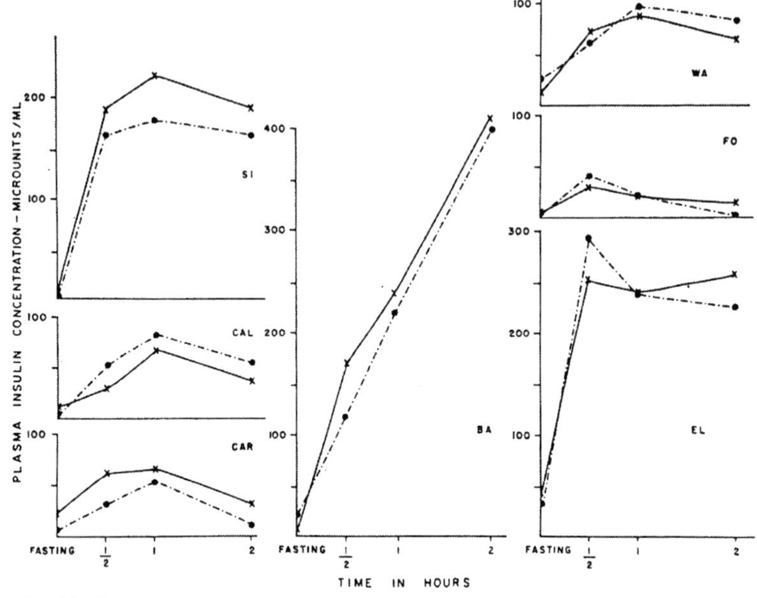

FIG. 10. REPRODUCIBILITY OF PLASMA INSULIN DETERMINATIONS ON THE SAME PLASMA SAMPLES PERFORMED ONE OR MORE MONTHS APART WITH DIFFERENT LOTS OF INSULIN-I^{131}. Plasmas were stored frozen between determinations. In these cases, the average values of the two determinations are presented in Table III.

yielded values ranging from 40 to 80 μU per ml (33) to as high as 4,600 μU per ml (34) in fasting plasmas and from about 130 to 800 μU per ml (33) to 9,000 to 22,000 μU per ml (35) after glucose in normal subjects. Measuring the increase in oxidation of glucose by rat epididymal adipose tissue *in vitro*, Martin, Renold and Dagenais (3) found that the insulin-like activity of fasting normal plasma in this preparation corresponded to 50 to 350 μU of insulin per ml. Pfeiffer, Pfeiffer, Ditschuneit and Ahn (36), using the same assay, found that plasma diluted 1:2 gave higher and more consistent insulin concentrations and reported normal fasting levels of 135 to 680 μU per ml in 15 normal human subjects, with concentrations frequently exceeding 2,000 to 4,000 μU per ml after tolbutamide and metahexamide. Employing the immunoassay method we have observed generally much smaller increases in peripheral insulin concentration after large doses of sodium tolbutamide, administered intravenously or by mouth, than after glucose given by the same routes to normal or diabetic men (37).

It is generally agreed (5, 34) that dilution of plasma or serum increases markedly the estimated insulin concentration in the diaphragm assay and similar observations have been made in the rat epididymal fat pad assay (36). This phenomenon has been either attributed to the presence of inhibitory substances in the plasma (5, 34) or interpreted as indicating that insulin-like activity of serum as measured by the isolated rat diaphragm is not specific for insulin per se. Randle has found that albumin and other proteins may exert a non-specific stimulation of glucose uptake by rat diaphragm (5) and that 1 ml of plasma exhibiting an insulin concentration of 13,000 μU per ml in the diaphragm assay had no effect on blood sugar when injected into alloxan-diabetic hypophysectomized rats, whereas 2,000 μU insulin produced a marked hypoglycemia (35).

The recent report by Leonards (6), that insulin-like activity in plasma, when tested on the rat epididymal fat pad, persists after total pancreatectomy and that insulin-neutralizing antiserum from guinea pigs has no inhibitory effect on the insulin-like activity of human serum in this system, has raised a serious question as to what part of the insulin-like effect on fat tissue is due to insulin itself.

In vivo insulin assays have also yielded variable estimates of plasma insulin concentration. Measuring the fall in blood sugar induced in adrenodemedullated alloxan-diabetic hypophysectomized rats, Anderson, Lindner and Sutton (38) were unable to detect circulating insulin in fasting plasma although the method was sensitive to 125 μU insulin. Bornstein and Lawrence (1) using adrenalectomized hypophysectomized diabetic rats reported plasma insulin concentrations 2 hours after glucose to average about 340 μU per ml in normal subjects and 100 to 320 μU per ml in diabetic patients not subject to ketosis, but Randle (5) was unable to confirm the suitability of these animals for insulin assay. More recently, Baird and Bornstein (39), employing adrenalectomized alloxan-diabetic mice, have found that normal fasting plasma extracted with acid ethanol-*n*-butanol-toluene (which is thought to separate insulin from insulin antagonists) contains about 1,000 μU per ml. Values about three times as high were observed after glucose feeding. Values as high or higher were found in four of six diabetic subjects.

At the present time it does not appear possible to resolve all the apparently divergent findings summarized here. It is necessary, however, to point out that plasma insulin concentrations determined by the immunoassay technique are in agreement with the lowest estimates derived from other methods of assay, notably the *in vivo* bioassays of Bornstein and Lawrence (1), and of Anderson and co-workers (38), and the diaphragm assay of Vallance-Owen and Hurlock (33). By comparison with the biological effects of exogenous insulin the lower concentrations appear most reasonable.

A rough estimate of the amount of insulin secreted can be derived from the insulin concentrations reported here according to the following considerations. From the area under the mean insulin curve in nondiabetic subjects it is found that the average insulin concentration during the 2 hour period following glucose administration was 117 μU per ml. It has been shown previously (22) that I^{131}-labeled insulin in man is metabolized at a rate of about 2 per cent per minute and is distributed into an apparent volume of distribution of about 37 per cent of body weight in about 45 minutes, distribution being about half completed at 15 minutes. If we now assume that the distribution and metabolism of endogenous insulin that reaches the peripheral circulation is similar quantitatively to that of exogenous insulin[9] and make the conservative estimate that, on the average, the endogenous insulin was distributed in a volume corresponding to 30 per cent of body weight (21 L) over the 2 hour period, we can calculate that 0.117 U per L x 21 L was being degraded at the rate of 2 per cent per minute during these 120 minutes. This computation leads to the estimate that approximately 6 U of insulin reached the peripheral circulation during the 2 hour glucose tolerance test. Madison, Combes, Unger and Kaplan (28) have found that approximately 50 per cent of insulin given into the portal vein is removed from the circulation during its first passage through the liver, and this value is in good agreement with the figure of 40 per cent given by Mortimore and Tietze in the rat (29). If we accept the 50 per cent value for the liver of man, it can be concluded that an average of about 12 U of insulin was secreted during the glucose tolerance test in nondiabetic subjects. This is what might be expected in each of three feedings per day. If, also, there is added into the calculation (on the same basis) the amount of insulin necessary to maintain a fasting level of 0.021 U per L for the other 18 hours, we arrive at the estimate of 36 U (postprandial secretion) plus 19 U (fasting secretion) = 55 U for the average total insulin secretion per day in nondiabetic subjects[10]. Since, even at the end of the 2 hour glucose tolerance test the insulin concentration was still above fasting levels, calculations over a more extended time period would yield even slightly higher estimates. These figures are certainly consistent with the insulin requirement of 30 to 40 U daily in totally depancreatized human subjects (40), since exogenously administered insulin does not experience the initial hepatic removal to which endogenously secreted insulin is subjected.

In order to resolve the much higher estimates of plasma insulin concentration given by Willebrands, van der Geld and Groen (34), Randle (35), and Pfeiffer and associates (36) with these considerations, we must assume either that the turnover rate of endogenous insulin is very much slower than that of exogenously administered insulin (in which event it is difficult to understand why human subjects do not remain in prolonged jeopardy of hypoglycemia from the high insulin concentrations that follow glucose administration) or that endogenous insulin is confined almost exclusively to the plasma. Even if the latter alternative (which also is in strong conflict with the results on distribution of exogenous insulin) were true, a fasting level as high as 4,600 μU per ml (34) would mean that there is almost 14 U of insulin in the circulation of fasting human subjects, a conclusion which is still difficult to accept. Randle's (35) values of 9,000 to 22,000 μU per ml in normal plasma 2.5 hours following glucose would mean a total of 27 to 66 U in plasma alone, neglecting insulin in extravascular space, at a time when the blood sugar is usually at a normal level. However, as already noted, Randle has indicated his conviction that this "insulin-like" activity is not due entirely to insulin alone (5).

To return now to the results of the present study, it will be noted that the high insulin concentrations observed in

[9] It has been established that exogenous unlabeled crystalline beef insulin and I^{131}-labeled crystalline beef insulin show virtually identical plasma disappearance curves in the rabbit (10). Furthermore, the precipitous fall in insulin concentration from peak levels, observed in many patients of the present study (Table IIIA), even when insulin secretion may be presumed to be continuing, is evidence that endogenous insulin also is rapidly removed from the circulation.

[10] These calculations ignore any increase in insulin secretion that would result from small feedings between meals.

diabetic subjects during the glucose tolerance test are not inconsistent with the less extensive data of Bornstein and Lawrence (1) and Baird and Bornstein (39). Very recently Seltzer and Smith (41), employing the rat diaphragm assay of Vallance-Owen and Hurlock (33), have reported insulin concentrations one hour after glucose, in tolbutamide-sensitive adult diabetics, almost in the normal range, but significantly lower values were observed in juvenile diabetics and adult tolbutamide insensitive diabetics. To resolve the present finding of a higher than normal integrated insulin output in diabetics during the glucose tolerance test with sustained hyperglycemia in these patients, it must be concluded that the tissues of the maturity-onset diabetic do not respond to his insulin as well as the tissues of the nondiabetic subject respond to his insulin. However, from these observations it cannot be concluded that the early diabetic has the same maximal potential insulin output as the nondiabetic, since in the latter the return of blood sugar to normal levels does not allow for the continued stimulus of prolonged hyperglycemia as in the diabetic. The attempt to produce a sustained stimulus to insulin secretion by repeated administration of glucose to a total of 250 g did result in a more marked insulin secretion in nondiabetic subjects. However, the response of diabetics was still greater indicating that their insulin reserve is not depleted during the 100 g glucose tolerance test. The experiment failed, however, to test maximal insulin secretory capacity of the nondiabetic subjects since a sustained hyperglycemia was not achieved in these patients.

Appreciation of the lack of responsiveness of blood sugar, in the face of apparently adequate amounts of insulin secreted by early maturity-onset diabetic subjects, is obviously of importance in the interpretation of the pathogenesis of this type of diabetes. However, the data at hand can only indicate that absolute insulin deficiency per se is not the cause of the hyperglycemia and suggest other possibilities that merit investigation, namely, 1) abnormal tissues with a high threshold for the action of insulin; 2) an abnormal insulin that acts poorly with respect to hormonal activity *in vivo* but reacts well immunologically *in vitro*; 3) an abnormally rapid inactivation of hormonally active sites [a suggestion in accord with the ideas expressed by Mirsky (42)] but not of immunologically active sites on the insulin molecules; and 4) the presence of insulin antagonists. The last suggestion has been made many times by previous workers. A joint attack on the problem, utilizing both the specific immunoassay for plasma insulin and an assay method that measures the net biological effect of insulin and its inhibitors would seem to be indicated.

The high fasting insulin concentrations observed in hypoglycemia associated with functioning islet cell tumors are not unexpected. However, the normal response to glucose in the one patient studied suggests that the insulin-producing tumor may be secreting insulin continuously or sporadically but that it is not stimulated specifically by hyperglycemia. The failure to detect high plasma concentrations of insulin in two cases can possibly be explained by the normally rapid turnover of insulin and the sampling at a time when insulin production by the tumor had been quiescent for an hour or two previously.

Leucine-induced hypoglycemia in children with idiopathic hypoglycemia was first reported by Cochrane, Payne, Simpkiss and Woolf (43) but a satisfactory interpretation of the disturbance has not been given. From the results of the present study it appears that leucine serves as an abnormal stimulus to insulin secretion in these subjects but may also have other effects. Most of the patients whose sera were assayed here have been studied in detail in other respects as well by the various investigators who supplied the sera and are to be reported by them individually.

SUMMARY AND CONCLUSION

1. An immunoassay for plasma insulin in man is presented, based on the reaction of human insulin, competing with beef insulin-I^{131}, with insulin-binding antibodies in the sera of guinea pigs immunized with beef insulin. The method is sensitive to less than 1 μU of insulin, permitting measurement of insulin concentrations in 10 to 20 μl of plasma.

2. Human insulin added *in vitro* to plasma is recovered quantitatively, and measured endogenous insulin concentrations decrease proportionately on dilution of plasma over the range 1:2 to 1:100.

3. Endogenous plasma insulin is destroyed by incubation with cysteine and endogenous insulin adsorption by cellulose columns is quantitatively similar to the adsorption of added beef insulin-I^{131}.

4. Repeat determinations of insulin concentrations on the same plasma samples (stored frozen in the interim) one or more months apart, with different lots of insulin-I^{131} were generally in good agreement.

5. Fasting plasma insulin concentrations in early maturity-onset diabetic patients who had never been treated with insulin, (mean, 27 μU per ml) and in nondiabetic subjects (mean, 21 μU per ml) did not differ markedly. Following 100 g of glucose by mouth, nondiabetic subjects usually showed peak insulin concentrations at 0.5 hour (mean, 143 μU per ml) or 1 hour (mean, 139 μU per ml) and a decline by 2 hours (mean, 106 μU per ml). In contrast, insulin concentrations in diabetic subjects showed a lesser increase at 0.5 hour (mean, 97 μU per ml) but continued to rise to a peak at 2 hours (mean, 243 μU per ml). The integrated average insulin concentration during the 2 hour glucose tolerance test was 26 per cent higher in diabetics (mean, 147 μU per ml) than in nondiabetics (mean, 117 μU per ml).

6. In a small series of patients subjected to additional glucose loading at 1.5, 2 and 2.5 hours, very high insulin concentrations were observed both groups, but levels in dia-

betic patients far exceeded those in nondiabetic subjects.

7. Fasting insulin concentrations were elevated in five of seven subjects with functioning islet cell adenomas but insulin secretory response to glucose was normal in the one patient studied.

8. Four of six subjects with leucine-sensitive hypoglycemia showed increased insulin concentrations following administration of leucine in six of nine experiments.

9. Insulin responses were generally in the high normal range in three patients with pituitary tumors (two associated with acromegaly) and in two patients with thyrotoxicosis.

10. Plasma insulin concentrations measured by immunoassay are compared with values obtained by other assay methods and found to yield the lowest estimates.

11. Calculation of the average normal daily insulin secretion rate, on the basis of the data presented, yields an estimate of about 55 U of insulin per day.

ACKNOWLEDGMENTS

We are indebted to the investigators mentioned, who sent us sera on the unusual cases reported here. We also wish to thank Mr. Manuel Villazon for technical assistance, Mr. Paul Newman for the charts, Mr. David Lubin, Mr. Glenn Harahan and Mr. Lawrence Steur for the figures, and Miss Eve Spelke and Mrs. Frieda Steiner for secretarial assistance. Finally, the cooperation of the Medical and Laboratory Services of the Bronx Veterans Administration Hospital is gratefully acknowledged.

REFERENCES

1. Bornstein, J., and Lawrence, R. D. Plasma insulin in human diabetes mellitus. Brit. med. J. 1951, 2, 1541.
2. Groen, J., Kamminga, C. E., Willebrands, A. F., and Blickman, J. R. Evidence for the presence of insulin in blood serum. A method for an approximate determination the insulin content of blood. J. clin. Invest. 1952, 31, 97.
3. Martin, D. B., Renold, A. E., and Dagenais, Y. M. An assay for insulin-like activity using rat adipose tissue. Lancet 1958, 2, 76.
4. Baird, C. W., and Bornstein, J. Plasma-insulin and insulin resistance. Lancet 1957, 1, 1111.
5. Randle, P. J. Insulin in blood. Ciba Found. Coll. Endocr. 1957, vol. XI, p. 115.
6. Leonards, J. R. Insulin-like activity of blood. What it is. Fed. Proc. 1959, 18, 272.
7. Berson, S. A., and Yalow, R. S. Cross reactions of human anti-beef pork insulin with beef, pork, sheep, horse and human insulins. Fed. Proc. 1959, 18, 11.
8. Berson, S. A., and Yalow, R. S. Species-specificity of human anti-beef, pork insulin serum. J. clin. Invest. 1959, 38, 2017.
9. Berson, S. A. *In* Resume of Conference on Insulin Activity in Blood and Tissue Fluids, R. Levine and E. Anderson, Eds. Bethesda, Md. 1957, p. 7.
10. Berson, S. A., and Yalow, R. S. Isotopic tracers in the study of diabetes in Advances in Biological and Medical Physics, J. H. Lawrence and C. A. Tobias, Eds. New York, Academic Press Inc., 1958, vol. VI, p. 349.
11. Berson, S. A., and Yalow, R. S. Recent studies on insulin-binding antibodies. Ann. N. Y. Acad. Sci. 1959, 82, 338.
12. Berson, S. A., and Yalow, R. S. Immunoassay of insulin *in* Hormones in Human Plasma, H. N. Antoniades, Ed. Boston, Little, Brown & Co. In press.
13. Berson, S. A., and Yalow, R. S. Immunologic reactions to insulin *in* Diabetes, R. H. Williams, Ed. New York, Paul B. Hoeber, Inc. 1960, p. 272.
14. Yalow, R. S., and Berson, S. A. Assay of plasma insulin in human subjects by immunological methods. Nature (Lond.) 1959, 184, 1648.
15. Yalow, R. S., and Berson, S. A. Plasma insulin concentrations in non-diabetic and early diabetic subjects determined by a new sensitive immunoassay technique. Diabetes. In press.
16. Bauman, A., Rothschild, M. A., Yalow, R. S., and Berson, S. A. Distribution and metabolism of I^{131} labeled human serum albumin in congestive heart failure with and without proteinuria. J. clin. Invest. 1955, 34, 1359.
17. Pressman, D., and Eisen, H. N. The zone of localization of antibodies. V. An attempt to saturate antibody-binding sites in mouse kidney. J. Immunol. 1950, 64, 273.
18. Yalow, R. S., and Berson, S. A. Effect of x-rays on trace-labeled I^{131} -insulin and its relevance to biologic studies with I^{131} -labeled proteins. Radiology 1956, 66, 106.
19. Berson, S. A., and Yalow, R. S. Radiochemical and radiobiological alterations of I^{131} -labeled proteins in solution. Ann. N. Y. Acad. Sci. 1957, 70, 56.
20. Ferrebee, J. W., Johnson, B. B., Mithoefer, J. C., and Gardella, J. W. Insulin and adrenocorticotropin labeled with radio-iodine. Endocrinology 1951, 48, 277.
21. Newerly, K., and Berson, S. A. Lack of specificity of insulin binding by isolated rat diaphragm. Proc. Soc. exp. Biol. (N. Y.) 1957, 94, 751.
22. Berson, S. A., Yalow, R. S., Bauman, A., Rothschild, M. A., and Newerly, K. Insulin-I^{131} metabolism in human subjects: Demonstration of insulin binding globulin in the circulation of insulin-treated subjects. J. clin. Invest. 1956, 35, 170.
23. Berson, S. A., and Yalow, R. S. Quantitative aspects of the reaction between insulin and insulin-binding antibody: Relation to problem of insulin resistance. J. clin. Invest. 1959, 38, 1996.
24. Field, J. B., Tietze, F., and Stetten, D., Jr. Further char-

acterization of an insulin antagonist in the serum of patients in diabetic acidosis. J. clin. Invest. 1957, 36, 1588.
25. Fisher, A. M. Personal communication.
26. Fajans, S. S., and Conn, J. W. The early recognition of diabetes mellitus. Ann. N. Y. Acad. Sci. 1959, 82, 208.
27. Somogyi, M. Determination of blood sugar. J. biol. Chem. 1945, 160, 69.
28. Madison, L. L., Combes, B., Unger, R. H., and Kaplan, N. The relationship between the mechanism of action of the sulfonylureas and the secretion of insulin into the portal circulation. Ann. N. Y. Acad. Sci. 1959, 74, 548.
29. Mortimore, G. E., and Tietze, F. Studies on the mechanism of capture and degradation of insulin-I^{131} by the cyclically perfused rat liver. Ann. N. Y. Acad. Sci. 1959, 82, 329.
30. Grodsky, G., and Forsham, P. An immunochemical assay of total extractable insulin in man. J. clin. Invest. 1960, 39, 000.
31. Arquilla, E. R., and Stavitsky, A. B. The production and identification of antibodies to insulin and their use in assaying insulin. J. clin. Invest. 1956, 35, 458.
32. Loveless, M. H. A means of estimating circulating insulin in man. Quart. Rev. Allergy 1956, 10, 374.
33. Vallance-Owen, J., and Hurlock, B. Estimation of plasma-insulin by the rat diaphragm method. Lancet 1954, 1, 68.
34. Willebrands, A. F., v. d. Geld, H., and Groen, J. Determination of serum insulin using the isolated rat diaphragm. The effect of serum dilution. Diabetes 1958, 7, 119.
35. Randle, P. J. Assay of plasma insulin activity by the rat-diaphragm method. Brit. med. J. 1954, 1, 1237.
36. Pfeiffer, E. F., Pfeiffer, M., Ditschuneit, H., and Ahn, C. Clinical and experimental studies of insulin secretion following tolbutamide and metahexamide administration. Ann. N. Y. Acad. Sci. 1959, 82, 479.
37. Yalow, R. S., Black, H., Villazon, M., and Berson, S. A. Comparison of plasma insulin levels following administration of tolbutamide and glucose. Diabetes. In press.
38. Anderson, E., Lindner, E., and Sutton, V. A sensitive method for the assay of insulin in blood. Amer. J. Physiol. 1947, 149, 350.
39. Baird, C. W., and Bornstein, J. Assay of insulin-like activity in the plasma of normal and diabetic human subjects. J. Endocr. 1959, 19, 74.
40. Goldner, M. G., and Clark, D. E. The insulin requirement of man after total pancreatectomy. J. clin. Endocr. 1944, 4, 194.
41. Seltzer, H. S., and Smith, W. L. Plasma insulin activity after glucose. An index of insulogenic reserve in normal and diabetic man. Diabetes 1959, 8, 417.
42. Mirsky, I. A. The etiology of diabetes mellitus in man. Recent Progr. Hormone Res. 1952, 7, 437.
43. Cochrane, W. A., Payne, W. W., Simpkiss, M. J., and Woold, L. I. Familial hypoglycemia precipitated by amino acids. J. clin. Invest. 1956, 35, 411.

CLASSICS IN OBESITY

HEREDITARY ADIPOSITY IN MICE

C. H. Danforth,
Department of Anatomy, Stanford University

BREEDERS have occasionally noted a tendency to adiposity in yellow mice, but thus far no one seems to have given much attention to this trait. Hereditary adiposity is of importance, however, not only for the geneticist, but for the bio-chemist, since mice with this characteristic are probably the only mammals known at present which, in the same cage with littermate controls, can be depended upon to develop an excess of fat without the intervention of any operative procedure or special dietary regime. Adiposity is of further interest since it furnishes readily available material to illustrate the interaction of hereditary and environmental factors in the production of a hereditary trait. The present fragmentary report is intended to do little more than draw attention to this interesting character, upon which further work must be done.

The material studied has come from a stock obtained originally by mating a few yellow males to females of various colors. Some of the descendants in later generations were yellow, others were not. The yellow ones were characterized by a marked degree of obesity*, developed soon after maturity, which differentiated them clearly from other mice, whether related or not. While this trait appears in both sexes, it is more marked in females† which occasionally attain a weight three times as great as normal adults of other strains. More frequently yellow females are about twice as heavy as others. A few yellow and non-yellow representatives of both sexes are shown in Figure 7. These specimens were etherized, then photographed, and weighed immediately. In Figure 8 one yellow and one non-yellow individual of each sex has been laid open to show the immense amount of fat which is deposited around the viscera of the yellow mouse. The subcutaneous fat is equally excessive. There is possibly some increase in other tissues, but this point needs further study, as does the question of fat within the different organs.

Danforth CH. Hereditary adiposity in mice. *J Hered.* 1927;18:153-162.
Reprinted by permission of Oxford University Press, Walton Street, Oxford OX2 6DP, UK.
Special thanks to Judy Willis of the Pennington Information Center for help in acquiring this document.

The Relation of Adiposity to Yellow Color

Since this pronounced adiposity was first observed in mice which were yellow, the question naturally arose as to whether or not the condition is necessarily associated with that color and experiments were made to test this point.

The genetics of yellow in mice has been extensively studied by a number of investigators‡, and its relation to other colors is now fairly well known. Yellow has been found to be epistatic to all the other self colors. The gene for dominant spotting usually restricts it somewhat, the homozygous genes for recessive spotting restricts it considerably more, and a combination of both these genes nearly, but never (?) entirely, eliminates it from the pelage. Ordinary albinism completely suppresses it. Its expression is also modified by a number of other factors which have given rise to such designations as sooty, black-and-tan, cream, and orange. All studies thus far reported seem to indicate that the principal gene, usually designated as A^y, is the same throughout the series and acts as a lethal when homozygous. Consequently all yellow mice are heterozygous and produce some yellow and some non-yellow young irrespective of how they are mated. This enables one to readily obtain inbred yellow and non-yellow littermates after any desired number of brother and sister matings.

The first step in testing the heredity of obesity was

*Briefly reported by the writer in the *Anatomical Record*, vol. 29, p. 354. 1925.

†While the male is generally larger in the Muridae, this is not always the case, even in wild species, as exemplified by *Peromyseus polionolus* (Summer; *Journal of Mammalogy*, 7, p. 149. 1926).

‡Most of the important papers in English are scattered through the last eight or ten volumes of the *American Naturalist*, *Genetics*, and the *Journal of Genetics*.

to compare weights of yellow and non-yellow individuals from the same litter. If adiposity and yellow color were due to independent genes in different chromosomes, the non-yellow young should become fat as often as the yellows; but they do not. If there were a gene for adiposity and another for yellow, both located in the same chromosome, the ease of demonstrating the fact would depend on the closeness of linkage between the two genes. One might expect if such were the case, that there would be an occasional cross-over*, especially since A^y probably belongs to a series of allelomorphs, the other members of which do cross over. If such a crossing-over between A^y and a possibly distinct gene for adiposity were to occur, there should be some lean yellow mice and some fat ones of other colors. But there have been no persistently slender yellow mice in which all question of pathological involvement could be definitely eliminated; and while fat mice sometimes occur "spontaneously" in other strains (and can be produced by operative procedure), none of these have appeared among the non-yellow descendants of yellow ancestors. Although these statements are based on only about two hundred fully adult individuals, which is not enough to definitely eliminate the possibility of linked genes – if indeed such a possibility can ever be entirely eliminated – the presumption is strong that only one gene is involved, and until evidence is obtained to the contrary, it may be assumed that it is the A^y gene itself which is responsible for adiposity.

The several yellow mice which failed to develop obesity cannot be counted as evidence for the crossing-over of genes because instead of being of normal weight, as would have been expected if crossing-over had occurred, these specimens were exceedingly thin. Such mice can be paralleled by sickly individuals of other strains, and it is probably that their condition was due to one or another of the maladies to which mice are susceptible. Nevertheless it is just possible that their emaciated condition was due not so much to external factors as to some inherent lack of metabolic stability in mice with the A^y gene. This is a question which needs to be definitely answered. It may be mentioned in passing that thus far all the individuals kept under controlled conditions have run true to form; the few puzzling cases have been those with inadequate records.

A further test of the relation of the A^y gene to adiposity consisted in making a number of out-crosses designed to introduce A^y into several different genotypic combinations. In this series yellows of two or possibly three grades of intensity were secured, as well as sooty yellows, yellows with dominant spotting, with recessive spotting, with both types of spotting in the same individual, and, finally, various classes of albinos carrying the A^y gene. The results of these experiments have been briefly reported elsewhere.† Suffice it to say here that the appearance of adiposity followed very strictly the distribution of the A^y gene, irrespective of the particular combination into which it had entered. The results strongly support the conclusion that the A^y gene, in addition to being lethal when homozygous, and producing yellow hair (except in albinos) when heterozygous, also endows its possessor with a strong tendency to an excessive deposition of fat.

If it should subsequently transpire that the hereditary element which we now designate as A^y is in reality a complex of three units, one a recessive lethal, one a dominant color factor, and one a dominant gene for adiposity, it would not materially affect the situation. It would simply mean the introduction of two new terms, and the loss of a supposed example fo multiple effects from a single gene. Such an eventuality is not likely.

The Development of Adiposity

One can not present an adequate picture of such a trait as adiposity without considering it from the viewpoint of anatomy, bio-chemistry, and genetics, three sciences which must ultimately combine in a joint attack on some of the problems which they now attempt to solve independently. Here it is hoped only to indicate in a very general way how this hereditary trait manifests itself. It is not present at birth, nor does it often become apparent until after puberty. From then on its development is clearly indicated by the typical weight curves shown in Figures 9 and 10.

The derivation of data for constructing these curves may be outlined in some detail. In the first case (Figure 9) the experiment was begun by mating a yellow female to a yellow male. The female was then isolated and given what was presumed to be an adequate diet and favorable surroundings. She produced (Aug. 10, 1924), nine young of which five were males. The latter were immediately discarded. The four females which remained were given distinctive marks on ears and tails, weighed, and returned to the nest. Subsequent weighings were made at frequent, but gradually increasing intervals. Three of the group proved to be yellow, the other black. One of the former escaped and one was used in another experiment. The two remaining, one yellow and one black, were observed for a period of 600 days. During this time they were always kept in the

*Cf. papers on linkage in rats and mice by Dunn, (Genetics, vol. 5, p. 149. 1920) and the important work of Detleisen and Castle and their collaborators, appearing mostly in later numbers of the same journal.

†Proceedings of the Society of Experimental Biology and Medicine, vol. 24, p. 69. 1926.

same cage and never in their whole lifetime were so much as twenty inches apart except for a few minutes now and then when they were being weighed. They were supplied throughout with an abundance of such food as was given to other members of the colony (cracked corn, oats, dog biscuit, lettuce, salt, and occasionally a little butter). The mother was removed on the 33rd day and an unrelated male was kept in the cage from the 231st to the 250th, and from the 356th to the 390th days. Throughout the entire period every effort was made to keep the external conditions favorable and, so far as these two mice were concerned, absolutely identical. Nevertheless the two weight curves are quite different. At birth the black mouse weighed 1.440 grams, the yellow one 1.325 grams. On the fifth day the black one weighed 3.115, the yellow one, 3.020. By the tenth day the yellow one was .17 gram heavier, and by the twentieth day it supassed the black one by .98 gram. When a month old the yellow one weighed 16.40 grams, the black one only 14.04 grams. At two months they weighed 23.5 and 20.0 grams, respectively. From this point on the relative trend of their weight curves can be followed from the figure. At the end of 600 days the yellow mouse weighed 55 grams, the black one 32 grams. The fact that the black mouse produced three young as a result of the first mating and two as a result of the second, while the yellow one did not produce any, is the only known point of difference in their whole life histories. Whatever the reason for this difference, it is clear that the production or non-production of young in this case did not appreciably alter the trend of the two curves. Figure 11 shows these two mice when about a year and a half old.

The upper curve in Figure 9 might suggest that the yellow female was sterile, which was possibly the case. However, the question of sterility in the yellow mouse presents several interesting ramifications which cannot be followed up at this time. As a rule yellow females probably produce fewer litters than do representatives of some other strians, and they also cease to reproduce at an earlier age. This may be due in part to purely mechanical effects of the fat. On the other hand, when they do have young, they usually have large litters, nine to twelve being common, and they are excellent mothers, with an apparently abundant milk supply. Their capacity in the latter respect makes them desirable foster mothers for the young of less vigorous parents.

Two other curves of a similar sort are shown in Figure 10. In this case the father of the two subjects was a black mouse, heterozygous for recessive spotting, and the mother a yellow mouse which carried genes for both types of spotting. The subjects themselves came from a litter of seven females and four males. One was yellow and white, the other brown and white. They were mated three times, the yellow and white one producing two litters of eleven each, the brown and white one three litters of six, eight, and two (?) young. In other respects the conditions were identical with those in the previous experiment.

When seven days old the brown and white mouse weighed 4.860 grams while the yellow and white one weighed only 4.425 grams. Nevertheless, in view of previous observations it was possible to predict on the basis of developing hair color that the latter would ultimately be much the larger. Such a prediction was indeed made at the time.

The results of these two tests, which are consistent with others conducted at the same time and subsequently, indicate the relative degree of adiposity commonly attained by mice having the Ay gene as contrasted with their littermates which lack this gene. The experiments show clearly that with these animals it is neither the environment nor abundance of food that primarily determines the production of fat.

Adiposity and Albinism

It has already been pointed out that albinos carrying A^y become adipose as do other mice with this gene. This fact might need no special emphasis were it not that albinism is often taken very seriously by workers in other fields than genetics. Indeed the varietal name albinus is frequently applied to both rats and mice, and the worker is apt to feel that by use of this term he has adequately characterized his material. But, although albinism undoubtedly involves much more than the mere lack of color, the term is after all rather non-committal. With reference to the genes relating to color the word "albino" fixes only one point, that the individual is homozygous for *c*, whereas "black," for example, tells us that the animal has both *C* and *B*, but does not have *A*, A^y, etc. In regard to such other traits as anemia* and adiposity "albino" is equally uninforming. While this is no argument against the use of this term when there is nothing any more explicit, it does suggest that the experimenter should not too complacently classify all individuals as albinos and others.

In the present series the A^y gene has been carried in pure albino stock for several generations. Whenever it is desired to test for the presence of A^y it can be done very readily by mating the albino with a mouse of some color other than yellow. If any yellow young are produced it shows that the albino parent carries A^y Such tests can often be made when the A^y individuals and their litter mates are of about the same size and practi-

3. B. de Aberle: Hereditary anemia in mice and its relation to dominant spotting, American Naturalist, vol. 59, p. 327. 1925.

cally indistinguishable. Drawing his material from such a stock, an unsuspecting experimenter might easily be misled by the apparently divergent responses of two seemingly identical, litter-mate sisters. Thus two albinos of albino ancestry for several generations were kept together from birth, except for a few days while they were having young and raising them to an age when the color could be determined. One was shown to carry A^y, the other not. When this test was amde they were of about the same weight and of similar appearance, but four months later the one carrying A^y was more than twice as heavy as her sister. One may speculate as to what conclusions might have been drawn if these two apparently admirably suitable individuals had been used as subject and control in an experiment involving some special procedure! Characteristic poses of two such mice after their genetic differences have had a change to manifest themselves are shown in Figure 12. The hump on the neck, shown there, is characteristic of mice with the A^y gene.

Utilization of the Excess Fat

Since on an ordinary diet mice carrying the A^ygene lay down much more fat than do mice without this gene, it is of interest to know if the fat is of such a nature as to be available in time of need. A few experiments have been made to test this point. The procedure followed was simply to put animals whose histories were fully known on a deficient diet, either lettuce or rice. In Figure 13 are represented the curves for two litter-mate sisters (the same used for the curves in Figure 10), which were kept for four weeks on a diet that, except for one day, consisted of lettuce in abundance, but nothing else except water. It will be seen that on such a diet the weights begin to fall promptly and that the slope of the curve is steep. In this instance on the twenty-eighth day the control animal had become comatose and was killed. During this period the yellow mouse had dropped in weight from 73 grams to 24 grams, a loss of 67 per cent. It was then returned to a normal diet and made a good recovery. The maximum loss thus far, followed by complete recovery has been 69.2 per cent.

The curves in Figure 13 are reproduced in preference to smoother ones because they show the interesting effect of a return to the regular diet for one day (the fifteenth).

Autopsies on yellow mice kept for a considerable period on such a restricted diet show the abdominal fat-masses reduced to small pinkish strands, which are largely blood vessels and connective tissue. In a mouse which has shrunken to less than half its original weight the skin often presents a grotesquely baggy appearance.

The result of a similar experiment in which polished rice was used in place of lettuce is shown in Figure 14. The two mice in this case were not sisters. The control was two days younger, but both had been kept together in the same cage for over sixteen months. After 39 days on this diet the control had become weakened beyond recovery. On the 41st day the yellow one, having lost 67 per cent of its original weight, was returned to a mixed diet on which it made a good recovery. The form of curve for mice on a rice diet differs from that obtained when lettuce is used, but the experiments agree in the important point that in either case the A^y mice tend to outlast the others and can make a good recovery after most of their fat has been used up.

A great deal of work needs to be done along these lines before conclusions of much value can be drawn. From the data in hand it appears that the excess fat is stored in a manner to make it readily available in time of need. Whether it is of the same value, gram for gram, as the fat of ordinary mice remains to be determined.

General Nature of the Trait

A trait of this sort presents many points of interest. One may wonder if similar mutations may not have been an important step in the evolution of hibernating animals – the appearance of individuals who in time of plenty can store in their own tissues material that may be utilized as needed in time of want. On the other hand one may ask if these families of fat mice are not closely analogous to those human families in which pronounced obesity also occurs as an hereditary* trait? But speculation along these lines is quite useless except in so far as it serves to suggest concrete questions for which definite answers may be sought.

With adiposity, as with a multitude of other traits, the real question is to explain the relation between a germinal condition and a somatic one – in short, what is the relation between A^y genes in the nuclei and fat in the tissues? At present the whole quesiton is before us, but it may be expected that various phases of it will be solved from time to time and the field of attack gradually narrowed. It would seem probable that the deposition of fat in A^y mice is due to some functional peculiarity which in turn is dependent, through few or many intermediate steps, on the ultimate constitution of the germplasm. The best mode of attack may be the isolation and analysis of these steps one by one.

It is of interest in this connection that a number of ordinary mice with both ovaries removed have developed weight curves very similar to those of unoperated yellow females. This in conjunction with the fact that the yellow females are possibly less fertile than others, and also even more obese than yellow males, might sug-

---

*See Davenport: Body Build and Its Inheritance, Carnegie Institute of Washington 1923.

gest that the ovary forms one link in the chain. But until spayed controls and unoperated yellow females can be fully compared, any conclusion to this effect would be hazardous. It is possible that the ovary and other members of the endocrine system are more or less involved in the production of the excess fat and these may have to be studied as one of the steps in the series, but at the same time it is not at all improbable that back of these is a controlling nervous factor which may perhaps eminate from the real anatomical expression of the A^y gene.

That there are other genes than A^y which have a slight influence on adiposity, increasing the weight of non-yellow mice and acting cumulatively in the yellows is a bare possibility suggested by observations which can not be reported at this time. If there be such other genes, it remains to determine whether they, along with the much more potent A^y, exert their influence on some particular organ or function connected with fat metabolism or whether their presence in the nuclei of areolar tissue cells makes these cells more active in the taking up and storage of fat. Perhaps it will require the cooperation of students in several fields to answer these questions satisfactorily.

From a purely didactic point of view a trait of this sort may serve to illustrate rather interestingly the interrelation between hereditary and environmental factors. Thus, under ordinary circumstances a mouse which carries the A^y gene becomes heavier than one which does not, but, by varying the diet, conditions may be made such that the reverse will be the case; or, again, by spaying the non-A^y individual both may be made to develop similar weight curves in identical surroundings. Further, since the trait does not appear until after birth, it presents another peculiarity which persons inexperienced in genetics often find difficult to associate with the idea of heredity.

Conclusions

In concluding this general account of adiposity in mice the following points may be enumerated by way of summary:

1. A pronounced form of adiposity, more marked in females, develops in certain mice at or subsequent to maturity and behaves in heredity as if due to a single gene which acts as a lethal when homozygous.
2. This gene seems to be identical with the one responsible for yellow color (A^y).
3. Its effect on adiposity is not influenced by albinism or other factors modifying color.
4. On an ordinary diet mice with the A^y gene lay down fat to an extent greatly in excess of control animals on the same diet.
5. Practically all of this fat can be utilized under adverse dietary conditions.
6. There are possibly other minor hereditary factors which influence adiposity to a slight degree.

OBESE, A NEW MUTATION IN THE HOUSE MOUSE*

ANN M. INGALLS MARGARET M. DICKIE AND G. D. SNELL
Roscoe B. Jackson Memorial Laboratory, Bar Harbor, Maine

OBESITY, other than that occurring in yellow mice, is relatively rare in mice. The obese yellow animals attain weights up to 75 or 80 grams but the average weight is around 60 grams and then there is a decrease in weight as age increases.† In the summer of 1949 some very plump young mice were found in the V stock.‡ Others occurred shortly after that among offspring of these V stock animals that had been outcrossed to the fuzzy sock.

Description of Character

Obese animals are first recognizable about four to six weeks of age (Figure 4). At that time they appear to have a slightly shorter body, are rather square and have expansive hind quarters. From that time on, they increase in weight rapidly, so by three months of age they weigh about twice as much as their non-obese litter-mates. The weight of the obese continues to increase, though not as rapidly as it did up to three months of age. At the present time there are two animals ten months of age that weight 90 and 75 grams (Figure 5B). They are still gaining. Figure 5A is a graph of weights of two obese and their non-obese sibs from birth to four months of age. The graph in Figure 5B shows the comparison of obese, fat yellows and normal animals.

As yet, we do not know the life span of the obese, but none have died up to 12 months of age.

Breeding Data

Obese animals, themselves, are sterile. Data obtained on offspring of heterozygotes show that out of 212 animals, 43 were obese. This approximates the 3 to 1 ratio expected for a recessive gene, with a slight deficiency of obese. It is suggested that this gene be designated by the symbol *ob*.

Summary

A new mutation called obese and designated by the symbol *ob*, occurred in the V stock at this laboratory in the summer of 1949. Obese animals increase rapidly in weight until they are about four times the weight of normal animals. This recessive gene causes sterility in the homozygote, but as yet, there seems to be no indication of any affect on the life span of the animals.

Ingalls AM, Dickie MM, Snell GD. Obese, a new mutation in the house mouse. *J Hered.* 1950;41:317-318.
Reprinted by permission of Oxford University Press, Walton Street, Oxford OX2 6DP, UK.
Special thanks to Judy Willis of the Pennington Information Center for help in acquiring this document.

*This work has been aided by grants to the Roscoe B. Jackson Memorial Laboratory from the Commonwealth Fund, Anna Fuller Fund, Jane Coffin Childs Memorial Fund for Medical Research and the National Advisory Cancer Council.

†DICKIE, M. M., and G. W. Woolley. *Jour. Hered.* 37:365-368. 1946.

‡V stock of Jackson Laboratory mice (*Mus musculus*) carries genes *aa lnln ss wa 1-wa-1 vv*.

Fat Accretion and Growth in the Rat[1]

THEODORE F. ZUCKER AND LOIS M. ZUCKER
Laboratory of Comparative Pathology, Stow, Massachusetts

ABSTRACT The normal course of fat accretion in male rats from birth to 3 years is described. The relative amount of fat and relative size of fat pads increased steadily throughout life (except for a brief cessation in fat accretion at weaning), in a manner closely related to body weight and independent of age. Several new rat strains with extremes of growth or fat accretion, fed the same diet, were used to define and illustrate courses of fat accretion: very large and very small non-obese strains and a hereditarily obese rat. Rats of different known strains fed a variety of more refined diets show a course of fat growth different from that obtained with stock diets. Several types of obesity are discussed: insulin obesity, nutritional obesity, and hereditary obesity. Hereditary size and growth of the rat were readily (in a few generations) altered up or down, by consistently using the largest or the smallest 25% of the population for breeders. It is probable that the large increase in size of some laboratory rats over the past 40 years has been accomplished not only by improvement in stock diets and colony conditions, but also by selection for increased hereditary size.

This report deals with the body fat of the rat both under conditions that would be called "normal" and conditions that justify classification as obesity. Relatively few data on "normal" fat accretion are available. We will reproduce some of these for comparison with our data.

On the subject of obesity in laboratory animals the following should be considered. In mice Fenton (1,2) found that some strains become obese when fed high fat diets, while others do not. Mickelsen et al. (3) studied such nutritional obesity in rats and more recently found[2] indications that in this species also a genetic predisposition is a factor. Extreme obesity can be produced in rats, mice, monkeys and dogs by surgical interference with the intactness of the hypothalamus (4). In mice hypothalamic lesions with resulting obesity also follow injection of goldthioglucose (5,6). Continued injection of protamine insulin in rats and mice causes increased lipogenesis and fat accretion (7). In some species (mouse and man, but not rat) corticosteroids can lead to hyperinsulinism with resultant obesity (8). In every case it appears that obesity is made possible by an increased caloric intake.

Besides the above instances which depend on conditions imposed by the experimenter, there are also obesities related to a cause entirely within the animal. Four mutations in mice are known which lead to obesity. Two of these are due to single recessive genes – the gene *ob*, called obese (9), and the gene *ad*, called adipose, which is at a different locus from *ob* (10). The yellow obese mouse depends on the dominant gene A^y which is an allele of agouti (11). These 3 types of obesities with genetically different mechanisms presumably

Zucker TF, Zucker LM. Fat accretion and growth in the rat. *J Nutr.* 1963;80:6-19.

Received for publication December 17, 1962.
[1]This investigation was supported in part by research grants C-4241 and A-4085 from the National Institutes of Health.
[2]Personal communication from Dr. Mickelsen.
[3]We are greatly indebted to Dr. James Q. Miller of the Neuropathology Laboratory at the Children's Hospital Medical Center, Boston, for his study of the hypothalamic region in two old and one young fatty. He reported: "The brains were removed, after sacrificing the animals, fixed in formalin and embedded in celloidin. Serial step sections were stained with cresyl violet and hematoxylin and eosin. Fat rat brains and controls were examined and compared to one another. No evidence of degenerative, neoplastic, or infectious desease was found, and there were no anatomical defect identified in the region of the hypothalamus in any of the specimens."

also operate through physiologically different mechanisms. With regard to Bielschowsky's (12) NZO obese mouse the genetic situation has apparently not been worked out.

Recently we described an obese mutation in the rat (13,14) which is dependent on a single recessive gene *fa*, called fatty. It was found that this obesity is not caused by any hereditary lesion of the hypothalamus.[3]

We are concerned in this report principally with three questions:

(1) Is fat accretion related to age or body weight?

(2) Is there, under conditions which can be considered "normal" for the laboratory rat, a definable controlled path of fat accretion?

(3) Can a reasonable distinction be made between "normal" fat accretion and obesity?

The first question is of importance since in most extant studies fat accretion has been related to age. To decide the question it is necessary to have rats that differ largely in weight for a given age. Widdowson and McCance (15), using early (preweaning) food restriction, conceded that fat is related to weight, not age. As appears below, we have used animals of hereditarily different growth rats, thus avoiding any further imposed experimental conditions. The third question deserves consideration because old rats have frequently been considered obese with the implication of a pathological state associated with senility.

METHODS AND MATERIALS

Random-bred rats. Male rats from a random-bred colony of Sherman origin, with body weights from 5 g (newborn) to 500 g (about 6 months old), were used for the carcass analysis data of figures 1, 7 and 8, as well as the data reported in the following paper (16). For older ages these were supplemented by rats of Sprague-Dawley (SD) origin in groups aged 5 months, 2 and 3 years; they came from the colony of Dr. H.S. Simms, a colony which is maintained for studies in aging. These particular old animals had remained in good physical condition and had shown no weight losses.

Rats selectively bred for body size. Two long-time experiments were carried out by breeding heavy to heavy rats and light-weight to lightweight rats over many generations with avoidance of inbreeding. The heaviest (or lightes) 25% of the available rats in each generation were used for breeders, and changes were very apparent within a few generations. The first of these experiments was carried out with the above-mentioned Sherman rat stock. The earlier results of this experiment have been described in a progress report (17). Three sizes of strains resulted: the small 9B strain, the medium size 13C, and the large 14C. These strains are the subject of figure 3. The second size selection experiment was carried out on a foundation stock made up by crossing 4 known rat stocks: 13C mentioned above; an albino strain of Wistar origin given to us by Dr. Oser of the Food Research Laboratories; long-Evans hooded rats from the colony of Dr. P.E. Smith at Columbia University; and a black strain from the Merck Institute for Medical Research. The purpose of setting up such a foundation stock was to provide a larger gene pool. The foundation stock and selective breeding scheme have been described together with some experimental data (18,19). The 2 strains resulting from this experiment are designated 4StS (small) and 4StL (large). Photographs and growth curves for these rats are shown in figures 5 and 6, and data on fat in figure 4 and table 1.

Spontaneous mutation to hereditary obesity. In building up the foundation stock for the size-breeding experiment, the 13C and Merck stock M were crossed to give 13M. This was carried on as a random-bred strain to serve as a control. Within this strain a spontaneous mutation occurred which produced obesity, always recognizable by 5 weeks of age and increasing steadily thereafter. The recessive mutant gene is called *fa* (fatty), and obese rats are designated as 13M strain, *fafa* genotype (13,14). Figure 5 includes a photograph, figure 6 mean growth curves, and figure 10 and table 1 show data on fat in these rats.

Since the fatty condition is due to a single recessive gene, fatty rats (genotype *fafa*) and normal rats (*FaFa* or *Fafa*) regularly occur in the same litter. There is no intermediate condition: a rat is either a fatty or of normal appearance. This is quite different from the result of selective breeding for large and small size, where the size difference is due to the accumulation of appropriate genes at many loci (thought to be of the order of 10 to 100). It is possible to have a continuous gradation in individual rat size from very large to very small; the cross of a large and a small rat will give intermediate-size rats. Random-bred closed colonies will vary around a stable mean size anywhere from large to small, generally in each case with a coefficient of variation of the order of 10. Very large and very small rat strains have mean sizes so far apart that there is no overlap.

Fat determinations. After washing out the intestines, the weighed body was cut into convenient pieces with large shears and ground in a meat grinder[4] with a known weight of Na_2SO_4 (1 to 3 time the carcass weight). The material was mixed by hand and again run through the grinder. It was left for approximately an hour to allow the mixture to set. The shears and grinder parts were scraped off and the mixture was given a final grinding, resulting in a sufficiently homogenous powdered mass. The mixture was airdried in a thin layer for several hours, thoroughly mixed, transferred to a bottle with well-fitting closure, and weighed. At this stage the mixture was by no means dry, in the sense of water-free, but was stable under refrigeration, did not suppor tmold growth, and could be sampled by weight. Total water loss to this point could be calculated as the difference between body weight plus Na_2SO_4, and air-dried weight. Aliquots of a few grams each were analyzed in duplicate for the remaining water (oven at 105°) and for total nitrogen and lipid components; sampling for all these constituents was quite satisfactory. Results on water,[5] nitrogen,[5] phosphatides and cholesterol (16) will be reported elsewhere. The samples for lipid analysis (4-g) were heated to boiling in an alcohol ether mixture (3:1), the suspensions were cooled, made to volume, and allowed to settle overnight. Aliquots of the supernatant solution were concentrated, transferred quantitatively to the apparatus of Stetten and Grail (20), and saponified. After acidification, the fatty acids and unsaponifiable matter (FAUns) were removed by continuous extraction with petroleum ether for 2 hours, and finally weighed after evaporating the solvent. All solvent evaporations w3ere carried out in a stream of CO_2. The rat Na_2SO_4 mixtures could be stored in the refrigerator for as long as 2 weeks before analysis. Data on rats below 15 g represent pooled carcasses of 2 to 5 individuals.

To show that the course of fat accretion is not related to conditions in one laboratory, we present quantitative comparisons of data from several other laboratories. In several such cases fat was determined by direct solvent extraction of a dried carcass or aliquot (without saponification). We have made reasonable reductions in such values in order to make them comparable with FAUns: for petroleum ether we used 15% (see fig. 12); for ethyl ether we used 20% (data of Pickens et al. (21) in fig. 8). In the following paper which deals with phosphatides and cholesterol (16) we suggest a reasonable correction of FAUns to approximate triglyceride values which more closely represent storage fat.

Diet compositions are given in the figure or table legends where they apply.

Fat in relation to body weight or age

As an example of the relation between body weight and carcass fat we have in figure 1 an allometric (i.e., log-log) plot of these two quantities in post-weaning male rats of our Sherman strain and the Simms SD strain, all fed the same commercial pelleted stock diet. Data for young and old rats overlap and all are closely related to body weight.

In a paper of Harned and Cole (22), body weight and percentage of fat (determined as FAUns) are given for rats of Wistar and Yale origin. The Yale rats were heavier for any given age than the Wistars. Since the animals had been bred for several generations in their laboratory under identical conditions including diet, they assumed – and gave their reasons for it – that the Yale rat had in the past been bred for larger body size. In groups of the 2 strains aged approximately 100, 160, 225 and 400 days, Yale rats had at each age a higher average percentage of body fat, and on this basis they designated the Yale rat as obese. For figure 2 we have calculated their data back to weight of FAUns and plotted as in figure 1. The line (slightly curved) drawn through the points is identical with the line of figure 1 fitted to our data. The average values for percentage of fat in the 2 strains were 13.14 and 8.63. In such a graph equal percentages of fat lie of necessity along a line of slope 1 (45°). The 2 dotted lines of this slope are drawn through the mean values for Yales and Wistars and indicate the percentage values at the abscissa for 100 g body weight. The observed much steeped slope corresponds to a constantly increasing percentage of fat, whereas the adherence to the same course by all 4 rat stocks of widely varying age for a given body weight (as shown in figs. 1 and 2) means that fat is closely related to body weight irrespective of age.

The relation of carcass fat to body size rather than to age has been verified in several other experiments. Figures 3 and 4 deal with the several strains bred for body size, and therefore differing greatly in growth rate, or body weight at a given age; fat is represented by the weight of the excised retroperitoneal fat pad. According to Hausberger (8): "Changes in body fat closely reflect the weight changes of dissectable adipose tissue." The rats of figure 3 are the 3 strains of different growth rate which resulted from our first size-selection experiment (see Methods and Materials section). As an illustration of the determining role of body weight rather than age, we note that at body weight of about 300 g all 3 strains are represented in figure 3; at this weight the mean ages for the 3 strains were 105, 75 and 58 days. Over the body weight range of 150 to 600 g the points fall on a single line of high slope irrespective of age.

Later we will deal with obese rats whose fat content was so large that it became a very appreciable part of body weight. To avoid any "spurious correlation' in using body weight as abscissa we substitute in figure 4 a skeletal measure of body size, namely the cube of the tibia length. These data were obtained from the rats of our second size-selection experiment, the 4StS and 4StL strains. Here again the fat pad data fall on a straight line of slope similar to that of figure 3. One-year-old 4StS rats and 9-week-old 4StL rats of the same skeletal size appear together, with the same fat in the graph of figure 4. In figures 5 and 6 the two left-hand parts show in photographs and growth curves the obvious differences between 4StS and 4StL rats.

Lifetime fat accretion

In figure 7 the data on carcass fat (FAUns) and (net) body weight of figure 1 are repeated, together with additional earlier points. Both colonies represented (Sherman and Simms SD) had been fed the same colony diet for generations. The break in the curve at about 10 g body weight may stand for some unknown change in developmental pattern. Alternatively the events surrounding birth may deplete the fat. The near horizontal section around weaning is also unexplained, but is quite widely observed and will be taken up later. From about 25 g body weight (about 15 days) the graph shows 2 diverging courses. The lower one represents animals that remained on the crude colony diet. In the upper curve are data for rats fed more concentrated or refined diets, the composition of which is given in the figure legend.

The upper curve of figure 7 has been drawn through 5 mean points; the rats represented in these means are shown individually by small crosses. The first mean (large circle with horizontal bar) represents 14 rats aged 19 to 28 days and not yet weaned. They received from the age of 2 weeks a past food supplement ad libitum, with stock diet pellets also available. The next mean (large filled circle) represents 7 rats that had received stock diet and past food ad libitum to the age of 25 days and were then weaned to a casein dextrin diet containing 38% of fat (7% of cottonseed oil, 31% of hydrogenated vegetable oil); they were killed at 37 days of age. The remaining rats received no paste food supplement preweaning. The open circle represents 6 rats with an aveage age of 163 days fed since weaning a casein glucose diet with only 2% of fat (cottonseed oil). The 2 half-filled circles represent rats fed a diet with 27% of fat (one-half cottonseed oil, one-half hydrogenated vegetable oil) isocalorically substituted for glucose in the preceding diet; average ages for the 2 points were 48 (2 rats) and 181 (3 rats).

The effect of preweaning supplements of the past food was rather transitory; such rats transferred to stock diet at 28 days of age were on the stock diet line by 40 days of age. Such rapid adjustment to a new body fat level either up or down has been illustrated by Peckham et al. (23).

All 4 of the experimental diets led to significantly fatter rats than stock diet; the significance ratio t was over 4 for each diet. For this calculation we used the curve drawn through the mean points for stock diet animals and measured the deviations of points for individual rats in the vertical direction.

In figure 8 we have repeated the lines of figure 7, and plotted some data from the laboratory of A.H. Smith (21) on his Yale rats. Each point represents the mean of 8 rats. The large circle with horizontal bar signifies a diet of paste food ad libitum in addition to stock diet. The first 2 such points (newborn and 14 days old) agree well with our preweaning curve. The later points are in excellent agreement with our upper curve for a variety of refined diets; these consist of a group at 21 days, 2 groups at 42 days (one of which got somewhat less than an ad libitum intake of paste), and groups at 110 and 230 days. They also had groups aged 110 and 230 days which had received paste food ad libitum to 21 days, one-half of the ad libitum intake to 42 days, and thereafter none, with stock diet fed ad libitum throughout. These 2 groups, represented by filled circles with horizontal and vertical bars, are approaching the stock line and are well below the upper experimental line. This upper course of fat accretion is also related to size and independent of age. The rats of Pickens et al. are the large Yale strain; they are much younger at any given weight than our Sherman strain. Yet both strains fed this type of diet lie on the same plotted course. Lying on the stock diet line in figure 8 are mean values for the Harned and Cole rats on stock diet (the same data shown individually in figure 2).

The data of Widdowson and McCance (15) give further confirmation of controlled fat accretion. These investigations were interested in body composition with varying growth rate which they produced by limiting some litters to 3 pups, while increasing others to 15 to 20 pups per dam. Figure 9 (data obtained as percentage of fat from their figure 11 and recalculated to absolute weight of fat) show that except for the near horizontal past around weaning, both the fast-growing and slow-growing rats show the steep slope for fat accretion. Also, rats weighing 200 g or more have body fat containing values that fall on the same line – for body weight determines fat contents. As soon as growth-inhibited rats had undergone enough realimentation, the fat content was determined by body weight independently of age. As far as fat is concerned, experimental differences disappear, although there are still large differences in body weight for a given age. Their data do not show the same absolute calories as presented in figure 7, presumably because of differences in experimental conditions. The curves clearly show periods when body fat does not increase even though body growth is continuing. This phenomenon, which is quite similar to the pause in fat accretion around weaning shown in figure 7, is also shown by data of Mayer and Vitale (24); groups of rats with mean body weights of 38 g at 21 days and 48 g at 24 days had 1.07 and 2.02 g of fat, respectively. Indications of the same thing are reported in a number of other papers.

Data so far shown demonstrate several points: (1) at all times except for a short period around weaning, the rate of fat accretion as shown by the steep slope of the lines is much greater than the rate of body growth (approximately twice); (2) rats as old as 3 years adhere to the same controlled path of fat accretion as rats 8 months old; (3) certain differences in the diet, independent of its fat content which varied between 2 and 38%, alter the course of fat accretion in the post-weaning period in a controlled manner.

Obesity

Hereditary obesity. The 13M *fafa* rat presents an obviously obese appearance (figure 5) and is even heavier as an adult than the skeletally very large 4StL strain, although it is skeletally not much larger than the very small 4StS strain (compare mean tibia lengths of figure 6). The fatty (genotype *fafa*) is also skeletally smaller than its normal 13M sibs (genotypes *FaFa* or *Fafa*) which are, judged by tibia length and body weight, about midway in size between 4StS and 4StL. One variety of obese mouse (genotype *obob*) also shows a smaller frame than its normal sibs (25). Figure 10 shows the state of adiose tissue on the hereditarily obese rat. Part of the line of figure 4, for the retroperitoneal fat pad in relation to the cube of tibia length, is repeated; the points represent individual *fafa* rats. All but one of these fatties were raised with the stock diet.[6] Due to hyperphagia (14) these rats deviate from the "normal" pattern and the longer this process goes on – the older the rats – the more obese they become. However, the fattest of all is a single *fafa* rat which was raised with a high-fat diet; obviously this was more efficient for fattening than the stock diet. The obese hyperglycemic mouse (*obob*) is said to do poorly with a high fat diet (26).

In a fat animal various fat depots may not all be enlarged to the same degree. It is well known for man that there are various characteristic patterns of excess fat distribution, some definitely associated with apricular causes of obesity (e.g. Cushing's syndrome). The fatty is characterized by emphasis on subcutaneous fat, especially about the neck, chest and upper back. Table 1 shows weights of various fat depots in a representative fatty, compared with a 4StL (a large non-obese rat) of the same body weight. From the ratio of fat pad weights in the 2 rats it appears that the retroperitoneal fat pad used in figure 10 to measure the obesity of fatties is of an intermediate degree of enlargement. Sibs of fatties which are normal in appearance but which carry one fatty gene (genotype *Fafa*) became somewhat obese when fed a high fat diet (14). Such rats displayed a different distribution of excess fat, with primary emphasis on retroperitoneal and mesenteric fat depots. In the obese mouse (*obob*) fat accumulation in the hind quarters is characteristic (25).

Insulin obesity. This is well delineated by data of Hausberger and Hausberger (7). Their experiment was performed with rats started at a body weight of 240 g; all experiments lasted 14 days and each group contained 4 to 6 rats. In figure 11 the groups representing initial and final untreated control rats (open circles) fit our line for stock diet animals. The rats treated with protamine insulin were but slightly heavier than the 14 day controls but had a much higher fat content. Cortisone alone did not increase fat but rather diminished it (unlike the situation with mice and men), but rats receiving cortisone and the standard insulin dose (lower asterisk) were obese, and when the inslin dosage was further increased (upper asterisk), the obesity was as great as on the lower dose of insulin alone.

Nutritional obesity. The demonstration by Mickelsen et al. (3) that immensely obese rats can be produced by feeding diets with as much as 60% of fat has opened up the study of nutritional obesity in the rat. Peckham et al. (23) set up 2 groups of weanling rats, one fed a peleted stock diet and the other Mickelsen's 60% fat diet. After 31 weeks the diet of one-half of each group was switched to the other diet; at 64 weeks a switchback was made. Both in body weight and body fat an adjustment to the new diet was apparent in a few weeks. To present the Peckham data in the form of a relation of fat to body weight, the fat-inflated body weight has to be considered. In figure 12 we show lines for the same rats as in figure 7, but based on fat-free net weight rather than net weight. Their 4 points for stock diet (open circles) fit our stock line quite well. Their points for rats fed the high fat diet (crosses) rise further and further above the line as the animals become older. We have also added to figure 12 some data from Mickelsen and Anderson (27). The 2 stock diet groups (filled circles) agree well enough with our line. The single rat fed a high fat diet (asterisk) with a fat-free carcass weight of 440 g had petroleum ether-soluble fat weighing 655 for comparison with our FAUns data. This marked obesity shows to what extent fat accumulation can progress above "normal" fat accretion.

DISCUSSION

It appears that under conditions of good health and good food, with no extraneously procedures, fat accretion in the laboratory rat is a controlled process characterized by a relative rate of fat increase about twice that of body weight increase. This is independent of age and, within limits, independent of fat content of the diet. Data from several laboratories for body weights above 150 g are in good agreement. The path of fat accretion at smaller body weights is not as well established and presents several unsolved problems.

We are concerned with 2 processes: increase in

body size and increase in fat. The most objective presentation results from using weight of fat as such (not percentage), or weight of a fat pad, plotted against a measure of body size. Body size can be measured by live weight, net weight, fat-free weight, or a skeletal measurement; if the latter is a length measurement it should be cubed. To visualize the relations most clearly, allometric (i.e. log-log) plotting is used. This type of plotting is based on the fact that growth is multiplicative, not additive. It results in a very uniform dispersion of individual points around the mean course over the entire life; the steadily increasing spread of individual points around the mean course when one uses observed values as such, rather than their logs, is a familiar feature of ordinary time-growth curves, and is illustrated for the bone-to-body weight relation by figure 2 of Zucker and Zucker (28). The reason that the various measures of body size are admissible is that they are all related to each other allometrically. The slope of the line will differ slightly according to which measure of body size is used.

In carcass analysis percentage composition has its place for many types of presentation. However, when we are interested in how much of each component is produced, the use of actual weights is recommended. Percentage values change without change in the actual amounts of the component under consideration, whenever any other component changes appreciably. Therefore expressing composition as percentage can be seriously misleading. Thus Widdowson and McCance (15), discussing a plot of percentage of fat, state: "All the animals gained fat during suckling and lost it afterwards." This hides the fact that fat content did not decrease, but merely remained constant, whereas other body components increased (see our figure 9 in comparison with their figure 12).

The effect on fat accretion produced by crude and more refined diets adds another example to the list of such unexplained differences that have been observed. Just as Ganther and Bauman (29) recently observed something in a crude stock diet that radically affects the metabolic paths involved in selenium excretion, so we may postulate an unknown factor which influences fatty acid metabolism.[7] Alternately, it may be that more rapid absorption fo soluble carbohydrate from refined diets stimulates insulin production which in turn leads to more fat accretion. Also the greater bulk of stock diets may spread out food intake and lessen any peaks of carbohydrate absorption. Measurements of food intake and fecal weight in adult rats have resulted in a figure of 31 g of fecal solids /100 g of food solids (32%) for the stock diet used in figure 7, as against 6% for the purified casein-sugar diet containing 2% of fat, and 10% for the purified diet containing 27% of fat.

Although we are concerned here only with laboratory rats, it may be asked whether the fat accretion described may apply only to animals confined in cages, not in their natural habitat. It may however be noted that many animals in the wild state store fat in the summer to have its energy available during the winter. For such a species the ability to store considerable amounts of fat may be a condition for survival.

Let us again consider the difference in body weight for a given age as seen in the data of Harned and Cole (22) and in our rat strains which were selectively bred for body size. Breeding practices involving the mating of large to large and small to small will, in succeeding generations, produce animals of distinctively different body sizes for a given age, and it will very quickly change the growth rate. This has been amply established for mice (discussion in Falconer (30)) and for rats (figure 6, and Zucker (19)). Since the inception of nutrition work with rats, there has been a steady increase in average body size of colony rats. This has been illustrated by Mendel and Hubbell (31) who describe the arduous task of impressing stock diets. In the handling of a colony it is an almost common practice that one selects the biggest and healthiest looking animals for breeders; thus it is almost inevitable that selection for large hereditary size will occur. In the Mendel and Hubbell paper it is stated that at an earlier time, definite but unsuccessful attempts were made to select for increased hereditary size. However, this was a period of when the rats were fed a distinctly inferior diet. Apparently at that time the inferior diet was growth limiting so that the genetic potential for growth could not assert itself. With the improvement in rations since then, the combined effect of hereditary size and good nutrition is quite apparent.

Falconer (32) notes that in mice, guinea pigs and rabbits there is an association between body size and litter size. With respect to rats, we have observed that in a large-size and small-size strains (4StL and 4StS) the first litters average 13.8 and 6.5 young per litter, with maximal numbers reaching 22 and 10, respectively. The repeated observation in independent experiments of such as association suggest that is geneticallly based. Thus the expectation that the frequent practice of breeding from females with numerous offspring per litter will also gradually increase body size suggests another path by which body size has increased through the years.

---

[7]Since submission of this manuscript, the paper by Di Giorgio, J., R. A. Bonanno and D. M. Hegsted (J. Nutrition, 78: 384, 1962) has appeared. They find that lipogenesis is less with stock diet than with purified diet when epididymal fat tissue is observed in vitro, and suggest the presence of an unknown food factor in stock diet.

ACKNOWLEDGMENTS

The authors are indebted to Dr. Warren Sperry in whose laboratory the lipid determinations on aliquots of the prepared carcass material were carried out, with the technical assistance fo Florence C. Brand, Viola Buniak and Marion Lucchino.

The authors wish to thank Dr. Henry S. Simms for his gift of rats.

LITERATURE CITED

1. Fenton, P.F. 1956 Growth and fat deposition in the mouse. A definition of obesity. Am. J. Physiol., 184: 52.
2. Fenton, P. F., and M. T. Dowling 1953 Studies on obesity. I. Nutritional obesity in mice. J. Nutrition, 49: 319.
3. Mickelsen, O., S. Takahashi and C. Craig 1955 Experimental obesity. I. Production of obesity in rats by feeding high-fat diets. Ibid., 57: 541.
4. Brobeck, J. R. 1946 Mechanism of the development of obesity in animals with hypothalamic lesions. Physiol. Rev., 26: 541.
5. Brecher, G., and S. H. Waxler 1949 Obesity in albino mice due to single injections of goldthioglucose. Proc. Soc. Exp. Biol. Med., 70: 498.
6. Marshall, N.B., R. J. Barnett and J. Mayer 1955 Hypothalamic lesions in goldthioglucose injected mice. Ibid., 90: 240.
7. Hausberger, F. X., and B. C. Hausberger 1958 Effect of insulin and cortisone on weight gain, protein and fat content of rats. Am. J. Physiol., 193; 455.
8. Hausberger, F. X. 1958 Action of insulin and cortisone on adipose tissue. Diabetes, 7: 211.
9. Ingalls, A. M., M. M. Dickie and G. D. Snell 1950 Obese, a new mutation in the house mouse. J. Hered., 41: 317.
10. Falconer, D. S., and J. H. Isaacson 1959 Adipose, a new inherited obesity of the mouse. Ibid., 50: 290.
11. Grueneberg, H. 1952 The Genetics of the Mouse, ed. 2. Martinus Nijhoff, The Hague, p. 40.
12. Bielschowsky, M., and E. Bielschowsky 1956 New Zealand strain of obese mice; their response to stilbestrol and to insulin. Austral. J. Exp. Biol. Med. Sci., 34: 181.
13. Zucker, L. M., and T. F. Zucker 1961 Fatty, a new mutation in the rat. J. Hered., 52: 275.
14. Zucker, T. F., and L. M. Zucker 1962 Hereditary obesity in the rat associated with high serum fat and cholesterol. Proc. Soc. Exp. Biol. Med., 110; 165.
15. Widdowson, E. M., and R. A. McCance 1960 Some effects of accelerating growth. I. General somatic development. Proc. Roy. Soc. (Ser.B), 152; 188.
16. Zucker, T. F., and L. M. Zucker 1963 Phosphatides and cholesterol in the rat body: effects of growth, diet and age. J. Nutrition, 80: 20
17. Zucker, T. F. 1953 Problems in Breeding for Quality, in Rat Qualtiy, a Consideration of Heredity, Diet and Disease, a symposium. National Vitamin Foundation, Inc., N. Y., p. 48
18. – 1957 Pantothenate deficiency in rats. Proc. Animal Care Panel, 7: 193.
19. Zucker, L. M. 1960 Two-way selection for body size in rats, with observations on simultaneous changes in coat color pattern and hood size. Genetics, 45: 467.
20. Stetten, D. W., Jr., and G. F. Grail 1942 Microextraction and microtitration of fatty acids. Ind. Eng. Chem., Anal. Ed., 15: 300.
21. Pickens, M., W. E. Anderson and A. H. Smith 1940 The composition of gains made by rats on diets promoting different rates of gain. J. Nutrition, 20: 351.
22. Harned, B. K., and V. V. Cole 1939 Evidence of hyperfunction of the anterior pituitary in a strain of rats. Endocrinol., 25: 689.
23. Peckham, S. C., C. Entenman and H. W. Carroll 1962 The influence of a hyper-caloric diet on gross body and adipose tissue composition in the rat. J. Nutrition, 77: 187.
24. Mayer, J., and J. J. Vitale 1957 Thermochemical efficiency of growth in rats. Am. J. Physiol., 189: 39.
25. Vlahakis, G., and W. E. Heston 1959 Relationship between recessive obesity and induced pulmonary tumors in mice. J. Hered., 50: 90.
26. Mayer, J. 1960 The obese hyperglycemic syndrome of mice as an example of "metabolic" obesity (see table 2). Am. J. Clin. Nutrition, 8: 712.
27. Mickelsen, O., and A. A. Anderson 1959 A method for preparing intact animals for carcass analysis. J. Lab. Clin. Med., 53: 282.
28. Zucker, T. F., and L. M. Zucker 1946 Bone growth in the rat as related to age and body weight. Am. J. Physiol., 146: 585.
29. Ganther, H. E., and C. A. Bauman 1962 Selenium metabolism. I. Effects of diet, arsenic and cadmium. J. Nutrition, 77: 210.
30. Falconer, D. S. 1953 Selection for large and small size in mice. J. Genetics, 51: 470.
31. Mendel, L. B., and R. B. Hubbell 1935 The relation of the rate of growth to the diet. III. A comparison of stock rations used in the breeding colony of the Connecticut Agricultural Experiment Station. J. Nutrition, 10: 557.
32. Falconer, D. S. 1960 The genetics of litter size in mice (see especially discussion by Wright and Falconer, p. 166). J. Cell. Comp. Physiol., 56: 153.

Body-Build and Its Inheritance

Charles B. Davenport

PART I. BUILD, ITS DEFINITION AND ITS ONTOGENY.

A. General Considerations.

If a hundred men of about the same stature be compared, it is seen that they vary greatly in weight. At the same time they vary in form, and especially in bulk. This variation is popularly recognized by the variety of terms applied to build. It may be of interest to pause a moment to consider popular terminology relating to build. We have, first, terms expressing a marked deviation below the normal build. We speak of persons as "slender," "thin," "gaunt," "slim," "slight," "spare," "lank," and "spindling." These terms are not exactly synonyms. "Lank" implies angularity; "gaunt" connotes the ravage of disease, "thin" connotes a loss of weight; "slight" connotes lightness and smallness of bone; "spindling" is used especially of youth in the period of rapid growth preceding adolescence; "slim" has a faint connotation of insufficiency; "slender" best expresses the idea which we shall want to use in this work where we have a relatively small interest in stature and where we wish to avoid connotation of disease, developmental changes, etc. In other languages there exists a series of terms which similarly differ slightly in connotation. Thus, in French, there is "maigre," in German "mager," which often connote a loss of weight through disease, "dünn," which connotes loss of a former more nearly average weight, and "schlank," which is close to the English "slender." On the other hand, the English language contains a variety of terms applicable to deviation in build above the average. Thus we have the words "stout," "portly," "fleshy," "corpulent," "thick-set," "obese," "chubby," and "fat." The word "stout" usually carries a connotation of vigor. The term "portly" connotes large size with a tendency to excessively great circumference. "Fleshy" is nearly synonymous with "portly" but has less connotation of majesty of size. "Corpulent" usually carries a connotation of abdominal enlargement. "Thick-set" implies a large bony frame. "Obese" frequently connotes excessive, strictly pathological, increase of build. "Chubby" is applied especially to infants. "Fat" connotes excessive production of fat in the body, as opposed to an unusually large muscular development. Perhaps of all of these terms "fleshy" is as satisfactory as any as an expression for build without connotation in respect to degree or source of great weight, whether due to fat, muscle, or bone. In the German language there are the terms "plump," and "schwerfällig," which serve to express large build. In the French language there are the terms "gros," "obese," and "embonpoint," which is near to the English equivalent "stout" or "fleshy." In the present work the term "fleshy" is used, despite its slight suggestion of muscular development merely, largely because it begins with a different letter from slender. The word "slender" will be used for the other extreme of build. It has been found convenient to indicate those terms by their initial letter "S" and "F" respectively.

Our main problem is, in how far does this difference in build between slender and fleshy persons depend on constitutional factors?

TYPES OF VARIATION IN BUILD

Two types of variation in build have to be distinguished: (a) the ontogenetic change in normal build during development with increasing stature, and (b) the change in weight in adults of relatively invariable stature. In type a, stature and other proportions are rapidly changing, but in type b, stature remains constant, and, throughout the race, stature does not differ as much in mature persons as it does from birth to maturity.

Davenport CB. *Body-Build and Its Inheritance.* Washington: Carnegie Institution of Washington; 1923.

Editor's Note: Selections from the monograph by Davenport have been chosen to provide the main arguments. Only certain tables and figures have been included. Those interested in additional details may consult the original.

Thanks to Judy Roberts of the Pennington Information Center for help in acquiring this document.

These two types follow different laws and must be studied by different methods. Consequently they are considered in distinct parts of the present paper.

THE MEASUREMENT OF BUILD

It is now necessary to consider how build may best be expressed quantitatively. The subject of the best index of build has been much discussed, but without sufficiently differentiating between the two types of variation in build, the ontogenetic and the adult. One of the latest authors to consider the matter is Bardeen (1920, p. 486), who mentions the desirability of recording the volume of the body as a whole, notes its impracticability, and concludes that we may estimate volume from weight. It may, however, be doubted if volume is really involved in the popular notion of build. At least, it is equally probable that the idea of build, as popularly conceived, is a relation of transverse to vertical diameters. When I look at a man, or a photograph of one as in plate 1, and think, "he is slender," it is because I make a mental comparison of his breadth (of shoulders or chest) with his height and find that his breadth in comparison with that of most men I know of that height is small; or if he is stout the diameter of the chest is large in relation to stature (plate 2). It seems probable that breadth in relation to height gives the best expression of the popular idea of build. By the use of this relation, build can be easily expressed for any age, since chest circumference (which bears a nearly constant relation to chest diameter) has been recorded for many persons of all ages.

Ontogenetic.–Since in so many children and young people the stature and chest circumference have been measured, it is possible to use these data in finding the law of normal ontogenetic changes in build from birth to maturity. This ratio, chest-girth÷stature, has thus been used in discussing this law, as more fully described in section B. This relation can be used for tracing the change in build of the same developing child or for tracing the average change of build.

Adult.–In the study of adult changes of build we start with the condition that in the individual the stature is fixed. Consequently, in an individual whose weight is changing, the relation of the build at *a* years is to that at another period *n* years later as chest-girth at a years: chest-girth at *a*+*n* years. Thus, in the adult period, changes of build are proportional to chest-girth In different persons, of differing stature, the stature has to be taken into account, and the differences in build are measured by the relation of relative chest-girth in children. Unfortunately, in our study of heredity in adult build, we usually do not know the chest-girth of the different members of the family, but only their stature and weight. Our problem is, then, to find a relation between chest-girth and weight that will enable us to infer the one from the other. This problem will be further considered in a later section.

SEXUAL DIFFERENCES IN BUILD.

Sex influences the body so profoundly that we have, first of all, to consider its influence on build, either in early or in adult stages. At birth there is, on the average, a difference between the sexes in weight. The male is about 2.5 per cent heavier than the female (3,310 : 3,230 grams in German children, Daffner, 1902, p. 125, quoting Hecker; 3,606 : 3,485 grams in American children, Benedict and Talbot, 1915). But this does not imply that the boy baby is the chubbier, since the boy baby is longer by about 1.7 per cent than the girl baby. There is no obvious difference in the chubbiness of the sexes at birth. Likewise, in later infancy no obvious difference has been detected, though no thoroughgoing studies have been made on this subject. In childhood and youth children of different sex differ in build on the average, but this is because the form of the ontogenetic curve of build is very different. After maturity and cessation of growth, there is a marked difference in form between the sexes. The female has more subcutaneous fat and appears plumper. If the criterion of weight be applied, the complication arises that the specific gravity of the female seems to be less than that of the male (Bardeen, 1920, p. 488, following Meeh, 1895). As found by Medico-Actuarial Mortality investigations of the Associated Life Insurance Medical Directors of the Actuarial Society of America, 1912, volume I, p. 251: "The difference in weight between men and women of the same height is slight under the age of 20, but above that age young men are distinctly heavier than young women, the difference becoming less marked as they grow older. The tall women are markedly lighter than men of the same height." The main reason for the greater weight of young men is their relatively much greater chest circumference.

Proceeding by a method to be developed later, I have divided adult build into five classes, and counted for the various matings the number of children falling into each. (See tables 1 and 2.) The average index of build, obtained from the individual indices of build, is 2.52 (metric system) or 35.81 ± 0.12 (English system) for males, and 2.43 (34.54 ± 0.13) for females, a difference of only 3.7 per cent in favor of the males, a difference that for our purposes can be neglected. A separation of the sexes in our studies will therefore be, ordinarily, not attempted, and this has the advantage in giving us larger frequencies in our tables.

RACIAL DIFFERENCES IN BUILD.

That there are marked racial differences in build is notorious. The slender Scotchman (plate 1, fig. 3) is in

TABLE 1.–*The distribution of frequencies of the various classes of build of offspring derived from the various types of matings.*
SUMMATION TABLE, MALES ONLY. BASED ON TABLE 11.

Type of mating.	No. of matings.	No. of children.	Build of male offspring.					Total No. male and female children.
			VS	S	M	F	VF	
VSxS	4	5	1	2	1	1	0	11
VSxM	8	11	0	2	7	2	0	28
VSxF	5	12	0	1	4	6	1	25
SxS	23	29	1	21	7	0	0	47
SxM	101	172	0	12	116	38	6	306
SxF	49	88	1	5	51	30	1	155
SxVF	11	23	0	3	8	10	2	34
MxM	92	178	0	18	117	40	3	327
MxF	114	194	0	9	118	58	9	340
MxVF	30	59	1	3	21	24	10	112
FxF	33	77	3	30	34	6	4	156
FxVF	30	57	0	0	22	28	7	100
VFxVF	7	21	0	0	9	3	9	30
Total..........	507	926	7	106	515	246	52	1,671
Average build..			25.00	29.03	33.64	39.15	49.09	....

Average male index of build, 35.81 ± 12. Standard deviation, 5.33 ± .084.

TABLE 2.–*The distribution of frequencies of the various classes of build of offspring derived from the various types of matings.*

SUMMATION TABLE, FEMALES ONLY. BASED ON TABLE 11a.

Type of mating.	No. of matings.	No. of children.	Build of female offspring.				
			VS	S	M	F	VF
VSxS	4	6	1	4	1	0	0
VSxM	8	17	1	5	10	0	0
VSxF	5	13	1	4	6	1	1
SxS	23	18	4	11	3	0	0
SxM	101	134	0	36	78	15	5
SxF	49	67	2	16	29	19	1
SxVF	11	11	0	1	6	4	0
MxM	92	149	2	21	81	41	4
MxF	114	146	0	19	90	30	7
MxVF	30	53	1	4	29	12	7
FxF	33	79	0	12	30	27	10
FxVF	30	43	0	3	16	14	10
VFxVF	7	9	0	0	5	3	1
Total............	507	745	12	136	384	167	46
Average build..			24.17	28.69	33.41	39.23	46.76

Average female index of build, 34.54 ± 13. Standard deviation, 5.13 ± .09.

striking contrast with the South Italian, Greek, or Russian Jew (plate 2, fig. 3). The Eskimo are noted for their fleshiness, but Arctic conditions seem to favor large build. (See Davenport and Love, 1921, p. 165.) Martin (1914, p. 248) gives an average body-build of 1.42 (2.3 our system) for South Russian Jews and 1.07 (1.7 our system) for Bushmen. Probably the Nilotic negroes are the slenderest race on earth (Martin, 191, p. 254; for photograph see Martin, p. 263, or Davenport, 1917, p. 347). The racial differences in body-build are so great that, when feasible, race should be taken into account in studies on body-build.

GEOGRAPHICAL DIFFERENCES IN BUILD.

Apart from race, it seems probable that climate influences build. The races that live in the north polar region are of stout build, but this may be a racial trait. On the other hand, the whites who come to live near the pole are heavier than those who live near the equator. This may be due to relative freedom in the subpolar area from certain diseases which reduce weight. There may, however, be a physiological response of the body to the long, cold winters. Whatever the explanation, men from Alaska were found, at mobilization of the United States Army in 1917-18, to have a much higher index of build than those from any other region, i.e., 2.28 (32.41);[a] North Dakota and South Dakota came next, with indices of 2.24 (31.85) and 2.23 (31.73) respectively. These were followed by Montana, Minnesota, and Wisconsin. Contrariwise, the recruits from the Gulf States had a low index of build. Whatever the determining causes, geographical differences in build do exist. Consequently, in studies of build, it is desirable to consider the residences of the persons studied.

PART II. MASS STUDIES IN HEREDITY OF ADULT BUILD.

It is a matter of common observation that in some families the parents and children are all slender; in others, there may be many examples of obesity. Worthington (1877, p. 50) cites a number of examples from C. Bouchard. A woman of 45 years weighs 107 kg. (236 pounds); her obesity began shortly after marriage; her father is very obese and her mother obese. A woman of 49 years, whose father is a Turk and whose mother is French, weighs 117 kg. or about 258 pounds; her mother was obese. A woman of 115 kg. or about 250 pounds has an obese mother and two sisters who were obese in infancy; also a gouty mother's father and father's father.

[a] The method of measuring build is discussed at page 24. The smaller index (usually lying between 1.5 and 4.5) is the metric index. The large index (20 up to 100) is the English system index, and is usually expressed without decimals.

The following, from Chambers (1850), show obesity "on both sides of the house": Male of 28 years, 120 kg. (266 pounds); woman of 48 years, 127 kg. (280 pounds); woman of 52 years, 98.4 kg. (217 pounds); man of 57 years, 227 kg. (500 pounds); woman of 58 years, 104 kg. (231 pounds); woman of 68 years, 118 kg. (260 pounds); woman of 70 years, 107 kg. (238 pounds). In many other cases cited by Chambers, one parent of the obese patient was obese. Howard (1908, p. 54) cites the case of a 7-year-old girl, 45.5 inches (115.6 cm.) tall, who weighed 40 kg. (88 pounds), had a pendulous abdomen, and was feeble-minded. Her sibs were not abnormal and her parents were of average build. One of her great uncles weighs 127 kg. (280 pounds), an uncle, at 40 years, about 109 kg., and an aunt of 31 years, 95 kg. (210 pounds). This case is instructive because of the skipping of a generation.

In the class of obese cases known as adiposis dolorosa, heredity is usually obvious. Price (1909) cites a case of an obese woman of 48 years and weighing 140 kg. (310 pounds) who belongs to a fraternity of 7; 1 was a miscarriage, 2 died young of accident, 1 died at 22 of typho-pneumonia, 1 died young of scarlet fever, and 1 brother is large and rheumatic. The father seems to have been of average build and the mother is stated to have been "very thin." Of her sibs, 6 were fleshy or very fleshy, 1 medium, and 1 slender; the children of these fleshy sibs of the mother are "all stout."

Lyon (1910, p. 68) discusses heredity in adiposis dolorosa and lipomatosis and cites a considerable number of cases of family recurrence in his cases and others. Thus he twice treated a father and his son for multiple fatty tumors; also twice a mother and daughter. Lyon's obese case No. 5 was like her 3 sisters and 1 daughter; a son of her father's brother showed similar fatty deposits. 10 other instances of family recurrence of abnormal fat deposit are cited.

Maranon and Bonilla (1920) cite the case of a girl of 18 years who was slender, like her parents, until after an attack of syphilis, when she came to weigh 157 kg. or 350 pounds, while her height was 160 cm., her chest-girth 130 cm., and that of her abdomen 150 cm. or 90 per cent of her height. She had a very large brother, and both mother's parents were obese, though the parents were not known to be so.

Such examples might be multiplied indefinitely.

Our problem is not what are all the causes of this diversity of build, but rather in how far do genetical factors play a part in this diversity. We are not oblivious to the fact that there are many factors responsible for the result–deviation from the average build. These we shall consider in detail in a later section, and the consideration will help us to see the limits to the action of the genetical factors. Before going on to that, we shall have to consider more in detail the nature of the facts for which an explanation has to be sought.

METHODS AND MATERIALS.

The method of analyzing the genetic factors in build is that of tabulating the distribution of abberant builds in the family network. There is required, first, a large mass of family data which includes many extreme or aberrant types of build, and which is as reliable and as accurately quantitative as possible; secondly, this has to be subjected to the ordinary methods of genetic analysis.

The available material has consisted of data on stature and weight given in the Records of Family Traits which constitute a fair sample of the population; and of quantitative data on special schedules giving stature and weight of a fraternity, its parents, uncles and aunts, and grand-parents. These special schedules had been mailed to an address list of overweight and underweight persons obtained through the kind cooperation of Mr. Arthur Hunter. Those who returned the schedules showed an especial appreciation of the requirements of our study. A third source was the A file of the Eugenics Record Office, where are gathered miscellaneous pedigrees of families showing aberrancy in build. A fourth and especially valuable source was the field work of Miss Louise A. Nelson, of the Eugenics Record Office; this started with selected, usually obese, cases.

After the data had been assembled and tabulated, a certain amount of correspondence and personal visitation was undertaken in order to secure a confirmation or revision of the records in hand. In some cases this brought to light errors in the records, in others, useful details. Naturally, it was not possible to secure a revision of all of the data used, but an attempt was made to select only records that had been compiled with care and conscientiousness, and these traits in the compiler reveal themselves pretty clearly to a person who has examined thousands of these records, just as carelessness is revealed also by slipshod speech or posture.

For our study we desire the data of stature and weight for children, parents, and grand-parents. With some exceptions only those families are studied in which all these data are accurately given. Also, only children who are above 18 years of age can be utilized, because stature changes so rapidly until that age. However, since it is build and not stature we are studying, the fact of increase of stature from 19 to 21 years of age affects the result very little. Finally, in a certain proportion of the cases the stature and weight of all of the grand-parents are not given quantitatively. Such families are utilized, nevertheless, with such quantitative data as may have been afforded.

The data were taken from the Records of Family Traits by Miss Miriam Kortright, who long assisted in our statistical work. The computations of index of build were made by Miss Kortright and Mr. William Kraus, Miss Laura Craytor, and Miss Margaret Andrus, who checked one another's work. The tabulation and seriations of the indices were done by Misses Margaret Babcock and Katharine Belzer.

THE ADULT INDEX OF BUILD.

In an earlier section of this paper the question of the best index of build has been discussed generally. It was pointed out that many regard it as a truism that build is a relation of volume to stature. Since the volume of a person's body is rarely known, and it is difficult to determine it, weight has been substituted for volume. However, this substitution assumes that specific gravity is the same for slender and for fat persons; but this is not at all the case. The specific gravity of a fat person is about that of water (0.978 to 1.079 in 4 children 7 to 13 years of age, Meeh, 1879, and 1.014 in a 61-year-old man of 98 km. weight, Mies, 1899); of a thin person it may be 5 to 8 per cent above that of water (1.049 to 1.082 for thin convicts, Mies, 1899). This variable specific gravity complicates the attempt to infer volume from weight. In view of these difficulties it were better to measure build by a relation of chest diameter (or circumference) to stature. But this ratio can not be used in our studies, since our data, for the most part, give only weight and stature and not chest-girth. It remains thus to determine the closest relation between weight and chest-girth. This determination I have attempted to make for 100 young men, 20 to 25 years of age, measured at Harvard University where they were students. If weight varied exactly with the chest-girth, then the ratio of the former to the latter should remain constant. Such a strict relation is hardly to be expected and, of course, is not found. The ratios obtained show a certain variability about the mean condition, and this variability is measured by the standard deviation. Similarly, if each weight be divided in turn by the second and third powers of stature, and the corresponding variability of the ratios be considered, we shall have a method of deciding whether weight varies more closely with the first, second, or third power of chest-girth, and which of those powers gives in its fluctuation the best measure of the corresponding fluctuations in weight.

A comparison of the standard deviations gives the following results for man:

Ratio:	$\frac{\text{weight}}{\text{chest-girth}}$	$\frac{\text{weight}}{(\text{chest-girth})^2}$	$\frac{\text{weight}}{(\text{chest-girth})^3}$
Standard deviation:	58.3	51.5	77.0

From these results the conclusion is drawn that since the variability (standard deviation) of weight÷(chest-girth)^2 is least, the square of the chest-girth varies more closely with weight than either the first or third power of chest-girth; consequently the square of chest-girth is the best measure of weight of the three.

By hypothesis, the chest-girth in persons of the same build varies very closely or exactly with stature; consequently we could substitute in the foregoing ratios for chest its average equivalent, $\frac{\text{stature}}{K}$, in which K is nearly 2, more precisely 1.9.

In any case it is thus clearly deducible that a better index of build is got by dividing weight by the square of stature than by its cube, as has been so often done. Accordingly, the ratio of weight to stature^2 has been adopted in this paper as the standard index of build. The correlation between this index of build and relative chest-girth is found by calculation to be about 0.45.

In any scale of index of build it is, of course, desirable to use the metric system. Unfortunately, most of our data are in English units, so that our indices were first obtained by the use of these units. We have in many cases transmuted the English into the equivalent metric measures. We have, however, retained the original English index, since a large portion of the more cultured part of the world uses that system in daily life.

To avoid decimals, the ratio, weight in pounds÷(stature in inches)^2 is multiplied in this book by 1,000; this gives a series of ratios running from 20 to 60 and over. To avoid confusion with the English system, the metric equivalents are taken as the ratio of weight in grams÷ (stature in centimeters)^2. This gives a series of index numbers of the order 1.5 to 4.0; in this case, at least, one decimal is always expressed. The small integral figure and the decimal at once indicate that the index is from metric units.

CLASSIFICATION OF BUILD.

For the purposes of analysis, it was found necessary to make a small number of classes of build. To decide upon the limits of these classes, a polygon of frequency of all indices of build was made, as shown in figure 7. It appeared plain at the outset that it is desirable to plot the data in this polygon by using as abscissæ the logarithms of the index of build rather than the absolute indices, since the range of weight above the mode is, for obvious reasons, very much greater than below the mode. Taking mean weight at 68 kg., or 150 pounds, the minimum weight is about 20 kg. (45 pounds), or 25 kg. (55 pounds) below the mean, and the maximum weight is about 150 kg. (330 pounds), or 182 kg. (400 pounds) above the mean. That is, the range of weight classes is three times as great above as below the mean. Plotting data in logarithmic fashion, it appears that the modal index of build is 2.3 (33). The range is from 1.4 (20) to 4.5 (64). Using the logarithms of abscissæ, the curve is more nearly a symmetrical one. It is more irregular above than below the mode, because the classes are more numerous and the frequency of each class smaller. The presence of two modes is suggestive of the hypothesis that the medium class and probably the fleshy classes are not strictly homogeneous, but, on the contrary, comprise groups of individuals whose build is due to dissimilar factors, or sets of factors.

To derive the desired classes from figure 7, the polygon was somewhat arbitrarily divided into five parts, as indicated. Taking 33.5 as a starting-point, an equal logarithmic distance was laid off, above and below this point, on the base-line. This was taken as the range of middle class. An equal logarithmic range was accorded the classes next above and below the median respectively. All of the remainders were thrown into the extreme classes to which are given, thus, a somewhat greater range than the interior classes. This seemed desirable, since their frequencies were so low. The adjusted classes finally adopted are as shown in table 9.

MASS STUDY OF VARIATION AND HEREDITY IN BUILD.

Having considered the classification and something of the causes of variation in build, we have now to consider the relation between the build of the parents and that of the progeny. This is the mass treatment of the data of "heredity" which was the prevailing method 25 years ago and earlier. It is still a useful method in the case of traits due to multiple factors, such as the present one.

There are 15 possible different combinations of

TABLE 9.–*The five standard classes of build; limits and middle points of each.*

Class.	Range of indices.		
	Metric.	English.	Middle of class (English).
Very slender (V.S.)	1.40 to 1.80	20 to 25.4	23.5
Slender (S)	1.81 2.14	25.5 30.4	28.0
Medium (M)	2.15 3.05	36.5 43.4	40.0
Very fleshy (V.F.)	3.06 4.50+	43.5 64 +	48.0

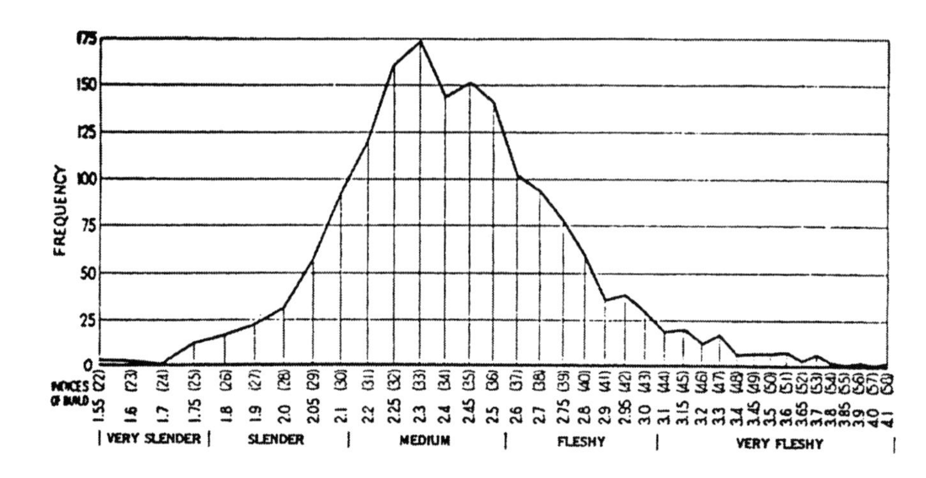

FIGURE 7.–Polygon of frequency of the various indices of build (weight ÷ stature^2). From last column of table 12, with slight modifications.

matings of the five grades. The first of these (VS X VS) is not represented in our data, and the fifth, VS X VF, is represented by only one mating and no column is devoted to it. Table 13 shows that there is a considerable correlation between the average build of the parentage and that of the progeny. From the matings of the fleshier parents the progeny are fleshier; from those of slender parents, slenderer. This relation may conceivably be due to family tradition handed down from parents to children. We shall see later that this hypothesis meets with formidable difficulties to acceptance. The most reasonable hypothesis is that there are, above all, hereditary family tendencies that help determine build.

Comparing the tables for male and female offspring, it appears, first, that there are, for some reason, more males than females about whom data of build are given, probably because more males than females know their stature and weight, or willingly record it; second,

TABLE 13.–*Distribution of progeny of the various matings, according to classes of build, absolute numbers, and proportions, based on Appendix table, including starred families.*

Type of mating.	Total No. of children.	Absolute numbers.					Proportional frequencies (per mile).				
		VS.	S.	M.	F.	VF.	VS.	S.	M.	F.	VF.
No. II VS x S	20	4	12	2	2	....	200	600	100	100	....
III VS x M	28	1	7	17	3	....	36	250	607	107	....
IV VS x F	25	1	5	10	7	2	40	200	400	280	80
VI S x S	51	5	35	11	....	....	98	686	215	....	....
VII S x M	313	....	49	200	53	11	....	157	639	169	35
VIII S x F	179	5	25	85	57	7	28	140	475	318	39
IX S x VF	50	....	7	18	17	8	....	140	360	340	160
X M x M	332	2	40	201	82	7	6	121	605	247	21
XI M x F	346	....	31	210	88	17	....	90	606	255	49
XII M x VF	112	2	7	50	36	17	18	63	446	321	152
XIII F x F	159	....	15	62	61	21	....	94	390	384	132
XIV F x VF	146	1	7	52	51	35	7	48	356	349	240
XV VF x VF	37	....	....	12	8	10	....	....	400	267	333
Total..................	1798	....	....	....	....	....	....	....	....	....	....

TABLE 14.–*Average number of progeny yielded by each type of mating (based on table 12).*

Mating.	No. of children.	Mating.	No. of children.
VS x F	5.00	S x F	3.16
F x F	4.72	S x VF	3.09
VF x VF	4.29	S x M	3.03
M x VF	3.70	M x F	2.98
M x M	3.55	VS x S	2.75
VS x M	3.50	S x S	2.04
F x VF	3.45		

there are relatively more females than males of very slender build (grades 22 to 31); there are recorded relatively more very fleshy males than females (grades of 50 and above); third, there are relatively more recorded daughters than sons derived from one very slender parent, and from the F X F and M X M matings. The male progeny are more variable than the female as 5.325 ± 0.084 is to 5.133 ± 0.089; but the difference is less than three times the probable error, and is, consequently, not very significant.

Considering next the table of total progeny of the various matings, it appears that the average number of children with recorded build from the recorded matings is variable. In descending order the fecundity of the matings is shown in table 14. This table shows that larger families, on the average, were derived from fleshy parents than from slender parents. Thus the F X F matings yield 2.3 times as many children, on the average, per mating as the S X S matings.

REGRESSION OF PROGENY TOWARD MEDIOCRITY.

Galton pointed out, in the case of stature, that, since correlation between parents and progeny is not perfect, the progeny of selected parents will tend to be less extremely selected and hence more nearly mediocre than their parents. It has, indeed, been shown in my studies on stature (1917, p. 341) that the progeny of tall parents do not show this regression to mediocrity as much as the progeny of short parents. This was regarded as evidence that the gametes of tall parents carried fewer recessive allelomorphs than those of short parents; hence were genetically "purer" and comprise more recessive factors. What is the condition in respect to the varying indices of build?

The answer to this question is given in table 15.

TABLE 15.–*Average build and regression from parental average of the progeny of the various types of mating: Also matings arranged in order of regression. Sexes combined (based on table 12).*

Type of mating.	No. of matings.	No. of progeny.	Avg. build of parents.	Avg. build of progeny.	Departure of parents from mediocrity.	Departure of progeny from mediocrity.	Regression.
VS x S	4	11	26.13	28.55 ± .86	- 8.73	- 6.69	+ 2.04
VS x M	8	28	28.38	32.18 ± .54	- 6.48	- 3.06	+ 3.42
VS x F	5	25	32.00	35.04 ± .83	- 2.86	- 0.20	+ 2.66
S x S	23	47	29.77	28.47 ± .24	- 5.09	- 6.77	- 1.68
S x M	101	306	30.90	34.01 ± .16	- 3.96	- 1.23	+ 2.73
S x F	49	155	33.85	34.39 ± .22	- 1.01	- 0.85	+ 0.16
S x VF	11	34	37.91	35.48 ± .51	+ 3.05	+ 0.24	+ 2.81
M x M	92	327	33.23	34.79 ± .15	- 1.63	- 0.45	+ 1.18
M x F	114	340	36.45	35.41 ± .16	+ 1.59	+ 0.17	+ 1.42
M x VF	30	112	40.68	36.53 ± .38	+ 5.82	+ 1.29	+ 4.53
F x F	33	156	39.21	37.56 ± .29	+ 4.35	+ 2.32	+ 2.03
F x VF	30	100	42.97	38.49 ± .36	+ 8.11	+ 3.25	+ 4.86
VF x VF	7	30	47.43	39.20 ± .78	+ 12.57	+ 3.96	+ 8.61
Total........	507	1671	34.86	35.24	....	....	....

Mediocrity for parents, 34.86. Mediocrity for progeny, 35.24

MATINGS ARRANGED IN ORDER OF REGRESSION.

S x S - 1.68	F x F + 2.03	VS x M + 3.42
S x F + 0.16	VS x S + 2.04	M x VF + 4.53
M x M + 1.18	VS x F + 2.66	F x VF + 4.86
M x F + 1.42	S x M + 2.73	VF x VF + 8.61
....	S x VF + 2.81	....

TABLE 16.–*Progeny of the various types of matings arranged in order of variability or standard deviation (S.D.), together with the probable errors (P.E.) of the means and deviations; also the coefficients of variation (based on table 12).*

Type of mating.	No. of progeny.	Mean build of progeny and (P.E.)	Standard deviaiton and (P.E.).	Coefficient of variability.
S x S................	47	28.47 ± 0.24	2.41 ± 0.17	8.97
M x M................	327	34.79 ± 0.15	4.06 ± 0.11	11.67
S x F................	155	34.39 ± 0.22	4.13 ± 0.16	12.01
S x M................	306	34.01 ± 0.16	4.20 ± 0.11	12.35
VS x S................	11	28.55 ± 0.86	4.21 ± 0.61	14.75
VS x M................	28	32.18 ± 0.54	4.22 ± 0.38	13.11
M x F................	340	35.41 ± 0.16	4.27 ± 0.11	12.06
S x VF.............	34	35.68 ± 0.51	4.44 ± 0.36	12.44
F x F................	157	37.56 ± 0.29	5.37 ± 0.20	14.30
F x VF.............	100	38.49 ± 0.36	5.38 ± 0.27	13.98
VS x F................	25	35.04 ± 0.83	6.18 ± 0.59	17.64
VF x VF.............	30	39.20 ± 0.78	6.31 ± 0.55	16.10
M x VF.............	112	37.64 ± 0.58	9.11 ± 0.41	24.17

This table shows for each of the 13 matings the average departure of the parents from mediocre build (which for the parents is 34.86) and the corresponding departure of their offspring from mediocre build (which for the progeny is 35.24). In the right-hand column of the table is given the difference between these two departures, which measures the amount of regression toward mediocrity on the part of the progeny.

Figure 8 shows clearly that, in spite of considerable irregularities, the line of regression descends from the matings of two very fleshy parents at the left, and in general from matings in which the average parental departure from the mean build of parents is positive, to the mating of two slender parents (or, less strikingly the VS X S mating) or in general to the matings in which the average parental departure is extremely negative. This result is most easily explained on the ground that whereas fleshy parents carry all sorts of gametes for build, slender parents carry a preponderance of gametes of their own kind; hence the progeny do not regress so much from the selected parental condition. This suggests that the slender parents are more nearly homozygous than the fleshy parents.

Still another test of the gametic composition of the parents is the variability of their offspring. The facts regarding such variability are given in table 16. From this table it appears that the mating that yields the least variable progeny is that of two slender consorts. The variability in their progeny is measured by 2.41± 0.17. The variability of the progeny of the VS X S mating is greater, 4.21 ± 0.61, but on account of the small number of the progeny the probable error is large, and it is possible that this difference in variability between S X S and VS X S progeny is not a significant one. Next to the least variable are the offspring of the M X M mating, 4.06 ± 0.11, and this leads to the conclusion that a large proportion of the M parents are not merely heterozygous, but constitute a "pure race" of medium build. The offspring of the S X F mating have a fairly small variability 4.13 ± 0.16, as befits a first generation (F_1) hybrid. On the other extreme, we have the M X VF mating with a standard deviation of 9.11 ± 0.41 This large standard deviation is due chiefly to the inclusion of one family (Ber-A) which contains 2 progeny of builds 79 and 103, weighing 180 kg. (400 pounds) and 215 kg. (475 pounds) respectively. Otherwise, the variability of this mating is not extreme. It is 5.25 ± 0.24. The next largest variability is from the VF X VF mating, 6.31 ± 0.55, a variability that is due to the absence of any important mode. The progeny of the VS X F mating are highly variable, 6.18 ± 0.59, but this standard deviation has the largest probable error of any except VS X S, so that great stress must not be laid upon its exact position. In general, the progeny of matings with 2 or 1 F or VF parents belong to the more variable group and those with S (or VS) parents to the less variable group. The meaning of this is clear to the geneticist who has dealt with multiple factors. It indicates that some or all of the factors that make for fleshy build dominate to a greater or less degree over the factors for slenderness. The test of the regression of progeny toward mediocrity and the test of the variability of the progeny of the various matings thus lead to the same result–the factors for fleshiness are imperfectly dominant over those for slenderness, and the latter probably lack some or all of those factors that make for fleshy build.

TABLE 19.–*Percentage distribution of parents of each sex among the various classes of build as found in 531 selected matings. Based on Appendix tables.*

Classes.	Males.		Females.	
	Frequency.	Per cent.	Frequency.	Per cent.
VS.....	22	.38	18	3.39
S........	97	18.27	127	23.92
M.......	230	43.31	210	39.55
F........	158	29.75	120	22.59
VF.....	44	8.29	56	10.55
Total..	531	100	531	100

HYPOTHESIS.

The foregoing brief studies of the progeny of classes of matings suggest the following hypothesis:

Fleshy build results from the action of several positive (dominant) factors that make for stoutness, while slenderness results from the absence of one or more of such factors, or is due to recessive factors. Fleshy parents may, and frequently do, carry gametes which lack the "fleshy" or carry the "slender" factor, while in slender parents for the most part the gametes carry only the slender factor, hence the gametes of slender parents are more nearly homogeneous. This hypothesis may be further developed as follows:

Assuming that there are two independent factors A and B for build, then these may be found in different zygotes in the following combinations:

AABB AaBB aABB aaBB
AABb AaBb aABb aaBb
AAbB AabB aAbB aabB
AAbb Aabb aAbb aabb

Or, disregarding order of the letters, and considering only the number and kind of genes in each kind of zygote, we have:

AABB 2AaBB aaBB
2AABb 4AaBb 2aaBb
AAbb 2Aabb aabb

in which the coefficients indicate the relative frequency of the different combinations.

We may assume that:

4 positive factors in a zygote correspond to a very fleshy person.
3 factors correspond to a fleshy person.
2 factors correspond to a person of medium build.
1 factor corresponds to a slender person.
0 factor corresponds to a very slender person.

MATE SELECTION IN BUILD.

Statistics on temperament and stature of consorts (Davenport, 1915, p. 106; 1917, p. 329) seem clearly to show that there is an assortative mating in respect to these traits. The question arises: Is there assortative mating in respect to build? The inquiry is rendered the more difficult, inasmuch as build changes to such an extent with age. Nevertheless, as there appears to be a considerable correlation (though not yet calculated) between build at 25 and at 50 years, it is fair to assume that some degree of the mature build is already indicated at the period just before marriage.

If, now, there is no assortative mating in respect to build, we should find that persons of any given build, say slender, would have very slender, slender, medium, fleshy, and very fleshy consorts in the respective proportions in which such classes of build occur in the whole population of parents. A marked deviation from this expectation would indicate the falseness of this hypothesis and that there is an assortative mating in respect to build.

To test the hypothesis we can make use of 531 matings, including those which are employed in the main tables. We find the male and the female consorts in these matings to occur in the different classes in the numbers and proportions shown in table 19.

In applying the test to the hypothesis we may assume in turn that the groom has done the selecting and that the bride has done the selecting. We then compare, in the selections made by the grooms, the expected proportion of the classes of build on the assumption of no assortative mating, with the proportions actually found in the brides. Similarly, with suitable changes for the selections made by the brides. The results are given in table 20 (not reproduced).

An inspection of tables 19 and 20 shows that the hypothesis that wives and husbands of men of each different class of build are merely random samples of the whole population of parents is not supported by the facts. Thus on the part of both very fleshy grooms and brides over 70 per cent more consorts who will ultimately be very fleshy are selected than are expected on the hypothesis of random sampling. Also, among fleshy fathers there is a marked excess of very fleshy wives. Slender parents have an excess of similar consorts. Medium parents have selected consorts nearly at random so far as regards build. Slender parents have selected a smaller proportion of very fleshy consorts than expectation on random choice, and very fleshy parents have selected less than the average of very slender and slender consorts. In a word, there is some degree of assortative mating and, indeed, a mating of similars. This result agrees with the findings in respect to stature;

similars tend to mate; while in the case of temperament, dissimilars tend to marry each other.

SUMMARY.

The progeny of the three matings may now be compared (table 26). While even very fleshy parents are sometimes heterozygous (perhaps carrying 5 or rarely even 4 zygotic factors for build), yet they do not produce any slender children. The merely "fleshy" parents, on the other hand, produce about 7 per cent slender. None would be expected on the 4-zygotic-factor hypothesis, but about 6 per cent would be on the 6-factor hypothesis.

A comparison of tables 23 (not shown) and 26 shows a profound difference in the distribution of build in the two sets of progenies. From the matings of slender parents come predominantly (84 per cent) slender and very slender offspring; from the mating of two fleshy or very fleshy parents come predominantly (67 per cent) fleshy and very fleshy offspring. The ranges of the offspring classes overlap somewhat, for the slender matings produce 16 per cent progeny who are above slender build; and the fleshy matings produce 32 per cent of progeny who are below fleshy build. The progeny of the slender matings are much less variable than those of fleshy matings. Thus, the standard deviation of the offspring in table 23 is only 3.13 ± 0.17; while the standard deviation of the offspring of the fleshy parents listed in table 24 (not shown) is 5.74 ± 0.39 and in table 25 (not shown) 4.70 ± 0.52. From the standpoint of genetics this indicates the presence of more genetical factors in the fleshy parents than in the slender.

However, there is one consideration that must not be overlooked. This is that the mean index of build of the slender offspring is lower than that of the fleshy ones. If we place the average index of the very slender and slender groups at 26, and of the pure fleshy at 40, then the coefficient of variability of the slender and very slender is 3.13 + 26, or 12 per cent, and that of the fleshy of table 24 is 4.70 + 40, or 14 per cent. Thus the fleshy offspring are not only absolutely but also relatively more variable than the slender offspring.

The standard deviation of the progeny of the S X S matings is 241; of the F X F matings is 5.37. The corresponding coefficients of variability are 2.41 + 28.47 and 5.35 + 37.56, or 8.46 per cent and 14.25 per cent respectively. That is, the coefficient of variability of build of the offspring of the F X F mating is 68 per cent greater than that of the S X S mating. The ranges of the logarithms of the indices of the S and the F groups is as near as possible the same, and the arithmetic range of the F is only 40 per cent greater than of the S group. Hence the greater variability of the offspring of the F X F as compared with the S X S matings can not be accounted for on a difference in the range of index values of the S and F classes. The most reasonable conclusion seems to be that the gametes of the fleshy parents are somewhat more variable than the gametes of the slender and the very slender parents.

PART III. FAMILY STUDIES IN HEREDITY OF BUILD.

C. GENERAL DISCUSSION

HEREDITY AND ENVIRONMENT IN BUILD.

That a tendency to slenderness or fleshiness of build "runs in families" and characterizes different races is a matter of common observation. But this fact is far from satisfying the clinician that heredity plays any part in this result. Thus, von Noorden, who occupies a leading position among Teutonic investigators of metabolism in general and obesity in particular, denies the importance of an hereditary anomaly of metabolism in different families and races. Rejecting "anomaly of metabolism" or "peculiarity of protoplasmic metabolism," he stresses "inheritance" of habits of life that favor obesity, the quantity and quality of food, and the ideals of bodily activity. For example, the Eskimo are fat because they eat blubber and huddle in narrow spaces, undergoing little movement throughout the long, dark winters. It is true that von Noorden speaks somewhat guardedly; he recognizes exceptions; suggests a possible hereditary hypofunction of the thyroid. But clearly constitutional peculiarities are, for him, exceptional as causes of overweight, and here is where he fails to recognize sufficiently the fact that usually only particular individuals of a fraternity are fleshy; the others may be slender.

But besides anomalies of protoplasm and family traditions of feeding, there are obviously other possibilities. It is well known that different varieties of cattle differ greatly in their capacity for fattening. Armsby and Fries (1911) have inquired into the influence of type upon the fattening of cattle. They used a pure-bred Aberdeen-Angus steer and a "scrub," part Jersey, steer for comparison. As is well known, the former belongs to the easily fattening beef type; the Jersey to the difficulty fattening milk type. During over 2 1/2 years, beginning at under 1 year of age, these steers were under nearly continuous observations. They were fed on ordinary growing rations, the same for each steer. The digestibility of the total ration was determined at intervals; four tests were made of each animal in the respiration calorimeter to determine the percentage availability of the energy of the feeds consumed by each. The results were as follows: Analysis of feces and urine failed to show any difference in percentage digestibility of the food by the two animals, and calorimeter tests failed to show any difference in the proportion of the food-energy which was being metabolized. But the two animals did not metabolize in the same way. Thus, in the scrub, a larger proportion of the gain made was of protein than in the case of the beef steer; and, conversely, the gain of the beef steer was more largely fat than in the case of the scrub. Reduced to common weight, the energy requirement for maintenance of the scrub steer was nearly 19 per cent greater than for the beef steer. Since the beef steer would eat more than the scrub and tended to store fat rather than protein, the greater tendency of the beef steer to fatten received a biochemical explanation. The results seem to show a difference between the two varieties in the working over of the assimilated materials.

Indeed, it is easily appreciated that steers of the beef and dairy types of cattle should metabolize differently when we consider the marked difference in the milk production of the cows of these two types. The cow of the highest dairy type is capable of manufacturing 20 kilograms of milk containing 1.2 kilograms of butter fat in one day, or 6 per cent (Bailey, Encl. Am. Agric., III, 365). The cow of the meat type, of larger size, produces up to 30 kilograms of milk, and this contains, perhaps, 1.3 kilograms of butter fat per day, or only 4.3 per cent (Sinclair, 1904, p. 740-42). There is here, obviously, a difference in the metabolic processes in the cows and this is reflected in the steers also.* There is an internal biochemical difference as well as a difference in the feeding instinct. The latter is not merely a matter of family tradition, of the family economics or mores; it is a physiological phenomenon as much as internal metabolism.

Indeed, even von Noorden (1907, III, p. 700) seems to be forced to this conclusion by cases of failure to reduce weight at a diet far below that which appears to be essential to maintenance. Thus a man of 39 years, who exercised freely in the open air, had a weight of 102 kg. For 3 months his diet never exceeded 1,720 calories (estimated at 1,000 calories short of normal requirements) and at the end of this period he weighed 101 kg.

That a relation between ingested food and activity is not the entire explanation of obesity is recognized by medical men of experience. Heckel (1920, p. 371), referring to recurrent obesity, remarks on its frequency and says: To constitute an obesity there must be organic and hereditary tendencies: "Ne devient pas obèse qui veut." "Aussi la guérison accidentelle ou thérapeutique d'une obésité n'indique-t-elle pas la disparition définitive des tendances personelles ou congénitale."

Gulick (1922) has lately undertaken experiments to throw light on the question why some persons fatten easily and some with difficulty. He had noted that he himself belongs to a non-fattening strain and that his inclination toward a very copious diet of predominantly starchy nature did not lead him to put on weight, even though his round of activity was moderate. So he undertook biochemical, nutritional studies on himself. His observation covered nearly 21 months. During part of this time his caloric intake was low, 1,875 to 2,780; during another part high, 3,400 to 4,100. He found that he fattened somewhat during the period of heaviest feeding. There was, however, always an excess of intake over predictable need, and this excess increased absolutely and probably even relatively as the intake increased. The fecal nitrogen was 2 1/2 to 3 1/2 times greater during over-feeding than under-feeding. The basal metabolism during maximum feeding was normal. Gulick concludes that a person belonging to the difficulty fattening type shows a wasteful rate of oxidation, whether under or over fed, but especially at the latter time. "It seems clear," concludes Gulick, "that throughout the entire experimental series there was some factor at work which caused fuel food to be burned more freely than in the average individual. This factor was not an over-active thyroid, as attested by the entirely normal basal metabolism." Gulick concludes that it was "some factor in the chemistry of nutrition" which caused extravagance. This he thinks may very possibly be comparable to the "secondary effect" of protein enrichment, which, according to Rubner, can raise the specific dynamic action of the food without raising the basal rate. It is also possible, he says, that the spare type may be accounted for by any factor that produces a high "cost of digestion," just as the obese may be supposed to suffer from an abnormally low "cost of digestion" (von Noorden).

Whatever the fundamental cause may be, the fact remains that in certain families there is a widespread inclination to the production of slender individuals, while in other fraternities certain proportions (though usually not all) of any fraternity are fleshy or even obese. Perhaps, as in the case of the Jersey as contrasted with the beef steer, the two kinds of individuals do not metabolize their food in the same way; some are spare and muscular, others lay on fat. In any case we can not disregard the constitutional factors in build.

Looking at the matter broadly, we can see that no other theory than that constitutional differences as well as nutritional differences determine build is sufficient to meet all the facts. In other species of animals we have precisely the same kind of differences between hereditary strains of slender and stout build that we have among humans. Thus, among dogs, the slender greyhound or Dachshund and the robust "Chow"; among horses the Thoroughbred and the stocky Percheron;

*I am indebted to Mrs. C.D. Walcott for calling my attention to this point.

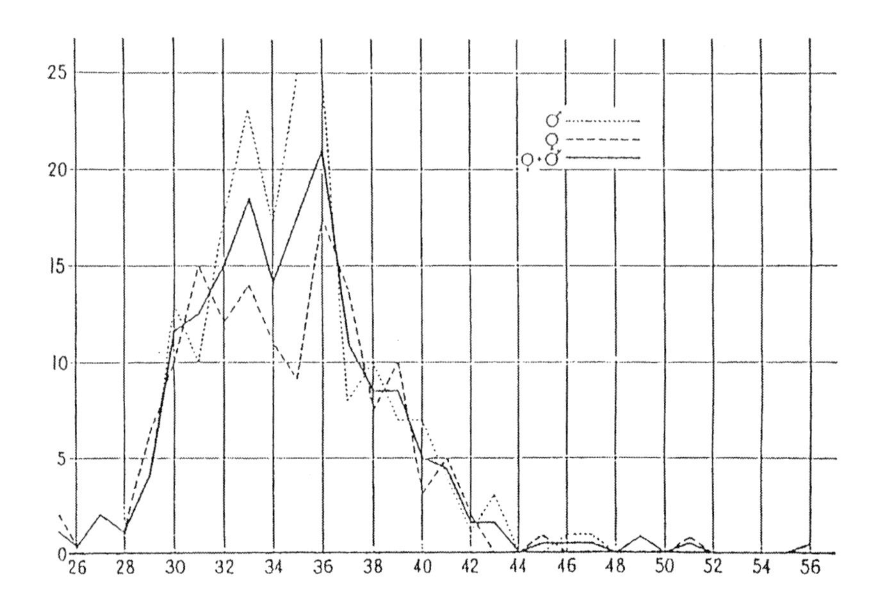

FIGURE 50–Polygon of distribution of offspring of M X M matings (from Appendix table X) for males, females, and sexes combined. Abscissæ:index of build, English system. Ordinates: absolute frequencies for males and females and their half sum for the sexes combined.

among swine the "razor-back" and the Berkshire; among poultry the slender Leghorn and the stocky Cochin. Slender and stocky as racial traits appear quite as white and black do and they doubtless have similarly a genetic basis.

A careful study of the families described in this paper must convince anyone, it seems to me, of the importance of the genetic factors. The Fun. family is of a wholly different type from the Thr-1 family. Even if the latter eat more, it is because of a constitutional urge like the constitutional urge that leads the Aberdeen-Angus steer to eat more than the Jersey steer. Very probably the Fun. family metabolizes in a different way from the Thr-1 family, building more protein and less fat.

In other cases it is not the whole fraternity that is fleshy or slender. This is well illustrated by the Wen. family, where 2 of 8 of the main fraternity are very fleshy and all the others of medium build. We have here to do not merely with a family habit of eating, but a differential constitution that provides one-quarter of the children with a large appetite that leads them to eat heavily and manufacture fat and provides three-quarters of them with a small appetite that leads them to eat lightly and to manufacture protein instead of fat. Constitutional differences in the appetite and method of metabolism are the essential factors; and these are the things that are inherited. Only on such an hypothesis can we account for the clear evidence presented of constitutional factors in build–not always one only, but sometimes three or more acting together to produce the end result of obesity.

A scientific man, interested in nutrition, who has a build of 3.6 (51) himself and one of whose sisters has a build of 3.1 (44), whereas his 4 other sibs have builds of 2.5 to 2.1 (35 to 30), writes that his brother (of medium build, but about 75 inches tall) consumes daily about 2,700 calories; he himself and his fleshy sister about 2,500, and the others of his fraternity, who are of medium build, 2,000 to 1,800. He is a professional man, who does a good deal of office or laboratory work. He drinks about 3 to 4 quarts of water per day. His son, who is nearly 11 years of age, weighs just over 120 pounds, is 63 inches tall, and fairly fleshy. Though he is active, "never still a minute," yet he has to be urged to eat, willingly misses a meal, and uniformly declines a second helping; "he eats much less than his 6-year-old cousins, who are actually under size for their age; he has never been a heavy eater from the time he was weaned."

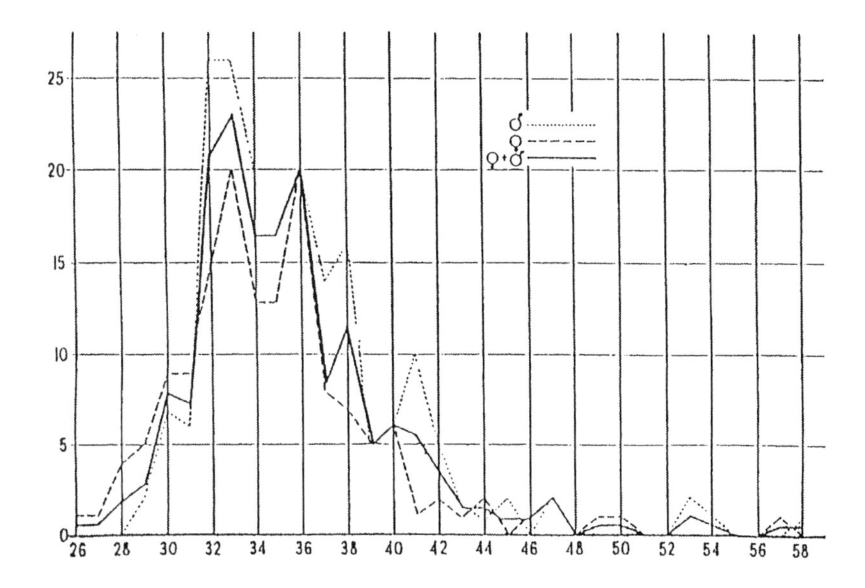

FIGURE 51.–Polygon of distribution of offspring of M X F matings (from Appendix table XI), sexes separate and combined. See also legend of Figure 50.

This boy, the son of a very fleshy man, seems to afford an example of the easily fattening type in whom the slight excess of calories produces a striking result in build.

EVIDENCE OF SEGREGATION IN THE HEREDITY OF BUILD.

The best single criterion of Mendelism in any hereditary distribution is segregation. If there is sufficient evidence of segregation in our study of build, then we are justified in concluding that build is inherited in "Mendelian fashion." There have been several occasions to refer to evidence of segregation in this work; some of this evidence may be brought together here and other added.

1. The difference in variability of the progeny of different matings. The offspring of slender parents are least variable, of fleshy parents most. This is evidence that the fleshy parents carry gametes for slenderness and thus that condition reappears in the offspring; but slender parents rarely carry gametes for fleshiness.

2. As a corollary of the above, regression takes place in the progeny of fleshy parents to a markedly greater degree than in the progeny of slender parents.

3. The progeny of heterozygous parents are significantly more variable than the progeny of parents belonging respectively to slender and to fleshy stock. This is evidence that the heterozygous parents carry a greater variety of gametes than those of "purer stock."

4. In different matings of the same type the variability of the progeny differs; apparently, because some parents belong to a special biotype and others simulate the biotype merely through heterozygosity. Thus, if the M X M mating be considered (table X), one finds some families characterized by slight variability of the offspring. The slight fluctuation in build of progeny of table 34 is obvious. The modal index of the progeny is close to 33. On the other hand, there are matings of this type which show a much greater variability.

These series of progeny fluctuate in build around 36. It seems probable that the variable progeny are the offspring of heterozygous parents, but this can rarely be proved, since the build of the grandparents is not often available in the present series.

That there are really at least two kinds of matings of the M X M type is shown more conclusively by figure 50, in which two modes, at 33 and 36, respectively, are clearly seen. The conclusion seems to be justified that the mode at 33 is that of progeny derived from the M biotype and the mode at 36 is that of the progeny of heterozygous M parents. The existence of these two modes in figure 50 is thus evidence of segregation.

Additional evidence is found in other matings, like-

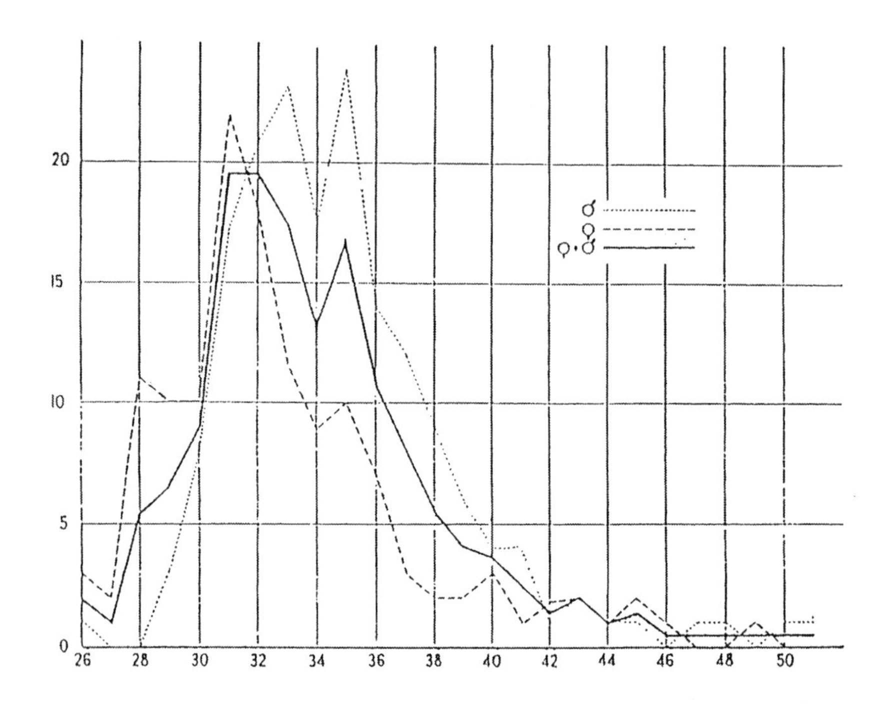

FIGURE 52.–Polygon of distribution of frequencies of build of offspring of S X M matings (from Appendix table VII), sexes separate and combined. See also legend to Figure 50.

wise. Thus the M X F mating shows two modes, at 33 and at 36 (fig. 51). There is also one other, possibly significant, mode, namely, at 38, in the fleshy group. Since F parents are sometimes homozygous, mating with M would tend to produce medium-fleshy progeny (i.e., 36). The F parents are, however, frequently heterozygous, containing both slender, medium, fleshy, and even very fleshy gametes; and, accordingly, we should expect somatic segregations at about the points 30, 33, 36, and 38 as centers, just where we find them.

Again, the S X M mating yields (fig. 52) modes at 32 and 35 respectively, a shade lower than those of the M X M or M X F matings; but the male offspring (taken alone) gives modes at 33 and 35. Where the mode is at 33 it is probable that an S and an M gamete have met; and this condition is relatively common just because M gametes are common. The mode at 35 may arise from an F gamete carried in a heterozygous M uniting with an S gamete. The S gamete carried in heterozygous M may be responsible for a probable mode which is hidden in the form of a hump at 28 in figure 52.

Attention is called to the probable influence of these modes on the two modes shown in figure 7, at 33 and 35 respectively. These two modes are strong evidence for a segregation in the factors for build. Thus the very irregularity of the polygon of figure 7 is evidence of the presence of segregating factors for build. Moreover, these two modes appear at every age from birth to maturity. This bimodality is easily accounted for on genetical grounds, but is inexplicable upon the bare nutritional hypothesis of build.

ON THE NUMBER OF FACTORS INVOLVED IN FLESHY BUILD.

It is by no means an easy matter to determine the number of independent factors which are active in the case of a trait that is due to multiple factors. This matter is still less easy if there is only very imperfect dominance approaching intermediacy of the trait in the progeny of the F1 mating. Yet that is the situation that has to be met in the study of heredity of build.

An attempt has been made in this paper to test the relative probability that there are only two, on the one hand, or three or more independent factors, on the other, involved. We have seen, in each of the various matings, that the result is, on the whole, more closely in accord with the 3-factor hypothesis than that of 2 factors. But this is not to insist that never more than 3 independent factors are involved in build, or never less than 3.

An attempt was made to apply Dr. Sewall Wright's formula (Castle, 1922, p. 22). The value for n (the number of factors) was calculated by the formula

$$N=\frac{D^2}{8(\sigma2^2 - \sigma1^2)}$$

where D is the difference between the means of parental pure races, s1 is the standard deviation of F1 and s2 is standard deviation of F2.

Substitution for the letters of their values given $n=(39.20-28.50)^2 + 8[(6.78)^2 - (5.02)^2] = 0.69$. We can only conclude that, owing to small numbers, this formula is not applicable here.

Returning, then, to our conclusion that the assumption of at least 3 gametic factors for some, probably most, cases of build accords best with the results of the various matings, we may inquire what is the nature of these factors. It seems probable that two of them may correspond to dystrophies of the pituitary and thyroid glands respectively and the other or others to other regulatory mechanisms of metabolism in the organism. It may well be that one of our factors is the same as that which causes hypothroidism; another as that which causes hypopituitarism, and the third that which inhibits the normal development of the genitalia, such as we see functioning in dystrophia adiposo-genitalis. This is, indeed, speculation. However, the speculation is an attempt to give a concrete form to the ideas of multiple factors in build.

If we assume three independent factors for build, it does not follow that these are present in all families. Just as it has been demonstrated that in different strains of mice there are in some cases 3, in others only 2 factors for susceptibility to cancer, so, apparently, it is with build. In certain families the distribution of build in the progeny is best accounted for on the hypothesis that, in such families, there are only two gametic factors for build. In other families there appears to be only one gametic factor for build.

It has been repeatedly pointed out that in many cases where multiple factors are invoked to explain the genetical results, the results can be equally well explained on the theory of blended inheritance. The advantage of the factorial theory is that it brings under one type of heredity even these most difficult cases of apparently blending inheritance. More than that, however, the theory of multiple factors explains a number of phenomena that the theory of blending inheritance does not, such as the greater variability of the F_2 as contrasted with the F_1 generation, and the skewness in distribution of progeny in the back-cross. Thus an F X S mating should produce a "medium" progeny with symmetrical distribution of deviating types on the theory of blending inheritance; actually it produces not only mediums, but an excess of fleshy over slender, which is readily accounted for on the hypothesis that fleshiness is partially dominant over slenderness. In this and other ways, especially in focussing attention on gametes, the doctrine of multiple factors is essential to an adequate interpretation of the results of mating between persons of dissimilar build.

D. SUMMARY OF CONCLUSIONS.

1. Two types of variation in build are to be distinguished: (1) the change in average build that accompanies ontogeny and (2) variations in adult build.

2. The popular idea of build is best expressed as the ratio of transverse chest diameter to stature, or (since the chest diameter is rarely known) chest-girth to stature. When only weight and stature are known, the closest approximation to the chest÷stature ratio is given by the weight÷(stature)^2 ratio, and this is taken as the standard index of build.

3. The correlation between the standard index of build and the relative chest-girth is, for males, about 0.45

4. The index of build of adult males is slightly greater than of females, because of the relatively greater chest-girth of males. The average index of build for males is 2.52 (35.8) and for females 2.43 (34.5).

5. There are marked racial differences in build; but they are not so great as the differences in ontogenetic stages.

6. There are geographical differences in build; the heavy build of northern peoples may be due to a physiological reaction or, in part, to a selective survival of the fleshier individuals or strains.

7. The ontogenetic curve of build, expressed by relative chest-girth, is expressed by figure 1 and (for infancy) figure 2. It shows that at birth chest-girth is about two-thirds of stature and diminishes in the male to the age of 12 years; thereafter, on the average, it rises to complete maturity.

8. Build declines temporarily during the first month of life, owing to the physiological difficulties attending adjustment to new conditions. It declines tem-

TABLE 26.–*Summary of selected fleshy mating, together with their progeny.*

	No.	Offspring. Frequency. S	M	F	VF	Proportion. S	M	F	VF
Mating 1. One parent VF; the other F, of F stock	50	2	11	23	14	4	22	46	28
Mating 2. Both parents F, of F stock	15	1	5	8	1	7	33	53	7
Mating 3. Other VF X VF matings	30	....	12	8	10	....	40	27	33

porarily, again, at about 8 months, probably due to the cutting of the incisor teeth.

9. The heavy build of the infant corresponds to that of the short-legged anthropoids. The long-legged, slender-build stage of the boy of 12 years persists in the Nilotic negroes and many low-grade feeble-minded.

10. In adult life the changes in build vary with families. In those characterized by slender build there is typically little change. In those characterized by fleshy build there is typically progressive increase in weight to 50 years. In some families weight fluctuates greatly at different periods of adult life. In general, though with numerous exceptions, a fleshy adult build is foreshadowed in plump build in childhood.

11. Mass studies on adult build give a polygon of distribution which is skew, the mode being toward the slenderer end of the polygon. There is evidence of more than one mode, and hence that there are two or more types of build. For purposes of description five classes of build are recognized–very slender, slender, medium, fleshy, and very fleshy.

12. The diseases associated with very slender and slender build are: tuberculosis, pneumonia, "nervousness," melancholia. The diseases associated with very fleshy or fleshy build are: diabetes, nephritis and dropsy, apoplexy, and arterio-sclerosis and paralysis accompanying it; also numerous diseases of the alimentary tract.

13. Fleshy parents have, on the average, in our data, larger families than slender parents.

14. Regression toward mediocrity is less striking in the offspring of slender than of fleshy parents, suggesting that fleshy parents carry not only genes for fleshiness but also for slenderness, while slender parents more rarely carry genes for fleshiness.

15. The offspring of two fleshy parents are twice as variable as those of slender parents.

16. The hypothesis is indicated that genetically build is controlled by multiple factors, with fleshiness tending slightly to dominate over slenderness.

17. There is a marked tendency for persons of similar build (or with potentialities for such) to intermarry. Dissimilar builds are selected against.

18. Two slender parents of slender stock have rarely any progeny whose index of build exceeds 2.2, or just above the upper limit of the slender group. In general, the progeny of slender parents are relatively slightly variable.

19. The slender parents are apparently of two kinds: those carrying only one kind of factor for fleshy build and the other two such gametic factors. The progeny of the former are very slightly variable; those of the latter more variable.

20. By comparing coefficients of variability instead of indices, and by making allowance for the greater range of the fleshy class than the slender class, it still appears that the progeny of fleshy parents are relatively and per unit range more variable than the progeny of slender parents. Absolutely the offspring of the fleshy parents are, as stated, twice as variable as of slender parents.

21. The matings of slender parents and fleshy parents of fleshy stock yield a variable progeny, such as is typically found in the F_1 generation when multiple factors are concerned. The variability is between that of the progeny of slender matings and that of the progeny of fleshy matings.

22. The F_1 generation has not a mode of build that is intermediate between that of the parental stocks, but one that is about the same as of the fleshy matings. This is evidence of partial dominance of fleshiness.

23. The mating of two heterozygous (F_1) parents produces, in general, an exceptionally variable progeny. This is one of the strongest evidences of the presence of genetical factors in build.

24. Many, if not most, parents of medium build belong to biotypes with 1 or 2 independent factors for build. Consequently the progeny of medium X medium matings is often strikingly invariable.

25. The "back-cross" of a heterozygous parent with a slender parent, on the one hand, or with a fleshy parent of fleshy stock, on the other, gives a variable progeny, whose mode is shifted toward fleshiness; but which shows a tendency to fall again into the slender (or fleshy) and medium-fleshy grandparental types.

26. Variations in build are not to be accounted for merely by variations in intake and out-go of calories, but also by the endogenous factors that determine the "economy of nutrition" or the cost in energy of adding

an additional kilogram of weight to the body. The factors involved in producing differences in these respects are hereditary factors.

27. The hereditary factors probably work through the intermediacy of special organs that influence metabolism, notably the endocrine glands. The latter thus intermediate between the chromosomal constitution, on the one hand, and control of metabolic processes, on the other.

28. The number of factors involved in very fleshy build is, in some cases at least, three independent ones. But the number is probably not the same in all biotypes. Probably in some there is only one, in others four or more.

29. The factors probably influence the functioning of the thyroid, pituitary, and perhaps other glands.

LITERATURE CITED:

Armsby H P, Fries JA. The influence of type and of age upon the utilization of feed by cattle. *U.S. Dept. Agriculture, Bureau of Animal Industry, Bulletin 128.* 1911.

Association of Life Insurance Medical Doctors and the Actuarial Society of America. *Medico-Actuarial Mortality Investigations.*New York; 1912:I.

Bardeen CR. The height-weight index of build in relation to linear and volumetric proportions, etc. Carnegie Inst. Wash. *Pub. No. 272.* 1920.

Benedict FG, Talbot FB. The physiology of the new-born infant. Carnegie Inst. Wash. *Pub. No. 233.* 1915.

Castle WE. Genetic studies of rabbits and rats. Carnegie Inst. Wash. *Pub. No. 320, 2 pls.* 1922.

Chambers TK. Corpulence, or excess of fat in the human body. *Lancet.* 1850;I.

Daffne F. *Das Wachstum des Menschen: Anthropologische Studien.* Leipzig: Englemann; 1902.

Davenport CB. The feebly inhibited: inheritance of temperament. Carnegie Inst. Wash. *Pub. No. 236.* 1915.

—. Inheritance of stature. *Genetics.* 1917;2:313-389. (Eugenics Record Office Bull. No. 18).

—. and Love AG. Army anthropology. Medical Dept. U.S. Army in World War. Gov't Printing Office. *Statistics, Part I.* 1921.

Gulick A. 1922. A study of weight regulation in adult human body during over-nutrition. *Amer. Journal of Physiology.* 1922;60: 371-395.

Heckel F. *Grandes et petites obésités; cure radicale.* Masson. 1920.

Howard –. Abnormal devlopment in a girl. Report for Soc. *Diseases of Children.* 1908;8: 54-56.

Lyon IP. Adiposis and lipomatosis. *Arch. of Inter. Med.* 1910;6:28-120.

Maranon G, Bonilla E. 1920. Histoire clinique et autopsie d'un cas d'obésité mortelle. *Rev. neurolog.* 1920;27:909-914.

Martin, R. *Lehrbuch der Anthropologie.* 1914;xvi.

Meeh K. Volummessungen des menschlichen Körpers und siener einzelnen Theile in den verschiedenen Alterstufen. *Ztsch. f. Biol.* 1895;31: 125-147.

Mies J. Über die Masse, den Rauminhalt und die Dichte des Menschen. Virchow's Arch. f. path. *Anat. u. Physiol.* 1889;157.

von Noorden C. Obesity. In: von Noorden C. *Metabolism and Practical Medicine.* London: Heinemann. 1907;III: 693-715.

Price GE. Adiposis dolorosa. *Amer. Jour. Med. Sci.* 1909;137: 705-715.

Rubner M. Die Gesetze des Energieverbrauchs bei der Ernährung. Leipzig & Wien. *F. Deuticke.* 1902.

Sinclair J. *History of Shorthorn Cattle.* London: Vinton; 1907.

Worthington LS. *De l'obésité, étiologie, thérapeutique, et hygiène.* Paris: Martinet; 1875.

Hereditary Biological Research

Otmar von Verschuer

Introduction

Those who are presently at the focus of the human heredity teachings for standard twin research have entered a phase that would perhaps be labeled as "critical reaction." In opposition to the original results, above all those of Siemens (1924a), which strongly oppose some elements of current opinion, are voices which have grown louder [Meirowsky (1924a, 1926b), J Bauer (1924), Leven (1924 a,b,c,e)], that raise serious methodological objections. Further advances in twin research can therefore only be achieved if we at once critically illuminate the biological foundations of twinship (formation and diagnosis of single-egg twins, questions of hereditary similarity and asymmetry) in the light of the latest research, in addition to seeking to enrich our knowledge through the most extensive research of twins possible. This double purpose shall serve the following task.

II. Twin Anthropology.

1. Anthropological Measurements.

In preparation for the anthropometric investigation of twins, I have suggested the calculation of deviation by percent and explained its advantages over the calculation of the correlation coefficients. The percent of deviation is obtained by calculating, for each pair of twins, the deviation of a measurement from the mean value as a percentage of the latter. The number thus obtained is the percent of deviation of the relevant pair of twins for the measurement. The middle value of the percent of deviation of a measurement, in a complete study of twins, is the middle percent of deviation (ε_E for MZ and ε_Z for DZ). It can be used as an expression of the difference of a measurement in comparison to another and to compare the variability of the same measurement in different groups. The calculation of the mean error of the mean percent of deviation can, as I have reasoned, follow the formula

$$f\varepsilon = \frac{\varepsilon}{\sqrt{2n}}$$

in the course of which ε stands for the mean percent of deviation and *n* stands for the number of twin pairs. The variability of body proportions in twins can be expressed in the same manner through the mean index of deviation.

Scheidt (1925a) compares groups of twins by how often the measurement differences for the relevant pairs of twins exceeds the probable false measurements. Through an adequate amount of data, one can receive in this manner enlightenment as to how often two groups of MZ and DZ twins in their body measurements agree within the margin for error and are respectively different. Alternately, if we want to determine the level of similarity in respect to differences in twin groups, in regard to any mixture, then the correlation may allow the calculation, or, due to its greater simplicity, the calculation of the mean percent of deviation may be given preference. It must be conceded that the difference between the twins' measurements is in part due to errors in measurement. Although I sought to limit such errors to the greatest possible minimum, so that I took each single measurement of the twins consecutively, the margin necessarily lies on the certainty of the measuring instruments).

The variability of the anthropological measurements and indices in the case of MZ twins, that I previously discussed, comes forward today with the reasonably greater material followed by the smaller mean errors; their difference for the single measurements in respect to the indices are more meaningful.

An excerpt from (Hereditary Biological Research) *Die Verebungsbiologische Zwillingsforschung. Ihre Biologischen Grundlagen.* Mit 18 Abbildungen. Ergebnisse der Inneren Medizin und Kinderheilkunde. Verlag Von Julius Springer: Berlin; 1927:31:35-120.

Reprinted with permission from Springer-Verlag Publishing Co., Postfach 10 52 80, D-69042, Heidelberg, Germany.

Translated by Scott R. Houghton, Baton Rouge, LA.

Editor's Note: The introduction and the section on anthropological measurements from von Verschuer's paper are translations. Relevant tables have also been edited and included. For more details, readers may wish to consult the original paper.

Special thanks to Judy Roberts of the Pennington Information Center for help in acquiring this document.

Table 6. The variability of the anthropological measurements of twins.

figure	single egg twins		same gender double egg twins	
	n	$\varepsilon_E \pm f_\varepsilon$	n	$\varepsilon_Z \pm f_\varepsilon$
Body weight	80	2.58 ± 0.20	38	4.56 ± 0.52
Body size	91	0.62 ± 0.05	43	1.55 ± 0.17
Length of the front torso	80	0.93 ± 0.07	34	1.80 ± 0.22
Shoulder span	87	0.77 ± 0.06	40	2.03 ± 0.23
Span of the iliac crests	83	1.19 ± 0.09	38	2.19 ± .025
Length of right arm	88	0.59 ± 0.04	40	2.04 ± 0.23
Length of right hand	87	0.63 ± 0.05	42	1.73 ± 0.19
Width of right hand	77	0.69 ± 0.06	41	1.70 ± 0.19
Length of right leg	80	0.70 ± 0.06	38	1.67 ± 0.19
Length of right foot	85	0.75 ± 0.06	40	1.95 ± 0.22
Width of right foot	69	0.43 ± 0.04	40	1.95 ± 0.22
Circumference of the neck	82	1.27 ± 0.10	42	1.75 ± 0.19
Circumference of the chest in normal breathing	74	1.03 ± 0.09	39	2.10 ± 0.24
Waist circumference	65	1.18 ± 0.10	36	2.11 ± 0.25
Horizontal circumference of head	91	0.62 ± 0.05	43	1.41 ± 0.15
Ear height of head	88	0.66 ± 0.05	42	2.00 ± 0.22
Height of whole head	90	0.62 ± 0.05	42	1.35 ± 0.15
Morphological face height	88	0.51 ± 0.04	43	1.71 ± 0.18
Greatest length of head	92	0.90 ± 0.07	43	1.70 ± 0.18
Greatest width of head	93	0.91 ± 0.07	43	1.58 ± 0.17
Cheekbone width	93	0.73 ± 0.05	43	1.70 ± 0.18
Angle of lower jaw	93	0.69 ± 0.05	43	1.75 ± 0.19
Height of nose	91	0.39 ± 0.03	43	1.84 ± 0.20
Width of nose	91	0.64 ± 0.05	43	1.86 ± 0.20
Width of mouth opening	91	0.74 ± 0.06	42	2.68 ± 0.29
Physiognomical length of ears	92	0.73 ± 0.05	43	4.43 ± 0.48
Physiognomical width of ears	92	0.54 ± 0.04	43	2.14 ± 0.23

Explanation : n = number of twin pairs. ε_E =mean percent of deviation of single egg twins. ε_Z =mean percent of deviation for double egg twins. f_ε=mean error of the mean percent of deviation.

The mean percent of deviation of DZ twins is shown in Table 6. The difference between the two columns is noteworthy.

The measurements from members of the same sex DZ solely would be used, and here the environmental proportion with our DZ are generally just as in agreement as with MZ, the great physical differences of DZ can only be explained through their hereditary differences. In the single measurements, the comparison of the mean percent of deviation of DZ (ε_Z) is very different from that of MZ (ε_E) : while, for example, for the length/width index of the head, the difference of the two values is one less, and for the body weight, pelvic width and neck circumferences, ε_Z is almost twice as great as ε_E, and ε_Z in respect to ι_Z for the body size, arm length, and ear index, is almost three times as great as ε_E in respect to i_E. This difference is conditional through differences in the paratypical and the genotypical variability. When a feature is subject to strong influence from its environment, then it will more often be different for MZ than a lesser variable feature. On the other hand, it is conceivable that, as for DZ, the concerned second feature is genotypically just as different, the paravariable feature could be more similar than the lesser variable, namely when stronger external influences have an effect on the two features in the same aspect.

I would like to illustrate an example of this: from a double-egged pair of twins, I has the hereditary disposition to greater body size and thicker layers of fat, and II has the hereditary disposition to smaller body size and thin layers of fat. The body weight (fat layers) are more variable than the body sizes. When both twins are allowed to be reared under the same external nutritional conditions, one would expect that the phenotypical development of the body size would not be influenced in the measurement; as with the body weights. Therefore, with I the tendency for thicker fat layers will be more obstructed than the tendency for greater body size, while with II the case is already conditional through the hereditary tendency for small body size and thinness. The result will be that the difference, by percent, of body size through the conditionally similar genotypical differences of the twins, will therefore be larger than in the case of body weight.

The differentials between the mean percent of deviations with DZ and MZ may be caused, although only predominantly, by differences in the genotypical variability of the single measurements. Various distinct genotypical predisposition probably also results in distinct variability. The extent of similar environmental effects of the hereditary mixtures of a double-egg pair of twins does not therefore need to be the same, as we generally accept in cases of single-egg pairs of twins.

The values of the mean percent of deviation with DZ depends, in large measure, upon the genotypical structure of the population, from which the twins came. Therefore, for a racially homogeneous population, the mean percent of deviation for DZ and for the hereditary characteristic, would be smaller than for a population with a strong racial mixture

In the population of Sweden, for example, that is for the most part a pure northern race, we would expect a lower average difference in body size or eye color

Table 8. Number of twins with a difference that is greater than their average amount of variability (greater than ε_E in respect to i_E).

	for MZ in %	for DZ in %
Body weight	33	69
Body size	39	79
Torso length	38	59
Arm length	36	80
Leg length	38	74
Shoulder width	41	78
Chest circumference	37	64
Length/width index of the head	44	49
Morphological face index	35	74

between two-egg twins than that for a mixed population in a modern metropolis. Our following explanation, therefore, is valid only for the Swabian population of Tubingen and the surrounding areas, where for the most part, our twins come from.

One can almost grasp the relationship between paratypically and genotypically associated proportions of variability if one proceeds following the given procedures of Lenz and von Verschuer (1926) (Method 1): The values of the percent of deviation of complete twins separated into MZ and DZ, will be ordered into variation classes, according to increasing percent of deviations, in the row of variation. The rows of variation and DZ will be converted into a numeric scale, with the highest being 100, and written one under another. By our requirements, the hereditary equalities of single-egg twins are portrayed according to the row of the percent of deviation of the MZ tvariability. We want to indicate this row as variations row, or *P*-Row (P_1, P_2, P_3 ... P_n). Three rows of the percent of deviation for DZ is alternately developed through typical and genotypical variability. Therefore, we designate this row as total variation row, or *G*-Row for short (G_1, G_2, G_3 ... G_n). As each singular value for *P*- and *G*-rows must correspond to the size of their percent of deviation, we must accordingly multiply them with the average percent of deviation of their variation class. (ε_1, ε_2, ε_3 ... ε_n).

The quotient of the sum of the products $P \cdot \varepsilon$ and $G \cdot \varepsilon$ indicates the proportion of the environment to the variability of DZ. We obtain therefore the following formula :

$$Q = \frac{P_1\varepsilon_1 + P_2 \cdot \varepsilon_2 + P_3\varepsilon_3 + \cdots P_n\varepsilon_n}{G_1\varepsilon_1 + G_2\varepsilon_2 + G_3\varepsilon_3 + G_n\varepsilon_n} = \frac{\Sigma P\varepsilon}{\Sigma G\varepsilon}$$

With encouragement from Lenz (1926b), I have in addition tried out the following modifications of the method:

1. (Method 2.) One adds together all distinctions (in this case deviations) of MZ according to their absolute value and divides by the number of pairs. Correspondingly one proceeds as for DZ. Then divide the mean difference (in this case deviation) of MZ through that of DZ and so directly obtain the proportion of the environment in the form of an actual fraction and respectively, when multiplied by 100, in percent.

2. (Method 3) One divides the mean percent of deviation of MZ directly through that of DZ.

For the indices, the three methods do not come into consideration, because as proportional numbers, they need not be expressed in terms of percent. By the

Table 9. The variability of the twins in alike and different environments.

	same environment	different environment
Single egg twins :		
Mean percent of deviation of body weight	1.39 ± 0.16	3.60 ± 0.41
" " " " " body size	0.52 ± 0.06	0.72 ± 0.08
" " " " " chest circumference	0.66 ± 0.08	1.43 ± 0.17
Mean deviation of arm length as a percent of body size	0.20 ± 0.02	0.25 ± 0.03
Mean deviation of leg length as a percent of body size	0.16 ± 0.02	0.23 ± 0.03
Mean deviation of chest circumference as a percent of shoulder width	0.57 ± 0.06	0.92 ± 0.11
Mean deviation of the length/width index of the head	1.05 ± 0.11	0.99 ± 0.11
Mean deviation of the height/width index of the nose	0.26 ± 0.03	0.82 ± 0.09
Mean deviation of the physiognomical ear index	0.39 ± 0.04	0.66 ± 0.07
Double egg twins :		
Mean percent of deviation of the body weight	4.70 ± 0.71	4.20 ± 0.80

Table 10. The variability of single egg twins of the same and different occupations.

	same occupation	different occupation
Mean percent of deviation for bodyweight	1.89 ± 0.31	4.50 ± 0.68
" " " " " body size	0.47 ± 0.08	0.82 ± 0.11
" " " " " chest circumference	0.91 ± 0.17	1.57 ± 0.25
Mean deviation of arm length as a percent of body size	0.24 ± 0.04	0.25 ± 0.03
Mean deviation of leg length as a percent of body size	0.11 ± 0.02	0.25 ± 0.04
Mean deviation of pelvic width as a percent of shoulder width	0.73 ± 0.13	0.75 ± 0.11
Mean deviation of the length/width index of the head	1.01 ± 0.16	0.88 ± 0.12
" " " the height/width index of the nose	0.63 ± 0.10	0.77 ± 0.10
" " " physiognomical ear index	0.28 ± 0.05	0.74 ± 0.10

absolute amounts, the values are calculated through the other two methods. This has a connection to the fact that the average age of MZ (19 years) in our material is higher than that of DZ (13 years); the variability (especially of the body weights) is greater in the higher age groups than in the lower ones. Moreover, the absolute body size increases with age, just as the absolute deviations do. Therefore, the mean deviation of body weight for MZ, for example, is 1.27kg (middle value for body weight 49kg), and for DZ is 1.51 kg (middle value .33kg); for the body size the mean deviation for MZ is 8.4 mm (middle value 153), for DZ is 20mm (mean value 129cm). From this it emerges that Method 2 is only applicable for data of the same approximate age and type in the calculation of the ratio of the environment to the variability.

Twins live mostly under very similar environmental conditions; for this reason the ratio of the environment is a smaller cause for differences between them than for other people. Only a few physical features (i.e., skull structure) can be accepted for twins (especially for MZ) as special intrauterine developmental conditions for greater variability than in other people. On the other hand it must not be forgotten that two-egg twins are different in their hereditary amounts at a maximum average of 50%. Therefore, for people who are in no way related, that are in great measure, as DZ, genetically different, their physical differences for the most part are based on their different hereditary dispositions.

The fore-mentioned numbers give us an approximate support for how broad a distinction is caused between two-egg twins on the average by hereditary disposition and environment. In order to formulate the generally operative ratio between hereditary disposition and environment for the phenotypical arrangement of the human body, a comparison of these results with the correlation of the body measurements between levels of relationships, as they were determined by Pearson, is most urgently necessary. The investigation concerning the variability of the human body, which we possess, for example, concerning the effects of war, specific occupations, and physical exercises on human physical development, must also be taken into account. While these two methods of research are only able to portray one side (the genotypical or the phenotypical) of the physical variability, the twins method is referred to as the connecting middle ground in development. If we compare the results of the different methods, then we will finally arrive at secured knowledge of the forming of the human body through hereditary disposition and environment.

One can assess the level of heritability or non-heritability of a feature, and then also how often the feature

Table 11. The influence the differences in birth weight have on the later variability in twins.

	birth weight differences under 250g	birth weight differences over 250g
Single egg twins :		
Mean percent of deviation of body weight	1.85 ± 0.31	2.50 ± 0.44
" " " " of body size	0.50 ± 0.08	0.80 ± 0.13
" " " the length/width index of the head	1.10 ± 0.17	0.90 ± 0.14
Double egg twins :		
Mean percent of deviation of body weight	2.90 ± 0.73	6.40 ± 1.50

Table 12. The variability of twins according to different ages.

	21/2 years	11-20 years	21-64 years
Single egg twins :			
Mean percent of deviation of body weight		1.78 ± 0.19	3.51 ± 0.41
Mean percent of deviation of arm length		0.61 ± 0.06	0.55 ± 0.06
Mean percent of deviation of pelvic width		1.07 ± 0.11	1.34 ± 0.16
Mean percent of deviation of chest circumference		0.70 ± 0.08	1.51 ± 0.19
Mean percent of deviation of head circumference		0.54 ± 0.05	0.72 ± 0.08
Mean percent of deviation of head length		0.90 ± 0.09	0.89 ± 0.10
Mean percent of deviation of head width		0.91 ± 0.09	0.89 ± 0.10
Mean percent of deviation of cheekbone width		0.58 ± 0.06	0.91± 0.10
Mean deviation of arm lengths as a percent of body size		0.23 ± 0.02	0.22 ± 0.02
Mean deviation of leg length as a percent of body size		0.20 ± 0.02	0.19 ± 0.02
Mean deviation of chest circumference as a percent of body size		0.35 ± 0.04	0.72 ± 0.09
Mean deviation of pelvic width as a percent of shoulder width		0.75 ± 0.08	0.71 ± 0.08
Mean deviation of the length/width index of the head		1.08 ± 0.11	0.90 ± 0.10
Mean deviation of the height/width index of the nose		0.39 ± 0.04	0.68 ± 0.08
Mean deviation of the physiognomical ear index		0.46 ± 0.05	0.57 ± 0.06
Double egg twins :			
Mean percent of deviation of body weight	3.30 ± 0.59	5.00 ± 0.83	—

is equally different for MZ and for DZ. This discovery easily concerns alternative features, and on the other hand is difficult with body measurements or proportions. I would like to retain two indices, with twins for alikeness (or difference), when their difference is smaller (larger) than the average amount of variability (ε_E in respect to i_E). In isolated cases this requirement is not always applicable, but with larger numbers it is indeed usable. I would prefer to give preference, however, to the above given calculation of the ratio of the environment to the variability.

In following I would like to investigate the general variability of twins in different environmental conditions for a few particular measurements.

We begin with the variability of the twins for different general environments. In this case two groups are formed. The first includes all twins, for which no environmental differences of any kind can be determined, or in other words having been born with the same birth weights and nourished in the same manner, always in the same village and lived in the same house, and participated in the same activities. The second group would include all twins for whom that anamnesis results in all sorts of differences. As we would expect, the general difference of the second group of MZ (ε_E in respect to i_E) is greater than those in the first group. In general, therefore, the physical variability of MZ is a function of the environment. When we observe, along with the corresponding values of DZ, then we see that these differences are not so distinct here.

The establishment of the effects of specific environmental influences is possible only through studies of a great deal of twin research. At any rate, we can come to interpretation through our investigation of the differences of variability in the similar and different careers of twins. For this, only certain twins were sought after, those who have finished with their schooling and have been in their career fields for at least one year, or, in other words, who are 14-15 years old. Under these requirements, 19 MZ pairs have the same careers and 27 have different careers. The same average index of deviation of the two groups is what I would like to bring in connection, with the smallness of the data and the absent differences in the skull measurements; in any case, no influences on body proportions through different career work can be provisionally determined from that data.

In order to assess the influence of birth weights on the altered development of the twins, the variability of the pair of twins with a birth weight difference, which was under 250g, would be compared to the one for pairs of twins who had a birth weight difference of 250g and above (Tab. 11). For MZ it shows a difference between these two groups just about as great a difference as for the two environmental groups. The conditions for DZ are also similar to the above. The intrauterine living conditions, as far as they are expressed in different birth weights, also appear in MZ to have an effect later in life.

When the physical variability of MZ is a function of the environment, then one would expect that the difference would increase with age. For that reason, the twins were broken up into three age groups: 2 1/2 - 10 years, 11 - 20 years, and 21 - 64 years. When we compare ε_E and i_E of the three groups to each other, (Table 12), then we see that the values gradually increase, which means that the average difference increases with age. We also find an increase of the average difference in DZ. In comparison the single measurements of MZ were depicted in only two groups of 2 1/2 - 16 years and of 17 years. For DZ, of the initial age groups that were left, only the third group was neglected due to small numbers.

The existing explanations stretch themselves solely across the variability in general, which as average of difference of all measurements in respect to indices would be calculated. The size of the investigated material allows us to consider the variability of singular amounts and indices closely. As an example, I would like to pick out the body weight, body size, and length/width index of the skull. The rest is presented on Tables 9-12.

The body weight stands with a mean percent of deviation of 2.6 by far at the peak of most of the variable amounts. On Tables 9-12 of investigated variability (environment, occupation, birth weight, age, gender) a difference is shown that greatly exceeds the extent of the averages. For example, in different environments- the difference between MZ is twice as large, and the difference of the body weight is more than twice as large. Every investigation confirms that the body weight is more dependent of the environment than the average of the researched amounts. When we investigate the two environmental groups of DZ twins, we find no detectable connection between environmental differences and body weight differences. The difference of the body weights of DZ increase with age and the differences in birth weights.

The body size belongs to the measurements with slight typical variability in MZ. It takes on accordingly in a somewhat weaker form the general differences of those on Tables 9-12 of the investigated variability. Only by age is the proportion reversed: the older twins are certainly within the middle margins for error; somewhat more closely related to body size than the younger twins. The cause here appears to lie in the growth rates, which again evens out after the conclusion of the rapid growth rate. In order to test this assumption more closely, I have begun with post-operative research situated in the growth rate age of twins.

The length and width and the length/width index of the skull belongs to the variable measurements of MZ. As for the cause here, Siemens and I have accepted only for twins the proper intrauterine conditions. Our renewed investigation gives us a further verification in that favor: with different environment and occupation, with different birth weight and with increasing age, the difference in the brain skull does not increase, in fact the values are somewhat smaller, at least within the middle of the margins for error. That speaks at once in favor that those other measurements of existing general cause of paravariability for the skull either do not or almost do not apply, and that it is a feature that in the later years of life is only a bit altered through environmental influences. It must consequently be that the established alteration of the skull develops already before the age of our youngest twins. From our findings about twins, the results show that presumably only during the fetal and infanthood periods, probably before bone covering of the fontanelle, can environmental influences cause the transformation of the skull.

CLASSICS IN OBESITY

Memoir on Heat

Read to the Royal Academy of Sciences, 28 June 1783

A-L Lavoisier, PS DeLaplace

This memoir is the result of experiments on heat which we have made together, M. de Laplace and I, in the course of last winter;[1] the moderate cold of that season did not allow us to make more of them. We had first proposed to wait, before publishing anything on this subject, until a colder winter could enable us to repeat them with all possible care, and to make more of them. But we decided to make this work public, although it is very imperfect, because the method that we have used may be of some use in the theory of heat, and because its precision and wide applicability could lead to its adoption by other scientists who, situated in the north of Europe, have winters very favorable for this kind of experiment.

We will divide this memoir into four sections. In the first, we will describe a new way of measuring heat. We will present in the second the results of the chief experiments we have made by this means. In the third, we will examine the conclusions that follow from these experiments. Finally, in the fourth section, we will treat combustion and respiration.

SECTION ONE
Description of a new means of measuring heat

WHATEVER may be the cause that produces the sensation of heat, it is able to increase and decrease; and, from this point of view, it can be treated quantitatively. It does not seem that it occurred to the ancients to measure these relative values, and only in the past century have men conceived of ways of doing so. Starting with the general observation that heat of greater or less intensity perceptibly varies the volume of a body, especially that of fluids, men built instruments capable of measuring changes in volume. Many natural scientists of this century have greatly improved these instruments, either by determining accurately certain fixed points of temperature such as the freezing point and the boiling point of water at a given atmospheric pressure, or by searching for the fluid whose changes in volume come nearest to being proportional to the variations of temperature so that there remains nothing more to wish for, relative to its measurement, except a sure means of determining the extreme degrees.

But the knowledge of the laws that heat follows when it is diffused through bodies is far from that degree of perfection necessary for analyzing the problems relating to the communication of heat and its effects in a system of unequally heated bodies, especially when their mixture breaks them down and forms new compounds. A great number of interesting experiments have been made, which show that, in the change from the solid to the fluid state, and from the fluid to the vapor state, a large quantity of heat is absorbed, either because it is combined in this transformation, or because the capacity of the substance to contain it increases. In addition it has been observed that, at the same temperature, the same volume of different substances does not contain an equal amount of heat, and that among them there are, in this respect, differences independent of their respective densities. Even the relative heat capacities of various substances have been determined; and since even the coldest bodies on the earth's surface are not entirely without heat, some have tried to discover the relations of absolute heat to its changes as shown by readings of the thermometer. But all these estimates, although very ingenious, are based on hypotheses which must be confirmed by a large number of experiments.

Before proceeding further, it is essential to establish precisely what we mean by the terms *free heat, heat capacity* or *specific heat of bodies.*

Scientists are divided about the nature of heat. A number of them think of it as a fluid diffused throughout nature, and by which bodies are more or less permeated according to their temperature and to their special faculty of retaining it.[2] It can combine with them and, in that state, it ceases to act on the thermometer and to pass from one body to another. It is only in the free state, when it can reach equilibrium among bodies, that it constitutes what we call *free heat.*

Lavoisier A-L, DeLaplace PS; Guerlac H, trans. Memoir on Heat. Read to the Royal Academy of Sciences, 28 June 1783. New York: Neale Watson Academic Publications, Inc; 1982.
Reprinted with permission from Watson Publishing Inc., P.O. Box 493, Canton, MA 02021. Special thanks to the Pennington Information Center for help in acquiring this document.

Other scientists think that heat is only the result of the imperceptible motions of the constituent particles of matter. We know that even the most dense bodies are filled with a great number of pores or tiny empty spaces whose volume can considerably exceed that of the matter that they enclose. These empty spaces allow the imperceptible particles to oscillate freely in all directions, and it is natural to think that these particles are in a constant agitation which, if it increases to a certain point, can break them apart and so decompose the bodies. It is this internal motion, according to these scientists we are speaking of, that constitutes heat.[3]

To develop this hypothesis, we shall point out that in all motions where there is no abrupt change, there exists a general law which the mathematicians have called the *principle of the conservation of vis viva*.[4] This law states that in a system of bodies that act on one another in any manner whatsoever, the *vis viva*, that is to say the sum of the products of each mass by the square of the velocity, is constant. If the bodies are acted upon by accelerative forces, the *vis viva* equals what it was at the onset of the motion plus the sum of the masses multiplied by the squares of the velocities due to the action of accelerating forces. In the hypothesis we are considering, heat is the *vis viva* resulting from the imperceptible motions of the constituent particles of a body. It is the sum of the products of the mass of each particle by the square of its velocity.

If you put in contact two bodies whose temperatures are different, the quantities of motion that they communicate to each other will at first be unequal; the *vis viva* of the colder will increase by the same amount as that of the other decreases; and this increase will take place until the quantities of motion communicated from one body to the other are equal. In this state the temperatures of the bodies will have become equal.

This manner of viewing heat easily explains why the direct impact of the sun's rays is undetectable, whereas they still produce a great heat. Their impulse is the product of their mass by their velocity. Now, although this velocity is excessively great, their mass is so small that the product is almost nil, while on the other hand their *vis viva* being the product of mass by the *square* of the velocity, the heat that it represents is very much greater than that of their direct impact. This impact on a white body, which reflects light abundantly, is greater than on a black body, and yet the solar rays communicate less heat to the former, because these rays, on being reflected, carry away their *vis viva*, whereas they communicate it to the black body which absorbs them.[5]

We shall not decide between these two hypotheses. Several phenomena seem favorable to the latter, such as, for example, the heat produced by the friction of two solid bodies. But there are other phenomena that are explained more simply by the first hypothesis. Perhaps both occur simultaneously. Whatever may be the case, since only these two hypotheses about the nature of heat can be devised, we should accept the principles common to both. Now, whichever one we follow, *in a simple mixture of bodies the quantity of free heat remains always the same.* This is evident, if heat is a fluid that tends to reach equilibrium and also if it is only the *vis viva* which results from the internal motion of matter, where the principle in question follows from the conservation of *vires vivae.* The conservation of free heat, in the simple mixture of bodies, is thus independent of any hypothesis about the nature of heat. It has generally been accepted by scientists, and we shall adopt it in the following investigations.

If heat is fluid, it is possible that during the combination of various substances, it combines with them or is evolved from them. Thus nothing indicates *a priori* that the free heat is the same before and after the combination; nothing, moreover, suggests it in the hypothesis that heat is only the *vis viva* of the particles of bodies, for in substances that combine together, acting on one another by virtue of their mutual affinities, their particles are subjected to the action of attractive forces that can alter the amount of their *vis viva*, and, consequently, the amount of heat. But one should accept the following principle as being common to the two hypotheses:

If, in any combination or change of state, there is a decrease in free heat, this heat will reappear completely whenever the substances return to their original state; and conversely, if in the combination or in the change of state there is an increase in free heat, this new heat will disappear on the return of the substances to their original state. This principle, moreover, is confirmed by experiment, and in what follows the detonation of saltpeter[6] will furnish us with visible proof. We can generalize it further, and extend it to all the phenomena of heat, in the following way. *All changes in heat, whether real or apparent, suffered by a system of bodies during a change of state recur in the opposite sense when the system returns to its original state.* Thus the changes of ice into water and of water into vapor cause the thermometer to show the disappearance of a very considerable amount of heat which reappears in the change of water into ice and in condensing the vapors. In general, you can turn the first hypothesis into the second by substituting for the words *free heat, combined heat,* and *evolved heat,* the words *vis viva, loss of vis viva,* and *increase in vis viva.*

Because of our ignorance as to the nature of heat, we can only observe carefully its effects, the chief of which consist in expanding bodies, turning them into fluids, and converting them into vapors. Among these effects we must choose one that is easy to measure and that is proportional to its cause. This effect will represent the heat just as in dynamics we represent force by the product of mass and velocity, although we are ignorant of the nature of the peculiar modification in virtue of which a body reaches successively different points in space. The effect through which we commonly measure heat is the expansion of fluids, and chiefly that of mercury. The expansion of this fluid, according to the interesting experiments of M. de Luc, is very nearly proportional to the heat, throughout the whole interval between the freezing point of ice and the boiling point of water;[7] it can obey another law at more extreme degrees of temperature. We shall indicate in what follows another effect of heat which is always proportional to it, whatever its intensity.

We shall use a mercury thermometer divided into eighty equal parts from the temperature of melting ice to that of boiling water at an atmospheric pressure of 28 inches of mercury. Each division marks a degree, and the origin of the degrees, or the zero of the thermometer, is the melting point of ice, so that the degrees below should be taken as negative. We shall imagine the scale of this thermometer extended indefinitely both below zero and above the boiling point of water, and divided in proportion to the heat. These divisions, which are nearly equal from 0 to 80 degrees, can be markedly unequal in the remote portions of the scale. But in any case each degree will always measure a constant amount of heat.[8]

If one imagines two bodies of equal mass brought to the same temperature, the quantity of heat necessary to raise the temperature by one degree may not be the same for these two bodies. And if one takes as unity the amount of heat which can raise the temperature of a pound of plain water by one degree, it is easy to see that all the other amounts of heat of different bodies can be expressed in terms of that unit. In what follows, we shall mean by *heat capacities*, or *specific heats*, the relative quantities of heat necessary to raise the temperature of equal masses the same number of degrees. These ratios can vary at different temperatures; if for example, the quantities of neat necessary to raise a pound of iron and a pound of mercury from 0 to 1 degree are in the ratio of 3 to 1, the amounts that must be used to raise these same substances from 200 to 201 degrees can be in a larger or smaller ratio. But one can suppose these ratios to be nearly constant from 0 to 80 degrees: at least experiment in this range has not led us to note any sensible difference. It is within this interval that we shall determine the specific heats of various substances.

To determine these quantities we used the following method. Let us consider a pound of mercury at 0 degrees and a pound of water at 34 degrees. On mixing them together, the heat of the water will pass to the mercury, and after a few moments the mixture will take on a uniform temperature. Let us suppose that is 33 degrees, and that in general, in a mixture of several substances which do not react chemically with one another, the quantity of heat always remains the same. According to these assumptions, the amount of heat lost by the water would have raised the temperature of the mercury 33 degrees; whence it follows that, to raise the mercury to a given temperature, there is only required the thirty-third part of the heat necessary to raise water to the same temperature, which is tantamount to saying that the specific heat of mercury is thirty-three times less than that of water.

From this we can infer a general and very simple rule for determining, by the method of mixtures, the specific heat of bodies; for if we call the mass of the warmer body m, expressed in fractions of the pound taken as unity; a the reading of the thermometer indicating its temperature; q the heat necessary to raise the temperature of 1 pound of this substance 1 degree; if one designates by m', a', q' the same quantities for the cooler body, and if finally one denotes by b the temperature of the mixture, when it has become uniform,[9] it is evident that the heat lost by the body m is proportional to the mass m and to the number of degrees $a - b$ by which the temperature has been decreased, multiplied by q, the quantity of heat which can raise the temperature of this substance 1 degree. Thus the expression for this quantity of heat lost will be $m\, q \cdot (a - b)$.

For the same reason, the quantity of heat acquired by the body m' is proportional to the mass m' and to the number of degrees $b - a'$ by which the temperature was increased, multiplied by its quantity q', which gives $m'q' \cdot (b - a')$ for this quantity of heat. But, since we presuppose that after the mixture the quantity of heat is the same as before, we must equate the heat lost by the body m to the heat gained by the body m', whence we obtain

$$m\, q \cdot (a - b) = m'q' \cdot (b - a')$$

This equation does not give the value of q or of q'; but it expresses their ratio as

$$\frac{q}{q} = \frac{m' \cdot (b - a')}{m \cdot (a - b)}$$

So in this manner we will have the ratio of the specific heats of the two bodies m and m', so that, if one compares the different substances in nature with one and the same substance, for example with ordinary water, one will be able by this means to determine the specific heats of these substances in terms of the specific heat of the substance to which we relate them.

This method, in practice, is subject to a large number of disadvantages which can cause appreciable errors in the results. The mixing of substances with very different specific gravities, such as water and mercury, is difficult to carry out so as to be certain that all its parts have the same temperature. Then it is necessary to take into account the heat that is lost to the vessels and to the atmosphere as the mixture reaches a uniform temperature, which requires a delicate computation that is subject to error. By this process, moreover, we cannot compare directly substances that act chemically upon each other. In that case we must compare them to a third substance with which they do not react; and if no such substance exists, we must compare them with two bodies, and even with a greater number, which by multiplying the ratios to be determined with respect to each other multiplies the errors of the results. Moreover, this method would be almost impossible to use to measure the cold or heat produced by chemical combinations, and it is absolutely inadequate for determining the heat given off in combustion and respiration. Since observing these phenomena is the most interesting part of the theory of heat, we have thought that a method capable of measuring them with percision would be of great use in this theory, since, without its aid, one could only formulate hypotheses concerning their cause which would be impossible to confirm by experiment. Because of this we decided to take up this problem first of all, and we shall now set forth the method we have arrived at and the train of thought that led us to it.

If you convey a mass of ice, cooled down to any degree whatever, into an atmosphere whose temperature is above zero, all its parts will be affected by the heat of the atmosphere until their temperature reaches zero. In this last state, the heat of the atmosphere will stop at the surface of the ice without being able to reach the interior. It will serve only to melt a first layer of ice, which will absorb it on turning into water. A thermometer placed in this layer will remain at the same temperature, and the only perceptible effect of the heat will be the transformation of the ice into a fluid. When afterwards the ice receives more heat, a new layer will melt and thus will absorb all the heat imparted to it. Because of this continued melting of the ice, all the interior parts of its mass will arrive successfully at the surface, and it is only here that they will begin to experience again the influence of the heat of the surrounding bodies.

Let us now imagine a hollow sphere of ice at zero degrees placed in an atmosphere whose temperature is above zero, and inside of which we place a body warmed to a given temperature. It follows from what we have just said that the external heat will not penetrate into the cavity of the sphere, and that the heat of the body will not be lost to the outside, and will stop at the interior surface of the cavity, of which it will continue to melt new layers, until the temperature of this body has reached zero. There is no reason to fear that the melting of the interior ice will be due to other causes than the heat lost by the thickness of the ice that separates it from the atmosphere. For the same reason, we can be confident that all the heat of the body, on being dissipated, is stopped by the interior ice and serves only to melt it. So if, when the temperature of the body has reached zero, we carefully collect the water enclosed in the cavity of the sphere, its weight will be exactly proportional to the heat that this body will have lost in passing from its original temperature to that of melting ice, for it is clear that double the amount of heat must melt twice as much ice. The quantity of melted ice, therefore, is a very accurate measure of the heat used to produce this effect[10].

Now nothing is simpler than the measurement of the phenomena connected with heat. Do you wish, for example, to know the specific heat of a solid body? You will raise its temperature a certain number of degrees, afterward placing it inside the sphere we have just metioned. You will leave it there until its temperature is reduced to zero, and you will collect the water produced by its cooling. This quantity of water, divided by the product of the mass of the body and the number of degrees its original temperature was above zero, will be proportional to its specific heat.

As to fluids, you will enclose them in vessels whose heat capacities you will be careful to determine, and the procedure will be the same as for solids, except that to obtain the amounts of water due to cooling the fluids, you must subtract from the amounts of water collected those which the vessels will have produced.

Do you wish to determine the heat given off in the chemical combination of different substances? You will bring them all, as well as the vessel which is to contain them, to a given temperature of zero. Then you will put their mixture inside the sphere of ice, being careful to keep it there until its temperature reaches zero. The amount of water collected in this experiment will measure the heat given off.

To measure the cold produced in certain reactions, as in the solution of salts, you will raise each of the substances to the same temperature, which we shall designate by m degrees. Afterwards you will mix them in the interior of the sphere, and you will observe the quantity of ice melted by cooling the mixture to zero. Let a be this quantity. To determine the number of degrees by which the temperature of the substances is lowered by their mixture below[11] their original temperature m, you will raise the temperature of this mixture by a certain number of degrees m', and you will determine the quantity of ice melted on cooling to zero. Let a' be this quantity. This granted, since to a quantity a' of melted ice there corresponds a temperature m' of the mixture, it is clear that the quantity a' of melted ice should correspond a temperature equal to am'/a'. This, then, is the temperature that results from the mixture of substances raised to the temperature m; accordingly on subtracting it from m, you will have $(a'm-am')/a'$ for the number of degrees of cold produced by the mixture.

We know that bodies in passing from the solid to the liquid state absorb heat and that in returning from the liquid to the solid state they restore it to the atmosphere and to the surrounding bodies. To determine it, let m be the temperature at which a body begins to melt. After being warmed to the temperature $m-n$, and then placed in the interior of the sphere, on cooling to zero it will melt a quantity of ice that we shall designate by a. After being warmed to the temperature $m+n'$, it will melt, on cooling, a quantity of ice we shall designate by a'; finally, when heated to the temperature $m+n''$, it will melt as it cools an amount of ice we shall call a''. This granted, $a''-a'$ will be the amount of ice that can be melted by the fluid body on cooling from n"–n' degrees. Whence it follows that in cooling by n' degrees it will melt a quantity of ice equal to

$$\frac{n' \cdot (a'' - a')}{n'' - n'}$$

Likewise we will find that the body, on cooling m degrees in the solid state, will melt the quantity of ice $ma/m-n$; so designating by x the quantity of ice that can be melted by the heat given off in changing from the fluid to the solid state, we will have, fot the total quantity of ice that should be melted by the body heated to $m+n'$ degrees,

$$\frac{n' \cdot (a'' - a')}{n'' - n'} + x + \frac{ma}{m - n}$$

the first term of this expression being due to the heat given off by the body before it passes into the solid state; the second term being the effect of the heat given off during this change of state, the third term being due to the heat lost by the solid body on being cooled to zero. If we equate the preceding quantity to the quantity a' of melted ice, we will have

$$\frac{n' \cdot (a'' - a')}{n'' - n'} + x + \frac{ma}{m - n} = a'$$

whence we derive

$$x = \frac{n''a' - n'a''}{n'' - n'} - \frac{ma}{m - n}$$

For precise results, it is advantageous to make n and n' very small.

Not only will this experiement give the value of x; in addition we will have the specific heats of the body in its two states of solidity and fluidity, since we know the quantities of ice that it can melt in these two states on cooling a given number of degrees.

To find the heat developed by combustion and respiration is no more difficult. You will burn the combustible bodies in the interior of the sphere. You let animals respire there. But, since the renewal of the air is indispensable in these two operations, it will be necessary to establish some communication between the interior of the sphere and the atmosphere surrounding it. And, so that the introduction of fresh air will not cause any perceptible error, it is necessary to perform these experiments at a temperature differeing only slightly from zero or at least to lower to this temperature the air you introduce.

The investigation of the specific heats of different gases[12] is more difficult because of thier low density; for, if you were content to enclose them in vessels like the other fluids, the amount of ice melted would be so small that the result of the experiment would become extremely unreliable. But if you place in the interior of the sphere a tube bent into a spiral[13] and send through the tube a stream of some sort of air, and then by means of two thermometers placed in this stream, one where it enters the sphere, the other where it leaves it, you measure the number of degrees by which the air is cooled during its transit, you can cool in this manner a considerable mass of the air and determine with percision its specific heat. The same method may be used to determine the amount of heat given off during the condensation of the vapors of different fluids.

You see, by the detail with which we have described matters, that the preceding method extends to all phenomena in which there is the production or absorption of heat. In these different cases you can always determine the quantities of heat that are produced or absorbed, and relate them to a common unit, for example, to the heat necessary to raise the temperature of a pound of water from 0 to 80 degrees; in this way you can determine and compare with each other the quantities of heat produced by the combination of oil of vitriol[14] with water, of the latter with quicklime, of quicklime with nitric acid, etc.; and those given off in the combustion of phosphorus, sulfur, carbon, pyrophore,[15] etc., in the detonation of saltpeter, in the respiration of animals, etc., all of which was impossible by the methods known up to now.

We have considered a sphere of ice only in order to make better understood the method we have used. It would be very difficult to obtain such spheres, but we have replaced them by means of the following device.

Figure I of Plate I represents a perspective view of this apparatus; Figure 3 shows a horizontal section; the vertical section, in Plate II, Figure I, shows its interior, which is divided into three parts. To make matters clearer, we shall distinguish them by the terms *inner space, middle space,* and *external space.* The inner space *ffff* (Figs. I and 3, Plate II) is a basket of iron wire held up by a few supports of the same metal. It is in this space that we place the bodies to be experimented upon. The upper part *LM* is closed by means of a lid *HG* separately shown (Plate II, Fig. 2); it is entirely open above, and the bottom is formed by a lattice of iron wire.

The middle space *bbbb* (Fig. I, Plate II) is intended to hold the ice which is to surround the inner space and be melted by the heat from the body in the experiment. This ice is supported and held in place by a screen *mm*, under which is a sieve *nn*; each is shown separately (Plate II, Figs. 4 and 5). As the ice is melted by the heat of the body put in the inner space, the water flows through the screen and the sieve; then it falls along the cone *ccd* (Plate II, Fig. I) and the tube *xy*, and is collected in the vessel *P* placed below the apparatus; *k* is a stopcock by means of which you can stop at will the outflow of the water from the inner space. Finally, the external space *aaaaa* is intended to hold the ice which is to block the effect of the heat from the atmosphere and surrounding bodies. The water produced by the melting of this ice flows along the tube *ST*, which can be opened or closed by means of the stopcock *r*. The entire apparatus is covered by the lid *FG* (Plate I, Fig. 2) fully opened at the top and closed at the bottom. It is made of tin covered with oil paint to insure it against rust.

To use it for an experiment, you fill with crushed ice the middle space and the cover *HG* of the inner space, the external space and the cover *FG* of the whole apparatus. Then you drain out the interior ice (thus we call the ice which is enclosed in the middle space and its cover, and which we must be careful to crush thoroughly and to press stongly into the apparatus). When it is sufficiently drained, you open the apparatus to place in it the body you wish to experiment upon, and close it again immediately. You wait until the body has completely cooled down and until the apparatus is sufficiently drained. Then weigh the water collected in the vessel *P*. Its weight exactly measures the heat given off by the body; for it is evident that the body is just as if it were in the center of the sphere of which we have just spoken, since all its heat is stopped by the interior ice, and since this ice is protected from any other source of heat by the ice enclosed in the lid and in the exterior space.

Experiments of this kind last fifteen, eighteen or twenty hours. Sometimes to speed them up, we place well-drained ice in the inner space, and cover with it the body we wish to cool down.

Figure 4 of Plate I shows a pail of sheet-iron intended to hold the body on which we wish to experiment; it is furnished with a lid *ab*, having a hole in the center and closed with a cork stopper pierced by the tube of a small thermometer.

Figure 5 of Plate I represents a round-bottomed flask whose stopper is pierced by the tube *cd* of the little thermometer *rs*. It is necessary to use flasks of this sort whenever one works with acids and, in general, with all substances that can react in any way with metals.

T (Fig. 6, Plate I) is a shallow hollow cylinder placed at the bottom of the inner space to support the round-bottomed flasks.

It is essential in this apparatus that there be no communication between the middle space and the external space, which can be easily tested by filling the external space with water. If there were a connection between these spaces, the ice melted by the atmosphere, whose heat acts on the envelope of the external space, could pass into the middle space, and then the water that runs out of that last space would no longer measure the heat lost by the body experimented upon.

When the temperature of the atmosphere is above zero, its heat can reach the middle space only with difficulty, because it is stopped by the ice of the lid and of the exterior space; but if the exterior temperature were below zero, the atmosphere could cool down the interior ice. It is therefore essential to experiment in an atmosphere whose temperature is not below zero; thus, in freezing weather, you must place the apparatus in a room you have been careful to warm. It is also necessary that the ice used not be below zero; in that case, it is necessary to crush it, spread it in very thin layers, and keep it thus for some time in a place where the temperature is above zero.

The interior ice always retains a small amount of water adhering to its surface, and one might think that this water would affect the result of our experiments; but it should be noted that at the beginning of each experiment the ice has already absorbed all the water that it can retain in this manner, so that, if a small portion of the ice melted by the body still adheres to the interior ice, the same quantity, or very nearly, of the water originally adhering to the surface of the ice should separate from it and flow into the vessel *P*, for the surface area of the interior ice changes very little during the experiment.

Whatever precautions we took, we found it impossible to prevent the outside air from penetrating the inner space. When the temperature is about 9 or 10 degrees, the air enclosed in this space has a greater specific gravity than the air outside; it flows out through the tube *xy*, and it is replaced by the outside air that enters through the upper part of the apparatus, and which gives up a part of its heat to the interior ice. There is thus produced in the contrivance a flow of air that is swifter when the outside temperature is greater, and this steadily melts the interior ice. To a large degree we can suppress the effect of this air flow by closing the stopcock *k*, but it is much better not to experiment except when the external temperature is no greater than 3 or 4 degrees, for we have noticed that then the melting of the interior ice, due to the atmosphere, is imperceptible. Thus at this temperature we can answer for the accuracy of our experiments on the specific heats of bodies close to 1 part in 40, and even 1 part in 60, if the room temperature is only 1 to 2 degrees.

We have had made two calorimeters[16] similar to that we have just described. One of them is intended for experiments in which it is not necessary to renew the interior air. The other apparatus is used in experiments in which the renewal of the air is absolutely necessary, such as those on combustion and on respiration. This second apparatus only differs from the first in that the two lids are each pierced by two holes through which pass two small tubes that provide a connection between the interior air and the atmosphere outside; by their means we can blow atmospheric air onto combustible substances. These tubes are shown in Figure 2 of Plate I.

We shall now describe the results of the chief experiments we have made with these devices (*b*).

(*b*) Since reading this memoir we have seen, in a very interesting paper by M. Vilke [*sic*] on heat, printed in the Stockholm Mémoires for the year 1781, that this learned scientist had the idea before we did of using the snow melted by bodies to measure their heat. But the difficulty of collecting the water produced by melting snow; the considerable time that bodies require to lose their heat in this fashion, and which according to our experiments can be twelve hours and even more; the heat that the snow receives in this period of time from the atmosphere and from the other bodies that surround it: all these reasons forced him to abandon this method and to resort to the method of mixutes, because he did not attempt to surround the snow which the bodies were supposed to melt with an external layer of snow or ice, to protect it from the heat of the atmosphere. It is in this external envelope that the chief advantage of our calorimeters consists, an advantage that made it possible for us to measure until now, such as the heat evolved in combustion and respiration. Moreover, in these experiments ice is preferable to snow.

SECTION FOUR

On combustion and respiration

Until very recently we had only vague and very imperfect ideas concerning the phenomena of the heat that is given off in combustion and in respiration. Experiment had taught us that bodies cannot burn or animals breathe without the participation of atmospheric air; but we did not know the way in which it influenced these two great processes of nature, and the changes they made it undergo. The most commonly held opinion attributed to this fluid no other functions than that of cooling the blood as it passes through the lungs, and by its pressure retaining the matter of fire at the surface of combustible bodies. The important discoveries made only a few years ago on the nature of aeriform fluids have greatly enlarged our knowledge of this subject[32]. It results from these discoveries that only a single kind of air, known by the names *dephlogisticated air, pure air*, or *vital air* is fitted for combustion, respiration, and the calcination of metals; that it makes up only about a fourth part of atmospheric air[33], and that this portion of the air is then absorbed, altered, or converted into fixed air by the addition of a principle that, to avoid all discussion concerning its nature, we shall call the *base of fixed air*. Thus air does not act in its operations as a simple mechanical cause but as a principle entering into new combinations. M. Lavoisier, having observed these phenomena, suspected that the heat and light which are given off were due, at least in great part, to the changes which the oxygen gas undergoes. Everything having to do with combustion and respiration is explained so naturally and simply by this hypothesis that he did not hesitate to propose it, if not as a demonstrated truth, at least as a most likely conjecture worthy, in every respect, of the attention of scientists. This is what he did in a Memoir on Combustion, printed in the Academy's volume for the year 1777, page 592 [34]. M. Crawford has offered a somewhat simiar explanation in a work on the same subject published in London in 1779 [35]. These two scientists agree in regarding oxygen gas as the principal source of the heat developed in combustion and respiration. There is however an essential difference between their views, in that M. Lavoisier thinks that the heat givem off in these two phenomena is combined with the oxygen gas, and that this fluid owes its aeriform state to the expansive force of the heat so combined, whereas according to M. Crawford, in the oxygen the matter of heat is in a free state; it is only given off from it because the oxygen, on combining, loses a large portion of its specific heat. M. Crawford bases this assertion on experiments in which he finds the specific heat of oxygen 87 times greater than that of ordinary water. If these experiments were accurate, it would be easy to show that the free heat of the oxygen more than suffices to produce all the phenomena of heat, and that even in combustions that evolve the most heat, as in that of phosphorus, a considerable amount of the free heat in the oxygen should combine. But these experiments are so ticklish it is necessary to have repeated them a great number of times before accepting them. Therefore we shall refrain from pronouncing on their exactness, until by our method we have determined the specific heats of the different gases. Here we will limit ourselves to comparing the amounts of heat that are evolved in combustion and respiration with the corresponding changes in the oxygen, without considering whether that heat comes from the air or from the combustible bodies and the animals that breathe. In order to determine these changes we performed the following experiments.

M (Plate II, Fig. 7) represents a large basin filled with mercury, over which we placed a bell jar *B*, filled with oxygen. This gas was not perfectly pure; 19 parts of it contained 16 parts of oxygen, and it included about 1/57 parts of its volume of fixed air. Under the bell jar we placed a small earthenware vessel *C*, filled with fine charcol which we had previously deprived of its inflammable air [36] by strong heat and which closely resembled that which we had used in the experiment on the heat evolved in the combusion of carbon. Above the charcol we placed a little tinder on which was a tiny bit of phosphorus, weighing at most 1/10 of a grain. The earthenware vessel, with all its contents, had been very precisely weighted; then by drawing out the contained air we caused by the mercury in the bell jar to rise to *E* so that the expansion of the air, caused by the combustion of the carbon, would not lower the mercury too far below the level of the mercury in the basin outside, which could have allowed the air under the bell jar to escape. After this, by means of a red-hot iron that we thrust rapidly through the mercury, we ignited the phosphorus, which set fire to the tinder and so lit the charcol. The combustion lasted 20 or 25 minutes, and, when the charcoal was extinguished, and all the air inside was cooled to atmospheric temperature, we made a second mark *E'*, where the mercury had risen through the decrease in volume of the air inside. Then we introduced some caustic alkali under the bell jar; all the fixed air was absorbed, and, after a lapse of time sufficient for this purpose, when the mercury had ceased to rise in the bell jar, we marked a line *E''* at the level of the surface of the caustic alkali. We were careful to note, at the three positions *E, E', E''*, the heights of the mercury above its level in the basin. Atmospheric air introduced under the bell jar by means of a glass tube lowered the mercury to the level of that outside in the basin. We then withdrew the vessel *C*, which we dried and weighed very precisely. Its loss of weight told us the quantity of carbon consumed. The outside temperature had varied but little in the course of the experiment, and the barometric reading was at about 28 inches of mercury.

To determine the volumes of air contained in the spaces *EBD, E'BD', E''BD''* we filled them with water, and the respective weights gave us, in cubic inches, the volumes of these spaces. But since the contained air was subject to different pressures, because of the different heights of mercury in the bell jar, we reduced each volume of air to that it would have occupied if it had been subject to a pressure of 28 inches of mercury. Finally we reduced the results of our experiments to those we would have obtained if the external temperature had been 10 degrees, invoking the fact that at a temperature of about 10 degrees, air expands 1/215 of its volume for each 1 degree of increased temperature[37]. Thus the gases whose volumes we shall give below should be thought of as having a temperature of 10 degrees and being under a pressure of 28 inches of mercury.

In the preceeding experiment there were 202.35 [cubic] inches of oxygen. By the combustion of carbon alone its volume was reduced to 170.59 inches and after the absorption of fixed air by the caustic alkali, the volume of air remaining was not more than 73.95 inches. The weight of carbon consumed, disregarding the ash, wa 17 2/10 grains; the weight of the tinder and the phosphorus together could have been half a grain. Moreover, we have found by numerous experiments that the weight of the ash formed by the charcol is about 10 grains per ounce. Thus we can infer that in this experiment there were very nearly 18 grains of carbon consumed, including its ash in this figure.

The oxygen which we used contained about 1/57 of its volume of fixed air, which had not been absorbed by the water over which it had remained for several months. This intimate adherence of fixed air to oxygen leads us to believe that, even after the absorption of the fixed air by the caustic alkali in our experiments, the remaining air still contained a little fixed air that we can evaluate, without appreciable error, at 1/57 of its total volume. On this assumption, to obtain the total volume of oxygen consumed by the carbon, it is necessary to take the difference between the volume of air before the combustion and the volume of air remaining after the absorption by caustic alkali, and reduce this difference by 1/57. Likewise on subtracting this same quantity from the volume of air absorbed by the caustic alkali, you will have the volume of fixed air produced by the combustion. Thus you will find that an ounce of carbon on burning consumes 4037.5 cubic inches of oxygen and produces 3021.1 cubic inches of fixed air. And if we call the volume of oxygen consumed unity, its volume, after combustion, will be reduced to 0.74828 [38].

To express as weights these volumes of oxygen and

fixed air, we must know the weight of a cubic inch of each of these gases. Now it has been found that oxygen is a little heavier than atmospheric air, approximately in the ratio of 187 to 185. The weight of atmospheric air has been very precisely determined by M. de Luc. On the basis of these measurements, we find that at a temperature of 10 degrees, and a barometric pressure of 28 inches of mercury, a cubic inch of oxygen weighs 0.47317 grains. M. Lavoisier has observed that at the same temperature and the same pressure, a cubic inch of fixed air weighs very nearly 7/10 of a grain. According to these results, an ounce of carbon, on burning, consumes 3.3167 ounces of oxygen and yields 3.6715 ounces of fixed air. Thus, for 10 parts of fixed air, there are about 9 parts of oxygen and 1 part of a principle contributed by the carbon and which is the base of fixed air[39]. But so fine a measurement requires a much greater number of experiments.

We saw above that an ounce of carbon, on burning, melts 6 pounds, 2 ounces of ice, whence it is easy to infer that when carbon burns, the transformation of one ounce of oxygen gas can melt 29.547 ounces of ice, and that the formation of an ounce of fixed air can melt 26.692 ounces of ice.

It is with the greatest caution that we present these results concerning the amounts of heat produced where carbon is burned in an ounce of oxygen gas. We were only able to make one experiment on the heat evolved in this combustion and, although it was carried out in quite favorable circumstances, we will be really convinced of its accuracy only after having repeated it a number of times. We have already said, and we cannot stress this fact too much, that it is less the result of our experiments than the method we have used that we offer to scientists[40], inviting them, if this method seems to offer some advantage, to check these experiments which we ourselves propose to repeat with the greatest care.

On burning phosphorus in the above apparatus, where the bell jar was filled with oxygen gas, we found that 45 grains of phosphorus absorbed on combustion 65.62 grains of oxygen gas; and since the product of this combustion is phosphoric acid, from this we may conclude that when this acid is formed, about 1 1/2 parts, or more precisely 1 4/9 parts, of oxygen gas combines with 1 part of phosphorus. This agrees with the result that M. Lavoisier was the first to obtain (*Mémoires of the Academy*, for the year 1777, page 69), and which subsequently M. Berthollet has confirmed by the method of chemical reactions.[41]

From this it follows that an ounce of phosphorus, on burning, absorbs 65.62/45 ounces of oxygen gas; now we have seen before that it can melt 6 pounds, 4 ounces, 48 grains of ice; therefore 1 ounce of oxygen gas, on being absorbed by the phosphorus, can melt 68.634 ounces of ice. But the same amount of gas, on becoming fixed air by the combustion of carbon, can melt 29 1/2 ounces, whence we draw the pretty remarkable conclusion *that the heat given off by oxygen gas, when it is absorbed by the phosphorus, is approximately two and one third times greater than when it is changed into fixed air.*

In the *Mémoires of the Academy* for the year 1777, page 597, M. Lavoisier was led to a similar result by his general theory of the formation of gases and vapors. According to this theory, oxygen gas, fixed air, and in general all gases and all vapors owe their gaseous state [*état aériforme*] to the large quantity of heat which is combined with them. Oxygen gas expecially seems to contain it in abundance; it releases it almost entirely when it passes into the solid state in the calcination of metals and in the combustion of sulfur, phorphorus, etc., but a considerable part of it is retained in the form of fixed air.

The absorption of oxygen gas by nitrous air[42] provides an exception to this general theory of the reactions of oxygen: the amount of heat given off in this particular reaction is very small, and incomparably less than that developed in the absorption of a similar volume of oxygen by phosphorus. It is therefore necessary to imagine in nitric acid, and consequently in saltpeter, a large amount of combined heat, which should reappear in its entirety when this substance is detonated, and this in fact is what experiment shows.

On strongly heating saltpeter, M. Berthollet was able to convert into oxygen nearly all the nitric acid that it contains[43]. In addition this able chemist has further observed that on detonating saltpeter with carbon, a large part of its acid changes into fixed air. Now an ounce of saltpeter contains 3 2/3 *gros* of nitric acid. So supposing that this acid consists wholly of oxygen, and that this is entirely converted into fixed air, we find, according to the preceding results on the combustion of carbon, that an ounce of saltpeter, on detonating with carbon, should melt 13 1/2 ounces of ice. Experiment gave us only 12 ounces of melted ice. But if you consider the uncertainty of the principles from which we started and the inevitable errors in the experiments, you will see that it is not possible to expect a more perfect agreement in these results. Therefore we may conceive the phenomenon of the detonation of saltpeter in this way: the oxygen contained in this substance was combined with it without the evolution of an appreciable amount of heat. Consequently it should produce only a small degree of cold on returning to the gaseous state. During the change of state the base of fixed air contained in the carbon takes up the oxygen and converts it into fixed air. When this occurs there should be given off a quantity of heat nearly equal to that which is evolved in the direct combination of carbon with oxygen gas. The cold resulting from the change of oxygen into the gaseous state, in the detonation of saltpeter, produces a small difference between these quantities of heat, and this difference is equal to the quantity of heat which is evolved from oxygen gas when it combines with nitric acid. We could determine it by the preceding experiment if the principles from which we started were exact, and we would find that in the combination of 1 ounce of oxygen gas to produce nitric acid the quantity of heat that is evolved can melt 3 1/4 ounces of ice. But these assumptions are too uncertain for us to be able in this way to determine with precision this amount of heat. However that may be, we can conjecture with some likelihood that saltpeter owes to the heat that is combined with it its property of detonating with substances that can combine with oxygen, a property not found in other substances, such as the phosphoric salts, which nevertheless contain a large amount of the same gas, but do not combine with it except with the evolution of considerable heat.

To ascertain the changes which the respiration of animals produces in oxygen gas, we filled the bell jar *B* of the previously described apparatus with this gas[44], and we put in it different guinea pigs, of about the same size as the one we used in our experiment on animal heat. In one of these experiments the bell jar contained, before putting in the guinea pig, 248.01 cubic inches of oxygen gas. The animal remained there for 1 1/4 hours. To introduce it under the bell jar we made it pass through the mercury; we withdrew it in the same fashion, and after having let the air inside the bell jar cool to room temperature, its volume was somewhat diminished and reduced to 240.25 cubic inches. Finally, after having absorbed the fixed air with caustic alkali, there remained 200.56 cubic inches of air. In this experiment there were 46.62 inches of modified oxygen gas and 37.96 inches of fixed air produced, a correction being made for the small amount of carbon dioxide contained in the oxygen gas of the bell jar. If one denotes by unity the volume of modified oxygen gas, the volume reduced by respiration will be 0.814. In the combustion of carbon, the volume of gas is diminished in the ratio of 1 to 0.74828. This difference may result, in part, from errors in measurement; but it also depends on a cause that we did suspect at first, and about which it is well to warn those who will want to repeat these experiments.

To stabilize the bell jar in the basin, we raised the level of the mercury inside slightly above the level of the mercury ourside. Now in putting the animal under the bell jar and in withdrawing it, we observed that the outside air penetrated slightly into the interior, along the body of the animal, although immersed partly in the mercury. The mercury does not adhere to the surface of the hair and the skin closely enough to prevent all contact between the outside air and that inside the bell jar; thus the gas appears less diminished by the respiration than in fact it is.

The weight of the fixed air produced in the preceding experiment is 26.572 grains; from which it follows that in the course of 10 hours the animal would have produced 212.576 grains of fixed air.

At the beginning of the experiment, the animal, breathing an air very much purer than that of the atmosphere, produced, perhaps in the same period of time, a much larger quantity of fixed air; but near the end it had difficulty breathing, because the fixed air settling by its weight [45] to the lower part of the bell jar, and probably also because the fixed air is in itself injurious to animals. We may therefore suppose without appreciable error that the quantity of fixed air produced is the same as if the animal had breathed atmospheric air whose goodness [46] is about the mean between that of the air in the lower part of the bell jar at the beginning and at the end of the experiment.

We then determined directly the amount of fixed air produced by a guinea pig when it is breathing atmospheric air. To do this we placed one of the animals under a large jar through which we passed a stream of air. The air, compressed in an apparatus very convenient for the purpose, entered the jar by a glass tube and issued from it by a second bent tube whose concave part was immersed in mercury and whose lower portion ended in a flask filled with caustic alkali. The air then passed out through a third tube, which ended in a second flask full of caustic alkali, and from there it spread into the atmosphere. The fixed air produced by the animal in the interior of the bell jar was trapped, in large measure, by the caustic alkali of the first flask, and that which escaped this reaction was absorbed by the alkali of the second flask. The increase in weight of the flasks gave us the weight of fixed air that was absorbed in them. In the course of 3 hours, the weight of the first flask increased by 63 grains; that of the second flask by 8 grains; thus the total weight of the two flasks increased by 71 grains. Assuming that this quantity of fixed air was solely due to the respiration of the animal, it would, during 10 hours, have produced 236.667 grains of fixed air, which differs by about one ninth from the result of the preceding experiment. This difference can be owing to the difference in the size and strength of the two animals and to the condition of each during the experiment.

If the vapors produced by respiration[47], carried by the flow of air, had been desposited in the flasks, the increase in weight of the caustic alkali would not have given the quantity of fixed air produced by the animal. To prevent this trouble we used a bent tube, whose concave portion dipped into the mercury. The vapors from the respiration condensed on the walls of this part of the tube, and collected in its concavity, so that on entering the first flask the gas was not perceptibly laden with them, for the part of the tube that entered the flask remained transparent. We can therefore suppose that if the weight of the flask was increased by these vapors, this increase was compensated by the evaporation of the water of the alkali they contained. One could fear, moreover, that a part of fixed air that was combined might be due to the atmospheric air. To reassure ourselves on this point, we repeated the same experiment with no guinea pig under the jar. In this case there was no increase in weight of the flasks. That of the second flask decreased by 4 or 5 grains, doubtless from the evaporation of the water of its alkali solution.

A third experiment made on a guinea pig in oxygen gave us 226 grains for the amount of fixed air produced in 10 hours.

On taking the average of these experiments and a few other similar ones made on a number of guinea pigs, both in oxygen and in atmospheric air, we estimated at 224 grains the quantity of fixed air produced in 10 hours by the guinea pig on which we experimented in one of our calorimeters to measure its animal heat.

Since these experiments were made at a temperature of 14 or 15 degrees, it is possible that the quantity of fixed air produced in respiration may be a little less than at zero degrees, which is the temperature inside our calorimeters. It should therefore be necessary, for greater percision, to determine the output of fixed air at the latter temperature. This is a precaution that we propose to observe in the new experiments we shall make on this subject.

The preceding experiments are contrary to the results of Messrs. Scheele and Priestley on the changes in oxygen gas caused by animal respiration. This produces, according to these two fine scientists, very little fixed air and a large amount of vitiated air which the latter has called *phlogisticated* air. But on examining with the greatest possible care, in a large number of experiments, the effect of the respiration of birds and of guinea pigs on oxygen gas, we have always observed that the change of this gas into fixed air is the most important alteration it experiences in animal respiration. On causing guinea pigs to breathe a large amount of oxygen, and absorbing by means of caustic alkali the fixed air produced by their respiration; then in making birds breathe the residual air, and again absorbing with caustic alkali the new fixed air that had been produced, we were able in this manner to convert into fixed air that had been produced, we were able in this manner to convert into fixed air a large part of the oxygen gas that we had used. That which remained had about the same goodness as it should have on the assumption that the transformation of oxygen gas into fixed air is the only effect respiration produces on this gas. It therefore seems to us certain that if respiration produces other changes in the oxygen gas, they are very small, and we do not doubt that scientists who make the same experiments with large devices using mercury will be led to the same result.

We saw above that in the combustion of carbon the formation of an ounce of fixed air can melt 26.692 ounces of ice. Starting from this result, we find that the formation of 224 grains of fixed air should melt 10.38 ounces. This amount of melted ice consequently represents the heat produced by the respiration of a guinea pig in the course of 10 hours.

In the experiment on the animal heat of a guinea pig, this animal came out of our apparatus with nearly the same body temperature with which it had entered; for we know that the body temperature of animals is always very nearly the same. Without the constant renewal of its heat, all that it had in the first place would be gradually dissipated, and we would have withdrawn it cold from the interior of the calorimeter, like all the inanimate bodies on which we have experimented; but its vital functions constantly restored to it the heat that it communicated to it surroundings and which, in our experiment, spread to the ice in the inner space, of which it melted 13 ounces in 10 hours. This quantity of melted ice, therefore, represents approximately the heat restored in the same length of time by the vital functions of the guinea pig. Perhaps we should diminish it by 1 or 2 ounces, or even more, because the animal's limbs were cooled down in the calorimeter, although the interior of its body kept nearly the temperature. Besides, the humors evaporated by its internal heat melted, on cooling, a small quantity of ice and joined with the water that flowed out of that apparatus.

If we decrease by about 2 1/2 ounces this quantity of ice, we will have the amount melted by the effect of the animal's respiration on the gas. Now if you consider the errors inevitable in these experiments and in the assumptions we made in our calculations, you will see that it is not possible to expect a more perfect agreement among these results. Thus we can consider the heat given off in the change of oxygen gas into fixed air by respiration as the principal cause of the preservation of animal heat, and if other causes contribute to maintain it, their effect is negligible.

Respiration is therefore a combustion, a very slow one to be sure, but moreover perfectly similar to that of carbon. It takes place inside the lungs,[48] without giving off any perceptible light, because the matter of fire, once liberated, is forthwith absorbed by the moisture of these organs. The heat developed in this combustion is imparted to the blood that flows through the lungs, whence it spreads throughout the animals's body. Thus the air we breathe serves two purposes equally necessary to preserve life: it removes from the blood the base of fixed air whose excess would be very harmful; and the heat which this reaction gives to the lungs makes up for our continual loss of heat to the atmosphere and surrounding bodies.

Animal heat is pretty much the same in the different parts of the body[49]. This effect seems to depend upon the three following causes: the first is the swiftness with which the blood circulates and promptly transmits even to the limbs the heat it receives in the lungs; the second cause is the evaporation produced in the lungs, and which lowers their temperature; finally, the third is related to the increase observed in the specific heat of the blood when, by contact with the oxygen gas, it is deprived of the base[50] of fixed air which it contains; a part of its specific heat developed when the fixed air is formed is thus absorbed by the blood, its temperature remaining always the same. But when, as it circulates, the blood take up again the base of fixed air, its specific heat decreases and it gives off heat; and since this process takes place in all parts of the body, the heat that it produces helps to maintain the temperature of the parts of the body remote from the lungs at about the same degree as that of the lungs[51]. Besides, however animal heat is restored, the cause that produces the formation of fixed air is the primary one. Thus we can lay down the following proposition: *whenever an animal is in a stable and resting state; whenever it can live for a considerable time, without suffering, in the medium which surrounds it; in general, whenever the circumstances in which it is found do not appreciably alter its blood and its bodily fluids, so that after several hours the animal's system experiences no sensible change, the maintenance of its animal heat is due, at least in large measure, to the heat produced by the combination of the oxygen gas breathed by the animal with the base of fixed air furnished by the blood.*

The method which has led us to this result is independent of any hypothesis, and that is its principal advantage. Whether the heat comes from the oxygen gas, or whether it comes from substances that combine with it, we cannot doubt that in the combination of oxygen gas with the base of fixed air there is developed a considerable amount of heat. This reaction offers, with respect to the heat, phenomena absolutely similar to those afforded by many other chemical reactions, and in particular, that of water with quicklime. And, which renders the identity more perfect, there is the fact that in the latter reaction [no] light is produced[52]. On comparing the heat given off by the combustion of carbon with the quantity of fixed air which is formed in this combustion, we have the heat developed in forming a given quantity of fixed air. If we then determine the quantity of fixed air that an animal produces in a given time, we will have the heat resulting from the effect of its respiration on the air. It is only a question of comparing this heat with that which maintains its animal heat and which is measured by the amount of ice that it melts in the interior of one of our calorimeters. And if, as we found in the preceding experiments, these two quantities of heat are very nearly the same, we can infer directly from this fact and without any hypothesis that the maintenance of animal heat is due, at least in large part, to the change of oxygen gas into fixed air during respiration. We intend to repeat and to vary these experiments by determining the quantities of heat renewed in different kinds of animals, and by inquiring whether, in all of them, this quantity of heat is always proportional to the quantities of fixed air produced in respiration[53]. Birds seem preferable to quadrupeds for this kind of experiment, because they produce, in the same length of time, and in equal volume, a larger quantity of fixed air. Thus, for example, we have observed two house sparrows consume nearly as much oxygen gas as a guinea pig.

To round out this theory of animal heat, we must explain further why it is that animals, although placed in environments differing widely in temperature and density, always maintain nearly the same body temperature, without however changing into fixed air amounts of oxygen gas proportional to these differences. But the explanation of these phenomena is related to the greater or lesser evaporation of the bodily humors, to their alterations, and to the laws according to which heat spreads to all parts of the body. Thus we shall wait, before concerning ourselves with this matter, until analysis[54], illuminated by a great number of experiments, shall have shown us the laws of the transmission of heat in homogeneous bodies, and when passing from one body to another of a different kind.

NOTES TO TRANSLATED TEXT

(Section One)

(1) This refers to the winter of 1782-1783. As printed in the *Oeuvres de Lavoisier* (Vol. II, Paris, 1862., pp. 283-333) the memoir is correctly described as reprinted from the *Mémoires d l'Académie des sciences* for the year 1780. This has confused several scholars, among them J. Rosenthal, translator of the German version in Ostwald's Klassiker. In fact, the Academy *Mémoires* for 1780 did not appear until 1784.

(2) See Introduction, p. x. This fluid "matter of fire" (*matière du feu*) was what Lavoisier and his disciples later called "caloric," a term first used in 1787 in the *Méthode de nomenclature chimique*, an English translation of which was published in London the following year.

(3) Some have gratuitously assumed that this anticipation of the modern dynamic theory of heat was particularly favored

by Laplace, who probably was responsible for the inclusion of these paragraphs. There is no supporting evidence for this conjecture. On the origin of this theory see my "Chemistry as a Branch of Physics: Laplace's Collaboration with Lavoisier," *Historical Studies in the Physical Sciences*, 1976, 7: 244-250.

(4) On *vis viva* (or *force vive*, as it was called in French) and the debates that this concept aroused, see René Dugas, *Histoire de la mécanique* (Paris and Neuchatel: Dunod, 1950), pp. 209-211 and Ch. II, "Querelle des Forces Vives"; also Thomas L. Hankins, "Eighteenth-Century Attempts to Resolve the *Vis Viva* Controversy," *Isis*, 1965, 56:281-297.

(5) The differential absorption of solar heat by objects of different colors was well known in the eighteenth century. See I.B. Choen, "Franklin, Boerhaave, Newton, Boyle, and the Absorption of Heat in Relation to Color," *Isis*, 1955, 46: 99-104; also the same author's *Franklin and Newton* (Philadelphia: American Philosophical Society, 1956), p. 234. Throughout this discussion of the absorption of heat from solar light, L.and L. give light rays mechanical properties that suggest their acceptance of the prevailing corpuscular theory of light. As they define "impulse" it is equivalent to our "momentum."

(6) Nitre or niter, which is potassium nitrate (KNO_3), today is better known as saltpeter, and this is the word I use.

(7) For Jean André Deluc (1727-1817) see *Dictionary of Scientific Biography*, Vol. IV (1971), pp. 27-29, and W.E. Knowles Middleton, *A History of the Thermometer* (Baltimore: Johns Hopkins University Press, 1966), pp. 117-126. The work of Deluc used by L. and L. was his *Recherches sur les modifications de l'atmosphère*, 2 vols. (Geneva, 1772).

(8) For Lavoisier's thermometer see Middleton, *op. cit.*, pp. 119-120. See also Maurice Daumas, *Lavoisier théoricien et expérimentateur* (Paris: Presses Universitaires de France, 1955), Ch. 6.

(9) That is, when it has reached thermal equilibrium.

(10) This abstract model of the sphere of ice was doubtless the device of Laplace, the physicist, rather than Lavoisier.

(11) In the text *au-dessus* ("above') is clearly a misprint for *au-dessous* ("below"), as the sense seems to indicate.

(12) In this paper L. and L. use the word *gaz* in our familiar sense of gas for the first time in print, but only in three places. More frequently L. and L. refer to "air" or "aeriform fluids." It is commonly accepted that the word originated with J.B. van Helmont (see the English version of his *Oriatrike*, London, 1662) whence it appeared in English in Stephen Blancard's *Physical Dictionary* (1693) and John Harris'*Lexicaon Technicum* (1704), in every case attributed to van Helmont and applied to "incoercible spirits," usually noxious, such as those produced by burning charcoal, "spiritous and putrid fermentations," and the "damps" of mines. In the eighteenth century it was also applied to the carbon dioxide in mineral waters, for example, by A. N. Monnet (1768), Pieter De Smeth (1772), P.-J Macquer (in the first edition of his *Dictionnnaire de chymie*, 1766), and in this older sense by Lavoisier in his *Opuscules* of 1774. As applied to all aeriform fluids the word appears here and there from this time on, but the chief influence leading to its adoption was the second edition (1778) of Macquer's *Dictionnaire*.

(13) The descriptive word in French is *serpentin*, usually meaning a spiral tube attached to an alembic which, passed through a trough of cold water, condensed the products of distillation.

(14) *Huile de vitriol*, or oil of vitriol, is concentrated sulfuric acid.

(15) Macquer calls it the "Pyrophore of Homberg." It was evidently a substance from animal excrement, probably phophorus-rich, which had the property of bursting into flame when exposed to the air.

(16) To avoid the word *machine*, by which the authors usually refer to their newly invented apparatus, I have translated it as calorimeter, a word they themselves (or Lavoisier) invented. See his *Traité élémentaire de chimie* (Paris, 1789), pp. vi and 387, where *calorimètre* is first used. It entered the English language soon after.

(Section Four)

(32)This, of course, applies chiefly to Lavoisier's own discoveries. See the Introduction and my *Antoine-Laurent Lavoisier, Chemist and Revolutionary* (New York: Scribner's, 1975), expecially Chs. 5-8.

(33) Early terms for oxygen gas. As J. Rosenthal remarked in a note to his German translation of this *Memoir on Heat*, Lavoisier's figures for the oxygen content of air varied from 1/4 to 1/6 of the total volume. An accepted modern figure is 21 percent by volume or 23 percent by weight.

(34)In reprinting the *Memoir on Heat* in his posthumous *Mémoires ds physique et de chimie*, Lavoisier added a note that the memoir on combustion had been initialed (*paraphé*) "by the Secretary of the Academy on September 5, 1777."

(35) For Adair Crawford (1748-1795), whose *Experiments and Observations on Animal Heat, and the Inflammation of Combustible Bodies* (London, 1779) is the work referred to, see J.R. Partington, *History of Chemistry*, Vol. III (London: Macmillan, 1962), pp.156-157. The misspelling of Crawford's name found in 1783 and 1784 was corrected (except for one place) when the *Memoir on Heat* was reprinted in the *Mémoires de physique et de chimie*.

(36) The authors (in this case chiefly Lavoisier) may have been referring to carbon monoxide (CO), which Priestley had discovered and called "heavy inflammable air," and which later (1800) William Cruickshank proved to be an oxide of carbon, determining its composition nearly correctly. Yet in 1792, when Lavoisier added a note to his *Mémoires de physique et de chimie*, his confusion is evidnet: "At that time [1783] we did not know that when it had not been stongly heated charcoal [*le charbon*] contains hydrogen gas, and that during the combustion some water is formed."

(37) How L. and L. obtained this figure has not been easy to

determine. It may have been an informal communication of the results of J.A.C. Charles (1746-1823). Gay-Lussac's experiments, published in 1801, could not have been performed before 1783. Perhaps the source was Guillaume Amonton's "Discours sur quelques propriétés de l'air," *Mémoires de l'Academie Royale des Sciences*, 1702, 155-174.
(38) See note 14 of J. Rosenthal's German translation of the *Memoir on Heat*.
(39) As is evident here, the elementary nature of carbon was not understood, nor had the precise composition of "fixed air" (CO_2) been determined.
(40) As before, I have translated *physicien* as "scientist." The use of the word "physicist" would have misleading overtones.
(41) Berthollet's experiments on the oxidation of phosphorus, performed by the "wet way" (that is, by reactions in solution) were reported in *Mémoires de l'Academie Royale des Sciences*, 1782 (1785), pp. 602-607. On Berthollet the most recent work is Michell Sadoun-Goupil's *Le chimiste Claude-Louis Berthollet 1748-1822, sa vie–son oeuvre* (Paris: Vrin, 1977).
(42) "Nitrous air" is nitric oxide (NO). This gas combines with oxygen to form the red gas nitrogen dioxide (NO_2), with a shrinkage of volume which provided, in eudiometers like those of Felice Fontana, a way of determining the "goodness" or *salubrità* of air.
(43) At high temperatures KNO_3 does in fact break down to yield oxygen, which was one of the ways that Scheele first produced this gas.
(44) Here again the authors use the word *gaz*. See the French text, p. 48.
(45) That is, by its greater specific gravity.
(46) See above, note 42. The authors' word is *bonté*.
(47) Almost entirely, of course, water vapor.
(48) It was only later that it was made clear that oxidation takes place in all the living tissues of the body, the blood being the medium that supplies the oxygen and takes up the carbon dioxide.
(49) That is, body temperature. While L. and L. understood perfectly well the difference between temperature and heat (see Introduction, p. xiii), this is one of several examples which show their language echoing an earlier confusion. On animal heat see Everett Mendelsohn, *Heat and Life: The Development of the Theory of Animal Heat* (Cambridge, Mass.: Harvard University Press, 1964).
(50) See above, note 27.
(51) It is now known that there is no marked difference in the specific heats of arterial and venous blood.
(52) Much heat (15.54 kilogram calories) but no light is given off when quicklime is moistened with water. As written, the statement does not amplify the previous sentence. Rosenthal was certainly correct when he suggested that a negative has been left out by the authors.
(53) Like other promises in the *Memoir on Heat* these projected experiments were never realized.
(54) The word does not mean chemical analysis. It is used in the Newtonian sense so popular in the eighteenth century. See my article "Newton and the Method of Analysis," in *Dictionary of the History of Ideas*, Vol. III (1973), pp. 378-91. This is reprinted in my *Essays and Papers*, pp. 193-216.

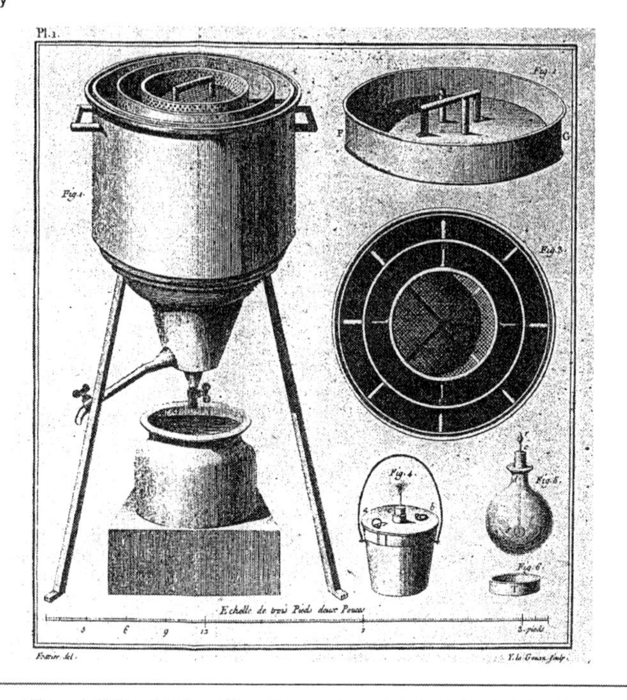
Pl. 1.
Fig. 1.
Fig. 2.
F
G
Fig. 3.
Fig. 4.
Fig. 5.
Fig. 6.
Echelle de trois Pieds deux Pouces
3 6 9 12
2
3 pieds

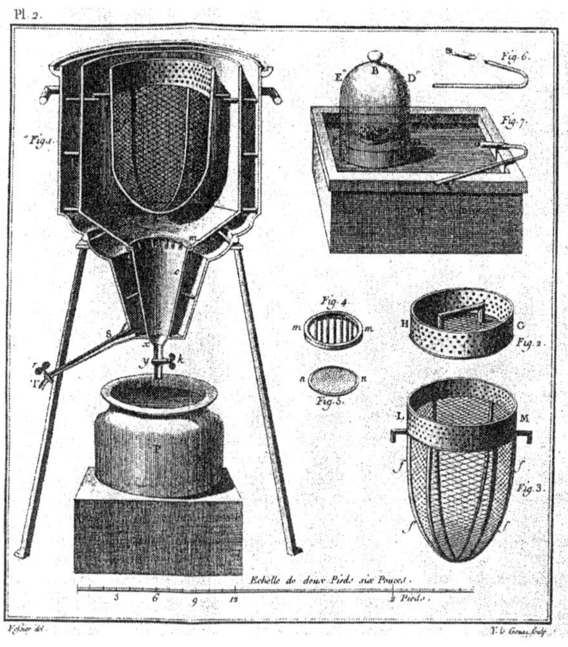
Pl. 2.
Fig. 1.
Fig. 6.
E
B
D
Fig. 7.
Fig. 4.
m
m
Fig. 5.
n
n
H
G
Fig. 2.
L
M
Fig. 3.
S
x
y
k
T
Echelle de deux Pieds six Pouces.
3 6 9 12
2 Pieds.

CLASSICS IN OBESITY

An Experimental Inquiry Regarding the Nutritive Value of Alcohol

W.O. Atwater and F.G. Benedict

Introduction

The present report gives the details of a number of metabolism experiments with men, in which the effects of diet with and without alcohol have been compared (a). The details of a number of digestion experiments, which form part of the same investigations, have also been included.

Purpose of the Experiments

The main purpose of the experiments has been to get light upon the effects of alcohol in the diet, with especial reference to the question of its nutritive value.

Food is used in the body to build and repair tissue and to furnish energy. Only the nitrogenous compounds (protein) of the food serve the first purpose; they also serve as a source of energy, but the main supply of energy is obtained from the fats and carbohydrates. The fuel ingredients may be burned at once or may be stored for future use.

Alcohol contains no nitrogen and therefore can not build or repair tissue; it is rather to be classed with the fats and carbohydrates, and if it has any food value, this must be as a fuel. It does not appear to be stored for any considerable time, but is disposed of soon after it is taken into the body.

Alcohol, however, differs from the protein, fats, and carbohydrates of food materials in that it may exert, and when taken in large enough doses does exert, an indirect action upon the brain and nerves and through them upon the nutritive and other processes to which the general term metabolism is applied. In this way its actual value may be either increased or diminished according as it aids or hinders digestion, or either accelerates or retards metabolism. We have then to consider not only its direct action as nutriment for the supply of energy, but also its indirect action upon the metabolism and utilization of other food. In the experiments here described the indirect action of alcohol has been studied only in so far as (1) through its influence upon the secretion of digestive juices or otherwise it has tended to increase or diminish the proportion of the other food digested, or (2) it has increased or decreased the metabolism of other food or body material.

The ulterior effects of alcohol do not come within the scope of this particular inquiry, which is limited to its use by the body as nutrient.

The Questions Actually Studied

It appears then that whatever value alcohol may have for nutriment must depend upon its ability to serve as fuel for furnishing energy to the body. Accordingly the main question proposed for study is this: What is the value of alcohol for fuel and how does it compare in this respect with sugar, starch, fats, and other nutrients of ordinary food materials? A collateral question is the

This work printed in 1902 is the sixth memoir in Volume 8 of the Memoirs of the National Academy of Sciences, printed at the government printing office in Washington. It is part of public domain. Special thanks to the Pennington Boimedical Research Center Information Center, Baton Rouge, LA, for help in acquiring this document.

[a]The inquiry was undertaken at the instance of the Committee of Fifty for the Investigation of the Drink Problem. The experimental work was done in the chemical laboratory of Wesleyan University. A large share of the expense was borne by the committee of fifty although contributions were also received from the Elizabeth Thompson and Bache funds and from private individuals. The experiments were parallel with others of similar character, which are conducted under the auspices of the United States Department of Agriculture. These latter experiments form a part of a general inquiry regarding the food and nutrition of man, which is authorized by Congress and prosecuted in differenct parts of the United States. The special inquiry into the nutritive action of alcohol was made possible by the generosity of Wesleyan University, which offered to the committee of fifty the use of laboratory and other facilities that have been made available to the Department of Agriculture and the Storrs Experiment Station for nutrition inquiries.

The investigation has been pursued with the active cooperation of a number of gentlemen, including especially Mr. A.P. Bryant, under whose direction the computations of the results have been made, and Mr. A.W. Smith, Dr. O.F. Tower, and Dr. J.F. Snell, all of whom have been intimately associated with the elaboration of the apparatus and methods. Mr. Smith and Dr. Snell served as subjects in several of the experiments reported beyond, though the subject of the larger number was Mr. E. Osterberg.

The details of the experiments without alcohol and of two of those with alcohol, Nos. 7 and 10, have been published in bulletins of the United States Department of Agriculture as stated beyond.

effect of alcohol upon the proportions of nutrients digested from the food with which it was taken.

Experimental research has shown several ways in which the ingredients of ordinary food and body material serve as fuel. They are oxidized in the body; in the oxidation, their potential energy becomes kinetic and is thus made useful to the body; part of this kinetic energy appears as heat; another part appears as muscular work; in yielding energy by its own oxidation, food protects the material of the body and of other food from consumption. We have then to consider how alcohol compares with the ordinary fuel ingredients of the food in these ways.

It is clear that the main problem is that of the metabolism of energy in the body. Accordingly, while the experiments here described bear upon the use of alcohol in each of the ways just mentioned and upon collateral topics also, the fundamental question studied has been this: To what extent is the energy of alcohol transformed and utilized in the body like the energy of the nutrients, especially the fats and carbohydrates, of ordinary food materials?

In studying these questions we go down to one of the fundamental principles of material science. The plan of the whole inquiry is based upon the principle that the chemical and physical changes which take place in the body, and to which the general term metabolism is applied, occur in obedience to the laws of the conservation of matter and energy. That the law of the conservation of matter applies within the living organism, no one would question. It might seem equally certain that the metabolism of energy within the body takes place in accordance with the law of the conservation of energy. In experiments with men in the respiration calorimeter described beyond, the close agreement between the income and the outgo of energy in the body, under various conditions of work and rest, may be regarded as practically demonstrating that the law holds in the living organism. Such demonstration had, indeed, been approximated by earlier investigations, notably those of Rubner with dogs.

Apparatus and Methods of Inquiry

The experiments here described were made with a respiration calorimeter especially devised for research of this kind. The apparatus serves to measure the materials received and given off by the body, including the products of respiration, and is thus a "respiration apparatus." It also serves to measure the heat given off by the body and hence is a form of calorimeter. To indicate this twofold purpose it is called a "respiration calorimeter." The apparatus and methods of its use have been described elsewhere; (a) a brief description will suffice here.

The chamber of the apparatus is so arranged that a man may spend a number of days in comparative comfort within it. It is lighted by a window, and is furnished with a folding chair, table, and bed, and, when the experiment involves muscular work, with a stationary bicycle also. The chamber is ventilated by a measured current of air, samples of which are taken for analysis before it enters and after it leaves the chamber. In this way the products of respiration are determined. Provision is also made for weighing, sampling, and analyzing all the food and drink, and the solid and liquid excreta as well. By comparing the chemical elements and compounds received by the body in food, drink, and inhaled air with those given off in the solid, liquid, and gaseous forms by the intestines, kidneys, lungs, and skin, it is possible to strike a balance between the total income and the total outgo of matter in the man's body. This serves as the measure of the metabolism of matter in the body.

In addition to this the metabolism of energy is also studied. To this end it is necessary to determine the potential energy of the food and drink taken into the body and of the solid and liquid excreta given off by the body, as well as the amounts of energy given off in the form of heat, external muscular work, and otherwise. The measurements of the potential energy of the food and excreta are made with the bomb calorimeter (b). The determination of the heat given off from the body is made by certain arrangements in connection with the respiration calorimeter. A current of water passing through a special coil of pipes suspended in the chamber absorbs the heat that is generated within it, and by measuring the quantity of water that passes through the coil and its rise in temperature the amount of heat absorbed may be determined. To this is added the latent heat of the water vaporized within the chamber.

So delicate are the measurements of temperature that the observer sitting outside and recording the changes every two or four minutes immediately detects a rise or fall of even one one-hundredth of a degree in the temperature of the inner copper wall or of the air inside the chamber. If the man inside rises to move about, the

[a] In the following bulletins of the Office of Experiment Stations of the United States Department of Agriculture: No.44, Report of Preliminary Investigations on the Metabolism of Nitrogen and Carbon in the Human Organism with a Respiration Calorimeter of Special Construction, by W.O. Atwater, Ph.D., C.D. Woods, B.S., and F.G. Benedict, Ph.D.; No.63, Description of a New Respiration Calorimeter and Experiments on the Conservation of Energy in the Human Body, by W.O. Atwater, Ph.D., and E.B. Rosa, Ph.D., pp. 94; No. 69, Experiments on the Metabolism of Matter and Energy in the Human Body, by W.O. Atwater, Ph.D., and F.G. Benedict, Ph.D., with the cooperation of A.W. Smith, M.S., and A.P. Bryant, M.S., pp. 112.; No.109, Further Experiments on the Metabolism of Matter and Energy in the Human Body, by W.O. Atwater, Ph.D., and F.G. Benedict, Ph.D., with the cooperation of A.P. Bryant, M.S., A.W. Smith, M.S., and J.F. Snell, Ph.D.

[b] For description of the bomb calorimeter see U.S. Dept. Agr., Office Expt. Stations, Bul. 21, pp. 120-126, and Storrs Conn. Experiment Station Report, 1897, p. 199.

increase in the heat given off from his body with this muscular work shows itself in a rise of temperature which is immediately detected.

In the work experiments the subject spends a certain portion of each day in muscular exercise upon an apparatus arranged as an ergometer, by which the amount of muscular work done may be measured. The ergometer consists of a stationary bicycle connected with a dynamo by which the power which the rider applies to the pedals, and which is not changed to heat by the friction of the machine, is converted into an electric current, which is passed through an electric lamp and is in turn changed to heat. The ergometer is arranged to measure the amount of muscular work done, in terms of heat, by determinations of the amount of energy converted into heat by friction and the amounts of electric current generated and changed to heat.

From the energy of food, drink, solid and liquid excretory products, and body material stored or lost the net income of energy may be computed. The net outgo is measured by the apparatus. By comparing these the balance of income and outgo of energy is found.

The data obtained as explained above, taken in connection with what is known of the physiologicial processes that go on in the body, give more accurate information than can be otherwise obtained regarding the ways in which the food is used in the body and the quantities of food ingredients that are needed to supply the demands of the body for the various purposes of work and rest and the comparative nutritive valve of different food materials.

Accuracy of Apparatus and Methods

Two methods of testing the accuracy of the apparatus are employed. By one method known amounts of heat are generated electrically within the chamber, and the heat is measured by the apparatus. In this way its accuracy as a calorimeter only is tested. By the second method known amounts of ethyl alcohol of known purity and composition are burned completely within the chamber, and the amounts of water, carbon dioxide, and heat resulting from the combustion of alcohol are determined by the apparatus. In this way its accuracy both as a respiration apparatus and a calorimeter is tested. In the average of five electrical tests the amount of heat measured by the calorimeter was 100.01 per cent of the amount generated by the electric current. The averages of the results obtained in seventeen alcohol tests are summarized in the following table:

Summary of results of tests in which alcohol was burned in the calorimeter.

	Carbon dioxide.	Water.	Heat.
	Grams.	*Grams.*	*Calories.*
Amount required	19,239.8	12,262.4	64,554.1
Amount found	19,206.9	12.379.1	64,513.3
	Per cent.	*Per cent.*	*Per cent.*
Ratio of amount found to amount required	99.8	[a]100.9	99.9

[a] After the completion of the later experiments a slight leak was found in the "valve box" through which the outgoing air current passed on its way to and from the "freezers," and by which water, condensed on the outside, may have entered. There is every reason to believe that the quantity of water actually found was thus made too large by a fraction of 1 per cent. In the average of the first nine experiments the amount of water actually found was 100.6 per cent of that required. As an alcohol check test was generally made between each two metabolism experiments or series of experiments we have a means of knowing when the leak began to effect the results and the amount of the error introduced. See Bulletin 109 of the Office of Experiment Stations, above referred to.

The results thus indicate that the respiration calorimeter is an instrument of precision and that the determinations of carbon dioxide, water, and heat produced within the chamber of the respiration calorimeter are sufficiently accurate for experiments with the living subject.

The Experiments

General Plan

For the subjects of the experiments men were selected who were in good health, had apparently normal digestion, and did not find the confinement in the chamber uncomfortable. A diet was chosen which provided materials as palatable and in as much variety as was consistent with convenient preparation, and with accurate sampling and analysis. The quantity and composition of the diet were generally such as to maintain the body nearly in nitrogen and carbon equilibrium under the conditions of the experiment, whether of work or of rest. In 13 of the experiments the diet included alcohol.

The alcohol amounted in general to about 72 grams (2 1/2 ounces) a day, or as much as would be contained in a bottle of claret or 3 or 4 glasses of whisky. In most cases pure (ethyl) alcohol, but in some whisky or brandy was used. It was mixed with either water or coffee, and was given in 6 small doses, 3 with meals and the rest at regular intervals between, in order to avoid as far as possible any effect upon the nerves. The alcohol supplied nor far from 500 calories of energy. In the experiments without external muscular work, the total energy of the diet was about 2,500 calories, so that the alcohol furnished one-fifth of the total energy. In the experiments in which the man was engaged in more or less active muscular work, the total energy of the food was larger, averaging about 3,900 calories, so that the alcohol furnished between one-seventh and one-eighth of the total energy of the diet.

In order that the subject might become accustomed to the diet and reach approximate nitrogen equilibrium with it before the experiment proper began, a preliminary digestion experiment of at least 3 days immediately preceded the metabolism experiment. Any change of diet found desirable or necessary was made during this period, and the preliminary experiment was continued until nitrogen equilibrium was supposed to be more or less nearly reached. In most cases the preliminary experiment continued 4 days. During this period the subject was, in general, engaged in his customary occupation, but conformed his muscular activity more or less to that of the coming experiment. Thus if it was to be a work experiment, he rode a bicycle or walked a considerable distance each day. If it was to be a rest experiment, he avoided all unnecessary exercise. For supper on the last day of this preliminary digestion experiment about .3 grams of lampblack was taken in a gelatin capsule with the food, in order to mark the separation of the feces of the preliminary experiment from those of the metabolism experiment proper. The subject entered the chamber about 7 o'clock on the evening of the last day of the preliminary digestion period and retired about 11 o'clock. At about 1 o'clock in the morning the heat measurements were begun.

The night sojourn in the chamber sufficed to get the temperature of the apparatus and its contents of carbonic acid and water into equilibrium, so that accurate measurements might begin at 7 o'clock on the first morning of the experiment proper. In some cases the experiment continued only 4 days; in other cases the experimental period consisted of 6 or 9 successive days spent within the apparatus, the entire period being divided into 3 experiments of 2 or 3 days each with changes in the diet as hereafter explained. The determinations of carbon dioxide, water vapor, and heat were made in 6-hour periods, so that complete data for an experiment showed the total amounts of these compounds given off from the body during the periods ending at 1 p.m., 7 p.m., 1 a.m., and 7 a.m. of each day of the experiment. As noted beyond, the urine was also collected and its nitrogen content determined for corresponding periods.

The daily routine of the subject within the chamber was indicated by a programme made up before the beginning of the experiment. A copy of the programme was furnished to the subject, who followed it with reasonable closeness, and other copies were posted in convenient places outside the apparatus for the benefit of those who had the experiments in charge.

Much care was necessarily taken in preparing the food materials selected for the diet and in taking samples for analysis. With the exception of milk and alcohol, the proper quantity of each kind of food, either for each meal or for the whole day, was put up in glass jars before the experiment began; and materials which might spoil during the course of the experiment, such as bread and meat, were thoroughly sterilized.

Special arrangements were made by which the mixed milk from a definite number of select cows was supplied for each experiment. But even with this precaution, the milk was not entirely uniform in composition from day to day.

The handling of the alcohol was much simpler. A quantity sufficient for several experiments was procured and analyzed, and the proper amounts were drawn each day as needed.

As stated above, the separations of the feces for each experiment were made by means of lampblack. The total feces for each experiment were analyzed, and the average per day used in the computations of results. It was assumed that when the food and exercise were so nearly uniform the undigested residues and metabolic products would not vary greatly from day to day, and such irregularities as might occur would hardly affect the average for an experiment.

The urine was collected in 6-hour periods, and the amount, specific gravity, and nitrogen determined for each period. Aliquot portions of the urine of the 6-hour periods were taken for preparation of a composite sample for the day, and in like manner aliquot portions of the composite sample of urine for each day were taken for the preparation of a sample for the whole experiment or series of experiments. The nitrogen and heat of combustion were determined in the urine for each day and in the composite for the whole experiment. The carbon and hydrogen were determined in the composite sample of urine for the whole experiment or series of experiments, and were divided among the different days in proportion to the amount of nitrogen (a).

Discussion of the Results of the Experiments

The special purpose of the experiments summarized on the preceding pages, in so far as they have had to do with the nutritive action of alcohol, has been the study of the metabolism of the energy of alcohol and its consequent value for fuel as compared with isodynamic amounts of carbohydrates and fats. Incidentally, its effects upon digestion, the completeness of its oxidation, and its action in protecting body fat and protein from oxidation have also been observed. The more important results may be discussed under the following topics:

1. Effects of alcohol upon the digestion of food.
2. Proportions of alcohol oxidized and unoxidized.

[a] For further explanation, see U.S. Dept. Agr., Office Exp. Stations, Bul. 69, pp. 21 and 35.

3. Metabolism of the energy of alcohol.
4. Protection of body material by alcohol.
   a, Protection of body fat.
   b, Protection of body protein.
5. Effect of alcohol upon the radiation of heat from the body.
6. Alcohol as a source of heat in the body.
7. Alcohol as a source of muscular energy.

Effect of Alcohol Upon the Digestion of Food–Digestibility Versus Availability of Nutrients

The term digestibility as applied to food has several meanings, which are not clearly distinguished in popular usage. It commonly refers to either the ease with which a given food material is digested, or the time required for the process, or the extent to which the material "agrees" or "disagrees" with different persons, or its effects upon bodily comfort and health. These factors depend largely upon individual peculiarities, vary widely with different persons and with the character of the food, and are difficult to measure.

The term digestibility is also used to designate the quantity or proportion of the food or of each of its different ingredients–protein, fats, carbohydrates, and mineral matters–actually digested and absorbed in the passage of the food through the digestive tract. Only this latter factor of digestibility is considered in these experiments. To determine what amount of each nutrient is actually digested it is necessary to know the quantity that is taken into the body in food and the quantity that has escaped digestion and is excreted in the feces. The latter quantity is not easily determined, however, because the feces contain, besides those portions of the food that have resisted the action of the digestive juices, other materials, the so-called metabolic products, which are mainly the residues of the digestive juices, and which are not easily separated fro the undigested portion of the food. For this reason it is difficult to determine the actual digestibility of food or of its several ingredients.

The availability of the food or of several ingredients, however, may be more accurately determined. By availability is here meant the quantity or proportion that can be used for the building and repair of tissue and the yielding of energy. The metabolic products, although derived originally from the digested food, are not used for either building material or fuel, and hence are not available in the sense in which the word is here employed. They may, therefore, be included with the undigested residue of the food and the small quantities of intestinal epithelium and other materials which make up the rest of the feces, and the amounts of available nutrients may be found by subtracting from the total ingredients of the food the total corresponding ingredients in the feces. These have often been called the digestible rather than the available nutrients, but the distinction here made is quite important.

The availability of the ingredients as thus determined is usually expressed by the percentage of the total amount of each in the food. This percentage is called the coefficient of availability. In the following table, which is a summary of a more detailed table given in the Appendix, the coefficients of availability of the protein, fats, and carbohydrates of the ordinary diet are compared with those of the alcohol diet, as actually found in the experiments. The average coefficients of availability of the nutrients of food as found in 93 experiments (a) with healthy men with ordinary diet under various conditions of work and rest are appended in the table for comparison.

It thus appears that the alcohol had little appreciable effect upon the availability of the other ingredients of the diet; the coefficients of availability of the nutrients of the ordinary food were practically the same with and without alcohol as part of the diet. The protein appears to have been slightly more available when the diet contained alcohol. The differences, especially in the more comparable experiments, are less than might be found with different subjects using the same ordinary food, or with the same subject using the same food at different times and under different conditions.

The conclusion from the results of these experiments would be to the effect that alcohol in moderate amounts tended to increase very slightly the availability of the nutrients of the diet, especially of the protein. In view, however, of the fact that there are often marked differences in the availability of the same diet with different persons and with the same person at different times, even this conclusion should be held with a degree of reserve. While it is statistically valid for these experiments, the extent to which it would be true in general experience is by no means certain.

Proportions of Alcohol Oxidized and Unoxidized

The difference between the amount of alcohol taken into the body in food and the amount given off unoxidized by the kidneys, lungs, and skin is taken as the amount oxidized in the body. For the determination of the amounts not oxidized in the body quantitative examination was made of the several excretory products for the presence of alcohol. No similar examination of the feces for alcohol was practicable; but, as it has been found in other experiments (b) that no alcohol was excreted through this channel, even when considerable quantities were ingested, it was here assumed that the

[a] See Atwater and Bryant, Availabiltiy and Fuel Value of Food Materials. Rept. Storrs (Conn.) Expt. Sta., 1899, p. 73.

[b] See Bodländer in Arch. Physiol. Pflüger, 32 (1883), p. 424.

TABLE 12.–*Coefficients of availability of food in the averages of experiments with and without alcohol.*

Kind and number of experiments.	Coefficients of availability.			
	Protein.	Fat.	Carbohydrates.	Energy.
Experiments more directly comparable.	*Per cent.*	*Per cent.*	*Per cent.*	*Per cent.*
Without alcohol, Nos. 9, 11, 26 and 28, 29, and 31, 32, and 34	92.6	94.9	97.9	91.8
With alcohol, Nos. 10, 12, 27, 31, 33	93.7	94.6	97.8	92.1
Experiments less directly comparable.				
Without alcohol, Nos. 5, and 13 and 14	92.6	94.1	98.1	90.3
With alcohol, Nos. 7 and 15 to 17	95.0	94.4	97.3	91.3
Average of other observations	93.0	95.0	98.0	[a]92.3

a Availability of energy based upon average proportions and amounts of nutrients found in dietaries of 38 families of farmers, mechanics, and professional men and 15 college boarding clubs in different parts of the United States. See article by A.P. Bryant on "Some Results of Dietary Studies." Yearbook U.S. Dept. Agriculture, 1898, p. 439.

feces would contain no appreciable amount of the alcohol taken with the food.

The alcohol eliminated by the kidneys would, of course, be found in the urine; that given off by the lungs and skin in the "drip" water collected from surface of the system of cooling tubes, or it might pass out of the chamber as vapor in the air current and be condensed in the "freezers," in which a large part of the water is collected from the outgoing air, or it might even pass through the freezers as vapor and be ultimately absorbed in concentrated sulphuric acid in an apparatus arranged for the purpose.

The determinations of the amounts of alcohol given off from the body unoxidized in experiment No. 7 were made according to the method described by BODLÄNDER (a). This method, however, does not give results sufficiently accurate when the amounts of alcohol are as small as were found in these experiments. In the latter experiments a modification (b) of this method was used, which has been shown to give very satisfactory results in the determination of extremely small quantities of alcohol.

The urine, drip water, and freezer water were distilled served times in order to separate the alcohol and other volatile and readily oxidizable organic matters and to obtain them in a more concentrated form. The amount of organic matter (here designated as reducing material) in the distillates was then determined by the method mentioned above. The amount of reducing material in the air current was estimated by passing the outgoing air through bulbs containing concentrated sulphuric acid, and determining the amount of reducing material in the acid. The total amount of reducing material thus determined in the various excretory products was calculated as alcohol.

Other investigators (c) have found evidence that such reducing materials are excreted by the body when no alcohol was ingested. In several experiments in which alcohol did not form part of the diet, examinations of respiratory and excretory products were made the same as when alcohol was given and reducing materials were found to be present (d). The average amount found in these experiments without alcohol was, therefore, deducted from the total amount determined in the experiments with alcohol and the difference taken as alcohol excreted, as shown below:

Alcohol ingested and excreted unoxidized.

Alcohol ingested, average 13 experiments	grams	72.3
Reducing material in excretory products:		
When alcohol was ingested, average 13 experiments	grams	1.6
When no alcohol was ingested, average 6 experiments	do	.3
Alcohol excreted	grams	1.3
Total alcohol metabolized	do	71
Do	per cent	98.2

From Table CXXII in the Appendix it will be observed that the quantities of alcohol eliminated by the lungs, skin, and kidneys varied from 0.7 to 2.7 grams, and averaged 1.3 grams per day. These quantities correspond to a range of from 1 per cent to 3.7 per cent and an average of 1.9 per cent of the total amount of alcohol ingested. We consider, therefore, that in general when alcohol is taken in small doses not more than 2 per cent is given off unoxidized, and the results of the later experiments indicate that this figure is really too large. Accordingly, the coefficient of availability of alcohol is taken as 98 per cent.

Comparing this with the coefficients of availability of protein, fat, and carbohydrates in the diet with alco-

[a] Loc. cit.

[b] See Benedict and Norris on "The Determination of Small Quantities of Alcohol," Jour. Am. Chem. Soc., 20 (1898), p. 299.

[c] Dupré, Proc. Roy. Soc. (London), 20 (1871-72), 268. See also Billings, Mitchell, and Bergy on "The composition of expired air and its effect upon animal life." Smithsonian Contributions to Knowledge, XXIX (1895), No. 989.

[d] See Table CXXI in the Appendix.

hol, as given in the Table 12, p. 257, it appears that the carbohydrates and larger than those of fats and protein of ordinary food. That is to say, it was found that 2 per cent or less of the total alcohl ingested in these experiments was given off unoxidized by the lungs and skin, while on the average about 2 per cent of the carbohydrates, 5 per cent of the fats, and 7 per cent of the protein of the ordinary diet appeared to be excreted unoxidized.

The conclusion is that in these experiments the alcohol was more completely consumed than are the nutrients of ordinary mixed diet.

Metabolism of the Energy of Alcohol

It was stated above that the experiments with men in the respiration calorimeter had shown a very close agreement between the income and outgo of energy in the body, and that this was regarded as practically a demonstration that the law of the conservation of energy holds in the living organism. Up to April, 1900, the results of 30 such experiments had been obtained. These covered, all told, 93 days; they were made with 4 different subjects, under various conditions of diet and occupation. When the figures for individual days or for individual experiments are considered, there appears to be more or less disagreement between the figures for income and those of outgo energy, though the differences are inside the natural range of error in such physiological experiments. When the results of all the experiments are averaged together, however, the differences counterbalance each other, and the daily income, 2,718 calories, is found to be practically identical with the daily outgo, 2,716 calories. This agreement is in accordance with the law of the conservation of energy, and thus confirms the belief that this law governs the metabolism of energy in the living organism.

In 13 of the 30 experiments referred to alcohol formed a part of the diet. The results of these experiments compared with those without alcohol imply very clearly that the law of the conservation of energy holds as well with the diet containing alcohol as with the ordinary diet. This may be seen from Table 13, which epitomizes the more detailed statistics given in Table CXX in the Appendix, and compares the averages of the results of the rest and the work experiments in which alcohol formed part of the diet with those of similar experiments without alcohol. Both those experiments that are strictly comparable and those less comparable, as explained on a preceding page, are here included

The energy of net income given in the table above represents the energy of the material actually oxidized in the body, as determined from the energy of the food, of the excretory products, and of the body material stored or lost. The energy of outgo is that given off from

TABLE 13.-*Metabolism of energy. Averages of results of experiments with ordinary and with alcohol diet.*

Experiments with and without alcohol.	Energy of net income.[a]	Energy of outgo measured as–		
		Heat.	Muscular work.	Total.
MORE DIRECTLY COMPARABLE.	*Calories.*	*Calories.*	*Calories.*	*Calories.*
Rest experiments.				
Without alcohol: Nos. 9, 24, 26, and 28	2,190	2,221	....	2,221
With alcohol: Nos. 10, 22, 27	2,191	2,221	....	2,221
Work experiments.				
Without alcohol: Nos. 11, 29 and 31, 32 and 34	3,660	3,451	220	3,671
With alcohol: Nos. 12, 30, 33	3,690	3,461	215	3,676
Average of rest and work experiments.				
Without alcohol	2,925	2,836	[b](1'10)	2,946
With alcohol	2,941	2,841	[b](108)	2,949
LESS DIRECTLY COMPARABLE.				
Rest experiments.				
Without alcohol: Nos. 13 and 14, 5,21	2,302	2,277	....	2,277
With alcohol: Nos. 7, 15 to 17, 18 to 20	2,358	2,358	....	2,358
Average of all above experiments.				
Without alcohol	2,717	2,650	[b](73)	2,723
With alcohol	2,746	2,680	[b](72)	2,752

[a] Estimated energy of material actually oxidized in the body.
[b] In this average the muscular work of the work experiments is distributed over both the work and the rest experiments, which is of course not strictly logical.

the body in the form of heat and external muscle work, as measured by the apparatus. According to the law of the conservation of energy, the income and the outgo must be equal. From the comparisons given in the table above it will be seen that, whether the diet did or did not contain alcohol, the outgo was sometimes greater and sometimes less than the income, but the difference in every case was far within the range of variation to be expected in physiological experiments of such nature as these, so that the results may be considered as showing practical agreement. If we counterbalance the variations by averaging the experiments in which alcohol formed part of the diet and those without alcohol, we get the following results:

Daily income and outgo of energy with and without alcohol

Diet.	Energy of material oxidized in the body.	Energy given off by the body.
	Calories.	*Calories.*
Average 13 experiments, without alcohol.......	2,717	2,723
Average 13 experiments, with alcohol...........	2,746	2,752

When the diet contained no alcohol, the energy of the proteids, fats, and carbohydrates burned in the body, averaging 2,717 calories per day, was practically identical with the energy given off by the body in the form of heat, or heat and (the heat equivalent of) the external muscular work, averaging 2,723 calories per day. When alcohol formed part of the diet the total energy of the proteids, fats, and carbohydrates burned in the body, added to the energy of the alcohol, averaged 2,746 calories per day, and the energy given off as heat, or heat and external muscular work, averaged 2,752 calories per day. The total kinetic energy of outgo is equal to the total potential energy of income, whether it be with ordinary diet alone, or with ordinary food and alcohol.

To these results there can be but one interpretation. The energy which was latent or potential in the alcohol was wholly transformed in the body, was actually given off from the body, and was exactly recovered as heat or heat and muscular work. Otherwise, how did the body dispose of the energy of the alcohol, and from what other source did it get an exactly equal amount to replace it?

The conclusions, therefore are:

1. The law of the conservation of energy obtained with the alcohol diet as with the ordinary diet.

2. The potential energy of the alcohol oxidized in the body was transformed completely into kinetic energy, and appeared either as heat, or as muscular work, or both. To this extent, at any rate, it was used like the energy of the protein, fats, and carbohydrates of the food.

The Protection of Body Material by Alcohol

General considerations. Precious experiments and their explanations.—The belief was formerly quite general that alcohol has a specific pharmacodynamic action in retarding the metabolism of body material, both fat and proteid. As much of the earlier experimenting implied that alcohol in moderate quantities tends to "prevent waste" or "conserve the tissues," and its oxidation in the body was not understood, this effect was naturally attributed to its action as a drug. Later, as the functions of the nonnitrogenous nutrients of food came to be better understood, and the fact that alcohol is oxidized as they are in the body became fully established, the view has become common that its effect in retarding or protecting metabolism is to be explained by a nutritive rather than a pharmacodynamic action–that, in other words, it tends, by its own oxidation, to prevent the oxidation of other materials. This latter function of alcohol, however, has been denied on two grounds:

1. The increased circulation of the blood through the peripheral capillaries and the fall of body temperature which follows the ingestion of alcohol have led to the theoretical inference that the energy supplied to the body by the oxidation of the alcohol is lost by the extra radiation of heat it causes, so that it can not do the work of the fats and carbohydrates in protecting food or body material from consumption. This ground, however, is hardly tenable since, as shown beyond, the fall of body temperature with ordinary doses is vary small, and the amount of extra heat radiated is only a fraction of that supplied by the alcohol.

2. The other ground for doubting the power of alcohol to protect body material from consumption is that of direct experiment. That it may protect fat is generally conceded, but there are a number of reliable experiments on record in which the replacement of the carbohydrates and fats of a ration by alcohol has been followed by an increased elimination of nitrogen. This has been explained by the assumption that alcohol tends to increase rather than diminish the catabolism of protein in the body. On the other hand there is a considerable amount of experimental evidence to the effect that alcohol may and at times does serve as a protector of protein.

As explained in a review of the experimenting upon this subject (a) it seems to us that the conflicting results may be explained by the hypothesis of two opposing tendencies of alcohol, the one pharmacodynamic and the other nutritive. This view makes the former a specif-

[a] Report of Physiological Subcommittee of Committee of Fifty for the Investigation of the Liquor Problem, Boston, Houghton, Mifflin & Co. (In press at the time of this writing.) See also a more detailed review of the subject by Rosemann. Der Einfluss des Alkohols auf den Eiweissstoffwechsel; Arch. f.d. ges. Physiol., Bd. 86, 1901, pp. 307-503.

ic, and sometimes, if not always, temporary action of alcohol, by which it increases the catabolism of protein, while the latter action is that resulting from its oxidation. According as the latter or the former action predominates the alcohol may protect protein or fail to do so. In favor of this theory is the fact that it explains and harmonizes the results of previous experimenting and those of our own experiments also.

In considering the efficiency of alcohol for the protection of body fat and protein it is important to distinguish between two questions. Does alcohol protect these materials at all? Is it equal in protecting power to the isodynamic amount of fats or of carbohydrates, or of a mixture of the two? The comparisons in these experiments are between nearly isodynamic amounts of alcohol and the other ingredients.

The evidence of the experiments here reported–Although the present experiments were not planned for the study of these particular questions, they throw some light upon them. The details, in their bearing upon the protection or nonprotection of body protein and fat, are brought together in Table CXX in the appendix, and the average results are summarized in Table 14 herewith, which shows the amounts of available protein and energy of the diet and the amounts of protein and fat gained or lost by the body in the experiments with and without alcohol.

The grouping in Table 14 is on the same basis as in the corresponding tables in the preceding pages and in the Appendix.

When the fuel value of the diet is in excess of the needs of the body, the latter often, though not always, increases its store of material. Sometimes this increase is in the form of protein, sometimes fat, and sometimes both protein and fat. When the body requires energy in excess of that supplied by the food, it will draw upon its previously accumulated store of fat or protein, or both, for fuel. Along with the gains and losses of protein and fat are changes in the carbohydrates (glycogen), but the total quantity of these substances in the tissues is relatively small. The present methods of experimenting do not suffice for accurate measurement of the changes of glycogen, and it is commonly left out of account in discussions such as that in which we are now engaged.

Protection of Body Fat

The figures for the individual experiments in Table CXX of the Appendix show in some cases a larger gain or smaller loss of fat without alcohol than with it; in other cases the results are reversed. When , however, the experiments are grouped together and the averages with and without alcohol are compared, it is clear that, except where the differences in fuel value of the diet were considerable, the differences of fat balance are hardly large enough to be of consequence. Taking the experiments altogether, the figures of the tables, and especially those of Table 14, show slight gains in fat both with and without alcohol, but the gain is slightly larger with the alcohol. Thus in Group I, in which the experiments are more directly comparable, the average gain in 9 experiments without alcohol is 1.1 grams, in 6 with alcohol 2.4 grams, making a difference in favor of the alcohol of 1.3 grams. In the less directly comparable experiments there is an average difference of 8.8 grams, and in Group III with all the experiments there is an average of 3.9 grams in favor of the alcohol. It is also to be noted that in general the total energy of the rations with the alcohol average somewhat larger than in those without alcohol. The figures for differences just cited are brought out more clearly in Table 17, beyond, in the discussion of the utilization of energy in the experiments with and without alcohol. The comparison as there made in detail shows on the whole an advantage of the ordinary diet over that with alcohol, though the difference is very small indeed.

A direct indication of the fat-protecting power of alcohol is found in the series of experiments with E.O., Nos. 22, 23, 24. These were practically three successive periods of 3 days each. In all there was a basal ration with 116 grams available protein and 2,290 calories of available energy. To this ration was added–in the first experiment, alcohol: in the second, nothing; in the third, sugar. The alcohol and sugar each furnished about 500 calories of energy. With the alcohol there was a daily gain of 63 grams of fat; with the basal ration this was reduced to 9 grams; with the sugar it rose again to 60 grams per day. With the sugar there was a loss of 1.7 and with the alcohol a gain of 1.4 grams, while with the basal ration alone there was a loss of 1.6 grams of protein. Leaving this slight gain or loss of protein out of account, the net gain of fat with the alcohol above that in the basal ration was 54 grams, which would make vary nearly 500 calories. The net gain of fat with sugar was 51 grams. In this particular case, therefore, with isodynamic quantities of sugar and alcohol, the gain of fat was practically the same with both.

An even more striking illustration of the fat-protecting power of alcohol is found in experiments Nos. 18-21, with A.W. S. as summarized on page 329 beyond. When alcohol was added to a basal ration of ordinary food, the body gained fat at the rate of 21-35 grams per day; but when the giving of alcohol was stopped and the body had only the basal ration, it lost 25 grams of fat per day.

A clearer demonstration of the power of alcohol to protect fat from consumption would be hardly possible than that given in the experiments with E.O. and A.W.S., just cited.

We thus have two kinds of tests of the power of

TABLE 14.–*Comparison of gains and losses of protein and fat in experiments with and without alcohol.*

Experiments compared.	Seriel numbers of experiments.	Total number of days	Average per day. Available food. Protein.	Energy.	Gain (+) or loss (-). Protein.	Fat.
MORE DIRECTLY COMPARABLE.			*Grams.*	*Calories.*	*Grams.*	*Grams.*
A and B:						
E.O., rest–						
Average, 2 experiments without alcohol.	9,24	7	114	2,618	-1.0	+39.0
Average, 2 experiments with alcohol	10,22	7	116	2,602	-2.8	+42.0
D:						
E.O., work–						
1 experiment without alcohol	11	4	110	3,510	-3.0	-39.7
1 experiment with alcohol	12	4	113	3,614	-1.0	-32.2
A,B, and D:						
E.O., rest and work–						
Average, 3 experiments without alcohol	9,24,11	11	112	2,915	-1.6	+12.7
Average, 3 experiments with alcohol	10,22,12	11	115	2,939	-2.2	+17.2
C:						
J.F.S., rest–						
Average, 2 experiments without alcohol	(26,28)	6	92	2,253	-4.0	+23.1
1 experiment with alcohol	27	3	92	2,264	-6.0	+18.2
E and F:						
J.F.S., work–						
Average, 4 experiments without alcohol	(29,31), (32,34)	12	95	3,251	-6.1	-27.5
Average, 2 experiments with alcohol	30,33	6	94	3,235	-14.5	-27.7
C,E, and F:						
J.F.S., rest and work–						
Average, 6 experiments without alcohol	(26,28), (29,31), (32,34)	18	94	2,918	-5.4	-10.6
Average, 3 experiments with alcohol	27,30,33	9	93	2,911	-11.6	-12.4
A to F (Group I):						
E.O. and J.F.S., rest and work–						
Average, 9 experiments without alcohol.	9,24,11,(26,28), (29,31), (32,34)	29	103	2,917	-3.5	+1.1
Average, 6 experiments with alcohol	10,22,12,27,30,33	20	104	2,925	-6.9	+2.4
LESS DIRECTLY COMPARABLE.						
G, H, and I (Group II):						
E.O. and A.W.S., rest–						
Average, 4[a] experiments without alcohol	(13,14), 5,21	14	100	2,239	-7.3	-2.3
Average, 7[a] experiments with alcohol	7,(15,16,17), (18,19,20)	16	98	2,400	-3.0	+6.5
AVERAGE OF ALL THE ABOVE EXPERIMENTS.						
A to I (Group III):						
E.O., J.F.S., and A.W.S., rest and work–						
Average, 13 experiments (3 with work) without alcohol.	(13,14),(26,28),(29,31),(32,34),5,9 11,21,24.	43	102	2,691	-4.8	-0.1
Average, 13 experiments (3 with work) with alcohol.	7,(15,16,17),(18,19,20),10,12,22,2 7,30,33	36	102	2,750	-5.6	+3.8

[a] When two or more similar experiments are grouped together, the group is counted as 1 experiment in drawing the average. Experiments thus treated are put in parenthesis in the second column; thus, (15 to 17).

alcohol as compared with that of isodynamic amounts of carbohydrates and fats of the food for the protection of body fat. In every individual case the protecting power of the alcohol is manifest. In some instances it is slightly inferior and in others it is slightly superior in this respect, and on the average it is just about equal to the nutrients which it replaced.

So far as we are áwarde these are the only experiments in which the power of alcohol to protect fats has been determined by direct quantitative tests. While there are numerous experiments on record which have seemed to indicate that alcohol has this power, we have found none which seem to us to imply the opposite (a). Fortunately this question, which is one of no little importance, thus seems to be so clearly settled as to require no further discussion. Such is not the case with the similar question regarding the power of alcohol to protect protein from consumption.

[a]See review of experiments on the effects of alcohol on the metabolism of carbon in the report of the Committee of Fifty referred to on page 261.

TABLE 15.–*Experiments with E.O.–Gains and losses of body protein and fat with and without alcohol*

Experiments	Total number of days.	Average per day.			
		In available food.		Gain (+) or loss (-).	
		Protein.	Energy.	Protein.	Fat.
MORE DIRECTLY COMPARABLE.					
Rest Experiments.		*Grams.*	*Calories.*	*Grams.*	*Grams.*
Without alcohol, Nos. 9, 24	7	114	2,618	-1.0	+39.0
With alcohol, Nos. 10, 22	7	116	2,602	-2.8	+42.0
Work experiments.					
Without alcohol, No. 11	4	110	3,510	-3.0	-39.7
With alcohol, No. 12	4	113	3,614	-1.0	-32.2
Rest and work experiments.					
Without alcohol, Nos. 9, 24, 11	11	112	2,915	-1.6	+12.7
With alcohol, Nos. 10, 22, 12	11	115	2,939	-2.2	+17.2
LESS DIRECTLY COMPARABLE.					
Rest experiments.					
Without alcohol, Nos. 13, 14[a]	7	99	2,294	-12.0	+25.7
With alcohol, No. 7	4	99	2,230	-12.0	-14.3
Average of All Above.					
Without alcohol	18	109	2,760	-4.2	+16.0
With alcohol	15	111	2,762	-4.6	+9.4

[a]Nos. 13 and 14 averaged as one experiment.

Protection of Body Protein

As regards the protection of body protein by alcohol, the results of the experiments are variable, but on the whole the catabolism of protein, as measured by the amount of nitrogen excreted by the kidneys, was slightly larger in the experiments with than in those without alcohol. In discussing the effect of alcohol upon protein metabolism, we must consider the variations from day to day in the amount of nitrogen excreted in the urine when alcohol forms a part of the diet, and compare them with the variations in similar experiments in which alcohol is not included in the diet. The data of the daily eliminations of nitrogen by the different subjects in experiments with and without alcohol are summarized in Table CXXIII in the Appendix.

What especially concerns us here is the influence of the substitution of alcohol for a portion of the ordinary food upon the gain or loss of body protein. As this seems to depend largely upon the individual, it will be well to discuss the experiments with the three subjects separately.

Experiments with E.O.–With this subject there was a marked tendency to excrete more nitrogen in the urine on either the day before or the day after he entered the respiration chamber. This tendency was as noticeable in the experiments without as in those with alcohol. This variation in nitrogen excretion is independent of either the character of the food or the activity of the subject, and appears to be due to a psychic cause that is little understood. Since this variation was often much larger than any which could be attributed to the alcohol, we hesitate to assign to the latter any definite and uniform effect upon the metabolism of nitrogen.

It is to be noted that there is no experiment with E.O. in which an alcohol diet immediately preceded or followed a diet furnishing the same amount of energy from ordinary food materials without alcohol. There are, however, a number of separate experiments which may be compared, as is done in Table 15.

In the less directly comparable experiments Nos. 13 and 14 are grouped together as one, since the average quantities of protein and energy are the same as in No. 7. The details, however, show that while the quantities of energy in the rations were the same in both, No. 13 had 110 and No. 14 only 89 grams of protein. Nevertheless the results as regards gain or loss of body material were almost identical. In each there was a loss of 12 grams of protein and in No.13 there was a gain of 27 grams and in No. 14 a gain of 24 grams of fat. The experiments were 40 days apart. We lay especial stress upon this circumstance, because it illustrates the futility of drawing final conclusions from a single experiment. In each of these cases the metabolism experiment was preceded by a period of 4 days with similar diet while the subject was outside the calorimeter, but in neither case was nitrogen equilibrium obtained. Neither one of these experiments, therefore, could be taken as a basis for conclusion as to the quantity of protein required for either nitrogen equilibrium or constant elimination of nitrogen. A special reason for citing them here with No.7 is that they were made with the same subject as the other experiments of the table.

The chief reliance is to be placed upon the more directly comparable experiments. In those in which the subject was at rest, the alcohol ration furnished 2 grams more protein and 16 less calories of energy per day than the nonalcohol ration. There was a larger loss of protein by 1.8 grams and a larger gain of fat by 3 grams with the alcohol. These differences are all very small, but in so far as they go they imply that the alcohol was somewhat less efficient as a protector of protein than the fats and carbohydrates which it replaced. In the work experiments the alcohol ration supplied 3 grams more of protein and 104 calories more of energy than the other. With both there was a loss of protein, the amount being 3 grams per day without and 1 gram per day with alcohol; but since the alcohol ration furnished 3 grams of protein more than any other, there remains a deficit of 1 gram of protein per day against the alcohol ration as compared with that without alcohol, and that notwithstanding the larger fuel value of the diet. Here again the alcohol ration is slightly inferior in protein protecting power.

Taking the rest and work experiments together, the alcohol rations, with an average of 3 grams of protein and 24 calories of energy per day more than the nonalcohol ration, show a greater loss of protein by 0.6 gram per day. On the other hand there is a slightly large average gain of fat with the alcohol.

If we reckon the less comparable experiments in the general average, we have 111 grams of protein with alcohol as against 109 grams without it, while the quantities of energy are the same in both rations. The average loss of protein is 0.4 gram greater and the gain of fat 5.6 grams less with the alcohol; but of course much less stress is to be laid upon the less comparable experiments.

On the whole it is clear that is these experiments with this subject the alcohol was not as efficient as isodynamic quantities of fats and carbohydrates in protecting protein. Notwithstanding the energy of the alcohol was actually larger than that of the fats and carbohydrates which it replaced, it did not equal them in protecting power. The difference is the more striking because of the slightly larger average quantities of protein in the alcohol rations. On the other hand, the differences between the amounts of protein and energy in the alcohol as compared with the nonalcohol experiments are so slight as to imply only a slight inferiority of the alcohol in the protection of protein.

While the alcohol was not isodynamically equal to the carbohydrates and fats in protecting power, it would be going very far to deny that the experiments imply a positive protecting action. Not only were the differences in favor of the protecting power of the carbohydrates and fats as compared with the alcohol very small, but the quantity of energy supplied by the alcohol was large. To claim that the alcohol has no protecting power would be to assume that the same reduction of fats and carbohydrates in the rations without any replacement by alcohol would have resulted in no greater differences in protein protection. This is in the highest degree improbable.

In this connection the results of experiments Nos. 22, 23, 24 above referred to are worthy of consideration. With the normal ration, plus alcohol, there was a gain of 1.4 grams of protein and 63 grams of fat per day; but when, in the period immediately following, the alcohol was removed, there was a loss of 1.6 grams of protein and a gain of only 9 grams of fat.

Experiments with A.W.S.–With this subject we have but one series of rest experiments. This consisted of a preliminary period of 4 days, followed by four experimental periods, during which the subject was in the respiration chamber. Throughout the preliminary and experimental periods there was a uniform basal ration of ordinary food, supplying about 90 grams of protein and 2,040 calories of energy. To this was added, in the preliminary period of 4 days, commercial alcohol, furnishing about 500 calories of energy. The nitrogen in the urine during the successive days was 12.2, 16, 19, 16.4 grams; that is to say, there was a marked increase of protein catabolism during the whole period. The first three experiments proper were of 2 days each. In the first of these periods commercial alcohol, in the second whiskey, and in the third brandy was added to the basal rations, the quantities being sufficient to furnish the same amount, about 500 calories of energy. The daily quantities of nitrogen in the urine were 17.4, 15.4, 14.7, 14.2, 13.8, and 14.4 grams.; that is to say, the rise in nitrogen excretion continued through the first day of the first period; thereafter it fell. During the fourth period of 3 days the basal ration was given without the alcohol. The natural inference is that with this subject, who had always been an abstainer, the rise in nitrogen excretion at first was due to the alcohol. The very evident fall after the fifth day implies that the action of alcohol in increasing the nitrogen was transitory, and that it had passed away at the end of the third period. The increase of nitrogen excretion in the fourth period was apparently due to the reduction of the ration by the removal of the alcohol.

The average gains and losses of protein and fat for the separate periods may be tabulated as follows:

Experiments with J.F.S.–Gains and losses of body protein and fat with and without alcohol.

Experiments.	Total days	Averages per day. In available food. Protein.	Energy.	Gain (+) or loss (-). Protein.	Fat.
Rest experiments.		*Grams.*	*Calories.*	*Grams.*	*Grams.*
Without alcohol, Nos. 26, 28	6	92	2,253	-4.0	+23.1
With alcohol, Nos. 27	3	92	2,264	-6.0	+18.2
Work experiments.					
Without alcohol, No. 29,31,32,34	12	95	3,251	-6.1	-27.5
With alcohol, No. 30,33	6	94	3,255	-14.5	-27.7
Average of all above.					
Without alcohol	18	94	2,918	-5.4	-10.6
With alcohol	9	93	2,911	-11.6	-12.4

Period.	Days.	Alcohol added to basal ration.	Gain (+) or loss (-) grams per day. Protein.	Fat.
First.	2	Commercial alcohol	-12	+25
Second	2	Whisky	-0	+35
Third	2	Brandy	+2	+21
Fourth	3	None	-3	-25

We thus have a gradual change from a loss of nitrogen to equilibrium and positive gain with the alcohol, and on its removal a positive loss. With the fat there is a constant gain with the alcohol and marked loss on its removal.

While it would be unwise to generalize from a single series of experiments, the indications here point clearly toward three conclusions: (1) The alcohol at first caused an increase of nitrogen metabolism and loss of body protein, but this effect was temporary; (2) thereafter the alcohol protected body protein; (3) the alcohol protected fat throughout

Experiments with J.F.S.–With the third subject there was opportunity to observe the immediate effect produced upon nitrogen metabolism by the substitution of alcohol for a part of the ordinary nutrients of the diet. Three series of experiments were made. Each included three periods of 3 days each. In each series the subject received the same basal ration throughout, but in addition thereto enough of either butter, sugar, or alcohol to furnish about 500 calories. In the first series the subject was at rest, and the order of addition was butter, alcohol, suger. In thesecond series the subject was at work and received a larger diet, the order being sugar, alcohol, butter. The third series was similar in all respects to the second except that the order was butter, alcohol, sugar.

These experiments were thus better adapted than any of those previously discussed to show the immediate effect of the substitution of alcohol for other nutrients in the diet, and in each case it will be seen that this substitution resulted in a loss (or an increased loss) of body protein, which loss continued through the 3 days of the alcohol period. The subject was unused to alcoholic beverages, and from what has already been said such a loss of protein during the first few days of the alcohol diet was to be expected from the results of other similar experiments. Whether this loss would have ceased on continuing the alcohol diet, as seems to have been the case with A.W.S., the experiments do not show.

Thus all of the experiments with this subject would indicate clearly that for periods of 3 days the alcohol was inferior to either fat or carbohydrates as a protector of protein. It should be stated, also, that the loss of body protein with the alcohol was greater than the figures in the table would indicate, for the nitrogen elimination of the period preceding the alcohol was in each case slightly increased by the entrance of the subject into the respiration chamber, while that of the period following the alcohol is increased by the lag in the excretion of the extra nitrogen metabolized under the influence of the alcohol. The lag would, of course, likewise prevent the effect of the alcohol from becoming fully apparent in the first day of the alcohol period. Hence a better idea of the actual effect of the alcohol would probably be obtained by omitting from consideration the first day of each period. The average elimination of nitrogen thus becomes, in the fore periods, 15.5 grams, in the alcohol periods, 17.1 grams, and in the after period, 15.5 grams per day, showing a difference in favor of the ordinary nutrients of 1.6 grams of nitrogen or 10 grams of protein instead of 6.2 grams, as shown in the preceding table.

It is also noticeable that the loss of body protein under the influence of alcohol was larger with this subject when at work than when at rest. the difference is not great and may be simply accidental. It might, however, be interpreted as indicating that the subject worked to better advantage on the ordinary diet than on the diet of which a part was alcohol. This would accord with the conclusions drawn by Chauveau from experiments on dogs (a) and by Parkes from extended observations on marching soldiers and workingmen (b).

Summary–In interpreting these experiments two things are to be considered. One it that the differences between the amounts of nitrogen excreted with and without alcohol are generally very small. The other is that there is good ground for the belief that with persons little accustomed to the use of alcohol it may have a tendency to increase nitrogen metabolism, which may counteract, to greater or less extent, the tendency to protect protein, though, with some persons at least, this action appears to be temporary. The results with the individual subjects may be briefly recapitulated as follows:

With E.O., who was accustomed to the use of moderate quantities of alcoholic beverages, the protein protecting power of the alcohol was apparent, but seemed to be somewhat inferior to that of fats and carbohydrates.

With A.W.S., an abstainer, there was an increase of nitrogen excretion during the first days after the beginning of the alcohol diet, with a resulting loss of body protein, but this action ceased after 5 or 6 days, and thereafter the alcohol apparently protected protein, though the experiments do not show how its efficiency in this respect compared with that of the carbohydrates and fats.

With J.F.S., who was also an abstainer, there was, in each case, an increase of nitrogen excretion and loss of body protein during the 3-day periods in which the alcohol replaced fat or sugar. There was thus a marked inferiority of alcohol in protecting power. The result is similar to that observed with A.W.S. during the first days with alcohol, but the experiments do not show what the effect of continuing the alcohol diet would have been, and they are, therefore, not decisive.

Taking the results of all the experiments together, it may be said that–

1. They offer no evidence to imply that alcohol can not protect protein, though they imply in some cases it may, at least for a time, fail to do so.
2. On the other hand, they give very marked indications of its protein protecting power.
3. They imply clearly that in this respect it was in some cases nearly or quite equal and in others decidedly inferior to the isodynamic amounts of carbohydrates and fats which it replaced.

Other experiments upon the protection of protein by alcohol.–It is clear that the experiments above described are not conclusive regarding the action of alcohol in protecting protein from consumption. They were not planned for the study of this subject. To make the results decisive the alcohol periods should be long enough to eliminate the more or less temporary action of alcohol as a drug; the available energy of the ration of the nonalcohol periods should equal in some cases the total available energy of the alcohol ration, while in other cases it should be repeated with different persons and under different conditions. These facts we did not fully understand when the experiments were begun, nor would it have been practicable with the means at our disposal to make such experiments with men in the respiration calorimeter as would be needed for the comprehensive study of the question. Experiments of from twenty to thirty consecutive days seem necessary for the most satisfactory results. For a man to spend so long a time in the respiration chamber of our apparatus would be, to say the least, very tedious, and the cost of such experiments, in labor and money, would have exceeded our available resources. Fortunately, the results obtained by a number of other investigators, while our experiments were being made and since, have done much to clarify the situation as regards the effects of alcohol upon protein metabolism.

Referring to the above-named reviews of the subject,(c) and especially to that of Rosemann for details and references to the original memoirs, it will suffice here to summarize the results. It appears that:

1. A large number of early experiments have brought conflicting results, some implying the protection of protein by alcohol; others the opposite. Of the former class those of Mogilianski are of especial interest. Of the latter those of Miura, made under the direction of Van Noorden, and those of Schmidt and of Schoeneseiffen, under the direction of Rosemann, have been much quoted. The general plan of experimenting followed by these three investigators consisted in giving the subject an ordinary diet for a time and observing the nitrogen balance. Thereafter, during a period of four to six days, alcohol was used. In Miura's case the alcohol was substituted for carbohydrates in a diet which had been adequate for maintaining nitrogen equilibrium; but with the alcohol the excretion of nitrogen increased and the body lost nitrogen. With Schmidt, alcohol was added to a diet with which nitrogen equilibrium had been maintained; the alcohol did not diminish the excretion of the nitrogen and the equilibrium continued. With Schoeneseiffen, alcohol was added to an inadequate diet with which there was loss of nitrogen; the loss continued with the alcohol.

[a]Compt. rend. Acad. d. Sc. Par. 132, pp. 65 and 110.

[b]Proc. Roy, Soc. 20 (1871-72), 402, and monograph "On the issue of a spirit ration during the Ashantee campaign, 1874," etc. London, 1875.

[c]Rosemann interprets two of our experiments, Nos. 7 and 10, the only ones then published, as not showing the protection of protein; an interpretation from which we should not dissent, since No. 7 was exceptional, and two experiments could hardly suffice for the establishement of the principle.

These experiments have furnished the chief basis for the contention that alcohol can not protect protein. In Miura's case the increase of nitrogen excretion with the alcohol was as large, and, indeed, in one instance very slightly larger, then when the carbohydrates were removed and no alcohol was used in their place. Miura, and after him Rosemann and others, inferred that alcohol was unable to protect protein from disintegration, and went so far as to ascribe to it a positive disintegrating action and to apply to it the term "proteid poison."

2. Neumann, in 1899, made experiments on a similar plan, save that the alcohol period was continued for sixteen days, during which part of the fat of the normal diet was replaced by alcohol. He found that during the first four days of the alcohol period there was no evidence of protein protection; the nitrogen excretion was increased and was as large as during another period when the ordinary ration was reduced and no alcohol was used in its place. Thereafter the nitrogen excretion diminished, and during the remaining twelve days of the alcohol period it was the same as with the normal ration. When the alcohol was removed and nothing substituted the excretion of nitrogen increased as before. Neumann concludes that in his own case the failure of the alcohol to protect protein at first was probably due to a specific though temporary action by which it tended to increase the disintegration of protein so that the tendency to protein protection was counteracted. Later this special action disappeared and the protecting action came into full play.

Neumann's interpretation of his experiments was questioned by Rosemann, who has been a most vigorous opponent of the theory that alcohol can protect protein, and a keen critic of the experiments which have seemed to favor this view. He maintained the disintegrating, but questioned the protecting action of the alcohol, alleging defects in the plans of Neumann's experiments. Neumann, without replying, repeated his experiments in such ways as to meet Rosemann's objections, and found conclusive evidence of the protecting power of the alcohol, these later results being published early in 1900. In 1901, Chotzen, working under the direction of Rosenfeld, and in 1901, Clopatt, each published results of inquiries which agreed with Neumann's. Meantime Rosemann made several series of experiments of his own, the outcome of which, to his surprise, clearly demonstrated the protecting power of alcohol, and confirmed the view maintained by Neumann. He has taken the pains to prepare an extensive summary of the experimenting in this field (a), in which he assents fully to the interpretation placed by Neumann, Rosenfeld, Chotzen, and Clopatt upon their experiments; believes that the protection of protein is shown by other experiments, as those of Mogilianski; considers it fully demonstrated by his own experiments; and comes to the definite conclusion that alcohol has a twofold influence upon the metabolism of protein, as previously suggested by Neumann. He is inclined to believe, with Neumann, that the disintegrating action is most apt to occur with persons little accustomed to the use of alcohol, and is of short duration, while in its action as a protector of protein it is analogous to the carbohydrates and fats, its influence being due to the utilization of its energy by the body. According to this view, the results obtained by Miura and others, in whose experiments the alcohol periods continued only from four to six days, are explained by the disintegrating action of the alcohol, which counteracted the protecting action, so that the resultant effect was an apparent failure of the alcohol to protect protein. With Neumann the alcohol periods continued after this disintegrating action ceased, and showed the more permanent protecting influence. The fact that in a number of the experiments the protecting influence was manifested from the start is explained by the absence or only partial action of the disintegrating tendency.

We have, then, a clearly defined theory regarding the influence of alcohol upon proteid metabolism. This theory assumes two different kinds of action of alcohol. In the one it is a direct protector of protein, and serves the body as food; in the other it tends to disintegrate protein, and acts as a drug. The belief in the first action follows as a corollary from the oxidation of alcohol in the body and the transformation of its energy. In undergoing these changes alcohol is similar to sugar, starch, and fat, which, by their own oxidation and consequent supply of energy to the body are able to protect the constituents of the food and of the body, including protein, from oxidation. That alcohol may and does protect protein is abundantly demonstrated by the experiments above cited.

The disintegrating influence of alcohol upon protein is less definitely proven. The theory is little more than a convenient hypothesis for explaining the failure of alcohol, under some circumstances, to protect protein. It is the only satisfactory hypothesis which has thus far been suggested. It is all the easier to accept because of the considerations that the breaking up of protein compounds in the body seems to be influenced, in some unexplained way or ways, by the nervous system, and this latter in turn is influenced by alcohol. In our own experiments, for instance, the excretion of nitrogen is apparently affected at times by the mental condition of the subject.

In large enough doses alcohol has a paralyzing effect, and may thus reduce general metabolism to a

[a]See page 261.

minimum and cause coma or even death. There is no proof that it can not, on the other hand, increase proteid metabolism.

The positive proof of the disintegrating action of alcohol upon protein is limited in amount. The experimental demonstration must be sought in cases in which more protein is broken down with alcohol than without it, the ration of ordinary food being otherwise the same in both cases. We have been able to find only three cases on record in which the amount of protein thus broken down with alcohol apparently exceeded by more than 0.1 gram of nitrogen per day the amount broken down without alcohol. They are discussed in the review above referred to. The first was in one of Miura's experiments, in which the excess with alcohol amounted to 0.5 gram of nitrogen (3.2 grams of protein) per day during an alcohol period of four days. The second was in one of Neumann's experiments, in which the excess during the first four days of an alcohol period of ten days was 0.9 gram of nitrogen per day. During the remaining six days of the same period the nitrogen excretion was less by 1.5 grams per day than in the corresponding period without alcohol. The third was in an experiment by Clopatt. During the first six days of an alcohol period of twelve days the nitrogen excretion exceeded that of a corresponding period without alcohol by 2 grams per day. During the remaining six days of the same alcohol period the nitrogen excretion was less by 1.4 grams per day than it was without alcohol.

It seems to the writers that in view of the unavoidable irregularities in nitrogen balance in such experimenting these data are insufficient to demonstrate the disintegrating action of alcohol, but, taken in connection with the need of an explanation for the occasional failure of alcohol to protect protein, they make the theory plausible.

Sources of uncertainty in this kind of experimenting.–One point which has hardly received the attention it deserves in discussions of this kind is the uncertainty of the nitrogen balance in any given case as a measure of the actual influence of a given condition upon nitrogen metabolism. This has been emphasized elsewhere in the present memoir (see pp. 393 and 394). Differences which look large in a table of figures are often far inside the unavoidable variations in actual experimenting.

Even when the differences are significant the interpretation may be erroneous. A striking illustration of the danger of such error is found in the current discussion of the question we are now considering. For a number of years past writers upon this subject have insisted most positively that alcohol, instead of being a protector of protein, is a protein poison. This theory is based almost wholly upon the experiments of Miura, Schmidt, and Schoeneseiffen. The experiments of Neumann, Rosenfeld-Chotzen, Clopatt, and Rosemann, not to speak of others, including our own, have shown that this theory was wrong and have given us a very plausible hypothesis to explain why it was wrong.

We can not insist too strongly upon the danger of drawing positive conclusions from figures for nitrogen balance as a measure of protein protection by either alcohol or sugar or starch in fat, Certainly comes only with careful planning and execution and manifold repetition of experiments.

Incidentally, it is to be noted that the excretion of nitrogen in the urine is not necessarily an exact measure of the amount of proteid broken down in short periods, since the time between the disintegration of the protein and the appearance of the nitrogen in the urine, the so-called nitrogen lag, varies widely. The longer the experimental period the less the error from this source.

Finally, there is the unsettled question as to how much of the protein metabolized is that of food and how much comes from organized tissue.

Final conclusions regarding the influence of alcohol upon protein metabolism–The experiments and considerations above cited seem to us to warrant the following conclusions:

1. The power of alcohol to protect the protein of food or body tissue, or both, from consumption is clearly demonstrated. Its action in this respect appears to be similar to that of the carbohydrates and fats; that is to say, in its oxidation it yields energy needed by the body, and thus saves other substances from oxidation. In this way alcohol serves the body as food. Just how moderate quantities of alcohol compare with isodynamic amounts of sugar, starch, and fat in the power to protect protein from catabolism is not yet settled. Apparently it is in some cases equal, in others inferior, to these substances. It is by no means certain that the fats and carbohydrates are always equal to each other in this power.

2. Alcohol appears also to exert at times a special action as a drug. In large quantities it is positively toxic, and may retard or even prevent metabolism in general and proteid metabolism in particular. In small doses it seems at times to have an opposite influence, tending to increase the disintegration of protein. This action, though not conclusively demonstrated, is very probable. It offers a satisfactory explanation for the occasional failure of alcohol to protect protein, the assumption being that the two tendencies counteract each other. The only justification for calling alcohol a proteid poison is found in this disintegrating tendency. This pharmacodynamic action of alcohol appears to be temporary and most apt to occur with people little accustomed to its use. The circumstances under which such action occurs can not now be fully defined.

Elimination of nitrogen in presence and absence of coffee.
[Quantities per day.]

Kind and number of experiments.	Days	Nitrogen. In food.	In feces.	In urine.	Gain (+) or loss (-) to body.
		Grams.	*Grams.*	*Grams.*	*Grams.*
I. With coffee:					
Average 4 experiments with alcohol [10,12,18,22]	13	18.6	1.2	18.2	-0.8
Average 4 experiments without alcohol [9,11,21,24]	14	18.6	1.5	17.5	-0.4
Increase (+) or decrease (-) with alcohol	....	0	-0.3	+0.7	-0.4
II. Without coffee:					
Average 5 experiments with alcohol [(19,20), 27,30,33]	13	15.8	1.0	16.1	-1.3
Average 7 experiments without alcohol [21, (26,28), (29,31), (32,34)]	21	15.9	1.0	15.7	-0.8
Increase (+) or decrease (-) with alcohol	....	-0.1	0	+0.4	-0.5
Increase (+) or decrease (-) in presence of coffee	....	+0.1	-0.3	+0.3	+0.1
III. Direct comparison, alcohol with and without coffee:					
Experiments 15,17,18, alcohol given with coffee	6	16.5	0.9	16.0	-0.4
Experiments 16,19,20, alcohol given without coffee	6	16.5	1.0	14.9	+0.6
Increase (+) or decrease (-) in presence of coffee	....	0	-1.0	+1.1	-1.0

Influence of coffee upon protein metabolism in these experiments.–In some of these experiments alcohol was administered with coffee, in others with water. It might be thought that the presence of the coffee would interfere with the action of the alcohol (a). The figures give no support for this view, as shown in the following tabular statement.

This table comprises all of the experiments that are directly comparable. The experiments in which the alcohol was given with coffee are averaged together and compared with the corresponding nonalcohol experiments, and the figures in the third line of category I show the effects of alcohol in presence of coffee. Under II a similar comparison is made of the experiments in which no coffee was given, the third line of figures here showing the effects of alcohol when taken alone. By subtracting the third line of figures under II from the corresponding figures under I we obtain values which may be taken as showing the influence of the coffee. A more direct comparison of results with and without coffee is given under III, but the number of experiments compared is necessarily smaller, and therefore individual variations have relatively much greater weight. While the differences which could be attributed to the coffee are probably within the limits of experimental error, it would seem that if there is any effect it is to increase rather than retard proteid metabolism.

[a]See Woodbury and Egbert, A Physiologic Consideration of the Food Value of Alcohol, Jour. Am. Med. Assc., Mar. 31, 1900.

Experimental Contributions to the Science of Human Daily Nutritional Needs With Particular Regard to the Necessary Amount of Protein (Author's Experiments)

by

Dr. med. & phil. R.O. Neumann,

University Lecturer, I. Assistant at Kiel Hygienic Institute

Introduction

The daily nutritional requirement represents a variable quantity which does not depend solely on bodily consumption, but which is also determined especially by the characteristics of the individual. Among these belong age, gender, lifestyle, type of profession and frame of mind, and especially body weight and activity level; climatic and social relations play a role as well.

The consequence of this is that the supply of nutrients and with it the most important components of nutrition, protein, fat and carbohydrates, suffers variations. If the fluctuations caused thereby remain within certain bounds, then no danger arises for the body, since a constant adjustment takes place; but if the absorption of combustible vital substances sinks continuously below a certain minimum amount, then the body is brought out of its equilibrium and suffers visible damage.

This proposition is especially valid when it has to do with a too small supply of protein. With this the related question arises: What is the smallest amount of protein that can keep the body in nitrogen balance? The answer is quite complicated, if not altogether impossible to give, since we must be aware that there is not just one protein minimum, but several minimums.

Daily experience shows that most people remain at body- and protein- equilibrium with their diet chosen under normal conditions, although their main nourishment consists in quite varied combinations, and so we will have to conclude that they can keep themselves in nitrogen balance also with varied amounts of protein. Rubner (page 126) has previously addressed the fact that we have to deal with several protein minimums, and also emphasized that because of this a search for one protein minimum would be unsuccessful. Of course that is just to say that a protein minimum suitable for all individuals is not to be found, but it can indeed be determined for a certain person and for certain foodstuffs.

While C. Voit required 118 grams of protein per day for the hardworking 70-kilo heavy woodworker, other researchers have found more, others nonetheless much less necessary. Hereby is created an abundance of contradictory material from which a compromise does not seem easy to extrapolate, and yet the results found can be explained, as we will see later, if one only: 1) pays attention to the factors noted above, which are involved in nutrition and 2) takes into consideration that the quantity of protein depends considerably on how much carbohydrate and fat are included in the food. Rubner (page 127) reports that through feeding of carbohydrates, protein conversion is depressed by 5%, while 95% of energy exchange is covered through carbohydrates. Also the very low numbers of Siven, who could remain in nitrogen balance with 30.1 grams per day, speak for this fact.

In the judgement of such extremely small numbers which vary so widely from Voit's norm we must admittedly ask ourselves whether these slight protein amounts

Neumann RO. Experimentelle beiträge zur Lehre von dem täglichen nahrungsbedarf des menschen unter besonderer berücksichtigung der notwendigen eiweifsmenge. *Arch Hyg.* 1902;45:1-4,69-78.
Reprinted with permission from The Williams & Wilkins Company, 428 E. Preston St., Baltimore, MD 21202.
Translated by April Armstrong, Baton Rouge, LA.

found in experiments should be significant for really practical nutritional proportions, or whether they just ought to prove that it is entirely possible to depress the quantity of protein so far for a short duration without danger to the body. The last result addresses doubtless high theoretical interests, but loses meaning in practice, since in reality there is no "normal" food combination which contains only a few grams of protein. It seems as if nature had already made provision so that with rational nourishment the organism does not need to be protein-impoverished. So indeed with the numerous compilations which have been made on the nutrition of individual persons or mass provisioning, we never find such skimpy amounts of protein. Also with metabolic experiments with an uncontrolled or a portioned diet, which were undertaken for practical nutrition purposes, higher numbers are constantly found.

Of course these also offer no uniform picture, since they were gained under the most varied hypotheses and conditions, and so it happens that the most important question about the necessary protein measurement still has found no conclusive answer.

Thus each contribution which is based on correct groundwork could be well-grounded and advance the solution of the matter.

The experiments which are to be recorded in the following comprise, as I will briefly indicate here, three segments and a period of 746 experiment days.

The three experimental segments should complement each other, since in the first and third experimental segments were conducted with freely chosen food, but in the second, metabolic experiments with measured nutrients are interpolated.

However, before I address my own experiments, we must take a look at the work which has been occupied with the same question and which is of interest here.

Experiments and Results of Earlier Researchers

With the so important question about a rational nutrition one should not be astonished that since the time when C. Voit established his normal diet principle, numerous researchers have occupied themselves with further research and further development of these things. The result of this was such an abundance of literature that after 27 years it is quite difficult to find one's way through the labyrinth. Moreover, individual researchers, in order to reach their goals, adopted varying methods, which unfortunately included various sources of error, which were able to advance the work only a little or not at all.

When we briefly bring to mind the known methods which can lead to determination of food proportions, they are the following:

1. Average freely chosen food:

a) with individuals of entire families:

One notes in the freely chosen, not ad hoc analysed foodstuffs, protein, fat and carbohydrate amounts according to known analyses for a protracted period and sees whether the individual remains at his body weight. From this one calculates the daily food allocation *According to Finkler one understands as food proportion the quantity which should be supplied; as food composition on the other hand the nourishment actually used in certain cases.

Comparison of Three Experiments with Each Other and With the Results of Other Researchers With the Conclusions Drawn Therefrom

If we subject the numbers gained from experiments conducted at various times to a test, an agreement in the main and most important points is unmistakable.

We had found (calculated for 70 kg):

	Protein	Fat	Carbo-hydrates	Alcohol	Calories
1st experiment:	69.1	90.2	242.0	45.6	2427.0
per kg:	0.99	1.3	34.5	0.56	34.7
2nd experiment:	79.5	163.0	234.0	-	2777
per kg:	1.1	2.3	33.4	-	39.7
3rd experiment:	74.0	106.0	164.2	5.3	1999
per kg:	1.0	1.5	23.4	0.07	28.5

It is self-evident that the determined values had to exhibit noticeable differences among them, but to some extent there were long pauses between the experiments, and the actual conditions under which the experiments were conducted were also not always exactly the same. But in one, and indeed the most decisive point all three experiments show the same conclusion: The low amount of protein with which the organism maintains nitrogen balance in the body, and indeed not just for a few days, but for a duration of very many months.

The protein figures 69.1 g, 79.5 g and 74 g lie way below Voit's normal limit of 118 g, for they amount to only about 3/4 of the protein amount he required; and if it is allowed to take an average of the numbers which in the first and third experiments were found by empirical methods, and from those which in the second experiment were found by experimental methods, then this average number- 74.2 g of protein- would also fall considerably below the 100 g amount desired by Munck and the 90 g which Demuth considered necessary.

On the other hand, they would come rather near the numbers found sufficient in food by Bohm (64 g), Rechenberg (79.8 g), Breisacher (83 g), Rumpf and

Schumm (83 g), Scheube (74 g).

Even lower numbers were found by Ritter (44.7 g), Hirschfeld (41.7 g), Klemperer (36.2 g), Lapique and Marette (34.7 g), Peschel (20.3 g), Voit (66.6 g), Siven (31.3 g) and Albu (34.1 g).

One must of course consider that in most cases these results are yielded only from short-term experiments, thus are not suitable for the drawing-up of a diet for practical purposes.

In consideration of this question Munck also says (p. 209)-

> "On the other hand it is not yet proven that in the long run 50-80 g of protein is sufficient for an adult. Up to now experiments only show that the body can maintain substance balance for a short while also with such a small amount of protein supply, but not that health and hardiness, as well as stamina do not suffer harm from a constant supply of such modest quantities of protein (even with an excessive supply of nitrogen -free substances)."

On the other hand I now believe to have shown through my three experiments that the body can not only maintain balance in the long run with protein amounts which lie between 70-80 g, but it also need suffer no loss of stamina, health and hardiness.

The body weight amounted in the ten-month first experiment to 66-67 kg, in the four-month second experiment to 67 kg and in the ten-month third experiment to 71 1/2 - 72 1/2 kg. No weight loss was confirmed, and well-being during the very long duration of the experiment was never disturbed.

But there is one point to take into consideration. Most authors who experimentally, even only for the short term, obtained such a scanty nitrogen quantity, purchased it with increased additions of carbohydrates or fats. Thus Breisacher for example
-calculated for 70 kg - consumed with 83 g of protein 665 g of carbohydrates; Demuth found with 59 g of protein 650 g of carbohydrates, Kellner and Mori with 102 g of protein 735 g of carbohydrates, Klemperer with 336.2 g of protein 514 g carbohydrates, Kumagava with 79.5 g protein 844 g carbohydrates, in two other experiments with 58 and 48 g of protein respectively 644 g carbohydrates, Rumpf and Schumm with 83 g protein 790 g carbohydrates, Schaube with 74 and 85 g protein 630 g carbohydrates.

In my experiments on the other hand the carbohydrate quantity not only did not remain at the normal quantity of 500 g required by Voit, but it even fell, in spite of the low protein intake, to less than half. The quantities amount in the first experiment to only 242 g, in the second 234 g, in the third 164 g.

From this it can be deduced, at least for my part, that a decrease in the 118 g protein quantity required b Voit can take place not only with the increase in carbo hydrates, but also with quite considerable decreases c the same under 500 g. This finding would suppo Siven's assertions. At any rate it cannot be passed ove in silence that in all my experiments the fat experience a considerable increase. The quantities amounted i the first experiment to 90 g, in the second to 163 g an in the third to 106 g. If we derive from the average c these amounts - 117 g - the normal quantity of 56 g then there remain 61 g of fat excess = 567 calories Thus in other words: the reduction of protein to 74 was possible without harm to the organism with a nor mal fat quantity of 56 g and a carbohydrate quantity c approximately 360 g.

The calorie quantities were not especially high i the experiments. They amounted in the first experimen to only 2427, in the second 2777 and in the third 199 The average number amounts to 2367 = 33.8 calorie per kg., an amount which however quite nearly reache the 34 calorie amount required by Rubner.

The calorie amount in the experiments of th authors mentioned above, who give large quantities c carbohydrates, is also accordingly more important, an almost without exception reaches or exceeds 3000 Only with Hamilton and Bowie do I find condition similar to mine. He (sic) found in the food of two men calculated at 70 kg - 90 protein, 77 fat and 257 carbohy drate = 2138 calories, with which they "could remai nearly in balance."

The proportion of protein-containing to protein-fre food in the individual experiments has already been dis cussed. In the first experiment it was 1:5.7, in the sec ond experiment 1:6.1, and in the third experiment 1:7.4 In comparison with the common average from all 30 investigations of other authors, which amounted t 1:5.2, we find our numbers from the second and thir experiment rather divergent, insofar as the percent pro portion of protein lags behind as compared to protein free nutrition.

Quite similar numbers result naturally if one calcu lates the calories which from 100 calories are allotted t protein, fat and carbohydrates.

The average of the three experiments amounts to:

	Protein	Fat	Carbohydrates
first experiment:	15.0	48.2	36.7
second experiment:	14.3	34.4	42.3
third experiment:	11.3	24.5	64.2

The numbers are not irregular among themselves but they also have one thing in common: The percent age ratio is quite low and it does not entirely correspon to the furnished requirements. In comparison with the calculations of all other investigations it is shown, however, that there too the greatest variations are to be found, so that one cannot with certainty draw usable conclusions therefrom.

The consumption of alcohol and the cost of food, both with as well as without beer, has been addressed in the respective experiments.

Since the experiments extended through both the summer and the winter months, there was an opportunity to observe whether a greater need for nutrients was shown in winter. Nothing was yielded in this regard, which would speak for or against this hypothesis, apparently because the body is not as adapted to the temperature changes so well as someone who works outdoors. The consumption and the store of nutrients was equally small.

It is not easy to say upon what this generally small supply of nutrients for a 70 kg heavy organism is based. The most probable basis is the habit of scanty consumption in general. I don't remember ever having eaten especially a lot. And it seems that the organism becomes accustomed to it and is able to manage with scanty, but otherwise sufficient fare. One knows precisely, on the other hand, that someone who otherwise "lives well" consumes more than ample nourishment, and in doing so extravagant consumption occurs in the organism.

Perhaps also the slight physical work plays an especial role as a reason for the small nutritional need, although standing and running about during the day also burn energy. Since my normally muscular body is covered with a tolerable padding of fat at 72 kg, so also is the conclusion unjustified that this nourishment is adapted only for a slender person.

Food distribution occurred as a rule every three hours.

I must confirm that this type of nutrient absorption seems thoroughly efficient and accurate, since the stomach has to work constantly but only a little, and an overexertion, as for example after a large meal, is excluded. The consequences of this overexertion, which are recognizable in great fatigue, are absent, so that one feels fresh and comfortable at any time of day. After these experiments I have adapted my lifestyle under normal conditions in this way, such that I eat more often, but less, and I continue to do very well.

After all the experiments and deliberations the question still remains open, which food proportion can be deduced from the cited material. Also here the answer must be: there is no precise measure, even for the individual person. We say of course that the body could regulate itself in 4 different balances, and each time a different food came into play. Only in general can an approximate, noteworthy food proportion be specified, and this could amount, first of all for my own self - 70 kg - to 70-80 protein, 80-90 fat and 800 carbohydrates.

Without wanting to generalize this food proportion, I am of the conviction that this amount suffices for most people who perform light and moderately heavy work.

Further long-term experiments, in which the sources of error as much as possible are eliminated, are necessary in order to obtain a conclusive judgement on this important question.

Summary

1. The compilation and uniform calculation of the bibliographical data on food proportions showed that of 307 investigations, conducted on families and individuals, Voit's protein amount of 118 g was not reached in 181 cases= 58.9%. In 126 cases it was exceeded = 41.1%.

In the experiments where protein figures lay below 118 g, 80.2 g per day was found as an average; in those over 118 g the average was calculated at 151.3 per day.

The total average for all 307 experiments is 109.7 g for protein.

2. The variations in the protein, fat, and carbohydrate intake in the named experiments are quite enormous. I cite here the two lowest and the two highest values:

	Protein	Fat	Carbohydrates
Lowest:	29,3 g; 30.1 g	3.5 g; 7.8 g	38 g; 83g
Highest:	212 g; 257 g	272 g; 289 g	907 g; 908 g

3. Since the experiments teach that under the most varied conditions and with the most different combined nutrition nitrogen balance occured, we see therein the already known fact that there is not one suitable food proportion for all individuals, but that the most varied organisms are capable of maintaining their state of balance with various food measures.

4. My own experiments were conducted with the aim of establishing food proportions and the necessary amount of protein chiefly for my own self, through the longest possible experimental duration and under the most possible avoidance of experimental sources of error with empirical as well as experimental methods.

The experiments stretched on the whole over a period of 746 days and broke down into three separate segments.

In the first and third segments, each of which lasted 10 months, I sought to establish the food amount empirically by the method of calculation. In the second segment, which all together comprised 120 days, the empirically found facts were to be controlled and completed through metabolic experiments.

5. The result was as follows:

Calculated for 70 kg, a daily requirement was determined for:

	Protein	Fat	Carbo-hydrates	Alcohol	Calories
1st experiment:	69.1	90.2	242.0	45.6	2427.0
per kilo	0.99	1.3	34.5	0.56	34.7
2nd experiment:	79.5	163.0	234.0	-	2777.0
per kilo	1.1	2.3	33.4	-	59.7
3rd experiment:	74.0	106.0	164.2	5.3	1999.0
per kilo	1.0	1.5	23.4	907(sic)	28.5

If the unresorbable components of the food are subtracted from the amounts found, then we obtain:

	Protein	Fat	Carbo-hydrates	Alcohol	Calories
1st experiment:	57.3	81.2	225.0	41.0	2199.0
2nd experiment:	63.5	140.0	205.0	-	2403.0
3rd experiment:	61.4	95.5	152.0	4.7	1766.0

Hence it follows chiefly from this that I was able to maintain myself in balance for long periods at various times with three different food amounts, and on the other hand, that this could occur with a relatively small amount of protein.

The average numbers from these three experiments amount to:

74.2 protein, 117 fat, 213 carbohydrates and 2367 calories.

The small protein amount lies far below Voit's normal amount of 118, and is situated also much lower than the 100 g required by Munk, and the 90 g of protein held as necessary by Demuth.

6. It arises even more as a result - since in all experiments only a small amount of carbohydrates was consumed, that the reduction of protein in nourishment is not necessarily dependent on an increase in the amount of carbohydrates, but that it is possible, with Voit's normal amount of 500 g and even with a considerable reduction of this amount, to reduce the protein proportion.

7. Body weight was maintained in all experiments, and in the last experiment even increased by 1 kg.

8. The ratio of protein-containing to protein-free food is set in the first experiment at 1:5.7, in the second experiment at 1:6.1 and in the third experiment at 1:7.4.

9. The breakdown of 100 calories is as follows:

	Protein	Fat	Carbohydrat
in the 1st experiment:	15.0	48.2	36.7
in the 2nd experiment:	14.3	48.4	42.3
in the 3rd experiment:	11.3	24.5	64.2.

10. The amount of beer in addition to food in th first experiment is also significant. The amount per da of course, comes to only about 1200 ccm, and yet th nutritional value amounts calculated therefrom come to

the protein, one eighth, 8.4:66.1

the carbohydrates, one fourth, 79.3:230 of the dai requirement.

The combustion of alcohol produces more than third of the calories provided by the fat, 314:776.

In comparison with total daily calorie requiremen the calories from beer likewise produce more than third: 678:2309.

11. The cost calculation showed that the total dail nutrients cost 0.71 marks in the first experiment, an 0.77 marks in the third.

This breaks down to:

	1st experiment	2nd experimen
non-alcoholic foods	0.43 marks	0.73 marks
beer..................	0.28 marks	0.04 marks

The alcohol cost, then, in the first experiment mo than half as much as the alcohol-free nourishment, fro which the conclusion must be drawn that it makes th food inordinately more expensive and as a consequenc is to be regarded as an unrational foodstuff. Beer is ju not "liquid bread," as is now and then gladly asserted.

12. With regard to all controlling conditions, th food measurement for my person was established as:

70-80 g protein 80-90 g fat and 300 g carboh drates.

In case these results are admissible for a generaliza tion, then this food measurement may also be consic ered as suitable and sufficient for other persons wit light work.

A STUDY OF WEIGHT REGULATION IN THE ADULT HUMAN BODY DURING OVER-NUTRITION

ADDISON GULICK

From the Laboratory of Physiological Chemistry, Department of Physiology, University of Missouri, Columbia

Received for publication December 3, 1921

In contrast to the brilliant successes that science has von in the study of nitrogen equilibrium, there is a ather discouraging inconclusiveness in the work that as been done on the factors that regulate the nutritive alance of the fat tissue of the body, and the balance etween the total intake and total output of potential and inetic energy in the adult warm-blooded organism. We o not yet know what mechanism there is to prevent the nlimited accumulation of potential energy in the form f an overload of adipose tissue. Is nerve regulation hrough changing appetite the only guide, or does the ody vary its destruction of fats and carbohydrates in ccordance with their fluctuating intake, somewhat after he manner that it varies its nitrogen exchange?

The best road to a true solution is probably in a tudy of selected contrasting individuals of the over-fat nd under-fat body habits, or better still, of the easily attening and difficultly fattening types.

The problem was first drawn to my attention by bservation of myself, and the experiments here report-d were performed upon myself as a selected example f the "spare" or apparently non-fattening type. I had ong noted my inclination toward a very copious diet of redominantly starchy nature, in spite of which my veight remained fairly constant, even on a moderate ound of activity, at a figure well below the average for ny stature. If the hereditary constitution is important in his connection, such family data as I possess seem to ndicate that I am derived largely from non-fattening trains.

ulick A. A study of weight regulation in the adult human body during over-utrition. *Am J Physiol.* 1922;60:371-395.

eprinted with permission from The American Physiological Society, 3650 ockville Pike, Bethesda, MD 20814.

It has long been recognized that food intake has a powerful effect on the rate of oxidation in the body. In the case of protein food, Rubner (1) distinguishes two such effects. The first of these is the oft discussed specific dynamic effect. The second is a change which appears more gradually, and is explained by him as a stimulus from plethora of nitrogenous products in the cell fluids. The specific dynamic effect occurs equally in well-fed and badly-fed animals, and so it cannot function as a safety valve for excessive intake. But the secondary or plethora effect may very well so function. According to Rubner, this effect shows itself as a cumulative increase in the specific dynamic effect of heavy protein meals, when they are administered on a series of days. He states that in spite of its cumulative character, this secondary effect is not in evidence during the hours when no food is being absorbed. Consequently a dog that has been over-fed in this manner shows no change in its basal metabolic rate, as ordinarily determined on an empty stomach (p. 260, loc. cit.).

Similar results are reported by Dengler and Meyer (2) in their study of the basal metabolism of a man who was over-fed with protein. They found the basal rate changed to a surprisingly slight degree as a result of nitrogen accumulation, and hence conclude that the excess of stored nitrogen was in a non-stimulating form.

A. Müller (3), in tests on a young man, found that the secondary rise on a high protein diet develops rapidly before much nitrogen storage can have occurred, and then fails to keep pace with the stored nitrogen, and is at best trivial in proportion to the quantity of nitrogen that is finally accumulated. So he does not look upon this heightened catabolism as a result of the stored nitrogen.

Grafe and Koch (4) experimented upon persons

who entered a clinic in an extremely under-nourished condition. The two principal subjects were both put through a heavy feeding period of 7 weeks duration to bring them back to normal weight. There resulted a very notable increase in the gaseous exchange. Thus the adult subject, at the initial weight of 40.3 kgm., showed a basal metabolism of 1081 cal. (26.8 cal. per kgm.) and a dynamic effect from eating a meal equal to 24 per cent of the calorie value of the meal. Seven weeks later at a weight of 60 kgm., the basal metabolism had risen to 1946 cal., (32.3 cal. per kgm.) and the dynamic effect had risen to 32 per cent of the fuel value of the meal. Most of the gain in basal metabolism occurred near the middle of the experiment. Although it appeared less rapidly than in Müller's experiment, it was of greater magnitude. The tests of the dynamic effect of the mixed diet fluctuated widely, and cannot be easily interpreted.

Atkinson and Lusk (5) experimented along lines similar to those followed by Rubner, but by over-feeding to a greater extreme were able to report that prolonged and excessive meat diet can cause a rise of the dog's basal metabolism which lasts for as much as two and one-half weeks after the special diet is ended. For their case, then, they conclude that the excess nitrogen was accumulated in a stimulating form.

The converse to the idea of increased or spendthrift oxidation during over-nourishment, is the idea of an especially economical oxidation during under-nutrition.

Anderson and Lusk (6) studied the respiration and the treadmill efficiency of a dog working with empty stomach, with definite meals, and during a prolonged fast. Among other things it was found that the markedly lowered basal metabolism of the fasting period, with its economy of nourishment, carried over into the period immediately following the fast. Eighteen hours after the first liberal meal the metabolism was at essentially the same base level as during the fast, showing that the total condition of the body, and not the question of a large or small influx of food on the previous day, determined the height of the basal metabolism. It is thus to be noted that this dog showed a persistent economy of metabolism after a period of fasting, comparable to the period of wasteful metabolism which Atkinson and Lusk's dog showed subsequent to a course of over-feeding.

The period of the World War has brought out a series of papers on gaseous metabolism during prolonged under-nutrition. Zuntz and Loewy (7), (8), who have a series of records of their basal metabolism since 1888, studies the effect on themselves of eating the German war ration, practically without any of the additions that free use of money could furnish. On this diet, which was inadequate in fuel value, and especially deficient in protein, they report in the case of Zuntz a 10 per cent fall of basal metabolism below the previous average, and in the case of Loewy a fall of 16 per cent. Th decrease is reported in terms of calories per day p square meter by the Meeh formula. The more accura DuBois formula would show even greater percenta changes in rate. Muscular efficiency on the treadmi had gone down in comparison to previous tests.

F.G. Benedict, Miles, Roth and Smith (9) work on the metabolism of volunteer squads of young me during experimental under-nutrition which covere three months of low diet. They found a very remarkab fall in the total fuel needs. Starting at an unknown hig level which was above 3000 cal., and may have been high as 3800 cal., they were finally able to hold the weight constant on an average net intake per person 1950 cal., the fecal and urinary calories being estimat and deducted. Meanwhile there had been a notable lo of nitrogen, 130 grams previous to the first serious inte ruption (at Christmas) and further losses to the end the experiment. The basal metabolism fell from a average of 1686 cal. at the start to 1367 cal. at the low est point, or from 940 per sq. m. to 788 per sq. m. Th the absolute figures fell 20 per cent and the rate p square meter came down 16 per cent. A remarkab slowing of the pulse accompanied this chang Efficiency in the tests of mechanical work was n impaired. The authors ascribe the changes to the wit drawal of the influence of dispensable nitrogen from t body, and argue that no great inroads had been made c the essential protoplasm.

Joffe, Poulton and Ryffel (10) report upon a case extreme under-nutrition in a vegetarian, who had prob bly previously habituated himself to a very meag intake. Throughout the tests the basal rate stayed in th neighborhood of 26.6 cal. per square meter per hour, 638 per square meter per day, calculated according DuBois. The increment of oxidation during work w about average, showing that the man had about the ave age of calorie efficiency in work. His pulse was alway below 50 in the reclining position.

Investigators agree, then, that when the diet is va ied downward there is a factor or group of factors tend ing to adjust the calorie output to the intake.

All the researches thus far reviewed follow th method of gas analysis, and judge the balance betwee intake and output so far as possible by a direct measure ment of both. Another plan of procedure is to depen upon the body weight as the criterion to show whether balance of intake and output has been established. I order to obtain convincing results by this plan it is nec essary to let the tests cover long periods of time, an also to have very large differences in the measure diets of the different experimental periods, so as to fa outweigh any variations in energy expenditure that ma come from uncontrolled factors. In the past this genera mode of experiment has been used, either with or without a supplementary study of the gas metabolism, chiefly by Neumann and by Grafe and his pupils.

Neumann (11) carried out upon himself one of the most prolonged quantitative diet experiments ever recorded, and showed a food intake which gave averages on different years of 2427 cal. and 2057 cal. respectively per 70 kgm. body weight. The actual weight in the former test (1895-96) averaged 66.5 kgm., and in the latter test (1900-01) average 72 kgm. In both years the weights were virtually stationary, tending slightly upward. Neumann's results seem to show ability of the organism to stabilize its weight on either low or medium intakes of fuel. But they do not deal in extreme differences of diet.

Grafe and Graham (12) carried out a prolonged experiment upon a dog, keeping full account of the nitrogen metabolism and weight during very marked over-feeding. From time to time the gas exchange was also determined. Although prevented from taking much exercise, this dog showed extraordinary constancy of body weight during both normal diet and excessive feeding. A puzzling feature is the fairly moderate gas exchange which the dog showed in all the tests.

It might be hoped that comparison of the metabolism in abnormally obese individuals and in persons of normal body habit might throw some light on the factors that prevent most persons from fattening indefinitely. This aspect of the problem was studied by Rubner (13), by A. Magnus-Levy (14) and by von Noorden (15). As summarized by von Noorden, the weight of evidence in these earlier papers is for a fairly comparable metabolic rate in these and the normal cases. DuBois and his colleagues improved this observation by applying new methods for determining the surface area of the human body. (See James H. Means (16), and F.C. Gebhart and Eugene F. DuBois (17).) Using DuBois' determinations of surface, it is easily shown that the great majority of over-fat subjects have a basal rate falling well within the normal rate per square meter of surface. This establishes the fact that the laying on of fat is not caused by a depression in the basal rate. The alternatives still left to account for an obese human type are *a,* an unproved possibility, referred to by von Noorden, that without having a lowered basal rate, the obese may still show an exceptionally low cost of digestion, perhaps by not showing the full normal specific dynamic effect of foods; or *b,* that they partially or entirely lack Rubbers' "secondary effect," which causes an upward shoving of the specific dynamic effect, and sometimes even of basal metabolism, whenever the protein over-nutrition becomes cumulative; or *c,* that control over fattening is not referable to any alteration of basal metabolism nor of the energy cost of digestion, but is to be sought in some such factor as a changed appetite.

We may sum up from the literature that under-nutrition (with loss of nitrogen) has a marked lowering effect on the basal metabolic rate and on the total metabolism of the twenty-four hours. Over-nutrition, coupled with heavy enrichment of the body with nitrogen, has at least in some instances an effect on the basal rate, and has been repeatedly found by Rubner and others to push up the specific dynamic or stimulating effect of protein during absorption, to higher and higher figures. Whenever these factors are at work they all tend to limit the fluctuation of the body mass, and especially to limit the accumulation of body protein. Grafe and his collaborators are the only one who have argued that a similar type of factors is powerful in preventing the immoderate accumulation of body fat.

OUTLINE OF EXPERIMENTS. The general intention of the experiments here reported was to attempt to establish constancy of weight at various levels of total intake. In order to insure the adequacy of the protein and accessories throughout the experiment, milk and eggs figure in all the dietaries used. Small amounts of fats were used but excesses were avoided because it is too easily conceivable that fats might be shunted into the adipose tissue, making a passive increase of body weight without in any way having shared in the metabolism. The main source of nourishment was carbohydrate, from rice, wheat and oats, and the experiments consisted chiefly in varying the quantity of starchy food from these sources.

The first test in March, April and May, 1916, was to find the minimum diet that would maintain an approximately normal body weight. After that the intention was to establish a constant weight on a high level of exchange. This attempt lasted with interruptions from May, 1916, to July, 1917.

At the height of this period of maximum weight and food intake the basal metabolism was determined by the analysis of gas exchange, conducted at the Carnegie Nutrition Laboratory, through the courtesy of Dr. F. G. Benedict and Dr. Thorne M. Carpenter. The body weight was then brought back rather abruptly to the initial level by means of a low calorie diet in July and August, 1917. To conclude the experiment another determination was made of the quantity of food necessary to hold the weight constant.

During several of the above periods records were made of general physical activity. Data were taken for the nitrogen balance during the period of rapid reduction. Analyses of foods were made for this period, but not for any of the other periods, nor were any tests made of combustion value. Instead the diet was limited to a very small selection of foods that would be as free as possible from erratic fluctuations in composition. This

TABLE I
Condensed outline of dietary

	EXPERIMENTAL PERIOD AND DATE								
	I	II		III and IV		V		VI	
	1916 March 4 to 29	1916 March 30 to April 22	1916 April 23 to May 9	1916 May 10 to June13	1916 June 14 to October 23	1916 October 24 to December 12	1916 December 13 to March 23	1917 March 24 to June 4	191 June to July
Rolled oats, gram (air dry)..	0	0	0	0	Ate heartily of varied and liberal diet; outdoor life for 2 1/2 months.	80	Od training; underslept, underate, and lost weight at first then regained gradually on a liberal diet.	100	Die irregu but essent lik Period (Respir analy
Rice, gram (air dry).............	300	300	300	325		200		200	
Milk, cc...............................	1450	1450	1450	1450		1450		1450	
Butter, gram.........................	30	30	35	50		50		50	
Rolls (40-50 grams each)....	Two	Two	Two	Six to Ten		Six to eight		Six to eight	
Eggs (45-55 grams each)....	Two	Two	Two	Two		Two		Two	
Sugar, gram.........................	0	0	0	30 grams some days		0		0	

	EXPERIMENTAL PERIOD AND DATE									
	VII	VIII		IX					X	X
	1917 July 8-14	1917 July 15-25	1917 July 26 to September 1	1917 September 2-5	1917 September 6-8	1917 September 9	1917 September 10 to October 3	1917 October 9-12	1917 October 13-23	O 2 N b
Rolled oats, gram (air dry)..	100	65.9	30	47.5	100	100	100	100	100	1
Rice, gram (air dry).............	200	96.4	60	95	200	200	200	200	200	2
Milk, cc...............................	402.7	1541.9	1417.5	1402	1393	1393	1393	1431	1431	14
Butter, gram.........................	40 (pure fat)	0	0	0	0	0	0	0	0	
Eggs (45-55 grams each)....	100.2 gm.	251.1 gm.	251.3 gm.	126.5 gm.	Two	Two	Two	Two	Two	Tw
Shredded wheat biscuit (about 30 grams each)........	375 gm.	6.8 gm. (av.)	0	0	0	One	Two	Three	Four	Fo

method is undoubtedly liable to a certain degree of inaccuracy, but not, we believe, to major errors or large systematic discrepancies that would alter the tenor of the conclusions.

The figures for the calorie values of the foods are taken consistently from Atwater and Woods' table published by the U.S. Dept. of Agriculture (18). These figures are based on Rubner's standard values for the physiologically available energy in protein, fat and carbohydrates when presented in the digestive tract in "perfectly digestible" form. Up to July, 1917, the foods were all of this "perfectly digestible" form, and it would be correct theoretically to use these fuel values without deducting for the loss by feces. After that date the use of shredded wheat in the diet caused a considerable increase in the moist weight of feces, but apparently not so great a change in the dry weight. The dry weight of a series of feces samples which were closely comparable to those of March and April, 1916 (ration of 2744 cal.), averaged 27 grams per day. This figure comes from an unreported preliminary test made in April, 1915. In June, 1916, it was about 51 grams per day (on 3800 calories), and in July, 1917, it was 78 grams (on 4113 calories with much shredded wheat). In August, 1917, it was about 22 grams (low diet), and in November about 35 grams (3200 calories with medium supply of shredded wheat).

The principal data obtained are the records of weight variation. Every effort was made to obtain reliable and comparable weighings. The regular hour was between 11:30 a.m. and 12:00 m. The fewest possible changes were made in the dietary of the breakfasts, in order to minimize the fluctuations that come from variation in the contents of the digestive tract. Defecation ordinarily occurred in the forenoon, and no weighings are included from the exceptional days on which it had not occurred before the hour for taking the weight. No laxative was used at any time. Care was taken that the bladder should be empty and that the stomach should not contain drinking water at the weighing hour. Whenever the weather was sultry, some water was drunk at about 9:30 to insure against shortage at 11:30. In spite of these precautions there were some rather disconcerting fluctuations of weight, that must be ascribed to variations of water metabolism. Some of the low weights that show abnormally low water content occurred in connection with temporary constipation, and were thus automatically excluded. In cases of insomnia (of which there were several instances toward the end of the experiments) there always resulted an abrupt transitory fall of weight, which is probably chiefly due to an accelerated renal activity. Some of these weights were recorded, but care was taken not to make unsuitable use of those particular figures. An abnormally low weight (500 grams below the previous day) was found on November 27, 1917, at the onset of a heavy nasal catarrh. It was discarded, leaving November 26 the last valid weighting. No weights were discarded for any other causes.

It must not be forgotten that body weight is only an approximate criterion for the equality of intake and output. A person who is oxidizing as much as 100 calories (11 grams) of body fat a day, may replace enough of that fat with water and have enough other fluctuations of his water metabolism to completely mask the fact for many days. This makes it very necessary for experiments upon the body weight to cover long periods of time.

Low level tests of 1916. The initial low level tests are not be understood as representing subnormal nourishment or any great degree of emaciation. At that time (age thirty-four) my weight had been fairly constant for a number of years, between 64 and 66 or possibly 66.5 kgm. This is below the average for the height of 181.2 cm., but if allowance is made for a rather short and narrowly built trunk, it does not necessarily indicate undernutrition.

No record of activity was made during this period, but the round of occupations corresponded very closely to the recorded activities of May and June, 1917, the schedule of duties, the plan of life and the daily habits being almost identical. This means about five miles a day by pedometer, about forty-five meters of staircases climbed per day, and a variety of light occupations connected with teaching and laboratory, many of which are already included in the estimated mileage. Night hours and habits of sleep were good, averaging not far from 8.2 or 8.3 hours rest per night. It should perhaps be mentioned that I am not a quiet sleeper. By fastening a pedometer to one ankle, it was found that in an average night 150 to 160 movements would be made, of sufficient vigor to be counted as steps by the pedometer. No sports, muscular games or pleasure walks were indulged in during any of the experimental periods upon measured diets. On this quite manner of life, starting at a weight (on March 3) of 64.16 kgm., it was attempted to establish a nutritive balance at about 2725 calories. This diet was probably a little less than was eaten before the experiments. As long as it lasted the sensations of hunger before meals were more than customarily acute.

For the entire duration of the test, till May 9, the tendency to lose weight was not entirely overcome. The 41-day period, March 30 to May 9, 1916 (period II), shows an average daily loss of 12 grams on 2744 calories of food, at an average weight of 61.81 kgm. Thus the body requires more than 2744 calories to sustain it at 62 kgm. even under the very moderate conditions of activity. Assuming that the 12 grams of flesh lost had a calorie value not higher than fat, the daily expenditure was more than 2744 and less than 2855 cal. A similar calculation from the last seventeen days of this period gives an expenditure of more than 2753 and less than 2827 cal.

These figures are distinctly larger than the ordinary expectation at the indicated degree of activity. Based on a height of 181.2 cm. and a weight of 61.8 kgm., the expected output of energy can be listed approximately as follows:

	calories
Basal metabolism, 24 hours[1]	1593.0
Added for 5.8 hours sitting, $\frac{5.8}{24}$ x 0.1 x 1595	38.5
Added for 10 hours standing, $\frac{10}{24}$ x 0.2 x 1595	132.1
Added for walking 5 miles, 5 x 0.6 x 65.4 (i.e., clothed weight.)	197.2
Added for estimated activities that fail to show on the pedometer (50 per cent of the walking)	98.6
Added for climbing 45 m. of stairs,[2] 45 x 4 x 65.4 x 0.002343	27.6
Added for descending 45 m. of stairs,[3] 45 x 2 x 65.4 x 0.002343	13.8
	2100.8
"Digestion cost" of 2711 cal. food (6 per cent)[4]	161.6
Predictable calorie output	2267.4
Food eaten	2744.0
Discrepancy of intake over predictable need	476.6 or 21 per cent

Where some of these items are problematical, they have been estimated at a rather liberal rate, e.g., the ten hours standing and the unknown activities equivalent to 2.5 miles of walking. The "digestion cost," and the increments of metabolism due to the sitting and standing positions have been placed at figures that may appear rather low, because the data upon these factors published in recent years by F.G. Benedict and his collaborators seem to call for a moderate estimate of their effect. (See Benedict and Murschhauser (20); Benedict and Carpenter (22).)

The failure to overcome the negative balance on an intake of 2744 calories indicates a physiological tendency, even at low weight levels, to expend more energy than is to be expected from the list of external activities. This physiological wastefulness left the system slightl under-nourished on a diet which ought otherwise t have been more than adequate.

High level tests. May, 1916, to June, 1917. Period III and IV of the experiments, covering May 10 to Jun 13, inclusive differ from the preceding in an increase amount of carbohydrate with a slight increase of butte (50 instead of 35 grams). In order to avoid overwhelm ing the stomach with an excessive volume of food, th additions were chiefly to the bread ration rather than th moist cereals. For two weeks (period III) a diet of 348 cal. was maintained, on which a gain was made of 2.2 kgm. As there was no promise of reaching a balanc quickly, a further increase of bread was made and th high feeding was kept up till June 13 (period IV, Ma 26 to June 13, inclusive). With an average diet of 380 calories, the daily gains continued about the same, to th final weight of 66.17 kgm.

Periods III and IV can count only as preliminar being too short to overcome the doubts that are neces sarily caused by the fluctuation of water metabolism. is well known (Bischoff and Voit (23); Voit (24) discus sion on page 347) that heavy feeding with a very starch diet will lead to a notable accumulation of water in th tissues. But we have no basis on which to predict th extent or duration of this process, and so have hardl any clue to the calorie value of the accumulated weigh in our experiment. If the accumulation during period I had been exclusively pure fat, –an assumption which i certainly contrary to fact, – it would have represented fuel accumulation of 1200 calories per day, or mor than the total daily excess of food in calories. The hig diet needs to be continued long enough to more near stabilize this factor of water intake.

The summer, from June 14 to October 23, was on liberal and hearty diet. Butter, meat, milk and especial ly all forms of carbohydrates were supplied unstintingl and were intentionally taken to the full limit that coul be relished. For 2 1/2 months the appetite was under th stimulus of an active outdoor life. The resulting weigh of 70.05 kgm. on October 24 was considerably th largest that I had ever reached.

There then followed a measured period of fifty day (period V) averaging 3376 calories per day, and wit daily activity at most only slightly greater than in th other experimental periods. The average gain during th fifty days was 30 grams per day. This must be interpre ed as showing a genuine plus balance, because the gai is distributed throughout the period, including its latte portion when water equilibrium must have been reason ably well established. The small size of the daily gair makes it seem probable that the fuel cost of maintenanc and activities had risen along with the body weight.

The period of over-nutrition was unavoidably inte

[1] Harris and Benedict's prediction for height, 181.2 cm.; weight, 71.81 kgm.

[2] Assuming a mechanical efficiency of 25 per cent.

[3] Assuming the descent to cost half as much as the ascent.

[4] Benedict and Carpenter (22).

rupted in the winter of 1916-1917 by a season of heavy duties, impaired sleep and consequent intolerance for an excessive diet. But there was no interruption of the record of essentially good health, and in February and March good nutritive conditions made it possible to recover the greater part of what had been lost.

On March 24, 1917, period VI was started with the initial weight of 71.20 kgm. It was continued 73 days with an average intake of 3545 calories of food and showed an average gain of 24 grams per day. As in the case of the preceding period, the weight curve does not suggest any modification of the water metabolism by the carbohydrate food. Its greater length renders it a comparatively safe period on which to base calculations. With an average weight only 1.03 kgm. above that of period V the additional 170 calories are carried with a smaller daily gain. There seems, then, to have been a definite although not very great growth of that extravagance in use of fuel food which was noted during period II.

This high expenditure of fuel food is much more pronounced in this period than in any previous test. This is not explained by activity, as the daily habits of period II and period VI are the nearest imaginable approach to duplicates of each other. It is likely that period V had slightly, but only slightly greater physical activity, on account of a slightly heavier schedule of university duties. In that case the relative metabolism of period VI above period V becomes the more noteworthy. Period V is the only one of the first six periods that differed perceptibly in its round of activities.

The record of activities with the aid of pedometers began to be taken that spring, and included about four weeks of period VI. Three pedometers were worn at the start, one at the belt, a second at the right ankle, intended to show minor movements of locomotion, and the third at the right forearm. The forearm position proved to be useless, because of the changes of posture, and because sudden motions were liable to jam the bob of the pedometer and make it stop recording. The ankle pedometer was also given up eventually. It seemed to be able to record more motions than the belt pedometer during the sitting and standing occupations, but it suffered from very nearly the same mechanical difficulties as the one on the arm. It was read night and morning for 14 days, and supplied the data on restless sleeping to which I have already referred. The belt pedometer was worn only during the waking hours, and was read once daily regularly through the remainder of the series of experiments.

The estimate of stairs climbed is a fairly accurate average, based on the extremely uniform round of places visited each day.

The record of hours devoted to sleep did not commence till July of that year. They vary from 8.20 to 8.35 hours in different months. I believe it probable that in period I to VI the hours were not less than the latter figures, but in order to insure against an under-estimate of activities, I have calculated on the basis of 8.2 hours.

A rather problematical point as regards activity is the number of hours in the standing position, and the amount of activity of gentler type than would record on the pedometer. Much time was spent standing, as I made but little use of chairs in the laboratory. In order to insure against an under-estimate, the figure has been set at ten hours for periods I to VI inclusive. In the same spirit I have assumed an arbitrary figure of half the energy of an average day's walking to cover the undeterminable lighter activities. These data give us the following estimate of the daily energy output that would fulfill the ordinary expectation for this period:

	calories
Basal metabolism, 24 hours[5]	1724.0
Added for 5.8 hours sitting, $\frac{5.8}{24}$ x 0.1 x 1724	41.7
Added for 10 hours standing, $\frac{10}{24}$ x 0.2 x 1724	143.7
Added for walking 4.82 miles, 4.82 x 0.6 x 75.4 (i.e., clothed weight.)	218.1
Added foractivities not shown on pedometer (estimated as 50 per cent of the walking)	109.0
Added for climbing 45 m. of stairs,[6] 45 x 4 x 75.4 x 0.002343	31.8
Added for descending 45 m. of stairs[7]	15.9
	2284.2
"Digestion cost" of 3545 cal. food (6 per cent)[8]	212.7
Predictable calorie output	2496.9
Food eaten	3545.0
Deduction for excess feces (21 grams excess above the normal 30 grams) 21 x 6.2 cal	130.2
Net cal. from diet	3414.8
Discrepancy of intake over predictable need	+37 per cent

This diet seems, from the calculation, to be no less than 37 per cent in excess of the predictable need, while the diet in period II showed an excess of 21 per cent. But it is necessary to allow for the difference between a falling weight in period II and a rising weight in the later period. If we assume that the calorie value of the

[5]Harris and Benedict's prediction for height, 181.2 cm.; weight, 71.81 kgm.

[6]Assuming a mechanical efficiency of 25 per cent.

[7]Assuming the descent to cost half as much as the ascent.

[8]Benedict and Carpenter (22).

flesh gained and lost does not exceed that of pure fat, then the total oxidation of material (food and body fat) in period II lies 21 per cent to 23 per cent above the predictable figure, and the oxidation in period VI is between 27 per cent and 37 per cent above the prediction. The discrepancy between the predictable and the observable expenditure had undergone an absolute increase and probably even a relative increase.

Basal metabolism during over-nutrition. In June, 1917, the courtesy of Dr. F.G. Benedict and of Dr. T.M. Carpenter and their collaborators in the Carnegie Nutrition Laboratory supplied me with three determinations of my basal metabolism by their usual routine methods. On June 12 and 16 the tests were in the bed respiration chamber, Miss Corson in charge, at the Deaconess' Hospital, Boston, and on June 20 by means of the large Tissot spirometer and Haldane gas analysis methods, carried out by Doctor Carpenter. These tests were all of them on the high diet, the average intake of three 2-day periods preceding these three tests being 3965 calories. As the experiments necessarily interrupted the diet, being taken at breakfast time on an empty stomach, and not being concluded for some hours, the average intake for the whole period of June 9 to 19 inclusive is only 3790 cal. On this diet of essentially 3965 calories representing the maximum intake up to that date, and at a body weight of 73.62 kgm., the recorded metabolism is very uniform with the single exception of the first respiration period of the first day, the period of introduction to the apparatus, when the psychic effects undoubtedly militated against complete relaxation. Rejecting this half-hour period, the average of the other results, by indirect calorimetry from the gas analysis, are 73.32 cal. per hour, or 1762 cal. per day for the waking basal metabolism. The prediction for weight 73.6 kgm., height 181.2 cm. and age thirty-five, made by Harris and Benedict (19) is 1749 cal., constituting an almost perfect agreement with the finding.

A very high respiratory quotient should be noted; the figures being 0.94, 0.93 and 0.89 on the three different days. In the first two of these cases the non-protein respiratory quotient was 0.98. Thus even thirteen to fifteen hours after the last meal, and although fats were by no means excluded from the high carbohydrate diet, the oxidative processes were limited practically to carbohydrate and protein.

In spite of this fact that the high carbohydrate of the previous evening is still exerting a great influence upon the respiratory quotient, the metabolic rate conform exactly to the prediction for the basal or post-absorbtive rate. The prolonged diet has *not raised the basal metabolic rate above the normal average.*

As I believe the figures have demonstrated that the metabolism as a whole is extravagant above the average, we shall have to look for the element of extravagance i some other factor than the basal rate.

Return to normal level. The return to a norma weight was accomplished in the summer months c 1917, while at the laboratories of the University c Illinois Medical School. During this period the foo urine and feces were analyzed for the determination c nitrogen balance. The urine analyses were continue most of the time to the end of the experiments o November 26 and the weighed diet up to that date wa limited to the same set of foods as were used in the sum mer period. Thus the nitrogen exchange was followe in full or in part during the whole of these 4 1/2 month Table 3 summarizes these analytical data.

The diet differed from that of previous periods i the substitution of shredded wheat in place of the mo difficulty analyzable white rolls, and also in the chang from soft boiled eggs to a form of custard, which cou easily be sampled for analysis when mixed and straine and ready to cook. Clear centrifuged butter fat was use in the summer months in place of commercial butte Head rice, Quaker brand rolled oats and whole mi completed the diet. The analysis of the milk was by ta ing equal daily samples. The shredded wheat was br ken small and mixed thoroughly in a large, moistur proof container, from which the daily portions and th sample for analysis were taken. The rolled oats and th rice were similarly mixed and sampled. All these cere samples were ground before dividing them into small portions for the analyses. The Kjeldahl-Gunnin method was used in all the nitrogen determinations.

The first week of this summer series, on a diet c 4115 cal., represents very nearly the maximum capacity c the subject for continuous consumption, unless fats we to be used more freely. A substantial plus balance i shown both in nitrogen and in body weight. The perio is too short to indicate the extent to which excess oxid tion may have developed, but it is clear that the proces had not gone fat enough to prevent further fattening.

Following this was a period of low nutrition, lastin 7 weeks, with a daily average of 1874 cal. The intentio was to dispose of the accumulated body fat without ru ning into the condition of depressed basal metabolis that will occur when there has been a heavy loss c nitrogen. Accordingly the quota of eggs was somewh increased, and the radical cut was confined to the cere foods and the butter fat, the latter being entirely disco tinued during most of the interval. It was impossibl however, to prevent a strongly negative balance of pr tein materials, so that the average daily weight loss approximately 200 grams for the rest of the summer accompanied by an average nitrogen loss of nearly 1 grams per day.

Final equilibrium. The attempts to reach a stab

TABLE 3
Summary of nitrogen exchange

	PERIOD AND DATE												
	VII		VIII				IX			X	XI	XII	XIII
	1917 July 8-9	1917 July 10-14	1917 July 15-24	1917 July 25 to August 7	1917 August 8-29	1917 August 30 to September 1	1917 September 2-12	1917 September 13 to October 8	1917 October 9-12	1917 October 13-23	1917 October 24-27	1917 October 28 to November 10	November 11-25
ration in days......	2	5	10	14	22	3	11	25	4	11	4	14	15
etary N..................	20.26	19.74	15.68	13.60	13.42	13.50	13.37	14.60	15.13	15.71	15.88	15.05	15.97
inary N................		14.30	16.02	14.16	13.23			12.17		12.80	12.09	11.13	12.16
cal N.....................		3.54	1.59	1.27	1.02								*2.00
ily N. balance.......		+1.89	-1.93	-1.82	-0.83								+1.81
balance for period..		+9.47	-19.34	-25.53	-18.35								+27.07
			Loss in 46 days 63.2 gm.										
lorie Intake............	4127	4110	2212	1811	1772	1788	2198	2537	2659				
r day......................	av. 4115		av. 1874				av. 2441			2781	3183	2970	3204
ange of weight during period..........	+0.64		-9.58				-2.83			-0.55	+0.25	-0.57	-0.05
ange of weight er day....................	+0.091		-0.196				-0.069			-0.05	+0.063	-0.044	-0.003

2.01 grams in 6 days, November 14-19, inclusive.

weight during September, October and November make it clear, first of all, that in spite of the considerable loss of nitrogen the body was by no means in a depressed metabolic state. It is impossible to tell whether the body was richer or poorer in protein constituents than it had been during the first equilibrium period (period II) of 1916. After more than a year of high calorie diet, with a fully adequate protein intake at all times, there can be no question that when the diet was changed in July the tissues were copiously stocked with protein materials. The figures obtained after July 15 can be extrapolated so as to show that between that date and the middle of September the body must have lost some 70 or 75 grams of nitrogen, – an amount that probably did not yet leave the body in any greatly depleted condition. When the diet was now increased to near 2500 calorie, this negative balance was checked, or possibly even changed to a small positive figure, but the loss of weight was not entirely overcome. The same was true in the period on 2780 calories in October, the nitrogen balance being somewhat further improved, but the weight still continuing to decline. A virtually steady weight was at last established on an appreciably higher diet, from October 24 to November 25 inclusive, but not till the nitrogen balance had become definitely positive. Judging from the final fortnight, (period XIII), 3200 calories were now necessary to maintain a body weight of about 61.3 kgm.

During September, 1917, it was impossible to make a satisfactory record of activity, because at that time the exigencies of changing to a new residence caused a temporary increase of manual labor. The October and November records are free from such complications, excepting that the use of a bicycle was commenced at this point, to get to and from work. Habits of sitting and standing were about as in the early months of experimentation. The recorded activities are as follows:

	PERIOD AND DATE			
	X October 13-23	XI October 24-27	XII October 28 to November 10	November 11-25
Duration in days	11	4	14	15
Sleep per day, hours	8.55	8.44	7.78	8.28
Walking per day, miles	4.76	7.62	3.58	4.35
Bicycle per day, miles	2.61	4.48	4.54	4.77
Stairs climbed per day (est.) meters	20	20	20	20

The bicycle route involved no steep grades, and always returned to the level of the original starting point. The bicycle was an exceedingly easy running one, capable of coasting freely on windless days on a gradient of 115 feet (35 m.) per mile, rider plus bicycle having a total weight of 83 kgm.

With out attempting to evaluate the energy used in bicycle riding, I believe it will be conceded to be insufficient to make the activities of the above periods appreciably greater than in periods II and VI. But the irregularities in sleep are probably a rather serious factor, and period XII is probably vitiated for purposes of comparison by the relatively poor "sleep" record. For this reason period XIII seems to be the principal one for a satisfactory comparison with period II, on the assumed basis that they represent essentially the same degree of muscle activity.

The summarized results of the last four periods are as follows:

PERIOD	DATES	INTAKE IN CALORIES	CHANGE OF WEIGHT PER DAY	REMARKS
			grams	
X	October 13-23	2781	-50	Maximum sleep. Activities below average
XI	October 24-27	3183	+63	Excellent sleep. Greater activities
XII	October 28-November 10	2970	-44	Imperfect sleep. Moderate activities
XIII	November 11-25	3204	-3	Excellent sleep. Moderate activities

I place beside these for comparison the earlier period:

II	March 30-May 9, 1916	2744	-12	Excellent sleep. Moderate activities

In spite of the inescapable irregularities inherent i human experimentation of this sort, a comparison of th forty-one days in 1916 with the final thirty-three days both of which were at practically identical average bod weights, brings out very definite evidence of a marke increase in the daily caloric requirement. It is not saf to attempt to calculate exactly how great this change ha been, but on the face of the results from the final fiftee days, the daily demand seems to have risen by some 30 to 400 calories.

DISCUSSION

The general results of these experiments are tha this example of a person belonging to the difficultly fat tening type was found to show a wasteful rate of oxida tion during all the feeding experiments, including bot the periods in which the diet was moderate or low an those in which a large excess of starch was superpose upon the normal diet. During the prolonged periods o high diet this wasteful oxidation became more pro nounced, and it continued so throughout the following periods of under-nutrition, so that even after the body had been brought down again to its original weight, i required more food to keep it at steady weight that ha been necessary at the start.

In a preliminary report of these experiments tha was made in 1917 (25) considerable uncertainty was expressed as to whether or not these figures could be used as evidence for a compensatory excess oxidatio during high feeding. This doubt was based on the fac that a comparison between the nutritive exchange during high feeding and that during the final low-weight periods could only lead to inconclusive results. In the present paper the final low-weight periods are not used fo this comparison, and the extravagance of the calorie exchange during over-nutrition is appraised by comparing it with the initial determination of minimum need, as made in 1916. It is believed that this plan of analysis is justified; firstly, because the calorie demand in the fina periods is so far above the need as found in 1916 that i seems to show a hangover effect from the months of excess nutrition; and, secondly, because even the initia need is noticeably in excess of the expectation by dead reckoning.

The basal rate of metabolism as determined in a reclining position before breakfast did not rise above the average expectation for the subject's age, weight and height. Pulse and blood pressure were also entirely normal.

It seems clear that throughout the entire experimental series there was some factor at work which caused fuel food to be burned more freely than in the average individual. This factor was not an overactive thyroid as attested by the entirely normal basal metabolism.

It is possible that a part of the waste is attributable to neuromuscular factors. During all the experimental periods the greater part of the daily activities were of the less intense variety, the calorific cost of which is always problematical, because it can never be predicted how much will be wasted in the increased tone of the unemployed muscles. This undeterminable expenditure may easily have varied from the average expectation, and may be responsible for some of the unexplained energy expenditure. But if this were the whole explanation, we ought to find a lessened wastefulness and not an increase during the months of over-feeding when there was a continued stuffed feeling and a disinclination to exertion. For this reason it seems more probable that the main factor is not to be sought in neuromuscular habits, but in some factor in the chemistry of nutrition.

The nitrogen balance may very easily be connected in some way with this problem, for although the actual intake of proteins was never abnormally high, the liberal calorie allowance of the experimental diets and of the subject's previous dietary habits was very favorable to an accumulation of nitrogen. Even the last tests, after there had been a loss of 70 grams or more of nitrogen, may have been under the influence of superabundant stores of protein materials, as that 70 grams were only removed after a maximum storage must have been attained, and by the time that the last experimental weeks had been reached, some of the lost nitrogen had been restored. If the factor causing extravagance is related to this supposed nitrogen enrichment, it is not to be compared with the plethora effect observed by Atkinson and Lusk (5), but it may very possibly be comparable to the "secondary effect" of protein enrichment, which according to Rubner (1) can raise the specific dynamic effect of the food without raising the basal rate. The present experiment differs from Rubner's in that the food for which the specific dynamic effect must be augmented is largely starch instead of protein.

It is also possible that nitrogen enrichment may not be the major explanation of the nutritive condition. For there is still the alternative that von Noorden's (15) suggestion respecting the obese type may have its converse, and the spare type can be accounted for by any factor that produces a high "cost of digestion," just as the obese may be supposed to suffer from an abnormally low "cost of digestion." The decision between these alternatives would only be possible after an extension of the tests beyond the limits that have been practicable in the present investigation.

SUMMARY

1. During periods aggregating about three hundred and seventy days on experimental diet, a person of the difficultly fattening type was investigated, first, to determine the minimum food required for maintenance of weight at the customary level; second, to ascertain whether and to what extent an excess of starchy food would be stored by this type of person as adipose in a long period of superabundant measured diet; and third, to ascertain whether after the body was returned to the initial weight with least possible loss of nitrogen, any change had occurred in the minimum requirement of food.

2. The person was found to owe his resistance against fattening to an extravagant calorie requirement which persisted at all times, despite a moderate daily round of activities.

3. This extravagance increased during the course of the excessive carbohydrate diet, and stayed above the initial level even after the return to normal weight.

4. The basal metabolic rate was not involved, but remained strictly normal.

5. The high calorie output and consequent resistance against fattening may find its explanation either in a condition of nitrogen enrichment, or in an upward variation of the "cost of digestion" (and assimilation) of starchy food.

Grateful acknowledgments are due to the Nutrition Laboratory of the Carnegie Institution, to Dr. F.G. Benedict, in charge of that laboratory, to Miss Corson, at the Deaconess' Hospital, Boston, and particularly to Dr. Thorne M. Carpenter for active interest in the determination of basal metabolic rate in June, 1917; and to the University of Illinois Medical School, Laboratory of Physiological Chemistry, Chicago, where I received liberal backing for the portions of the work done in July and August, 1917, through the generous recommendation of Dr. W.H. Welker. All other parts of the experiments here reported are from the Laboratory of Physiological Chemistry, Department of Physiology, University of Missouri.

BIBLIOGRAPHY

(1) RUBNER: Gesetze des Energieverbrauchs, 1902.
(2) DENGLER AND MEYER: Zentrbl. f.d. gesammt. Physiol. u. path. d. Stoffwechsels., 1906, 288.
(3) MÜLLER: Zentrbl. f. d. gesammt. Physiol. u. Path. d. Stoffwechsels., 1911, 617.
(4) GRAFE AND KOCH: Deutsch. Arch. f. Klin. Med., 1912, cvi, 564.

(5) ATKINSON AND LUSK: Journ. Biol. Chem., 1919, xli, p. xiii.
(6) ANDERSON AND LUSK: Journ. Biol. Chem., 1917, xxxii, 421.
(7) LOEWY AND ZUNTZ: Berl. Klin. Wochenschr., 1916, 825.
(8) ZUNTZ AND LOEWY: Biochem. Zeitschr., 1918, xc, 244.
(9) BENEDICT, MILES, ROTH AND SMITH: Carnegie Instit. Pub. 280, 1919.
(10) JOFFE, POULTON AND RYFFEL: Quart. Journ. Med. (Oxford), 1918, xii, 334.
(11) NEUMANN: Arch. f. Hyg., 1902, xlv, 1.
(12) GRAFE AND GRAHAM: Zeitschr. f. physiol. Chem., 1911, lxxiii, 1.
(13) RUBNER: Beiträge zur Ernährung im Knaebenalter mit besonderer Berücksichtigung der Fettsucht, Berlin, 1902.
(14) MAGNUS-LEVY: Zeitschr. f. Klin. Med., 1906, lx, also xxxiii, and other references.
(15) VON NOORDEN: Metabolism and practical medicine; see discussion on p. 693-715, esp. p. 698; also full liter-ature references on obesity.
(16) MEANS: Journ. Med. Research, 1915, xxvii, 121.
(17) GEBHART AND DUBOIS: Archives of Int. Med., 1916, xvii.
(18) ATWATER AND WOODS: U.S. Dept. Agric. O.E.S. Bull. no. 28, 1896.
(19) HARRIS AND BENEDICT: Carnegie Instit. Pub. no. 279, 1919.
(20) BENEDICT AND MURSCHHAUSER: Carnegie Instit. Pub. no. 231, 1915.
(21) BENEDICT AND CATHCART: Carnegie Instit. Pub. no. 187, 1913.
(22) BENEDICT AND CARPENTER: Carnegie Instit. Pub. no. 261, 1918.
(23) BISCHOFF AND VON VOIT: Gesetze der Ernährung des Fleischfressers, 1860.
(24) VON VOIT: Handb. d. Physiol. d. allg. Stoffwechsels, (Vol. vi, pt. 1, of Hermann's Handbuch), 1881.
(25) GULICK: This Journal, 1918, xlv, 549.

THE DOUBTFUL NATURE OF "LUXUSKONSUMPTION"[1]

BY F. H. WILEY[2] AND L. H. NEWBURGH
(From the Department of Internal Medicine, Medical School, University of Michigan, Ann Arbor)

(Received for Publication May 22, 1931)

In 1911, and several times thereafter, Grafe and his associates (1) stated that the fasting, resting metabolism of an individual is not proportional to the surface area, but is significantly affected by the calorific value of the food previously ingested. They also postulated that the total metabolism is influenced in the same way by the total intake of energy. According to them, normal animals, including man, maintain a constant weight, almost without regard to the energy intake, and obesity is often nothing more than the failure of this alleged mechanism to respond normally to the stimulus of food. Finally, leanness is an over-response to a normal stimulus.

They supported these views by the following type of experiments: A dog was starved for a long time, and its resting, fasting metabolism was then determined. This value was used as the basis for comparison. The dog was now offered an abundance of food, and gained weight rapidly. The metabolism was repeatedly determined in the fasting, resting state. The metabolic rate thus determined showed a progressive increase out of proportion to the increase in body surface. Table I sets forth their data in detail, rearranged by us.

This increase in metabolic rate of the overfed animal beyond that of the starved animal was accepted by them as proof that the resting, fasting metabolism of the normal animal is increased by previous overfeeding. But the metabolic rate obtained after prolonged starvation should not have been accepted as a proper basis for comparison, since Schondorff (2) had previously shown that starvation caused a decrease in this rate. Zuntz (3) later showed that this decrease might be as much as 30 per cent below the normal. In spite of the demonstration by Schondorff, that a starved dog has a greatly depressed rate, Grafe accepted the heat production of his dog, after 21 days' starvation, as a proper value for the basis of his calculations. The 24 hourly heat production of 672 Calories was thus erroneously used as the norm with which to compare the metabolism of overnutrition. When the animal was normal, in the usual sense of the word (i.e. after 2 months of food ad libitum), its heat production was 1,005 Calories. Starvation had accordingly reduced it 26 per cent. Liberal feeding permitted the basal metabolism to return to approximately the normal value, which at its height was 62 per cent above the starvation level but only 11 per cent more than the normal value.

In 1912, Grafe and Koch (4) reported the study of a man whose normal weight was 62.62 kgm. and whose height was 156.2 cm. He was 35 years old. He came to the hospital suffering from stenosis of the pylorus accompanied by persistent vomiting. His weight had fallen to 40 kgm. His fasting, resting metabolism was determined, the stenosis was then relieved by operation, and ten days later a period of overnutrition was begun. It lasted seven weeks, at the end of which time the patient's weight had again become 60 kgm.

Inspection of Table II makes it clear that the undernourished patient exhibited the usual depression of the metabolic rate. When the operation had made it possible for him to absorb food in large quantities, the ingestion of 100 Calories per kilogram caused him to gain in the neighborhood of 22 kgm. in less than two months,

Wiley FH, Newburgh LH. The doubtful nature of "luxuskonsumption." *J Clin Invest.* 1931;10:733-744.

Special thanks to Judy Willis of the Pennington Information Center for help in acquiring this document.

[1] The expenses of this investigation were defrayed in part by a fund for the study of nutrition, created by Mr. W.K. Kellogg, of the Kellogg Corn Flake Company, Battle Creek, Michigan.
[2] National Research Council Fellow in Medicine.

TABLE I

Effect of different degrees of nutrition upon basal metabolism, according to Grafe

Diet and length of period	Body weight	Basal heat production per 24 hours		Basal metabolic rate	
		Determined	Predicted*	After Gräfe	Standard
	kgm.	*Calories*	*Calories*	*per cent*	*per cent*
Beginning	20.15	1056	987	+ 54	+ 7
21 days Starvation 21st day	15.00	672	905	± 0	- 26
7 days 2243 Calories per day 4th day	18.50	816	963	+ 19	- 15
29 days 2580 Calories per day 29th day	20.25	1047	992	+ 53	+ 5
11 days 1659 Calories per day 11th day	20.17	1112	989	+ 62	+ 11
19 days 1120 Calories per day 19th day	20.00	1061	980	+ 55	+ 8
10 days 882 Calories per day 10th day	18.50	839	963	+ 22	- 13
7 days Starvation 6th day	17.50	856	946	+ 25	- 9
2 months Unrestreicted	21.00	1005	1005	+ 48	± 0

*Predicted heat production was obtained from heat production determined after the animal had led an unrestricted life for two months. This value was corrected for changes in surface area as indicated by change in weight from 21.00 kgm.

and in addition merely permitted the oxidative rate to return to the normal level. There is, then, no evidence that "Luxuskonsumption" increased the fasting, resting metabolism.

It should be recalled that Grafe had said that the normal animal maintained a constant weight in spite of overfeeding, because the extra food stimulated the total metabolism to such an extent that the excess was oxidized, but he published no data that dealt with the total metabolism.

We have, accordingly, reinvestigated this questio[n]. In a recent publication from this laboratory (5), we ha[ve] shown that quantitative data regarding the total metab[o]lism may new be secured, and such data are included [in] our study.

The subject was a very thin young man, wh[o] weighed 57.5 kgm. (nude), and whose height was 18[...] cm. (6 feet). He was 28 years old at the time the expe[...]

TABLE II

Effect of different degrees of nutrition upon basal metabolism, according to Grafe

Sex–M. Height–156.5 cm. Age–35 years

Condition of patient	Weight	Surface area	Calories per square meter per hour		Basal metabolic rate
			Determined	Predicted	
	kgm.	square meters			per cent
Before operation	40.0	1.34	30.5	39.0	- 22
	40.0	1.34	29.5	39.0	- 24
After operation and period of overnutrition.	60.2	1.59	40.1	39.0	+ 2
(100 Calories per kilo)	60.2	1.59	41.4	39.0	+ 5

ment was undertaken. At the age of 17 he had attained his full height and weighed only 150 kgm (110 lb.). by the time he was 20 years old he had attained his present weight. During his twenty-first year, for a period of 3 months, he happened to be eating food that tasted unusually good. He was fully aware of eating much more food than usual, and feeling unusually indolent. During these 3 months his weight increased about 11 kgm. (25 lbs.). Following this unusual experience, he again partook of food which made no unusual appeal to him. In spite of his unusual height and leanness, he was quickly satiated and did not indulge in the common custom of eating before retiring. He failed to derive the usual pleasure from sweets and pastries. His mother diligently tried, without success, to get him to eat what she considered a sufficient amount. She even forced him to take a variety of "tonics" with the hope of increasing his weight. Hence on the basis of his food habits, his leanness might as easily be attributed to an unusually small intake of energy as to an abnormally great oxidative rate.

On November 5, 1930, he began to eat all of his food in the hospital diet kitchen. His dietetic prescription was protein 91 grams, fat 186 grams, and carbohydrate 241 grams, giving about 3,000 Calories. To avoid monotony the dietitian fed these materials in the form of different foodstuffs for three consecutive days, and used precisely the same foodstuffs for every subsequent three day period. The occupation of the subjects was that of a professional chemist, and he made no conscious alteration in the routine of his life. On November 23, 1930, the diet prescription was changed to protein 89 grams, fat 413 grams, and carbohydrate 445 grams, giving about 5,000 Calories. The food was fed according to the above described plan. During part of the second period his activity was slightly, but definitely, increased due to pressure of extra work. The second diet was continued through December 7, 1930. Thereafter, until January 5, 1931, he made a serious effort to continue to gain weight by overeating. From the latter date until March 19 he took food according to his desires.

Sample diets of each period covering the three day cycle, and intended to be identical with those served to the subject, were prepared by the dietitian except that the milk, cream, butter and sugar were omitted. The milk, cream and butter are regularly analyzed by the hospital chemist, and are found to conform with standard value. The sample diets were dried over a steam bath, weighed and ground to a fine powder. A thoroughly mixed sample was then ignited in a bomb calorimeter to obtain its heat value. In addition, the nitrogen, fat and ash content were determined.

The nude, fasting weight of the subject was recorded every third morning. The total weight of the ingesta, and of urine and stools were analyzed for nitrogen and total solids, and the heat value of the dried stool was obtained by means of the bomb calorimeter. The basal metabolism was measured three times during the first period, five times during the second period, and several times thereafter.

The actual total energy of the diet for the eighteen day period was obtained as follows: milk, cream, butter and sugar were found to contain, by calculation, 33,246 Calories. The energy value of the remainder of the diet, as determined by means of the calorimeter, was 23,436 Calories, giving a total of 56,682 Calories. The dried stool contained 2,450 Calories, and the urine contained 1,644 Calories (urinary nitrogen X 8). The subtraction

TABLE III
Data from our subject on maintenance diet

Diet–3,000 Calories

Date	Body weight at beginning of period	Weight of ingesta	Weight of urine and stool	Insensible loss of weight	Surface area	Basal metabolism		Basal metabolic rate	Respira-tory quotient
						Predicted	Determined		
	grams	*grams*	*grams*	*grams*	*square meters*	*Calories*	*Calories*	*per cent*	
November 1930									
5-6-7	57,562	7,227	3,348	3,863	1.73	1,640	1,470	- 10.4	.854
8-9-10	57,578	7,285	3,031	4,413					
11-12-13	57,439	6,894	2,853	3,537	1.73	1,640	1,510	- 8.0	.811
14-15-16	57,943	7,466	3,750	3,801					
17-18-19	57,858	6,960	2,619	4,104	1.73	1,640	1,450	- 11.5	.776
20-21-22	58,122	7,457	4,132	3,899					
23	57,548							- 10.0	
				Total 23,617			Average 1,4775		

of the energy lost by excretion from the total potential energy of the diet left 52,588 Calories available to the organism.

The weights of the subject, ingesta, stool and urine, contained in Table III, permit the calculation of the insensible loss of weight. By subtracting from the body weight at the end of the period the weight of the ingesta, and adding to this value the weights of the urine and stool, and subtracting this modified final weight from the initial weight, the insensible loss of weight was obtained (5). The total insensible loss for the eighteen days was 23,617 grams. In the earlier publication (5), we have shown that the total dissipation of heat may be calculated from the insensible water. Its weight in turn may be calculated by subtracting the difference between the weight of the exhaled carbon dioxide and that of the absorbed oxygen from the insensible loss of weight. A discussion of the method for determining these values may be found in the previous paper (5). In this instance they were 17,674 grams of carbon dioxide and 16,021 grams of oxygen, giving a difference of 1,653 grams. Thus the insensible water was 21,964 grams. The heat removed by it was obtained by multiplying it by 0.58. This heat represents 24 per cent of the total heat dissipated (5). The heat dissipation calculated in this manner was 53,087 Calories for eighteen days, or 2,947 Calories per twenty-four hours. Accordingly, it is true that this subject, leading his usual life, transformed energy at the rate of 2,947 Calories per day when he was receivin[g] 2,922 Calories per day.

Will he, then, transform more energy merel[y] because he ingests more food?

The subject was, accordingly, fed the second die[t] the calorific value of which was roughly 5,000 Calori[es] per day, for 15 days. Accurate information wa[s] obtained for this period in the same manner as has bee[n] described for the first period. It was found that the tot[al] energy of the diet was 75,125 Calories for the perio[d]. The stools for the period contained 2,745 Calories, an[d] the urine contained 1,056 Calories, giving a total [of] 71,324 Calories available to the organism.

Table IV gives the weights of the subject, ingest[a,] stool and urine for the second period. The total insens[i]ble loss calculated from the table was 21,763 gram[s]. The total nitrogen of the urine was 132 grams. Th[e] metabolic mixture was calculated from the carbohydra[te] of the diet, the nitrogen excretion and the insensible lo[ss] of weight by the method described in the earlier pap[er] (5). It was found to consist of 871 grams of protei[n,] 1,928 grams of fat, and 6,315 grams of carbohydrate f[or] the period of fifteen days. The corresponding carbo[n] dioxide and oxygen values were respectively 16,35[.] grams and 13,752 grams. The difference, 2,605, su[b]tracted from the total insensible loss 21,763, ga[ve] 19,158 grams of insensible water for the period. Th[e] total heat dissipation indicated by this value was 46,29[.]

TABLE IV

Data from same subject on supermaintenance diet

Diet–5,000 Calories

Date	Body weight at beginning of period	Weight of ingesta	Weight of urine and stool	Insensible loss of weight	Surface area	Basal metabolism		Basal metabolic rate	Respiratory quotient
						Predicted	Determined		
	grams	*grams*	*grams*	*grams*	*square meters*	*Calories*	*Calories*	*per cent*	
November 1930									
23-24-25	57,548	8,324	2,258	4,143					
26-27-28	59,471	8,218	3,463	4,227	1.76	1,651	1,560	- 5.5	.869
29-30-December 1	59,999	7,991	3,189	4,369	1.77	1,660	1,545	- 6.9	.875
2-3-4	60,432	8,292	2,739	4,691	1.77	1,660	1,575	- 5.1	.843
5-6-7	61,294	7,391	2,414	4,313	1.78	1,670	1,600	- 4.2	.903
8	61,958				1.79	1,679	1,610	- 4.1	.880
				Total 21,743					

Calories for fifteen days, or 3,082 Calories per day. Accordingly, the subject transformed 135 more Calories of energy per day when he was ingesting about 5,000 Calories than when the intake of energy was about 3,000 Calories, an increase of about 4.5 per cent in total metabolism.

The average surface area for the second period was 2.3 per cent greater than for the first period. Other things being equal, this would call for an average increase of 67.5 Calories per day in the second period, leaving 68 Calories per day thus far unaccounted for. These 68 Calories may be properly attributed to the specific dynamic effect of the extra fat and carbohydrate of the diet in this period, since there is a quantitative relationship between the amount of material ingested and its dynamic effect. Lusk (6) has recently stated that the metabolism is increased after the ingestion of fat and carbohydrate by four per cent and six per cent respectively of the Calories furnished by these foodstuffs. In the second period the fat was 116 grams and the carbohydrate 180 grams greater per day than in the first period. Four per cent of the extra Calories in the fat is 42, and six per cent of the extra Calories in carbohydrate is 43. Thus the total metabolism should have increased in the second period 85 Calories, due solely to the extra food ingested. It will be recalled that the calculations required us to account for 68 Calories in this way. Thus all of the increase in the total metabolism is disposed of without recourse to "Luxuskonsumption".

From Tables III and IV it may be seen that the basal metabolic rate in the second period was about 5 per cent higher than in the first period.

An inspection of the respiratory quotients for each period shows that they were markedly higher when the subject was taking the excessive diet. It is generally conceded that this phenomenon indicates that the disposal of the previously ingested food is still going on: in other words, that the metabolism has not yet fallen to its basal level because of the continued specific dynamic action.

In the third period when the subject was still overeating, as evidenced by continued gain in weight, the basal metabolism quickly fell to its original level. This was to have been expected since the diet was now only moderately excessive and its specific dynamic action was complete before the determination of the basal metabolism on the following morning.

Here again there is no need of postulating a "Luxuskonsumption" to account for the facts.

Further information in regard to the response of the subject may be obtained from an analysis of the gain in weight during this period. The actual addition of body weight was 4,410 grams. It is conceivable that all of it might have been due to the retention of that amount of

TABLE V
Return of subject to maintenance diet

Date	Diet	Body weight at end of period	Surface area	Basal metabolism		Basal metabolic rate	Respiratory quotient
				Predicted	Determined		
		grams	*square meters*	*Calories*	*Calories*	*per cent*	
December 8-15	Deliberate intake of food greater than desire	62,610	1.79	1,679	1,580	- 6.1	.842
December 15-22	Same as above	62,984	1.80	1,6888	1,490	- 11.7	.857
December 22-January 13	Food according to desire	62,256	1.79	1,679	1,490	- 11.3	.765
January 13-February 13	Same as above	61,574					
February 13-March 19	Same as above	60,943					

water. If this were true, it would necessarily also be true that he had burned all of the diet. However, an analysis of the data gives a quite different answer (7). The comparison between the available energy of the diet and the transformation of energy shows that the subject acquired 24,830 Calories deposited as 179 grams of protein and 2,499 grams of fat. These materials in the form of body tissue amounted to 3,465 grams. In addition to this weight there should have been a water retention of 945 grams to account for the total gain in weight. The determination of the water exchange for the period accounted for the retention of 897 in addition to that deposited with the protein and fat. These considerations offer further evidence to demonstrate that the extra energy absorbed form the excessive diet was, in the main, stored and not burned.

DISCUSSION

About 20 years ago, Grafe stated that the oxidative rate in the animal organism was significantly affected by the amount of energy taken in. It had already been clearly demonstrated by several different investigators that the heat production in the basal state falls as much as 30 per cent due to prolonged starvation. Much later, F.G. Benedict (8) fed a group of men, who were habitually ingesting 3,200 to 3,600 Calories, a diet containin 1,400 Calories. After three weeks the average weight c the subjects had declined 12 per cent and their basa metabolism had fallen 18 per cent. They were now abl to maintain this new low weight on 1,950 Calories, an the basal metabolism remained low. It is true then tha the organism can reduce its rate of oxidation in respons to underfeeding and, if the latter is not too extreme weight may be maintained after an initial loss. This i clearly an adaptation capable of prolonging the life c the organism in the face of famine. On the other hand it is not easy to picture any advantage obtainabl through the ability to dispose of an over abundance c food rather than to store it so that it would be availabl in time of need.

Grafe, however, tried to prove that the norma mammalian organism did automatically dispose o excessive food through the mechanism of an increase metabolic rate. We have shown above that his data d not support his hypothesis, for when the fasting, restin metabolic rate of his dogs obtained during a period o over nutrition is compared with this rate obtained whe the dog was apparently normal, no significant increas is found. He obtained an apparent increase by firs pushing the rate down by means of a long period of sta vation. He thus obtained a metabolic rate 26 per cent lower than the normal but, nevertheless, he accepted this value as a proper basis for compensation. The same criticism applies to the study of the patient whose rate was 22 per cent below normal when he was emaciated and in whom very marked "Luxuskonsumption" permitted the rate to return to the usual level for such an individual in health.

Even though the fasting, resting metabolism does not appear to be stimulated by previous over nutrition, it may still be true that the total transformation of energy can be increased by this factor. Grafe did not deal with this phase of the subject at all. However, due to the development of a method in this laboratory, such data are now obtainable without the use of a calorimeter.

The subject whom we studied belonged to the group of persons alleged to be pathologically lean because, accepting the dictum of Grafe, they oxidize all of the food taken into the body without regard to quantity. The slight increase observed in both the basal and total metabolism, on a super-maintenance diet, was found to be entirely attributable to the increase in surface area plus the extra specific dynamic effect of the greater diet. It was equally clear that this subject was quite capable of gaining weight when he took food in excess of his habitual desire. A scrutiny of his life brought out the important fact that he had always been indifferent in regard to food, and that he had consequently eaten sparingly. However, during a short period of his life he had food set before him which was so attractive that it overcame his indifference and he gained a large amount of weight during this interval. A recognition of the fact that he habitually ate less than the usual amount of food for his group is sufficient reason for his thinness.

Clearly the body weight is affected on the one hand by the individual metabolic requirement and on the other hand by the total intake of energy. Evidently the mechanism, commonly called appetite, functions to maintain a balance between the supply and the demand. This is hardly the place to discuss the well known factors that influence appetite and individual metabolic requirements. Observations and special studies on appetite (9) in this clinic have convinced us that the abnormalities of body weight are regularly due to failure of the appetite to make a complete adjustment between the inflow and outflow of energy.

SUMMARY

(1) The basal metabolism and the total transformation of energy of an unusually thin subject were recorded when (1) he was on a maintenance diet and (2) when he was being vigorously overfed.

(2) It could not be shown that either the basal or the total transformation of energy per square meter of body surface was increased by more than the increment due to the extra specific dynamic action of the additional food.

(3) On the other hand, the subject added about 4.5 kilograms to his weight in 15 days when he was being overfed.

(4) No support for the "Luxuskonsumption" hypothesis of Grafe was secured.

BIBLIOGRAPHY

1. Grafe, E., and Graham, D., Ztschr. f. physiol. Chem., 1911, lxxiii, 1. Uber die Anpassungsfahigkeit des tierischen Organismus an uberreichliche Nahrungszufuhr.
2. Schondorff, B., Arch. f. d. ges. Physiol., 1897, lxvii, 430. Ueber den Einfluss der Schilddruse auf den Stoffwechsel.
3. Zuntz, N., Biochem. Ztschr., 1913, lv, 341. Einfluss chronischer Unterernahrung auf den Stoffwechsel.
4. Grafe, E., and Koch, R., Deutsches Arch. f. klin. Med., 1912, cvi, 564. Uber den Einfluss langdauernder, starker Uberernahrung auf die Intensitat der Verbrennungen im menschlichen Organismus (Untersuchungen bei Mastkuren).
5. Newburgh, L.H., Wiley, F.H., and Lashmet, F.H., J. Clin. Invest., 1931, x, 703. A Method for the Determination of Heat Production Over Long Periods of Time.
6. Lusk, G., J. Nutrition, 1931, iii, 519. The Specific Dynamic Action.
7. Wiley, F.H., and Newburgh, L.H., J. Clin. Invest., 1931, x, 723. An Improved Method for the Determination of Water Balance.
8. Benedict, F.G., Miles, W.R., Roth, P., and Smith, H.M., Carnegie Inst. of Wash., 1917, Pub. No.280. Human Vitality and Efficiency under Prolonged Restricted Diet.
9. Harrington, M.M., J. Am. Dietet. Assoc., 1930, vi, 101. Appetite in Relation to Weight.

Measurement of Total Carbon Dioxide Production by Means of D_2O^{18} [1]

Nathan Lifson, George B. Gordon[2] and Ruth McClintock
From the Department of Physiology, University of Minnesota School of Medicine, and Radioisotope Unit, Veterans Administration Hospital, Minneapolis, Minnesota

THIS PAPER describes a method using D_2O^{18} for measurement of total CO_2 production in the intact animal. The method was suggested by the finding that the oxygen of respiratory CO_2 and the oxygen of body water are in isotopic equilibium with one another (I). It is unique in that it may permit determination of total CO_2 output (and hence an estimate of energy expenditure) over long periods merely by isotopic analysis of initial and final blood samples.

Methods

Theoretical Basis of the Method

The turnover rate of the oxygen of the body water is greater than that of the hydrogen. This is chiefly due to the fact that the oxygen but not the hydrogen is lost via respiratory CO_2. If the body water is labeled with D_2O^{18}, the difference between the two turnover rates can be measured and employed to calculate the rate of CO_2 production as follows:

Deuterium is removed from the body almost entirely via water, permitting one to write $-dN_D^*/dt = r_{H_2O}(N_D^*/N) = r_{H_2O}S_D$, where N is the number of water molecules in the body, N_D^* is the number of D_2O molecules in the body, r_{H_2O} is the rate of loss of water molecules from the body, S_D is the specific activity (excess) of deuterium in the body water, and t is the time. Dividing through by N yields: $-dS_D/dt = (r_{H_2O}/N)S_D = K_DS_D$; r_{H_2O}/N is thus the fractional turnover rate of the deuterium of body water, which we have called K_D.

The O^{18} is removed from the body not only by the same routes as is the deuterium but also by respiratory CO_2. For the loss of O^{18} from the body water, one can write $-dN_O^*/dt = r_{H_2O}(N_O^*/N) + 2r_{CO_2}(N_O^*/N) = (r_{H_2O} + 2r_{CO_2})S_O$ where N_O^* is the number of H_2O^{18} molecules in the body water, r_{CO_2} is the rate of CO_2 production, and S_O is the specific activity (excess) of the H_2O^{18} in the body water. The factor of 2 must be used because each molecule of CO_2 contains 2 atoms of oxygen whereas each molecule of water contains only 1 atom of oxygen. Dividing through by N yields in this case: $-dS_O/dt = ((r_{H_2O} + 2r_{CO_2})/N)S_O = K_OS_O$. K_O is the fractional turnover rate of the O^{18} of the body water. Now, since $K_O - K_D = (r_{H_2O} + 2r_{CO_2})/N - r_{H_2O}/N$, $K_O - K_D = 2r_{CO_2}/N$ *and* $r_{CO_2} = (N/2)(K_O - K_D)$; or CO_2 output $= (N/2)(K_O - K_D)dt$.

If N, K_O, and K_D remain constant with time,

$$\text{Total } CO_2 \text{ output} = (N/2)(K_O - K_D)\Delta t_{CO_2}. \quad (1)$$

K_O and K_D can be evaluated by the logarithmic rate of decrease of the concentration of O^{18} and D, respectively, in the body water: $-dS/dt = KS$;

$$(-dS/S)/dt = K = -d\ln S/dt.$$

which for finite periods of time with K constant becomes $\Delta \ln S/\Delta t = 2.3\ (\Delta \log S/\Delta t)$. N can be obtained in the intact animal by the volume of dilution principle or, if the animal is killed, by desiccation of the carcass.

In the application of this equation, isotopic fractionation effects must be taken into account. If f_1 is the fractionation factor, D_2O (gas)/D_2O (liquid), f_2 is the fractionation factor, H_2O^{18} (gas)/H_2O^{18} (liquid), f_3 is the fractionation factor, CO_2^{18} (gas)/H_2O^{18} (liquid), and r_G is the rate of evaporative water loss, then equation 1 is modified to

Total CO_2 output

$$= \left[\frac{N}{2f_3}(K_O - K_D) - \frac{(f_2 - f_1)r_G}{2f_3}\right]\Delta t_{CO_2}. \quad (2)$$

[1] This investigation was supported in part by a research grant (G-3483-Phys.) from the National Institutes of Health, Public Health Service and by a research grant (NR 115-366) from the Office of Naval Research.
[2] At present on active duty, Medical Corps, United States Army.

Reprinted with permission of the American Physiological Society. J Appl Physiol. 1955;7:704–710.

[3] Little error arises from applying the usual fractionation factors to excess isotopic concentrations in the concentration ranges employed in this study

By substituting values of .93 for f_1 (2), .99 for f_2, and 1.04 for f_3 (3) in equation 2, one obtains[3]

$$\text{Total } CO_2 \text{ output} = [(N/2.08)(K_O - K_D) - .03\ r_G]\Delta t_{CO_2}. \quad (3)$$

This is the equation used to calculate total CO_2 outputs. The assumptions of the derivation will be considered in the DISCUSSION.

Experimental Procedure

A comparison has been made in 15 unfasted mice between the total CO_2 output calculated from equation 3 and the measured CO_2 output. The body water was enriched with D_2O^{18}. In some experiments 0.3 cc each of 100% D_2O and 10 atom % excess H_2O^{18} were injected intraperitoneally and at least 1 hour allowed before initial sampling for isotopic analysis.[4] In others the animals drank dilute D_2O^{18} (3% D_2O and 1.4 atom % excess H_2O^{18}) for several days. In still others the mice drank the H_2O^{18} for several days and were given an intraperitoneal injection of 0.3 cc of 100% D_2O 1 hour before the initial sampling. The initial S_D was determined on urine or tail blood. The initial S_O was measured on respiratory CO_2, collected for a few minutes as shown in figure 1*A*, or on tail blood or both. The D_2O concentrations of urine and blood agreed satisfactorily, as did the O^{18} concentrations of respiratory CO_2 and blood. The mouse was then placed in a metabolism chamber in which it had access to food and water (4) and which was arranged as shown in figure 1*B* for collection in NaOH of the total CO_2 output for periods of 1–3 days. After this total CO_2 collection the mouse was transferred to the chamber of figure 1*A* and another short-time sample of CO_2 was obtained, following which the animal was decapitated for a final blood sample. The head and carcass were minced and dried to constant weight at 105°–110° C for measurement of total body water. The final S_D was determined on the blood, the final S_O on the CO_2 or blood or both.

Analytical Procedures

The NaOH in which the total CO_2 production was collected was diluted to a known volume with water and the CO_2 concentration of an aliquot was determined in the manometric Van Slyke apparatus. A correction was applied for the amount of CO_2 contained in the NaOH and diluting water. The isotopic analyses on blood and urine were performed in duplicate or triplicate on samples of approximately .05 cc each. The D_2O and H_2O^{18} abundance ratios were measured as previously described (1,5) by means of the mass spectrometer. In the later experiments, closely bracketing standards were employed to increase the accuracy of the isotopic analyses. The abundance of O^{18} in normal mouse CO_2 did not differ significantly from that in CO_2 equilibrated with distilled water.

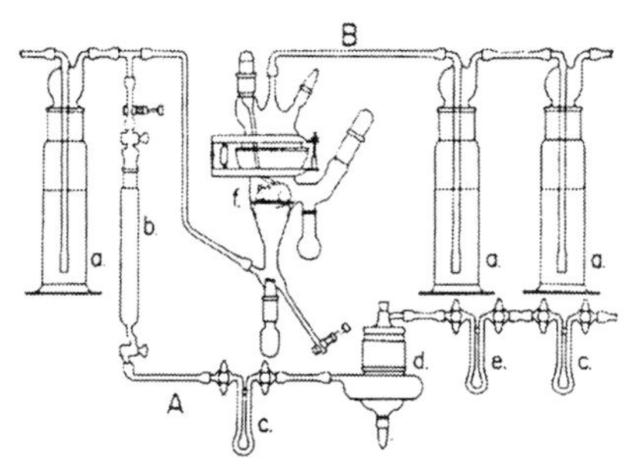

Figure 1: *A*, train for collection of initial and final CO_2 samples for isotopic oxygen analysis. *B*, train for collection of total CO_2. *a*) traps containing 250 cc 7.5 N NaOH for removal or collection of CO_2; *b*) $Mg(ClO_4)_2$ (Anhydrone) tube to remove water vapor; *c*) U-tubes immersed in liquid O_2 to freeze out CO_2; *d*) small chamber; *e*) U-tube in dry ice-acetone mixture to freeze out water vapor; *f*) large chamber. Gas flow was provided by a compressed air tank, or room air was drawn through the train by a suction pump.

The terms of equation 3 were thus obtained as follows: N from the product of the average weight of the mouse during the time of the total CO_2 collection and the percentage water content as estimated by desiccation of the carcass and head; K_O from $(2.3[(\log S_O)_{\text{initial}} - (\log S_O)_{\text{final}}])/\Delta t_O$, where Δt_O is the time between the initial and final samples for O^{18} analysis; K_D from $(2.3[(\log S_D)_{\text{initial}} - (\log S_D)_{\text{final}}])/\Delta t_D$ where Δt_D is the time between the two corresponding samples for D analysis; r_G by subtracting the amount of urine collected per unit time from the total water turnover rate, $(K_D N)$; and Δt_{CO_2} from the time for the total CO_2 collection.

Results

In table 1, a protocol is given for one mouse. Table 2 shows a comparison for 15 mice between the observed total CO_2 outputs and those calculated from equation 3. In addition, the values which were substituted into this equation are listed. In figure 2 the comparison between the calculated and observed total CO_2 outputs is presented graphically. The average absolute difference between the CO_2 output as calculated from equation 3 and the CO_2 actually collected is seen to be 7 (± 7)%.[5] When account is taken of algebraic

[4] All values given under Methods for volumes and isotopic concentrations are approximate.

[5] Standard deviation of the distribution.

sign, the average discrepancy is −3 (± 10)%. This latter mean is not significantly different from zero. Therefore, the method as employed yields reasonable estimates for the total CO_2 output of mice.

The values of K_O (per day) vary from .414 to .643, K_D from .256 to .419, and K_O–K_D from .146 to .224. Since the average discrepancy between the observed and calculated CO_2 outputs for the mice represented by these extremes is 3% (maximum −4%), this method of calculation of total CO_2 output applies as well to mice with quite different rates of D_2O and H_2O^{18} turnover.

Discussion

Magnitude of Analytical Errors

In order to interpret the magnitude of the discrepancies indicated in table 2 between the observed and calculated values for total CO_2 output, some estimate is necessary of the uncertainty of the analytical procedures themselves, exclusive of biological factors.

The calculated CO_2 output involved measurement of Δt, N, K_O, K_D and r_G. Errors in the measurement of Δt were negligible. The value for N was determined from the product of the average body weight and the percentage of water content of the carcass and head, as estimated by desiccation. Each of these determinations was accurate to better than 1%.

In computing K_O and K_D the major error was introduced in the determination of the final S_O because this sample had the smallest absolute isotopic abundance. Even when bracketing standards were employed, the value for S_O probable was uncertain to approximately .003 atom % excess. An error of this magnitude would in itself have produced an error of some 4% in the calculated CO_2 output. When bracketing standards were not employed, the error could have been much greater. For example, in the case of mouse 11, in which the final S_O was .123 atom % excess, the discrepancy of −21% could be accounted for by an error of less than 0.01 atom % excess. Thus, the sensitivity of the result to small errors in the final S_O could explain much of the observed discrepancy between calculated and observed values. The 2 mice in which the largest discrepancies were encountered (+20% for mouse 6 and −21% for mouse 11) were among the 11 studied before bracketing standards were used, whereas the maximum discrepancy in the case of the 4 mice in which bracketing standards were employed was −8%.

In the estimation of r_G, the evaporative water loss was taken as the difference between the total water turnover per day, ($K_D N$), and the urine collected per day. The urinary volume may have been in error because of evaporation of the urine or dilution by spilled drinking water. However, even if the evaporative loss is taken to be equal to the total water turnover, the average error would be increased by only 3% over that obtained by employing the estimated r_G of table 2. The uncertainty in the value for r_G is, therefore, not likely to have been important.

The accuracy of the observed value for total CO_2 output was also considered. Three experiments were carried out in which CO_2 was released by lactic acid from a known amount of $BaCO^2$ placed in a reaction chamber just ahead of, or in place of, the large metabolism chamber. In three such experiments the CO_2 collected amounted to 98–100% of that released.

It is concluded that the errors of the analytical procedures could in large part explain absolute discrepancies between calculated and observed values for total CO_2 output of the magnitude shown in table 2.

Assumptions of the Method

The assumptions involved in the derivation and application of equation 3, with a discussion of each, follow.

1) One assumption is that N remains constant during the period of measurement and can be ascertained by desiccation. If N is equal to the body water content, constancy of body weight over the time intervals employed could be considered as indicating constancy of N for the purpose in question. In those experiments in which body weight did change, N has been calculated from the arithmetic mean of the initial and final weights. If the weight change were not uniform with time, the arithmetic mean weight could differ from the true integrated mean body weight. During these experiments the body weights of the mice changed an av-

TABLE 1. SAMPLE PROTOCOL (MOUSE 20)

Wt., gm—before chamber	26.12	
final av.	26.14	
	26.13	
Carcass wet wt, gm	24.99	
Carcass dry wt, gm	9.95	
Carcass water, gm	15.04	
Water content, %	60.2	
Av. N. mM	874	
	D_2O	H_2O^{18}
Initial S (atom % excess)	1.622	.599
Final S (atom % excess)	.625	.135
Log initial S	1.210	.777
Log final S	.796	.130
Δ log S	.414	.647
Δt, days	2.84	2.81
K, days^{-1}	.336	.531
K_O-K_D, days^{-1}	.195	
Δt_{CO_2}, days	2.76	
Total CO_2 (calc.), mM	207	
Total CO_2 (obs.), mM	226	
Error, %	−8	

TABLE 2. SUMMARY OF DATA INCLUDING COMPARISON BETWEEN OBSERVED CO_2 OUTPUT AND THAT CALCULATED ACCORDING TO EQUATION 3

Mouse No., Strain	Av. N	K_O	K_D	r_G	Δt_{CO_2}	Total CO_2* (Calc.)	CO_2 (Obs.)	Error
	mM	days⁻¹	days⁻¹	mM/day	days	mM	mM	%
3, C₃H	1025	.513	.321	170	.92	82	82	0
4, C₃H	1023	.498	.311	210	.92	70	81	−2
5, C₃H	1136	.506	.345	270	.92	73	84	−13
6, C₃H	1036	.448	.204	150	.95	83	69	+20
7, C₃H	1055	.643	.419	273	.95	100	98	+2
8, C₃H	1028	.523	.308	210	1.72	121	136	−11
9, C₃H	980	.536	.333	131	.97	80	91	−2
10, C₃H	953	.484	.287	218	1.90	150	165	−4
11, C₃H	1040	.560	.300	308	2.84	215	273	−21
12, C₃H	971	.414	.268	216	2.88	178	186	−4
14, C₃H	1108	.581	.393	357	2.83	253	235	+8
15, C₃H	1007	.530	.353	277	2.83	219	211	+4
16, C₃H	1085	.597	.397	347	2.95	277	302	−8
18, BOb	949	.424	.256	205	2.87	202	207	−2
20, BOb	874	.531	.336	234	2.76	207	226	−8

Mean absolute error 7 ± 7%
Mean algebraic error −3 ± 10%

Bracketing standards were employed for *mice 15–20*. All but *mouse 12* were males.
* Corrected for fractionation.

erage of 4%. If this were to reflect an error in the average N of 2%, which appears improbably large, an approximately equal error in calculation of total CO_2 output would result.[6]

The more serious question is whether or not the desiccation 'space' in which the D and O^{18} respectively distribute themselves. The true 'space' would be larger if there is exchange of D or O^{18} with compounds other than water, or smaller if there are compartments of water which do not mix with the administered labeled water. To include a correction for true 'space' as well as fractionation effects, equation 3 must be modified to the following:

$$\text{Total } CO_2 \text{ output} = \left[(BN/2f_3)(K_O - K_D) - \frac{(A-B)r_L + (Af_2 - Bf_1)r_G}{2Af_3} \right] \Delta t_{CO_2}. \quad (4)$$

where A=true mean D_2O 'space'/N; B=true mean H_2O^{18} 'space'/N; r_L=rate of loss of water as liquid; r_G=rate of loss of water as vapor. The other symbols are as defined for equation 3.

If A=B=1, this equation reduces to equation 3. When A and B are calculated from the initial volumes of dilution of the injected D_2O and H_2O^{18}, values for A of 1.03–1.12 (average 1.06) and for B of 1.00–1.03 (average 1.02) are obtained (table 3).[7] When the mean values for A and B are substituted in equation 4, the calculated CO_2 outputs average 3% lower than those corrected for fractionation alone. If the individual values for A and B given in table 3 for mice 3 to 8 are used, each calculated CO_2 output in these six mice is practically the same as that obtained from use of the average values except in the case of one mouse (mouse 4).

Even though the volumes of dilution of D_2O and H_2O^{18} provide values for the respective initial 'spaces,' these 'spaces' are no doubt expanding at different rates during the experimental period by incorporation of D and O^{18} from body water into other constituents. The calculated CO_2 output would be erroneously low if the true mean H_2O^{18} 'space' is being underestimated relative to the mean D_2O 'space' by the initial volumes of distribution.

The procedures used for determination of the volume of dilution of D_2O were checked by adding the labeled water to a known volume of ordinary water. The water volume estimated from the isotopic concentration of the mixture agreed to within 2% of the actual volume (table 3).

2) A second assumption is that the only loss of D and O^{18} from the body occurs via H_2O and CO_2. Loss of any exchangeable D and O^{18} present in excreted compounds in the same ratios as in body water would result in no error. The effect would then be merely to add to the apparent water turnover, increasing K_O and K_D equally without

[6] An equation which takes account of a changing N can be derived if N is expressed as a function of time. With uniformly changing N, the arithmetic mean N is practically equal to the correct value which should be used.

[7] These data suggest that H_2O^{18} is a better substance than is D_2O for measuring total body water by the volume of dilution principle.

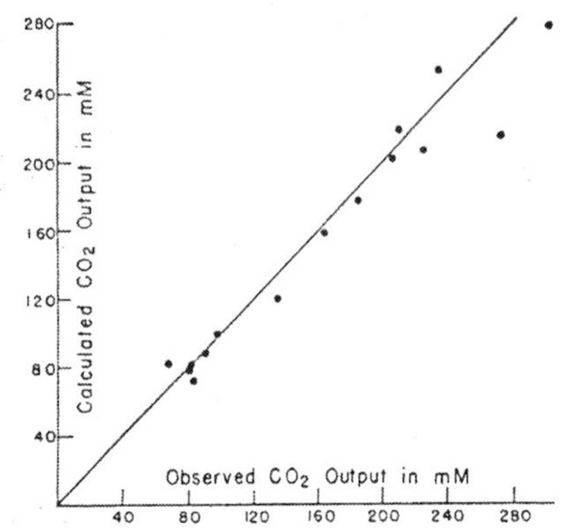

Figure 2: Graphical comparison between observed total CO_2 output of mice and total CO_2 output calculated from *eq. 3*.

changing $(K_O - K_D)$. For example, on the assumption that the 4 H atoms and one O atom of urea, (the urinary constituent most important in the present considerations) are in isotopic equilibrium with body water, the loss of 2 of the H atoms and the O atom would be included in the water turnover. Thus, the influence on $(K_O - K_D)$ and the calculated CO_2 output would correspond to the loss of the D equivalent of 1, not 2 molecules of water for each molecule of urea.

If r_O represents the rate of loss of oxygen atoms from the body at the specific activity of body water by routes other than H_2O and CO_2, and r_H represents one-half the corresponding value for hydrogen (the rate of loss of the H equivalent of 1 H_2O molecule) then equation 4 becomes modified to the following:

$$\text{Total } CO_2 = [(BN/2f_3)(K_O - K_D) - ((A-B)r_L + (Af_2 - Bf_1)r_G + (Ar_O - Br_H)/2Af_3)]\Delta t_{CO_2}. \quad (5)$$

In the case of a mouse with a rate of CO_2 production of 100 mM per day, on a diet of fox chow containing 20% protein, about 5 mM would appear in the urine. The r_O due to urea excretion would amount similarly to 5mM per day and r_H to 10 mM per day; hence $(r_O - r_H)^8$ equals −5. The other important route of loss is via the feces. For example, the hydrogens of the hydroxyl groups of cellulose can exchange with those of water. The diet of the mice contained 5–6% 'fiber.' If this is assumed to be cellulose, each monosaccharide unit of which has 3 exchangeable hydrogens one

^{8} $(Ar_O - Br_H)$ is approximately equal to $(r_O - r_H)$ since A and B are both close to unity.

TABLE 3. COMPARISON OF VOLUMES OF DILUTION OF D_2O AND H_2O^{18} WITH TOTAL BODY WATER AS MEASURED BY DESICCATION

Mouse No.	Wt.	1 Vol. Dilut., D_2O	2 Vol. Dilu., H_2O^{18}	3 BW by Desiccation	A Col. 1/ Col. 3	B Col. 2/ Col. 3
	gm	*cc*	*cc*	*cc*		
3	20.2	19.0	18.7	18.3	1.09	1.02
4	30.2	20.8	18.6	18.6	1.12	1.00
5	32.5	21.8	20.8	20.7	1.05	1.00
6	29.6	20.3	19.2	18.9	1.07	1.02
7	30.4	20.6	19.4	18.9	1.09	1.03
8	26.9	20.0	18.6	18.1	1.10	1.03
18	30.5	20.0		18.2	1.10	
20	27.5	18.1		16.5	1.10	
E1	29.5	18.4		17.9	1.03	
E2	28.2	16.9		16.2	1.04	
E3	23.8	15.0		14.8	1.07	
E4	26.9	17.3		16.6	1.04	
E5	26.6	16.4		15.8	1.04	
E6	32.6	18.5		17.9	1.03	
E7	30.2	17.7		17.2	1.03	
E8	25.9	16.3		15.8	1.03	
					1.06 ±.03†	1.02 ±.01
Cont.*				Vol. H_2O		
1		10.2		10.0	1.02	
2		19.6		19.7	.995	
3		20.2		20.3	.995	
4		16.1		16.1	1.00	
5		17.5		17.5	1.00	
					1.00 ±.01	

* D_2O added to known volume of H_2O (see text).
† Values are means ± S.D.

can compute r_H due to this loss to be about 2 mM per 100 mM of CO_2 output. On this basis, the calculated CO_2 outputs would be increased by more than 3% due to urinary urea and fecal 'fiber' loss alone. The magnitude of $(r_O - r_H)$ attributable to other fecal constituents has not as yet been evaluated.

Table 4 presents the values for total CO_2 output obtained in the following ways: *a)* observed; *b)* calculated from equation 1, i.e. uncorrected; *c)* calculated from equation 3, i.e. corrected for fractionation effects only; *d)* calculated from equation 4, i.e. corrected for both fractionation and the mean initial volumes of dilution; and *e)* calculated from equation 5, i.e. corrected for fractionation, initial volume of dilution, and the above estimated loss in urea and

TABLE 4. COMPARISON OF OBSERVED VALUES FOR CO_2 OUTPUT WITH THOSE CALCULATED IN VARIOUS WAYS AS INDICATED

Mouse No.	Total CO_2 obs.	CO_2 Calculated According to							
		Equation 1[a]		Equation 3[b]		Equation 3[c]		Equation 3[d]	
		Total	Error	Total	Error	Total	Error	Total	Error
	mM	*mM*	%	*mM*	%	*mM*	%	*mM*	%
3	82	90	+10	82	0	80	−2	82	0
4	81	88	+9	79	−2	76	−6	79	−2
5	84	84	0	73	−13	70	−17	73	−13
6	69	91	+32	83	+20	81	+17	87	+26
7	98	112	+14	100	+2	97	−1	100	+2
8	136	137	+1	121	−11	114	−16	110	−12
9	91	97	+6	89	−2	86	−5	89	−2
10	165	178	+8	159	−4	156	−5	161	−2
11	273	252	−8	215	−21	205	−25	214	−22
12	186	205	+10	178	−4	173	−7	178	−4
14	235	295	+26	253	+8	244	+4	251	+7
15	211	253	+20	219	+4	211	0	218	+3
16	302	320	+6	277	−8	267	−12	277	−8
18	207	220	+11	202	−2	198	−4	204	−1
20	226	235	+4	207	−8	201	−11	208	−8
			+10 ± 10[e]		−3 ± 10		−6 ± 10		−2 ± 11

[a] Uncorrected. [b] Corrected for fractionation. [c] Corrected for fractionation and space; av. values for A and B used, A = 1.00, B = 1.02. [d] Corrected for fractionation, space and estimated loss in urea and 'fiber.' [e] Values are means ±S.D.

'fiber.' The average discrepancy between observed CO_2 outputs and those calculated as indicated in (*e*) above is −2 (± 11)%. The inclusion of corrections both for initial 'space' and for loss in urea and 'fiber' does not change appreciably the values obtained from equation 3. These two corrections are approximately equal but opposite in sign. Thus the major correction of the simple relationship of equation 1, total CO_2 output=$(N/2)(K_O - K_D)\ \Delta t$, arises from fractionation effects.

3) A third assumption is that K_O and K_D are constant. This assumption is obviously contrary to fact, since the CO_2 output and the intake and excretion of water occur at changing, rather than constant rates. However, it can be shown that if the relationship $-dS/dt=KS$ holds for all intervals within the experimental period, where K is an explicit function of t and not of S, the mean K over the total time interval is equal to that obtained by using the initial and final points only.

4) A fourth assumption is that the specific activity of D and O^{18} in any water lost from the body is the same as that in blood, and that the specific activity of the O^{18} in CO_2 is also the same as that in blood. The results of the comparison of the isotopic concentrations of CO_2 and blood confirm the previous report (1) of equality between the two, after correction for fractionation effects. Similarly, urinary water is isotopically a sample of body water and the same is undoubtedly true of respiratory water loss. We have not as yet performed the necessary determinations on fecal water. We have ascertained that for a few hours after the injection of D_2O and H_2O^{18}, the water lost by evaporation has a lower concentration than does blood water, at least when the animal is placed in a stream of dry air. Apparently the water initially given off by the hair and skin has not reached isotopic equilibrium with the blood water. However, error would occur in the calculated CO_2 output only if the ratio of D to O^{18} in the water lost were different from that in the blood water. Equality in absolute concentrations is not essential.

In summary, it would appear that use of the above assumptions has not introduced serious error in the calculated CO_2 output compared to the analytical error. Thus there is some reason *a*) for believing that the errors resulting from employing the first and second assumptions approximately cancelled each other and *b*) for minimizing those due to the third and fourth assumptions.

Variations and Applications of the Method

The experiments described in this paper represent only one variation of a general method of approach, some further examples of which will be mentioned.

If an animal drinks doubly-labeled water until the isotope concentration in the body water reaches a steady state, the rate of CO_2 production can be calculated from the water intake and the ratios of the concentrations of each isotope in the drinking water (*DW*) to that in the body water (*BW*), according to the following equation (in which the same assumptions are included as in *eq. I*):

$$r_{CO_2} = \frac{r_{DW}}{2}\left[\left(\frac{S_{DW}}{S_{BW}}\right)_O - \left(\frac{S_{DW}}{S_{BW}}\right)_D\right]$$

Here r_{DW} is the rate of total water intake. This equation has been tested on only one animal, with 1% difference (probably fortuitously small) between observed and calculated CO_2 outputs. The chief difficulty at present is in accurate measurement of the water intake. In the single experiment of this type performed intraperitoneal injections of water were employed; food water was negligible.

With an animal drinking doubly-labeled water, the values of K_O and K_D for substitution in equation 1, and therefore the CO_2 output, can also be obtained from the rates at which the body water concentration of each isotope increases before the steady state is reached.

If an animal breathes oxygen containing O^{18}, the rate of oxygen consumption can be calculated, without use of deuterium, from the rate at which the body water becomes labeled.

The method of determining total CO_2 production described in the present paper provides a means of estimating the total energy metabolism of an animal. While the relationship of the CO_2 output to energy liberation is more dependent upon R.Q. than is that of the O_2 consumption, the energy output may be approximated by assuming a value for the R.Q. If the composition of the diet is known, a more accurate value can be obtained. An estimate of the total energy expenditure of an animal with unrestricted activity would be useful in a variety of situations, even with the present accuracy of the method.

This approach is not restricted to the study of a single animal body, but could be applied to any aqueous system in which CO_2 is produced, such as a bacterial culture or a purely chemical system. If water loss is negligible, the deuterium measurements become unnecessary.

In the study of the CO_2 output of species other than the mouse, the suitable time intervals will depend mainly on the absolute and relative magnitudes of the turnover rates of D and O^{18} respectively. Optimum periods are those which produce decreases in S such that log ($S_{initial}$ S_{final}) can be accurately measured. In humans, intervals of 2–3 weeks would correspond, in this respect, to those of 2–3 days in mice. Moreover, since any percentage error in (K_O–K_D) will reflect itself in a similar percentage error in the calculated CO_2 output, accuracy is favored by a high ratio of K_O to K_D. In the mice K_O/K_D was of the order of 1.6. Where this ratio is of the order of 1.4, as might be expected for the 'typical' adult human, K_O and K_D will have to be determined with somewhat greater accuracy to make the method useful, even if uncertainty is introduced for no other reasons. Aside from theoretical considerations, the use of this approach in metabolic studies of larger animals, such as man, is at present limited because of the cost of H_2O^{18}.

Summary

A simple formula (equation 1) has been derived by which the total CO_2 output of an animal can be calculated from the total body water and the difference between fractional turnover rates of the D and O^{18} of body water labeled with D_2O^{18}. In applying the formula isotopic fractionation factors were taken into account, which involved a very crude estimate of urinary volume (eq. 3). The turnover rates of D and O^{18} were estimated by initial and final sampling. In a series of 15 mice the calculated CO_2 outputs were compared with the observed CO_2 outputs. The average absolute discrepancy between calculated and observed CO_2 outputs was 7 (± 7)%. The average algebraic discrepancy was –3 (± 10)%. The sources of error, assumptions, and variations of the method are discussed.

Acknowledgments

We are indebted to John Saari, Bailey Donnally, Charles Bollenbacher, and Harold Liemohn for performing the mass spectrographic isotope analyses under the supervision of Dr. A. O. Nier. We also wish to thank Dr. Robert L. Evans for mathematical assistance.

References

1. **Lifson, N, Gordon, GB, Visscher, MB, Nier, AO.** *J Biol Chem.* 1949;180:803.
2. **Kirshenbaum, I.** *Physical Properties and Analysis of Heavy Water.* New York: McGraw-Hill, 1951.
3. **Dole, M.** *Science* 1949;109:77.
4. **Roth, LJ, Leifer, E, Hogness JR, Langham, WH.** *J Biol Chem.* 1948;176:249.
5. **Johnson, JA, Cavert, HM, Lifson, N, Visscher, MB.** *Am J Physiol.* 1951;165:87.

CLASSICS IN OBESITY

Microscopial Researches into the Accordance in the Structure and Growth of Animals and Plants

Theodore H. Schwann

SECTION III.
REVIEW OF THE PREVIOUS RESEARCHES-THE FORMATIVE PROCESS OF CELLS-THE CELL THEORY.

The two foregoing sections of this work have been devoted to a detailed investigation of the formation of the different tissues from cells, to the mode in which these cells are developed, and to a comparison of the different cells with one another. We must now lay aside detail, take a more extended view of these researches, and grasp the subject in its more intimate relations. The principal object of our investigation was to prove the accordance of the elementary parts of animals with the cells of plants. But the expression "plant-like life" (pflanzen-ähnliches Leben) is so ambiguous that it is received as almost synonymous with growth without vessels; and it was, therefore, explained at page 6 that in order to prove this accordance, the elementary particles of animals and plants must be shown to be products of the same formative powers, because the phenomena attending their development are similar; that all elementary particles of animals and plants are formed upon a common principle. Having traced the formation of the separate tissues, we can more readily comprehend the object to be attained by this comparison of the different elementary particles with one another, a subject on which we must dwell a little, not only because it is the fundamental idea of these researches, but because all physiological deductions depend upon a correct apprehension of this principle.

When organic nature, animals and plants, is regarded as a Whole, in contradistinction to the inorganic kingdom, we do not find that all organisms and all their separate organs are compact masses, but that they are composed of innumerable small particles of a definite form. These elementary particles, however, are subject to the most extraordinary diversity of figure, especially in animals; in plants they are, for the most part or exclusively, cells. This variety in the elementary parts seemed to hold some relation to their more diversified physiological function in animals, so that it might be established as a principle, that every diversity in the physiological signification of an organ requires a difference in its elementary particles; and, on the contrary, the similarity of two elementary particles seemed to justify the conclusion that they were physiologically similar. It was natural that among the very different forms presented by the elementary particles, there should be some more or less alike, and that they might be divided, according to their similarity of figure, into fibres, which compose the great mass of the bodies of animals, into cells, tubes, globules, &c. The division was, of course, only one of natural history, not expressive of any physiological idea, and just as a primitive muscular fibre, for example, might seem to differ from one of areolar tissue, or all fibres from cells, so would there be in like manner a difference, however gradually marked between the different elementary particles, in the way required by its physiological function. It might be expected that there would be a definite mode of development for each separate kind of elementary structure, and that it would be similar in those structures which were physiologically identical, and such a mode of development was, indeed, already more or less perfectly known with regard to muscular fibres, blood-corpuscles, the ovum (see the Supplement), and epithelium-cells. The only process common to all of them, however, seemed to be the expansion of their elementary particles after they had once assumed their proper form. The manner in which their different elementary particles were first formed appeared to vary very much. In muscular fibres they were globules, which were placed together in rows, and coalesced to form a fibre, whose growth proceeded in the direction of its length. In the blood-corpuscles it was a globule, around which a vesicle was formed, and continued to grow; in the case of the ovum, it was a globule, around which a vesicle was developed and continued to grow, and around his again a second vesical was formed.

The formative process of the cells of plants was clearly explained by the researches of Schleiden, and

Schwann TH; Smith H, trans. Microsccopical researches into the accordance in the structure and growth of animals and plants. London: Sydenham Society 1847:117-118,161-185.

appeared to be the same in all vegetable cells. So that when plants were regarded as something special, as quite distinct from the animal kingdom, one universal principle of development was observed in all the elementary particles of the vegetable organism, and physiological deductions might be drawn from it with regard to the independent vitality of the individual cells of plants, &c. But when the elementary particles of animals and plants were considered from a common point, the vegetable cells seemed to be merely a separate species, co-ordinate with the different species of animal cells, just as the entire class of cells was co-ordinate with the fibres, &c., and the uniform principle of development in vegetable cells might be explained by the slight physiological difference of their elementary particles.

The object, then, of the present investigation was to show, that the mode in which the molecules composing the elementary particles of organisms are combined does not vary according to the physiological signification of those particles, but that they are everywhere arranged according to the same laws; so that whether a muscular fibre, a nerve-tube, an ovum, or a blood-corpuscle is to be formed, a corpuscle of a certain form, subject only to some modifications, a cell-nucleus, is universally generated in the first instance; around this corpuscle a cell is developed, and it is the changes which one or more of these cells undergo that determine the subsequent forms of the elementary particles; in short, that there is one common principle of development for all the elementary particles of organisms.

In order to establish this point it was necessary to trace the progress of development in two given elementary parts, physiologically dissimilar, and to compare them with one another. If these not only completely agreed in growth, but in their mode of generation also, the principle was established that elementary parts, quite distinct in a physiological sense, may be developed according to the same laws. This was the theme of the first section of this work. The course of development of the cells of cartilage and of the cells of the chorda dorsalis was compared with that of vegetable cells. Were the cells of plants developed merely as infinitely minute vesicles which progressively expand, were the circumstances of their development less characteristic than those pointed out by Schleiden, a comparison, in the sense here required, would scarcely have been possible. We endeavoured to prove in the first section that the complicated process of development in the cells of plants recurs in those of cartilage and of the chorda dorsalis. We remarked the similarity in the formation of the cell-nucleus, and of its nucleolus in all its modifications, with the nucleus of vegetable cells, the pre-existence of the cell-nucleus and the development of the cell around it, the similar situation of the nucleus in relation to the cell, the growth of the cells, and the thickening of their wall during growth, the formation of cells within cells, and the transformation of the cell-contents just as in the cells of plants. Here, then, was a complete accordance in every known stage in the progress of development of two elementary parts which are quite distinct, in a physiological sense, and it was established that the principle of development in two such parts may be the same, and so far as could be ascertained in the cases here compared, it is really the same.

But regarding the subject from this point of view we are compelled to prove the universality of this principle of development, and such was the object of the second section. For so long as we admit that there are elementary parts which originate according to entirely different laws, and between which and the cells which have just been compared as to the principle of their development there is no connexion, we must presume that there may still be some unknown difference in the laws of the formation of the parts just compared, even though they agree in many points. But, on the contrary, the greater the number of physiologically different elementary parts, which, so far as can be known, originate in a similar manner, and the greater the difference of these parts in form and physiological signification, while they agree in the perceptible phenomena of their mode of formation, the more safely may we assume that all elementary parts have one and the same fundamental principle of development. It was, in fact, shown that the elementary parts of most tissues, when traced backwards from their state of complete development to their primary condition are only development to their primary condition are only developments of cells, which so far as our observations, still incomplete, extend, seemed to be formed in a similar manner to the cells compared in the first section. As might be expected, according to this principle the cells, in their earliest stage, were almost always furnished with the characteristic nuclei, in some the pre-existence of this nucleus, and the formation of the cell around it was proved, and it was then that the cells began to undergo the various modifications, from which the diverse forms of the elementary parts of animals resulted. Thus the apparent difference in the mode of development of muscular fibres an blood-corpuscles, the former originating by the arrangement of globules in rows, the latter by the formation of a vesicle around a globule, was reconciled in the fact that muscular fibres are not elementary parts co-ordinate with blood-corpuscles, but that the globules composing muscular fibres at first correspond to the blood-corpuscles, and are like them, vesicles or cells, containing the characteristic cell-nucleus, which, like the nucleus of the blood-corpuscles, is probably formed before the cell. The elementary parts of all tissues are formed of cells in an analogous, though very diversified manner, so that it may be asserted, *that there is one universal principle of development for the elementary parts of organisms, however different, and that this principle is the formation of cells.* This is the chief result of the foregoing observations.

The same process of development and transformation of cells within a structureless substance is repeated in the formation of all the organs of an organism, as well as in the formation of all the organs of an organism, as well as in the formation of new organisms; and the fundamental phenomenon attending the exertion of productive power in organic nature is accordingly as follows: *a structureless substance is present in the first instance, which lies either around or in the interior of cells already existing; and cells are formed in it in accordance with certain laws, which cells become developed in various ways into the elementary parts of organisms.*

The development of the proposition, that there exists one general principle for the formation of all organic productions, and that this principle is the formation of cells, as well as the conclusions which may be drawn from this proposition, may be comprised under the term *cell-theory,* using it in its more extended signification, whilst in a more limited sense, by theory of the cells we understand whatever may be inferred from this proposition with respect to the powers from which these phenomena result.

But though this principle, regarded as the direct result of these more or less complete observations, may be stated to be generally correct, it must not be concealed that there are some exceptions, or at least differences, which as yet remain unexplained. Such, for instance, is the splitting into fibres of the walls of the cells in the interior of the chorda dorsalis of osseous fishes, which was alluded to at page 14. Several observers have also drawn attention to the fibrous structure of the firm substance of some cartilages. In the costal cartilages of old persons for example, these fibres are very distinct. They do not, however, seem to be uniformly diffused throughout the cartilage, but to be scattered merely here and there. I have not observed them at all in new-born children. It appears as if the previously structureless cytoblastema in this instance became split into fibres; I have not, however, investigated the point accurately. Our observations also fail to supply us with any explanation of the formation of the medullary canaliculi in bones, and an analogy between their mode of origin and that of capillary vessels, was merely suggested hypothetically. The formation of bony lamellæ around these canaliculi, is also an instance of the cytoblastema assuming a distinct form. But we will return presently to an explanation of this phenomenon that is not altogether improbable. In many glands, as for instance, the kidneys of a young mammalian fœtus, the stratum of cells surrounding the cavity of the duct, is enclosed by an exceedingly delicate membrane, which appears to be an elementary structure, and not to be composed of areolar tissue. The origin of this membrane is not at all clear, although we may imagine various ways of reconciling it with the formative process of cells. (These gland-cylinders seem at first to have no free cavity, but to be quite filled with cells. In the kidneys of the embryos of pigs, I found many cells in the cylinders, which were so large as to occupy almost the entire thickness of the canal. In other cylinders, the cellular layer, which was subsequently to line their walls, was formed, but the cavity was filled with very pale transparent cells, which could be pressed out from the free end of the tube.

These and similar phenomena may remain for a time unexplained. Although they merit the greatest attention and require further investigations, we may be allowed to leave them for a moment, for history shows that in the laying down of every general principle, there are almost always anomalies at first, which are subsequently cleared up.

The elementary particles of organisms, then, no longer lie side by side unconnectedly, like productions which are merely capable of classification in natural history, according to similarity of form; they are united by a common bond, the similarity of their formative principle, and they may be compared together and physiologically arranged in accordance with the various modifications under which that principle is exhibited. In the foregoing part of this work, we have treated of the tissues in accordance with this physiological arrangement, and have compared the different tissues with one another, proving thereby, that although different, but similarly formed, elementary parts may be grouped together in a natural-history arrangement, yet such a classification does not necessarily admit of a conclusion with regard to their physiological position, as based upon the laws of development. Thus, for example, the natural-history division, "cells," would, in a general sense, become a physiological arrangement also, inasmuch as most of the elementary parts comprised under it have the same principle of development; but yet it was necessary to separate some from this division; as, for instance, the germinal vesicle, all hollow cell-nuclei, and cells with walls composed of other elementary parts, although the germinal vesicle is a cell in the natural-history sense of the term. It does not correspond to an epithelium-cell, but to the nucleus of one. The difference in the two modes of classification was still more remarkable in respect to fibres. The mode of their origin is most varied, for, as we saw, a fibre of areolar tissue is essentially different from a muscular fibre; while, on the other hand, a whole primitive muscular fasciculus is identical in its mode of origin with a nervous fibre, and so on. The existence of a common principle of development for all the elementary parts of organic bodies lays the foundation of a new section of general anatomy, to which the term *philosophical* might by applied, having for its object-firstly, to prove the general laws by which the elementary parts of organisms are developed; and, secondly, to point out the different elementary parts in accordance with the general principle of development, and to compare them with one another.

SURVEY OF CELL-LIFE

The foregoing investigation has conducted us to the principle upon which the elementary parts of organized bodies are developed, by tracing these elementary parts, from their perfected condition, back to the earlier stages of development. Starting now from the principle of development, we will reconstruct the elementary parts as they appear in the matured state, so that we may be enabled to take a comprehensive view of the laws which regulate the formation of the elementary particles. We have, therefore, to consider-1, the cytoblastema; 2, the laws by which new cells are generated in the cytoblastema; 3, the formative process of the cells themselves; 4, the very various modes in which cells are developed into the elementary parts of organisms.

Cytoblastema.- The cytoblastema, or the amorphous substance in which new cells are to be formed, is found either contained within cells already existing, or else between them in the form of intercellular substance. The cytoblastema, which lies on the outside of existing cells, is the only form of which we have to treat at present, as the cell-contents form matter for subsequent consideration. Its quantity varies exceedingly, sometimes there is so little that it cannot be recognized with certainty between the fully-developed cells, and can only be observed between those most recently formed; for instance, in the second class of tissues; at other times there is so large a quantity present, that the cells contained in it do not come into contact, as is the case in most cartilages. The chemical and physical properties of the cytoblastema are not the same in all parts. In cartilages it is very consistent, and ranks among the most solid parts of the body; in areolar tissue it is gelatinous; in blood quite fluid. These physical distinctions imply also a chemical difference. The cytoblastema of cartilage becomes converted by boiling into gelatine, which is not the case with the blood; and the mucus in which the mucus-cells are formed differs from the cytoblastema of the cells of blood and cartilage. The cytoblastema, external to the existing cells, appears to be subject to the same changes as the cell-contents; in general it is a homogeneous substance; yet it may become minutely granulous as the result of a chemical transformation, for instance, in areolar tissue and the cells of the shaft of the feather, &c. As a general rule, it diminishes in quantity, relatively with the development of the cells, though it seems that in cartilages there may be even a relative increase of the cytoblastema proportionate to the growth of the tissue. The physiological relation which the cytoblastema holds to the cells may be twofold: first, it must contain the material for the nutrition of the cells; secondly, it must contain at least a part of what remains of this nutritive material after the cells have withdrawn from it what they required for their growth. In animals, the cytoblastema receives the fresh nutritive material from the bloodvessels; in plants it passes chiefly through the elongated cells and vascular fasciculi; there are, however, many plants which consist of simple cells, so that there must also be a transmission of nutrient fluid through the simple cells; blood-vessels and vascular fasciculi are, however, merely modifications of cells.

Laws of the generation of new cells in the cytoblastema.- In every tissue, composed of a definite kind of cells, new cells of the same kind are formed at those parts only where the fresh nutrient material immediately penetrates the tissue. On this depends the distinction between organized or vascular, and unorganized or non-vascular tissues. In the former, the nutritive fluid, the liquor sanguinis, permeates by means of the vessels the whole tissue, and therefore new cells originate throughout its entire thickness. Non-vascular tissues, on the contrary, such as the epidermis, receive the nutritive fluid only from the tissue beneath; and new cells therefore originate only on their under surface, that is, at the part where the tissue is in connexion with organized substance. So also in the earlier period of the growth of cartilage, while it is yet without vessels new cartilage-cells are formed around its surface only, or at least in the neighbourhood of it, because the cartilage is connected with the organized substance at that part, and the cytoblastema penetrates from without. We can readily conceive this to be the case, if we assume that a more concentrated cytoblastema is requisite for the formation of new cells than for the growth of those already formed. In the epidermis, for instance, the cytoblastema below must contain a more concentrated nutritive material. When young cells are formed in that situation, the cytoblastema, which penetrates into the upper layers, is less concentrated, and may therefore serve very well for the growth of cells already formed, but not be capable of generating new ones. This constitutes the distinction which was formerly made between a growth by apposition and one by intussusception; "growth by apposition" is a correct term, if it be applied to the generation of new cells, and not to the growth of those already existing, the new cells in the epidermis for example, are formed only on its under surface, and are pushed upwards when other new ones are formed beneath them; but the new cells are generated throughout the entire thickness of the organized tissues. The cells, however, grow individually by intussusception in both instances. The bones occupy, to a certain extent, a middle position between the organized and unorganized tissues. The cartilage in the first instance has no vessels, and the new cells are, therefore, formed in the neighbourhood of the external surface only; at a subsequent period it receives vessels, which traverse the medullary or Haversian canals, the latter, however, are not sufficiently numerous to allow of the entire tissue becoming equably saturated with the fluid parts of the blood, a process which would be still further impeded by the greater firmness of cartilage and bone. According to the above law, then, the formation of new cytoblastema and new cells may take place partly upon the surface and partly around these medullary canals. Now the structure of bone becomes most simple, if we assume that, in consequence of the firmness of the osseous substance, this process goes on in layers, which do not completely coalesce together. It must consist of a double system of layers, one being concentric to each of the medullary canals, and the other to the external surface of the bone. When the bone is hollow, the layers must also be concentric to the cavity; and when small medullary cavities exist in the place of canals, as in the spongy bones, the layers must also be concentric to them. The difference in the growth of animals and plants also rests upon the same law. In plants, the nutritive fluid is not so equably distributed throughout the entire tissues, as it is in the organized tissues of animals, but is conveyed in isolated fasciculi of vessels, widely separated from one another, more after the manner of bone. These fasciculi of vessels are also observed to be surrounded with small (most likely younger) cells, so that, in all probability, the formation of their new cells also takes place around these vessels, as it does in bones around the medullary canaliculi. In the stem of dicotyledonous plants the sap is conducted between the bark and the wood, and on that account the new cells are generated in strata concentric to the layers of the previous year. The variety in the mode of growth, as to whether the new cells are developed merely in separate situations in the tissue, or equally throughout its whole thickness, does not, therefore, constitute any primary distinction, but is the consequence of a difference in the mode in which their nutritive fluid is conveyed.

The generation of cells of a different character, such as fat-cells, in the interior of a non-vascular tissue (in cartilage which does not as yet contain vessels, for example), appears at first sight to form an exception to the law just laid down. But such is not really the case; the circumstance is capable of two explanations, either the cytoblastema for this kind of cells is furnished by the true cells of the tissue only when they have attained a certain stage of their development, or, the cytoblastema which penetrates into the depth of the tissue contains the nutritive material for the true cells of the tissue in a less concentrated state, whilst it is still sufficiently impregnated with the nutritive material for the other kind of cells.

According to Schleiden, new cells are never formed in the intercellular substance in plants; in animals, on the contrary, a generation of cells within cells is the less frequent mode, but this does occur, and in such a way, that a threefold or fourfold generation may take place in succession within one cell. Thus, according to R. Wagner's observations (see the Supplement), the Graafian vesicle appears to be an elementary cell; the ovum is developed within it in like manner as an elementary cell; within this, again, according at least to observations made upon the bird's egg, cells are generated, some of which contain young cells. It appears also, that a formation of true cartilage-cells can sometimes take place within those which already exist, and that yound cells (fat-cells?) may be generated within them again. Several such examples might be brought forward; but by far the greater portion of the cells of cartilage are formed in the cytoblastema on the outside of the cells already present, and we never meet with a generation of cells within cells in the case of fibre, muscle, or nerve.

General phenomena of the formation of cells. Round corpuscles make their appearance after a certain time in the cytoblastema which, in the first instance, is structureless or minutely granulous. These bodies may either be cells in their earliest condition (and some may be recognized even at this stage), that is, hollow vesicles furnished with a peculiar structureless wall, cells without nuclei, or they may be cell-nuclei or the rudiments of cell-nuclei, round which cells will afterwards be formed.

The cells without nuclei, or, more correctly, the cells in which no nuclei have as yet been observed, occur only in the lower plants, and are also rare animals. For the present, however, the following must be regarded as such, viz.: the young cells contained within others in the chorda dorsalis (see p. 13), the cells of the yelk-substance in the bird's egg (p. 50), the cells in the mucous layer of the germinal membrane of the bird's egg (p. 60), and some cells of the crystalline lens (p. 88). Pl. I, fig. 10, *c*, represents one of these cells without nuclei. Thus the mode of growth, in this instance, is similar to that of the nucleated cells, after the formation of their cell-membrane.

By far the greater portion of the animal body, at least ninety-nine hundredths of all the elementary parts of the bodies of mammalia are developed from nucleated cells.

The cell-nucleus is a corpuscle, having a very characteristic form, by which it may in general be easily recognized. It is rather round or oval, spherical or flat. In the majority of fully-developed animal cells its average size would be about 0•0020-0•0030 Paris inch; but we meet with nuclei which are very much larger, and others, again, much smaller than this. The germinal vesicle of the bird's egg may be regarded as the largest cell-nucleus; the nuclei of the blood-corpuscles of warm-blooded animals afford examples of very small cell-nuclei. If the latter were but a very little smaller they would escape observations altogether, and the blood-corpuscles would then appear to be cells without nuclei. No other structure can be detected in these very small nuclei, nor can their characteristic form be further demonstrated. On the other hand, that of the large blood-corpuscles may be distinctly recognized as a cell-nucleus.

The cell-nucleus is generally dark, granulous, often somewhat yellowish; but some occur which are quite pellucid and smooth. It is either solid, and composed of a more or less minutely granulated mass, or hollow. Most nuclei of animal cells exhibit more or less distinct trace of a cavity, at least, their external contour is generally somewhat darker, and the substance of the nucleus seem to be somewhat more compact at the circumference. The nucleus may often be traced through its progressive stages of development from a solid body to a perfect vesicle; this may be observed in the nuclei of the cartilage-cells in the branchial cartilages of tadpoles. The membrane of the cell-nucleus and its contents may be distinguished in those which are hollow. The membrane is smooth, structureless, and never of any remarkable thickness, that of the germinal vesicle being the thickest. The contents are either very minutely granulous, especially in the small hollow cell-nuclei, or pellucid, as in the germinal vesicle, and the larger nuclei in the cells of the branchial cartillages of the tadpole, or larger corpuscles may be subsequently formed in the interior of hollow nuclei, for instance, the innumerable corpuscles in the germinal vesicle of the fish, and fat-globules in the nucleus of the fat-cells in the cranial cavity of fishes.

The nucleus, in most instances, contains one or two, more rarely three or four small dark corpuscles, *the nucleoli.* Their size varies from that of a spot which is scarcely discernible to that of Wagner's spot (*macula germinativa*) in the germinal vesicle. Nucleoli cannot be distinctly recognized in all cell-nuclei. They may be distinguished from the larger corpuscles, which are sometimes developed in certain hollow nuclei, from the circumstance of their being formed at a much earlier period; they exist, indeed, before the cell-nucleus. They are placed eccentrically in the round nuclei, and in the hollow ones are distinctly seen to lie upon the internal surface of the wall. It is very difficult to ascertain their nature; it may also vary very much in different cells. They sometimes appear to be capable of considerable enlargement, as in the nuclei of the fat-cells in the cranial cavity of the fish, and in such instances often have the appearance of fat. According to Schleiden, hollow nucleoli also frequently occur in plants.

Most cell-nuclei agree in the peculiarity of not being dissolved, or rendered transparent by acetic acid, at least not rapidly so, whilst the cell-membrane of animal cells is in most cases very sensitive to its action. Some cells, (such as those of the yelk-cavity of the egg, plate II, fig. 3,) which have no perceptible nucleus of the ordinary form, exhibit a globule having the appearance of a fat-globule, which grows as the cell expands, though not in the same proportion, and was probably formed previous to the cell. Whether such a globule have the signification of a nucleus or not, must remain an undecided question.

The formation of the cell-nucleus. In plants, according to Schleiden, the nucleolus is first formed, and the nucleus around it. The same appears to be the case in animals. According to the observations of R. Wagner on the development of ova in the ovary of Agrion virgo,[1] the germinal spot is first formed, and around that the germinal vesicle, which is the nucleus of the ovum-cell, Eizelle.[2] The youngest germinal vesicle there represented by Wagner, appears to be hollow. This is not generally the case, however, in the formation of cell-nuclei. Plate III, fig. 1, *e*, appears to be a cell-nucleus of a cartilage-cell in the act of forming. A small round corpuscle is there seen, surrounded by some minutely granulous substance, whilst the rest of the cytoblastema is homogeneous. This granulous substance is gradually lost around the object; at a subsequent period it begins to be sharply defined, and then exhibits the form of a cell-nucleus, which continues to grow for a certain period. (See pl. III, fig. 1, *a,b.*) Such a nucleus usually appears solid in the first instance, and many nuclei remain in this condition; in others, on the contrary, the portion of the substance situated nearest to the external surface continually becomes darker, and not unfrequently at last forms a distinctly perceptible membrane, so that the nucleus is hollow in such instances. The formative process of the nucleus may, accordingly, be conceived to be as follows: A nucleous is first

1 See Wagner, Beiträge zur Geschichte der Zeugung und Entwickelung; Erster Beitrag., tab. II, fig. 1.
2 See the Supplement.

formed; around this a stratum of substance is deposited, which is usually minutely granulous, but not as yet sharply defined on the outside. As new molecules are constantly being deposited in this stratum between those already present, and as this takes place within a precise distance of the nucleolus only, the stratum becomes defined externally, and a cell-nucleus having a more or less sharp contour is formed. The nucleus grows by a continuous deposition of new molecules between those already existing, that is, by intussusception. If this go on equably throughout the entire thickness of the stratum, the nucleus may remain solid; but if it go on more vigorously in the external part, the latter will become more dense, and may become hardened into a membrane, and such are the hollow nuclei. The circumstance of the layer generally becoming more dense on its exterior, may be explained by the fact that the nutritive fluid is conveyed to it from the outside, and is therefore more concentrated in that situation. Now if the deposition of the new molecules between the particles of this membrane takes place in such a manner that more molecules are deposited between those particles which lie side by side upon its surface than there are between those which lie one beneath another in its thickness, the expansion of the membrane must proceed more vigorously than its increase in thickness, and therefore a constantly increasing space must be formed between it and the nucleolus, whereby the latter remains adherent to one side of its internal surface.

I have made no observations on the formation of nuclei with more than one nucleolus. But it is easy to comprehend how it may occur, if we conceive that two nucleoli may lie so close together that the layers which form around them become united before they are defined externally, and that by the progressive deposition of new molecules, the external limitation is so effected that two corpuscles are enclosed by it at the same time, and then the development proceeds as though only one nucleolus were present.

When the nucleus has reached a certain stage of development, the cell is formed around it. The following appears to be the process by which this takes place. A stratum of substance, which differs from the cytoblastema, is deposited upon the exterior of the nucleus. (See pl. III, fig. 1, *d.*) In the first instance this stratum is not sharply defined externally, but becomes so in consequence of the progressive deposition of new molecules. The stratum is more or less thick, sometimes homogeneous, sometimes granulous; the latter is most frequently the case in the thick strata which occur in the formation of the majority of animal cells. We cannot at this period distinguish a cell-cavity and cell-wall. The deposition of new molecules between those already existing proceeds, however, and is so effected that when the stratum is thin, the entire layer-and when it is thick, only the external portion-becomes gradually consolidated into a membrane. The external portion of the layer may begin to become consolidated soon after it is defined on the outside; but, generally, the membrane does not become perceptible until a later period, when it is thicker and more defined internally; many cells, however, do not exhibit any appearance of the formation of a cell-membrane, but they seem to be solid, and all that can be remarked is that the external portion of the layer is somewhat more compact.

Immediately that the cell-membrane has become consolidated, its expansion proceeds as the result of the progressive reception of new molecules between the existing ones, that is to say, by virtue of a growth by intussusception, while at the same time it becomes separated from the cell-nucleus. We may therefore conclude that the deposition of the new molecules takes place more vigorously between those which lie side by side upon the surface of the membrane, than it does between those which lie one upon another in its thickness. The interspace between the cell-membrane and cell-nucleus is at the same time filled with fluid, and this constitutes the cell-contents. During this expansion the nucleus remains attached to a spot on the internal surface of the cell-membrane. If the entire stratum, in which the formation of the cell commenced, have become consolidated into a cell-membrane, the nucleus must lie free upon the cell-wall; but if only the external portion of the stratum have become consolidated, the nucleus must remain surrounded by the internal part, and adherent to a spot upon the internal surface of the cell-membrane. It would seem that the portion of the stratum which remains may be disposed of in two ways: either it is dissolved and forms a part of the cell-contents, in which case the nucleus will lie free upon the cell-wall as before; or it gradually becomes condensed into a substance similar to the cell-membrane, and then the nucleus appears to lie in the thickness of the cell-wall. This explains the variety in the position of the nucleus with respect to the cell-membrane. According to Schleiden, it sometimes lies in the thickness of the membrane in plants, so that its internal surface, which is directed towards the cell-cavity, is covered by a lamella of the cell-wall. In animals it also sometimes appears to be slightly sunk in the cell-membrane; but I have never observed a lamella passing over its inner surface; on the contrary, in almost all instances it lies quite free, adherent only to the internal surface of the cell-membrane.

The particular stage of development of the nucleus at which the cell commences to be formed around it varies very much. In some instances the nucleus has already become a distinct vesicle ere it occurs; the germinal vesicle, for example; in others, and this is the most common, the nucleus is still solid, and its development into a vesicle does not take place until a later period, or perhaps the change never occurs at all. When the cell is developed, the nucleus either remains stationary at its previous stage of development, or its growth proceeds, but not in proportion to the expansion of the cell, so that the intermediate space between it and the cell-membrane, the cell-cavity, is also constantly becoming relatively large. If the growth of a cell is impeded by the neighbouring cells, or if the new molecules added between the existing particles of the cell-membrane are applied to the thickening of the cell-wall instead of to its expansion, it may occur that the nucleus becomes more vigorously expanded than the cell, and gradually fills a larger portion of the cell-cavity. An example of this was brought forward at page 23, from the branchial cartilages of the tadpole; on the whole, however, such instances are very rare. As the nuclei, in the course of their development, and especially in such instances as that just mentioned, continually lose their granulous contents and become pellucid, and as in some cases, the germinal vesicle for example, other corpuscles, such as fat-globules, &c. may be developed in these contents of the nucleus (a circumstance which never occurs with respect to the cell-cavities) it is often difficult to distinguish such enlarged nuclei from young cells. The presence of two nucleoli is often sufficient to enable us to distinguish such an enlarged hollow nucleus. The observation of the stages of transition, between the characteristic form of the cell-nucleus and these nuclei which so much resemble cells, will also aid us in obtaining the information desired. As in the case of the germinal vesicle, however, a positive decision can only be obtained by demonstrating that such a nucleus has precisely the same relation to the cell that an ordinary cell-nucleus has; that is to say, that such a nucleus is formed before the cell, that the latter is formed as a stratum around it, and that the nucleus is afterwards surrounded by the cell. Whether the nucleus undergoes any further development, as the expansion of the cell proceeds, or not, the usual result is that it becomes absorbed. This does not take place, however, in all cases, for, according to Schleiden, it remains persistent in most cells in the Euphorbiaceæ, and the blood-corpuscles may be quoted as an example to the same effect in animals.

The fact that many nuclei are developed into hollow vesicles, and the difficulty of distinguishing some of these hollow nuclei from cells, forms quite sufficient ground for the supposition that a nucleus does not differ essentially from a cell; that an ordinary nucleated cell is nothing more than a cell formed around the outside of another cell, the nucleus; and that the only difference between the two consists in the inner one being more slowly and less completely developed, after the external one has been formed around it. If this description were correct, we might express ourselves with more precision, and designate the nuclei as cells of the first order, and the ordinary nucleated cells as cells of the second order. Hitherto we have decidedly maintained a distinction between cell and nucleus; and it was convenient to do so as long as we were engaged in merely describing the observations. There can be no doubt that the nuclei correspond to one another in all cells; but the designation, "cells of the first order," includes a theoretical view of the matter which has yet to be proved, namely, the identity of the formative process of the cell and the nucleus. This identity, however, is of the greatest importance for our theory, and we must therefore compare the two processes somewhat more closely. The formation of the cell commenced with the deposition of a precipitate around the nucleus; the same occurs in the formation of the nucleus around the nucleolus. The deposit becomes defined externally into a solid stratum: the same takes place in the formation of the nucleus. The development proceeds no farther in many nuclei, and we also meet with cells which remain stationary at the same point. The further development of the cells is manifested either by the entire stratum, or only the external part of it becoming consolidated into a membrane; this is precisely what occurs with the nuclei which undergo further development. The cell-membrane increases in its superficies, and often in thickness also, and separates from the nucleus, which remains lying on the wall; the membrane of the hollow cell-nuclei grows in the same manner, and the nucleolus remains adherent to a spot on the wall. A transformation of the cell-contents frequently follows, giving rise to a formation of new products in the cell-cavity. In most of the hollow cell-nuclei, the contents become paler, less granulous, and in some of them fat-globules, &c., are formed. (See pages 173,4.) We may therefore say that the formation of cells is but a repetition around the nucleus of the same process by which the nucleus was formed around the nucleolus, the only difference being that the process is more intense and complete in the formation of cells than in that of nuclei.

According to the foregoing, then, the whole process of the formation of a cell consists in this, that a small corpuscle (the nucleolus) is the earliest formation, that a stratum (the nucleus) is first deposited around it, and then subsequently a second stratum (substance of the cell) around this again. The separate strata grow by the reception of new molecules between the existing ones, by intussusception, and we have here an illustration of the law, in deference to which the deposition takes place more vigorously in the external part of each stratum than it does in the internal, and more vigorously in the entire external stratum than in the internal. In obedience to this law it often happens that only the external stratum becomes condensed into a membrane (membrane of the nucleus and membrane of the cell), and the external stratum becomes more perfectly developed to form a cell, than the nucleus does. When the nucleoli are hollow, which, according to Schleiden, is the case in some instances in plants, perhaps a threefold process of the kind takes place, so that the cell-membrane forms the third, the nucleus the second, and the nucleolus the first stratum. Probably merely a single stratum is formed around an immeasurably small corpuscle in the case of those cells which have no nuclei.

Varieties in the development of the cells in different tissues. Although, as we have just seen, the formative process of the cells is essentially the same throughout, and dependent upon a formation of one or many strata, and upon a growth of those strata by intussusception, the changes, on the other hand, which the cells, when once formed, undergo in the different tissues, are, in their phenomena at least, much more varied. They may be arranged in two classes according as the individuality of the original cell is retained (independent cells), or as it is more or less completely lost (coalescing cells, and cells which undergo division).

The varieties which occur amongst the independent cells, are partly of a chemical nature, and partly have reference to a difference in the growth of the cell-membrane, by which means a change in the form of the cell may be produced.

The cell-membrane differs in respect to its chemical qualities in different kinds of cells. That of the blood-corpuscles, for instance, is dissolved by acetic acid, whilst that of the cartilage-cell is not. The chemical composition of the cell-membrane differs even in the same cell according to its age, so that a transformation of the substance of the membrane itself takes place in plants; for, according to Schleiden, the cell-membrane of the youngest cells dissolves in water, the fully-developed cells not being acted upon by that fluid. The simple cells are still more remarkable for their cell-contents. One cell forms fat, another pigment, a third etherial oil; and here also a transformation of the cell-contents takes place. A granulous precipitate is seen to form gradually in what was in the first instance a pellucid cell, and this usually takes place first around the cell-nucleus; or, *vice versâ*, during incubation, the granulous (fatty) contents of the cells of the yelk-substance gradually undergo partial solution. According to Schleiden, this transformation of the substance of the cell-contents proceeds in accordance with a certain rule; I have not made any investigations upon the subject in animals.

We should also include under this head the formation of the secondary deposits upon the internal surface of the cell-membrane, so very frequently met with in plants. If a firm cohering substance be formed from the cell-contents, it may be deposited upon the internal surface of the cell-membrane. In plants this deposition generally takes place in layers, a stratum being formed in the first instance upon the internal surface of the cell-membrane, upon the internal surface of that one a second, and so on until at last the entire cavity may be almost filled by them. According to Valentin, these surrounding deposits always take place in spiral lines which are subject to great varieties in their arrangement, for there may be one or many of them, and they may either completely cover the internal surface of the cell-membrane, or not be in contact with each other at all. I have not observed any such secondary stratified depositions in animals.

The variations which may occur in the growth of the cell-membrane in simple cells, depend upon the circumstance as to whether or not the addition of new molecules takes place equably at all parts of the cell-membrane. In the first case the form of the cell remains unchanged, and the only other distinction possible would be grounded upon the fact as to whether the greater part of the new molecules were deposited between the particles which lay side by side upon the superficies of the cell-membrane, or between those which lay one behind another in its thickness. The first mode of growth produces an expansion of the cell-membrane, the effect of the second is more especially to thicken it. Both modes are generally combined, but in such a manner that the expansion of the cell-membrane prevails in most instances.

A great variety of modifications in the form of the cells may be produced by the irregular distribution of the new molecules. The globular, which is their fundamental form, may be converted into a polyhedral figure, or the cells may become flattened into a round or oval or angular tablet, or the expansion of the expansion of the cells may take place on one or on two opposite sides, so as to form a fibre, and these fibres again may either be flat, being at the same time in some instances serrated, or lastly, the expansion of the cells into fibres may take place on different sides so as to give them the stellate form. Some of these changes of form are, no doubt, due to mechanical causes. Thus, for example, the polyhedral form is produced by the close crowding of the spherical cells, and these, when separated from one another, sometimes assume their round figure again, such is the case with the yelk-cells. Some of the other changes would seem to be capable of explanation by exosmosis. If, for example, the contents of a round cell be so changed, that a fluid is generated in it which is less dense than the surrounding fluid, the cell will lose some of its contents by exosmosis, and must, therefore, collapse, and may become flattened into a table as in the blood-corpuscles. Such explanations, however, are unsatisfactory in by far the greatest number of instances, and we are compelled to assume, that the growth does not necessarily proceed equably on all sides, but that the new molecules may be deposited in greater abundance in certain situations. Let us take the instance of a round cell, the cell-membrane of which is already developed, and suppose the deposition of new molecules to be confined to one particular part of the cell-membrane, that part would become expanded, and so a hollow fibre would grow forth from the cell, the cavity of which would communicate with the cell-cavity. The same result would take place, but more easily, if the new molecules were disposed unequally previous to the period when the external stratum of the precipitate, which is formed around the nucleus, had become condensed into a distinctly perceptible cell-membrane. The hollowing out of the fibre would then be less perfect, and the growth of the fibre must advance, particularly as regarded its thickness, before any manifest distinction between wall and cavity could be perceived.

The cause of this irregular disposition of the new molecules may, in some instances, be due to circumstances altogether external to the cell. If, for instance, a cell lay in such a position that one side of it was in contact with a concentrated nutritive material, one could conceive that side of the cell growing more vigorously, even though the force, which produces the growth of the cell, should operate equably throughout the entire cell. Such an explanation cannot, however, be received at all in most instances, but we must admit modifications in the principle of development of the cells, of such a nature, as that the force, which affects the general growth of the cells, is enabled to occasion an equable disposition of new molecules in one cell, and an unequal one in another.

Amongst the changes which more or less completely deprive the original cells of their individuality, are to be classed, in the first place, the coalescence of the cell-walls with one another, or with the intercellular substance; secondly, the division of one cell into several; and, thirdly, the coalescence of several primary cells to form a secondary one.

A coalescence of the cell-membrane with the intercellular substance, or with a neighbouring cell-wall, appears to take place in some cartilages for example. At first the cell-membrane has a sharply-defined external contour, by degrees the boundary line becomes paler, and at last is no longer perceptible with the microscope. We cannot, at present, lay down any general law respecting the circumstances under which such a coalescence occurs; it presupposes the cell-membrane and intercellular substance are homogeneous structures, and may perhaps always take place when such a state exists.

As regards the subdivision of the cells, we have already seen how a jutting out of the cell-membrane may be produced by its more vigorous growth in certain situations. <But a jutting inwards into the cavity of the cell may also result from the very same process. <Now, if we imagine this jutting inwards to take place in a circular form around a cell, as the consequence of a partial increase in the force of its growth, it may proceed to such an extent, that one cell may be separated into two, connected together only by a short peduncle, which may afterwards be absorbed. This would illustrate the most simple form of subdivision in a cell. In the animal cells, however, which undergo subdivision, that is, the fibre-cells, the process is more complicated; firstly, because when an elongated cell subdivides, it splits into many fibres; and, secondly, because the cells are so very minute. The process, therefore, cannot for these reasons be accurately traced, and the following is all that we can detect; a cell becomes elongated on two opposite sides into several fibres; from the angle, which the fibres on either side form with each other, a striated appearance gradually extends over the body of the cell; this formation of striae becomes more and more distinct, until the body of the cell splits entirely into fibres.

The coalescence of several primary cells to form a secondary cell is, to a certain extent, the opposite process to the last. Several primary cells, of muscle for instance, are arranged close together in rows, and coalesce into a cylinder, in the thickness of which lie the nuclei of the primary cells. This cylinder is hollow and not interrupted by septa, and the nuclei lie upon the internal surface of its wall. These are the facts of the process, so far as they have as yet been observed. One can form a conception of so much as is yet required to render them complete. If two perfectly-developed cells coalesce together, their walls must first unite at the point of contact, and then the partition-wall between the cavities must be absorbed. Nature, however, does not by any means require that these acts should occur at precisely defined periods. The coalescence may take place before the cell-wall and cell-cavity exist as distinct structures, somewhat in the following manner: the nuclei are formed first, around them a new stratum of substance is deposited, the external portion of which, in accordance with the course of formation of an ordinary simple cell, would become condensed into a cell-membrane. But in this instance the nuclei lie so close together, that the strata forming around them and corresponding to the cells, flow together, to form a cylinder, the external portion of which becomes condensed into a membrane, just in the same manner as in simple cells, where merely the external portion of the stratum formed around the nucleus, becomes hardened on the outside into a membrane, in consequence of the reception of new molecules. There is, therefore, nothing in this which differs so very materially from the course of development of a simple cell; indeed, we seemed to be compelled to assume a similar process for the formation of the nuclei furnished with two or more nucleoli. (See page 176.) It is possible that there may be stages of transmission between the ordinary simple cell and these secondary cells. It has been already mentioned at pages 117-118, that fat-cells occur in the cranial cavity of fishes, many of which contain two nuclei. It is possible that only one of them is the cytoblast of the cell, and that the second is a nucleus which has formed subsequently; but they resemble one another so completely in their characteristic position on the cell-membrane (see pl. III, fig. 10,) that perhaps they may both be cytoblasts of a cell which has been formed around both nuclei, in consequence of the external stratum of the precipitate having become condensed in such a manner that the membrane enclosed both nuclei. Meanwhile observation affords no demonstrative proof on the subject, and the similarity in the position of the two nuclei may be explained in another way. Fat thrusts all bodies which have imbibed water towards the outside of the cell, in order that it may assume its own globular form. If now a second nucleus should form in one of these fat-cells, it will be thrust towards the outside, and must gradually raise the cell-membrane into a prominence. It may also be observed, that opportunities of demonstrating the actual absorption of the fully-developed partition-wall between two cells do occur in the spiral vessels of plants.

b. Adipose cells. In the later periods of foetal existence, adipose cells occur in many situations in addition to the fibrecells before described. They are usually first seen in small groups between the fibre-cells. They are round cells of very various sizes, which are generally completely filled by a single fat-globule. The cell-membrane which closely encompasses the contents, is most minutely granulous, or, according to Gurlt, homogeneous. It is in most instances very thin, being about half the thickness of a blood-corpuscle, but sometimes it is much thicker, and in the subcutaneous areolar tissue of the thigh of a rickety child, at the age of twelve months (probably in connexion with the disease), was almost as thick as the breadth of a human blood-corpuscle. In the early stage, this cell-membrane encloses a very distinct nucleus of a round or oval form, which is sometimes flattened. When the former is thin, the nucleus presents itself externally as a little prominence upon the round fat-globule, which is closely encompassed by the cell-membrane; but when thick, the nucleus lies embedded in it. It contains one or two nucleoli. It is not uncommon for adipose cells to contain a number of small globules instead of *one* fat-globule, in such instances, one of them is generally remarkable for its larger size. The adipose cells are best seen in the fat found in the cranial cavity of a young carp, before it has attained the length of six inches. (See pl. III. fig. 10.) They there lie in so soft a substance, that they may be insulated without any difficulty, and float singly in the water in which they are examined. Some are so large as to be visible even with the unaided eye. When examined under the microscope with a magnifying power of 450, the cell-membrane is readily recognized, it is very thin, and closely encompasses the contents. It rises into a little prominence on one side, within lies a proportionately large, and very beautiful cell-nucleus, which is oval, but not flattened, and contains one or two very distinct nucleoli. Some of these fat-cells have two such nuclei, which have precisely similar relations to the cell, and both elevate the cell-membrane into a prominence at the points where they are attached. When one of these cells is pressed under the compressorium, the cell-membrane is at first remarkably expanded, and then tears to a very limited extent, allowing the fat to flow our. When the pressure is discontinued, it contracts again strongly. It has a minutely granulous aspect, is soft and very elastic, but not fibrous.

In close apposition, the cells become flattened against one another into polyhedral shapes, and, as Gurlt remarks, they then resemble vegetable cells in their appearance. We, however, may go further and regard them as corresponding in signification also, In them the fat forms the cell-contents, as the pigment does in its cells, and the ethereal oil, &c. in those of plants. In its physiological signification of nutritive deposit it has more analogy with starch than with any other substance. I know not whether the nucleus is the part first formed in these cells, or not. Nuclei without any investing cells are found in the cranial cavity of the carp, lying with the adipose cells in the surrounding cytoblastema; these, however, may be nuclei of fibre-cells of areolar tissue. Sooner or later the nuclei become absorbed. They were stillquite distinct in the adipose cells of the subcutaneous areolar tissue in the thigh of the before-mentioned rickety child twelve months old, whilst I could not detect any in the neck of a foetus at the seventh month. The absorption of the nucleus proceeds in one of two ways; either its external contour becomes gradually indistinct, some granulous substance merely being left in its place, which substance also disappears at a later period, or small fat-globules are formed both within the nucleus itself, and in its immediate proximity, which go on increasing in size, whilst the nucleus gradually disappears. The cell-membrane probably remains, even in the mature condition of the tissue, and Gurlt has made the very interesting observation, that in emaciated persons, the ordinary adipose cells are filled with serum.

Observations on the Development of the Fat Vesicle

Arthur Hassall

When the difficulty of determining the exact structure of the fat vesicle is considered,-a difficulty arising from the extreme tenuity of its cell-wall, and the opacity of its contents,-it is scarcely surprising that we should yet be without any consistent account of the modes of development and growth of the fat vesicle.

This hiatus in the structural history of that peculiar animal tissue, fat, the present brief remarks are intended in some measure to fill up.

When the little fatty masses which are met with so abundantly in the neck, in the neighbourhood of the thyroid and thymus glands, as also in some other situations in a fœtus nearly or quite arrived at maturity, are examined, it will be composed of a number of distinct and opaque bodies of various sizes, presenting a smooth outline, having a more or less rounded or oval form, and held loosely together by fibrocullular tissue, the extension of which forms the envelope which invests each of these bodies. It will also be further noticed, that each mass of fat is supplied with one or more bloodvessels, and that these break up into numerous lesser branches, one of which goes to each of the previously described bodies, being conveyed to it by the connecting fibrous tissue; and that, having reached this body, it undergoes a further subdivision, the branches extending over its entire surface.

In continuation of these observations, it will be remarked, that each of these peculiar bodies bears a close resemblance, in its general aspect, to a lobe of a sebaceous gland-a resemblance which, as will be seen almost immediately, extends even to its internal structure.

If a number of these bodies be torn into fragments with fine needles, and be examined with a half or quarter inch object glass, it will be observed that the cavities of some of them are filled with cells of a large size, and which again are occupied with numerous globules of various dimensions, presenting many of the characters of oil globules, but being of greater consistence. These cells, save by their somewhat larger size, it is impossible to distinguish from the perfect cells of sebaceous glands; so complete, indeed, is this resemblance, that at first sight I did not hesitate to regard them as belonging to some sebaceous gland, and which I was much astonished to encounter in such a situation. Others of these peculiar bodies, which may be termed "fat cysts," contain a mixture, in variable proportions, of these compound cells and of free globules, which, however, it is observed are generally of larger size than those contained within the compound or parent cells. Lastly, others of these bodies enclose no compound cells, but are filled with globules of still larger size.

Now the curious part of this history is, that is these globules which go on increasing in size, and bursting the envelopes which contain them, ultimately become what are ordinarily regarded as the true fat vesicles.

In the article Fat, in an early number of the "Microscopic Anatomy," I noticed the fact that the fat vesicles of children are not so large as those of the adult; this fact it then appeared to me had an evident relation to the growth of the fat vesicle, and it suggested the idea that the fat corpuscle was of very slow growth, not attaining its full dimensions until near the adult age, and that it was permanent in its character, enduring throughout life. This idea gathers increased weight, and indeed its correctness is rendered almost certain, by the additional observations just cited on the development and growth of the fat vesicle.

It would appear, therefore, taking into consideration all the foregoing particulars, that the principal development of fat vesicles takes place in the advanced fœtus and in the early years of life, (for I now remember having met with "fat cysts" in the great omentum of children of five and six years of age, although at the time of observing them I did not know their nature and meaning,) that what are usually regarded as the true fat vesicles or cells, are first contained in parent cells, and lastly, that they are slow in their growth and persistent throughout life.

I infer also further, from the foregoing facts, that the ordinary fat vesicles are incapable of acting as parent cells and of reproducing their like; an inference which might be fairly entertained on other grounds-viz.,

Hassall A. Observations on the development of the fat vesicle. *Lancet* 1849;I:63-64.

the difficulty, not to say impossibility, of detecting nuclei in them, and the absence of those granules amongst their contents which are so characteristic of true cells, and which there is so much reason to believe are the real germs of the future generations of cells.

From comparative observations it would appear that the development and growth of fat proceeds at different rates in different localities of the same body, it being more advanced in one situation than in another; and also in the same parts in different children of the same age; so that an exactly similar condition of things to that which I have described as existing in the masses of fat which occur in the region of the neck in the mature fœtus, must not in all cases be looked for.

The structural resemblance which I have shown to exist between fat cells in an early condition of their development and the cells of sebaceous glands is most interesting, the latter appearing to be, in fact, simply fat in a rudimentary and imperfect state of its development.

Figures illustrative of the above observations will be given in the concluding number of the "Microscopic Anatomy."

An Explanation of Hunger[1]

Walter B. Cannon, Anton L. Washburn
(From the Laboratory of Physiology in the Havard Medical School)

Hunger and appetite are so intimately interrelated that a discussion of either requires each to be clearly defined. According to one view the two experiences differ only quantitatively, appetite being a mild stage of hunger.[2] Another view, better supported by observations, is that the two experiences are fundamentally different.[3]

Appetite is related to previous sensations of the taste and smell of food; it has therefore, as Pawlow has shown, important psychic elements. It may exist separate from hunger, as, for example, when we eat delectable dainties merely to please the palate. Sensory associations, delightful or disgusting, determine the appetite for any edible substance, and either memory or present stimulation can thus arouse desire or dislike for food.

Hunger, on the other hand, is a dull ache or gnawing sensation referred to the lower mid-chest region and the epigastrium. It is the organism's first strong demand for nutriment, and, not satisfied, is likely to grow into a highly uncomfortable pang, less definitely localized as it becomes more intense. It may exist separate from appetite, as, for example, when hunger forces the taking of food not only distasteful but even nauseating. Besides the dull ache, however, lassitude and drowsiness may appear, or faintness, or headache, or irritability and restlessness such that continuous effort in ordinary affairs becomes increasingly difficult. That these states differ with individuals–headache in one, faintness in another, for example–indicates that they do not constitute the central fact of hunger, but are more or less inconstant accompaniments, for the present negligible. The dull, pressing sensation is the constant characteristic, the central fact, to be examined in detail.

Of the two theories of hunger–(1) that it is a general sensation with a local reference, and (2) that it has a local peripheral source–the former has been more widely accepted. The support for that theory can be shown to be not substantial. The wide acceptance of the theory, however, warrants an examination of it in some detail.

HUNGER NOT A GENERAL SENSATION.

Underlying the idea that hunger arises from a general condition of the body is the consideration that, as time passes, food substances disappear form the blood, and consequently the nerve cells, suffering from the shortage of provisions, give rise to the sensation.[4]

In support of this view the increase of hunger as time passes has been pointed out. There is abundant evidence, however, that the period of increase is short, and that during continued fasting hunger wholly disappears after the first few days.[5] On the theory that hunger is a manifestation of bodily need, we must suppose that the body is mysteriously not in need after the third day, and that therefore hunger disappears. The absurdity of such a view is obvious.

Continued hunger soon after eating (when stomach is full), especially in cases of duodenal fistula,[6] and satisfaction when the escaping chyme is restored to the intestine, have been cited as ruling out the peripheral and thus favoring the central origin of the sensation. As

[1]The indicative evidence of the results here reported was presented to the Boston Society of Medical Sciences, January 17, 1911. See CANNON: The mechanical factors of digestion, London and New York, 1911, p. 204. The full account was presented to the Harvey Society, New York City, December 16, 1911.

[2]BARDIER: Richet's Dictionnaire de physiologie, article "Faim," 1904, vi, p.I; HOWELL: Text-book of physiology, fourth edition, Philadelphia and London, 1911, p. 285.

[3]See STERNBERG: Zentralblatt für Physiologie, 1909, xxii, p. 653. Similar views were expressed by BAYLE in a thesis presented to the Faculty of Medicine in Paris in 1816.

[4]SCHIFF: Physiologie de la digestion, Florence and Turin, 1867, p. 40.

[5]See LUCIANI: Das Hungern, Hamburg and Leipzig, 1890, p. 113; TIGERSTEDT: Nagel's Handbuch der Physiologie, Berlin, 1909, i, p. 376; JOHANSSON, LANDERGREN, SONDÉN, and TIGERSTEDT: Skandinavisches Archiv für Physiologie, 1897, vii, p. 33; CARRINGTON: Vitality, fasting and nutrition, New York, 1908, p. 555; VITERBI: quoted by BARDIER, *loc. cit.*, p. 7.

[6]See BUSCH: Archiv für pathologische Anatomie und Physiologie und für klinische Medicin, 1858, xiv, p. 147.

will be seen later, however, other possible peripheral sources of hunger exist besides the stomach. Further consideration of this point will be given in due course.

Because animals eat, sometimes eagerly, when the gastro-intestinal tract is wholly separated from the central nervous system,[7] the conclusion has been drawn that hunger must be a general sensation and not of peripheral origin. But appetite as well as hunger may lead to eating. As Ludwig stated many years ago, even if all afferent nerves were severed, psychic reasons still could be given for the taking of food.[8] Indeed, who accepts dessert because he is hungry? Evidently, since hunger is not required for eating, the fact that an animal eats is no testimony whatever that the animal is hungry, and therefore, after nerves have been severed, is no proof that hunger is of central origin.

Further objections to the theory that hunger is a general sensation lie in the weakness of its main assumption and in its failure to account for certain well-known observations. Thus no evidence exists that the blood has in fact changed when hunger appears. Moreover in fever, when bodily stores are being most rapidly destroyed, and when therefore, according to this theory, hunger should be most insistent, the sensation is wholly absent. And the quick absolution of the pangs soon after food is taken, before digestion and absorption can have proceeded far, as well as the quieting effect of swallowing indigestible stuff, such as moss and clay, further weakens the argument that the sensation arises directly from lack of nutriment in the body.

Many have noted that hunger has a sharp onset. If this abrupt arrival of the characteristic ache corresponds to the general bodily state, the change in general bodily state must occur with like suddenness, or have a critical point at which the sensation is instantly precipitated. No evidence exists that either of the conditions occurs in metabolism.

Another peculiarity of hunger which we have noticed is its intermittency. It may come and go several times in the course of a few hours. Furthermore, during a given period, the sensation is not uniform in intensity, but is marked by ups and downs, sometimes changing to alternate presence and absence without alternation of rate. Our observations have been confirmed by psychologists, trained to introspection, who have reported that the sensation has a distinctly intermittent course.[9] In the experience of one of us (C.) the hunger pangs came and went on one occasion as follows:

Came	Went
12-37-20	12-38-30
40-45	41-10
41-45	42-25
43-20	43-35
44-40	45-55
46-15	46-30

and so on, for ten minutes longer. Again in this relation, the intermittent and periodic character of hunger would require, on the central theory, that the bodily supplies be intermittently and periodically insufficient. During one moment absence of hunger would imply abundance of nutriment in the organism, ten seconds later presence of hunger would imply hat the stores had been suddenly reduced, ten seconds later still absence of hunger would imply sudden renewal of plenty. Such zigzag shifts of the general bodily state may not be impossible, but, from all that is known of the course of metabolism, they are highly improbable. The periodicity of hunger, therefore, is further evidence against the theory that the sensation has a general basis in the body.

The last objection to this theory is its failure to account for the most common feature of hunger, – the reference of the sensation to the epigastric region. Schiff and others[10] have met this obligation by two contentions. First, they have pointed out that hunger is not always referred to the stomach. Schiff interrogated ignorant soldiers regarding the local reference; several indicated the neck or chest, twenty-three the sternum, four were uncertain of any region, and two only designated the stomach. In other words, the stomach region was most rarely mentioned.

The second contention against the importance of local reference is that such evidence is fallacious. Just as the reference of tinglings to fingers which have been removed from the body does not prove that the tinglings originate in those fingers, so the assignment of the ache of hunger to any special region does not demonstrate that the ache arises from that region.

Concerning these arguments we may recall first Schiff's admission that the soldiers he questioned were too few to give conclusive evidence. Further, the testimony of most of them that hunger seemed to originate in the region of the sternum cannot be claimed as unfavorable to a peripheral source of the sensation. The description of feelings which develop from disturbances within the body is almost always indefinite; the testimony is not, therefore, dismissed as worthless. On the contrary, such testimony is used constantly in judging internal disorders.

The force of the contention that reference to the

[7]See SCHIFF: *Loc. cit.*, p. 37; also DUCCESCHI: Archivio di fisiologia, 1910, viii, p. 582.

[8]LUDWIG: Lehrbuch der Physiologie des Menschen, Leipzig and Heidelberg, 1858, ii, p. 584.

[9]We are indebted to Prof. J.W. BAIRD of Clark University, and his collaborators, for this corroborative testimony.

[10]See SCHIFF: *Loc. cit.*, p. 31; BARDIER: *Loc. cit.*, p. 16.

periphery is not proof of the peripheral origin of a sensation depends on the amount of accessory evidence which is available. Thus, if an object is seen coming into contact with a finger, the simultaneous sensation of touch referred to that finger may reasonably be assumed to have resulted from the contact, and not to have been a purely central experience accidently attributed to an outlying member. Similarly in the case of hunger–all that is needed as support for the peripheral reference of the sensation is proof that conditions occur there, simultaneously with hunger pangs, which might reasonably be regarded as giving rise to those pangs. In the fasting stomach may not conditions, in fact, be present which would sustain the theory that hunger has a local peripheral source?

Certain assumptions have been made regarding the state of the fasting stomach, and certain references have been drawn from these assumptions which must be considered before the results we have to present will have a proper setting.

OBJECTIONS TO SOME THEORIES THAT HUNGER IS OF LOCAL ORIGIN

Hunger is not due to emptiness of the stomach, for Nicolai found after gastric lavage that the sensation did not appear in some instances for more than three hours.[11] This testimony confirms Beaumont's observation on Alexis St. Martin, that hunger arises some time after the stomach is evacuated.[12]

Hunger is not due to hydrochloric acid secreted into the empty stomach. The gastric wash-water from hungry subjects is neutral or only slightly acid.[13] Furthermore, persons suffering from achylia gastrica declare that they have normal feelings of hunger.

Hunger is not due to turgescence of the gastric glands. This theory, propounded by Beaumont,[14] has commended itself to several recent writers. Thus Luciani has accepted it, and by adding the idea that nerves distributed to the mucosa are specially sensitive to deprivation of food, he accounts for the hunger pangs.[15] Also Valenti declared two years ago that the turgescence theory of Beaumont is the only one possessing a semblance of truth.[16] The experimental work reported by these two investigators, however, does not necessarily support the turgescence theory. Luciani severed in fasting dogs the previously exposed and cocainized vagi, and Valenti merely cocainized the nerves; the dogs, eager to eat a few minutes previous to this operation, now ran about as before, but when offered food, licked and smelled it, but did not take it. This total neglect of the food lasted varying periods up to two hours. The vagus nerves seem, indeed, to convey impulses which affect the procedure of eating, but there is no clear evidence that those impulses arise from distention of the gland cells. The turgescence theory would also meet difficulties in an attempt to explain the disappearance of hunger after the swallowing of indigestible material; for such material, not being appetizing, does not cause any secretion of gastric juice.[17] Furthermore, Nicolai found that the sensation could be abolished by simply introducing a stomach tube. The turgescence of the gastric glands would not be reduced by either of these procedures. The turgescence theory, finally, does not explain the quick onset of hunger, or its intermittent and periodic character, for the cells cannot be repeatedly swollen and contracted within periods a few seconds in duration.

HUNGER THE RESULT OF CONTRACTIONS

There remain to be considered, as a possible cause of hunger pangs, contractions of the stomach and other parts of the alimentary canal. This suggestion is not new. Sixty-six years ago Weber declared his belief that "strong contraction of the muscle fibres of the wholly empty stomach, whereby its cavity disappears, makes a part of the sensation which we call hunger."[18] Vierordt drew the same inference twenty-five years later (in 1871);[19] and since then Knapp and also Hertz have declared their adherence to this view. These writers have not brought forward any direct evidence for their conclusion, though Hertz has cited Boldireff's observations on fasting dogs as probably accounting for what he terms "the gastric constituent of the sensation."[20]

The argument commonly used against the contraction theory is that the stomach is not energetically active when empty. Thus Schiff stated "the movements of the empty stomach are rare and much less energetic than during digestion."[21] Luciani expressed his disbelief by asserting that gastric movements are much more active during gastric digestion than at other times, and cease almost entirely when the stomach has discharged its contents.[22] And Valenti stated only year before last: "We know very well that gastric movements are exag-

[11] NICOLAI: Ueber die Entstehung des Hungergefühls, Inaugural-Dissertation, Berlin, 1892, p. 17.
[12] BEAUMONT: The physiology of digestion, second edition, Burlington, 1847, p. 51.
[13] NICOLAI: *Loc. cit.*, p. 15.
[14] BEAUMONT: *Loc. cit.*, p. 55.
[15] LUCIANI: Archivio di fisiologia, 1906, iii, p. 542.
[16] VALENTI: Archives italiennes de biologie, 1910, liii, p. 97.

[17] See PAWLOW: The work of the digestive glands, London, 1902, p. 70; HORNBORG: Skandinavisches Archiv für Physiologie, 1904, xv, p. 248.
[18] WEBER: Wagner's handwörterbuch der Physiologie, 1846, iii^2, p. 580.
[19] VIERORDT: Grundriss der Physiologie, Tübingen, 1871, p. 433.
[20] KNAPP: American medicine, 1905, x, p. 358; HERTZ: The sensibility of the alimentary canal, London, 1911, p. 37.
[21] SCHIFF: *Loc. cit.*, p. 33.
[22] LUCIANI: *Loc. cit.*, p. 542.

gerated while digestion is proceeding in the stomach, but when the organ is empty they are more rare and much less pronounced," and therefore they cannot account for hunger.[23]

CONTRACTIONS OF THE ALIMENTARY CANAL IN FASTING ANIMALS.–Evidence opposed to these suggestions has been in existence for many years. In 1899 Bettmann called attention to the contracted condition of the stomach after several days' fast.[24] In 1902 Wolff reported that after forty-eight hours without food the stomach of the cat may be so small as to look like a slightly enlarged duodenum.[25] The anatomist His has also observed the phenomenon.[26] Seven years ago Boldireff demonstrated that the whole gastro-intestinal tract has a periodic activity while not digesting.[27] Each period of activity lasts from twenty to thirty minutes, and is characterized in the stomach by rhythmic contractions 10 to 20 in number. These contractions, Boldireff reports, may be stronger than during digestion, and his published records clearly support this statement. The intervals of repose between periodic recurrences of the contractions last from one and a half to two and a half hours. Especially noteworthy is Boldireff's observation that if fasting is continued for two or three days the groups of contractions appear at gradually longer intervals and last for gradually shorter periods, and thereupon the gastric glands begin continuous secretion, and all movements cease. All these testimonies to increased tone and periodic pulsations definitely prove, contrary to previous statements, that the empty stomach may be the seat of vigorous muscular activities.

Boldireff considered hunger in relation to the activities he described, but solely with the idea that hunger might *provoke* them; and since the activities dwindled in force and frequence as time passed, whereas in his belief they should have become more pronounced, he abandoned the notion of any relation between the phenomena.[28] Did not Boldireff misinterpret his own observations? When he was considering whether hunger might cause the contractions, did he not overlook the possibility that the contractions might cause hunger? A number of experiences have led to the conviction that Boldireff did, indeed, fail to perceive part of the significance of his results. For example, in auscultation of the alimentary canal relatively loud borborygmi have been noted as the hunger pangs were disappearing. Again the sensation can be momentarily abolished a few seconds after swallowing a small accumulation of saliva or a tablespoonful of water. Since the stomach is in high tonus in hunger, this result can be accounted for as due to the momentary inhibition of the tonus by swallowing.[29] Thus also could be explained the disappearance of the ache soon after eating is begun, for repeated swallowing results in continued inhibition.

THE CONCOMITANCE OF CONTRACTIONS AND HUNGER IN MAN.–Although the evidence above mentioned had led to the conviction that hunger results from contractions of the alimentary canal, direct proof was still lacking. In order to learn whether such proof might be secured, one of us (W.) determined to become accustomed to the presence of a rubber tube in the oesophagus.[30] Almost every day for several weeks W. introduced as far as the stomach a small tube, to the lower end of which was attached a soft-rubber balloon about 8 cm. in diameter. The tube was thus carried about each time for two or three hours. After this preliminary experience the introduction of the tube, and its presence in the gullet and stomach, were not at all disturbing. When a record was to be taken, the balloon, placed just below the cardia, was moderately distended with air, and was connected with a water manometer ending in a cylindrical chamber 3.5 cm wide. A float recorder resting on the water in the chamber permitted registering any contractions of the fundus of the stomach. On the days of observation W. would abstain from breakfast, or eat sparingly, and without taking any luncheon would appear in the laboratory about two o'clock. The recording apparatus was arranged as above described. In order to avoid the possibility of an artifact, a pneumograph, fastened below the ribs, was made to record the movements of the abdominal wall. Between the records of gastric pressure and abdominal movement one electromagnetic signal marked time in minutes, and another traced a line which could be altered by pressing a key. All these recording arrangements were out of W's sight; he sat with one hand at the key, ready, whenever the sensation of hunger was experienced, to make the current which moved the signal.

When W. stated that he was hungry, powerful contractions of the stomach were invariably being registered. The record of W's introspection of his hunger pangs agreed closely with the record of his gastric contractions. Almost invariably, however, the contraction nearly reached it's maximum before the record of the sensation was started (see Fig. 1). This fact may be regarded as evidence that the contradiction precedes the sensation, and not *vice versa*, as Boldireff considered it. The contractions were about a half-minute in duration,

[23]VALENTI: *Loc. cit.*, p. 97.
[24]BETTMANN: Philadelphia monthly medical journal, 1899, I p. 133.
[25]WOLFF: Dissertation, Giessen, 1902, p. 9.
[26]HIS: Archiv für Anatomie, 1903, p. 345.
[27]BOLDIREFF: Archives biologiques de St. Petersburg, 1905, xi, p. I. See also Ergebnisse der Physiologie, 1911, xi, p. 182.
[28]BOLDIREFF: *Loc. cit.*, p. 96.
[29]CANNON and LIEB: this Journal, 1911, xxix, p. 267.
[30]NICOLAI (*Loc. cit.*) reported that although the introduction of a stomach tube at first abolished hunger in his subjects, with repeated use the effects became insignificant.

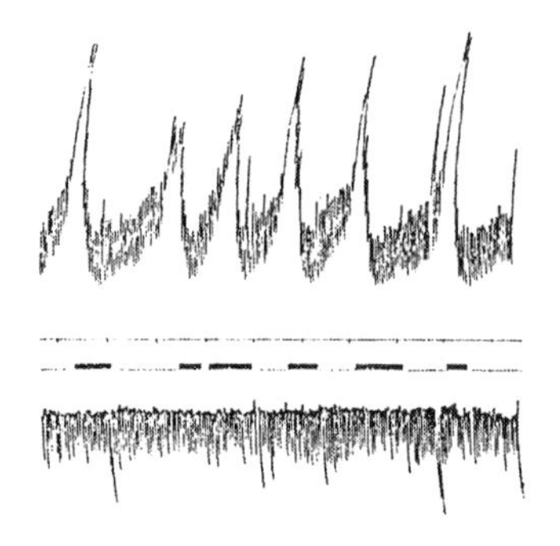

Figure 1: One half the original size. The top record represents intragastric pressure (the small oscillations due to respiration, the large to contractions of the stomach); the second record is time in minutes (ten minutes); the third record is W's report of hunger pangs; the lowest record is respiration registered by means of a pneumograph about the abdomen.

and the intervals between varied from thirty to ninety seconds, with an average of about one minute. W's augmentations of intragastric pressure ranged between 11 and 13 in twenty minutes; C. had previously counted in himself 11 hunger pangs in the same time (see ten-minute record, p. 444). The rate in each of us, therefore, proved to be approximately the same. This rate is slightly slower than that found in dogs by Boldireff; the difference is perhaps correlated with the slower rhythm of gastric peristalsis in man compared with that in the dog.[31]

Before hunger was experienced by W. the recording apparatus revealed no signs of gastric activity. Sometimes a rather tedious period of waiting had to be endured before contractions occurred, and after they began they continued for a while, then ceased (see Fig. 2). The feeling of hunger, which was reported while the contractions were recurring, disappeared when they stopped. The inability of the subject to control the contractions eliminated the possibility of their being artifacts, perhaps induced by suggestion. The close concomitance of the contractions with hunger pangs, therefore, clearly indicates that they are the real source of those pangs.

Boldireff's studies proved that when the empty stomach is manifesting periodic contractions the intestines also are active. Conceivably all parts of the alimentary canal composed of smooth muscle share in these movements. The lower oesophagus in man is provided with smooth muscle. It was possible to determine whether this region in W. was active during hunger.

To the oesophageal tube a thin-rubber finger cot (2 cm. in length) was attached and lowered into the stomach. The little rubber bag was distended with air, and the tube, pinched to keep the bag inflated, was gently withdrawn until resistance was felt. The air was now released from the bag, and the tube further withdrawn about 3 cm. The bag was again distended with air at a manometric pressure of 10 cm. of water. Inspiration now caused the writing lever, which recorded the pressure changes, to rise; and a slightly further withdrawal of the tube changed the rise, on inspiration, to a fall. The former position of the tube, therefore, was above

[31] CANNON: The mechanical factors of digestion, London and New York, 1911, P. 54.

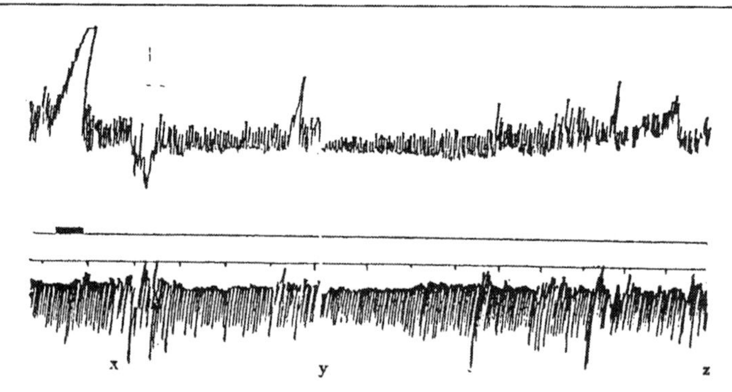

Figure 2: One half the original size. The same conditions as in Fig. 1 (fifteen minutes). There was a long wait for hunger to disappear. After *x*, W. reported himself "tired, but not hungry." The record from *y* to *z* was the continuance, on a second drum, of *x* to *y*.

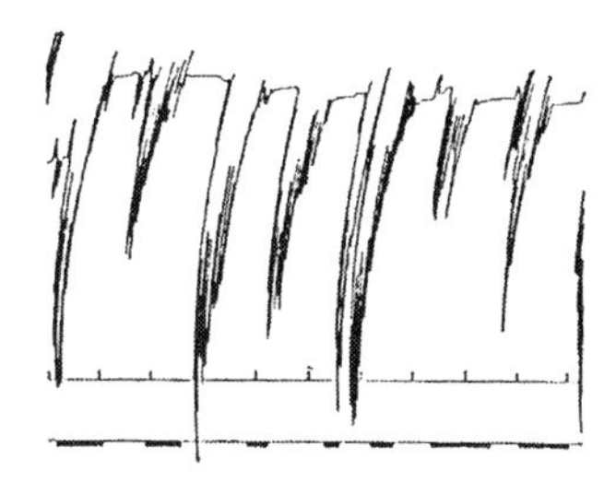

Figure 3: One half the original size. The top record represents compression of a thin-rubber bag in the lower oesophagus. The pressure in the bag varied between 9 and 13 cm. of water. The cylinder of the recorder was of smaller diameter than that used in the gastric records. The oesophageal contractions compressed the bag so completely that, at the summits of the large oscillations, the respirations were not registered. When the oscillations dropped to the time line, the bag was about half inflated. The middle line registers time in minutes (ten minutes). The bottom record is W's report of hunger pangs.

the gastric cavity and below the diaphragm. In this position the bag, attached to a float recorder (with chamber 2.3 cm. in diameter) registered the periodic oscillations shown in Fig. 3. Though individually more prolonged than those of the stomach, these contractions, it will be noted, occur at about the same rate. It is probable that the periodic activity of the two regions is simultaneous, for otherwise the stomach would force its gaseous content into the oesophagus with the rise of intragastric pressure.

What causes the contractions to occur has not been determined. From evidence already given they do not seem to be directly related to bodily need. Habit no doubt plays an important role. For present considerations, however, it is enough that they do occur, and that they are abolished when food, which satisfies bodily need, is taken into the stomach. By such indirection are performed some of the most fundamental of the bodily functions.

Peculiarities of hunger explained by contractions.–If these contractions are admitted as the cause of hunger, most of the difficulties confronting other explanations are readily obviated. Thus the occurrence of hunger at meal-times is most natural, for, as the regularity of defecation indicates, the alimentary canal has habits. Activity returns at the usual meal-time as a result of custom. By taking food regularly at a definite hour in the evening for several days, a new hunger period can be established. Since at these times the empty stomach, as Boldireff showed, has stronger contractions than the filled organ, hunger is aroused.

The contractions furthermore explain the sudden onset of hunger and its peculiar periodicity–phenomena which no other explanation of hunger can account for. The quick development of the sensation after taking a cold drink is possibly associated with the well-known power of cold to induce contraction in smooth muscle.

The great intensity of hunger during the first day of starvation, and its gradual disappearance till it vanishes on the third or fourth day, are made quite clear, for Boldireff observed that gastric contractions in his fasting dogs went through precisely such alterations of intensity and were not seen after the third day.

In fever, when bodily material is being most rapidly used, hunger is absent. Its absence is understood from an observation reported four years ago, that infection with systemic involvement is accompanied by a total cessation of all movements of the alimentary canal.[32] Boldireff observed that when his dogs were fatigued the rhythmic contractions failed to appear. Being "too tired to eat" is thereby given a rational explanation.

Another pathological form of the sensation–the inordinate hunger (bulimia) of certain neurotics–is in accord with the well-known disturbances of the tonic innervation of the alimentary canal in such individuals.

Since the lower end of the oesophagus, as well as the stomach, contracts periodically in hunger, the reference of the sensation to the sternum by the ignorant persons questioned by Schiff was wholly natural. The activity of the lower oesophagus also explains why, after the stomach has been removed, or in some cases when the stomach is distended with food, hunger can still be experienced. Conceivably the intestines also originate vague sensations by their contractions. Indeed the final banishment of the modified hunger sensation in the patient with duodenal fistula, described by Busch, may have been due to the lessened activity of the intestines when chyme was injected into them.

The observations recorded in this paper have, as already noted, numerous points of similarity to Boldireff's observations on the periodic activity of the alimentary canal in fasting dogs. Each period of activity, he found, comprised not only widespread contractions of the digestive canal, but also the pouring out of bile, and of pancreatic and intestinal juices rich in ferments. Gastric juice was not secreted at these times; when it wa secreted and reached the intestine, the peri-

[32]Cannon and Murphy: Journal of the American Medical Association, 1907, xlix, p. 840

odic activity ceased.[33] What is the significance of this extensive disturbance? Recently evidence has been presented that gastric peristalsis is dependent on the stretching of gastric muscle when tonically contracted.[34] The evidence that the stomach is in fact strongly contracted in hunger–i.e., in a state of high tone–has been presented above.[35] Thus the very condition which causes hunger and leads to the taking of food is the condition, when the swallowed food stretches the shortened muscles, for immediate starting of gastric peristalsis. In this connection the recent observations of Haudek and Stigler are probably significant. They found that the stomach discharges its contents more rapidly if food is eaten in hunger than if not so eaten.[36] Hunger, in other words, is normally the signal that the stomach is contracted for action; the unpleasantness of hunger leads to eating; eating starts gastric secretion, distends the contracted organ, initiates the movements of gastric digestion, and abolishes the sensation. Meanwhile pancreatic and intestinal juices, as well as bile, have been prepared in the duodenum to receive the oncoming chyme. The periodic activity of the alimentary canal in fasting, therefore, is not solely the source of hunger pangs, but is at the same time an exhibition in the digestive organs of readiness for prompt attack on the food swallowed by the hungry animal.

[33]BOLDIREFF: *Loc. cit.*, pp. 108-111.

[34]CANNON: this Journal, 1911, xxix, p. 250.

[35]The "empty" stomach and œsophagus contain gas (see HERTZ: Quarterly journal of medicine, 1910, iii, p. 378; MIKULICZ: Mittheilungen aus dem Grenzgebieten der Medicin und Chirurgie, 1903, xii, p. 596). They would naturally manifest rhythmic contractions on shortening tonically on their content.

[36]HAUDEK and STIGLER: Archiv für die gesammte Physiologie, 1910, cxxxiii, p. 159.

Cannon WB, Washburn AL. An Explanation of Hunger. Am J Physiol 1912;29:441-454.

This article was reprinted with permission from the American Physiological Society, Bethesda, MD.

Contributions to the Physiology of the Stomach. –II. The Relation Between the Contractions of the Empty Stomach and the Sensation of Hunger[1]

Anton J. Carlson
(From the Hull Physiological Laboratory of the University of Chicago.)

I.

In view of the fact that the literature on the nature of the sensation of hunger is exhaustively reviewed in the recent paper by Cannon and Washburn[2] an extended critique of the facts and theories at this time is superfluous. But the main theories, together with the facts adduced in their support, may be recounted here for the purpose of orientation.

(1) HUNGER IS A GENERAL SENSATION DUE TO CERTAIN CONDITIONS OF THE METABOLISM IN ALL THE TISSUES, OR MORE PARTICULARLY IN THE NERVE CELLS.[3] – In support of this view have been cited such facts as the uncertainty of the peripheral reference of the sensation; the alleged persistence of hunger after total excision of the stomach or after section of the vagi and high spinal transection; the alleged persistence of hunger when the stomach is filled with food, etc. As regards total excision of the stomach, this is, strictly speaking, impossible, or at least has not yet been made. Some stomach tissue is invariably left below the diaphragm in order to render continuity of the digestive tract possible, and this stomach remnant has a tendency to hypertrophy or dilate into a considerable stomach pouch. Moreover, in the clinical cases it is not clear that the observer has differentiated between *appetite* and *hunger*. In the case of experimental animals the criterion for hunger has been the interest in or eagerness for food. This is a criterion for appetite, but does not necessarily involve hunger. The persistence of hunger when the stomach is filled with food should be recognized as a special pathological condition ("polyphagia").

The most cogent objections to the above theory are the practically universal reference of the hunger sensation to the stomach or epigastrium; the intermittency of the sensation, at least in moderate hunger; the temporary abolition of the hunger, in normal persons, by anything, even indigestible materials, introduced into the stomach.

(2) HUNGER IS CAUSED BY THE STIMULATION OF AFFERENT NERVES IN THE STOMACH BY THE DISTENTION OF THE TUBULES OR DUCTS OF THE GASTRIC GLANDS OWING TO THE ACCUMULATION IN THEM OF GASTRIC JUICE.–This is the "turgescence theory " of Beaumont. It would account for the reference of the hunger sensation to the stomach, but I know of no other fact that can be adduced in its support. Accurate knowledge of the structure of the gastric glands would have rendered the promulgation of the hypothesis impossible. The hypothesis has lived, because linked with the name of Beaumont. The peculiar and sudden pouring out of gastric juice during or after states of hunger described by Beaumont in connection with the statement of his theory of hunger is an error of observation, or pathological. At least I have never observed this phenomenon in V.

(3) HUNGER IS DUE TO THE STIMULATION OF AFFERENT NERVES IN THE STOMACH BY THE CONTRACTION OF THE STOMACH MUSCULATURE (WEBER).–In support of this view have been cited the contracted condition of the empty stomach; the periodic contraction of the empty stomach described by Boldireff in the dog; the cessation of hunger by the introduction of indigestible material into the stomach, as this is known to cause temporary inhibition of the stomach tonus; the rumbling noise (borborygmi) frequently heard in the stomach in hunger. This rumbling noise, frequently loud enough to be heard by the hungry person himself without auscultation or special attention, must be due to contractions in some region of the digestive tract.[4]

But we owe the actual demonstration of the syn-

[1]The reader is referred to the first article (this Journal, 1912, xxxi, p. 151) for an account of the methods, etc., employed in the experiments reported in this paper.

[2]CANNON and WASHBURN: this Journal, 1912, xxix, p. 441.

[3]This view is elaborated in great detail by TURRO in a series of articles in Zeitschrift für Psychologie und Physiologie des Sinnesorganes, 1910-1911, xliv and xlv.

[4]My colleague, Dr. A. B. LUCKHARDT, has called my attention to the fact that in "nervous" persons borborygmi may be very pronounced without being associated with hunger.

chrony of the hunger sensations with the strong contractions of the empty stomach to Cannon and Washburn. These observers recorded the subjective sensation of hunger simultaneously with the intragastric pressure, and found that the stomach contractions and the hunger sensations run parallel. The fact that the beginning of the stomach contractions is in evidence before the hunger sensation is felt and that the sensation lasts longer than the active phase of the contraction is adduced in support of the view that contractions in some way stimulate afferent nerves in the stomach, and these impulses give rise to the hunger pangs. Cannon and Washburn also demonstrated the synchrony of the hunger sensations with similar contractions in the lower end of the esophagus.

The beautiful demonstration of Cannon and Washburn leaves undecided the nature of the stimuli causing the "hunger contractions" and the peculiar periodicity of these contractions. There can be no further question of the parallel between the stomach contractions and the hunger sensation, but the evidence for the view that the former are the cause of the latter seems to me still incomplete. I do not appreciate the force of Cannon's argument that no other condition than the contractions as the cause can account for the periodicity or intermittency of the hunger sensations. Assuming that the stomach contractions constitute the primary stimuli in the genesis of hunger, does that really solve the problem of periodicity? It would seem that the problem is only shifted a little; for these stomach contractions must depend on corresponding rhythmical activities of central or peripheral nervous mechanisms. Such a nervous rhythm giving rise to the hunger sensations indirectly through contractions in the digestive tract is just as difficult to explain as a similar nervous rhythm giving rise to or constituting the hunger sensation directly.

2. Without having done any special work in this field, the writer has for a number of years inclined to the view that motor activities are an expression or a result of the state of hunger rather than the cause of hunger. Considered biologically, it would seem that in motile organisms the expression or result of hunger ought to be motion or locomotion – to bring the organism into new environments and thus increase the chances of obtaining food. For this purpose movements of the legs, wings, fins, or cilia would be more serviceable, of course, than movements of the digestive tract. This locomotor action as an unconscious expression of hunger is beautifully illustrated in decerebrated mammals and birds. The reader will recall Goltz's classical experiments on decerebrated dogs. Prolonged absence of food and hence a state of hunger led to restlessness and incessant locomotion in the dog without the cerebrum, while, other things being equal, a filled stomach resulted in rest and quiet. These phenomena are very striking in decerebrated pigeons, as most physiologists know from personal observations. Six years ago the writer kept a completely decerebrated pigeon for nearly a year. When the crop was empty, the pigeon would keep in incessant motion (walking) until fed, and even coo. This is true at least for periods up to sixteen hours. A few grains of corn or wheat put on the tongue and swallowed lead at once to repose in an attitude of sleep for a short period. The larger the meal the longer the period of repose. In view of what is known of the function of the cerebrum in mammals and birds it seems clear that these motor phenomena in hunger are primary and fundamental reflexes, or an automatism independent of conscious hunger states. The cessation of restlessness and locomotion in birds immediately following the introduction of a few grains of wheat or even a few grains of sand into the crop is capable of two interpretations. The restlessness and locomotion may be a reflex phenomenon, the primary stimulus being the contraction of muscular mechanism of the oesophagus and the stomach, which contractions are inhibited by mechanical stimulation of nerves in the oesophagus and the crop. Or the locomotion is an expression of a fundamental automatism inhibited by afferent impulses from nerves distributed to the crop. There has been no decisive evidence in favor of either of these two hypotheses.

II.

The subject of the present experiments, Mr. V., was not told of the nature of the experiments till near the end of the series. This was done to avoid errors from conscious interference, both in the way of inhibition and excitation. When seated or lying down during the experiments, his position was such that he could not see the kymograph or any of the recording apparatus. The signal key or keys for recording the hunger sensation were placed in his hand, and he was instructed to press the key as soon as he felt hunger and to keep on pressing it till the hunger was no longer felt. There was no difficulty in keeping his attention fixed on this for shorter periods of one or two hours and under conditions of hunger of moderate intensity. But when the observations were continued without interruption for five to six hours and therefore during several periods of intense hunger, V. would usually become restless, apparently somewhat tired, and therefore unable to give undivided attention to the introspection. It may be stated that the man had no previous training in introspection or subjective analysis.

Most of the observations were made in a period of from four to ten hours after meals, and only a few as long as twenty-four hours after a meal, for the reason that the hunger pains in most instances became gradually more severe to the point of discomfort, and the man became restless and tired.

As a check on the intragastric respiratory pressure, records of the respiratory movements (Chest pneumograph) were always taken simultaneously with that of the stomach movements.

III.

1. CONFIRMATION OF THE OBSERVATIONS OF CANNON AND WASHBURN.– The general results are in complete accord with those of Cannon and Washburn. When the empty stomach showed strong contraction, V. invariably replied that he felt the hunger in his stomach. There is, on the whole, a fairly close correspondence between the duration of stomach contractions and duration of the subjective sensations of hunger. On days when the stomach did not exhibit strong contractions, V. stated that he did not feel hungry, even though in two cases the observations were continued to within twenty-four hours after the previous meal. These "hunger contractions" of the empty stomach are primarily those of the strong periodic rhythm described and illustrated in the first communication, so that further discussion at this time is superfluous.

2. THE RELATION BETWEEN THE STRENGTH OF THE STOMACH CONTRACTIONS AND THE INTENSITY OF THE HUNGER SENSATIONS. –Data on the above point were obtained in the following manner. Three signal magnets were arranged to record on the drum perpendicular to the recording point of the bromoform manometer, and the three corresponding keys placed in V.'s hand. He was then instructed to press key No. 1 when he felt, without a question, even the faintest hunger; No. 2 when he felt hunger of moderate strength; and No. 3 when he felt the strongest hunger. In view of the fact that V. had no training in subjective analysis, the results are remarkably uniform and accurate.

In general V. would press key No. 1 (weak hunger) at the beginning of a contraction period when the individual contractions were relatively feeble. Then, as the contraction increased in strength, there came a period of vacillation between key No. 1 and key No. 2 (moderate hunger). As the contractions grew still stronger, key No. 2 would be used for a while without any change. Then followed a period of alternation between key No. 2 and key No. 3, and in the final stage of maximum activity of the contraction period the signal was made with key No. 3 exclusively. In other words, *there is a fairly close correspondence between the strength of the stomach contractions and the degree of hunger sensations experienced simultaneously.*

The above account applies particularly to the first hunger period appearing after a meal and for the milder hunger periods in general. On more prolonged fast, that is, after having experienced several hunger periods, V. usually did not signal with key No. 1 at all, and sometimes not even with key No. 2, but would start in with key No. 3 (strongest hunger) at the very beginning of a period, despite the fact that *the strength of the stomach contractions was not greater (or might even be less) than that designated as very mild or moderate hunger a few hours earlier.* This seems to indicate either an increased excitability of the afferent nerves in the stomach, or an increased excitability of some parts of the brain.

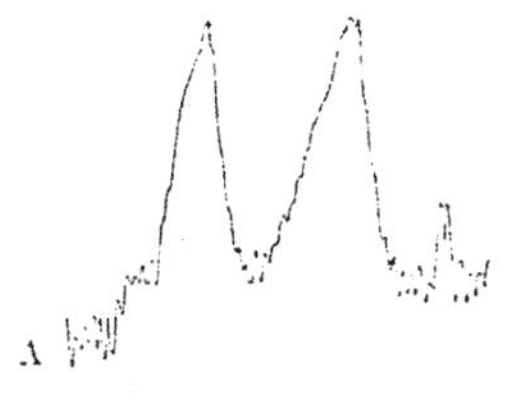

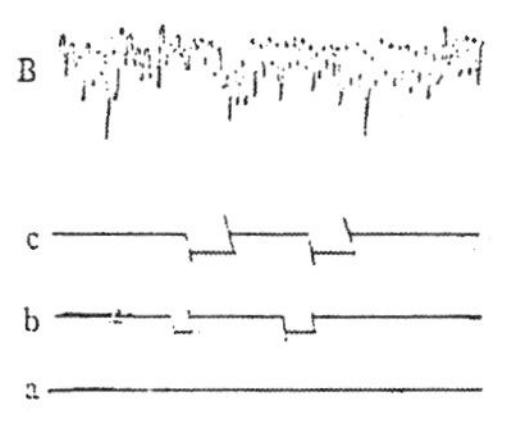

Figure1: Two thirds the original size. *A*, tracing of stomach contractions; *B*, respiratory movements; *a*, signal for weak hunger; *b*, signal for moderately strong hunger; *c*, signal for strong hunger. Showing the increase in the intensity of the hunger sensation during single contractions.

The close parallel between the degree of the stomach contractions and the intensity of the hunger sensations is further shown by the fact that the beginning of a strong contraction was frequently signalled by key No. 2 (moderate hunger), and then a shift made to key No. 3 (strong hunger) nearer the apex of the contraction. This is illustrated in Fig. I. *Evidently V. was able to distinguish a gradually increasing intensity of the hunger sensation during and parallel with the individual stomach contraction.* But this distinction was never made in very strong hunger and corresponding contractions. Very rarely was the beginning of a strong contraction signalled with key No. 1 (weak hunger). Whenever this happened, V. would shift to key No. 2, and finally to key No. 3 *pari passu* with the increase in the amplitude

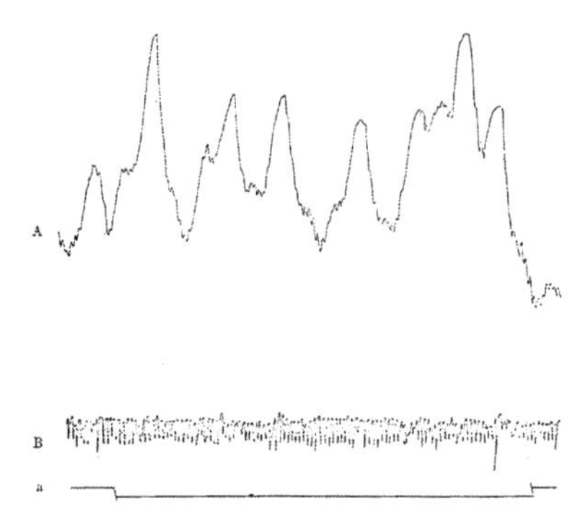

Figure 2: Four fifths the original size. *A*, stomach contractions; *B*, respiratory movements; *a*, hunger signal. Showing complete fusion of the hunger sensations (hunger tetanus) during incomplete tetanus of the stomach contractions.

of the contraction.

The weaker contractions of the stomach that appear between the stronger contractions during a period of moderate hunger or at the beginning of a period of strong hunger are nearly always correctly signalled with key No. 1 or key no. 2, usually the latter. This discrepancy must be noted, however, that these weaker contractions always recognized and usually signalled with key No. 2, may not show a greater degree of shortening of the muscle than the contractions present during the pauses between the strong hunger periods, and these latter contractions are usually not recognized even as mild hunger. This is a further indication of a change either in the brain or in the excitability of the nerves of the stomach during the periods of strong hunger.

3. FUSION OF THE HUNGER SENSATIONS INTO HUNGER TETANUS PARALLEL WITH STRONG AND RAPID CONTRACTIONS OR TETANUS OF THE STOMACH CONTRACTIONS. – The essential features and conditions of the incomplete tetanus of the stomach contraction at the end of the period of very vigorous contractions were described in the first communication, to which the reader is referred. These tetanus periods of the stomach are invariably accompanied by a similar fusion or tetanus of the hunger sensation. The fusion of the hunger sensation appears to be more complete than the fusion of the stomach contractions. When the rate of the strong stomach contractions approaches two per minute, the fusion of the hunger sensations is practically complete. V. is at least unable to distinguish any rhythmical variations in the hunger intensity. These phases of the stomach contractions are always signalled with key no. 3 (strongest hunger). A typical record illustrating this tetanus of hunger parallel with the gastric tetanus (usually incomplete) is reproduced in Fig. 2. The greater fusion of the hunger sensations than is shown by the synchronous stomach contractions is probably due to the fact that the strong individual sensations lag or persist longer than the corresponding stomach contractions.

The abrupt cessation of the gastric tetanus at the end of a strong contraction period is accompanied by an equally abrupt and complete cessation of the hunger sensations (Fig. 3).

4. THE RECOGNITION OF INDIVIDUAL CONTRACTIONS OF THE "TWENTY-SECONDS RHYTHM" AS "HUNGER CONTRACTIONS."–The special character of the "twenty-seconds rhythm" of the empty human stomach is sufficiently described in my first communication. It will suffice to restate that it is not yet decided whether this rhythm, which is continuous, is due to the antrum or is also characteristic of the body of the stomach. This seems of particular importance in connection with the fact that even these contractions may induce hunger states.

The individual contractions signalled as mild or moderate hunger are usually stronger than those not definitely recognized in consciousness (Fig. 4). But occasionally there may be no marked difference in the amplitude of the contractions. Each consecutive contraction of the "twenty-seconds rhythm" is never signalled as a hunger contraction unless the contractions are very strong, in which case they can hardly be distin-

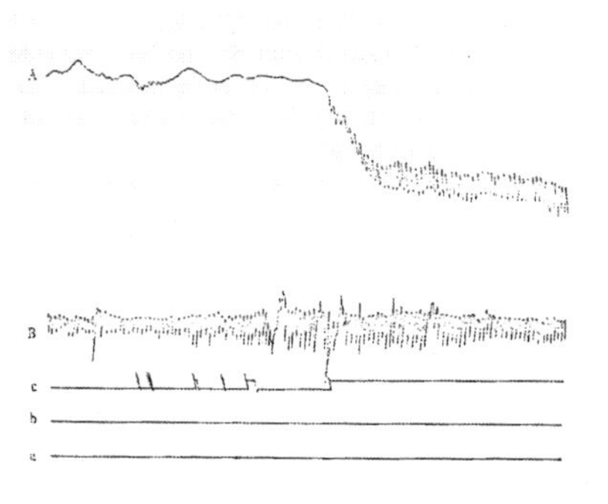

Figure 3: Four fifths the original size. *A*, stomach contractions; *B*, respiratory movements; *a, b,c,* signals for weak, moderate, and strong hunger respectively. Record of the end of a period of strong hunger and hunger tetanus, showing abrupt cessation of the hunger sensation parallel with the abrupt cessation of the stomach tetanus.

guished from the moderate contraction of the periodic or "thirty-seconds rhythm."

Assuming that the "twenty-seconds rhythm" is an antrum rhythm, and that the stomach contractions cause the hunger sensations, it follows that strong contractions of the pyloric region should cause hunger. Now, such strong contractions of this region of the stomach occur during vomiting, yet vomiting is, to my knowledge, never accompanied by hunger sensations. Of course, it is possible that the change in the physiological condition of the gastric nervous mechanism usually present in vomiting may account for the absence of hunger.

The recognition of only an occasional contraction of the "twenty-seconds rhythm" as a hunger contraction when all the contractions are of nearly uniform intensity is probably due to variations in attention.

5. THE SIGNIFICANCE OF THE TIME RELATIONS BETWEEN THE STOMACH CONTRACTIONS AND THE HUNGER SENSATIONS. –It was pointed out by Cannon and Washburn that the time relations between the stomach contractions and the hunger sensations might serve to determine the nature of their causal relationship. It is doubtful, however, whether the data secured by the methods so far employed are of much significance as regards this point. Unless the balloon in the stomach completely fills the stomach cavity and the pressure in the balloon is very slight, it is clear that the manometer does not register the very beginnings of the contractions. And on the subjective side we have the fluctuation of attention as a source of error. Nevertheless, a number of days were devoted to this phase despite these obvious defects in our method.

The recognition of a stomach contraction as a hunger pang depends not only on the strength of the contraction, but also on the rapidity of development of the contraction phase; that is, two contractions may indicate equal degrees of shortening of the stomach musculature, but if the contraction phase of one covers a minute or more while that of the other half a minute or less, the latter contraction only is accompanied by a definite hunger sensation. The stomach may thus exhibit slow tonus undulations of considerable magnitude without any attendant hunger state. The reader will recall that the above relation of the rate of the contraction to the hunger sensation is in accord with one of the general "Laws of Stimulation." The fact would seem to strengthen the view that the sensation is the result of the contraction.

In no instance out of the numerous tests made did V. indicate feeling hungry *before* the beginning of the stomach contractions. But when the balloon and the manometer were adjusted as delicately as possible, the hunger signal and stomach contractions appeared nearly simultaneously. But inasmuch as the manometer probably does not register the very beginning of the contractions, it is evident that some seconds of the contraction phase always precede the hunger feeling.

When the stomach contraction is of moderate strength and hunger sensation of correspondingly moderate intensity, the hunger sensation usually ceases at the height of the contraction, but when the contractions are very strong the hunger sensation persists also during the relaxation phase. In other words, the sensation lags both at the beginning and at the end of the contraction.

6. THE RELATION OF "HUNGER" TO "APPETITE." – During the intervals of the strong contraction periods, when the keys for the hunger signals are left undisturbed despite the presence of feeble rhythms in the stomach,

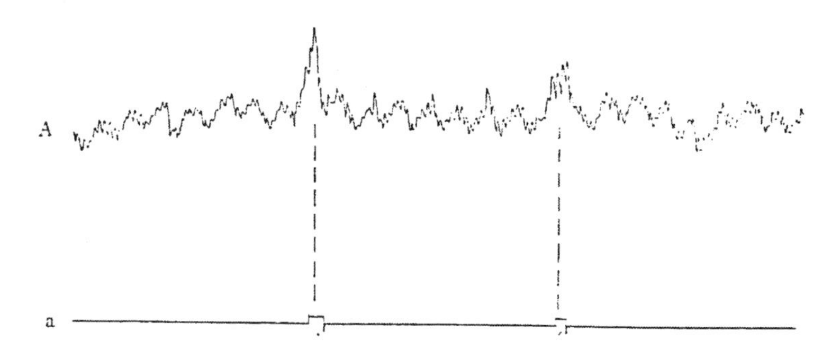

Figure 4: Four sevenths the original size. *A*, stomach contractions; (twenty-seconds rhythm); *a*, hunger signal. Showing recognition of the stronger contractions of the twenty-seconds rhythm as hunger pangs.

V. was frequently asked if he would like to eat or if he felt hungry. His answer was invariably that he would like to eat or felt a desire for food, and not infrequently he would say, "I feel hungry, but I don't feel the contractions." When pressed for an explanation of this statement, he always insisted that he "felt this hunger in the stomach." This explanation of this situation is not very clear to me. The results reported in the previous pages show conclusively that the strong stomach contractions are recognized as hunger pangs, and that the rhythms of the stomach movements and the hunger sensations run parallel. Now, is the weaker but more or less persistent "hunger," referred to the epigastrium, but not definitely associated with the stomach contractions, even though the stomach shows some activity, due to confusion of *appetite* with *hunger?* Or are the feeble stomach contractions correlated with or capable of giving rise to a feeble but rather persistent hunger sensation? V. is not able to make any definite distinction between hunger (Bohemian, *hlad*) and appetite (Bohemian, *chut*). This does not appear to be due to unfamiliarity with the language, because through an interpreter he is equally unable to make clear distinction in his native language. This is not surprising in view of the fact that the terms "hunger" and "appetite" are used interchangeably by most people, including physiologists. Howell[5] states that "hunger in its mild form is designated as 'appetite,'" and on this basis appetite in its strong form would be designated as hunger. Cannon and Washburn support the opposite view, that hunger and appetite are fundamentally different sensations, appetite having an agreeable character depending on previous sensations of taste and smell of food, that is, on certain memories, while hunger is essentially a painful sensation referred to the epigastrium and not dependent on previous experience with food.

According to this view, hunger is the more fundamental and primitive sensation, while appetite requires a nervous organization capable of associated memory. Is this conception of appetite adequate? Must we not look for the primary basis of appetite in a desire for food as the expression of an inherited mechanism, primarily independent of, but subsequently modified by, the individual experience? In other words, have we not in appetite for food conditions as primitive and essentially fixed by inheritance as in the case of the sexual desires or "instincts"? Pure hunger, not accompanied by "appetite," can be experienced, if during hunger the attention is fixed on the hunger pangs themselves, or if it is occupied with other processes that will completely exclude the ideas of food and eating and their associations. When this is done, hunger in its various stages becomes different degrees of pain. The cry of the newborn child for food is, in all probability, due to this pure hunger pain (plus the inherited "desire for food") and the quieting effect of feeding due to its abolition. Pain as such, however, has no special correlation with the feeding reflexes.

The elements in appetite due to the individual's experience with foods can be experienced in the absence of hunger only, as in the contemplation of one's favorite dish shortly after a full and satisfying meal. The sensations aroused by this contemplation are agreeable and may even lead to salivation, but these sensations are not (or at least not necessarily) associated with a desire to eat. The inheritance factor in appetite, the desire to eat, is in some way caused by the hunger pains. This desire minus the individual's memories of previous experience with foods appears to be in evidence in extreme hunger states when unpalatable or disgusting foods, straw, sticks, etc., are chewed and swallowed.

In the adult, in normal health, the hunger pains, the desire for foods, and pleasant memories of the taste and smell of foods are ordinarily present simultaneously; they mutually reinforce one another, and lead to a common goal, the taking of food. These facts probably account for the common view that hunger and appetite designate different degrees of the same sensation.

The mutual "reinforcing" or "facilitation" action of the two sensations is seen in the universal experience of increased appetite, or the initiation (more correctly the recognition) of hunger by seeing, smelling, or tasting palatable food. It can be shown on V. that this sudden recognition of or increase in the intensity of the appetite sensation has no counterpart in a sudden initiation or increase in the hunger contractions of the stomach.[6] The phenomena are evidently concerned with central processes, the association processes initiated by the olfactory and visual impulses affecting the paths and centres concerned in conscious hunger in such a way that subconscious hunger states enter consciousness.

If the above analysis of the elements of appetite and hunger approach the actual conditions, there appears to be no contradiction in V.'s statement of "feeling hungry," but not feeling the contractions, or hunger pangs. If during relative quiescence of the stomach the attention is not fixed on food or eating, one does not "feel hungry," because the feeble hunger processes remain subconscious. But when the attention is fixed on food or eating, the cerebral processes involved in their memories render the weak hunger state conscious, one experiences a peculiar uncomfortable feeling of tension (not distinct pain) in the epigastrium, and the ear is cocked for the dinner bell. In strong hunger the sequence of

[5] Howell: Textbook of physiology, 1911, p. 285.

[6] Later work on dogs seems to show that the seeing and smelling of foods lead to strong contractions of the œsophagus.

events is reversed, the strong stomach contractions giving rise to the hunger pains and the desire for food, which in turn starts the memory processes of taste and smell of foods.

7. THE STOMACH CONTRACTIONS GIVE RISE TO THE HUNGER SENSATIONS.–The consideration of the cause of the hunger contractions will be taken up in a later paper, but the simpler question of the action of the contractions may be briefly dealt with now. Assuming, for the present, that the stomach contractions give rise to the hunger sensations through the action of afferent nerves from the stomach, in what way does the contraction act as the stimulus to these nerves? Does the hunger sensation arise (1) from the stimulation of nerves in the mucosa; (2) from the stimulation of nerves in the muscular coats and in the connective tissue; (3) or is it due to an inter-central discharge from the Auerbach's plexus to the brain, associated with the motor discharge from the same plexus to the stomach musculature?

As regards the first possibility, the following experiments have been made, with negative results. It would seem that the only way in which contraction of the stomach musculature could stimulate nerve endings in the mucosa is by *mechanical pressure.* This I have tried to imitate in the following way. During the period of relative quiescence of the stomach between two periods of strong hunger, when the afferent nerves concerned are in such condition that their stimulation will give rise to hunger, mechanical pressure on the mucosa by distention of the balloon or rubbing the mucosa by the closed end of a test tube never causes sensations of hunger unless these procedures lead to contraction. V. always stated that he felt these pressures, but the sensations were not like hunger. The objection might be raised against these experiments that the pressure is not sufficiently strong, and, in the case of the test tube, does not touch a sufficiently large area of the mucosa. I admit that a more intense mechanical stimulation of the mucosa could be produced by Pawlow's method of blowing sand into the stomach by bellows. But I have not felt justified in using similar procedures on V. The methods used do not, of course, produce the strongest possible mechanical stimulation of the mucosa, but these stimulations were sufficient to affect consciousness. They were perceived, but not as hunger sensations. It seems therefore highly probable that the afferent nerves in the mucosa are not primarily concerned in the genesis of the hunger sense. *They are, however, concerned in the inhibition of hunger.*

The hunger sensation seems to be produced by the contractions only. When the empty stomach is normal, strong contractions, however caused, cause hunger. Thus, is the balloon in the stomach is rather suddenly distended, this may produce one, two, or three strong contractions of the previously quiescent stomach, and these are recognized as hunger contractions identical with those of the "spontaneous" hunger periods. It seems to me that this experiment constitutes *a demonstration of the peripheral genesis of hunger,* as the subjective state clearly is induced by the peripheral change. A tracing illustrating this phenomenon is reproduced in Fig. 5.

But how do the contractions stimulate the afferent nerves in the muscle layers? None of my observations on V. throw any light on this question. Contraction in skeletal muscle stimulates afferent nerve fibres in the muscle. But it seems to me that the pain experienced from contractures or "cramps" in skeletal muscles and in the intestines is different from the hunger pangs, even though pain is inherent in hunger. The difference may be only an apparent one, due to the fact that the latter pains arouse the memories of previous agreeable experiences with food. Because of the folding of the mucosa and the sub-mucosa into rugæ and the changes in the arrangement of the cells in the muscle layers in the stomach during contractions,[7] there must be a great variation in tension on the nerve fibres in the contracted and in the relaxed condition of the stomach wall. This variation in tension, rather than actual pressure, may constitute the stimulus, in so far as the stimulus is a

[7]MÜLLER, cited from CANNON: The mechanical factors in digestion, 1911, p. 60.

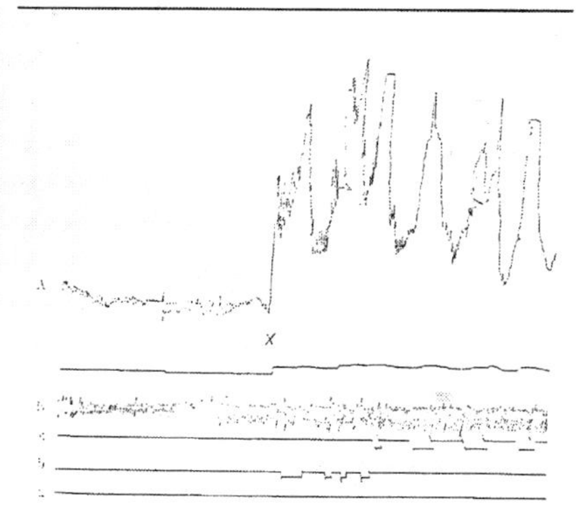

Figure 5: Two thirds the original size. *A*, stomach contractions; *B*, respiratory movements; *a, b,c,* signals for weak, moderate, and strong hunger respectively. The pressure in the balloon is slight. There is no evidence of strong stomach contractions, and V. feels no hunger. At *c* the pressure in the balloon is suddenly increased. This distention of the balloon indicates a few strong stomach contractions, which in turn cause the hunger states. A demonstration of the gastric genesis of hunger.

mechanical one. It would therefore seem that hunger contains elements of kinæsthetic sensation as well as pain, the latter predominating in strong hunger.

8. I HAVE BEEN STRONGLY IMPRESSED BY V.'S ABILITY TO RECOGNIZE FEEBLE STOMACH CONTRACTIONS AS HUNGER STATES.– It is probable that very strong stomach contractions can be recognized as separate hunger pangs by most men. The writer has at least no difficulty in doing this. But the delicate analysis disclosed in these experiments on V. is beyond the writer's ability in introspection. On many days I denied myself food for periods similar to those imposed on V. so as to bring the stomach of subject and observer in conditions as nearly alike as possible. But even with the stomach rhythm and the hunger rhythm of V. being recorded before my eyes and convinced that my own stomach was engaged in a similar rhythm, as hunger was present, the most that I could determine was the fact that the moderate hunger sensations were more or less discontinuous.

Two explanations of V.'s unusual ability in recognizing the stomach activities have occurred to the writer. (1) Since early boyhood the stomach has been to V the object of special care and attention. In consequence of this special attention to the stomach the afferent nervous impulses from the stomach may have attained a clearer definition in consciousness analogous to the remarkable development of analysis in the tactile or pressure senses in the absence of vision. If this hypothesis is correct, afferent impulses from the stomach other than those concerned in hunger ought to show a similar marked influence on consciousness in V. (2) At the point of gastrostomy V.'s stomach adheres to the parietal peritoneum. There may be adhesions of greater extent in consequence of the operation. The hunger sensation of V. may therefore include a greater degree of pain than is the case in normal men, as the contracting stomach may pull on the parietal peritoneum, which, according to many observers, is very sensitive to painful stimuli. The weaker stomach contractions may thus be recognized as hunger because more painful than under normal conditions. I have questioned V., but he is unable to recollect any difference in his hunger sensation before his accident and after the completion of the gastrostomy. Confirmatory evidence (or the opposite) ought to be obtainable without much difficulty, as cases of gastrostomy are fairly common. Clinicians having such case in hand would do a service to physiology if they could determine whether gastrostomy invariably augments the hunger sensations or makes the hunger pangs more painful.

Two other possibilities have been suggested. There may be an increased excitability of the afferent nerves of the stomach as a result of the constant presence of the rubber tube. But there seems to be no evidence of this in the appearance or in the sensibility of the gastric mucosa. My colleague, Professor Lingle, suggested that cutaneous sensory nerve fibres may have grown into the stomach wall in consequence of the union of the stomach and the body walls. In such case there may be elements of epicritic pain and touch in V.'s hunger pangs.

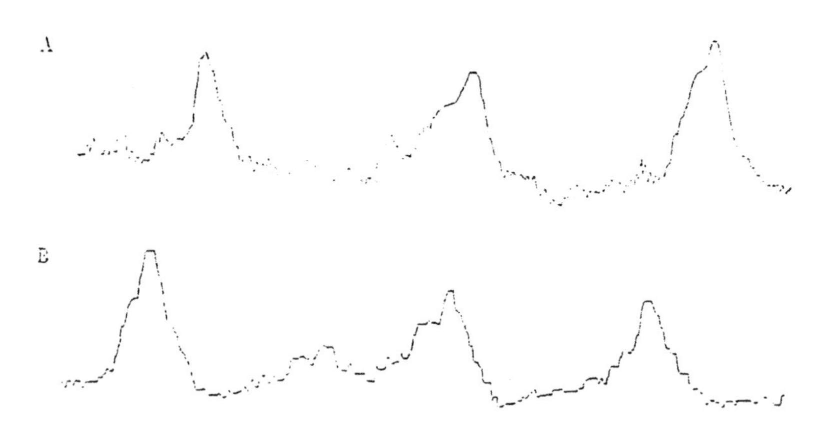

Figure 6: Two fifths the original size. *A*, tracing of the hunger contractions of the empty stomach in man (Mr. V.); *B*, tracings of the contractions of the empty stomach of a dog with a gastric fistula. Showing practical identity of the rhythms of the empty stomach in man and dog.

This seems improbable in view of what is known of the specific character of the regeneration of nerve fibres after lesion, and I have not been able to obtain any "tactile" sensations from the gastric mucosa in proximity to the gastrostomy.

9. THE SIMILARITY OF THE HUNGER CONTRACTIONS OF THE EMPTY STOMACH OF MAN TO THE STRONG CONTRACTIONS OF THE EMPTY STOMACH IN THE DOG.–The work on dogs with a fistula in the fundus for the introduction of the ballon as originally employed by Boldireff has been carried far enough to establish the practical identity in character of the contractions of the empty stomach in man and dog. The rapid or continuous rhythm shown by the stomach of V. is also shown by the dog's stomach. The rate of the rhythm is different, however. But it is the strong stomach contractions that are of interest in this connection. When the size of the ballon is adjusted approximately to the difference in capacity of the human and canine stomachs, the records obtained from man and dog can scarcely be told apart (Fig. 6). The man tells us that a sensation of strong hunger is felt synchronously with the contraction. We have a right to conclude that the dog experiences the same sensation simultaneously with the corresponding contraction. *We have, then, in the strong contractions of the empty stomach an objective criterion for the presence or absence of hunger in experimental animals.*

It may be noted in this connection that dogs will show a lively interest in and great desire for food during periods when the strong contractions of the empty stomach are absent. And conversely, if the dog suspects that he will be allowed to see and smell the food only, he may show no interest in the food, despite the presence of strong stomach contractions with the attendant strong hunger sensations. Interest in and desire for food are therefore no criterion for hunger in experimental animals.

Carlson AJ. Contributions to the Physiology of the Stomach–II. The Relation Between the Concentrations of the Empty Stomach and the Sensation of Hunger. Am J Physiol 1912;31:175-192.

This article was reprinted with permission from the American Physiological Society, Bethesda, MD.

GLUCOSTATIC MECHANISM OF REGULATION OF FOOD INTAKE*

Jean Mayer, Ph.D., D.Sc.

BOSTON

The regulation of energy intake is fundamental to all homeostatic mechanisms. Yet this basic process has received less attention than many of the physiologic regulations that it makes possible.

Before this century, three theories were advanced to account for the phenomenon of hunger. The theories of peripheral origin (Haller, Erasmus, Darwin, Johannes Müller and Weber) held that the taking of food resulted from the stimulation either of all afferent nerves by some change in the tissues or of a strictly local group of sensory nerves, mainly in the stomach. The theory of central origin (Magendie, Tidewald and Milne-Edwards) postulated that a hunger center was sensitive to a starvation state of the blood. The theories of general sensation (Roux and Michael Foster) considered that the hunger center of the blood was stimulated not only by the hunger state of the blood but also indirectly by afferent impulses from all organs of the body.

After Cannon and Washburn, as well as Carlson, had shown that epigastric sensations of "hunger pain" coincided with waves of contractions of the empty stomach, Carlson[1] suggested that hypoglycemia, mediated by its effect on the stomach, might be responsible for inducing these hunger sensations. Although hunger pangs are found in most persons, the idea that the sensations elicited by stomach contractions due to hypoglycemia[2] were at the basis of the regulation of food intake was abandoned for the following reasons: it was repeatedly shown, in particular by Sherrington, that total denervation and surgical removal of the total denervation and surgical removal of the stomach did not fundamentally alter the characteristics of food intake regulation. Adolph[3] demonstrated, by diluting the ration of laboratory animals with inert material, that differences in the bulk of the diet had only a transient influence. Scott and his collaborators[4] were unable to correlate spontaneous fluctuations of blood sugar levels with a desire for food. The existence of diabetic hyperphagia and of the phenomenon of hunger diabetes also presented seemingly insurmountable difficulties. Even the increase in spontaneous intake due to insulin-induced hypoglycemia was held by some authors to be of no general significance because of the abnormal "unphysiologic" circumstances in which the organism was placed.[5]

The demonstration by Hetherington and Ranson[6] that destruction of parts of the medioventral nuclei of the hypothalamus leads to obesity and the work of Anand and Brobeck[7] showing that more lateral lesions cause anorexia reopened the problem of the nature of the physiologic mechanism of the regulation of food intake.

Experimental work on rats, mice, dogs and human subjects culminated in the proposal of a "glucostatic mechanism" of regulation of food intake.[8-10] The initial reasoning was as follows: the regulation of food intake proceeds by relatively frequent partaking of food (meals). It appears improbable that hypothalamic centers are sensitive to decrease of the body content in fat or protein — during the short interval between meals, this decrease is proportionally very small. On the other hand, the body stores of carbohydrate are limited. The postprandial liver glycogen content in man is approximately 75 gm. — only 300 calories' worth. In the postabsorptive period, in spite of gluconeogenesis (the synthesizing of glycogen from body proteins), glycogen stores become rapidly depleted. This synthesis of glycogen from proteins and the shifting of metabolic oxidation in non-nervous tissues from glucose to fat (as measured by the lowering of the respiratory quotient) tend to minimize the drop in blood glucose resulting from depletion of liver glycogen stores. Thus, minimum levels necessary for the survival of the central nervous system are maintained. Only partaking of food,

Mayer J. Glucostatic mechanism of regulation of food intake. N Engl J Med. 1953;249 (1):13-16.
Reprinted with permission the Massachusettes Medical Society, 1440 Main St. Waltham, MA 02154.

however, can restore full homeostasis of the central nervous system. It appeared, as a working hypothesis, that the central nervous system, dependent exclusively on a continued supply of glucose in blood, should maintain "glucoreceptors" sensitive to fluctuations of available blood glucose. (That glucoreceptors do in fact exist in the central nervous system has been implicitly recognized by surgeons; a common method for testing the completeness of vagotomies consists in administering insulin and ascertaining that the resultant hypoglycemia fails to elicit or delays gastric secretion of hydrochloric acid.)* In this "glucostatic" view, hunger would be integrated among the mechanisms through which the central nervous system ensures its homeostasis.

A first (and rather crude) test of this hypothesis was provided by a systematic survey of the effect of administration of various metabolites[9] on the food intakes of groups of normal animals. Increases in levels of reducing sugar in blood were obtained by injections of glucose or fructose or small doses or epinephrine. Decreases were obtained by injections of small, graded doses of insulin. Levels below normal fasting values were avoided, so as to stay within physiologic limits. The effects of the injection of substances without influence on blood glucose levels, like sucrose and fat emulsions, were also studied. It was found that temporary increases in blood glucose levels corresponded to decreases in food intake and vice versa, even when the calorie equivalent of injected metabolites was taken into account. Substances without effect on blood glucose did not influence food intake over and beyond caloric value, if they were metabolizable. Although significant, variations in food intake induced by these variations in blood sugar were small because of the efficiency of homeostatic mechanisms concerned with blood glucose levels. To demonstrate more clearly the inhibitory effect of high blood glucose levels on food intake, animals of the "Houssay" type, in this case alloxan-treated by pophysectomized rats, were injected with glucose. (Although these animals do not normally present hyperglycemia, they have been deprived of the mechanisms that ensure the rapid removal of injected glucose; hyperglycemia can thus be conveniently maintained for a much longer period. Two daily glucose injections were found to reduce food intake by half; three such injections, maintaining hyperglycemia around the clock, caused death of these animals from inanition in spite of the presence of food in their cage.

The apparent paradoxes afforded by the hyperphagia of diabetes mellitus, by the phenomenon of hunger diabetes, in which a previously fasted person will continue to eat in spite of a blood glucose reaching abnormally high levels, by the hyperphagia accompanying tendency to higher glucose levels in the obese, still had to be resolved before it could be concluded that blood glucose levels regulate food intake. It appears that all these conditions may have one factor in common — namely that whereas absolute levels of blood glucose are increased, utilization is decreased. For variation of blood sugar levels to influence hypothalamic glucoreceptors, glucose has to cross the membranes of these cells. This presumably implies phosphorylation through the hexokinase reaction. If phosphorylation is impaired, "effective sugar levels" will be in fact lower than absolute values as measured.

This concept was tested and put on a quantitative basis in a series of experiments performed on human subjects.[10, 12] Because of the inaccessibility of the hypothalamic centers, peripheral arteriovenous differences were determined as an index of rates of glucose utilization. These differences (designated as "Δ-glucose") were measured in the antecubital region (between finger blood and antecubital-vein blood). With one exception, discussed in some detail below, Δ-glucose values were found to correlate closely with the caloric intake of the subject and with hunger feelings (Fig. 1).

Diets calorically adequate were associated with Δ-glucose values that remained large throughout the day, decreasing only at mealtime. By contrast, submaintenance diets were followed by rapid shrinkage of Δ-glucose after meals; at the same time, hunger returned. When hunger diabetes was present, blood glucose values rose until a difference appeared between arterial and venous levels — only then was hunger assuaged. Generally speaking, there appeared to be a quantitative relation between food intake and the area represented by the Δ-glucose as a function of time. There was also a quantitative relation between Δ-glucose values and the incidence of hunger feelings; antecubital arteriovenous differences of more than 15 mg. per 100 cc. were never associated with hunger; values staying near 0 for any length of time were always associated with hunger.

In uncontrolled diabetes mellitus, a similar picture was obtained; blood sugar values had to be forced up through ingestion of food to levels where arteriovenous differences were introduced for ravenous hunger feelings to be satisfied. Cortisone administration accompanied by increased appetite caused an elevation of absolute glucose levels but a decrease in Δ-glucose.

The effect of epinephrine deserves special mention since it represents an apparent exception to the general rule. Administration of epinephrine caused an immediate increase in blood glucose; it drastically reduced or

*This phenomenon was recently analyzed experimentally by Porter et al.[11] It was shown specifically that in monkeys the anterior hypothalamus was responsible for the secretion of hydrochloric acid after insulin administration.

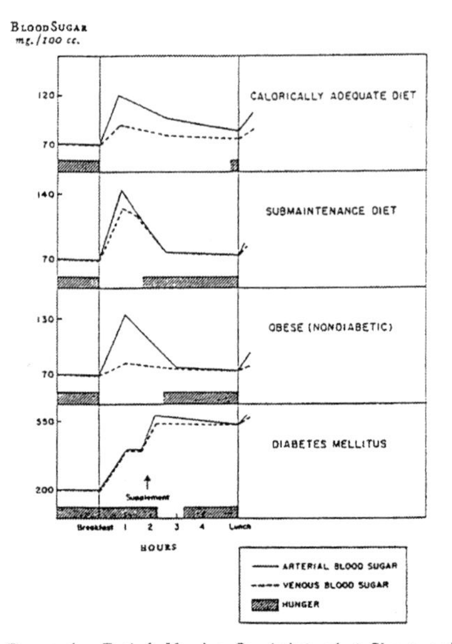

FIGURE 1. *Typical Morning Correlations of Δ-Glucose and Hunger Feeling.*
The size of the Δ-glucose (peripheral glucose arteriovenous difference) correlates with hunger feelings. No hunger feeling appears if the Δ-glucose is greater than 10 mg. per 100 cc.

eliminated any effect of hunger. However, at the same time, it decreased peripheral Δ-glucose to levels near 0. Although it may be an oversimplification to ascribe this seeming contradiction to one of the many physiologic effects of epinephrine, it is worth noting that epinephrine introduces a differential between peripheral and central blood flow.[13] By the same token, experiments conducted on animals demonstrate that, whereas it decreases peripheral Δ-glucose values, it increases carotid-jugular glucose differences; thus it not only produces hyperglycemia but also increases the proportion of glucose made available to the nervous centers.*

Insulin treatment first causes a fall in blood sugar owing to increased peripheral utilization of glucose. In a second phase, a compensatory rise takes place that is secondary to decreased utilization of glucose in the periphery.[15] Delta glucose values rapidly decline when the blood sugar falls to or below post-absorptive levels. The occurrence of increased hunger after insulin administration is therefore easily interpreted if hunger is seen as a direct response to carbohydrate deprivation.

In hyperthyroidism, alimentary hyperglycemia typically occurs and is followed regularly by a postalimentary hypoglycemia. It has been suggested[16] that accelerated metabolism of glucose takes place in the hyperthyroid patient and that the alimentary hyperglycemia may be only a manifestation of starvation diabetes that follows rapid depletion of carbohydrate stores. It appears that the metabolic hypoglycemia of hyperthyroidism may thus be related to the increased food intake characteristic of this condition.*

The possibility that the "feeding centers" in the lateral hypothalamus represent the sensitive area with facilitatory properties in terms of eating mechanisms has been discussed by Brobeck.[18] In the glucostatic view proposed here these centers would represent the glucoreceptors. There is an obvious need for a mechanism that would translate available blood glucose into variations in the physiologic state of the tissues. Such a mechanism is suggested by the observation that a drop in serum inorganic phosphate and in potassium consistently accompanies large Δ -glucose values.[12, 20, 21] It is possible that the passage of potassium ions into the glucoreceptor cells along with the glucose phosphate represents the point at which effective glucose level is translated into an electric or neural mechanism.

It is recognized that hypothalamic impulses still have to be interpreted, integrated and acted upon by the cerebral cortex; that other afferent impulses (gastric hunger pangs, in particular) also play a role in determining conscious states of hunger; and that other psychologic and physiologic factors may intervene to modify appetite at least temporarily. Conditioned reflexes, particularly in the dog, and habits in man also play an important role. Still, although feelings involving desire for food or satiety are not in any sense quantifiable, they represent a conscious expression of one of the most precise regulatory devices in biology. The glucostatic mechanism suggested here seems to provide a basis for such a precise regulation. It may be added that, because of the established decrease by available glucose of the rate of fat[22] and amino acid[23] utilization in non-nervous tissue, and probably of the rate of gluconeogenesis as well,[24] the regulation of food intake is easily integrated into the general regulation of metabolism.

Finally, it may be noted that the glucostatic theory seems to permit interpretation of certain types of alteration of the regulation of energy intake, in particular

*Keller and Roberts[14] recently demonstrated that glucose consumption of hypothalamic tissue is increased in vitro within a few minutes of the administration of epinephrine.

*It has recently been shown[17] that, in the cold, carbohydrate metabolism is also accelerated and glycogen reserves are decreased. A similar situation is known to prevail in growth.

†It was later demonstrated that electric stimulation of this lateral area causes an increase in food intake.[19]

hypothalamic obesity,[25] the hereditary obese hyperglycemic syndrome of mice[26] and at least one form of human obesity.[27] The demonstration[28] that, in the hereditary obese-hyperglycemic syndrome of mice, the alpha cells of the islands of Langerhans oversecrete a hormone with hyperglycemic, glycogenolytic and anti-insulin properties opens the possibility that this hormone plays a major role in the regulation of food intake and in the etiology of obesity.

REFERENCES

1. Carlson, A. J. The Control of Hunger in Health and Disease. 320 pp. Chicago: University of Chicago Press, 1916.
2. Bulatao, E., and Carlson, A. J. Contributions to physiology of stomach: influence of experimental changes in blood-sugar levels on gastric hunger contractions. Am. J. Physiol. 59:107-115, 1924.
3. Adolph, E. F. Urges to eat and drink in rats. Am. J. Physiol. 151:110-125, 1947.
4. Scott, W. W., Scott, C. C., and Luckhardt, A. B. Observations on blood sugar level before, during and after hunger periods in humans. Am. J. Physiol. 123:243-247, 1938.
5. Janowitz, H.D., and Grossman, M. I. Hunger and appetite: some definitions and concepts. J. Mt. Sinai Hosp. 16:231-240, 1949.
6. Hetherington, A. W., and Ranson, S. W. Hypothalamic lesions and adiposity in rat. Anat. Rec. 78:149-172, 1940.
7. Anand, B. K., and Brobeck, J. R. Localization of "feeding center" in hypothalamus of rat. Proc. Soc. Exper. Biol. & Med. 77:323,1951.
8. Mayer, J., and Bates, M.W. Mechanism of regulation of food intake. Federation Proc. 10:389, 1951.
9. Idem. Blood glucose and food intake in normal and hypophysectomized, alloxan-treated rats. Am. J. Physiol. 168:812-819, 1952.
10. Mayer, J. Glucostatic theory of regulation of food intake and problem of obesity. Bull. New England M. Center 14:43-49, 1952.
11. Porter, R. W., Longmire, R. L., and French, J.D. Neurohumoral influence on gastric hydrochloric acid secretion. Federation Proc. 12:110, 1953.
12. Van Itallie, T. B., Beaudoin, R., and Mayer, J. Arteriovenous glucose differences, metabolic hypoglycemia and food intake in man. J. Clin. Nutrition 1:208-217, 1953.
13. Somogyi, M. Studies of arteriovenous differences in blood sugar. Effect of epinephrine on rate of glucose utilization. J. Biol. Chem. 186:513-526, 1950.
14. Keller, M.R., and Roberts, S. Epinephrine stimulation of pituitary metabolism. Federation Proc. 12:76, 1953.
15. Somogyi, M. Studies of arteriovenous differences in blood sugar. Effect of epinephrine on rate of glucose utilization. J. Biol. Chem. 193:859-871, 1951.
16. Peters, J. P., and Van Slyke, D. D. Quantitative Clinical Chemistry. Vol. 1. Interpretations. 1041 pp. Baltimore: Williams and Wilkins, 1946. P. 328
17. Baker, D. G., and Sellers, E. A. Carbohydrate metabolism in rat exposed to low environmental temperature. Federation Proc. 12:8, 1953.
18. Brobeck, J. R. Physiology of appetite. In Overeating, Overweight and Obesity: Proceedings of the Nutrition Symposium held at the Harvard School of Public Health, Boston, October 29, 1952. 151 pp. New York: National Vitamin Foundation, 1953. Pp. 36-51.
19. Delgado, J. M. R., and Anand, B. K. Increase of food intake induced by electrical stimulation of lateral hypothalamus. Am. J. Physiol. 172:162-168, 1953.
20. McCullagh, D. R., and Van Alstine, L. Phosphates in sugar tolerance test. Am. J. Clin. Path. 2:277-287, 1932.
21. Levine, R., Loube, S. D., and Weisberg, H. F. Nature of action of insulin on level of serum inorganic phosphate. Am J. Physiol. 159:107-110, 1949.
22. Geyer, R. P., Bowie, E. J., and Bates, J. C. Effects of fasting and pyruvate on palmitic acid metabolism, J. Biol. Chem. 200:271-274, 1953.
23. Winzler, R.J., Moldave, k., Rafelson, M.E., Jr., and Pearson, H.E. Conversion of glucose to amino acids by brain and liver of newborn mouse. J. Biol. Chem. 199:485-492, 1952.
24. Engel, f. L., Schiller, S., and Pentz, E. I. Studies on nature of protein catabolic response to adrenal cortical extract. Endocrinology 44:458-0475, 1949.
25. Mayer, J., Bates, M. W., and Van Itallie, T. B. Blood sugar and food intake in rats with lesions of anterior hypothalamus. Metabolism. 1:340-348, 1952.
26. Mayer, J., Russell, R. E., Bates, M. W., and Dickie, M.M. Metabolic, nutritional and endocrine studies of hereditary obesity - diabetes syndrome of mice and mechanism of its development. Metabolism 2:9-21, 1953.
27. Beaudoin, R., Van Itallie, T. B., and Mayer, J. Carbohydrate metabolism in "active" and "static" human obesity. J. Clin. Nutrition 1:91-99, 1953.
28. Mayer, J., Silides, D. N., and Bates, M.W. Possible role of pancreatic alpha cells in hereditary obese-hyperglycemic syndrome of mice. Federation Proc. 12:423, 1953.

A Fall in Blood Glucose Level Precedes Meal Onset in Free-Feeding Rats

J. LOUIS-SYLVESTRE AND J. LE MAGNEN

Laboratoire de Neurophysiologie Sensorielle et Comportementale, Collège de France 11, place Marcelin Berthelot, 75 231 Paris Cedex 05, France

LOUIS-SYLVESTRE, J. AND J. LE MAGNEN. A fall in blood glucose level precedes meal onset in free feeding rats. NEUROSCI. BIOBEHAV. REV. 4 Suppl. 1,13-15, 1980.- It has been suggested for a long time that the metabolic stimulation to eat or the hunger arousal of eating, originated from a fall in the blood glucose level induced by the periodic failure of hepatic glucose production to match the peripheral glucose uptake. However, this suggestion has not been substantiated directly by the results of periodic blood glucose evaluations performed during intermeal intervals in free-fed rats. In this experiment, a technique involving a continuous blood glucose determination over several hours was used in free-feeding, undisturbed rats. it was shown that all nocturnal and diurnal meals were preceded by a 6 to 8% fall of blood level, starting 5 to 6 min prior to meal onset. The overall consequences of these findings are discussed.

LOUIS-SYLVESTRE, J. AND J. LE MAGNEN. Chez les rats se nourrissant librement, une chute de glycémie précède chaque repas. NEUROSCI. BIOBEHAV. REV. Suppl. 1, 13-15, 1980 - L'hypothèse selon laquelle la stimulation à manger ou éveil spécifique de faim a pur origine une chute de glucémie induite par le déficit périodique entre production hépatique et utilisation périphérique du glucose est ancienne. Cependant, jusqu'a present, les résultats de déterminations épisodiques de la glycémie, pratiquées au cours des intervalles interprandiaux, chez le rat se nourrissant ad libitum n'ont pas apporte de preuve directe. Une technique permettant une détermination continue, de longue durée, de la glycémie chez le rat se nourrissant librement a été mise au point. Son utilisation a permis de montrer que 5 à 6 minutes avant tout repas, diurne ou nocturne, se produit une chute de glycémie de 6 à 8%.

Pre-prandial blood glucose decrease Blood glucose level

ALL the energy used by animals is ultimately derived from the food they eat. While tissue metabolism requires continuous supplies of utilizable fuels, nutriments are ingested only during feeding episodes or meals. Thus, food intake serves to replenish various fuel reserves: ingested foods remaining in the gastrointestinal tract, liver glycogen or fat depots. It seems reasonable to assume that the internal stimulus to eat might be related to exhaustion of at least one of these reserves. The exact nature of this internal stimulus is still controversial: the importance of the role of glucopenia has long been suggested by the demonstration that different conditions of cytoglycopenia produced for example by the administration of insulin [5,9,10,12,14,17,] or 2-deoxy-D-glucose [3,4,15,16,18,20] or by diabetes [1] led to an increase in feeding.

Since the essential goal of research in this field is to account for normal spontaneous eating, it seemed appropriate to investigate the evolution of metabolic parameters along with the concomitant time patterning of meals in undisturbed free-feeding animals. In a recent study, Strubbe et al. [19] measured blood glucose (BG) and plasma immunoreactive insulin (IRI) during meals and during meal-to-meal intervals in the rat. To determine these parameters under normal conditions they took blood samples at 20 min intervals as long as the rat did not begin to eat. After the start of the meal (time zero) samples were taken at +5,+15, +25 min etc... All the determinations falling within 5±4 min before

Louis-Sylvestre J, Le Magnen J. A fall in blood glucose level precedes meal onset in free-feeding rats. Neurosci Biobehav Rev. 1980;4:13-15.

time zero were pooled and called the level of glucose or IRI at -5 min. With this method, they found that in the pre-meal period, there was no decrease in the BG level and that the insulin level was lower than at any other time.

In the present work, a sensitive method of continuous in vivo determination of BG was used, and it was found that every meal was preceded by a decrease in BG.

METHOD

Male Wistar rats (300-350 g) were housed individually and maintained under a 12 hr dark-light cycle with lights on at 12 a.m. for the first group of animals, and 12 p.m. for the second group. The cages were equipped with a food-cup weighing device which permitted the continuous recording of food intake.

The rats were surgically implanted with both a Y-shaped cardiac (see below) and a femoral vein catheter. The ends of the catheters terminated in stainless steel tubes fixed on the rats' head. Five days were allowed for recovery. To allow a longer lasting efficiency of the catheters, the rats were infused continuously (except during the experiment) via both catheters with a sodium chloride (9%) and geparin (15 U/ml) solution at a rate of 40 ul/hr. The infusion device (double swivel joint) was set so as to allow the rats complete freedom of movement in their home cages.

BG level was measured by means of a glucose-oxidase method using a Technicon Autoanalyzer (GOD PAP method Boehringer). The temporal resolution was 30 sec for 10% changes. The recording noise never exceeded 1.25%, with standard glucose and 2.6% with rat blood.

The glucose analyzer and pen recorder were set so that a 10mg/100ml difference was translated into a pen deviation of 15 mm.

The mean time course of the blood glucose was obtained by averaging continuous individual curves. The standard error of the mean (SEM) was calculated for selected times. The Mann-Whitney U Test was used for statistical evaluation.

For this study, it was important to obtain a continuously uncoagulated sample of blood without a general heparinization of the animal. As it is well known, heparin interferes with lipid metabolism and we observed that general heparinization abolished food intake. The Y-shaped cardiac catheter had two long side branches and a very short common branch (3mm) at the cardiac end. It allowed an inward infusion of a heparin solution (10000 U/ml) at a rate of 1 μl/min, and outward withdrawal of uncoagulated blood at a rate of 25 μl/min.

In order to extend the recording period and to increase the physiological relevance of the results, it was important to avoid the stress due to loss of blood. So, concomitantly with the blood sampling, a continuous transfusion (15 ul/min) of fresh decalcified (1.5 mg/ml EDTA) rat blood was performed via the femoral catheter.

Procedure

At the time of the experiment, the ends of the rats' catheters were connected via long tygon tubes to the corresponding calibrated tubes of a proportioning pump These tubes allowed the rats freedom to move and feed. Each animal underwent only one long-lasting blood glucose determination. It was begun one hour before the lights were turned on or off and lasted between 3 and 5 hours.

RESULTS

In free-feeding undisturbed rats, when food intake and blood glucose level were recorded simultaneously and continuously, a preprandial, a prandial and an inter-prandial phase could by distinguished and examined.

No statistical difference between the day and the night could be detected in any characteristic of the three phases, so the results were pooled.

A fall in blood glucose preceded each meal; it began some five minutes (5±0.3 min) before the meal and continued for three minutes after the start of the meal. Whatever the size of the meal, the fall was identical (6.5%). From the initial level of the inter-prandial phase, which was 92±2 mg/100 ml, the lowest value obtained at the end of the progressive decrease was 86 mg/100 ml (see Fig.1). Then, during the prandial episode, the blood glucose level increased. Whatever the size of the meal. the peak value was identical: 109±0.4 mg/100 ml, and was reached 17±0.5 min after the beginning of the meal. The BG level then decreased and reached the inter-prandial level some 40 min (41±1 min) after the beginning of the meal. After that, some oscillations usually occurred.

The descending portion of the prandial blood glucose curve had an inflexion point and, in each record, two different BG disappearance rates could be evaluated by the Conard's K coefficient. the first part lasted about 8 min and was found to be different according to the size of the meal: K=2.2±0.3 on the average for meals larger than 2 g (2.8±0.2 g; n=7) and K=1.7±0.2 for the smaller meals (1.5±0.2 g; n=8). No such difference was seen for the second part, which lasted about 16 min: K=0.85±0.1.

Between prandial episodes, the blood glucose level remained at a constant level in all rats. It was 92± 2mg/100 ml (n=15) during the night and 91±2mg/100 ml (n=12) during the day (N.S.). Random variations never exceeded 5.7%.

DISCUSSION

The prominent finding of this work is the observation of a fall in BG preceding each meal by 5 to 6 min in the night as well as in the day.

In rats maintained in a 12 hr dark-light cycle and in a steady state condition, the observation of the night and day periodicity of meals and intermeal intervals led to the conclusion that the meal-to-meal periodicity is modulated by a superimposed 12 hr mechanism. It is now well established that a neuroendocrine metabolic pattern is the basis of the nocturnal energy storage and diurnal energy mobilization and utilization. This pattern involves: hyperinsulinemia, increased rate of glucose utilization, lipogenesis and glycogen storage in the night period, and hypoinsulinemia, glucose intolerance, lipolysis and glycogenolysis during the day. A meal usually provides the animal with nutriments in amounts that far exceed its immediate requirement. Because of the large capacity of the gastro-intestinal tract and the relatively slow absorption of metabolites, the length of time during which metabolites are provided by a feeding bout extends well beyond the meal itself. According to the time of day, ingested fuels are utilized in a different manner. At night, the neuroendocrine conditions are such that the absorbed fuels cover the current metabolic requirements and the need for storage. During the day, the absorbed metabolites are added to the metabolic fuels mobilized from internal reserves; both sources are utilized to cover the metabolic requirements.

In a recent experiment [7], it was shown that at night, in rats, an increment in liver glycogen occurs from meal to meal. So liver glycogen, just like fat, is stored during the night and mobilized during the day. Therefore, the only reserve to be involved in meal periodicity is the gastrointestinal content. A fall in blood glucose level is induced by the failure of gepatic glucose production to match the peripheral glucose uptake; so the pre-prandial BG decrease might be due to the exhaustion of the intestinal supply to the portal vein and to its consequences on the hepatic glucose discharge into the general circulation. This assumption could be verified easily by a "continuous" determination of the portal vein BG from meal to meal.

The occurrence of a BG decrease before each meal does not necessarily demonstrate that it per se is the internal stimulus to eat. It might not by the true signal but rather is consequence. An increase in insulin level or a decrease in glucagon level could be candidates as true signals from which the BG decrease would result. These hypotheses are highly doubtful since it is well demonstrated that insulin secretion diminishes while glucagon secretion increases as the gastro-intestinal tract empties [2,11]. If the pre-prandial BG decrease is the source of the actual signal, then either hypoinsulinemia or hyperglucagonemia could be candidates. Recent experiments from Strubbe et al. [19] do not support the view that under normal ad lib condition, insulin provides and important signal for the initiation of feeding.

Evidence outlined in the overview of this volume [6] supports the notion that a neuronal network, including the LH area as a critical site, is involved exclusively in the feeding mechanism. Moreover, it has been shown [13] that the glucosensitive by insulino-independent sites in the LH area. These sites would respond by activating the efferent motor program of eating.

As a whole, the prandial hyperglycemic episode which is identical by night and day does not seem to vary according to the amount eaten. It is noteworthy that the maximum level of Bg is reached before the end of the meals which are somewhat larger than 2.5 g in size. However, the initial descending phase of the hyperglycemic phenomenon varies in slope as a function of meal size. This could be related to the amount of insulin secreted during the meal and more precisely during the preabsorptive period. It has been shown recently [8] that the preabsorptive insulin release varies as a function of the differential palatability of foods as measured by the amount eaten until satiation.

From the end of the prandial hyperglycemic episode, until the following pre-prandial BG decrease, the BG level was found strikingly constant. Therefore, it should be proposed to replace the notion of basal or resting BG level with the notion of an euglycemia represented by the BG level regulated accurately in the interprandial intervals. The present finding points out, once more, the accuracy of the short-term regulation of BG level (see[6]). This regulation is insured by well known internal mechanisms involving insulin and glucagon secretions. Another agent of this regulation might be a somatostatin induced modulation of the rate of absorption. In a recent paper, Unger et al. [20] hypothesized that a possible role for somatostatin secreted by D cells in the islets could be to adjust precisely the rate of metabolite absorption to the rate of the current metabolite needs. Moreover, the possible modulation of the absorption rate by metabolic requirements via somatostatin (in conjunction with the slower glucose uptake) could explain the lengthening of intermeal-intervals during the day. The mobilization of glucagon and fat stores could decrease the need for nutriments from the intestinal reserve. By contrast, at night, absorption could be accelerated by an increased need for nutriments due to both immediate and storage needs.

REFERENCES

1. Booth, D.A. Some characteristics of feeding during streptozotocin-induced diabetes in the rat. J. comp. physiol. Psychol. 80:238-249, 1972.
2. Cahill, G.F. Hormone-fuel interrelationships during fasting. J. Clin. Invest. 45:1751-1769, 1966.
3. Houpt, T. R. and H. E. Hance. Stimulation of food intake in the rabbit and rat by inhibition of glucose metabolism with 2-deoxy-D-glucose. J.comp. physiol. psychol. 76:395-400, 1971.
4. Jones, R. G. and D. A. Booth. Dose-response for 2-deoxy-D-glucose induced feeding peripheral factors. physiol. behav. 15:85-90.
5. Larue-Achagiotis, C. and J. Le Magnen. The different effects of continuous night and day-time insulin infusion on the meal pattern of normal rats: comparison with the meal pattern of hyperphagic hypothalamic rats. physiol. Behav. 22:435-439,1979.
6. Le Magnen, J. The body energy regulation: the role of the three brain responses to glucopenia. Neurosci. biobehav.Rev.4 Suppl. 1, 65-72, 1980.
7. Le Magnen, J. and M. Devos. Parameters of the meal pattern in rats: Their assessment and physiological significance. Neurosci. Biobehav. Rev. 4: Supple 1, 1-11, 1980.
8. Louis-Sylvestre, J. and J Le Magnen. Palatability and preabsorptive insulin release. Neurosci. Biobehav. Rev.4: Suppl.1, 43-46, 1980.
9. Lotter, E. C. and S. C. Woods. Injections of insulin and changes of bodyweight. physiol. behav. 18:293-298, 1977.
10. MacKay, E.M., J. W. Callaway and R. H. Barnes. Hyperalimentation in normal animals produced by protamine insulin. J . Nutr. 20: 59-66, 1940.
11. Marliss, E. B., T. T. Aoki, R. H. Unger, J. S. Soeldner and G. F. Cahill. Glucagon levels and metabolic effects in fasting man. J. clin. Inves. 49:2256-2270, 1097.
12. May, K.K. and J.R. Beaton. Hyperphagia in th einsulin-treated rats. Proc. Soc. exp. Biol. Med. 127: 1201-1204, 1968.
13. Oomura, Y. Significance of glucose, insulin and free fatty acid on the hypothalamic feeding and satiety neurons. In:Hunger: Basic Mechanisms and Chemical Implications., edited by D. Novin, W. Wyrwicka and G. Bray, New York: Raven Press, 1976, pp.145-158.
14. Panksepp, J. A., K. Pollack, R. Krost, R. Meerer and M. Ritter. Feeding in response to repeated protamin zinc insulin injections. Physiol. Behav.14:487-594, 1975
15. Rezek, M. and E. A. Kroeger. Glucose antimetabolites and hunger(theoretical article). J. Nutr. 106:143-157, 1976.
16. Smith, G. P. and A. N. Epstein. Increased feeding in response to decreased glucose utilization in the rat and monkey. Am. J Physiol. 217:1083-1087.
17. Steffens, A. B. The influence of insulin injections and infusions on eating blood glucose level in the rat. Physiol. Behav. 4:823-828, 1969.
18. Stricker, E.M. and N. Rowland. Hepatic versus cerebral origin of stimulus for feeding induced by 2-deoxy-D-glucose in rats. J. comp. physiol. Psychol. 92:126-132, 1978.
19. Strubbe, J. H., A. B. Steffens and L. DeRuiter. Plasma insulin and the time pattern of feeding in the rat. Physiol. Behav. 18: 81-86, 1977.
20. Thompson, D. A. and R. G. Campbell. Metabolic hormonal and gehavioral correlates of 2-deoxy-D-glucose induced experimental hunger in man. 59th A. Meeting of the Endocrine Soc. Abstract n 108, 1977.
21. Unger, R.H., R. E. Dobbs and L. Orci. Insulin, glucagon and somatostatin secretion in the regulation of metabolism. A. Rev. Physiol. 40:307-343, 1978.

Relationship Between Serum Amino Acid Concentration and Fluctuations in Appetite[1]

Sherman M. Mellinkoff, Marjorie Frankland, David Boyle and Margaret Greipel
From the Department of Medicine, School of Medicine, University of California Medical Center, and Wadsworth Veterans Administration Center, Los Angeles, California

A number of observations suggest that amino acid metabolism may have something to do with the regulation of hunger. If amino acid solutions are infused too rapidly, anorexia or nausea may appear (1, 2), and gastric peristalsis has been found to cease during the intravenous administration of amino acids (3). In this laboratory measurements of the serum amino acid and blood sugar concentrations have been made under a variety of circumstances (4, 5). Simultaneously, crude estimations of appetite have been attempted.

Method

Just before each blood sample was taken the subject was asked whether or not he was 'hungry.' An attempt was made to interpret his response according to the following scale: nauseated, minus I; no desire for food, 0; might eat if offered food, but not very hungry, I plus; ravenous, 4 plus; and 2 plus and 3 plus graded between I plus and 4 plus.

In all of the experiments reported here the subjects were either normal volunteers or patients with no disease known to affect protein or carbohydrate metabolism. In *experiment I* nine subjects ate a standard breakfast containing approximately 20 gm of protein: two eggs, a glass of milk and a piece of toast. Venous blood was collected in the fasting state and at hourly intervals after the breakfast for 4 hours. The serum amino acid nitrogen concentration of each blood sample was determined in duplicate by the method of Albanese and Irby as previously described (4). The standard deviation in 230 such pairs was 0.16 mg%.

In *experiment II,* with II subjects, 500 cc of 5% amino acids and 5% glucose[2] were infused in 45 minutes. Blood specimens were obtained in the fasting state and at hourly intervals for a period of 4 hours after the beginning of the infusion. In five instances blood samples were also obtained ½ hour after the start of the infusion. Serum amino acid nitrogen was determined as described above, and the blood sugar concentration of each sample was determined by the Mattice modification of the Folin-Wu method (6). For 286 such paired determinations the standard deviation was 2.7 mg%.

In *experiment III,* with 13 subjects, 250 cc of a 10% aqueous solution of enzymatically digested casein[3] were infused in 45 minutes. Blood specimens were obtained immediately preceding the infusion and after the beginning of the infusion at the following intervals: 10 minutes, 30 minutes, 1 hour, 2 hours, 3 hours and 4 hours. Blood sugar concentration of each specimen was determined as described above, and serum amino acid concentration of each specimen, except those drawn at 10 and 30 minutes, was estimated as described above.

In *experiment IV* each of 13 subjects drank 250 cc of the same 10% amino acid mixture used in *experiment III.* Both serum amino acid nitrogen and blood sugar were estimated in the fasting state and at ½-hour intervals for 2 hours and for another 2 hours at 1-hour intervals.

Results

For a long time we were unable to decide how these data could best be analyzed. In fact, it seemed unlikely that such crude estimations of the desire to eat could be tabulated or pooled at all. Nevertheless, simple graphic representation of the data from individual subjects seemed usually to follow this pattern: in all four experiments the appetite diminished when the amino acid concentration rose, and when the amino acid concentration fell the appetite increased. This tendency is illustrated in figures 1 and 2. Unfortunately, blood sugar determinations were not made in

Received for publication August 29, 1955.

[1] This investigation was supported by a research grant from the United States Office of Naval Research, Contract Nonr-233(26).

[2] Five per cent Amigen and 5% glucose and 10% Amigen generously supplied by Mead Johnson and Co.

[3] Ten per cent Amigen generously supplied by Mead Johnson and Co.

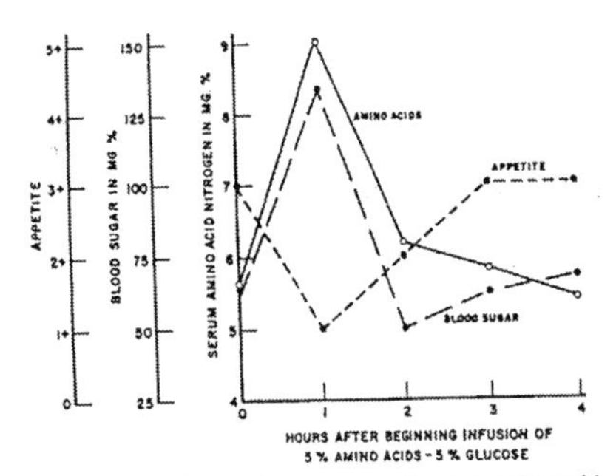

Figure 1: Appetite and blood sugar and serum amino acid concentrations in *JK* following infusion of 500 cc of distilled water containing 5% amino acids and 5% glucose in 45 min.

Table 1. Correlation between fluctuations in appetite and changes in serum amino acid and blood sugar concentrations

Exp.	r* for change in serum amino acid nitrogen conc. and in appetite	*P*	r* for change in blood sugar conc. and in appetite	*P*
1	−0.595	<0.01		
2	−0.405	<0.01	−0.318	<0.05
3	−0.509	<0.01	+0.232	<0.05
4	−0.526	<0.01	+0.297	<0.05

*Correlation coefficient.

experiment I (test meal), but in the three experiments in which the blood sugar concentration was measured there seemed again to be a general pattern (figs. 1 and 2): when amino acids were infused with glucose, the appetite appeared to vary inversely with both the amino acid and blood sugar concentrations, but when amino acids were administered alone, whether by mouth or by vein, the appetite appeared to vary inversely with the amino acid concentration but directly with the blood sugar.

There was considerable variation, however, from subject to subject, and not all of the appetite responses behaved in the manner described above.[4] Each individual's fasting 'appetite level' was arbitrarily called 0, and deviations from this point were measured in terms of the number of 'plusses' separating any subsequent 'appetite level' from the fasting one. Thus, if *subject 1* had been thought to be 2 plus hungry in the beginning, and 0 at 1 hour, the appetite level at 1 hour was called minus 2. In the same way each fasting amino acid and sugar concentration was called 0, and deviations from this point expressed in mg% plus or minus. Correlation coefficients were then calculated for the association of fluctuations in appetite with changes in the amino acid and sugar concentrations (table 1). There were statistically significant negative correlations between changes in the serum amino acid nitrogen concentration and appetite in all four experiments. In *experiment II* (i.v. amino acids with glucose) there was a negative correlation between changes in the blood sugar concentration and the appetite, but in *experiments III* and *IV* (i.v. and oral amino acids) there was a positive correlation between changes in the blood sugar concentration and appetite. Some of these data are depicted in a scatter graph (fig. 3).[5]

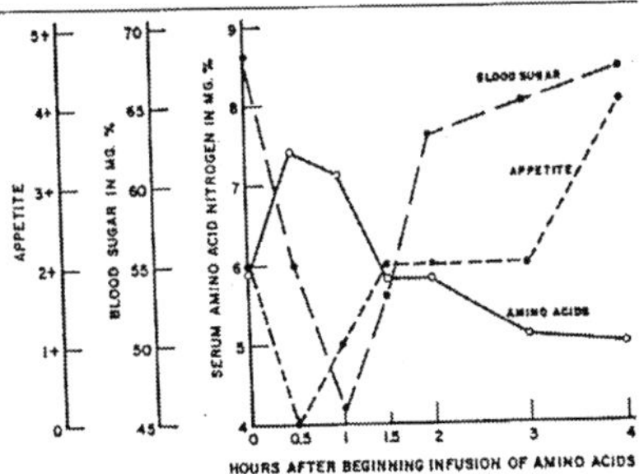

Figure 2: Appetite and blood sugar and serum amino acid concentrations in *AR* following infusion of 250 cc of 10% amino acids in 45 min.

Discussion

Whether induced by feeding of protein or of amino acids, or by infusing amino acid mixtures, a rise in the serum amino acid concentration appears to be accompanied by a waning of appetite. The subsequent increase of appetite

[4] We are indebted to Dr. Victor Hall for suggesting a method that proved helpful in the statistical analysis of all the data.

[5] Five additional figures have been deposited as document number 4767 with the ADI Auxiliary Publications Project, Photoduplication Service, Library of Congress, Washington 25, D.C. Copies may be secured by citing the document number and by remitting with the order $1.25 for photoprints, or $1.25 for 35 mm microfilm. Make checks or money orders payable to: Chief, Photoduplication Service, Library of Congress.

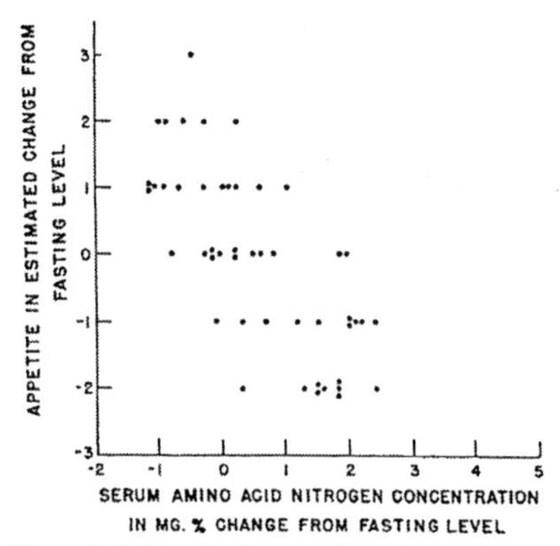

Figure 3: Relationship between change in appetite and change in serum amino acid concentration in 13 subjects following ingestion of 250 cc of 10% amino acids.

is accompanied by a fall in the amino acid concentration. Although the measurements of appetite were very rough and undoubtedly inaccurate, it seems unlikely that the correlations found here so consistently would have occurred by chance. Inaccuracy in measuring appetite would not of itself produce such correlations, unless the errors were somehow similar and consistent. The latter possibility seems very remote indeed, since almost all of the subjects knew nothing about the objectives of the study, nor were they in any way prejudiced as to the type of response expected.

When in *experiment I* it appeared that appetite varied in a direction opposite to the serum amino acid concentration, it seemed possible that factors responsible for appetite and the normal emptying of the stomach were correlated, and that the emptying of the stomach in turn regulated the rate at which protein was digested and absorbed as amino acids. If this hypothesis were correct, the amino acid blood level per se would have nothing to do with appetite. In *experiment II*, however, it became evident that intravenously induced amino acid blood levels were similarly related to appetite, and hence the emptying time of the stomach would not seem to be an essential factor in these relationships.

In *experiment II* (amino acid-glucose infusions) the appetite appeared to diminish with a high blood sugar concentration and to flourish with low blood glucose levels. Such an association was in keeping with classical ideas about the blood sugar and hunger (7). The correlation coefficient relating blood sugar and appetite was less (–0.318) than the correlation coefficient relating the serum amino acids to appetite (–0.405). Nevertheless, the possibility remained that the causal correlation was between the blood sugar and the appetite, and that the amino acids happened to wax and wane along with the sugar. To test this hypothesis a method was needed to make the blood sugar and the amino acids change in opposite directions.

This opportunity presented itself with the chance discovery that the infusion of amino acids created a reciprocal relationship between the serum amino acid and blood sugar concentrations (5). Accordingly, it was found in *experiments III* and *IV* that the administration of hydrolyzed casein by vein or by mouth diminished appetite as the amino acid concentration rose and the blood sugar fell. That the appetite should be at its nadir when the blood sugar concentration was low is particularly surprising because some of the blood sugars attained were below 40 mg% and produced signs of hypoglycemia, such as sweating, torpor and tachycardia. Similarly, the recovery of appetite was associated with a fall in the serum amino acids and a rise in the blood sugar.

These data by no means prove that the blood sugar has nothing to do with the control of appetite. Neither do they establish a causal relationship between the serum amino acid concentration and the appetite. As a matter of fact, it seems unlikely that the serum amino acid concentration per se is an important determinant of appetite because the fasting amino acid concentration does not reflect the degree of hunger. Diabetics, for example, have in general a relatively high fasting blood amino acid concentration (8), despite the well-known diabetic polyphagia. In hepatitis, a disease notorious for anorexia, the postprandial serum amino acid concentration is relatively low (4).

How, then, can these relationships be explained? Only further experiment can answer this question. At present one can only observe that after the consumption of protein some metabolic change associated with waxing and waning of the serum amino acid concentration appears to affect appetite, and that this effect seems to be independent of changes in the blood sugar concentration.

Summary

In normal volunteers and patients without diseases known to affect protein or carbohydrate metabolism crude estimations of appetite were correlated with the serum amino acid and blood sugar concentrations in four circumstances: *a*) after a 20-gm protein breakfast, *b*) after infusions of hydrolyzed casein and glucose, *c*) after infusions of hydrolyzed casein alone and *d*) after the ingestion of hydrolyzed casein. In all four experiments there was a reciprocal relationship between the serum amino acid concentration and appetite. A similar relationship between the blood sugar concentration and appetite was found after infusions of glucose and hydrolyzed casein, but the administration of hydrolyzed casein alone caused the blood sugar concentration and the appetite to diminish simultaneously.

References

1. Smyth, C. J., A. G. Lasichak and S. Levy. *J. Clin. Investigation* 26: 439, 1947.
2. Learner, N., H. W. Robinson, E. M. Greisheimer and M. J. Oppenheimer. *Gastroenterology* 5: 201, 1945.
3. Crider, R. J. and S. M. Walker. *Arch. Surg.* 57: 10, 1948.
4. Mellinkoff, S. M., D. J. Jenden and M. Frankland. *Arch. Int. Med.* 94: 604, 1954.
5. Mellinkoff, S. M., M. Frankland, D. Boyle and M. Greipel. *Stanford M. Bull.* 13: 117, 1955.
6. Lauber, F. V. and M. R. Mattice. *J. Lab. & Clin. Med.* 29: 113, 1944.
7. Bard, P. *Macleod's Physiology in Modern Medicine.* St. Louis: Mosby, 1941, p. 960.
8. Peters, J. P. and D. D. Van Slyke. *Quantitative Clinical Chemistry.* Baltimore: Williams & Wilkins, 1946, p. 806.

CLASSICS IN OBESITY

Neuropeptide Y Stimulates Feeding but Inhibits Sexual Behavior in Rats*

John T. Clark,† Pushpa S. Kalra, and Satya P. Kalra
Department of Obstetrics and Gynecology, University of Florida College of Medicine, Gainesville, Florida 32610

Abstract

The effects of neuropeptide Y (NPY), a tyrosine-rich peptide found in the rat brain, on feeding and sexual behavior were studied in male and female rats. Intraventricular (ivt) injections of NPY during the final hours of the light period induced feeding in a dose-related manner. While the lowest dose tested (0.02 nM) was without effect, higher doses (0.12, 0.47, 2.3 nM) uniformly elicited feeding with a latency of about 15 min in male rats. With the most effective dose, 0.47 nM, the increased food intake was due to an increased local eating rate. In contrast, the pattern of feeding behavior after a related peptide, rat pancreatic polypeptide (rPP), was quite different and less impressive. During the first hour, only one ivt dose of rPP (0.45 nM) evoked an increase in food intake, due to an increased time spent eating. Further, the effects of NPY on food intake were greater during the nocturnal period. Interestingly, increased food intake in nocturnal tests (4 h) was due solely to augmented intake during the first 60 min after ivt administration.

In mating tests, initiated 2 h after the onset of darkness and 10 min after ivt administration of peptide, all but the lowest dose of NPY (0.01 nM) drastically suppressed ejaculatory behavior. Most rats treated with higher doses of NPY (0.02, 0.12, or 0.47 nM) mounted and intromitted only a few times before the cessation of sexual activity, and elongated latencies to the initial mount and intromission were observed. In contrast to the dramatic NPY-induced suppression of ejaculatory behavior, rPP (0.11 and 0.45 nM) was without effect on copulatory behavior. To substantiate further that the impairment of sexual behavior seen in NPY-treated rats was not due to an attenuated sexual ability, an additional experiment was performed. Penile reflexes, including erection, were monitored 10 min after ivt injection of NPY (0.12 nM), rPP (0.11 nM), or saline. No effect of NPY or rPP was observed on the proportion of rats showing erection or latency to initial erection, or in the number of erections per test. In fact, a slight facilitation of penile dorsiflexion responses was seen after NPY. These findings suggest that NPY selectively depresses sexual motivation in the male rat.

In ovariectomized female rats responding to estrogen plus progesterone with a good level of sexual receptivity (lordosis quotient > 70), ivt saline and 0.01 nM NPY were without effect on sexual behavior. However, higher doses of NPY (0.12 and 0.47 nM) promptly suppressed sexual behavior in tests initiated 10 min after treatment. A significant 50% decrement in receptivity and a virtual elimination of proceptive behavior were observed. Further, although a low level of mounting (one to five mounts in 15 min) was seen in both the saline (33% mounting) and the 0.01 nM NPY (38% mounting) treated groups, none was observed in animals treated with the higher NPY doses. These observations indicate that NPY may also suppress female sexual behavior.

These studies demonstrate that NPY, a novel hypothalamic peptide, stimulates feeding in male rats in both diurnal and nocturnal tests and suppresses sexual behavior in male and female rats. We suggest that NPY may be an endogenous neurochemical signal that decreases sexual motivation and subsequently increases the appetite for food in the rat. (*Endocrinology* 117: 2435–2442, 1985)

Although it is commonly recognized that disorders of feeding behavior are associated with altered reproductive function and behavior (1–9), convincing experimental evi-

Received May 20, 1985.
*Presented in part at the Washington Spring Symposium, Neural and Endocrine Peptides and Receptors '85, Washington DC, May 1985 (Exps 1, 2, and 4) and the 67th Annual Meeting of the Endocrine Society, Baltimore, MD, June 1985 (Exp 5).
This research was supported by NIH Grant HD-11362.
†Recipient of NIH Postdoctoral Fellowship HD-06660.
Adapted from the *Endocrinology* 1985;117(6):2435–2422.

dence to support these clinical observations is lacking. However, a perusal of studies with laboratory animals indicates that feeding and sexual behavior may be inversely regulated (10–13). For example, a stimulation of feeding behavior is reported after treatment with adrenergic agonists (14,15) or opioid peptides (16,17) in doses which elsewhere have been shown to inhibit sexual behavior (18–21). Despite this suggestive line of evidence and some degree of overlap in the anatomical disposition of the neural circuitries controlling the two behaviors (22,23), the possibility that a common neural system (or systems) may modulate these two basic appetitive behaviors has not been carefully explored.

Neuropeptide Y (NPY), a 36-amino acid peptide isolated from porcine brain (24), is also widely distributed in the rat brain (25–28). Extensive mapping of neural pathways by immunocytochemical techniques has revealed NPY-like immunoreactivity in diencephalic areas implicated in the regulation of feeding (25–27) and sexual (25,28) behaviors. Further, NPY has considerable amino acid sequence homology with other members of the pancreatic polypeptides (PP) family of hormones (29,30). We have recently reported that intraventricular (ivt) administration either of NPY or the closely related human PP (hPP) increased feeding in ovarian steroid-pretreated ovariectomized (31) and intact (32) rats. We reasoned that if overeating and sexual behaviors are inversely related then NPY should attenuate sexual performance. This report describes in detail the effects of NPY and the structurally related rat pancreatic peptide (rPP) on feeding and sexual behaviors in normal male rats, and of NPY on female sexual behavior, in an attempt to uncover a possible underlying commonality in the neural mechanisms integrating sexual and feeding behaviors.

Materials and Methods

Adult male and female Sprague-Dawley rats [Charles River Breeding Laboratories, Wilmington, MA; CRL:CD[(R)] (SD)BR] were maintained in wire bottom cages under controlled light (lights on, 1100–0100 h) and temperature (22–23 C) with ad libitum access to food and water. All animals were implanted with permanent cannulae in the third cerebral ventricle of the brain under pentobarbital anesthesia (40 mg/kg) (31,33). Female rats were ovariectomized immediately after the implantation of ivt cannulae. On the day of the experiment only those rats which displayed efflux of cerebrospinal fluid were used for the experiments. NPY (porcine) and rPP were obtained commercially from Peninsula Laboratories, Inc. (Belmont, CA). Peptide purity varied from 72–77% for NPY (porcine) and was 88% for rPP.

Exp 1: effects of ivt NPY and rPP on daytime feeding behavior in male rats

Eleven to 13 days after implantation of ivt cannulae, food and water were removed at 0800–0830 h. One hour later, the effects of ivt injection of saline (3 μl), NPY (0.02, 0.12, 0.47, or 2.3 nM), or rPP (0.11 and 0.45 nM) in saline were assessed. Immediately after injection, rats were returned to their home cages where a preweighed amount of rat chow was placed. The rats were continuously observed for 60 min. From the record, together with the food weighing, the following parameters were derived: total food intake (grams), latency to initial feeding response (minutes), total time eating (minutes), local eating rate (grams per min, an index of food consumed per unit time spent eating), and total time spent grooming (minutes). Additionally, the number of animals displaying feeding behavior during the first 60-min period and in the subsequent period from 60–120 min and cumulative food intake during the entire 120 min were recorded.

Exp 2: effects of ivt NPY on nocturnal feeding in male rats

In this experiment, 11–13 days after ivt cannulae implantation, food and water were removed 1 h before lights off (1000 h). Two hours later, animals were injected with either NPY (0.12 nM or 0.47 nM) or saline. Immediately after injection, rats were returned to their home cages which contained a known amount of rat chow. Water was freely available, although no attempt was made to quantify water intake. Food intake was determined by weighing the remaining food along with the spillage at 30, 60, 90, 120, and 240 min after injection.

Exp 3: effects of NPY and rPP on male rat sexual behavior

All males were tested for the expression of male sexual behavior before ivt cannula implantation. Copulatory test consisted of exposure to a receptive female (receptivity induced by 100 μg estradiol benzoate followed 48 h later by 500 μg progesterone and verified using nonexperimental male rats and monitoring all mounts, intromissions, and ejaculations. Measurements derived from the record were: mount and intromission latencies (ML, IL), time from introduction of the female to the initial mount or intromission; ejaculation latency (EL), time from initial intromission to ejaculation; postejaculatory interval (PEI), time from ejaculation to the subsequent intromission; and mount and intromission frequencies (MF, IF), the number of mounts and intromissions preceding ejaculation. Additionally, a measure of intromissive success, or copulatory efficacy, was calculated as IF/(MF + IF) (18). Tests were terminated if intromission did not occur within 30 min of female introduction, EL exceeded 30 min, PEI exceeded 15 min, or immediately after the postejaculatory intromission. Copulatory tests were initiated 2 h after the onset of darkness and only rats that had ejaculated on three successive copulatory tests were used in this study.

Seven and 14 days after ivt implantation, rats were

again tested for the display of male copulatory behavior. Only those rats ejaculating on both these tests were used in the experiment thus males had at least five tests with ejaculation before ivt peptide administration. The effects of NPY (0.012, 0.024, 0.12, and 0.47 nM), rPP (0.11 and 0.45 nM), or saline (17 and 22 days after surgery) were determined in a counterbalanced design so that each rat received peptide and saline treatments and served as its own control. Copulatory tests were initiated 10 min after ivt injection of the peptide or saline.

Exp 4: effects of NPY or rPP on penile reflexes

In order to identify further whether the decreased sexual performance observed in Exp 3 was due to an imposed deficit in sexual motivation or sexual ability, an additional experiment was performed. Thirteen days after implantation of ivt cannulae, rats were injected with NPY (0.12 nM), rPP (0.11 nM), or saline (3 μl). Ten minutes later the rats were tested for the display of penile reflexes. The procedure for evoking and the criteria for scoring the penile reflex response were the same as previously described (34). Briefly, the rat was placed on its back and gently restrained in a clear plastic cylinder with the penile sheath retracted using a wooden applicator. All penile responses which occurred within 20 min of the first erection were scored as follows: erection—increased tumescence of the penis, partial or complete, with subsequent detumescence; cup—intense erection with flaring of the engorged glans penis; and flip—a dorsiflexion of the penis.

Exp 5: effects of NPY on female sexual behavior

Starting 2 weeks after cannulae implantation and ovariectomy, rats were injected sc with estradiol benzoate (100 μg) followed 48 h later by progesterone (500 μg) once a week. Basal levels of female sexual behavior were recorded in tests initiated 4 h after progesterone treatment. Once a good level of sexual receptivity was achieved [lordosis quotient (LQ) > 70] in basal tests, the effects of ivt NPY (0.012, 0.12, or 0.47 nM) or saline (3 μl) were assessed in behavioral tests initiated 10 min after ivt injection (and 5 h after progesterone treatment). Testing was conducted in plexiglass arenas (12 × 12 × 24 in) with a cage-adapted sexually vigorous male rat. Feminine sexual behavior was recorded until the male had mounted 10–15 times. The males were allowed occasional intromissions with a separate group of highly receptive females in order to maintain their sexual interest at a high level. The receptivity responses were expressed as an LQ (ratio of mounts to mounts eliciting lordosis × 100). Proceptive behavior (soliciting) was recorded on a scale of 0–2 as follows: 0, no proceptive behavior; 1, low level of proceptive behavior (hopping-darting or ear wiggles); or 2, moderate to high levels of proceptive behaviors. Similarly, rejection behavior (directed toward the male) was recorded as follows: 0, no rejection or evading the male; 1, a low level of rejection or avoidance; and 2, a moderate to high level of rejection and avoidance. Twenty minutes after the ivt injection of NPY or saline, a sexually receptive (nonexperimental) female was introduced into the behavioral arena containing the cage-adapted experimental female, and parameters of masculine sexual behavior were monitored for 15 min. The occurrence of each mount, intromissive pattern, and ejaculatory pattern were recorded on an Esterline-angus event recorder (Esterline Angus Instrument Corp., Indianapolis, IN), and the following parameters were calculated from the record: ML, IL, MF, IF, and total number of copulatory attempts (mounts + intromissions).

To assess a possible stimulatory effect of NPY on sexual behavior, female rats prepared as above but displaying low levels of sexual receptivity (mean LQ, 11.6 ± 3.8, n = 19) were used. Parameters of female sexual behavior were assessed in tests initiated 10 min after ivt injection of NPY (0.024 or 0.048 nM) or saline (3 μl). Tests were terminated after 10–15 mounts by the male, with a different male substituted whenever more than 2 min elapsed between successive mounts. Mounting behavior was assessed as above.

Statistical analyses

Feeding behavior. Data are presented as mean ± SEM and are given only for those animals initiating feeding. The number of rats initiating feeding was evaluated using the Fisher exact probability test (comparing to saline-treated rats), and the parameters of feeding behavior were evaluated by Dunnett's tests (comparison with a common control) followed by Mann-Whitney U tests. Comparisons of food intake were made for discrete time intervals after ivt injection as well as for cumulative food intake.

Male sexual behavior. Data are presented as mean ± SEM and were analyzed by Friedman two-way analysis of variance (comparing pretest to peptide and saline tests) followed by post hoc Wilcoxon matched pairs-signed ranks tests. The proportion of males mounting, intromitting and ejaculating, or showing penile reflexes were evaluated using the McNemar test for significance of changes. Penile reflex data were evaluated using the Mann-Whitney U test to compare peptide to saline values.

Female sexual behavior. The data were analyzed in two ways: results of 4-h tests (basal) were compared to results of 5-h tests using Wilcoxon matched pairs-signed ranks tests; and further, results of 5-h tests were compared for peptide and saline groups using Dunnett's test (comparison with a control) followed by post hoc Mann-Whitney U tests.

Results

NPY potently stimulates diurnal feeding in male rats

NPY evoked feeding in a dose-related manner with 100% of the rats eating in the first hour after injection of 0.47 or 2.3 nM (Fig. 1a) with a latency to onset of feeding varying between 12–15 min (Fig. 1c). Cumulative food in-

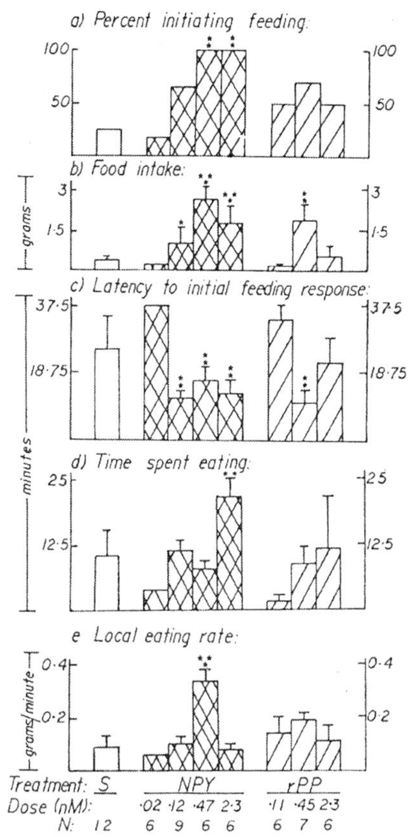

Fig. 1. Effect of ivt administration of NPY, rPP, or saline on feeding behavior of adult male rats in the 60-min after treatment. Panel a): ★★, $P < 0.025$, Fisher exact probability test compared to saline-treated rats; panel b): ★, $P < 0.05$; ★★★, $P < 0.01$, Mann-Whitney U test; panel c): ★★, $P < 0.025$, Mann-Whitney U test; panel d): ★★★, $P < 0.01$, Mann-Whitney U test; panel e): ★★★, $P < 0.01$, Mann-Whitney U test.

take during the first hour was enhanced by NPY with a dramatic response apparent at 0.47 nM (Fig. 1b), which appears to be due solely to an increased local eating rate (Fig. 1e). Although a similar increment in food intake was seen after 2.3 nM, this increase was apparently due to increased time spent eating (Fig. 1d) and not an increase in local eating rate (Fig. 1e). The pattern of feeding behavior elicited by rPP was quite different and less impressive. During the first hour, only a single dose of rPP (0.45 nM) evoked an increase in food intake, with a latency to response equivalent to that seen after 0.47 or 2.3 nM NPY (Fig. 1). Interestingly, by the second hour all rats treated with a lower dose of NPY (0.12 nM) and rPP (0.11 and 0.45 nM) displayed feeding, and significant increases in cumulative food intake were seen (Table 1).

Effects of NPY on nocturnal feeding

NPY induced increased food intake in a dose-related manner over that normally seen during the initial hours of darkness (Fig. 2). This NPY-induced stimulation of nocturnal feeding occurs mainly during the first 30 min after ivt injection (Fig. 2A), although cumulative food intake is elevated for at least 4 h (Fig. 2B).

Effects of NPY or rPP on male copulatory behavior

Doses of NPY which evoked feeding (Fig. 1) produced a dramatic suppression of male copulatory behavior (Fig. 3). Although the majority of rats mounted, fewer intromitted and only a few ejaculated in mating tests initiated 10 min after the ivt injection of 0.02, 0.12, or 0.47 nM NPY. All rats ejaculated in control tests, and most ejaculated after the lowest dose of NPY (0.012 nM). This low dose of NPY had no effect on any of the parameters of male copulatory behavior, while the higher doses significantly increased ML and IL (Fig. 3). The suppression of ejaculatory behavior was apparently not due to the increased latency to initiate copulation since in most rats that displayed mounting or intromissive behavior (but failed to ejaculate), all sexual activity ceased after one to five mounts within 5 min after the initial

TABLE 1. Cumulative food intake for the 2-h period after ivt administration of NPY and rPP

	Intake during interval from 60–120 min after ivt injection (g)	Cumulative 2-h intake (g)
Saline	0.39 ± 0.12	0.60 ± 0.19
NPY (nM)		
0.02	0.13 ± 0.04	0.19 ± 0.05
0.12	0.36 ± 0.18	0.94 ± 0.33[a]
0.47	1.32 ± 0.36[a]	3.96 ± 0.23[a]
2.3	1.00 ± 0.24[a]	2.74 ± 0.82[a]
rPP (nM)		
0.11	0.23 ± 0.08	0.29 ± 0.1
0.45	0.85 ± 0.24[a]	2.39 ± 0.48[a]
2.3	0.69 ± 0.15[b]	0.92 ± 0.27[b]

[a] $P < 0.01$ compared to saline.
[b] $P < 0.05$ compared to saline.

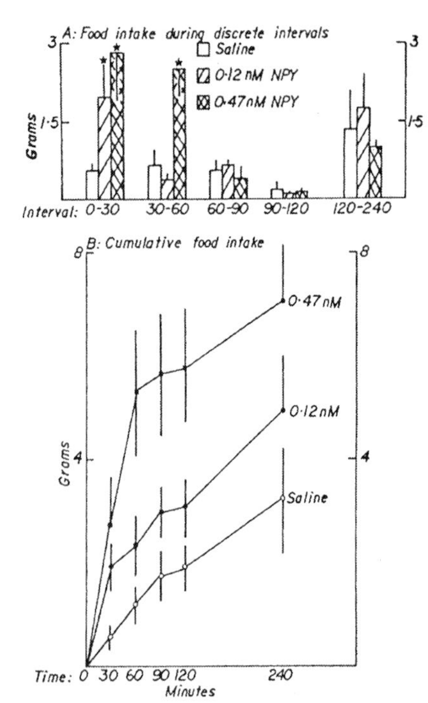

Fig. 2. Effects of ivt NPY or saline on nocturnal feeding in adult male rats. ★, 0.47 nM > 0.12 nM > saline, $P < 0.05$; ★★, 0.47 nM > 0.12 nM = saline, $P < 0.01$; A, 0.12 nM > saline, $P < 0.01$; B, 0.47 nM > saline $P < 0.01$; $n = 6$ per group. Cumulative food intake was significantly greater after NPY than after saline at each time point.

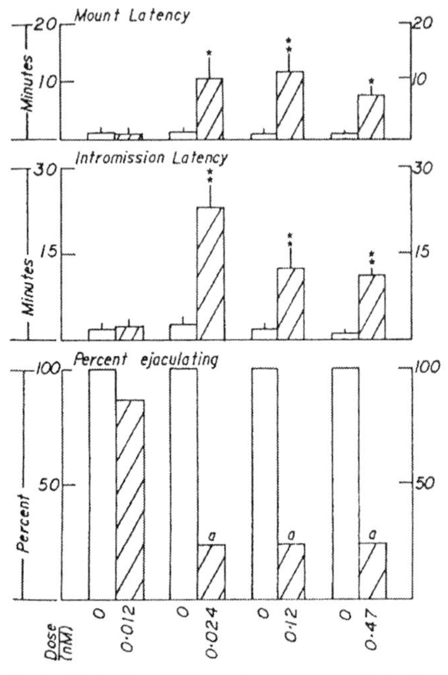

Fig. 3. Effects of ivt NPY or saline on mount and intromission latencies (in minutes) and on the number of males achieving ejaculation in tests initiated 10 min after injection [0 test (open bars) after saline injection, others (hatched bars) after various doses of NPY; ★, saline values are significantly lower than NPY values, $P < 0.05$; ★★, saline values are significantly lower than NPY values, $P < 0.01$; a, significantly fewer males ejaculated after NPY than after saline treatment, $P < 0.01$, $n = 7$ for 0.012 nM and $n = 9$ for 0.024, 0.12, and 0.47 nM].

copulatory act. Of the two males ejaculating after 0.024 nM NPY, one showed an increased and the other a decreased EL, whereas both showed increased MF, IF, and PEI and a reduced ejaculation frequency. Similar data were obtained from the males ejaculating after 0.12 nM ($n = 2$ of 9) or 0.47 nM ($n = 2$ of 9).

In marked contrast to the suppressive effects of NPY, there was no effect of rPP (0.11 or 0.45 nM) on any parameter of male rat copulatory behavior (Table 2).

Effect of NPY and rPP on penile reflexes

A dose (0.12 nM) of NPY, which stimulated feeding (Fig. 1) and suppressed sexual (Fig. 3) behavior, did not adversely affect penile reflex activity (Table 3). In fact, there was a significant increase in the number of cups and flips per test and a nonsignificant trend toward a decreased latency to the initial erection. A similar dose of rPP failed to significantly alter any parameter of reflexive activity (Table 3).

Effects of NPY on female sexual behavior

As depicted in Fig. 4, ivt administration of saline or 0.012 nM NPY did not affect either receptive or proceptive aspects of feminine sexual behavior. In fact, a slight in-

TABLE 2. Effects of ivt administration of rPP (0.11 or 0.45 nM) on male sex behavior

	rPP (0.11 nM)	Saline	rPP (0.45 nM)	Saline
Proportion of rats mounting	7/8	8/8	6/6	6/6
Proportion of rats intromitting	7/8	8/8	6/6	6/6
Propotion of rats ejaculating	7/8	8/8	6/6	6/6
ML (min)	1.6 ± 1.3	0.3 ± 0.08	0.9 ± 0.5	1.6 ± 1.2
IL (min)	3.8 ± 1.9	1.1 ± 0.6	1.1 ± 0.5	2.9 ± 1.8
EL (min)	10.2 ± 1.8	11.5 ± 1.7	6.3 ± 1.0	7.8 ± 1.7
PEI	6.4 ± 0.3	6.8 ± 0.5	5.6 ± 0.5	6.4 ± 0.6
Intercopulatory interval	0.53 ± 0.06	0.59 ± 0.07	0.60 ± 0.06	0.57 ± 0.11
MF	14.2 ± 2.9	14.7 ± 6.1	11.5 ± 1.7	13.0 ± 2.8
IF	19.3 ± 2.6	22.3 ± 4.2	9.5 ± 0.8	12.8 ± 1.2
Copulatory efficacy	0.59 ± 0.04	0.62 ± 0.04	0.47 ± 0.05	0.52 ± 0.04
Ejaculation frequency (in 30 min)	1.8 ± 0.2	2.0 ± 0.3	2.8 ± 0.3	2.5 ± 0.2

crease in receptivity was evident (comparing 4-h to 5-h tests; $P < 0.01$). Higher doses of NPY significantly suppressed receptivity and virtually eliminated proceptive behaviors (Fig. 4). Rejection behavior was not significantly affected, but a trend toward increased rejection rates was seen after the higher NPY doses (rejection scores of 0.83 ± 0.31 and 0.67 ± 0.31 for 0.47 and 0.12 nM NPY vs. 0.33 ± 0.20 for 0.12 nM NPY and saline-treated rats).

Although a low level of mounting (one to five mounts in 15 min) was seen in both the saline and 0.012 nM NPY-treated females (38% and 33% showed mounting behavior, respectively), none was observed in females treated with the higher NPY doses.

NPY (0.024 or 0.048 nM) did not improve the behavioral response of those female rats which displayed a low basal level of sexual behavior in previous tests (data not shown).

Discussion

These studies clearly show that NPY potently enhanced ingestive behavior in a dose-related manner in male rats. These observations corroborate our findings of stimulation of feeding in intact (32) and ovariectomized, steroid-treated female rats (31). In the present studies we also found that NPY was effective in stimulating feeding during the nocturnal period. The increments in cumulative food intake at the end of 4 h may be due to the dramatic increase in feeding shortly after NPY injection. In contrast to the effects of NPY, we found rPP less effective in stimulating feeding behavior. Thus, emerging evidence that NPY uniformly elicits vigorous feeding in ovariectomized steroid-treated females (31), intact female rats (32), and male rats, while two closely related members of the PP family of hormones, rPP and hPP (31), are far less effective, implies that NPY, or NPY-like peptide, discharged from the neuronal network (31–33) in critical areas of the rat brain may normally stimulate feeding behavior.

Additionally, we have now observed that NPY can drastically suppress male and female copulatory behavior in the rat. The decreased sexual performance of male rats after NPY administration was apparently due to an imposed deficit in sexual motivation since NPY produced no obvious adverse effect on penile reflexes, including erection, in ex copula tests. Thus, most males initiated mating but failed to sustain a sufficient level of sexual arousal to allow for the maintenance of full sexual performance until ejaculation. Further, NPY suppressed steroid-induced proceptive and receptive sexual behaviors in ovariectomized rats. The suppressive effects of NPY on sexual behavior in male and female rats and the relative ineffectiveness of rPP, as seen in males, suggest that NPY-containing neural elements may be

TABLE 3. Effects of ivt administration of 0.12 nM NPY, 0.11 nM rPP, or 3 μl saline on penile reflex activity

	NPY	rPP	Saline
Proportion of rats with erection	9/12	8/11	14/20
Latency to first erection[a]	5.0 ± 1.7	7.0 ± 1.0	7.4 ± 1.0
Number of erections per test[a]	20.0 ± 5.1	21.3 ± 2.2	22.8 ± 4.3
Number of cups per test[a,b]	1.3 ± 0.6[c]	0.3 ± 0.2	0.4 ± 0.3
Number of flips per test[a,b,d]	3.8 ± 1.3[c]	2.3 ± 0.8	0.8 ± 0.5

[a] Only values for those rats showing erection within 15 min of sheath retraction were used.

[b] Those rats showing erection, but failing to display cups or flips, were assigned a value of zero.

[c] NPY-treated rats showed significantly more cups and flips than did saline-treated rats ($P < 0.05$, Mann-Whitney U test).

[d] Number of flips is the number of quick flips plus long flips.

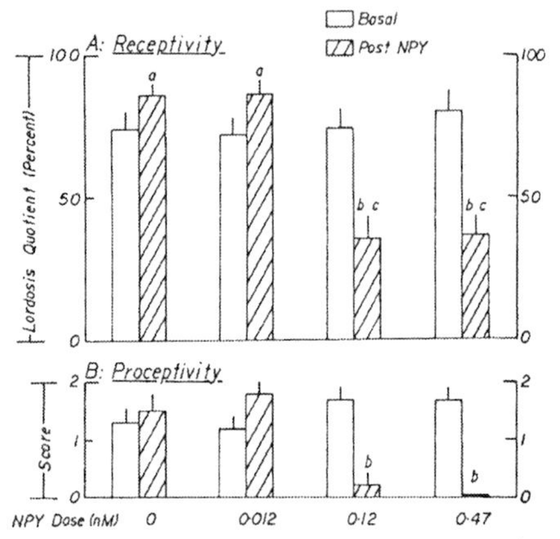

Fig 4. Effects of ivt administration of NPY on estrogen plus progesterone-induced sexual behavior in ovariectomized rats. Receptivity (A) is indicated by LQ and proceptivity (B) was scored by methods described in text. Basal tests were conducted 4 h after progesterone, and post-NPY tests were conducted 10 min after NPY (and 5 h after progesterone). a, Basal test values less than post-NPY test values, $P < 0.01$; b, basal test values greater than post-NPY test values, $P < 0.01$ c, 0.12 and 0.47 nM test values less than 0 or 0.012 nM test values; n = 8 for saline; n = 6 rats per NPY dose.

a component of the neuronal circuitry which terminates sexual behavior in both male and female rats.

Our observations also shed light on the commonality of NPY involvement in regulating the two behaviors. We have reported that NPY stimulated feeding behavior in steroid-primed ovariectomized rats (31). These observations, along with the current findings of suppression of female sexual behavior and the stimulation of diurnal and nocturnal feeding concomitant with suppression of sexual behavior in male rats, raise the intriguing possibility that NPY may be an endogenous neurochemical signal which simultaneously turns off the neural circuitry controlling sexual behavior and turns on the neural circuits that regulate appetite for food in both male and female rats. The two other members of the PP family of hormones, which have been tested to date, stimulate feeding to a lesser degree than NPY. Moreover, despite a high degree of amino acid sequence homology between NPY and rPP, we did not observe overlapping effect of these peptides on male sexual behavior. Thus, it seems that either a unique amino acid sequence(s) and/or a conformational change in the NPY molecule imparts such profound, discriminating effects on the two behaviors.

A comparison of the behavioral effects and endocrine effects (31–33, 35,36) of NPY revealed a marked difference in the threshold of responsiveness. We observed that low doses of NPY (0.02 nM in males and 0.12 nM in females) were highly effective in suppressing sexual behavior, primarily (in the male at least) by suppressing sexual motivation. On the other hand, higher doses were needed to evoke maximal feeding and LH release responses (33,35,36). A low threshold of sexual response to NPY implies that, normally, sexual motivation must be suppressed in order for feeding to occur. These derivations are especially interesting in light of the reported hierarchical organization of behaviors, with sexual behavior normally taking precedence over feeding (37). In food-deprived male rats given simultaneous access to a sexually receptive female and food, feeding has been observed to occur almost exclusively during periods when sexual arousal is decreased (38–40), as after ejaculation. Conversely, and in line with a few known clinical disorders (5–9), it has also been shown that transection of discrete neural pathways in the rat hypothalamus produces hyperphagia accompanied by markedly impaired copulatory behavior (41,42). While it is possible that hunger and sex may be subserved by separate drive systems (43–45), our studies are in accord with the view that acute stimulation by NPY of neural centers that enhance ingestive behavior may lead to decrements in sexual motivation.

The precise location of central NPY-sensitive neuronal elements involved in these behavioral responses is unknown. It is possible that there may be distinct anatomical sites of NPY action modulating the two behavior responses. Perhaps, they may be coextensive in areas which have been implicated in the regulation of these two basic behaviors. The hypothalamic paraventricular nucleus is thought to be of considerable significance in controlling ingestive behavior (46), and in line with our findings (31,32,35), local injection of NPY in that region stimulated feeding (47). However, since the latency to feeding (10–15 min) was similar after either ivt or local injection of NPY in the paraventricular nucleus, it is more likely that a complex interaction, possibly involving other neuronal systems, may underlie the action of NPY. On the other hand, evidence suggests that NPY neurons innervate the medial preoptic area and ventromedial nucleus (25–28), sites known to mediate the male and female sexual behaviors, (48,49). Further, sequential treatment of ovariectomized rats with estrogen plus progesterone effected decreases in NPY immunoreactivity in the preoptic area at a time when sexual behavior is maximal, suggesting that the effects of NPY on female sexual behavior may be mediated via an action in this area of the brain (50).

In conclusion, the present experiments clearly demonstrate that NPY potently stimulates feeding in male rats in both diurnal and nocturnal tests, whereas rPP is less effective, and that NPY suppresses sexual behavior in male and female rats. We, therefore, suggest that NPY may be an endogenous neurochemical signal that decreases sexual motivation and subsequently increases the appetite for food.

Acknowledgments

The excellent technical assistance of D.L. Heaton-Jones and S. Myrick, and the cheerful secretarial support of Ms. S.C. McDonnell are gratefully acknowledged.

References

1. Herzog DB, Norman DK, Gordon C, Pepose M 1984 Sexual conflict and eating disorders in 27 males. Am J Psychiatry 141:989
2. Margules DL 1984 Central and peripheral opioid peptides in learned helplessness; feeding, drinking and obesity, male and female running behavior; and immunocompetence. In: Muller EE, Genazzani AR (eds) Central and Peripheral Endorphins: Basic and Clinical Aspects. Raven Press, New York, p 203
3. Huhner M 1925 A Practical Treatise on the Disorders of the Sexual Function in the Male and Female. FA Davis Co, Philadelphia
4. Kennedy WP 1926 Diet and sterility. Physiol Rev 6:485
5. Kley HK, Deselaers T, Peerenboom H 1981 Evidence for hypogonadism in massively obese males due to decreased free testosterone. Horm Metab Res 13:639
6. Schneider G, Krischner MA, Berkowitz R, Ertel NH 1979 Increased estrogen production in obese men. J Clin Endocrinol Metab 48:633
7. Amatruda JM, Harman SM, Pourmotabbed G, Lockwood DH 1978 Depressed plasma testosterone and fractional binding of testosterone in obese males. J Clin Endocrinol Metab 47:268
8. Glass A, Swerdloff R, Bray G, Dahms W, Atkinson R 1977 Low serum testosterone and sex-hormone-binding-globulin in massively obese men. J Clin Endocrinol Metab 45:1211
9. Barbato AL, Landau RL 1974 Testosterone deficiency of morbid obesity. Clin Res 22:647A
10. Edmonds ES, Withyachumnarnkul B 1980 Sexual behavior of the obese male Zucker rat. Physiol Behav 24:1139
11. Withyachumnarnkul B, Edmonds ES 1981 Plasma testosterone levels and sexual performance of young obese male Zucker rat. Physiol Behav 29:773
12. Chelich AM, Edmonds ES 1981 Copulatory behavior and reproductive capacity of the genetically obese female Zucker rat. Physiol Behav 27:331
13. Stone CP, Ferguson L 1938 Preferential responses of male albino rats to food and to receptive females. J Comp Psychol 26:237
14. Leibowitz SF 1975 Role of alpha and beta receptors in mediating effects of hypothalamic adrenergic stimulation. Physiol Behav 14:743
15. Ritter S, Wise CD, Stein L 1975 Neurochemical regulation of feeding in the rat: facilitation by α-noradrenergic, but not dopaminergic, receptor stimulants. J Comp Physiol Psychol 88:778
16. Grandison L, Guidotti A 1977 Stimulation of food intake by muscinol and beta endorphin. Neuropharmacology 16:533
17. Morley JE, Levine AS, Yim GK, Lowy MT 1983 Opiod modulation of appetite. Neurosci Biobehav Rev 7:281
18. Clark JT, Smith ER, Davidson JM 1985 Evidence for the modulation of sexual behavior by α-adrenoceptors in male rats. Neuroendocrinology 41:36
19. McIntosh TK, Vallano MC, Barfield RJ 1980 Effects of morphine, β-endorphin and naloxone on catecholamine levels and sexual behavior in male rats. Pharmacol Biochem Behav 13:435
20. Meyerson BT 1981 Comparison of the effects of β-endorphin and morphine on exploratory and socio-sexual behavior in the male rat. Eur J Pharmacol 69:453
21. Svensson L, Hansen S 1984 Spinal monoaminergic modulation of masculine copulatory behavior in the rat. Brain Res 302:315
22. MacLean PD 1959 The limbic system with respect to two basic life principles. In: Brazier MAB (ed) The Central Nervous System and Behavior. Josiah Macy Foundation, New York, pp 31–118
23. Myers RD 1974 Handbook of Drug and Chemical Stimulation of the Brain: Behavioral, Pharmacologic and Physiological Aspects. Medical Economics (Division of Van Nostrand Reinhold Co), New York
24. Tatemoto K, Carlquist M, Mutt V 1982 Neuropeptide Y—a novel brain peptide with structural similarities to peptide YY and pancreatic polypeptide. Nature 296:659
25. Emson PC, DeQuidt ME 1984 NPY—a new member of the pancreatic polypeptide family. Trends Neurosci 7:31
26. Allen YS, Adrian TE, Allen JM, Tatemoto K, Crow TJ, Bloom SR, Polak JM 1983 Neuropeptide Y distribution in the rat brain. Science 221:877
27. Guy J, Allen YS, Polak JM, Pelletier G 1983 Immunocytochemical localization of neuropeptide Y (NPY) in the rat brain. Soc Neurosci Abstr 9:291
28. O'Donohue TL, Chronwall BM, Dimaggio DA 1983 Distribution of neuropeptide Y-like immunoreactivity in rat brain. Soc Neurosci Abst 9:290
29. Kimmel JR, Pollock HG, Hazelwood RL 1968 Isolation and characterization of chicken insulin. Endocrinology 83:1323
30. Lin T-M 1980 Pancreatic polypeptide: isolation, chemistry and biological function. In: Glass GBJ (ed) Gastrointestinal Hormones. Raven Press, New York, p 275
31. Clark JT, Kalra PS, Crowley WR, Kalra SP 1984 Neuropeptide Y and human pancreatic polypeptide stimulate feeding behavior in rats. Endocrinology 115:427
32. Clark JT, Kalra SP 1985 Neuropeptide Y (NPY)-induced feeding: comparison with rat pancreatic polypeptide (rPP), human NPY, and peptide YY (PYY) in male and female rats. Soc Neurosci Abstr 11:619
33. Kalra SP, Gallo RV 1983 Effects of intraventricular administration of catecholamines on luteinizing hormone release in morphine treated rats. Endocrinology 113:23
34. Davidson JM, Stefanick ML, Sachs BD, Smith ER 1978 Role of androgens in sexual reflexes of the male rat. Physiol Behav 21:14
35. Allen LG, Kalra PS, Crowley WR, Kalra SP 1985 Comparison of the effects of neuropeptide Y and adrenergic transmitters on LH release and food intake in male rats. Life Sci 37:617
36. Kalra SP, Crowley WR 1984 Norepinephrine-like effects of neuropeptide Y on LH release in the rat. Life Sci 35:1173

37. Hinde RA 1970 Animal Behavior. McGraw Hill, New York
38. Sachs BD, Marsan E 1972 Male rats prefer sex to food after 6 days of food deprivation. Psychonomic Sci 28:47
39. Sachs BD 1965 Sexual behavior of male rats after one to nine days without food. J Comp Physiol Psychol 60:144
40. Brown RE, McFarland DJ 1979 Interaction of hunger and sexual motivation in the male rat: a time-sharing approach. Anim Behav 27:887
41. Paxinos G, Bindra D 1973 Hypothalamic and midbrain pathways involved in eating, drinking, irritability, aggression and copulation in rats. J Comp Physiol Psychol 82:1
42. Paxinos G, Bindra D 1972 Hypothalamic knife cuts: effects of eating, drinking, irritability, aggression and copulation in the male rat. J Comp Physiol Psychol 79:219
43. Olds JE 1958 Effects of hunger and male sex hormone on self stimulation of the brain. J Comp Physiol Psychol 51:320
44. Jarmon H, Gerall AA 1961 The effect of food deprivation upon the sexual performance of male guinea pigs. J Comp Physiol Psychol 54:306
45. Paxinos G 1973 Midbrain and motivated behavior. J Comp Physiol Psychol 85:64
46. Leibowitz SF 1978 Paraventricular nucleus: a primary site mediating adrenergic stimulation of feeding and drinking. Pharmacol Biochem Behav 8:163
47. Stanley BG, Leibowitz SF 1984 Neuropeptide Y: stimulation of feeding and drinking by injection into the paraventricular nucleus. Life Sci 35:2635
48. Hart BL, Leedy M, Neural bases of sexual behavior: a comparative analysis. In: Adler NT (ed) Handbook of Behavioral Neurobiology. Plenum Press, New York, in press
49. Barfield RJ, Glaser JH, Rubin BS, Etgen AM 1984 Behavioral effects of progestin in the brain. Psychoneuroendocrinology 9:217
50. Crowley WR, Tessel RE, O'Donohue TL, Adler BA, Kalra SP 1985 Effects of ovarian hormones on concentrations of neuropeptide Y in discrete brain nuclei of the female rat. Endocrinology 116:1151

Cholecystokinin Decreases Food Intake in Rats[1]

James Gibbs,[2] Robert C. Young, and Gerard P. Smith
From the Edward W. Bourne Behavioral Research Laboratory, Department of Psychiatry, New York Hospital—Cornell Medical Center, Westchester Division, White Plains, New York

Abstract
Partially purified cholecystokinin (CCK) was injected intraperitoneally into fasted rats prior to food presentation. The hormone produced a large dose-related suppression of intake of solid and liquid diets. Identical doses of the synthetic terminal octapeptide of cholecystokinin produced identical results. An effective dose of CCK did not suppress drinking after water deprivation. Treated animals did not appear ill and were not hyperthermic; neither CCK nor the octapeptide produced learning of a taste aversion in bait-shyness tests. The effect of CCK is not a property of all gut hormones, since injections of secretin did not affect feeding. These studies raise the possibility that CCK plays an inhibitory role in the short-term control of feeding behavior.

An unidentified blood-born factor appears to act as a "satiety signal" (Davis, Campbell, Gallagher, & Zurakov, 1971). Gut hormones released by ingested food might play such a role in the short-term control of food intake. This idea is not a new one. In 1937, MacLagan reported decreased feeding in rabbits following injections of a crude extract of canine intestine. The extract was called enterogastrone because it was thought to contain the substance which mediated the inhibition of gastric secretion observed after a fatty meal (Kosaka & Lim, 1930). More recently, crude intestinal extracts also inhibited food intake in rats (Glick & Mayer, 1968; Ugolev, 1960). Using a partially purified preparation of porcine enterogastrone, Schally, Redding, Lucien, and Meyer (1967) reduced food intake of mice; injections of secretin or pancreatic glucagon were not effective.

Cholecystokinin (CCK), the other available intestinal hormone, has enterogastrone activity in the dog (Johnson & Grossman, 1970; Nakajima & Magee, 1970). Glick, Thomas, and Mayer (1971) reported that CCK failed to affect food intake in rats. We report here, however, that CCK significantly decreased food intake in rats under different experimental conditions. Part of this work has been reported previously in the form of a preliminary communication (Gibbs, Young, & Smith, 1972).

Experiment 1

Method

The subjects were 29 adult male Sprague-Dawley rats (Hormone Assay, Chicago, Illinois) weighing 450–550 gm. They were housed and tested in individual cages on an artificial 12-hr. light cycle and were maintained on Purina Rat Chow pellets and tap water.

The rats were deprived of food for 5 ½ hr. (10 a.m.–3:30 p.m.) each day. Fifteen minutes prior to presentation of a weighed amount of Purina pellets, the rats were injected intraperitoneally (ip) with 1 ml. of either .15 M saline or partially purified porcine CCK (10% W/W, GIH Research Unit, Karolinska Institutet, Stockholm, Sweden) in doses of 2.5, 5, 10, 20, or 40 Ivy dog U/kg body weight dissolved in .15 M saline.[3] Food consumption was calculated by subtracting the weight of the remaining pellets and crumbs from the initial weight at 30-min. intervals for 150 min. Tap water was available throughout the test period.

Experiments were designed in a crossover pattern; food consumption of each rat after CCK administration was compared with consumption after saline administration on the preceding or following day. Statistical comparisons were made with a matched-pairs *t* test.

Results

The extract containing CCK inhibited food intake (Table 1). The effect was large—a 50% suppression at 30

[1]The authors thank Frank P. Brooks, Alan N. Epstein, William T. Lhamon, Paul R. McHugh, and Eliot Stellar for their interest and encouragement. Joseph Antin and Jonathan Holt gave expert technical assistance. This research was supported by National Institutes of Health Career Development Award 7K04 NS38601 and Grant NS08042 to Gerard P. Smith.
[2]Requests for reprints should be sent to James Gibbs, Edward W. Bourne Behavioral Research Laboratory, Department of Psychiatry, New York Hospital—Cornell Medical Center, Westchester Division, 21 Bloomingdale Road, White Plains, New York 10605.
[3]Ivy dog unit of CCK (Ivy & Janacek, 1959): "that amount of vasodilantin-free cholecystokinin which when dissolved in normal saline solution and injected intravenously in the dog during 10–15 seconds causes within 1–5 minutes a rise in intra-gall-bladder pressure of 1 cm. of bile."
Adapted from the *Journal of Comparative and Physiological Psychology*, 1973;84(3): 488–495.

min. by the 40 U/kg dose. The magnitude of the inhibition was dose related over the range of doses tested, and the lowest effective dose of CCK was 5 U/kg.

The inhibition occurred within the first 30 min. of the test period; furthermore, an analysis of the amounts eaten during each 30-min. interval (Figure 1) demonstrates that the effect of CCK was in fact limited to this first 30 min. even with the largest dose (40 U/kg) of the hormone. The CCK-injected rats compensated for their early deficit in food intake by eating more than saline-injected controls late in the test period. By the time of the 150-min. measurement, only rats which had received the largest dose of CCK still had a significant decrease of cumulative food intake (Table 1).

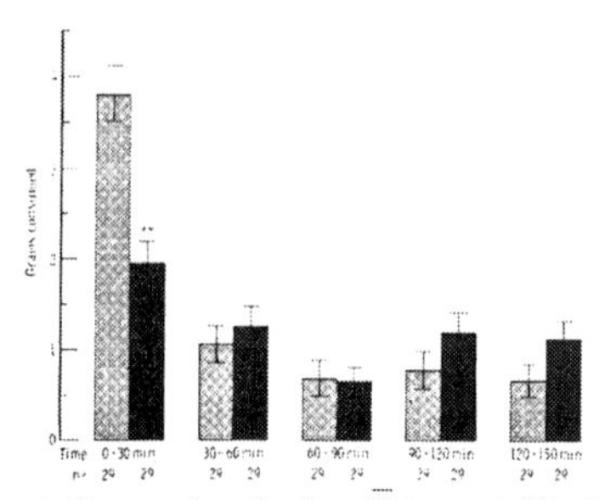

Figure 1: Consumption of pellets (X in gm. ± SE_M during 30-min. intervals following intraperitoneal injection of saline (light bars) or 40 U/kg of cholecystokinin (CCK) dissolved in saline (dark bars). (CCK significantly inhibited food intake only for the 0–30 min. interval; double asterisk indicates $p < .001$.)

Experiment 2

The inhibition of feeding produced by the 10% preparation of CCK could have been due to impurities in the extract and not the hormone itself. We tested this possibility by using 2 purified compounds: (*a*) the synthetic C-terminal octapeptide of CCK (SQ 19,844, the gift of M. Ondetti, Squibb Laboratories, New Jersey) and (*b*) caerulein (the gift of A. Anastasi, Farmitalia, Milan, Italy). Caerulein is a decapeptide extracted from the skin of the frog (*Hyla caerulea*). The C-terminal heptapeptide amides of caerulein and CCK differ by only 1 amino acid. Anastasi, Bernardi, Bertaccini, Bosisio, de Castiglione, Erspamer, Goffredo, and Impicciatore (1968) reported that caerulein was 15 times as potent by weight as CCK in stimulating pancreatic volume flow in the dog, and this factor was used to calculate doses.

Method

The 28 subjects for the octapeptide tests were from the same group used in Experiment 1. They were injected with 1 ml. of either .15 M saline or octapeptide of CCK in doses of 2.5, 20, or 40 Ivy dog U/kg body weight dissolved in .15 M saline.

Twelve adult male Sprague-Dawley rats (Hormone Assay, Chicago, Illinois) weighing 450–550 gm. were subjects for the caerulein tests. They were injected with either .15 M saline or caerulein in amounts of .1, .4, .8, and 1.2 μg/kg

TABLE 1

CUMULATIVE FOOD CONSUMPTION (AS PERCENTAGE OF CONTROL) OF RATS AFTER TREATMENT WITH CHOLECYSTOKININ (EXPERIMENT 1) OR SYNTHETIC C-TERMINAL OCTAPEPTIDE OF CHOLECYSTOKININ (EXPERIMENT 2)

Treatment dose (in Ivy dog U/kg)	Time after food presentation (in min.)				
	30	60	90	120	150
2.5, CCK	94	94	87	97	111
2.5, octapeptide	98	103	105	99	100
5.0, CCK	74*, ****	80****	92	95	99
10.0, CCK	68***, ****	72****	73****	91	97
20.0, CCK	68****	74****	77****	90	92
20.0, octapeptide	74****	75****	81****	97	94
40.0, CCK	50****	65****	69****	79****	87**
40.0, octapeptide	51****	70****	75****	84****	93**

Note. Mean control intakes for all tests ranged 5.4–7.7 gm. at 150 min. and were measured on the day immediately preceding or following a treatment day. Each percentage was obtained from a minimum of 20 rats.

* $p < .05$, significantly different from 10 U/kg percentage at 30 min.

** $p < .02$, significantly different from saline controls, matched-pairs t tests, 2-tailed.

*** $p < .01$, significantly different from 40 U/kg percentage at 30 min.

**** $p < .002$, significantly different from saline controls, matched-pairs t tests, 2-tailed.

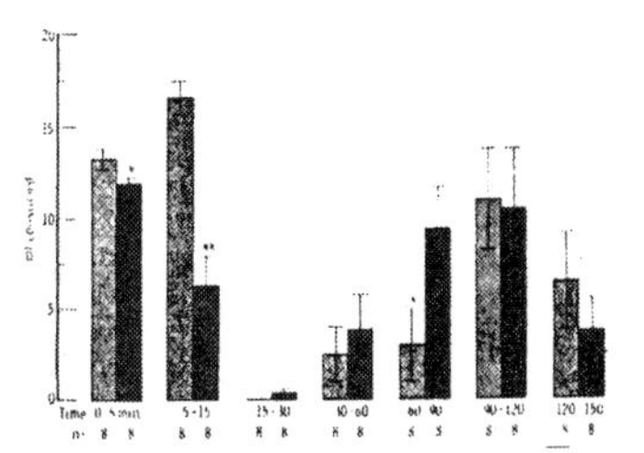

Figure 3: Consumption of diluted liquid diet ($\bar{X}$ in ml. ± SE_M) during intervals following intraperitoneal injection of saline (light bars) or 10 U/kg of cholecystokinin (CCK) dissolved in saline (dark bars). (CCK significantly inhibited food intake during the 0–5 min. [$p < .05$] and 5–15 min. [$p < .001$] intervals. The CCK-treated rats ate significantly more than controls during the 60–90 min. interval [$p < .05$].)

Method

The subjects were 25 adult male Sprague-Dawley rats weighing 450–550 gm. They were housed and maintained as described in Experiment 1. The rats were deprived of water for 12 hr. (10:00 p.m.–10:00 a.m.). One-half hour before water presentation, food was removed from the cages for the duration of the test. Fifteen minutes prior to water presentation in graduated drinking tubes, rats were injected ip with 1 ml. of either .15 M saline or partially purified CCK in a dose of 20 U/kg body weight dissolved in .15 M saline. Measurements of consumption were made at 5 and 15 min. from the time of water presentation. As in Experiment 1, a crossover design was used.

Results

The CCK did not suppress drinking. There were no significant differences in the amounts drunk during the 0–5 min. period: Saline-injected rats drank 9.8 ± .5 ml. ($\bar{X}$ ± SE_M) and CCK-injected rats drank 9.2 ± .5 ml. ($p > .05$, matched-pairs t test, 2-tailed). Hormone-injected rats showed a slight increase in water intake during the 5–15 min. interval, drinking 2.0 ± .3 ml., while saline-injected rats drank 1.1 ± .3 ml. ($p < .005$). This 5–15 min. interval is the period when CCK is most effective in suppressing liquid diet consumption (see Experiment 3).

Figure 4: Cumulative consumption of diluted liquid diet ($\bar{X}$ in ml. ± SE_M) following intraperitoneal injection of saline (light bars) or 38 U/kg of cholecystokinin—CCK—(dark bars). (The CCK limited meal size. Intake of hormone-treated rats was significantly depressed during the 5–15 min. and 15–30 min. [$p < .001$], and the 30–60 min. [$p < .05$] intervals.)

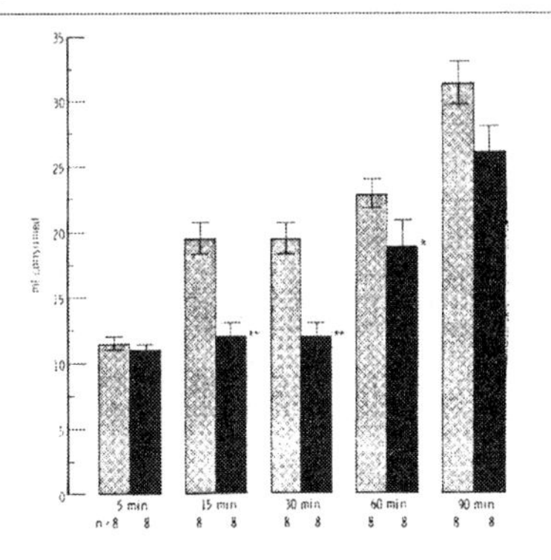

Experiment 5

It is possible that CCK inhibited feeding by making the rats sick, but this possibility is not likely: (*a*) Rats ate rapidly following injections of even large doses of CCK, but simply stopped eating sooner (see Figure 4); (*b*) they maintained control intakes of both solid food and liquid diet during 8 mo. of frequent CCK injections; and (*c*) they did not have elevated body temperatures following injections of 40 U/kg of CCK. Temperature measurements were made with a rectal probe thermometer under conditions identical to the feeding-test situation. Saline-injected rats had a body temperature of 97.8 ± .2°F. ($\bar{X}$ ± SE_M), while CCK-injected rats had a temperature of 97.7 ± .2°F. ($n = 8$, $p > .05$, t test for means of 2 samples, 2-tailed).

In addition, we tried to detect any inapparent distress by attempting to induce learning of a taste aversion with CCK. We employed the experimental design of Nachman (1970), using lithium chloride to make rats ill in temporal association with the novel taste of saccharin, resulting in bait shyness to saccharin on a subsequent presentation.

Method

The subjects were 34 adult male Sprague-Dawley rats (Hormone Assay) weighing 450–550 gm. They were housed and maintained as described in Experiment 1. The animals were deprived of water and given a daily 10-min. test of water consumption, measured in graduated drinking tubes, in their home cages. After being trained for 4 days to drink all their daily water during this limited period, rats were presented on Day 5 with a .25% sodium saccharin solution instead of water. One minute following this 10-min. exposure to the novel taste of saccharin, rats were injected with either (*a*) .15 M NaCl; (*b*) .15 M LiCl, .6% body weight; (*c*) partially purified CCK, 40 U/kg body weight dissolved in .15 M NaCl; or (*d*) synthetic terminal octapeptide of CCK, 40 U/kg body weight dissolved in .15 M NaCl. On Days 6 and 7, all rats were provided with water for the usual 10-min. test period and, without interruption, 20 min. of additional drinking time. On Day 8, all rats were again offered the .25% sodium saccharin solution for 10 min. Amounts drunk by each treatment group on each day were statistically compared with a t test for means of 2 samples.

Results

Neither CCK nor octapeptide of CCK produced learning of a taste aversion as measured by the amount of saccharin drunk at the second offering (Table 3).

None of the treatments immediately following the first saccharin offering produced overt symptoms such as diarrhea. Furthermore, on Test Days 6 and 7, there were no statistically significant differences in amounts of water drunk by groups treated with saline, LiCl, CCK, and octapeptide; thus, the animals were not made chronically ill by the treatments. Nevertheless, rats injected with LiCl on Day 4 displayed a marked aversion for saccharin on Day 8.

Experiment 6

This experiment asked 2 questions: First, is the inhibition of feeding demonstrated with CCK a property of other gut hormones? Secretin, another polypeptide hormone released from the duodenal mucosa as a consequence of food intake, was used for this test. Second, does secretin potentiate the action of CCK on feeding? To answer this question, the 2 hormones were administered together in a range of dose combinations and the results compared with the effects of CCK injections alone.

TABLE 3

WILLINGNESS OF RATS TO DRINK SACCHARIN SOLUTION AT SECOND OFFERING WHEN INJECTIONS OF VARIOUS CHEMICALS FOLLOWED FIRST OFFERING

Treatment	n	Saccharin intake at second offering ($\bar{X}$ in ml. $\pm SE_M$)
CCK effect		
.15 M LiCl	6	.7 ± .5
CCK[a] in .15 M NaCl	6	16.5 ± 1.5[b], *
.15 M NaCl	6	14.2 ± 1.5*
Octapeptide effect		
.15 M LiCl	5	0.0 ± 0.0
Octapeptide[a] in .15 M NaCl	6	16.8 ± 2.0[b], *
.15 M NaCl	5	18.6 ± 1.6*

[a] 40 Ivy dog U/kg.

[b] Not statistically different from NaCl-injected rats.

* $p < .001$, different from LiCl-injected rats, t test for means of 2 samples, 2-tailed.

Method

The 12 subjects for the secretin tests were fully grown male rats similar to those used in the previous experiments. They were injected ip on different experimental days with 1 ml. of either (*a*) .15 M saline; (*b*) pure natural porcine secretin (4,000 clinical U/mg, GIH Research Unit, Stockholm, Sweden) in doses of 2.5, 5, 10, or 40 clinical U/kg body weight dissolved in .15 M saline; or (*c*) partially purified CCK in doses of 2.5, 5, 10, or 40 Ivy dog U/kg body weight.

The same rats were subjects for the combination experiment. They were injected with 1 ml. of either (*a*) partially purified CCK in doses of 2.5, 10, or 40 Ivy dog U/kg body weight or (*b*) 1 of the following combinations of CCK (Ivy dog units) plus secretin (clinical units): 2.5 U/kg CCK+10 U/kg secretion; 2.5 U CCK+40 U secretin; 10 U CCK+10 U secretin; or 40 U CCK+10 U secretin. All animals in these procedures were maintained with diluted liquid diet on the deprivation schedule described in Experiment 3.

Results

Secretin did not significantly affect feeding (Figure 5). The 10 clinical U/kg dose of secretin produced the largest suppression of feeding (10%), but this was not statistically significant.

No combination of secretin and CCK produced a suppression of food intake significantly greater than the decrease after CCK in the same dose administered alone.

Discussion

This work demonstrates that the gut hormone CCK suppresses feeding in the rat.

Figure 5: Consumption of diluted liquid diet (expressed as percentage of control consumption) during first 15 min. of the test period following intraperitoneal injection of cholecystokinin (Ivy dog units, dark bars) or secretin (clinical units, hatched bars) in various doses. (Mean control intakes ranged 28.7–35.4 ml. Single and double asterisks indicate statistical differences from saline controls at $p < .01$ and $p < .001$, respectively.)

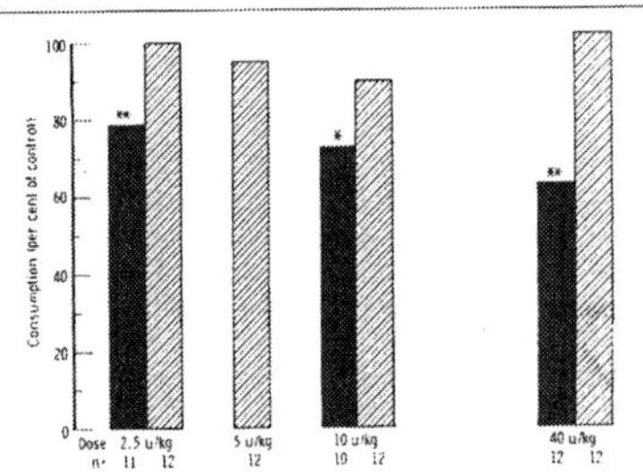

A partially purified preparation of CCK decreased intake of both solid and liquid food (Experiments 1 and 3), but did not decrease water intake (Experiment 4). The suppression of food intake by this preparation was a property of the CCK molecule and was not due to impurities present in the extract, because the synthetic C-terminal octapeptide of CCK and the decapeptide caerulein suppressed food intake (Experiment 2). Both the octapeptide (Rubin, Engel, Drungis, Dzelzkalns, Grigas, Waugh, & Yiacas, 1969) and caerulein (Stening & Grossman, 1969a; Stening, Johnson, & Grossman, 1969; Vagne & Grossman, 1968) have the physiological spectrum of action of the whole CCK molecule.

We also tested the effect of secretin on feeding. Like CCK, secretin is a polypeptide gut hormone released by ingested food. Its chemical structure is different from CCK and, in particular, it does not share the C-terminal heptapeptide sequence of CCK. Secretin failed to suppress food intake (Experiment 6). Despite their strucural differences, secretin potentiates several of the gastrointestinal effects of CCK (Henriksen & Worning, 1967; Spingola, Meyer, & Grossman, 1970; Stening & Grossman, 1969b). Under our experimental conditions, however, secretin did not potentiate the inhibition of food intake by CCK (Experiment 6).

A humoral factor which is proposed as an inhibitory signal regulating meal-taking behavior must meet certain criteria:

1. The proposed signal should be activated as a consequence of feeding. CCK, a polypeptide hormone, is released from the duodenal mucosa by ingested food: Measureable increases in CCK activity in the plasma occur in the anesthetized dog and cat following duodenal perfusion with emulsified fat, long- and short-chain fatty acids, peptones, and hydrochloric acid (Berry & Flower, 1971; Ivy & Oldberg, 1928).

If the proposed inhibitory signal were released in proportion to the amount of food ingested, this would account for the observation of Le Magnen ande Tallon (1966) that meal size of rats is correlated with the length of the next intermeal interval but not with the length of the preceding interval.

2. The proposed signal, administered exogenously prior to a meal, should significantly decrease meal size. Experiments 1 and 3, respectively employing solid and liquid foods, clearly fulfill this criterion (see Tables 1 and 2). If the relationship between the signal and feeding inhibition is an orderly one, a dose-response relationship will be obtained; the inhibition of feeding caused by CCK was large and dose related in both experiments. The finding that CCK significantly decreases food intake in the rat contrasts with the results of Glick et al. (1971). These authors injected rats intraperitoneally and intraaortically with CCK or secretin and studied the effect of each hormone on the rate of bar pressing for pellets or undiluted liquid diet. They found no effect of secretin and a trend, not statistically significant, toward decreased bar pressing after CCK. Differences between their experiments and the work reported here include the dose of CCK, length of deprivation, and measure of motivation (operant task vs. consumption). Which of these factors is the important difference is unclear.

3. The proposed inhibitory signal, in order to account for the frequency of meal-taking behavior, should have a relatively rapid onset and brief duration of action. As measured by its ability to contract gall-bladder strips, CCK is released and metabolized rapidly. It appears in the portal circulation of the cat 1–3 min. after introduction of emulsified fat into the duodenum and has a half-life of 10–15 min. (Berry & Flower, 1971). The behavioral effects of CCK seen in Experiment 1 were also rapid and brief: Feeding was decreased 15–20 min. following injection, and this effect was limited entirely to the 0–30 min. interval of the test period with solid food (see Figure 1) and to the 0–15 min. interval with liquid food (see Figure 3).

4. The effect of the proposed signal should not be due to illness. There was no indication that rats were toxic after administration of CCK in the doses used in this study. Appearance, eagerness to eat, maintenance of control food intake over several months, and lack of body temperature elevation after CCK treatment all indicated that the animals were not made ill by injections. However, it was possible that nausea or other discomforts were temporarily present and that feeding was inhibited by such disturbance.

Following Rzóska's (1953) description of bait shyness, Garcia, Kimeldorf, and Hunt (1961) established that rats will learn to shun novel taste stimuli which are followed by treatments that cause illness. We used this observation in Experiment 5 to search for behavioral evidence of any subclinical discomfort caused by CCK. We were unable to demonstrate any conditioned taste aversion.

5. The proposed inhibitory signal or group of signals should be effective in physiological doses. The amount of CCK employed in the lowest effective dose of these experiments appears to be of the same order of magnitude as the available measurements of plasma levels: Berry and Flower (1971) reported maximum concentrations of 10 mU/ml of plasma CCK activity following hydrochloric acid perfusion of the duodenum in the dog and cat; the 2.5 U/kg dose of CCK, which gave a clear suppression of liquid food intake (Table 2), is approximately equivalent to an extracellular fluid concentration of 12.5 mU/ml, assuming instant and homogeneous distribution in an extracellular space equal to 20% body weight.

From the data presented in this study, however, it cannot be concluded that the effect of CCK is a physiological one. It is important to note that the design of Experiments 1 and 3 does not eliminate the release of endogenous signals which suppress feeding. Figure 4 demonstrates this by showing that saline-injected control rats also stopped eating 15–30 min. after feeding began. Exogenous CCK may interact with these endogenous signals (endogenous CCK or other humoral or neural factors) to suppress feeding. Until such signals are known and their effects and interactions controlled, the threshold dose of CCK for the inhibition of feeding must be considered provisional.

Our results with exogenous CCK fulfill 4 of 5 criteria for a humoral inhibitory signal which participates in the short-term control of food intake. Whether these results represent a natural function of the endogenous hormone remains to be determined.

References

ANASTASI, A., BERNARDI, L., BERTACCINI, G., BOSISIO, G., DE CASTIGLIONE, R., ERSPAMER, V., GOFFREDO, O., & IMPICCIATORE, M. Synthetic peptides related to caerulein. *Experientia*, 1968, **24**, 771–772.

BERRY, H., & FLOWER, R. J. The assay of endogenous cholecystokinin and factors influencing its release in the dog and cat. *Gastroenterology*, 1971, **60**, 409–420.

DAVIS, J. D., CAMPBELL, C. S., GALLAGHER, R. J., & ZURAKOV, M. A. Disappearance of a humoral satiety factor during food deprivation. *Journal of Comparative and Physiological Psychology*, 1971, **75**, 476–482.

GARCIA, J., KIMELDORF, D. J., & HUNT, E. L. The use of ionizing radiation as a motivating stimulus. *Psychological Review*, 1961, **68**, 383–395.

GIBBS, J., YOUNG, R. C., & SMITH, G. P. Effect of gut hormones on feeding behavior in the rat. *Federation Proceedings*, 1972, **31**, 397.

GLICK, Z., & MAYER, J. Preliminary observations on the effect of intestinal mucosa extract on food intake of rats. *Federation Proceedings*, 1968, **27**, 485.

GLICK, Z., THOMAS, D. W., & MAYER, J. Absence of effect of injections of the intestinal hormones secretin and cholecystokinin-pancreozymin upon feeding behavior. *Physiology and Behavior*, 1971, **6**, 5–8.

HENRIKSEN, F. W., & WORNING, H. The interaction of secretin and pancreozymin on the external pancreatic secretion in dogs. *Acta Physiologica Scandinavica*, 1967, **70**, 241–249.

IVY, A. C., & JANACEK, H. M. Assay of Jorpes-Mutt secretin and cholecystokinin. *Acta Physiologica Scandinavica*, 1959, **45**, 220–230.

IVY, A. C., & OLDBERG, E. A. A hormone mechanism for gallbladder contraction and evacuation. *American Journal of Physiology*, 1928, **86**, 599–613.

JOHNSON, L. R., & GROSSMAN, M. I. Analysis of inhibition of acid secretion by cholecystokinin in dogs. *American Journal of Physiology*, 1970, **218**, 550–554.

KOSAKA, T., & LIM, R. K. S. Demonstration of the humoral agent in fat inhibition of gastric secretion. *Proceedings of the Society for Experimental Biology and Medicine*, 1930, **27**, 890–891.

LE MAGNEN, J., & TALLON, S. La periodicité spontanée de la prise d'aliments ad libitum du rat blanc. *Journal de Physiologie (Paris)*, 1966, **50**, 323–349.

MACLAGAN, N. F. The role of appetite in the control of body weight. *Journal of Physiology*, 1937, **90**, 385–394.

NACHMAN, M. Learned taste and temperature aversions due to lithium chloride sickness after temporal delays. *Journal of Comparative and Physiological Psychology*, 1970, **73**, 22–30.

NAKAJIMA, S., & MAGEE, D. F. Influences of duodenal acidification on acid and pepsin secretion of the stomach in dogs. *American Journal of Physiology*, 1970, **218**, 545–549.

RUBIN, B., ENGEL, S. L., DRUNGIS, A. M., DZELZKALNS, M., GRIGAS, E. O., WAUGH, M. H., & YIACAS, E. Cholecystokinin-like activities in guinea pigs and in dogs of the C-terminal octapeptide (SQ 19,844) of cholecystokinin. *Journal of Pharmaceutical Sciences*, 1969, **58**, 955–959.

RZÓSKA, J. Bait shyness, a study in rat behavior. *British Journal of Animal Behaviour*, 1953, **1**, 128–135.

SCHALLY, A. V., REDDING, T. W., LUCIEN, H. W., & MEYER, J. Enterogastrone inhibits eating by fasted mice. *Science*, 1967, **157**, 210–211.

SPINGOLA, L. J., MEYER, J. H., & GROSSMAN, M. I. Potentiated pancreatic response to secretin and endogenous cholecystokinin (CCK). *Clinical Research*, 1970, **18**, 175.

STENING, G. F., & GROSSMAN, M. I. Gastrin-related peptides as stimulants of pancreatic and gastric secretion. *American Journal of Physiology*, 1969, **217**, 262–266. (a)

STENING, G. F., & GROSSMAN, M. I. Potentiation of cholecystokinetic action of cholecystokinin (CCK) by secretin. *Clinical Research*, 1969, **17**, 528. (b)

STENING, G. F., JOHNSON, L. R., & GROSSMAN, M. I. Effect of cholecystokinin and caerulein on gastrin- and histamine-evoked gastric secretion. *Gastroenterology*, 1969, **57**, 44–50.

UGOLEV, A. M. The influence of duodenal extracts on general appetite. *Doklady Akademii Nauk SSSR*, 1960, **133**, 632–634.

VAGNE, M., & GROSSMAN, M. I. Cholecystokinetic potency of gastrointestinal hormones and related peptides. *American Journal of Physiology*, 1968, **215**, 881–884.

Eating or Drinking Elicited by Direct Adrenergic or Cholinergic Stimulation of Hypothalamus

S.P. Grossman
From the Department of Psychology, Yale University, New Haven, Connecticut

Abstract
A double cannula system, allowing repeated stimulation of central structures with crystalline chemicals, was developed. This technique was employed to study the effects of adrenergic and cholinergic stimulation of the lateral hypothalamus of rats. Drug-specific effects on the feeding and drinking mechanisms, respectively, were observed.

The exploration of the central nervous system by means of electrical stimulation has provided a wealth of information of great interest to physiologists and psychologists alike. The usefulness of this technique is limited, however, because the effects of stimulation are not restricted to synaptic junctions but affect fibers of passage, causing conduction in both normal and antidromic directions.

It has long been recognized that chemical stimulation avoids these problems, but the technique has in the past been plagued by the problem of uncontrolled spread, which raises a serious objection to the injection of chemicals in solution. Attempts to control for this factor by minimizing the injected quantities have apparently not been completely successful in preventing the escape of the fluid along the shank of the needle, following the path of least resistance.

Depositing chemicals in solid form has been shown to reduce this problem greatly (1), but this method has not allowed repeated stimulation of a selected locus. In the present study, a technique was developed which avoids this objection.

A double cannula system, consisting of two modified syringe needles, was permanently implanted unilaterally, by means of a stereotaxic instrument, into the lateral hypothalamus of each of 12 albino rats. Histological verification of the intended placements showed the tip of the cannula to be located in a circumscribed perifornical region at the same rostrocaudal coordinate as the ventromedial nucleus (see Fig. 1), an area corresponding to the ventral portion of Anand and Brobeck's "feeding area" of the lateral hypothalamus (2).

After 5 days of postoperative recuperation, the inner cannula was removed and minute amounts (1 to 5 μg) of crystalline chemicals were tapped into its tip before it was returned to its usual position. Successive treatments were administered to all animals in a counterbalanced order, with a minimum of 3 days between injections. Both food and water were freely available throughout the experiment. The food and water consumption of satiated rats was recorded for 1 hour immediately following stimulation and compared with the consumption in a comparable period immediately preceding the injection. Daily food and water consumption records were maintained.

None of the animals ever consumed food or water in measurable quantities during the prestimulation period. The injection of epinephrine or norepinephrine resulted in highly significant ($p<.01$) food consumption beginning 5 to 10 minutes after stimulation and persisting with variable intensity for 20 to 40 minutes. Food consumption averaged 3.0 gm under epinephrine and 4.3 gm under norepinephrine.

The injection of acetylcholine (capped by physostigmine) or carbachol into the identical loci in the same animals resulted in highly significant drinking ($p<.01$), the latency, duration, and magnitude of the effect being comparable to those obtained for eating after the injection of adrenergic substances. Water consumption averaged 7.4 ml after the injection of acetylcholine and 12.8 ml after the injection of carbachol, this difference being highly significant ($p<.01$). There was no significant food consumption after cholinergic stimulation (see Fig. 2).

The injection of adrenergic substances resulted in significantly less water intake than cholinergic stimulation ($p<.01$). Since in all but one animal the drinking occurred

Reprinted with permission from *Science*, 1960;13:301–302.

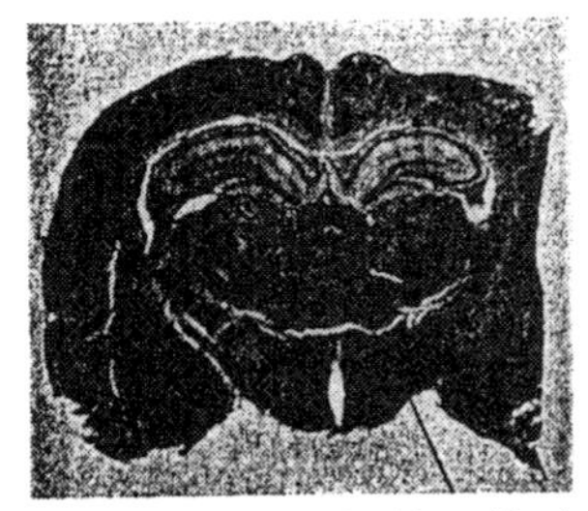

Figure 1: End of needle tract in the right perifornical region of the rat brain. Stimulation at this point, as well as at loci slightly more medial and ventral, produced the effects described in the text.

only after a considerable amount of dry food had been consumed, water consumption seemed to be secondary to the food intake rather than a direct consequence of stimulation. To establish further the specificity of the adrenergic effect, norepinephrine was deposited in the lateral hypothalamus of six food- and water-satiated animals, which were then placed in observation cages containing only water. For 30 minutes after the injection none of the animals consumed measurable quantities of water, though four of them repeatedly sampled the drinking tube very briefly. Food was then introduced, and all animals ate almost immediately, though total food consumption was lower than that normally observed, since the food was introduced only toward the end of the period previously established as the duration of the adrenergic effect.

In order to control for the effect of osmotic stimulation, comparable amounts of NaCl were deposited in all the animals. No significant food or water intake was observed. In order to control for general excitation effects, strychnine in comparable quantities was deposited in six animals which also showed the above-described effects of adrenergic and cholinergic stimulation. No consumatory behavior was observed following this stimulation.

The daily consumption records indicate that the amount of food or water consumed during the 1-hour period after stimulation, totaling as much as 40 percent of the animal's normal daily intake, appeared to be consumed above and

Figure 2: Food and water intake during 1 hour following stimulation. (The intake during a comparable control period was zero in all cases and is not shown.)

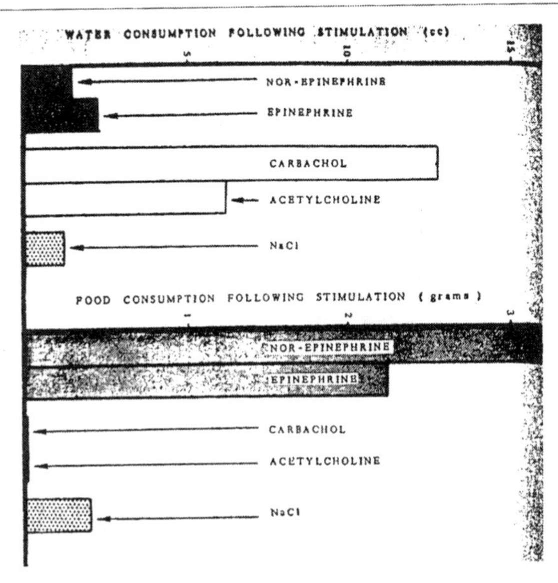

beyond the normal daily intake. Because of the variability of these records, no statistical evaluation of this effect can be presented, but the conclusion is supported, at least for eating, by the consistent weight gain observed on the day following adrenergic stimulation.

A control for the specificity of the localization of the observed effects was obtained in a preliminary study designed to yield optimal stereotaxic coordinates for the study reported here. It was found that very small deviations from the optimal position, shown in Fig. 1 sufficed to eliminate the effects completely.

The results of this investigation indicate that (i) cell concentrations active in the regulation of both food and water intake are present in the lateral hypothalamus; (ii) cell concentrations exerting this control appear to be highly localized but not clearly separate from each other, since stimulation of "identical" loci in the same animal can evoke both forms of behavior; and (iii) the feeding mechanism appears to be selectively activated by adrenergic stimulation, while the drinking mechanisms appear to respond selectively to cholinergic stimulation (3).

References and Notes

1. **P.D. MacLean,** *A.M.A. Arch. Neurol Psychiat.* 78, 113 (1957).
2. **B.K. Anand and J.R. Brobeck,** *Proc. Exptl. Biol. Med.* 77, 323 (1951).
3. This investigation was supported by a Public Health Service research fellowship (MF-101 597), as well as by funds from Dr. Neal E. Miller's grant (M647) from the National Institute of Mental Health, U.S. Public Health Service.

CLASSICS IN OBESITY

Brain Serotonin Content: Physiological Regulation by Plasma Neutral Amino Acids

John D. Fernstrom, Richard J. Wurtman
Laboratory of Neuroendocrine Regulation, Department of Nutrition and Food Science, Massachusetts Institute of Technology, Cambridge

Abstract
When plasma tryptophan is elevated by the injection of tryptophan or insulin, or by the consumption of carbohydrates, brain tryptophan and serotonin also rise; however, when even larger elevations of plasma tryptophan are produced by the ingestion of protein-containing diets, brain tryptophan and serotonin do not change. The main determinant of brain tryptophan and serotonin concentrations does not appear to be plasma tryptophan alone, but the ratio of this amino acid to other plasma neutral amino acids (that is, tyrosine, phenylalanine, leucine, isoleucine, and valine) that compete with it for uptake into the brain.

We have shown that when plasma tryptophan concentrations rise in rats receiving low doses of tryptophan (*1*) or subconvulsive doses of insulin (*2*), or in rats consuming a carbohydrate diet (*3*), brain tryptophan and serotonin concentrations also increase. Such variations in amine concentration reflect the general dependence of the rate of serotonin formation on the degree of saturation of tryptophan hydroxylase, the enzyme that catalyzes the rate-limiting step in serotonin biosynthesis (*4*). We suggested that the brain tryptophan elevations were direct responses to the increases in plasma tryptophan, and that, generally, any perturbations which increased plasma tryptophan would similarly increase brain tryptophan and serotonin (*3*). Since dietary protein should elevate plasma tryptophan both by eliciting insulin secretion and by providing new tryptophan, we anticipated (*3*) that its consumption should also elevate brain tryptophan and serotonin.

We now report that the elective consumption of protein-containing diets may or may not be followed by increases in brain tryptophan and 5-hydroxyindoles, and that this effect of food consumption on the brain is best correlated not with plasma tryptophan concentration, per se, but with the ratio of plasma tryptophan to five other neutral amino acids that presumably compete with it for uptake into the brain.

Male Sprague-Dawley rats (Charles River Breeding Laboratories) were housed as described in (*3*). At 9 p.m. the evening before an experiment, the rats were placed in clean cages and deprived of food. Between noon and 3 p.m. the next day, groups of six to eight animals were given free access to one of the following diets: (i) diet 1, a carbohydrate diet (*3*); (ii) diet 2, diet 1 supplemented with 18 percent casein, dry weight; (iii) diet 3, diet 1 supplemented with an artificial amino acid mixture similar to casein in amino acid content (*5*), 18 percent dry weigh; (iv) diet 3, but lacking specific amino acids as described below. In all experiments, animals consumed approximately 5 to 7 g of food during the first hour and 3 to 5 g during the second hour. Control rats were fasted and were killed at the beginning of the first hour of the experiment (0-hour control), or 1 or 2 hours later (1-hour and 2-hour controls, respectively). Experimental rats were killed 1 or 2 hours after diet presentation. Blood and brains were collected and prepared as described (*3*). Tryptophan (*6*), serotonin (*7*), and 5-hydroxyindoleacetic acid (*8*) were assayed fluorimetrically. Other plasma amino acids were measured by means of a Beckman model 121 amino acid autoanalyzer.

If rats ate diet 2 (18 percent casein), plasma tryptophan concentrations increased 60 percent above those of fasted controls in 2 hours (0-hour control, 11.44 μg/ml; 2-hour control, 10.46 μg/ml; 2-hour casein, 16.44 μg/ml; $P < .001$); however, brain tryptophan concentrations did not increase (0-hour control, 4.08 μg/g; 2-hour control, 5.07 μg/g; 2-hour casein, 3.47 μg/g). Brain serotonin also failed to rise (0-hour control, 0.58 μg/g; 2-hour control, 0.53 μg/g; 2-hour casein, 0.53 μg/g). The consumption of a standard rat chow (Big Red Laboratory Animal Chow, 24 percent protein, dry weight) produced similar results, that is, a 70 percent increase in plasma tryptophan ($P < .001$) after 2 hours, but no elevations in brain tryptophan or serotonin.

Other investigators, using brain slices (*9*) or animals eated with pharmacologic doses of individual amino acids (*10*), have shown that groups of amino acids (for example, neutral, acidic, basic) are transported into brain by different carrier systems, and that within a given group, the member amino acids compete with each other for common transport sites. Since protein ingestion introduces variable amounts of all amino acids into the blood, brain tryptophan could fail to increase after protein ingestion because the plasma concentrations of other competitor amino acids increase more than does the concentration of tryptophan. To test this hypothesis, we allowed groups of six animals to eat either diet 3 (carbohydrate diet containing the complete amino acid mixture) or diet 3 minus five of the amino acids thought to share a common brain transport system with tryptophan (tyrosine, phenylalanine, leucine, isoleucine, and valine). Both diets significantly increased plasma tryptophan above concentrations in fasted control rats (Fig. 1). The plasma concentrations of most other amino acids measured (for example, serine, proline, threonine, and alanine) also increased, except for those omitted from the diet. However, only when the competing neutral amino acids were deleted from the diet did large increases occur in brain tryptophan, serotonin, or 5-hydroxy-indoleacetic acid (Fig. 1).

To rule out the possibility that the differences between 's consuming diet 3 and this diet minus the five competitor ino acids were simply nonspecific effects resulting from the lack of any group of amino acids, we repeated the above experiment omitting aspartate and glutamate from the complete amino acid mixture. These two amino acids comprise approximately the same percent of the total alpha-amino nitrogen in casein as the five competing amino acids. Because they are charged at physiologic *p*H, they are transported into the brain by a different carrier system from that transporting tryptophan (*9*). Hence, their absence should not alter the postprandial competition for brain uptake between tryptophan and other amino acids within its transport group. At 1 and 2 hours after presentation of this diet or of diet 3 (complete amino acid mixture), plasma tryptophan concentrations again increased 70 to 80 percent above those of fasted controls ($P < .001$). However, the ingestion of either diet resulted in no increases in brain tryptophan, serotonin, or 5-hydroxyindole-acetic acid.

These results show that brain tryptophan and 5-hydroxyindole concentrations are not simply a reflection of plasma tryptophan, but also of the plasma concentrations of other neutral amino acids. To illustrate this relation, we performed a correlation analysis between brain tryptophan and the ratio of plasma tryptophan to the five competing amino acids among individual rats given the diets shown in Fig. 1 (Fig. 2). This analysis gave a correlation coefficient .95 ($P < .001$ that $r = 0$), whereas a correlation of brain tryptophan with plasma tryptophan alone was less striking ($r = 0.66$; $P < .001$ that $r = 0$). Further, a correlation between brain 5-hydroxyindoles (serotonin plus 5-hydroxyindoleacetic acid) and the plasma amino acid ratio gave a coefficient of 0.89 ($P < .001$), whereas a correlation with plasma tryptophan alone was less noteworthy ($r = 0.58$; P

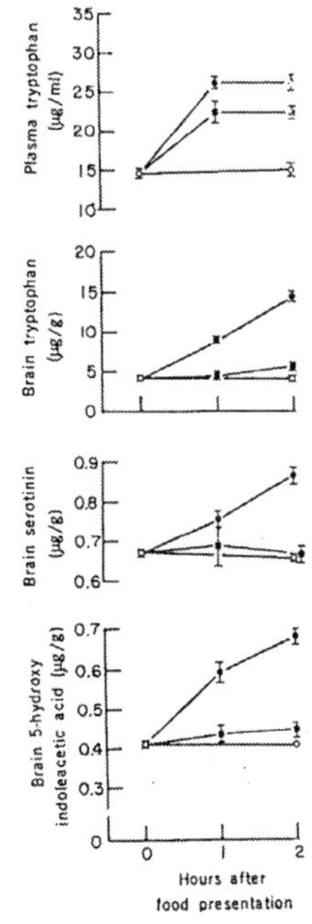

Fig. 1. Effect of the ingestion of various amino acid-containing diets on plasma and brain tryptophan, and brain 5-hydroxyindoles. Groups of eight rats were killed 1 or 2 hours after diet presentation. Vertical bars represent standard errors of the mean (○—○), Fasting controls; (■—■), complete amino acid-mixture diet; (●—●), mixture diet minus tyrosine, phenylalanine, leucine, isoleucine, and valine. The 1- and 2-hour plasma tryptophan concentrations were significantly greater in animals consuming both diets ($P < .001$) than in fasting controls. All brain tryptophan, serotonin, and 5-hydroxyindoleacetic acid concentrations were significantly greater in rats consuming the diet lacking the five amino acids than in fasting controls ($P < .001$ for all but 1-hour serotonin, $P < .01$). Among animal eating the complete amino acid mixture, the 2-hour brain tryptophan concentration was significantly above that of the corresponding fasting controls ($P < .001$).

< .001) (Fig. 2). Thus, the brain concentrations of both tryptophan and the 5-hydroxyindoles more nearly reflect the ratio of plasma tryptophan to competing amino acids than the plasma tryptophan alone. Tryptophan in plasma is divided between a larger, albumin-bound pool and a smaller, free pool (*11*). If brain tryptophan is in equilibrium with free rather than total plasma tryptophan, these correlations may be improved even further by substituting free for total tryptophan in the plasma ratio (*12*).

The effect of food consumption on brain 5-hydroxyindoles may now be modeled as in Fig. 3. Since carbohydrate ingestion elicits insulin secretion, it simultaneously raises

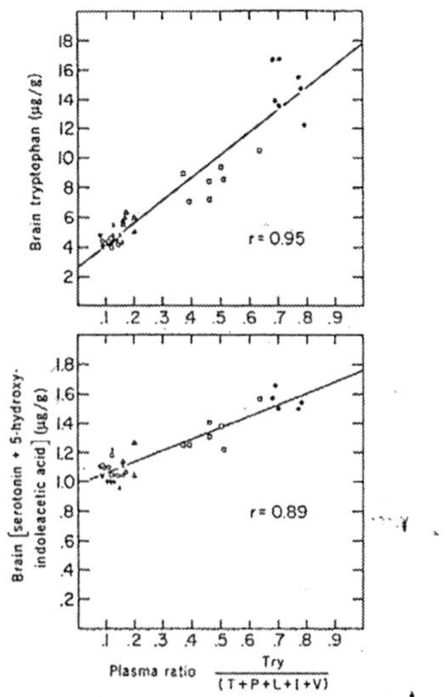

Fig. 2. (*A*) Correlation between brain tryptophan (*Try*) concentration and the plasma ratio of tryptophan to the five competing amino acids in individual rats studied in the experiment described in Fig. 1 ($r = 0.95$, $P < .001$ that $r = 0$). (B) Correlation between the sum of brain serotonin and 5-hydroxyindoleacetic acid, and the plasma ratio of tryptophan to the five competitor amino acids (*T*, tyrosine; *P*, phenylalanine; *L*, leucine; *I*, isoleucine; *V*, valine) in individual rats studied in the experiment described in Fig. 1 ($r = 0.89$, $P < .001$ that $r = 0$). (○) The 1- and (▼) 2-hour controls; (X) 1-hour complete amino acid mix diet; (△) 2-hour complete amino acid mix diet; (□) 1-hour complete mixture diet minus five competing amino acids; (●) 2-hour complete mixture diet minus five competing amino acids.

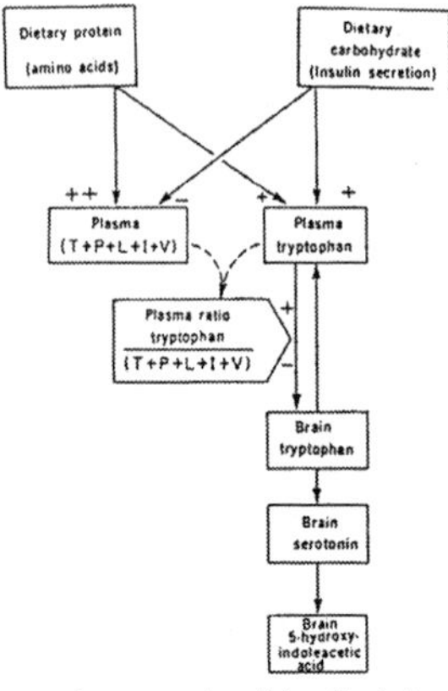

Fig. 3. Proposed sequence describing diet-induced changes in brain serotonin concentration in the rat. The ratio of tryptophan to tyrosine (*T*) plus phenylalanine (*P*) plus leucine (*L*) plus isoleucine (*I*) plus valine (*V*) in the plasma is thought to control the tryptophan concentration in the brain.

plasma tryptophan and lowers the concentrations of the competing neutral amino acids in rats (*2*); hence, the ratio of plasma tryptophan to competing amino acids increases, leading to elevations in brain tryptophan and serotonin. Protein consumption provides the plasma with a source of all the amino acids; however, the ratio of tryptophan to competitor amino acids in dietary proteins is almost always lower than this ratio in plasma (*5*). Probably for this reason, protein ingestion increases plasma tryptophan less than it does the plasma concentrations of competing amino acids, thereby decreasing the ratio. The insulin secretion elicited by protein consumption will, by itself, produce an opposite change in this ratio. Thus, brain tryptophan and 5-hydroxyindoles could decrease, increase, or remain unchanged after protein consumption, depending on the amino acid composition of the dietary protein, and the proportion of protein to carbohydrates.

Studies of the competitive among various amino acids for uptake into the brain have largely utilized brain slice preparations, or animals treated with pharmacologic doses of one or two amino acids (*9, 10, 13*). Our data provide evidence that such competition occurs in the concentration ranges that normally exist in untreated animals consuming natural proteins; further, this action appears to control the content of a putative neurotransmitter, serotonin in the brain. Since a wide variety of dietary and hormonal inputs probably can influence the ratio of plasma tryptophan to its ompetitor amino acids, our data suggest that serotonin-containing neurons provide the rest of the brain with information about a broad range of metabolic states (*14*).

References and Notes

1. J. D. Fernstrom and R. J. Wurtman, *Science* 173, 149 (1971).
2. ——, *Metabolism* **21**, 337 (1972).
3. ——, *Science* **174**, 1023 (1971).
4. W. Lovenberg, E. Jequier, A. Sjoerdsma, *Advan. Pharmacol.* **6A**, 21 (1968).
5. Composition of amino acid mixture (grams per 100 g of mixture): tryptophan, 1.07; threonine, 4.45; isoleucine, 5.51; leucine, 8.35; lysine, 7.48; methionine, 2.58; cysteine, 9.27; phenylalanine, 4.53; tyrosine, 5.69; valine, 6.57; arginine, 3.74; histidine, 2.85; alanine, 2.94; aspartate, 6.48; glutamate, 20.04; glycine, 1.78; proline, 9.70; and serine, 5.70. Mixture taken from M. L. Orr and B. K. Watt, *Home Economics Research Report No. 4* (U.S. Department of Agriculture, Washington, D.C., December 1957).
6. W. D. Denckla and H. K. Dewey, *J. Lab. Clin. Med.* **69**, 160 (1967).
7. J. H. Thompson, Ch. A. Spezia, M. Agnulo, *Experientia* **26**, 327 (1970).
8. B. T. Ho and D. Taylor, *Biochem. Med.* **5**, 521 (1971).
9. R. Blasberg and A. Lajtha, *Arch. Biochem. Biophys.* **112**, 361 (1965).
10. G. Guroff and S. Udenfriend, *J. Biol. Chem.* **237**, 803 (1962).
11. R. H. McMenamy and J. L. Oncley, *ibid.* **233**, 1436 (1958).
12. It has recently been shown that in human subjects carbohydrate ingestion causes a selective decline in free (that is, non-albumin-bound) plasma tryptophan, coincident with insulin-mediated reduction in plasma free fatty acids (D. Lipsett, B. K. Madras, R. J. Wurtman, H. N. Munro, in preparation).
13. A. Yuwiler and R. J. Louttit, *Science* **134**, 831 (1961); A. Yuwiler and E. Geller, *Nature* **208**, 83 (1965); S. Roberts, *Progr. Brain Res.* **29**, 235 (1968).
14. The precise uses to which the brain puts this information await identification. However, in collaboration with Dr. Loy Lytle, we have obtained some evidence that the increase in brain serotonin induced by an injection of L-tryptophan is associated with dose-related decreases in food consumption and motor activity. Similar injections of D-tryptophan or L-lysine, which do not increase brain serotonin, fail to modify food consumption and activity.
15. Supported in part by grants from the John A. Hartford Foundation and the National Aeronautics and Space Administration (NGR-22-009-627).

CLASSICS IN OBESITY

On Hysterical Anorexia (a)

Dr. Lasègue
Professor of Clinical Medicine in the Faculty of Medicine of Paris Physician to La Pitié Hospital

In my opinion we shall never succeed in composing the history of hysterical affections but by the separate study of each symptomatic group. After this preliminary analytical labour, we may collect the fragments, and from them reproduce the whole disease. Regarded in its entirety, hysteria has too many individual phenomena and hazardous incidents to allow of the particular being found in the general.

This procedure, very questionable when applied to diseases limited as to time, as to space and localisations, and as to the modality of phenomena, here finds its legitimate employment. I have already endeavoured to characterise cough and temporary catalepsy of a hysterical nature; and others have devoted valuable monographs to hemiplegia, transitory or permanent contractions, anæsthesia, etc. On the present occasion I wish to treat of a symptomatic complexus too often observed to be a mere exceptional occurrence, and which possesses the further advantage of enabling us to penetrate into the intimacy of the mental dispositions of hysterical subjects.

The disturbances of the digestive organs which supervene during the course of hysteria are numerous. They consist in repeated and sometimes almost incoercible vomiting, in gastric pains, hæmatemeses, in constipations, or diarrhœas, which are singular, whether by their evolution or by some of their characters. Among the more serious symptoms, vomiting of blood has chiefly attracted the attention of physicians. Gastralgias—purely subjective phenomena—are ill understood, and disturbances of the intestinal canal give rise to much uncertainty.

Attention has been paid in preference to the curious perversions of appetite, examples of which superabound in almost innumerable varieties. While relating singular cases of strange appetite, the true condition of the patients has not been investigated: and the whole is reduced to the profitless notion that hysterical patients are liable to the most out-of-the-way disorders of the digestive functions. Nevertheless, it would not be impossible to attempt a classification of this description of anomalies; but although I have had the opportunity of observing a great number of these, I do not intend to speak of them here, even incidentally.

The object of this memoir is to make known one of the forms of hysteria of the gastric centre which is of sufficient frequency for its description not to be, as too readily happens, the artificial generalisation of a particular case, and constant enough in its symptoms to allow of physicians who have met with it controlling the accuracy of the description, and to prevent those who have yet to meet with it in their practice being taken unawares. The term "anorexia" might have been replaced by "hysterical inanition," which would better represent the most characteristic of the accidents; but I have preferred the former term, without otherwise defending it, precisely because it refers to a phenomenology which is less superficial, more delicate, and also more medical.

Of the different stages of which digestion consists, the best analysed by patients, and the least easily investigated by the physician, is the appetite for food. If the term "anorexia" is generally adopted to represent a pathological condition, it has no physiological correspondent, and the word "orexia" does not exist in our language. The consequence is that we are defective in expressions for the degrees or varieties of inappetence—the poverty of our vocabulary corresponding to the insufficiency of our knowledge.

In certain cases there is suppression of appetite, without the patient exhibiting aught else than regret at the absence of a stimulus for taking food. Repugnance is not present, and frequently the proverb *l'appetit vient en mangeant* receives its justification. Under other conditions, the patient has a more or less decided repugnance for certain aliments, while in other cases any alimentary substance whatever excites disgust. However general the inappetence may be, it always has its graduated scale, so that aliments are not indiscriminately rejected with the same insistance.

On the other hand, there are affections, whether of the stomach or of the central nervous system, whether localised or diathetic, which are accompanied by an illusory sense of appetite, occurring at unequal or quasi-regular intervals. In certain hysterical and in certain diabetic patients these false appetites become exacting and imperious. Almost always

(a) *Archives Générales de Mèdecine.* April, 1873.

Adapted from *Medical Times and Gazette.* Sept. 6, 1873, pp. 265–266; Sept. 27, 1873, pp. 367–369.

such patients, in obedience to a theoretical hypothesis, entertain the idea that their uneasiness is due to inanition, and that it may be overcome by the aid of nutriment, however reduced in quantity this may be. Experience shows us that two drops of laudanum succeed better in appeasing this imaginary hunger than does the ingestion of aliments.

Exactly opposed to this exaggeration is the diminished appetite and the conviction that food will prove injurious, the patient here, as in the former case, acting in conformity to an instinctive hypothesis. When she is docile, and desirous of being delivered from her fears, she makes the effort, and acquires the conviction either that her health is improved under the employment of alimentation, even though it does cause suffering, or that her apprehensions have been ill-founded. When indocile, and anxious before all things to avoid pain, which, although hypothetical, is dreaded in advance, she persists in her abstinence from food. This is the case with the hysterical patients whose history I shall now endeavour to depict. Cases which persist for years are not suitable for narration, and I believe that it will be better, in place of particular facts, that I should present a somewhat diagrammatic sketch of the disease.

A young girl, between fifteen and twenty years of age, suffers from some emotion which she avows or conceals. Generally it relates to some real or imaginary marriage project, to a violence done to some sympathy, or to some more or less conscient desire. At other times, only conjectures can be offered concerning the occasional cause, whether that the girl has an interest in adopting the mutism so common in the hysterical, or that the primary cause really escapes her.

At first, she feels uneasiness after food, vague sensations of fullness, suffering, and gastralgia *post-prandium*, or rather coming on from the commencement of the repast. Neither she nor those about her attach any importance to this. The same sensations are repeated during several days, but if they are slight they are tenacious. The patient thinks to herself that the best remedy for this indefinite and painful uneasiness will be to diminish her food. Up to this point there is nothing remarkable in her case, for almost every sufferer from gastralgia has submitted to this temptation, until he has become assured that such relative inanition is not only profitless but aggravates his suffering. With the hysterical things take another course. Gradually she reduces her food, furnishing pretexts sometimes in a headache, sometimes in temporary distaste and sometimes in the fear of a recurrence of pain after eating. At the end of some weeks there is no longer a supposed temporary repugnance, but a refusal of food that may be indefinitely prolonged. The disease is now declared, and so surely will it pursue its course that it becomes easy to prognosticate the future. Woe to the physician who, misunderstanding the peril, treats as a fancy without object or duration an obstinacy which he hopes to vanquish by medicines, friendly advice, or by the still more defective resource, intimidation. With hysterical subjects a first medical fault is never reparable. Ever on the watch for the judgments concerning themselves, especially such as are approved by the family, they never pardon; and considering that hostilities have been commenced against them, they attribute to themselves the right of employing these with implacable tenacity. At this initial period, the only prudent course to pursue is to observe, to keep silent, and to remember that when voluntary inanition dates from several weeks it has become a pathological condition, having a long course to run.

It is necessary, in order to appreciate at their value the various elements which concur in the development of the disease, to submit each of these to a minute analysis. The gastric pain, which is, or appears to be, the point of departure of the accidents, requires especially that we should dwell upon it. It varies in intensity from a confused sense of pressure to a kind of stomachal cramp, accompanied by fainting, pallor, sweats, or even shivering. There is neither vomiting nor any real desire to vomit even in extreme cases, the patient only asserting that a degree beyond would induce this. In mere appearance these painful paroxysms in nowise differ from those which are so frequently met with in all affections of the digestive organs. Food induces them, and they do not occur except after meals. If this were really so, we should want any distinctive signs, and should be reduced to adding gastralgia to the already too long list of localised hysterical neuroses.

But the painful sensation persists more or less during the intervals of the repasts, being sometimes insignificant, sometimes more considerable, and now and then so attenuated in degree that the patient complains of a general uneasiness without being able to indicate a fixed point. Whatever may be its form, seat, or degree, is this painful sensation due to a stomachal lesion, or is it not only the reflex impression of a perversion of the central nervous system? I cannot believe that the solution can rest doubtful from the moment that the question is put. At the commencement of a great number of cerebro-spinal diseases we meet with præcordial suffering, a sense of epigastric pressure, or contractions, which also attend even transitory emotions. All of us have felt this kind of uneasiness while referring it to the definite moral cause that has given rise to it; but supposing an individual suddenly seized with this epigastric constriction, without any obvious cause, the uneasiness becomes such as to give rise to anxiety. The patient seeks from whence so strange an impression can arise, and it is often in such a search that the *délire des persecutés* commences. Supposing that the cephalic affection does not lead to such serious consequences, the first and most natural hypothesis that occurs to the patient is that he is suffering from disease of the stomach. All præcordial anxiety, with apprehension and the semi-vertigo it entails, becomes exaggerated by food, which forms an additional reason for attributing it to gastric irritation.

The characteristics of this gastralgia from reflex causes are not impossible of discernment, the circumstances under which they may exist being by no means of rare occurrence. It is distinguished from painful irritation of the stomach because it is not exactly located, and is accompanied by an entirely special inqueitude, it is sudden, the way not having been prepared for it by gradually increasing indigestions; it is not followed by dyspeptic accidents; the intestinal functions remain unimpaired save by habitual constipation, which is easily overcome; the nature of the food taken exercises no influence on the paroxysms; and the character of the pain, when it really exists, bears no analogy to the gastric suffering determined by a lesion, however superficial.

From the moment that the nature of this *malaise* has been ascertained, important progress has been made in the establishment of the diagnosis. I cannot too strongly insist on these splanchnic neuroses, and on their relations to certain cerebral conditions.

The hysterical subject, after some indecision of but short duration, does not hesitate to affirm that her only chance of relief lies in an abstinence from food; and, in fact, the remedies appropriate to other gastralgias are here absolutely inefficacious, however zealously both physician and patient may employ them. The repugnance for food continues slowly progressive. Meal after meal is discontinued, one of these, whether breakfast or dinner, alone being alimentary; and almost always some article of diet is successively suppressed, whether this be bread, meat, or certain vegetables—sometimes one alimentary substance being replaced by another, for which an exclusive predilection may be manifested for weeks together. Things may be thus prolonged during weeks or months without the general health seeming to be unfavourably influenced, the tongue being clean and moist and thirst entirely absent. The persevering constipation readily yields to mild laxatives, the abdomen is not retracted, and sleep continues more or less regular. There is no emaciation, although the amount of detriment scarcely amounts to a tenth of that habitually required by the patient. The power of resistance of the general health in the hysterical is too well known for astonishment being excited at seeing them support without injury a systematic inanition to which robust women could not be exposed with impunity. Moreover, this diminution of aliment is made not suddenly, but by degrees, so that the economy more easily habituates itself to the decrease. Another ascertained fact is, that so far from muscular power being diminished, this abstinence tends to increase the aptitude for movement. The patient feels more light and active, rides on horseback, receives and pays visits, and is able to pursue a fatiguing life in the world without perceiving the lassitude she would at other times have complained of. There are no visible signs of chlorosis or anæmia, or, at least, inanition cannot be accused of having induced them, for most of the patients were already in a chloro-anæmic condition.

If the situation has undergone no change as regards the anorexia and refusal of food, the mental condition of the patient is brought out more prominently, while the dispositions of those surrounding her undergo modification as the disease becomes prolonged. If the physician had promised rapid amendment, or if he has suspected a bad disposition on the part of his patient, he has long since lost all moral authority. Nevertheless, the patient only exceptionally resists the administration of medicines. Just as she is invincible in regard to food, she shows herself docile even for the least attractive remedies. I have seen one chewing morsels of rhubarb whom no consideration would have induced to taste a cutlet. The most active gastric stimuli, purgatives whether mild or drastic, mineral waters, produce no effect, good or bad. The same may be said of diffusible stimuli, fetid gums, valerian, hydro-therapeutics, douches at different temperatures, as also of tonics, preparations of iron, cutaneous derivatives, etc. Laxatives alone are of use by removing constipation, none of the other agents even producing a diminution of the anorexia. When after several months the family, the doctor, and the friends perceive the persistent inutility of all these attempts, anxiety and with immoral treatment commences; and it is now that is developed that mental perversion, which by itself is almost characteristic and which justifies the name which I have proposed for want of a better—hysterical anorexia.

The family has but two methods at its service which it always exhausts—entreaties and menaces,—and which both serve as a touchstone. The delicacies of the table are multiplied in the hope of stimulating the appetite; but the more the solicitude increases, the more the appetite diminishes. The patient disdainfully tastes the new viands, and after having thus shown her willingness, holds herself absolved from any obligation to do more. She is besought, as a favour, and as a sovereign proof of affection, to consent to add even an additional mouthful to what she has taken; but this excess of insistance begets an excess of resistance. For it is a well known law conformable to the experience of all that the best way to double the obstinacy of the hysterical is to allow the supposition, explicitly or implicitly expressed, to transpire that if they would they could dominate their morbid impulses. A single concession would transfer them from the position of the patients to that of capricious children; and to this concession, in part from instinct and in part from obstinacy, they will never consent.

The anorexia gradually becomes the sole object of preoccupation and conversation. The patient thus gets surrounded by a kind of atmosphere, from which there is no escape during the entire day. Friends join counsels with relatives, each contributing to the common stock, according to the nature of his disposition or the degree of his affection. Now, there is another most positive law that hysteria is subject to the influence of the surrounding medium, and that the disease becomes developed and condensed so much the more as the circle within which revolve the ideas and sentiments of the patient becomes more narrowed. The fault does not altogether lie in a pathological vitiation of disposition. Under the influence of sensations, which in more than one particular resemble the impressions of hypochondriacs and the delirious ideas of the insane, the hysterical constantly find themselves unable to resist this domination by a voluntary effort. At the most, distraction of attention enables them to forget at intervals, and these are the sole respites they obtain. The more their attention is intensified, the more does their idea of *malaise* become developed, and at the end of a variable time of this mischievous concentration the patient enters upon a new phase, and, systematising after the manner of certain of the insane, she no longer troubles herself in search of arguments. The responses become still more uniform than the questions.

Tired of supplications, if the endeavour be made to insist, the attempt will be still more fruitless than those which preceded it. In fact, what is to be said? The patient, when told that she cannot live upon an amount of food that would not support a young infant, replies that it furnishes sufficient nourishment for her, adding that she is neither changed nor thinner, and has never refused encountering any task or labour. She knows better than anyone what she requires, and, moreover, it would be impossible for her to tolerate a more abundant alimentation. When told that this inanition will at last induce disease of the stomach, she says that she never was better, and suffers in nowise, her state of good health contradicting all these fears. And, in fact, the pains attendant on the early stages have diminished or disappeared or only return at long intervals—an amelioration attributed by her to the regimen she has pursued. The fasting, indeed, is not absolute, and in nowise resembles the refusal of food in melancholia. The anorexia has not increased, and especially, it has not become transformed into the analogous disgust for food felt by some phthisical and many cancerous patients. The patient willingly joins her family at meals, on the condition that she is allowed to take only what she wishes.

What dominates in the mental condition of the hysterical patient is, above all, the state of quietude—I might almost say a condition of contentment truly pathological. Not only does she not sigh for recovery, but she is not ill-pleased with her condition, notwithstanding all the unpleasantness it is attended with. In comparing this satisfied assurance to the obstinacy of the insane, I do not think I am going too far. Compare this with all the other forms of anorexia, and observe how different they are. At the very height of his repugnance, the subject of cancer hopes for and solicits some aliment which may excite his appetite, and is ready for all kinds of trials, although incapable of triumphing over his disgust. The dyspeptic, without organic lesion, exhausts his ingenuity in varying his regimen, and complains with all the bitterness habitual to those who suffer from affections of the stomach. Here we have nothing like this, but, on the contrary, an inexhaustible optimism, against which supplications and menaces are alike of no avail: "I do not suffer, and must then be well," is the monotonous formula which has replaced the preceding, "I cannot eat because I suffer." So often have I heard this phrase repeated by patients, that now it has come to represent for me a symptom—almost a sign.

If I attach to this mental condition an importance that perhaps will appear exaggerated, it is that in fact the whole disease is summed up in this intellectual perversion. Suppress this, and you have an ordinary affection which at last yields to the classic procedures of treatment. Carry it to its extreme—and you will never go too far—and then you have a dyspepsia bearing no resemblance to others, which pursues a foreknown course, and which will not be relieved by habitual means. Moreover, I do not believe that gastric hysteria is any exceptional occurrence, for in other hysterical localisations we meet with at least an equal indifference, however inconvenient and painful their manifestations may be. The subject of hysterical convulsive cough does not demand relief from a spasm which is so irritating, and sometimes so ridiculous. She joins in the chorus of those who are pitying her; but when active treatment is in question, she is more indifferent than zealous in the matter. It is the same with paraplegic patients condemned to absolute repose, and who are willing to live in this way, without ever insisting that their attendants, exhausted in useless attempts, should have recourse to heroic measures.

[Professor Lasègue, after adducing some interesting examples of other hysterical localisations, for which we have not space, continues thus]—

In the end the tolerance of the economy, marvellous as this is, becomes exhausted, and the disease enters upon its third stage. Menstruation, which up to then had been insufficient and irregular, now ceases, and thirst supervenes. An examination shows retraction of the abdomen, which has not been observed before, and palpation indicates a progressive diminution of its elasticity, an habitual symptom in prolonged inanition. The epigastric region has become tender to pressure, although the patient complains of no spontaneous pains. An obstinate constipation no longer yields to purgatives. The skin is dry, rugous, and without suppleness. The pulse is frequent. Emaciation makes rapid progress, and with it the general debility increases. Exercise becomes laborious, the patient remaining willingly lying down; and when she rises she suffers from vertigo, a tendency to sickness, or even attacks of syncope. The countenance is pale, without the lips being colourless. An anæmic cardio-vascular souffle is almost constant, and which, often existing in advance of the affection, rarely fails to appear at its late period. This sketch is far from representing exactly the individual diversities that are observed. Sometimes it is the emaciation, sometimes the debility, sometimes the anæmia, with its accompanying local or general accidents, that is most prominent; while exceptionally nervous spasmodic disturbances, neuralgias, etc., arise, the active symptoms seeming to become effaced in proportion as the strength of vital resistance is diminished.

The appearance of these signs, the import of which can escape no one, redoubles anxieties, and the relatives and friends begin to regard the case as desperate. It must not cause surprise to find me thus always placing in parallel the morbid condition of the hysterical subject and the preoccupations of those who surround her. These two circumstances are intimately connected, and we should acquire an erroneous idea of the disease by confining ourselves to an examination of the patient. Whenever a moral element intervenes in a disease, as here it does without any doubt, the moral medium amidst which the patient lives exercises an influence which it would be equally regrettable to overlook or misunderstand. True and sincere affliction has succeeded to remonstrances. By the force of sentiments as much as by the necessities caused by new sufferings, the hysterical subject has been constituted really a sick person, no longer taking part in the free movements of common life. It seems to me that this unconscious change in the respective positions of the patient and her friends plays here a considerable part. The young girl begins to be anxious from the sad appearance of those who surround her, and for the first time her self-satisfied indifference receives a shock. The moment has now arrived when the physician, if he has been careful in managing the case with a prevision of the future, resumes his authority. Treatment is no longer submitted to with a mere passive condescendance, but is sought for with an eagerness that the patient still tries to conceal. The struggle thus established between the past and the present is a curious one to observe, and easy of proof providing that the investigation is in nowise allowed to be suspected.

Two courses are now open to the patient. She either is so yielding as to become obedient without restriction, which is rare; or she submits with a semi-docility, with the evident hope that she will avert the peril without renouncing her ideas and perhaps the interest that her malady has inspired. This second tendency, which is by far the more common, vastly complicates the situation. It is no easy thing to re-establish the regular function of a stomach which has so long been condemned to repose. We meet with alternatives of success and failure, and frequently only obtain a very insufficient result. I know patients who ten years after the origin of the affection have not yet recovered the aptitude of eating like other people. Their health is not deeply affected, but their amendment is very far from representing a cure.

Sometimes some unexpected event comes to break through the course of the disease—a marriage, grief, or some great moral perturbation. At others it is some physical occurrence, as a pregnancy or a febrile affection; but there are cases which resist both classes of these modifying agents. As a general rule we must look forward to a change for the better only taking place slowly—by successive starts; and we should be on our guard against affirming beforehand the amount of amelioration with which we must rest content.

Well founded as anxiety in these cases may be, I have never yet seen an anorexia terminate directly in death; but, in spite of this experimental assurance, I have passed through repeated perplexities. It is probable that the pathological sensation—the primary cause of the inanition—disappears by the fact of the increasing cachexia. It is not only of fever that we may say that it resolves spasmodic action, for the same property appertains to a great number of other morbid conditions. Delivered of her sub-delirious preoccupation, the hysterical patient passes into the condition of other dyspeptic patients, and only presents the same difficulties in her cure that we are accustomed to meet with. Hysteria, whatever extreme violence it may attain, is not itself mortal, but it may become the occasional or indirect cause of fatal diseases; and first among these is pulmonary tubercle. The hysterical anorexia itself is always cured more or less completely at the end of years, passing through the period of decrease with an appetite that is limited or exclusive, and occasionally fantastical. I attended with Trousseau a young woman who, having been thoroughly hysterical from the time of puberty, became, without appreciable cause, the subject of an invincible anorexia. She had reached such a state of emaciation and debility that she could no longer leave her bed. Her food consisted exclusively of some cups of tea with milk. Obstinate constipation had led to serous diarrhœa, with pseudo-membranous exudations. Nevertheless she became pregnant, and under the influence of that condition she set her wits to work to find out some article of food agreeable to her stomach. During six months she lived only on *café au lait,* into which she cut slices of pickled cucumbers, only adding very gradually some feculents to this singular diet. At the present time she is in a most satisfactory state of health, although always remaining excessively lean. Generally the appetite limits itself to aliments less singularly chosen, and then a free career is given to the fancy. I remember a patient 26 years of age, who, living in a distant province, neither would nor could eat anything but a biscuit made by a particular Paris baker. Many confine themselves to a particular kind of vegetable, refusing both meat and bread; while others will only take viands, the taste of which is disguised by spices. Although these capricious restrictions are a favourable sign, the patients continue to submit themselves without any desire to the diet they have chosen for want of a better. The anorexia persists indefinitely for long after they have returned to the ordinary regimen. I have never known the disease relapse, and, once established, the relative or complete cure is maintained. At the period when the hysterical affection had yielded, or had assumed other forms, I have endeavoured to obtain from the patients some more precise information concerning the sensations they had experienced, and which had induced them to avoid food. None of them have been able to furnish me with anything more exact than what I have reported. The typical formula employed during the course of the disease was reproduced—"I could not; it was too strong for me, and, moreover, I was very well."

The cases which have served me as a basis for this memoir are eight in number, all women, the youngest being 18, and the eldest 32. Hysteria manifested its presence in all by various symptoms, and in one only there had not been paroxysms. She was chloro-anæmic, and her mother had suffered from two attacks of hysterical hemiplegia. It was easy enough to assign the date of the commencement of the affection, but the anorexia was lost while passing through such insensible shades that the precise period of its termination could not be fixed. Speaking as nearly to the truth as possible, we may say that the affection, comprising the various phases that have been indicated, has never persisted for a less time than from eighteen months to two years.

Although these cases are few in number, they so much resemble each other that the latter ones found me in no indecision in regard either to diagnosis or prognosis, and, in fact, all passed on according to rule. In describing this variety, I proposed to myself, as I said at the commencement, to detach a species or a fragment, but especially to signalise the considerable part that is played in certain forms of hysteria by the mental disposition of the patient, and to point out yet once more the intimate relation that attaches hysteria to hypochondriasis.

V.—Anorexia Nervosa (Apepsia Hysterica, Anorexia Hysterica)

William Withey Gull, M.D., Bart.
Read October 24, 1873

In an address on medicine, delivered at Oxford in the autumn of 1868,* I referred to a peculiar form of disease occurring mostly in young women, and characterised by extreme emaciation, and often referred to latent tubercle, and mesenteric disease. I remarked that at present our diagnosis of this affection is negative, so far as determining any positive cause from which it springs; that it is mostly one of inference from our clinical knowledge of the liability of the pulmonary or abdominal organs to particular lesions, and by proving the absence of these lesions in the cases in question. The subjects of this affection are mostly of the female sex, and chiefly between the ages of 16 and 23. I have occasionally seen it in males at the same age.

To illustrate the disease I may give the details of two cases, as fair examples of the whole.

Miss A., æt. 17, under the care of Mr. Kelson Wright, of the Clapham Road, was brought to me on Jan. 17, 1866. Her emaciation was very great. (*Vide* Woodcuts † Nos. 1 and 2.) It was stated that she had lost 33 lbs. in weight. She was then 5 st. 12 lbs. Height, 5 ft. 5 in. Amenorrhœa for nearly a year. No cough. Respirations throughout chest everywhere normal. Heart-sounds normal. Resps. 12; pulse, 56. No vomiting nor diarrhœa. Slight constipation. Complete anorexia for animal food, and almost complete anorexia for everything else. Abdomen shrunk and flat, collapsed. No abnormal pulsations of aorta. Tongue clean. Urine normal. Slight deposit of phosphates on boiling. The condition was one of simple starvation. There was but slight variation in her condition, though observed at intervals of three or four months. The pulse was noted on these several occasions as 56 and 60. Resps. 12 to 15. The urine was always normal, but varied in sp. gr., and was sometimes as low as 1005. The case was regarded as one of simple anorexia.

Various remedies were prescribed—the preparations of cinchona, the bichloride of mercury, syrup of the iodide of iron, syrup of the phosphate of iron, citrate of quinine and iron, &c.—but no perceptible effect followed their administration. The diet also was varied, but without any effect upon the appetite. Occasionally for a day or two the appetite was voracious, but this was very rare and exceptional. The patient complained of no pain, but was restless and active. This was in fact a striking expression of the nervous state, for it seemed hardly possible that a body so wasted could undergo the exercise which seemed agreeable. There was some peevishness of temper, and a feeling of jealousy. No account could be given of the exciting cause.

Miss A. remained under my observation from Jan. 1866 to March 1868, when she had much improved, and gained in weight from 82 to 128 lbs. The improvement from this time continued, and I saw no more of her medically. The Woodcut, Miss A., No. 2, from photograph taken in 1870, shows her condition at that time. It will be noticeable that as she recovered she had a much younger look, corresponding indeed to her age, 21; whilst the photographs, taken when she was 17, give her the appearance of being near 30. Her health has continued good, and I add a fourth photograph taken in 1872.

It will be observed that all the conditions in this case were negative, and may be explained by the anorexia which led to starvation, and a depression of all the vital functions; viz., amenorrhœa, slow pulse, slow breathing. In the stage of greatest emaciation one might have been pardoned for assuming that there was some organic lesion, but from the point of view indicated such an assumption would have been unnecessary.

This view is supported by the satisfactory course of the case to entire recovery, and by the continuance of good health.

Miss B., æt. 18, was brought to me Oct. 8, 1868, as a case of latent tubercle. Her friends had been advised accordingly to take her for the coming winter to the South of Europe.

*'Lancet,' August 1868.

†The woodcuts illustrating this Paper are fac-similes of the original photographs exhibited at the time the Paper was read.

Adapted from *Transactions of the Clinical Society of London.* 7:22–28. 1874.

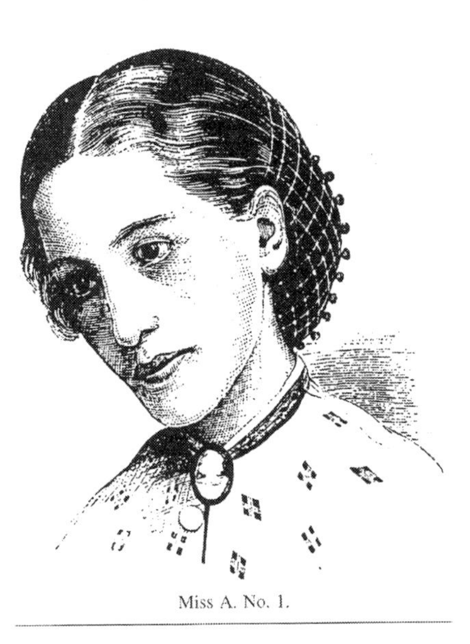

Miss A. No. 1.

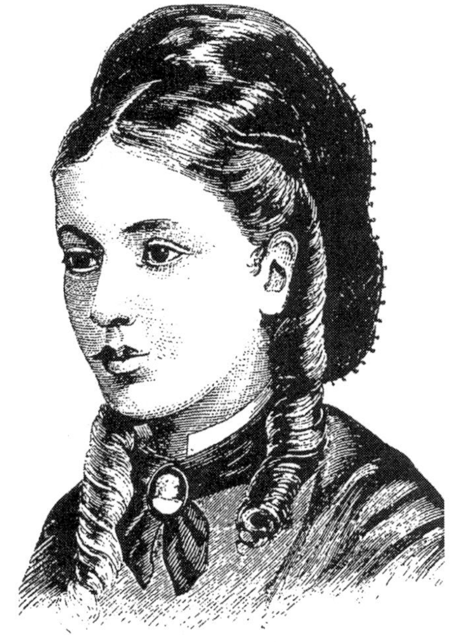

Miss A. No. 2.

The extremely emaciated look (*vide* Woodcut, Miss B., No. 1), much greater indeed than occurs for the most part in tubercular cases where patients are still going about, impressed me at once with the probability that I should find no visceral disease. Pulse 50, Resp. 16. Physical examination of the chest and abdomen discovered nothing abnormal. All the viscera were apparently healthy. Notwithstanding the great emaciation and apparent weakness, there was a peculiar restlessness, difficult, I was informed, to control. The mother added, 'She is never tired.' Amenorrhœa since Chrismas 1866. The clinical details of this case were in fact almost identical with the preceding one, even to the number of the pulse and respirations.

I find the following memoranda frequently entered in my note-book:—'pulse 56, resp. 12; January 1868, pulse 54, resp. 12; March 1869, pulse 54, resp. 12; March 1870, pulse 50, resp. 12.' But little change occurred in the case until 1872, when the respirations became 18 to 20, pulse 60.

After that date the recovery was progressive, and at length complete. (*Vide* Woodcut, Miss B., No. 2.)

The medical treatment probably need not be considered as contributing much to the recovery. It consisted, as in the former case, of various so-called tonics, and a nourishing diet.

Although the two cases I have given have ended in recovery, my experience supplies one instance at least of a fatal termination to this malady. When the emaciation is at the extremest, œdema may supervene in the lower extremities—the patient may become sleepless—the pulse become quick, and death be approached by symptoms of feeble febrile reaction. In one such case the *post-mortem* revealed no more than thrombosis of the femoral veins, which appeared to be coincident with the œdema of the lower limbs. Death apparently followed from the starvation alone. This is the clinical point to be borne in mind, and is, I believe, the proper guide to treatment. I have observed that in the extreme emaciation, when the pulse and respiration are slow, the temperature is slightly below the normal standard. This fact, together with the observations made by Chossat on the effect of starvation on animals, and their inability to digest food in the state of inanition, without the aid of external heat, has direct clinical bearings; it being often necessary to supply external heat as well as food to patients. The best means of applying heat is to place an india-rubber tube, having a diameter of 2 inches and a length of 3 or 4 feet, filled with hot water along the spine of the patient, as suggested by Dr. Newington, of Ticehurst.

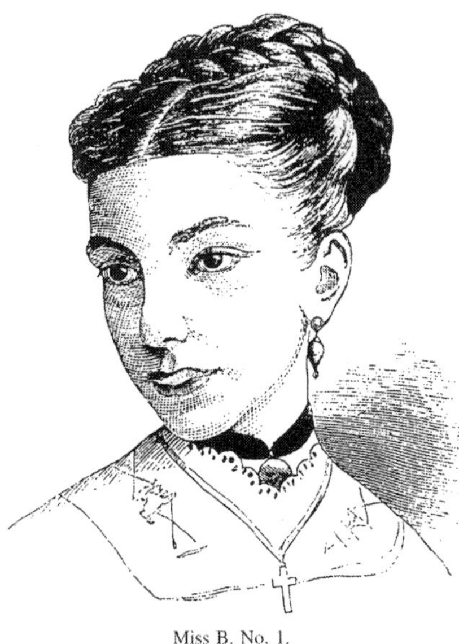

Miss B. No. 1.

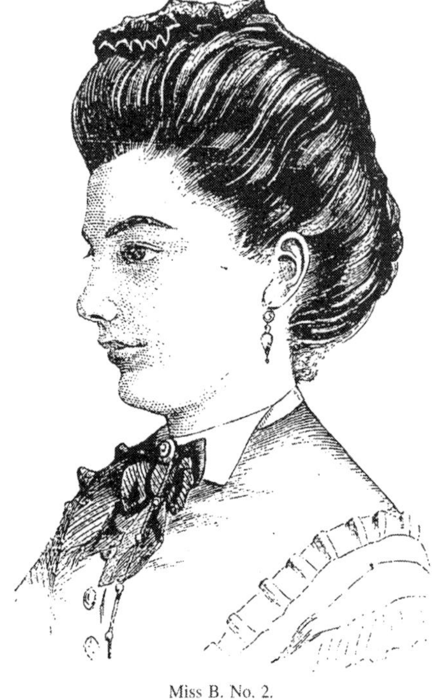

Miss B. No. 2.

Food should be administered at intervals varying inversely with the exhaustion and emaciation. The inclination of the patient must be in no way consulted. In the earlier and less severe stages, it is not unusual for the medical attendant to say, in reply to the anxious solicitude of the parents, 'Let her do as she likes. Don't force food.' Formerly, I thought such advice admissible and proper, but larger experience has shown plainly the danger of allowing the starvation-process to go on.

As regards prognosis, none of these cases, however exhausted, are really hopeless whilst life exists; and, for the most part, the prognosis may be considered favourable. The restless activity referred to is also to be controlled, but this is often difficult.

It is sometimes quite shocking to see the extreme exhaustion and emaciation of these patients brought for advice; yet, by warmth and steady supplies of food and stimulants, the strength may be gradually resuscitated, and recovery completed.

After these remarks were penned, Dr. Francis Webb directed my attention to the Paper of Dr. Laségue (Professor of Clinical Medicine in the Faculty of Medicine of Paris, and Physician to La Pitié Hospital), which was published in the 'Archives Générales de Médecine,' April 1873, and translated into the pages of the 'Med. Times,' Sept. 6 and 27, 1873.

It is plain that Dr. Laségue and I have the same malady in mind, though the forms of our illustrations are different. Dr. Laségue does not refer to my address at Oxford, and it is most likely he knew nothing of it. There is, therefore, the more value in his Paper, as our observations have been made independently. We have both selected the same expression to characterise the malady.

In the address at Oxford I used the term *Apepsia hysterica*, but before seeing Dr. Laségue's Paper, it had equally occurred to me that *Anorexia* would be more correct.

The want of appetite is, I believe, due to a morbid mental state. I have not observed in these cases any gastric disorder to which the want of appetite could be referred. I believe, therefore, that its origin is central and not peripheral. That mental states may destroy appetite is notorious, and it will be admitted that young women at the ages named

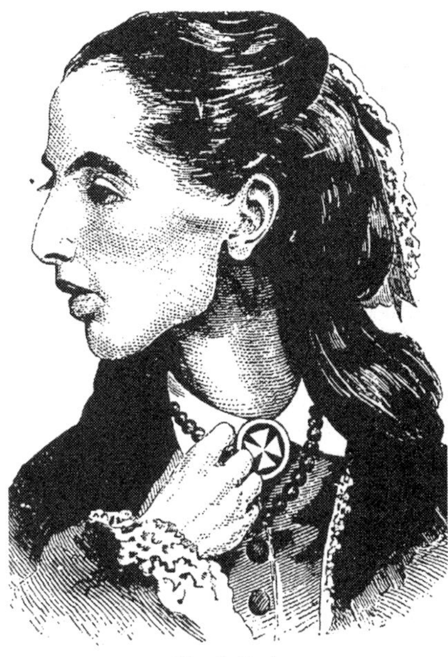

Miss C. No. 1.

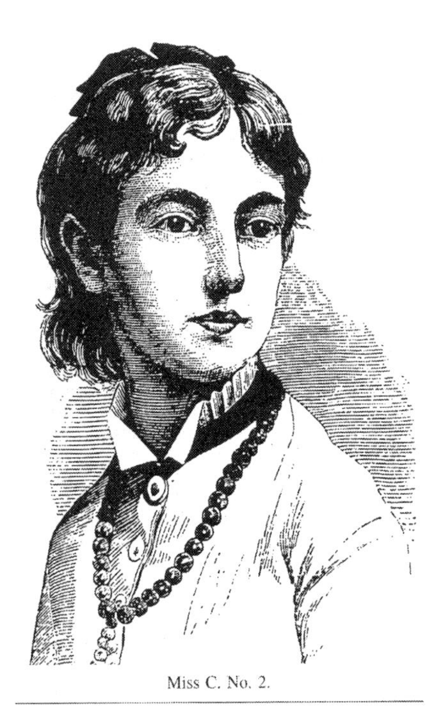

Miss C. No. 2.

are specially obnoxious to mental perversity. We might call the state hysterical without committing ourselves to the etymological value of the word, or maintaining that the subjects of it have the common symptoms of hysteria. I prefer, however, the more general term 'nervosa,' since the disease occurs in males as well as females, and is probably rather central than peripheral. The importance of discriminating such cases in practice is obvious; otherwise prognosis will be erroneous, and treatment misdirected.

In one of the cases I have named the patient had been sent abroad for one or two winters, under the idea that there was a tubercular tendency. I have remarked above that these wilful patients are often allowed to drift their own way into a state of extreme exhaustion, when it might have been prevented by placing them under different moral conditions.

The treatment required is obviously that which is fitted for persons of unsound mind. The patients should be fed at regular intervals, and surrounded by persons who would have moral control over them; relations and friends being generally the worst attendants.

Addendum.

As a further illustration, I may add the following correspondence on one of these cases with Dr. Anderson, of Richmond.

Miss C., æt. 15 years 8 months, was sent to me in April 1873. The clinical history was that she had been ailing for a year, and had become extremely emaciated. (Woodcut, Miss C., No. 1.) The catamenia had never appeared. Pulse 64, resp. 16. Very sleepless for six months past. All the viscera healthy. Urine normal. Lower extremities œdematous. Mind weakened. Temper obstinate. Great restlessness. No family history of disease beyond the fact that the maternal grandmother had had peculiar nervous symptoms. I wrote the following letter to Dr. Anderson:—

> 'DEAR DR. ANDERSON,—I saw Miss C. to-day. The case appears to be an extreme instance of what I have proposed to call "Apepsia hysterica," or "Anorexia nervosa." (*See* "Address on Medicine at Oxford," 1868.) I believe it to be essentially a failure of the powers of the gastric branches

of the pneumogastric nerve. It differs from tuberculosis, though that state may subsequently arise, by the pulse, which I found to be 64, by the breathing, 16, the cleanness of the tongue, &c. In fact, the disease will be most correctly interpreted if it is remembered that no symptom more positive than emaciation is presented in and throughout its course.

'I would advise warm clothing, and some form of nourishing food every two hours, as milk, cream, soup, eggs, fish, chicken. I must only urge the necessity of nourishment in some form, otherwise the venous obstruction, which has already begun to show itself by œdema of the legs, will go on to plugging of the vessels. With the nourishment I would conjoin a dessert-spoonful of brandy every two or three hours. Whilst the present state of weakness continues, fatigue must be limited, and if the exhaustion increases beyond its present degree the patient should for a time be kept in a warm bed. I do not at present prescribe medicines, because the nursing and the food are more important than anything else. Such cases not unfrequently come before me; but as the morbid state is not yet generally recognised, I should be glad if you would second my wish of having a photograph taken of Miss C. in her present state, that we may compare it with some later one, if, as I hope, our plan of treatment is successful, as in my experience it generally is. I would, as I say, enclose a prescription, but I feel it most necessary to insist on food and stimulants, at least for a time.

'Yours truly,

'April 30, 1873.'

On May 24 I received the following note from Dr. Anderson:—

'DEAR SIR WILLIAM,—I enclose photograph of Miss C. . . . There is rather an improvement in one respect, viz. there is less aversion to food. Want of sleep and swelling of the feet are the two great troubles. You have given us all new hope, however, and I trust I may one day send you a *plump* photograph, like what she was two years ago. With renewed thanks, I am, dear Sir William, yours very truly,'

On Oct. 23, 1873, I received a further report.

'DEAR SIR WILLIAM,—Miss C. is now at Shanklin, but returns very soon. I hear she is much better. She had a bad slough on the leg near the ankle, from persisting in wearing a tight boot.

'The great difficulty was to keep her quiet, and to make her eat and drink. Every step had to be fought. She was most loquacious and obstinate, anxious to overdo herself bodily and mentally. I will give you particulars when they return, but I am told she is-much improved. Rest, and food, and stimulants as prescribed, undoubtedly did her a great deal of good. She used to be a nice, plump, good-natured little girl. Believe me, &c.'

The last report I received was on April 15, 1874.

'DEAR SIR W.,—I am sure you will be delighted to hear that Miss C., in whose case you were so kindly interested, . . . has now made a complete recovery, and is getting plump and rosy as of yore.. . . .' (*Vide* Woodcut, Miss C., No. 2.)

Obesity, Social Class, and Mental Illness

Mary E. Moore, Ph.D., Albert Stunkard, M.D., Philadelphia, and Leo Srole, Ph.D., Brooklyn, N.Y.
From the Departments of Psychiatry and Medicine, University of Pennsylvania (Drs. Moore and Stunkard), and the Department of Psychiatry, State University of New York, Downstate Medical Center (Dr. Srole).

Abstract
The relationship between obesity and mental health was investigated, using data obtained from 1,660 persons selected as representative of 110,000 inhabitants of a residential area of New York City. In addition to confirming the previously noted relationship between obesity and age, preliminary analysis revealed a striking relationship between obesity and socioeconomic status of origin. The prevalence of obesity was 7 times higher among women reared in the lowest social class category as compared with those reared in the highest category. Scores made by the obese respondents on 9 mental health indices were compared with scores made by individuals of average weight. The obese respondents made more pathological scores on 8 of the 9 measures and on 3 of these the difference was statistically significant ("immaturity," "rigidity," and "suspiciousness").

This communication describes the relationship of obesity to mental health. It is based upon the reanalysis of data from a representative sample of 1,660 adults living in a residential area of New York City. In the course of this analysis, a striking relationship between obesity and social class was discovered.

It is widely believed that obesity is closely associated with certain mental disturbances and even that such disturbances may be a major cause of obesity. Most of the evidence in support of these views is derived from case reports of patients in psychotherapy or from surveys of obese patients in medical facilities.[1-5] Studies conducted with increasing methodological rigor, however, have not only often failed to support these clinical impressions, but have also contradicted each other.[6-11] The need for broadly based samples and comparable control groups has thus become compelling. The present investigation was designed to meet this need. It possesses, in addition to some unique qualities of the sample, an unusual advantage. The data were not collected for the purpose of relating obesity and mental health, and the bias introduced into data collection by the investigators' prejudices has thus been obviated.

Read at the Annual Meeting of the American Psychosomatic Society, April 1, 1962
Adapted from *JAMA*. 181:962–966. 1962.
Reprinted with permission.

Methods and Materials

The data reported here were collected as part of the Midtown Manhattan Study, a comprehensive survey of the epidemiology of mental illness. The Midtown Study has been described elsewhere in great detail,[12] but its methodology will be briefly reviewed. The segment of the population under study was a group of 110,000 individuals that constituted all of those adults between 20 and 59 years of age who occupied a certain residential area of New York City. The group was homogenous in race—99% were white—but it represented extremes in socioeconomic status that ranged from extremely high to extremely low. It was made up of about equal proportions of native-born New Yorkers, American-born persons who had migrated to New York, and foreign-born immigrants. A cross-section of 1,900 individuals was selected as representative of the 110,000 by means of systematic probability sampling, and interviews were conducted with 1,660, or 87%, of those selected. Analysis of demographic factors indicated that the 13% not included in the study did not differ significantly from the rest of the sample.

Subjects were queried in their homes by trained field workers. The interviews took about 2 hours and covered such areas as social and ethnic background, history of certain somatic disorders, and a large number of items designed to assess the individual's psychological and interpersonal functioning. A series of 8 psychological scores was constructed from these items. These were: childhood anxiety, withdrawal, neurasthenia, frustration-depression, tension-anxiety, rigidity, suspiciousness, and immaturity. The higher the scores, the greater the pathology.

A general mental health rating was given each respondent, in addition to his psychological scores. This rating was a composite of ratings made independently by 2 psychiatrists who did not see the respondents personally, but who made their evaluation in terms of a 6-point scale, which was later collapsed into 4 main categories: symptom free, mild symptom formation, moderate symptom formation, and impaired.

A major focus of the Midtown Study was the relationship between social class and mental illness. Previous studies which had investigated this relationship had not established controls for its reciprocal nature: while mental illness may in part depend on social class, it may also have an effect on social class, particularly in a downward direction. Instead of using the respondent's own socioeconomic status, therefore, the Midtown researchers used a measure based on the social class of the respondent's father when the respondent was entering adulthood. The father's occupation and education formed the basis for an 11-point scale of parental socioeconomic status. This constituted a measure of important social influences on the respondent which was in no sense a product of the respondent's mental health.

Verbal reports of the heights and weights of the respondents were obtained and recorded by the interviewers in terms of precoded intervals. Figure 1 shows the distribution of height by weight of the 690 males and 969 females in the sample. (One female under 4 ft. in height was omitted from further analysis.)

When the present analysis of obesity was undertaken, a height-weight rating was constructed by slicing these height-weight distributions into the 7 diagonal layers which are indicated in Figure 1. (It should be noted that since the distributions for the sexes differ, the cutting points also differ. Therefore the height-weight rating does not permit direct comparisons between the sexes.)

This rating can be put into the more familiar setting of the figures on desirable weight,[13] derived from the *Build and Blood Pressure Study* of 1959,[14] if the midpoint of the height and weight intervals is considered to represent the heights and weights of all the individuals in that interval, and if it is assumed that all respondents were of medium frame. (Arbitrary values were assumed for the 2 men and 3 women whose heights or weights fell into the extreme open-ended categories.) Table 1 shows this comparison between the height-weight rating and desirable weight. Desirable weights are those for a given height and body build, for which the mortality rate among insured persons was the lowest. The men in our sample run from 37% under to 62% over desirable weight and the women's weights range from 30% under to 68% over the so-called desirable figures.

Average weights in the national sample of 5,000,000 persons on which the *Build and Blood Pressure Study* was based, ran from about 5% to 15% over the desirable weights. We have, therefore, designated individuals who received height-weight ratings 5, 6, and 7 as obese and will contrast them with the normals—those who received height-weight ratings of 3 or 4 and whose weights were close to the national average.

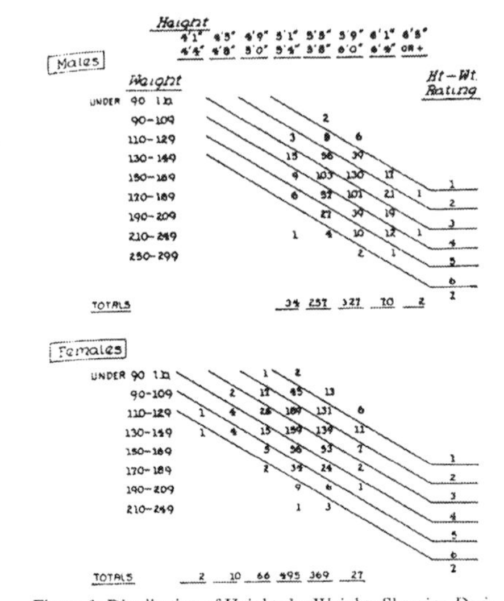

Figure 1: Distribution of Heights by Weights Showing Derivation of Height-Weight Rating. Shown are heights and weights of sample under study. Diagonal lines indicate which height and weight categories are combined to form 7 height-weight ratings. These ratings range from 1 (severely underweight) to 7 (grossly overweight).

Table 1.—Relationship of Height-Weight Rating to Desirable Weight

Height Weight Rating	Men		Women	
	Frequency in Sample	% Plus or Minus Desirable Weight	Frequency in Sample	% Plus or Minus Desirable Weight
1	8	−37	21	−30
2	63	−14	168	−11
3	210	+ 2	352	+ 3
4	239	+15	242	+21
5	117	+29	100	+37
6	44	+44	50	+52
7	7	+62	16	+68

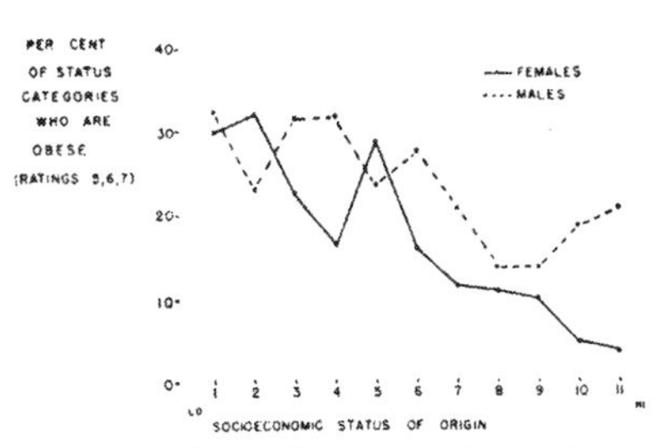

Figure 2: Chart shows striking relationship between socioeconomic status and obesity.

It should be recalled that actual measurements of height and weight were not obtained in the Midtown Study. The error introduced by using the reports of the respondents is probably in the direction of a regression toward the mean. The effect would be to cause us to classify in the normal weight categories some persons who were actually either underweight or overweight. It is not clear what the effect would be of erroneously including some underweight persons in the normal weight categories. The erroneous inclusion of some obese persons in the normal weight categories, on the other hand, would obscure any real differences between obese persons and those of normal weight. Such a tendency to obscure differences permits greater confidence in any positive findings which may emerge.

Results

In the Midtown Study, the 2 variables that were found to be most important in evaluating the psychological functioning of various segments of the sample were age and parental socioeconomic status. Those of lower socioeconomic status and those in the older age groups were more likely to be mentally ill. The relationship between the height-weight rating and each of these variables was, therefore, examined.

A striking relationship between socioeconomic status and obesity was discovered (Fig. 2). Some 30% of the women in the lowest socioeconomic category were obese and this percentage tended to decrease with increasing socioeconomic status until, in the highest socioeconomic status category, only 4% were obese. For men, the same tendency existed, although to a lesser extent.

Age, as well as socioeconomic status, is related to obesity. Figure 3 indicates the percentage of each 5-year age category who are obese (received ratings of 5, 6, or 7 on the height-weight rating). Women show a low percentage in the younger age groups—only 5% of the 20- to 24-year-old group are obese. The percentage of obese women rises sharply after age 40, reaches a peak of 34% at age 50 to 54, and drops to 26% in the oldest category. For men, a positive relationship between age and obesity is also apparent, although it is less pronounced and the peak occurs somewhat earlier.

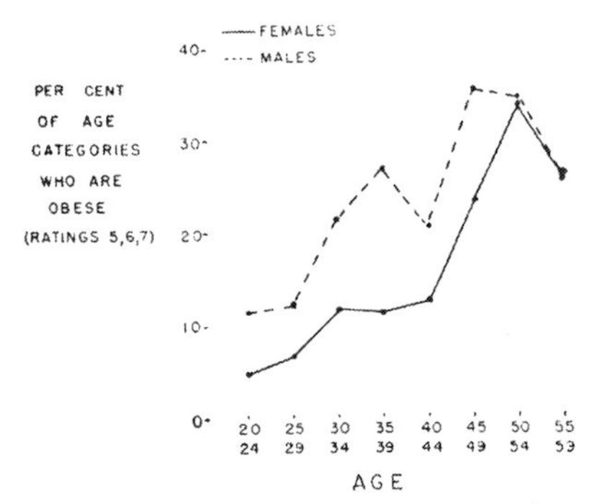

Figure 3: Percentage of each 5-year age category who are obese.

Since obesity was related to age and to socioeconomic status, and since both of those variables are, in turn, related to mental health, any investigation of the relationship between obesity and mental health must control for the age and social class of the respondents. For this purpose, the sample of male and female obese and normals was each divided into 6 subgroups, according to their social class (low—categories 1 through 3, medium—categories 4 through 7, high—categories 8 through 11) and age

Table 2.—Size of Subgroups When Sample of Males and Females Was Broken Down by Age and Parental Socioeconomic Status

Sex	Status	Age	Obese	Normals
Male	Low	Yng.	17	61
		Old	38	58
Male	Middle	Yng.	30	82
		Old	51	112
Male	High	Yng.	9	64
		Old	28	72
Female	Low	Yng.	21	91
		Old	55	85
Female	Middle	Yng.	15	96
		Old	53	134
Female	High	Yng.	3	86
		Old	19	101
(Age was not available on 1 normal-weight individual.)		Total	334	1,042

(young—20 through 39, and old—40 through 59). Table 2 shows the size of the resulting subgroups. Fifteen of these groups contain at least 50 cases and only 2 contain less than 15 cases. These 2 are the male and female obese who are young and who have a high socioeconomic status of origin.

The 8 psychological scores and the evaluation of symptomatology made by psychiatrists (psychiatrists' rating) provide measures of various aspects of mental health. In order to test whether obese persons were more likely than those of normal weight to score abnormally on these measures, the percentage of each subgroup of obese who made a pathological score was compared with the comparable percentage of the corresponding subgroup of normals. Table 3 shows these comparisons in terms of the differences between the percentages obtained from the normal and obese subgroups. This table also indicates the probabilities (obtained by using a 2-tailed Wilcoxon matched-pairs signed-rank test) that these differences are statistically significant.

Eight of the 9 measures showed the obese to be less healthy than their controls. Significant results were obtained for "rigidity," "immaturity," and "suspicion." Although not achieving the 0.05 level of significance, the results for "withdrawal," "frustration-depression," "neurasthenia," "tension-anxiety," and the psychiatrists' rating also went in the same direction. The only exception to the general trend was in the case of "childhood anxiety" in which the obese group made slightly less pathological scores than the controls; this difference, however, was so small as to be indistinguishable from chance.

Comment

One of the most interesting findings of this study is the high correlation between obesity and social class. Clinical investigations had previously suggested such a relationship,[13] but this is the first controlled study, as far as we know, that has demonstrated it. The fact that obesity is 7 times more frequent in lower-class than in upper-class women has profound implications for theory and for therapy. For it means that whatever its genetic and biochemical determinants, obesity in man is susceptible to an extraordinary degree of control by social factors. It suggests that a broad-scale assault on the problem need not await further understanding of the physiological determinants of obesity. Such an assault might be carried out by a program of education and social control designed to reproduce certain critical influences to which society has already exposed its upper-class members.

Much of our understanding of social and psychological factors in obesity has been derived from the psychotherapy of obese persons. Such persons, however, as a result of the selective process in recruitment for psychotherapy, tend to be from the upper or upper-middle classes—groups which in the Midtown Study, at least, do not contribute significantly to the total obese population. The problem of obesity in the Midtown Study is rather one of lower- or lower-middle-class persons—groups whose response to weight control measures has been less carefully studied. Perhaps some of the pessimism about the control of obesity and the preoccupation with individual psychological factors which has stemmed from the study of upper-class obese persons is not justified when considering the numerically far more important lower-class groups. Perhaps, for example, simple but energetic information programs directed to the appropriate groups could achieve far more than has been thought possible. Agencies for this purpose are plentiful. Well-baby

Table 3.—Comparison Between Obese and Normals on Mental Health Measures

Sex	Status	Age	Immaturity	Suspiciousness	Rigidity	Frustration-Depression	Withdrawal	Tension-Anxiety	Neurasthenia	Psychiatric Rating	Childhood Anxiety
Male	Low	Yng.	+ 3	+ 3	+ 2	− 2	− 0	+ 6	+ 5	− 1	− 9
		Old	+ 1	+ 9	+ 2	+ 1	+ 24	+ 8	+ 6	− 9	− 17
Male	Middle	Yng.	+ 4	+ 7	+ 11	+ 4	+ 2	+ 1	− 15	+ 6	− 9
		Old	+ 15	+ 21	+ 27	+ 2	+ 11	− 13	+ 5	+ 6	− 8
Male	High	Yng.	+ 15	+ 21	+ <1	+ <1	+ 14	+ 24	+ 5	+ 11	+ 17
		Old	+ 25	+ 18	+ 13	+ 9	+ 14	− 9	− 3	+ 16	− 6
Female	Low	Yng.	+ 3	+ 13	− 9	− 12	− 8	+ 4	+ 3	− 9	+ 19
		Old	+ 1	+ 6	+ 13	+ 10	− 1	+ 4	+ 21	+ 7	+ 3
Female	Middle	Yng.	+ 38	+ 25	+ 46	+ 6	+ 11	+ 9	+ 13	+ 13	− 3
		Old	+ 15	+ 20	+ 26	+ 9	+ 19	+ 7	+ 23	+ 12	− 7
Female	High	Yng.	+ 1	+ 21	+ 13	+ 21	+ 5	+ 45	− 13	− 12	− 5
		Old	+ 18	+ 5	+ 25	+ 6	− 2	+ 4	+ 10	+ 9	− 28
		P	<.008	<.008	<.007	<.055	<.055	<.108	<.137	<.204	<.478

Figures are differences between percentages of normals and obese who responded pathologically. Pathologically is defined as answering more than one of items in score in pathological direction or being classified as impaired in psychiatrists' rating. Plus (+) means that higher percentage of obese group fell into pathological category, minus (–) means that higher percentage of normals did. Probability (P) that obese and normals do not differ was determined, using 2-tailed Wilcoxon test, for each of mental health measures.

clinics and child care centers deal with precisely the social groups in which the problem is most pronounced and with just those persons who determine the family eating patterns. Union, company, and municipal health programs reach a significant part of the men in the crucial social classes. A program directed toward these groups could bring the control of obesity, for the first time, within the capacity of traditional public health measures. And the economy in shifting the emphasis from individual medical to public health measures would make an informed large-scale attack on the problem feasible.

The finding that age is positively related to obesity has been reported in several previous studies. The results are similar to those found in the Midtown Study—an increased prevalence with increasing age and a decline among older age groups, probably due to the increased mortality rates among older obese persons. The similarity in findings from different samples supports the notion that increase in body weight with increasing age is a biological characteristic of man, as of so many mammals.

When age and socioeconomic variables were held constant, the obese persons scored lower on mental health measures than their nonobese controls. Statistically significant differences were found for 3 of these measures: immaturity, rigidity, and suspiciousness. Of all the mental health measures utilized in this study, immaturity accords most closely with the conventional view of the characteristics of obese persons. According to this view, a key trait of obese persons, and one frequently ascribed an etiological importance in their overeating, is a defect in impulse control. The finding of immaturity in this study supports this theory. The finding of rigidity, on the other hand, is not a conspicuous feature of the usual clinical descriptions of obese persons, and might even be considered at the opposite pole from immaturity. A possible explanation is that this rigidity is a means of coping with the untoward effects of defective impulse control.

The greater prevalence of suspiciousness among obese persons is likewise not a generally accepted correlate of obesity. A recent investigation, however, has found that some obese persons suffer from a body-image disturbance which involves an exaggerated self-consciousness and "the feeling that others can look upon them only with horror and contempt."[16] These findings suggest that factors such as suspiciousness may be more important in the personality of obese persons than has heretofore been suspected.

This study has correlated obesity with a variety of other factors. But correlations alone cannot tell us which, if any, of the factors are primary. Our results do not indicate whether the mental health factors are causes of obesity or the results of being obese in a society that devalues obesity. The answers to such questions can perhaps be determined only by longitudinal investigations. The findings of the present study give one ample reasons to believe that such longitudinal investigations might be most fruitful.

Summary

Data on a representative sample of 1,660 adults living in a central residential area of New York City were reanalyzed to ascertain the relationship between obesity and mental health. In the course of this analysis, a striking relationship between obesity and social class was discovered—obesity is 7 times more frequent among women of the lowest socioeconomic level than it is among those of the highest level; among men the same relationship exists, although to a much lesser degree. In common with other studies, the prevalence of obesity was found to increase with increasing age. The relationship of obesity and 9 measures of mental health was investigated, holding constant age and socioeconomic variables. The obese persons made more pathological responses than did those of normal weight; and for 3 of the measures, immaturity, suspiciousness, and rigidity the results were statistically significant.

Piersol 203, University Hospital, 3400 Spruce St., Philadelphia (Dr. Moore).

Data from the Midtown Study were made available by the director, Dr. Alexander Leighton, Department of Social Psychiatry, Cornell University Medical College.

Supported in part by a grant from the National Institutes of Mental Health, National Institutes of Health, U.S. Public Health Service.

References

1. Bruch, H.: *Importance of Overweight*, New York City: W. W. Norton Co., 1957.
2. Hecht, M.: Obesity in Women, Psychiatric Study, *Psychiat Quart* **29**:203–231 (Jan.) 1995.
3. Huckel, H.: More Than Bread: 6 Cases of Compulsive Eating, *Psychoanalysis* **4**:53–62, 1955.
4. Fromm, E.: Dynamics in Case of Obesity, *J Clin Exp Psychopath* **19**:292–302 (Dec.) 1958.
5. Richardson, H.: Obesity and Neurosis; Case Report, *Psychiat Quart* **20**:400–424 (July) 1946.
6. Feiner, A.: Study of Certain Aspects of Perception of Parental Figures and Sexual Identification of Obese, Adolescent Female Group, *Amer J Dig Dis* **21**:298–299 (Oct.) 1954.
7. Friedman, J.: Weight Problems and Psychological Factors, *J Counsel Psychol* **23**:524–527 (Dec.) 1959.
8. Fry, P.: Comparative Study of 'Obese' Children Selected on Basis of Fat Pads, *Amer J Clin Nutr* **1**:453–467 (Sept–Oct.) 1953.
9. Kotkov, B., and Murawski, B.: Rorschach Study of Personality Structure of Obese Women, *J Clin Psychol* **8**:391–396 (Oct.) 1952.

10. Suezek, R.: Personality of Obese Women, *Amer J Clin Nutr* **5**:197–202 (March–April) 1957.
11. Weinberg, N.; Mendelson, M.; and Stunkard, A.: Failure to Find Distinctive Personality Features in Group of Obese Men, *Amer J Psychiat* **117**:1035–1037 (May) 1961.
12. Srole, L., et al.: *Mental Health in the Metropolis: Midtown Manhattan Study,* Vol. 1, New York: McGraw-Hill Book Co.; 1962.
13. Metropolitan Life Insurance Company: New Weight Standards for Men and Women, *Statis Bull* **40:** (Nov.–Dec.) 1959.
14. Society of Actuaries: *Build and Blood Pressure Study,* 1959.
15. Bruch, H.: Psychiatric Aspects of Obesity in Children, *Amer J Psychiat* **99**:752–757 (March) 1943.
16. Stunkard, A., and Mendelson, M.: Disturbances in Body Image of Some Obese Persons, *J Amer Diet Ass* **38**:328–331 (April) 1961.

CLASSICS IN OBESITY

Obesity in Childhood and Personality Development*

Hilde Bruch, M.D.
New York

It is a matter of common knowledge that obese people show certain similarities of character and behavior. According to popular opinion, fat people are cheerful and easygoing. They enjoy life in general, and good, rich food in particular. This popular concept has been challenged as incorrect for the obese adult by Newburgh (1) and Rennie (2). It certainly is not true for the obese child. On the contrary, obese children are fundamentally unhappy and maladjusted. Timid and retiring, clumsy and slow, they are not capable of holding a secure place among other children. Oversensitive and unable to defend themselves, they are helplessly exposed to the jeers and heckling of their more active comrades. Thus they shun healthy play and exercise, and become miserable and seclusive. However, their lack of interest and fearfulness can generally be traced to a time before a marked degree of obesity existed. Although it is obvious that obesity tends to set a child apart and to interfere with his social life, these are secondary changes which do not in themselves give a satisfactory clue to the development of obese children.

The peculiar behavior of obese children in which immaturity, overdependence and lack of aggressiveness are described as outstanding features, has been recognized by several observers (3,4,5). These earlier reports are limited to observations on obese boys who were classified as suffering from "adipose-genital dystrophy" or as exhibiting the "Froehlich Syndrome." Existence of endocrine dysfunction is taken for granted and, accordingly, personality traits are explained as the result of direct influences of some disturbed physiologic function, such as "a low basal metabolic rate," as the reaction of the total personality to the deficiencies (5), as "determined by the endocrine factors basic to the syndrome" (4), or they are simply attributed to "hormonal deficiency" (3).

My own approach to the behavior problems of obese children has been somewhat different. They were not labelled with an elaborate but generally unfounded and misleading endocrine diagnosis. The condition of obesity, that is, the excessive accumulation of subcutaneous fat tissue, has been contemplated in its significance as a symptom. An attempt has been made to understand the meaning of this symptom in relation to the growth and development of the total personality, that is, in respect to physical, mental, social, and emotional maturation.

One may define obesity as a variation of body build which is characterized by excessive growth in volume. This somatic expression of growth, the expansion in space, stands in contrast to the apparent absence of aggressiveness in the behavior. Some discrepancies in the growing-up process may be suspected as the basic disturbance in the development of the obese personality. This approach to the problem presupposes a concept of "growth" which refers not only to the increase in bodily size and to physical maturation, but includes also the emergence of an integrated new individual who is capable of independent and responsible action.

The phases of bodily growth which are not expressed by weight are also increased in obese children. Advanced growth in stature, accelerated skeletal maturation, and normal or frequently early puberty are the rule for both boys and girls who grow obese before the age of adolescence (6). These observations have been made on more than 200 children who were from 25 to 150 per cent overweight. The group includes many diagnosed by some other observer, as having obesity of the hypopituitary, hypothyroid, or some other endocrine type. The finding of intensive growth and rapid development is not consistent with the diagnosis of endocrine hypofunction. The basal metabolism has been found to be higher than that of non-obese children (7). In view of these findings, it is obvious that the peculiar behavior cannot have resulted from hormonal deficiency or adjustment to it. Furthermore, the intellectual development, as determined by the Stanford Binet test, is frequently ad-

---

* Presented at the 1941 meeting.

From the Department of Pediatrics, College of Physicians and Surgeons, Columbia University, and the Pediatric Division of the Vanderbilt Clinic and the Babies Hospital. Aided by a grant from the Josiah Macy, Jr., Foundation.
From Am. J. Orthopsychiat. 1941:11:467–473.

vanced. Children with severe mental defects were not included in this study since it was felt that they offered problems of a different type. No patient in our series had symptoms of an intracranial tumor.

In contrast to the expansive growth and accelerated physical and mental development stands the marked retardation of the social and emotional maturation. The overt expression of this immaturity takes manifold forms. The most obvious manifestation is a continued dependence upon the mother, even at an advanced age, for the simplest services of physical care and for the satisfaction of emotional needs. Many, even older, obese children are not capable of dressing themselves nor of any other task of self-care. The lack of independence may extend to every detail of daily life and bodily function. There are children, ten years of age or more, who never had a bowel movement without being coaxed, or even accompanied, to the bathroom. Enuresis persists in about 40 per cent of such children above six years of age. Some of eight years or more continue to be spoon-fed. Persistence of bottle feeding and unwillingness to chew are not unusual up to five years.

Sometimes young obese children express a desire to do things for themselves. Without encouragement and opportunity, they fail to develop motor skill according to their age, and gradually lose interest in becoming independent and passively accept the services of others. If demands are made upon them later on, they are so slow and incompetent that they become discouraged and soon give up, especially when nagged and driven to greater hurry.

As an example, I wish to cite David, a boy of ten, who was brought for examination because the school urged it. He was markedly overweight and so slow and unskilled that he could not do such simple things as hanging up his coat, using the scissors, or opening a closet door. His achievement in the intellectual field was good and he was a proficient reader. The mother continued to accompany him to school which was only one block away, and led him by the hand like a two-year-old. During the medical examination he accepted dressing and undressing by his mother with such inactivity that he resembled a wooden mannequin. The mother did not consider his lack of skill unusual. She resented the fact that the school authorities had interfered and drawn her attention to it. It had never occurred to her that David might do anything for himself, or that he might do small jobs around the house or run errands for her. She had never allowed him to play with other children.

It is not surprising that children of this type do not find much enjoyment and satisfaction in active games and in association with other children. Usually they are frankly afraid of new experiences or contacts. When asked if he ever enjoyed running a race, one boy answered in surprise: "I have nothing to run for." Another said wistfully that he would like to if he could win. "I have to carry all this fat around with me everywhere I go. I could run a race with it but I could never win." So he went to the movies five or six times a week, or listened to the radio by the hour, and always found comfort in eating.

Delay in acquiring the usual muscular skills, and fear of active exercise, can be traced to lack of training and opportunity. Many children have been kept away from all contacts with other children, and have been constantly impressed with the possible dangers of exercise. Thus play and athletics, the source of enjoyment and recreation for other children, have been charged with the concept of threat and danger for the obese child.

The marked inactivity is of importance for the development of obesity as the amount of energy released through muscular activity is very small (8). This would not lead to obesity if the food intake were proportionately small. In the obese child, however, the ingestion of food is far in excess of that of normal children (9). It is not unusual to receive the explanation that the child overeats because he is bored and has nothing else to do. From a quantitative point of view the large intake of food is of greater importance than the inactivity. It is present with even greater regularity. There is a general tendency of obese patients to minimize the extent of overeating. A few freely admit they like to eat enormous quantities. An eleven-year-old Italian boy weighing 255 pounds came for treatment because he could no longer bend down and tie his shoes. He had eaten about two loaves of bread per day, more than a pound of spaghetti at each meal, and whatever else he could get hold of. In addition, he had trained all his school friends to bring an extra sandwich for his lunch. He had consumed something like 12 to 15 sandwiches in school in one day. In this way he had doubled his weight during the last $2\frac{1}{2}$ years. More amazing than this gluttony was his ability to accept an entirely different and restricted diet without complaining of hunger or suffering from physical discomfort during the period of weight reduction.

The food intake of obese children is not only excessive, but also shows an astonishing preference for starches or sweets. Practically all fat children overeat on bread, cake, candy, ice cream and soups. In some younger children large quantities of milk are the main dietary item; in a few cases excessive amounts of meat are taken. Not one child in our group had learned to eat a mixed, well balanced diet. Vegetables and salads lead in the series of foods which are disliked. Fruits, with the exception of bananas and orange juice, come next. In many cases there is a marked resistance against any change in the composition of meals. On the whole, the pronounced likes and dislikes for certain foods may be described as a persistence of taste development at an early, infantile level.

Even more conspicuous than the huge quantities and one-sided composition of food is the high emotional significance for obese children and their parents. The unwillingness to change the established faulty feeding habits points to the exaggerated importance which food has in the life of these families. A mother who brought her child for treatment because he was too fat objected, quite distraught, when a diet was discussed: "Does that mean he would lose his appetite and eat less? No, I wouldn't like that."

In order to recognize the factors within the home which have contributed to the development of overdependence and overeating, a study of the family background has been made. An extensive report has been previously published (10). I can mention here only some general aspects. Many fathers of obese children were found to be weak and unaggressive, with little drive and ambition. They are unable to give positive guidance to their children and to counteract the overindulgent and retarding influence of the mothers. With few exceptions the mothers are domineering in the life of the families. Many mothers had suffered great poverty and often hunger in their childhood and were thrown upon their own resources at an early age. They had reacted to their early experiences with self-pity and resentment and were blocked in emotional development. They continued to look upon life in the light of their early disappointments and failures and were unable to loosen the ties to their past. In a primitive way they try to create for their children that "normal" carefree childhood of which, they feel, they had been deprived and which is represented for them in a life of idleness and in abundance of food.

The manifestation of this maternal attitude is an overt display of protectiveness and overemphasis on feeding. However, this expression of affection and devotion cannot hide the underlying insecurity, possessiveness and often hostility in relation to the child. The basic insecurity expresses itself in profound fears for the life and safety of the child, with constant apprehension of injury and death. Only when the child is in her presence does she find relaxation and peace of mind. Many far reaching over-protective measures are devised to spare the mother the anguish of her own fears, with complete disregard of the child's needs and wishes. At the same time the mother is irritated by the child's presence and the demands he makes upon her. Quite often she resorts to beating, constant nagging and criticizing to find relief from her own irritation.

There is also an urgent need on the part of the mother to keep the child dependent and to possess his love and loyalty exclusively. Dissatisfied in her marital relation and without community outlets for her ambition, she concentrates on her home and her child in her strivings for personal satisfaction and achievement. By keeping her child in close personal contact and by ministering to him, she fosters in him the need for her continued attention. With threats of withholding her affection she tries' to control and mould him to her will. By so doing she prevents him from developing personal independence and establishing satisfying relations to an outside world in which she herself has not found security. The mother of a 12-year-old boy stated, "I don't mind him being babyish as long as he does not get into bad company," and considered every child he might meet to be "bad" and below her standards. Growth and maturation of the child are dangers to be warded off since they remove the basis for a relationship which the mother desires to perpetuate.

Mothers of obese children express a definite preference for girls, and voice their disappointment of sons in their presence. They explain the preference for girls by such statements as: "They are better companions," "They stay closer to you," "You can dress them nicely," and "You don't lose them when they get married." They consider their children a possession to be shown off or preserved, and not as individuals in their own right.

The manifestation of the ambivalent attitude of such mothers varies widely from case to case. The individual development and experiences to which these attitudes can be traced are equally manifold. A common factor is the mother's fundamental inability to give of herself, and substitutes concrete offerings as an expression of her affection. It is because of her own immaturity and insecurity that she cannot permit the child to grow away from her into a separate, self-reliant and independent being.

The study of the family frame of obese children thus reveals the existence of factors which retard personal development of the child and lead to inactivity and overeating. The home does not fulfill his basic needs of being loved and accepted for his personal value, and of growing and developing in harmony with his innate capacities. Yet the environmental influences do not in themselves explain why a child grows obese. Observations in our large group suggest that obesity represents a form of the child's response to these influences. It is the somatic expression of this response, fundamentally determined by forces within the child. This specific responsiveness of the child may be approached from different angles. I shall consider it here as a variation of his growth, and disregard the wide variety of individual reactions.

Growth is an active process, an intrinsic quality of each living organism. It is the creative power which differentiates one individual from the other. It implies for the child constant changes in his potentialities and in his personal relationships. With progressing maturity he becomes more and more self-reliant, assumes responsibilities for himself and finds satisfaction through expressing his creative drives. This development is grossly distorted in the obese child. One may consider as a basic weakness in his behavior the fact that he does not rebel against excessive feeding and prolonged overprotection. He accepts them because his fundamental attitude toward the environment is demanding. He indulges in the continued and excessive gratification at this primitive level, and is unwilling to give up the pleasures and safety of infancy. He does not conform to the changes which growing-up implies and fails to direct his energies to other achievements. It is as if he sells his birthright of becoming an independent and mature person for the continued abundance of nourishment and protection.

Obese children have been described as submissive and unaggressive. This description is correct as far as it relates to overt behavior and activities. Yet it is not correct for an understanding of the basic attitudes. The obese child is not passively resigned; he makes his claims and does not tolerate that his demands remain unsatisfied. Since his demands tally with his mother's need of offering food and services so lavishly, they find appeasement and gratification. There is a certain balance in the mother-child relationship in which food stands for love and satisfaction and thus represents an important tie. It is a precarious balance, however, contrary to the natural process of biological and emotional maturation.

Sooner or later the child must meet social demands and assert himself as an individual in relation to other children. Quite often the entry into school represents the first contact with the outside world, for which the child is entirely unprepared. Patients are frequently brought for examination not because the parents consider the appearance or behavior of the child as unusual, but because the school finds that he does not fit into the group. The conflict involved in social adjustment increases with age. The child exposed to rejection and unable to hold his own, resorts to overeating since he knows food as a never failing source of comfort and satisfaction. It is not infrequent that the development of a severe degree of obesity occurs after entry into school. In overeating, the obese child finds an outlet for his aggressive and hostile feelings. It is the weapon with which he meets traumatic experiences, failure and disappointment.

Yet, not only external influences disturb the peace in the relationship between the mother and her obese child. He progressively increases his demands and always wants immediate satisfaction. "Gimme, gimme, gimme, is all I ever hear from him," complained one mother. Another described the demanding attitude of her son: "If he wants something he wants it badly. Whatever he sees other boys have, he wants too. He wants it as badly and cries for it like a baby cries for his bottle." Both these boys were eleven years old. In other respects they were perfect examples of quiet submissive behavior. They were polite, would not talk back, were unable to defend themselves against the heckling and attacks of other boys, and did not protest against persistent maternal protection.

Even if complete satisfaction of increasing wants can be secured, the child's innate power for growth and maturity cannot be indefinitely suppressed. The obese child may fight the continued infantilization and make an effort to assert himself. His weapons for the struggle are inadequate; he uses temper tantrums, crying spells and stubborn sulkiness. In relation to schoolmates, he may attempt to attract their attention by boisterous behavior, clowning and talkativeness; or, he may become bossy and aggressive against younger and weaker children. Yet, he has not the courage of developing true personal independence by giving up his infantile pleasures.

The creative component of the growth of the obese child expresses itself in exaggerated bodily size and early sexual maturation. This rapid rate of physical development belies all attempts to keep him small and dependent, and contradicts his immature and babyish behavior. Deposition of fat is not a passive process; it is more than the mechanical sequel of a positive energy balance. Storage fat is regulated through the vegetative nervous system and is controlled through impulses from the midbrain. In view of these facts it is not inconceivable that an individual can give material expression to the inner picture of his own self. The child, through the excessive accumulation of fat tissue, achieves an aggrandizement of his bodily appearance. At the same time he perpetuates, or even exaggerates the preponderance of fat over muscle development, a relationship which is normal during infancy. The very existence of obesity in a child is a concrete illustration that the conflicts which Allen (11) calls the "dilemma of growth" have not yet found a solution.

I cannot go into detail of how somatic expression of psychic experiences might be achieved, but refer to the work of Schilder (12). He has developed the concept of the "body image," which is derived from all sensory and psychic experiences. This "body image" is in constant integration in the central nervous system. Its conception is a way of seeing life and personality as a whole. According to Schilder, one may look upon "our own body as an image, which is built up in ourselves in accordance with our instinctive attitudes." Coghill (13), starting from embryological observations, speaks of man as "a mechanism which, within the limitations of life, sensitivity and growth, is creating and operating himself." Through this process of self-operation and self-creation, and through appeasement of the infantile instinct of deriving satisfaction exclusively from food, the obese child, impeded in the dynamic expression of his self, manifests his creative strivings in the static form of bodily largeness. The inordinate expansion reveals the inmost desire of the child to be big and powerful. Although passive and quiet, he is by no means inconspicuous; on the contrary, he makes an impression on his environment through his very size and appearance. In his insecure and unstable relation to his surroundings, physical size gives him a certain feeling of safety and strength. The heavy layer of fat acts like a wall behind which the child seeks protection against a threatening outside world.

Homburger (14) has reported that obese children, in a play situation, construct buildings which resemble the outlines of their bodies, a finding he has not observed in any other group. Our own material of Rorschach records (15) reveals, besides many other features, the preoccupation of the obese child with the problem of "size," and suggests the emotional and symbolic importance of obese largeness. Another finding in Rorschach tests, which seems limited to obese children, is an interpretation of symmetrical figures as "a man and a woman," or "boy and a girl." This type of interpretation is given more often by boys than girls, and points to their confusion about sex. Close dependence upon and strong identification with the mothers invariably leads to conflicts about their masculinity.

Obesity in childhood may thus be understood as a disturbance in the maturation of the total personality and as a somatic compensation for thwarted creative drives, whereby the total size of the body becomes the "expressive organ" of the conflict. It thus becomes clear why obese children show so much resistance against treatment, even if they suffer from the handicap of obesity and are anxious to lose weight. They are not only unwilling to give up the immediate satisfaction of eating, but fear even more the possibility of becoming small and weak. Treatment consisting only of mechanical reduction of food intake, is often doomed to failure. Endocrine treatment, with extremely rare exceptions, has no justifiable place in the management of obesity in childhood. It is not only useless, it may even be harmful through the implication of sexual maldevelopment or some mysterious abnormality. To be of real value, therapy should help the child grow independent and self-reliant, and make constructive use of his good physical and mental endowment, so that he can find more dynamic outlets for his creative drives than the static form of physical largeness.

Bibliography

1. Newburgh, L. H. *The Cause of Obesity.* J.A.M.A., 97: 1659 (Dec. 5), 1931.
2. Rennie, T. A. C. *Obesity as a Manifestation of Personality Disturbance.* Dis. of the Nerv. Syst., 1: 238, 1940.
3. Lurie, L. A. *Endocrinology and the Understanding and Treatment of the Exceptional Child.* J.A.M.A., 110: 1531 (May 7), 1938.
4. Levy, D. M. *Aggressive-Submissive Behavior and the Fröhlich Syndrome.* Arch. Neurol. and Psychiat., 36: 991 (Nov.), 1936.
5. Mittelmann, B. *Juvenile Adiposogenital Dystrophy: Neurologic and Psychopathologic Aspects.* Endocrinology, 23: 637, 1938.
6. Bruch, H. *Obesity in Childhood. I. Physical Growth and Development of Obese Children.* Am. J. Dis. Child., 58: 457 (Sept.), 1939.

7(a). ———. *Obesity in Childhood.* II. *Basal Metabolism and Serum Cholesterol of Obese Children.* Am. J. Dis. Child., 58: 1001 (Nov.), 1939.

7(b). Talbot, N. B., and Worcester, J. *The Basal Metabolism of Obese Children.* J. Pediat., 16: 146 (Feb.), 1940.

8. Bruch, H. *Obesity in Childhood.* IV. *Energy Expenditure of Obese Children.* Am. J. Dis. Child., 60: 1082 (Nov.), 1940.
9. ———. *Obesity in Childhood.* III. *Physiologic and Psychologic Aspects of the Food Intake of Obese Children.* Am. J. Dis. Child., 59: 739 (Apr.), 1940.
10. Bruch, H., and Touraine, G. *Obesity in Childhood.* V. *The Family Frame of Obese Children.* Psychosom. Med., 2: 141, 1940.
11. Allen, F. H. *The Dilemma of Growth.* Arch. Neurol. and Psychiat., 37: 859 (Apr.), 1937.
12. Schilder, Paul. *The Image and Appearance of the Human Body.* Psyche Monographs, London, 1935.
13. Coghill, G. E. *Anatomy and the Problem of Behaviour.* Cambridge University Press, 1929.
14. Homburger, E. *Traumatische Konfigurationen im Spiel.* Imago, 23: 447, 1937.
15. Bruch, H. *Rorschach Tests of Obese Children* (unpublished).

Emotional Aspects of Obesity

*Walter W. Hamburger, M.D.**

INTRODUCTION

The Cause of Obesity. The medical literature contains many reports of careful clinical and experimental studies on obese patients. These studies have failed so far to reveal any constant etiologic cause for the usual case of obesity. Repeated metabolic studies of obese children and adults have revealed no abnormality.[1–7] Nor do obese persons usually have a demonstrable endocrine disorder. Pancreatic islet cell tumors can lead to obesity via hyperinsulinism, but such lesions are not found in the usual case of obesity. The obesity formerly associated with hypothyroidism and Cushing's syndrome has been shown to be due to water retention or to a redistribution of fat deposits rather than the development of true obesity.[2,3,7–9] Similarly, obese patients do not usually have a demonstrable lesion in the central nervous system, although both clinical and animal observations indicate that hypothalamic lesions can in certain instances produce obesity.[2,3,7,8,10,14–16] The concept of juvenile obesity as a manifestation of a pituitary lesion (Fröhlich's syndrome) has been largely abandoned.[3,7,10–12] Miscellaneous biochemical causes for obesity such as hypoglycemia, hypercholesterolemia or the presence of a lipophilic substance in the blood stream[2,3,5,7] have not been consistently identified.

The frequent occurrence of familial obesity would seem to implicate hereditary factors but proven data of genetic transmission in humans is meager.[2,3,8] Twin studies are inconclusive. Danforth[17] did demonstrate a gene connected with yellow hair color which bred obesity in wild mice, but how this may relate to human obesity is not yet clear.

Most modern authors have concluded that obesity is due to excessive inflow of energy exceeding the outflow, such disproportion being caused primarily by overeating[1–4,6–8]. When the total intake of solids and water is accurately recorded, the body weights of obese persons correspond with the inflow and outflow of energy in normal fashion.[1–3] Muscular inactivity, as well as overeating, may, of course, contribute to the disproportion between intake and outflow of energy. Bruch[6] reported that 72 per cent of 140 obese children were physically inactive, but the degree of inactivity could not be correlated with the severity of the obesity. Calorically speaking, the obese person's relative inactivity seems to be of less importance than his overeating.[3,6] Bruch[16], by as quantitative methods as possible in both home and clinic, demonstrated that 142 obese children overate during periods of weight gain and ate a normal amount during stationary weight periods. Most clinicians dealing with obese patients have reached the same conclusion by more random observations, namely, that most of their obese patients do overeat. Conversely, if and when their patients adhere to a diet reasonable for their energy needs, they do lose weight.

Thus, we arrive at the conclusion that the one consistent and demonstrable finding in obesity is overeating. Whatever the predisposition to obesity may ultimately prove to be, the symptom of hyperphagia seems to be a necessary component. Hereditary, constitutional or hypothalamic factors may all play a part and need further elucidation, but without overeating the predisposed individual will not develop obesity. In this connection it is interesting that Danforth's obese bred mice ate more than their controls.[18] Similarly the rats which Brobeck and his associates made fat by hypothalamic lesions, also first developed hyperphagia.[14,15] If their diet was restricted they failed to become obese. Brobeck concluded that hypothalamic lesions abolish the animals' usual controls over eating. These experiments indicate that the symptom of hyperphagia may itself be under the influence of hypothalamic, hereditary or constitutional factors. This has been clearly summarized in Friedgood's recent discussion [19], but needs further study.

Hunger versus Appetite. It may be pertinent to emphasize the difference between hunger and appetite as regulators of food intake. This difference has been stressed by Cannon[20], Harrington[21], Newburgh[3] and others. Hunger is the physiological expression of the body's need for energy (food) which operates involuntarily in the healthy individual. As suggested above, this need (hunger) may well be under the control of inherited, constitutional or hypothalamic regulation. It is noteworthy that hunger is an uncomfortable sensation localized to the epigastrium. The discom-

From the Department of Psychiatry, University of Rochester School of Medicine and Dentistry, and the Strong Memorial and Rochester Municipal Hospitals, Rochester, New York.
* Assistant Professor of Psychiatry, University of Rochester School of Medicine and Dentistry; Assistant Psychiatrist, Strong Memorial and Rochester Municipal Hospitals.
From Med. Clin. N. A. 1951:35:483–499.
Reprinted with permission of W.B. Saunders Company.

fort of hunger is relieved by eating. Appetite, on the other hand, is a psychological desire to eat and gives a distinct anticipatory pleasure. Normally hunger produces appetite, but appetite also exists independently and can be stimulated by other means. For example, discussing or reading about liked food stimulates appetite. Overseas soldiers spend many a bull session discussing steak and french fries—even after a full meal of C-rations. Appetite is conditioned by the sight, smell and memory of certain foods and individual experiences while eating. Eating is well understood as an important esthetic, social and emotional experience in daily life. Food and restaurant advertisements rely on these relationships for their appeal. Thus a particular individual's appetites, taste for specific foods and his eating habits are conditioned by his entire life experiences with food and eating.

Appetite and the Emotions. A particular factor in appetite is the person's emotional state. It is common knowledge that when a person is upset or under some emotional tension there is often a reflection in his appetite. Interestingly enough, this may be either in the direction of an increase or decrease. The ubiquitous emotional experiences of love and grief are particularly well known for their disturbing effects on appetite. Anger too may disturb appetite, as every parent knows. The child may refuse to eat as an angry or defiant gesture toward the parent. In morbid emotional states, particularly the depressions, eating disturbances are usually cardinal symptoms. Often the neurotically depressed person will overeat and gain weight, whereas the psychotically depressed person often refuses food. Thus in sickness and in health there is an intimate interrelationship of appetite and the person's emotional state.

With such widespread knowledge concerning the relationship of emotions to appetite, it is odd that we, as physicians, have only recently turned our attention to the interaction of appetite and emotions in obese patients. The following clues have long been in evidence: (1) Despite violent protestations against their obesity, and despite the exhortations and diets of their physicians, many fat people continue to overeat. This paradox suggests the possibility that overeating subserves some strong emotional need. (2) If we take a detailed history regarding the eating habits of obese patients, we often learn that they themselves are aware that when they are emotionally aroused, they overeat and that eating makes them feel better emotionally. Freed[22] asked 500 obese patients, "When you are nervous or worried do you eat more or less?" Three hundred and seventy replied that they ate larger meals or ate more frequently. An additional ninety-five stated that they ate more when "idle, bored or tired." Only thirty-five had noted no connection between appetite and their emotional state.

This reaction in obese persons does not seem to be qualitatively different from that of normal people whose appetite may increase during the experience of love, grief or other universal feelings. Closer scrutiny of obese patients' eating patterns might reveal that quantitatively, however, their appetite response to an emotional stimulus is greater than that of the healthy person. One thing that has interferred with progress in this direction has been the traditional concept of a fat person as a jovial, happy and well-adjusted individual. In the series of patients to be described in this paper, we found this to be usually untrue. When it was superficially true, more prolonged study revealed this attitude to be a psychological protection against underlying emotional upsets of a potentially neurotic or psychotic nature.

CLINICAL MATERIAL

The author therefore determined to investigate the role of emotional factors in the hyperphagia (overeating) of obese patients. The clinical data comes from the detailed psychiatric study of eighteen obese patients seen in the medical and psychiatric clinics of a general hospital* (1946–50), and in the author's private psychiatric practice (1948–50). These patients do not represent consecutive cases of obesity, but were selected because they had adequate psychological study to reveal some of their motives for overeating. In the majority of instances these obese patients were referred to Psychiatric Clinic after adequate medical study, either because of known emotional illness or because of their failure to lose weight with diet and drugs. These patients were studied from one to 398 hours (Table 1), a total of approximately 900 diagnostic and therapeutic hours. Several of my colleagues† contributed detailed data on several of the clinic cases they have been treating. Also random reference will be made to published case reports of other authors.

Overeating as a Response to Nonspecific Emotional Tensions. Twelve patients in the present series of eighteen had been aware of marked changes in appetite accompanying transient, nonspecific emotional upsets. Two of these were in the direction of eating less. The other ten reported eating more than usual when upset. For example, Patient 10 said, "When I feel mad or blue I eat a big piece of pie and feel better." Patient 14 noticed that when she was upset she went to the kitchen and took a little bite ". . . whether I wanted it or not" (whether she was hungry or not) Patients 11 and 15 both spoke of the "soothing" effect of eating when nervous. The medical interne wrote in his history of Patient 13: "With anxiety her hunger (appetite) increases." This data points up how likely obese patients are to experience a disturbance in appetite, usually in the direction of

† The author wishes to thank Doctors Robert L. Roessler, Instructor in Psychiatry, Owen Otto, Rockefeller Foundation Fellow in Psychiatry; Philipp C. Sottong and Albert W. Sullivan, Veteran Postgraduate Fellows in Psychiatry, for their helpful data.
* Strong Memorial Hospital, Rochester, New York.

overeating, when emotionally disturbed. Although feelings of upset, nervousness, anger, anxiety and boredom were mentioned by various patients in this connection, the most frequently named emotional stimulus to overeating was feeling blue or depressed. This suggests that overeating in obese patients may often be a reaction to the specific mood of depression. Data to be discussed under "Treatment" and "Discussion" seem to confirm this possibility.

It should be mentioned that questionnaires such as Freed's[22] on the relationship of emotions to eating are of limited value because often patients are not fully conscious of any connection between the two. For example, Patient 12, who was treated for 398 hours, originally had stated there was no connection between her feelings and her eating habits. Later in psychotherapy when more aware of her reactions, she reported repeatedly observing herself eating more when unhappy or upset.

Overeating as a Substitute Gratification in Intolerable Life Situations. Seven patients (Cases 2, 3, 5, 9, 12, 13, 18) gave a history of reacting to intolerable or frustrating life situations with chronic overeating. If a person can respond to a transient mood or an acute emotional experience with overeating, is it not logical that he might continue to overeat if the emotional stimulus itself continued over a long period? These seven patients, in some way predisposed to hyperphagia, reacted to intolerable life situations by overeating, apparently gaining some sort of substitute emotional gratification and relief of tension. Let me give some examples:

Patient No. 3, Mrs. T. B., is a 47 year old 233 pound woman who developed obesity at age 25, shortly after her marriage and the birth of her first child. Physical examination was normal except for patient's obesity and excess hair on the upper lip. B. M. R. was +6 per cent; glucose tolerance test and other laboratory studies were normal. Patient's mother was described as a domineering, strict woman who told patient nothing of sex, childbirth and marital relationships. In her youth patient made poor family and social adjustments, and remained immature. She was therefore poorly prepared for marriage and parenthood, had constant friction with her husband, and in-laws. Early in her marriage, patient and her husband were separated for a year and a half. Patient was unable to solve these marital problems in any mature or realistic manner, had frequent crying spells.

Diagnosis other than obesity: none.

Comment. This woman began to overeat in reaction to a disturbed marital relationship which she was unable to improve. Because of her inability to make a realistic change in her situation she reacted to her continuing unhappiness and frustration with chronic overeating. In some way the eating served as a substitute emotional gratification, and a release from tension. The factors which predisposed her to this reaction and to obesity are not known.

Patient No. 9, Mr. W. H., a 45 year old married man weighing 243 pounds, consulted the psychiatric clinic because of repetitive business failures. Patient had noted his inability to assert himself, be independent and get along with bosses. He also attributed failure to his obesity. He had been overweight since childhood, as were his parents. Father was a disciplinarian. Mother was overly protective and overly solicitous of patient who was the only child. She always feared he wasn't eating enough and pushed sweets at him. Patient periodically became discouraged and depressed over his business failures and at such times ate more. In the past six years, with increasing financial worries, he has gained 55 pounds.

Diagnosis other than obesity: Character disorder, passive-dependent type with depressive trends.

Comment. This man had been overweight since childhood and thus predisposed to overeating and obesity in reaction to life stresses. Hereditary and constitutional factors are suggested by the parental history of obesity. A psychological fixation on eating may have occurred in childhood due to mother's known tendencies to overprotect and overfeed her only child. In any event, when faced with repetitive business failures which he was unable to do anything about, he reverted to a childhood gratification, overate and gained an additional 55 pounds.

Overeating as Symptom of an Underlying Emotional Illness, Especially Depressions and Hysteria. Patients 1, 4, 6, 11, 12, 14, 15 and 16 developed hyperphagia as only one of many symptoms of an underlying emotional illness. This symptomatic overeating led to an increase in weight. It seems warranted in these cases to stress the underlying psychological illness because such patients may well present themselves first at an Endocrine or Medical Clinic with the complaint of obesity, the underlying emotional illness not being apparent. In Table 1 it can be seen that sixteen patients had some demonstrable psychological disorder warranting a psychiatric diagnosis. Of these sixteen cases, nine consisted of so-called character disorders, seven of definitive psychoneuroses. This, of course, does not necessarily mean that obesity is part of that disease process as they could be separate entities occurring independently in the same person. Sometimes the obesity antedated the known psychological illness. At other times the emotional illness bore a reciprocal relationship to the obesity and appeared when the patient lost weight. However, the eight patients mentioned above overate and gained weight simultaneously with the development of a demonstrable emotional illness. In these cases the symptomatic hyperphagia was found to have a specific unconscious meaning to the sick person. The underlying illnesses were neurotic depres-

TABLE 1

EIGHTEEN PATIENTS WITH OBESITY AND VARIOUS EMOTIONAL DISORDERS

Patient	Sex	Age	Maximum Weight in Pounds	No. of Hours Studied	Diagnosis Other Than Obesity
1	F	20	178	3	(1) Hysterical psychopath (2) Attempted suicide
2	F	21	235	25	(1) Reactive depression, attempted suicide (2) Character disorder: inadequacy, periodic alcoholism
3	F	47	233	1	None
4	F	24	185	25	Anxiety-hysteria
5	F	16	178	22	(1) Character disorder: inadequacy, antisocial behavior (2) Attempted suicide
6	M	25	?	1	Neurotic depression
7	M	20	265	7	Character disorder: inadequacy, emotional instability, latent homosexuality
8	M	32	250	56	(1) Character disorder: passive-dependent type with impotence and latent homosexuality (2) Essential hypertension
9	M	45	243	25	Character disorder: passive-dependent type with depressive trends
10	F	22	170	44	(1) Conversion hysteria (2) Anxiety-hysteria (3) Frigidity
11	F	19	166	213	(1) Anorexia nervosa (2) Mixed psychoneurosis, obsessive - compulsive and hysterical features
12	F	30	225	398	(1) Conversion hysteria (2) Character disorder: immaturity reactions
13	F	33	156	1	Sterility, cause unknown
14	F	48	240	1	(1) Hypochondriasis (2) Neurotic depression
15	F	23	243	2	Anxiety-hysteria
16	F	22	205	29	(1) Character disorder (2) Possible hypothyroidism
17	F	38	365	2	(1) Character disorder; inadequacy with episodic alcoholism (2) Borderline intelligence (3) Chronic cholecystitis
18	F	20	210	23	Character disorder: inadequacy with emotional instability

sions in Cases 6 and 14, obsessive-compulsive and hysterical neurosis in Case 11, while hysterical features were predominant in Cases 1, 4, 12, 15 and 16.

It should be stressed that of the entire series of eighteen patients, twelve exhibited depressive features in their histories; three of these had made suicidal attempts. These histories included transient depressive feelings, neurotic or reactive depressions, characterological depressive traits, but no instance of frank depressive psychosis. Others, as we will discuss under "Treatment," became depressed as they lost weight in treatment. The frequency of depressive trends in other obese patients has been pointed out several times.[23-27] Mittleman too mentioned this in his psychological study of sixteen boys with the so-called adiposogenital dystrophy (Fröhlich's syndrome.[28]

In patients 1, 4, 11, 12, 15 and 16, all hysterical women, overeating was associated with a sexual conflict, either phantasied or realistic. More often than not, an external sexual temptation or upsetting sexual experience could be demonstrated. Patient 15, for example, obese all her life, had an exacerbation of hyperphagia and gained an additional 50 pounds when she began to date steadily for the first time in her life. The constant feature of all women in this group was marked difficulty in adjustment to men, leading either to shyness and retirement, or to promiscuity. In marriage they were usually frigid. They often demonstrated other hysterical features in their histories. Several gave a story of preexisting hysterical conversion symptoms or anxiety-hysteria (phobias). Patient 12, for example, had a fourteen year history of conversion symptoms in almost every system of the body: hysterical aphonia, globus hystericus, fainting, abdominal pain, headaches. For various reasons these women failed to mature emotionally and were incapable of enjoying an adult sexual life. This has happened to some because they have remained emotionally, and in a childlike way, attached to their fathers. Patients 12 and 16 gave a history of childhood sexual assaults which also served as traumatic sexual fixations. In any event, sexual impulses are inacceptable to these people and a sexual phantasy, temptation or experience provokes displeasure and symptom formation. These hysterical patients all reacted to their sexual conflicts by overeating. Inasmuch as they could not accept genital gratification they displaced their sexual impulses (from below, above) to overeating. To them eating had an unconscious (repressed) sexual significance.

The proof of this formulation is given explicitly by Patients 11 and 12, both of whom disclosed childhood oral impregnation phantasies. They both had thought that a woman became pregnant by taking something by mouth and that the baby grew in the stomach. Patient 12 had thought that women became pregnant by eating an egg. Since childhood she had had an irrational disgust and felt nauseated at the sight of a poached egg! These oral impregnation phantasies are well-known in young children and in hysterical patients who do not have obesity. Overeating is thus a classical hysterical symptom: whereas sexual impulses were rejected (repressed), the symptom itself symbolically contained the repressed sexual impulse, i.e., the desire to become pregnant.

In this particular subgroup, where the hyperphagia is an hysterical symptom, the obesity itself has taken on an unconscious secondary symbolic significance. On the one hand it stands for physical unattractiveness and hence a protection against men, consistent with these women's rejection of their own sexuality. Patient 16, for example, at age 22 had never dated, could not dance, was shy and ill at ease with men. In psychotherapy she associated her fears with a sexual assault at age 7. In treatment she discovered how her obesity was a protection against men, and as she herself put it, "an escape from the problems of sex." At the same time as she discussed her sexual conflicts in treatment she began to go steady with a young man, became more confident of herself, lost 22 pounds.

On the other hand, obesity itself may unconsciously symbolize pregnancy due to the childhood association that a pregnant woman is a fat woman. Patient 11 demonstrated hysterical features. When she was fat this 18 year old girl said "I feel as big now as if I'm carrying someone around with me." Again she said her abdomen puffed out after eating, "like a pregnant woman's." It was this patient who had previously had anorexia nervosa starting after a friend had jokingly said she looked pregnant in a certain photograph. Both her overeating and her obesity thus had an unconscious symbolic meaning of oral impregnation and pregnancy itself.

This secondary symbolic meaning of the obesity itself as either a protection against physical attractiveness and men or as an unconscious equivalent of pregnancy has been pointed out by a number of authors.[23,24,25,29] Reeve[29] cites the case of a female college student who gained weight when a suitor became attentive, lost weight when he became disinterested. This may help to explain the original paradox of why many fat female patients consciously complain of their weight and wish to be thin and attractive, while actually they do not adhere to their diets and do not make healthy heterosexual adjustments.

Overeating As an Addiction to Food. Still another motive for overeating was disclosed in Patients 1, 6, 7, 8, 10, 14, 17 and 18. This type of hyperphagia seems to be the most malignant type, characterized by a compulsive craving for food, often starting in earliest childhood and apparently independent of external precipitating events. However, external stresses may aggravate the preexisting obesity. This overeating might well be regarded as an addiction to food. These patients have a constant craving for food, especially candy, ice cream and other sweets. This craving is frequently uncontrollable and must be satisfied. Three patients in this series (Cases 5, 7, 11) stole food or money with which to go on candy and ice cream sprees. Patient 18 lied to her parents to escape their discovery of candy and other goodies hidden in her room. Similarly Lurie[31] in describing children with Fröhlich's syndrome cites a 15 year old boy referred from the Juvenile Court for stealing money from relatives and friends. It was learned that his sole purpose in stealing was to have money with which to buy huge quantities of ice cream. The compulsive, uncontrollable quality of appetite in these food addicts can thus be seen.

These patients crave food like an alcoholic addict craves drink. Over and over Patient 11, during psychotherapy, spontaneously compared her compulsive eating jags to the behavior of an alcoholic. She said she could no more eat one piece of food than an alcoholic can take one drink. On an eating spree she would go from drugstore to restaurant "like an alcoholic making his rounds." She was afraid to take a cocktail for fear her compulsion would switch from food to alcohol. This patient was the one who stole candy from other patients' rooms while institutionalized.

The similarity of this craving for food to the alcoholic's craving for alcohol has been noted by a number of clinicians[23,24,27,32,33] Fenichel in his *Psychoanalytic Theory of Neurosis* 32 actually discusses the psychological aspects of obesity under addiction (pp. 241, 381–382).

In this connection, it may be more than chance that two patients in this series were known alcoholics at one time or other. Patient 17 had a period of alcoholism when her weight was 270. When she stopped drinking in 1947, she promptly gained to 365, suggesting that food was a substitute for the alcohol. Benedek[34] reported a case of obesity (later inability to eat) in a female alcoholic.

The most revealing example of a food addict is Patient 18, a 20 year old woman who became obese at age 5 to a high in young adulthood of 210 pounds. The endocrinologist recorded in his history that in addition to a constant craving for sweets, she hoarded candy and other food which she hid in her room, enjoying their presence without necessarily eating them. When I asked why she hoarded the food and candy, tears came to her eyes and in a desperate and defiant tone of voice said simply, "They're mine." It was learned that she also hoarded all the letters she had ever received, playing cards from a grade school collection, and as an adult collected different kinds of stationery. Food seemed to be invested with the attributes of personal property, and as such enhanced this patient's self-esteem.

This unhappy young woman had felt unwanted and unloved her entire life. She was the only child raised in a troubled home of constant discord between neurotic parents and a paternal aunt and grandmother who also lived there. Patient had become the emotional whipping post for all members of this unhappy family. There had always been an overemphasis on food. A Kosher table was kept; grandmother was diabetic and dieted and there was constant wrangling among the three adult women as to who should do the cooking. Patient was thin until age 5. Mother was alleged to have had a "nervous breakdown" when patient hadn't eaten well as an infant. Father used to stand on his head to get patient to eat. Since patient got fat, mother threatens to have another "nervous breakdown" because of patient's overeating. Patient's food habits are a constant source of family discussion and not eating is used as a bribe for parental demonstrations of affection.

Comment. In this case it would seem that the possession and eating of food served as a substitute emotional satisfaction for the love and affection which she basically craved. Hence, we postulate that the food addict may unconsciously be substituting a craving for food for a primary craving for love, affection and security. Not only did Patient 18 give a lifelong history of feelings of rejection, loneliness and lack of love, but eight others in this series of eighteen patients similarly had severe emotional deprivations in earliest childhood (Cases 1, 5, 6, 7, 9, 12, 15, 17). The parents in these cases were usually either dead, divorced, rejecting, alcoholic or badly neurotic. This explains why Patient 18 who so desperately wanted a mother's love, gave her doctor a diet history of liking orange juice "when mother fixed it," but not when grandmother did. Bruch[13,38], and others have stressed the point that the very physical fact of obesity, the "bigness," is itself a symbol of strength and security, and may represent a symbolic defense against feelings of rejection, loneliness and insecurity.

Actually there was no patient among the eighteen who did not give a history of some type of disturbed intrafamilial relationships in his or her home during the formative years. Interestingly enough, this did not always take the form of a broken home or openly rejecting parents, but as in Cases 7 and 8 (both men), there was a history of a doting, overprotective, "smothering" type of mother. This particular type of overprotecting mother has been noted before in the family history of obese patients. Bruch has particularly stressed this in her studies of the family backgrounds of obese patients.[13,16,37–40] Olga Lurie[41] and Selling[42] pointed out the same thing in the background of children with a variety of eating problems. David Levy[43] and Mittleman[28] commented on the frequent overprotective mothers found in their studies of boys with the so-called Fröhlich syndrome. Usually, such overprotective mothers are overcompensating for underlying tendencies toward hostility, competitiveness or rejection of their children and the child may sense this as inadequate love.

PSYCHOLOGICAL ASPECTS OF TREATMENT

Although treatment was not the primary aim of this study, and those patients who were in psychotherapy were not necessarily seeking help for their obesity, it is noteworthy that only three patients lost any weight while under observation. Some were receiving diet and drugs in addition to psychotherapy, others not. Therefore, the role of the psychotherapeutic intervention is not clear. It is clear that in this particular series, psychotherapy was not generally effective in achieving weight reduction.

Our clinical material furnishes one suggestion as to why the traditional treatment of obese persons with diet, exercise and drugs has often been difficult and sometimes of no avail. The data indicated that the obese patients in this series overate in relation to underlying emotional problems. Sometimes the hyperphagia was a symptom of an underlying psychological illness, sometimes in reaction to an acute or chronic emotional stress, sometimes as a substitute gratification for other unsatisfied longings. Usually there were multiple emotional factors in the hyperphagia of any one patient. In any event, we would say psychologically that these obese patients seemed to have an "emotional need" to overeat. It is thus logical to assume that these patients might cling to their overeating as long as their underlying emotional conflicts continued or unless some other substitute gratification could be utilized.

In this connection, let us listen to how some of the patients in this series had responded to treatment in the past. Patient 17 said to her endocrinologist—and I quote from her chart—"When I go on the diet I feel weak. When I eat what I want, I feel fine. So why should I stick to the diet?" When Patient 7 dieted in 1947 and lost 67 pounds in six months, he became progressively depressed and agitated. This reached such a degree of upset that his physician finally suggested he regain some weight. He regained it all and lost his nervous symptoms. Patient 4 had gone on a voluntary diet and lost 55 pounds. She developed globus hystericus, fears of being alone and dying, wished she were fat again as she felt happier. Patient 10 gave a history of "nervous symptoms" appearing every time she lost weight by dieting: ringing in the ears, weakness, dizziness, irritability and headaches. This was documented on four separate dietary occasions.

Six patients in this series had developed emotional upsets when they lost weight (Patients 3, 4, 7, 10, 12, 15). This response to weight reduction might well be termed a negative therapeutic reaction. It is logical in terms of the preceding formulations. In addition, Patients 12 and 18 became frankly depressed in psychotherapy, not related to weight loss, but apparently because psychotherapy threatened to undermine the defensive meaning of their overeating and disclose the patient's underlying emotional conflicts. At one point it was necessary to inform the colleagues of Patient 12 that she was suicidal, and hospitalization was considered. Case 18 had to be terminated when patient became so depressed that she cried through each interview (and had gained an additional 13 pounds).

The outlook for reducing or eliminating the obese patients' hyperphagia should theoretically depend upon the underlying emotional conflicts of which the hyperphagia is thought to be a symptom. If the overeating is in reaction to an acute or chronic external stress or frustration, the need to overeat should disappear if the stress can be eliminated. If the hyperphagia is but one symptom of an underlying psychological disease, the prognosis for symptom relief should depend on the prognosis of the underlying illness. If the overeating, for example, is an hysterical symptom, the prognosis should be that of hysteria in general. We would anticipate that the patient addicted to food as a substitute gratification for cravings of love, affection and security, would be the least reversible, for these underlying emotional needs are the most difficult to satisfy. This entire theoretical prognosis can refer only to the emotional aspects of hyperphagia. The reversibility of hereditary, constitutional, hypothalamic or biochemical factors in obesity is still less clear, and beyond the scope of this paper.

DISCUSSION

Application of the Psychoanalytic Concept of Orality to Obesity. Fortunately, psychoanalytic psychology provides us with a theoretical frame of concepts which make the preceding clinical observations more meaningful. In Freud's libido theory, the concept of orality has been validated by a generation of psychoanalysts working in many different countries.[32,44,45] I would like to enumerate in simple terms some of the various meanings of this concept and try to relate them to the preceding clinical data.

1. Mouth activities play a large role in the earliest part of human life. These activities have great emotional significance for the infant. Through suckling at the mother's breast, the infant associates the receiving of food with the warmth of mother's love. As Alexander puts it, "The first relief from physical discomfort the child experiences during nursing, and thus the satisfaction of hunger becomes deeply associated with the feeling of well being and security. . . ."[37] Babcock[30] has stressed the early nursing process as the infant's first interpersonal experience with the mother, and as such a nonverbal means of communication between mother and child. Certain children become fixated at this oral stage of emotional development due to either inadequacy or, at times, an excess of maternal love. In later life these individuals may have excessive oral-receptive needs. Sometimes we actually speak of these individuals as "oral characters" or "unweaned sucklings." They are very dependent, childlike, demanding people. Their craving for love and security, if not satisfied, may be translated into a craving for food because of this unconscious infantile association of being fed with being loved. This intimate association of eating with love and security continues throughout our lives. Later in childhood it is still the loving parents who supply the food. Patient 11 dwelled at length in psychotherapy on her jealousy of her father and brother because mother had always served them their food first at meal time and patient felt this meant mother "loved

them more." Another patient not included in this series spoke of competing with his siblings at table for the largest food servings as a symbol of parental affection. Even the advertiser whose slogans "Pies like mother makes," and "Home Cooking," is relying on the consumer's appetite being stimulated by associating the food appeal with the love appeal. Alexander's discussion of this relationship between eating and being loved is particularly clear and convincing.[35–37]

2. In infancy, stimulation of the oral cavity, whether by suckling on the breast, pacifier or thumb, is a pleasurable (erotic) activity divorced from the nutritional aspects of eating. As the normal child develops, the nutritional aspects of eating become separated from the erotic ones and the erotic component gradually shifts to the genitals. However, traces of oral eroticism normally persist into adult life. These are evident in the oral gratification of kissing, smoking and chewing. The individuals who were in some way fixated at the oral stage of emotional development may in the face of adult emotional conflict, return to that stage. This seems to be the case in hysterical hyperphagia where the patients react to a sexual threat or experience not with genital excitation but by displacement to hyperphagia where eating again becomes highly erotized. An important paper in this connection is Coriat's[46] which discusses the relationship of sexual and nutritional cravings.

3. The particular psychological illness characterized by a return to this oral stage of emotional development is the depression.[32,45,47,48] This furnishes a theoretical common denominator to the somewhat random clinical observations that overeating often seems to be a specific defense against depression and that when some fat people lose weight they become depressed. The common denominator is this concept of orality. It is also generally agreed among psychoanalytic investigators that oral fixations are prominent psychological features in alcoholism and other drug addictions. More recently it has been correlated with certain cases of peptic ulcer.

Other Evidences of Oral Fixations Besides Overeating. In view of this application of the psychoanalytic concept of orality to obese persons, might we not expect to find other evidences of oral fixation in addition to that of overeating? The case material reveals that seven patients (Cases 2, 5, 8, 11, 12, 17, 18) had other excessive or inappropriate oral traits in childhood or adult life. These included alcoholism, excessive finger sucking or nail biting, gnashing of the teeth, and one patient who repetitively bit her arm during sleep. Patient 17 was interesting as she repeatedly smacked her lips and drooled during her interview. Four of Mittleman's "Fröhlich" cases[28] were described as excessive nail biters and chewers of sand, pencils, wood, and in one case, plaster.

Predisposing Factors. If the concept of oral fixations applies to depressions, alcoholism, drug addictions and possibly peptic ulcer, then we are faced with the question "Why do fat people overeat and become obese rather than developing any of these other syndromes?" In other words, what predisposes these people to hyperphagia and obesity rather than another of these illnesses? Here we are on increasingly unsteady ground. The possible hereditary, constitutional, biochemical, hypothalamic or metabolic factors are not known at the present time.

Psychosocial Predisposition to Eating Disturbances. If we continue to restrict our attention to the data at hand, we learn that in at least five of our patients, a psychological predisposition to eating disturbances was apparent in the undue emphasis placed on food and eating in the patient's childhood. Patient 18's history is a good example: (1) Her family kept an Orthodox Jewish table with great emphasis on the traditional religious rituals and prohibitions. (2) The paternal aunt and grandmother lived in the home and they and the mother were in constant battle as to who should do the cooking, and what and how they cooked. (3) The paternal grandmother was diabetic and on a diet. (4) Patient was told that as a young child she often refused her food, that father "stood on his head to make her eat," and mother had to go to a sanitarium, she worried so about patient's not eating.

The possibility that family attitudes, habits and customs about food and eating predispose children to hyperphagia in later life is given support by Bruch's study of a larger number of obese patients. She reports[39] that many mothers of obese children overvalued food, especially immigrant mothers who had themselves been deprived of food abroad. Forty per cent were Jewish families where food had a deep emotional and religious significance. In many instances a disproportionate amount of income was spent for food. Many of these mothers were overprotective and oversolicitous and they too may have substituted the giving of food for real affection. Such psychological factors may well contribute to the predisposition to overeating.

Nonpsychological Factors in Overeating. This investigation has been devoted exclusively to the study of the emotional aspects of obesity. It seems probable that genetic, constitutional, metabolic or other factors are necessary to convert simple overeating into the syndrome we know as obesity. Similar nonpsychological factors, especially hypothalamic regulation, may abnormally influence the appetite of obese persons. The ultimate demonstration of such factors will not necessarily invalidate the emotional elements discussed. Alexander's concept of "multicausality"[36], may well apply to obesity as to other psychosomatic syndromes.

The purpose of this paper is to report only on some of the emotional meanings of overeating which were discovered in the psychiatric study of eighteen obese patients. This series of cases is not necessarily a true cross section of obese patients, inasmuch as many of them had selectively been referred to Psychiatry. As a group they are unquestionably very sick emotionally. Nevertheless, it is hoped that by studying even a few obese patients intensively, we can learn more directly why some obese patients overeat and seem to cling to their symptom of hyperphagia. It will be necessary to apply some of the findings to consecutive obese patients, preferably in a Medical or Endocrine Clinic setting.

SUMMARY

1. A review of the pertinent literature on obesity fails to reveal any intrinsic metabolic, endocrinologic or central nervous system abnormality in the usual case. The symptom of hyperphagia has been the only consistent finding in obese patients.

2. The hyperphagia of eighteen selected obese patients was studied by psychiatric interviewing and multiple emotional meanings to overeating were discovered: in response to nonspecific emotional tensions; as a substitute gratification in reaction to intolerable life situations; as a symptom of an underlying emotional illness, especially depressions and hysteria: as a malignant addiction to food.

3. Obesity is a psychosomatic syndrome, the cardinal symptom of which is hyperphagia. Whatever metabolic, genetic or biochemical factors may play a role in either the symptom or the syndrome, emotional elements, of which the patient is often unaware, contribute a large part.

REFERENCES

1. Newburgh, L. H.: The Cause of Obesity. J.A.M.A. *97*:1659, 1931.
2. Newburgh, L. H.: Obesity. Arch. Int. Med. *70*:1033, 1942.
3. Newburgh, L. H.: Obesity (Chapter 11) in Williams, Textbook of Endocrinology, W. B. Saunders Co., Philadelphia, 1950.
4. Newburgh, L. H.: Obesity. I. Energy Metabolism. Physiol. Rev. *41*:18, 1944.
5. Bruch, Hilde: Obesity in Childhood: II. Basal Metabolism and Serum Cholesterol of Obese Children. Am. J. Dis. Child. 58(2):1001, 1939.
6. Bruch, Hilde, "Obesity in Childhood: IV. Energy Expenditure of Obese Children," Am. J. Dis. Child., *60*(2):1082, 1940.
7. Rynearson, E. H. and Gastineau, C. F.: Obesity. Springfield, Ill., C. C. Thomas 1949.
8. Conn, J. E.: Obesity: II. Etiological Aspects. Physiol. Rev. *41*:31, 1944.
9. Evans, Frank A.: Obesity (Chapter X) in Duncan, Diseases of Metabolism, W. B. Saunders Co., Philadelphia, 1947.
10. Bruch, Hilde: The Fröhlich Syndrome. Am. J. Dis. Child., *58*(2):1282, 1939.
11. Bruch, Hilde: Obesity in Childhood: I. Physical Growth and Development of Obese Children. Am. J. Dis. Child. *58*(1): 457, 1939.
12. Bruch, Hilde: Obesity in Relation to Puberty. J. Pediat., *19*:365, 1941.
13. Bruch, Hilde: Obesity in Childhood and Personality Development. Am. J. Orthopsychiat. *11*:467, 1941.
14. Brobeck, John R., Tepperman, Jay, and Long, C. N. H.: The Effect of Experimental Obesity Upon Carbohydrate Metabolism. Yale J. Biol. & Med. *15*:893, 1942–43.
16. Bruch, Hilde: Obesity in Childhood: III. Physiologic and Psychologic Aspects of the Food Intake of Obese Children. Am. J. Dis. Child., *59*(2):739, 1940.
17. Danforth, C. H.: Hereditary Adiposity in Mice. J. Hered. *18*:153, 1927.
18. Rytand, D. A.: Hereditary Obesity of Yellow Mice. Proc. Soc. Exper. Biol. & Med. *54*:340, 1943.
19. Friedgood, Harry B.: Neuroendocrine and Psychodynamic Aspects of the Endocrinopathies (Chapter X) in Williams, Textbook of Endocrinology, W. B. Saunders Co., Philadelphia, 1950.
20. Cannon, Walter B.: The Wisdom of the Body. New York, W. W. Norton & Co., 1932.
21. Harrington, M. M.: Appetite in Relation to Weight. J. Am. Diet. A. *6*:101, 1930.
22. Freed, S. C.: Psychic Factors in the Development and Treatment of Obesity. J.A.M.A. *133*:369, 1947.
23. Schick, Alfred: Psychosomatic Aspects of Obesity. Psychoanalyt. Rev. *34*:173, 1947.
24. Richardson, H. B.: Obesity as a Manifestation of Neurosis. M. Clin. North America *30*(2):1187, 1946.
25. Richardson, H. B.: Obesity and Neurosis. Psychiat. Quart. *20*:400, 1946.
26. Richardson, H. B.: Psychotherapy of the Obese Patient. New York State J. Med. *47*:2574, 1947.
27. Rennie, T. A. C.: Obesity as a Manifestation of a Personality Disturbance. Dis. Nerv. System *1*:238, 1940.
28. Mittlemann, Bela: Juvenile Adiposogenital Dystrophy. Endocrinology *23*:637, 1938.
29. Reeve, George H.: Psychological Factors in Obesity. Am. J. Orthopsych. *12*:674, 1942.
30. Babcock, Charlotte G.: Food and Its Emotional Significance. J. Am. Dietet. A. *24*:390, 1948.
31. Lurie, L. A.: Endocrinology and the Understanding and Treatment of the Exceptional Child. J.A.M.A. *110*:1531, 1938.
32. Fenichel, Otto: The Psychoanalytic Theory of Neurosis. New York, W. W. Norton & Co., 1945.
33. Weiss, Edward, and English, O. Spurgeon: Psychosomatic Medicine. 2nd ed. Philadelphia, W.B. Saunders Co., 1949.
34. Benedek, Therese: Dominant Ideas and Their Relation to Morbid Cravings. Internat. J. Psychoanaly. *17*:1936.
35. Alexander, Franz: The Influence of Psychologic Factors Upon Gastrointestinal Disturbances. Psychoanalyt. Quart. *3*:501, 1934.
36. Alexander, Franz: Psychosomatic Med. New York, W. W. Norton & Co., 1950.
37. Alexander, Franz: Gastrointestinal Neurosis (Chapter VI), in Portis, Diseases of the Digestive System, Lea & Febiger, Philadelphia, 1941.
38. Bruch, Hilde: Psychiatric Aspects of Obesity in Children. Am. J. Psychiat. 99:752, 1943.
39. Bruch, Hilde, and Touraine, Grace: Obesity in Childhood. V.

The Family Frame of Obese Children. Psychosom. Med. *2*:141, 1940.
40. Bruch, Hilde: Psychological Aspects of Obesity. Bull. New York Acad. Med. *24*:71, 1948.
41. Lurie, Olga R.: Psychological Factors Associated with Eating Difficulties in Children. Am. J. Orthopsych. *11*:452, 1941.
42. Selling, L. S.: Behavior Problems of Eating. Am. J. Orthopsychiat. *16*:163, 1946.
43. Levy, D. M.: Aggressive-Submissive Behavior and the Fröhlich Syndrome. Arch. Neurol. & Psychiat. *36*:991, 1936.
44. Freud, Sigmund: Three Contributions to the Theory of Sex. New York, N. M. D. Pub. Co., 1910.
45. Abraham, Karl: A Short Study of the Development of the Libido (1924), (Chapter 26) in Selected Papers of Karl Abraham, Hogarth, London, 1927.
46. Coriat, I. H.: Sex and Hunger. Psychoanalyt. Rev. *8*:375, 1921.
47. Freud, Sigmund: Mourning and Melancholia (1917), Coll. Papers, Vol. IV, Hogarth, London, 1925.
48. Abraham, Karl: The First Pre-Genital Stage of the Libido (1916), (Chapter 12) in Selected Papers of Karl Abraham, Hogarth, London, 1927.
49. Gill, Dorothy J.: The Role of Personality and Environmental Factors in Obesity. J. Am. Dietet. A. *22*:398, 1946.
50. Rascovsky, A., de Rascovsky, M. W. and Schlossberg, T.: Basic Psychic Structure of the Obese. Int. J. Psychoanal., *31*:144, 1950.

VARIANT REACTIONS TO PHYSICAL DISABILITIES *

NORMAN GOODMAN
Queens College

SANFORD M. DORNBUSCH
Stanford University

STEPHEN A. RICHARDSON
Association for the Aid of Crippled Children

ALBERT H. HASTORF
Stanford University

In an earlier study, a consistent preference pattern in the rank-ordering of various types of physical disabilities was demonstrated among children aged 10 and 11. We suggested this pattern reflected a widespread cultural value in our society. In the present paper we postulate two factors significant in the acquisition of a value: (1) the child's exposure to the value, and (2) the child's ability to learn the value. From the first factor we predicted that adults hold the same preference pattern to the various disabilities; and that Jewish and Italian children, coming from subcultures which, we believed, held different values related to physical appearance, would hold a different preference pattern. From the second factor we predicted that mentally retarded and emotionally disturbed children would hold preference patterns that differ from the normative. The results supported these hypotheses.

IN an earlier paper we demonstrated that children aged 10 and 11 exhibited a remarkably consistent preference pattern in rank-ordering various types of physical disabilities.[1] We suggested that this pattern reflected a widespread cultural value in our society. Our use of the term value in this paper follows Kluckhohn's carefully reasoned definition: "A value is a conception, explicit or implicit, distinctive of an individual or characteristic of a group, of the desirable which influences the selection from available modes, means and ends of action."[2] It involves in essence "choice behavior." Empirical studies have already demonstrated that this kind of behavior is related to the social and personal characteristics of the individual involved.[3] Here we shall consider how values are acquired in the socialization process and test predictions derived from this analysis.

Children are not taught explicitly that a child with one kind of disability is more likable than a child with another kind of disability. The prevalence of the types of disabilities we have examined is so low that few children will have had contact and experience with such disabled children. Hence these values are likely to be implicit and are learned in the socialization process largely in the absence of first-hand experience. "Implicit values will [often] be manifested only in behavior and through verbalizations that do not directly state the pertinent values."[4] That "children detect and incorporate cultural uniformities even when these remain implicit and have not been reduced to rules" has been pointed out by Merton,[5] who also notes that the children themselves may be largely unaware of these cultural uniformities.[6] Indeed, most adults are largely un-

* We gratefully acknowledge the assistance of James Block, Caroline Conklin, Anne L. Constant, Matthew Friedman, Baha Abu-Laban, Abraham Ross, and Rebecca Vreeland in the collection and analysis of a portion of the data. Barbara F. Dornbusch drew the pictures used as stimuli. In addition we wish to express our gratitude to the agencies and institutions which made this work possible. This research was supported by the National Institute of Mental Health (Grant No. M-2480) and the Association for the Aid of Crippled Children.

[1] Stephen A. Richardson, Norman Goodman, Albert H. Hastorf and Sanford M. Dornbusch, "Cultural Uniformity in Reaction to Physical Disabilities," *American Sociological Review,* 26, (April, 1961), pp. 241–247.

[2] Clyde Kluckhohn, "Values and Value-Orientation in the Theory of Action: An Exploration in Definition and Classification," in Talcott Parsons and Edward A. Shils (eds.), *Toward A General Theory of Action,* Cambridge, Mass.: Harvard University Press, 1951, p. 395.

[3] Orville G. Brim, Jr., David C. Glass, David E. Lavin and Norman Goodman, *Personality and Decision Processes: Studies in the Social Psychology of Thinking,* Stanford, California: Stanford University Press, 1962.

[4] Kluckhohn, *op. cit.,* p. 398.

[5] Robert K. Merton, *Social Theory and Social Structure,* Glencoe, Ill.: The Free Press, 1957, p. 158.

[6] Our attempt to elicit verbal explanations for the ranking we reported in our earlier paper illustrates this point.

aware of the cultural and other bases for much of their values and behavior.[7]

The subjects for the earlier study were Catholic and Protestant, white, Negro and Puerto Rican, boys and girls, lower and middle class, and lived in urban, suburban, or rural areas. Hence they are likely to have different reference groups from which they learned, and to which they refer, their attitudes and behavior. Despite these differences and despite the fact that the study was conducted in both schools and summer camps, there was uniformity in ranking between groups as well as statistically significant consensus within each of the groups.

These three factors: (1) the children's difficulties in verbalizing the values; (2) the significant consensus both between and within the classes of children studied; and (3) the diversity of backgrounds of the children suggest that we had uncovered an implicit value in our society which relates to preferential selection of different physical handicaps.

As a basis for predicting which child will conform to or deviate from the implicit values reflected in the rankings of different forms of disability, we postulate two factors that are significant in the acquisition of cultural values. These are:

1. The child's exposure to the value.
2. The ability of the child to learn the value.

We suggest that the absence of either or both of these factors will retard or prevent the child's acquisition of a value.[8]

Let us examine each of these factors. We would expect to find some continuity between the 10-to-11-year-old children and adults in their preference patterns for the various disabilities. This expectation follows from our understanding of how culture is learned, since socialization of the young is largely in the hands of adults. In other words, adults expose their children to their values and communicate these values through their own behavior. From this we deduce that adults would hold the same preference order toward different disabilities as the 10-to-11-year old children expressed in the earlier study, since presumably the children acquired them from the adults.

One class of children who would deviate from the established value toward disability would be those who in the socialization process have little or no exposure or an ambivalent exposure to the majority value. To test this we chose children belonging to subcultures which we believed were likely to differ from the majority culture in values relevant to the evaluation of visible handicaps.

In this group we would place Jews and Italians of low socio-economic status. We restrict our prediction to the lower class since there is evidence that subcultural differences are especially marked at this level and tend to disappear as one ascends the socio-economic ladder; this is especially true for Jews.[9] Data obtained on a very small sample of Jewish children in our earlier study suggested that this group differed from the others in its preferences toward drawings of handicapped children. The differences were elicited primarily by two drawings—the obese child and the child with a facial disfigurement.

We hypothesized that the reaction to the obese child was probably influenced by Jewish cultural practices and values associated with eating, which are generally believed to differ from general American practices and values.

Further, Jews are generally thought to be readily identifiable on the basis of distinct facial characteristics.[10] In our society, these two groups rank low on the scale of social status. If this is true, it is not unreasonable

[7] For an excellent discussion of the cultural and other bases of behavior with specific reference to parent-child relations see Orville G. Brim, Jr., *Education for Childrearing*, New York: Russell Sage Foundation, 1959, Chapter III.

[8] Note the similarity to Brim's intervening variables in a sociological approach to a theory of personality. Orville G. Brim, Jr., "Personality Development as Role-Learning," in Ira Iscoe and Harold Stevenson (eds.), *Personality Development in Children*, Austin: University of Texas Press, 1960.

[9] Fred L. Strodtbeck, "Family Interaction, Values and Achievement," in David C. McClelland, Alfred L. Baldwin, Urie Bronfenbrenner and Fred L. Strodtbeck, *Talent and Society*, Princeton, New Jersey: Van Nostrand, 1958, pp. 135–194.

[10] Hans H. Toch, Albert I. Rabin and Donald M. Wilkins, "Factors Entering into Ethnic Identifications: An Experimental Study," *Sociometry*, 25 (September, 1962), pp. 297–312.

to expect that the norms of Jews would tend to play down the significance of deviant facial appearance. In fact, it is likely that their norms would stress that this type of disability is not an appropriate cue to be considered in social interaction. Hence, we expect Jewish children to report a greater preference than others for the facially disfigured child. We added low-income Italian children because their similar eating practices and distinguishing facial appearance might cause them to react to disability in the same way as Jewish children. With respect to the ability of the child to learn the value (our second postulated factor) we predicted that mentally retarded children would not have acquired the established norm because of their intellectual limitations. We also predicted deviance in children who were severely psychiatrically disturbed since, from a social psychological viewpoint, they have failed to internalize adequately the societal values relating to appropriate forms of interpersonal behavior due to their deficient mental functioning. For both classes of children the deficiency in learning is especially marked when we consider those values which are largely implicit.

Stated in order, the four hypotheses to be tested in this paper are as follows:

Hypothesis 1. Adults will report a rank order of preferences for drawings of children with various types of visible handicap and without a handicap which are identical with the ranking obtained from children who share their culture. This rank order of preferences will be:

Rank 1. A child with no visible physical handicap (drawing A).
Rank 2. A child with crutches and a brace on the left leg (drawing L).
Rank 3. A child sitting in a wheelchair with a blanket covering both legs (drawing W).
Rank 4. A child with the left hand missing (drawing H).
Rank 5. A child with a facial disfigurement on the left side of the mouth (drawing F).
Rank 6. An obese child (drawing O).

Hypothesis 2. Jewish and Italian children from families of low socio-economic status will report a preference pattern different from that stated in Hypothesis 1, since they will rank the facially disfigured child (drawing F) and the obese child (drawing O) higher.

Hypothesis 3. The rank order of preferences for the stimulus drawings reported by children who are mentally retarded will differ from that of children who are not retarded.

Hypothesis 4. The rank order of preferences for the stimulus drawings reported by children who are psychiatrically disturbed will differ from that of children who are not disturbed.

METHODS

The subjects of this study are divided into seven groups, six of which consist of boys and girls 10 and 11 years of age. The seventh—the adult group—consists of persons with varying degrees of training in the medical, social, or behavioral sciences (e.g., nurses, physical and occupational therapists, physicians, psychologists, social workers). We selected adults who work with children having physical disabilities to emphasize the pervasiveness of these culturally acquired values even in individuals who are medically, socially, and psychologically sophisticated about physical disabilities. None of the subjects (children or adults) in the study is physically handicapped. A description of each set of subjects follows:

Set 1. Boys and girls attending a summer camp which provides underprivileged children of various races and religions from New York City with a two- or three-week vacation. The set contains white, Puerto Rican, and Negro children who are Catholic or Protestant. This set taken from our earlier study is hereafter called the normative group.[11] As we earlier pointed out there were no differences in the findings which were systematically related to these background characteristics[12] (N=104).

[11] Since our earlier study revealed no differences among the groups studied we could have chosen any of them as a standard. This one was the largest lower class set of children without handicapped members. In the earlier study, this was Set 3.

[12] In fact, however, some *minor* intra-set variability may be attributable, at least in part, to internal differences on these variables. We discuss one of these—sex differences—later since it alone

Set 2. White Jewish boys and girls of low socio-economic status in New York City who attended a summer camp. This camp has no connection with the one attended by Set 1 (N=69).

Set 3. Italian Catholic boys and girls of low socioeconomic status attending public and parochial schools in New York City (N=63).

Set 4. White Negro and Puerto Rican boys and girls mostly of low socioeconomic status confined to a residential psychiatric institution. The children were mostly Catholic and Protestant. Approximately three-fifths of the group have been diagnosed as exhibiting what has been termed the "passive-aggressive" syndrome. Most of the remainder of the group has been diagnosed as either schizophrenic or as having schizoid tendencies (N=50).

Set 5. White, Negro and Puerto Rican boys and girls mainly from upper income families in two residential institutions for the mentally retarded. The children were mostly Catholic or Protestant. Approximately 20 per cent had I.Q.'s of 65 or below, most of the remaining subjects having I.Q.'s between 66 and 100 (N=70).

Set 6. Mentally retarded white boys and girls from lower income families in two camps—one a day camp and the other a "sleep-away" camp. These were mainly Catholic and Protestant children. These children are not institutionalized. Approximately 25 per cent had I.Q.'s of 65 or below, most of the remaining subjects having I.Q.'s between 66 and 100 (N=26).

Set 7. Male and female adults concerned with the rehabilitation of the physically disabled. Among the subjects are nurses, physical and occupational therapists, physicians, psychologists, and social workers (N=72).

The uniform stimulus for all subjects was a set of six drawings of a child identical in all respects except for the presence or absence of various types of visible handicaps. To hold constant the relationship between the sex of the subjects and that of the child in the drawing, identical sets of male and female drawings were prepared and, in the children's groups, subjects were shown drawings only of children of their own sex. To obtain a preferential rank-ordering, the drawings were placed in random order from left to right in front of the subject and the following instructions were given: "Look at all of these pictures." After the child was given sufficient time to examine all pictures, the experimenter said, "Tell me which boy [girl] you like best." The subject would point at a drawing, which was then removed. "Which boy [girl] do you like next best?" This procedure was continued until the complete ranking was obtained. The procedure was modified for group administration for the adult group.

distinguished groups large enough to permit separate analyses. (See footnote 14.)

RESULTS

Hypothesis 1. Adults will report a rank order of preferences for drawings of children with various types of visible physical handicaps and without a handicap which is identical with one obtained from children who share their culture. This rank order of preferences will be: A, L, W, H, F, O.[13]

Confirming evidence for this hypothesis is found in Table 1. The rank order between the normative group (Set 1) and the adult group (Set 7) is identical.

Hypothesis 2. Jewish and Italian children from families of low socio-economic status will report a preference pattern different from that stated in Hypothesis 1 since they will rank the facially disfigured child (drawing F) and the obese child (drawing O) higher.

The data presented in Table 1 indicate partial confirmation of the hypothesis. The Jewish children (Set 2) do in fact prefer the facially disfigured child and the obese child to a greater degree than do the children in the normative group. However, for the Italian children (Set 3), though the facially disfigured child is decisively preferred to any of the other handicapped children,[14] the obese child remains conspicuously last.

[13] For a full description of these symbols see above, p. 431.

[14] Both the Jewish and Italian girls (but especially the latter) report less of a preference for the facially disfigured child than do the boys in these groups. This sex difference stemming from the differential importance placed upon appearance by boys and girls at this age was expected in light of our earlier work (*op. cit.*, p. 245). However, the magnitude of the difference in the Italian group (the girls placed drawing F in fifth position, the boys in second) was surprising.

TABLE 1. RANK ORDER OF DRAWINGS FOR ALL SETS OF SUBJECTS

	Sets of Subjects *						
Rank Position	Set 1	Set 2	Set 3	Set 4	Set 5	Set 6	Set 7
1	A	A	A	A	A	L	A
2	L	F	F	F	F	O	L
3	W	H	L	L	H	A	W
4	H	O	W	O	L	W–F	H
5	F	L	H	W	O	W–F	F
6	O	W	O	H	W	H	O
Coefficient of concordance	.20	.37	.17	.22	.17	.02	.27
Significance level	<.001	<.001	<.001	<.001	<.001	N.S.	<.001
Number of subjects	104	69	63	50	70	26	72

* Set 1=Normative Group.
Set 2=Jewish group.
Set 3=Italian group.
Set 4=Institutionalized psychiatric group.
Set 5=Institutionalized mentally retarded group.
Set 6=Non-institutionalized mentally retarded group.
Set 7=Adult group.

The difference between the Jewish and Italian children is further revealed in Table 2, which shows that the rank order of the Italian group more closely approximates that of the normative group and the adults (Tau=.60) than it does the Jewish group (Tau=.47). Moreover, there is no relationship whatsoever between the normative group (or adults) and the Jewish group (Tau=.07).

This lack of agreement between the Jews and the normative and adult groups is even more striking when one notes that the concordance measure of the Jewish group is somewhat higher than any of the others. Apparently the Jewish children show internal consistency on these rankings, but not with the general population.

Hypothesis 3. Children who are mentally retarded will report a different rank order of preferences for the stimulus drawings than will children who are not retarded.

Once more Table 1 provides confirmatory evidence for this hypothesis. The rank orders of preferences of the two mentally retarded groups (Sets 5 and 6) are distinctly different from that of the normative group (Set 1). This finding is further bolstered by the data presented in Table 2, which indicate that the rank correlation between each of the two mentally retarded groups is low.

We tested two alternate explanations which would have made the results trivial —namely that the lack of a normative ranking by mentally retarded children results from (1) their inability to comprehend the task or (2) their unreliability in perceiving the physical handicap portrayed in the draw-

TABLE 2. TAU CORRELATIONS BETWEEN PREFERENTIAL ORDERING FOR ALL SETS OF SUBJECTS

	Sets of Subjects						
Sets of Subjects	Set 1	Set 2	Set 3	Set 4	Set 5	Set 6	Set 7
Set 1 Normative group	—	.07	.60	.33	.20	.13	1.00
Set 2 Jewish group	—	—	.47	.47	.87	.13	.07
Set 3 Italian group	—	—	—	.73	.60	.17	.60
Set 4 Institutionalized psychiatric group	—	—	—	—	.60	.26	.33
Set 5 Institutionalized mentally retarded group	—	—	—	—	—	.00	.20
Set 6 Non-institutionalized mentally retarded group	—	—	—	—	—	—	.13
Set 7 Adult group							

ings. The first possibility was tested by having mentally retarded children rank three pictures of food in terms of their liking of them—a chocolate pudding dessert with whipped cream, a pile of stringbeans, and a piece of plain unbuttered toast. The assumption underlying this procedure—which was confirmed with a sample of children of normal intelligence—was that most children would rank the dessert first and that there would be no decided preference for either of the other two. Except for those few in the lowest I.Q. range (65 or below) these results were obtained, and hence the first alternate hypothesis was rejected.

Next, we took a duplicate set of the standard stimulus drawings and asked each child to match them with the drawings of the original set. Once more the task was accomplished by most of the children except the few in the lowest I.Q. group and hence the second alternate hypothesis was also rejected.

Hypothesis 4. Children who are psychiatrically disturbed will report a rank order of preferences for the stimulus drawings different from that of children who are not disturbed.

Table 1 provides supporting data for this hypothesis. We note that the rank order of the drawings by the psychiatric group (Set 4) is clearly different from that of the normative group (Set 1). This fact is also apparent in Table 2, where the correlation between the normative group and the psychiatric group is low.

DISCUSSION

Two factors were postulated as significant in the acquisition of cultural values: the child's exposure to the value, and his ability to learn the value. On the basis of the first factor we predicted that because children acquire values largely through exposure to the values of adults, adults would hold the same preference order toward handicaps that we had found in children. This prediction was confirmed. It is of particular interest that the normative preference order toward differing handicaps is present also in those adults who are engaged in the rehabilitation of the physically disabled.

A further prediction from the exposure factor in the acquisition of values was made by selecting children whose immediate social environment or subculture we believed exposed them less to the dominant cultural values and more to different and conflicting values. The data on children from low-income Jewish and Italian families in New York City largely support the prediction that their values would differ from the normative pattern. The prediction of a higher ranking of the obese child for Jewish and Italian children was confirmed only for the Jewish children. Although Jewish and Italian families do not differ significantly in their eating behavior, perhaps they do differ in their *values* associated with food. Psychiatrists have long perceived a relationship between eating practices and affection and have stated that this is especially marked in the Jewish culture. The well-fed stockily built Jewish child is often viewed by other Jews as one who is both healthy and *loved*. It is perhaps significant that the association between feeding and affection has not been observed in Italians. The affective quality of the learning situation may be related to this differential transmission.

We noted earlier that the concordance measure was higher for the Jewish children than for any of the others. This is in accord with other studies that have shown Jews are more homogeneous in the expression of certain values than many other religious or ethnic groups.[15] The significance of these data is not that they replicate and confirm this general information, but that they suggest that this cultural homogeneity is apparently the result of learning experiences which take place in childhood.

The second factor in a child's acquisition of a cultural value—his ability to learn from exposure—led us to select children who were mentally retarded or severely emotionally disturbed. Our results showed these children differed as predicted from the normative values which related to disability.

[15] For example, see Charles F. Westoff, "The Social-Psychological Structure of Fertility," *Proceedings of the International Population Conference*, Vienna, 1959, p. 362.

The postulate of exposure may also be called into play in interpreting these results. The absence or reduction of exposure to the outside dominant culture is likely to occur for the two institutionalized sets of children (Sets 4 and 5). They are intensively exposed to their peers in the institution, who share their difficulty in learning and probably have greatly reduced exposure to children who hold the normative values. Unlike the non-institutionalized retarded, they do achieve some
deviant rankings.

In conclusion, the evi
postulates that a child
through exposure to the v
to learn. The differentia
dren from low-income J
neighborhoods lead us t
affective component of
may be a phenomenon
ploration.

Cursory Remarks

On

CORPULENCE;

By

A Member of the Royal College of Surgeons

[William Wadd, Surgeon]

Thank not, ye candidates for health,

That ought can gain the wish'd-for prize;

(Or pills or potion, power or wealth,)

But temperance and exercise.

London:

Printed for J. Callow, Medical Bookseller

No 10 Crown Court, Princes Street, Soho

By J. and W. Smith, King Street, Seven Dials.

1810

INTRODUCTION

A Gentleman with whom I was early in the habit of having frequent discussions on professional subjects, had often introduced his tendency to corpulence, expressing his fears, lest his pursuits which were sedentary, should increase, what he already felt a growing inconvenience. On this account he addressed a letter, earnestly requesting my reference, to such authors as might satisfy his curiosity, or give him some information, on a subject which so much engrossed his thoughts. At the same time he stated stating, some circumstances of his life connected with and, illustrative of his complaints' with observations on the effect a vegetable diet had on them.

He had approached his thirtieth year before he experienced any great inconvenience from his increase of bulk. From this period his mind was deeply impressed with the apprehension of becoming corpulent. Inactivity, somnolency, depression of sprits, that train of symptoms usually called nervous an inaptitutde for study, were symptoms which could not but produce much anxiety. By an abstemious mode of living, and a vegetable diet, he became lighter, more capable of mental exertion, and in every respect improved in health - but whenever he resumed his former habits, his complaints returned in full force.

The variation in this gentlemen's health and feelings, from an alternate change in his regimen, was not less decided and remarkable, than the alteration the declining strength of Cornaro experienced, when the return of the vintage enabled him to take his usual quantity of new wine.

I employed a few leisure hours in bringing together the opinions of different writers, on what appears to me not only an interesting subject, but one which has been most neglected, when from circumstances, it most required attention. As it is probably, that the following pages may chiefly attract the attention of those whose "embonpoint" appearance denotes good temper, no apology need be made for offering a few observations to their consideration. The rules by which Cornaro repaired his constitution, greatly injured by an irregular course of life, until he was forty years old, were successfully adopted by the celebrated Miller of Billericay; and should I be fortunate enough to lead a single individual, labouring under similar infirmities, to attempt the restoration or his health, by the same means, I shall feel amply gratified.

CURSORY REMARKS,
&c. &c. &c.

If the increase of wealth and the refinement of modern times, have tended to banish plague and pestilence from our cities, they have probably introduced to us the whole train of nervous disorders, and increased the frequency of corpulence.

Hollingshed, who lived in Queen Elizabeth's reign, speaking of the increase of luxury in those days, notices, "the multitude of chimnies lately erected; whereas in the sound remembrance of some old men, there were not above two or three, if so many, in most uplandish towns of the realm." (* footnote: *Hollingshed's Chronicles*, vol. II). How far corpulency has kept pace with the number of chimnies, I pretend not to determine; certain it is that Hollingshed and his contemporaries, furnish no account of the front of a house, or the windows, being take away, to let out, to an untimely grave, some unfortunate victim, too ponderous to be brought down the staircase.

The English nation has at all times been as famous for beef, as her sons have been celebrated for bravery; and that they understood good living, even in the earliest ages, we may learn from Caesar, who, speaking of the diet of Britons says, "*Lacte et carne vivunt.*"

It has been conjectured by some, that for one fat person in France or Spain, there are a hundred in England. I shall leave others to determine the fairness of such a calculation.

That we have however approach, or even exceed it, no one will doubt, who reflects on the increasing improvements in the art of grazing, and the condescension of some modern physicians, who have added the culinary department to the practice of physic. And it ought not to be omitted, amongst the great events of the present aera, that the combined efforts, of art and nature, produced, in the jubilee year 1809, the fattest ox, and the most corpulent man, ever heard of in the history of the world.

It is undoubtedly a singular circumstance, that a disease which had been thought characteristic of the inhabitants of this island, should have been so little attended to. Dr. Thomas Short in 1727, published a discourse on Corpulency, which, with a small pamphlet by Dr. Flemyng, and some occasional remarks in a few systematic works, will, I believe, be found to comprise all that has been said by physicians in this country, on what Dr. Fothergill termed, "a most singular disease."

In answer to this, we may be told that sufficient has been written, for any man to be his own physician and his complaint, and that *"le regime maigre,"* and Dr. Radcliffe's advice, of keeping " the eyes open and the mouth shut," contains the whole secret of the cure.

That Lewis Cornaro and Thomas Wood believed in this doctrine, and acted up to its principles, by a rigid perseverance in temperance, undoubtedly is true; and it is equally true, that the one emerged from a state of constant torment, and the other from the oppression of a load of fat.

There may be others, and probably many, in private life, who have had good sense and courage enough to adopt this line of conduct; but the instances on record are rare.

To account for this is difficult; since from the days of Hippocrates downwards, dietetics, and the efficacy of abstinence, have been the constant theme of physicians and moralists.

The history of persons who have been brought to a premature death by the excessive accumulation of fat, in general, does little more than excite our astonishment at the trespass nature has endured: but an accurate account of those who have succeeded in opposing, and conquering this disease, would form a very useful and interesting narrative.

The extraordinary case of the late Mr. Lambert, is a forcible example in point. From the detail of his life, it does not appear, that any decided attempt was made, to arrest the progress of the disease, which from an early period, seemed rapidly to increase.

Whether this arose from ignorance of the fatality of it, or from the common prejudice, that the complaint is so connected and interwoven with the constitution, as to be irremediable, is matter of conjecture; and we are only left to wonder that this prodigy of clogged machinery, should have continued to move so many years.

It may be useful to some of my readers to be informed of a few circumstances relative to the anatomy and physiology of the parts concerned, and of the nature and properties of the substance, the encreased deposit of which is so injurious to the functions of life. This I shall do as concisely as possible.

The manner in which fat is distributed over the body, is now generally understood to be by the texture of the cellular membrane. Formerly it was supposed, that it merely adhered in clusters or lumps to the parts where it was found.

This membrane is thicker in some parts than in others, and is composed of a number of cells communicating with each other. Some have thought that the fat was contained in cells peculiar to itself; on which account, the name of adipose has been given to that part of the membrane in which it is found. The other has been called reticular cellular substance, and is considered as the universal connecting medium between the larger and smaller parts, extending itself to inconceivable minuteness, and constituting, according to the opinion of Dr. Hunter, one half of the whole body.

That celebrated anatomist, in his lectures, always described the fat as contained in little bags of its own, not communicating with each other. He observed, that if pressure was made on the adipose membrane, the oil did not recede into the surrounding cells, as water did in anascarca - and that water was often seen in parts of the membrane where fat was never found. An instance is mentioned, however, by Mons. Lorry, in "*Memoires de l'Academie de Medicine*,"* of the fat falling down to the foot and forming a tumor. (*footnote: In this paper Mons. Lorry gives an account of diseases he supposed were produced of fat, from its mixture with various other substances, as milk, pus, &c. He contends, there is a reciprocity of action between fat and bile, by which he endeavors to account for many of the appearances met with in bilious diseases.)

There is another membrane which ought also to be noticed, namely, a duplicature of the peritoneum, called the omentum,* situated in the front of the abdomen, immediately before the intestines. (* Footnote: A great many fanciful conjectures have been entertained concerning the uses of the omentum. Some have questioned whether it was not the common root of fat, having an undiscovered communication with the membrana adiposa. Others have thought it subservient to the liver, and that it co-operated in the formation of the bile, &c. Perhaps there was as much probability in such notions, as in some modern opinions concerning the spleen - end of footnote) This is generally known by the term caul, and is a conspicuous receptacle of fat in elderly people. In a healthy state it seldom weighs more than half-a-pound, but it has been found increase to many pounds. Boerhaave mentions a case of a man whose belly grew so large, that he was obliged to have it supported by a sash; and had a piece of the table cut out to enable him to reach it with his hands. After death his omentum weighed thirty pounds.

A preternatural accumulation of fat in this part, cannot fail to impede the free exercise of the animal functions. Respiration is performed imperfectly, and with difficulty; and the power of taking exercise is almost lost - added to which from the general pressure on the large blood vessels, the circulation through them is obstructed, and consequently the accumulation of blood encreased in those parts, where there is no fat, as the brain, lungs, &c. Hence we find the pulse of fat people weaker than in others, and from these circumstances also, we may easily understand how the corpulent grow dull, sleepy and indolent.

The quantity and quality of fat varies according to the age, and the parts in which it is deposited. It is firmer and higher colored in old persons, than in young ones. It is also more condensed and solid in parts liable to compression, than in the omentum, about the heart, stomach and intestines. In children the fat is distributed over the surface of the body, but as they grow up, it is more generally disposed as it becomes deeper seated.

Malpighi and other anatomists have thought that there was a glandular apparatus superadded to the cellular apparatus superadded to the cellular membrane, to assist in the formation of fat. But this has never been discovered.

The accumulation of fat, or what is commonly called corpulency, and by nosologists denominated *polysarcia*, is a state of body very generally met with in the inhabitants of this country; and though it may exist to a certain degree * without (*Footnote: It is supposed, that a person weighing one hundred and twenty pounds, general contains twenty pounds of fat), being deemed worthy of attention, yet when excessive, is not only burthensome, but predisposes to disease, particularly scurvy, * and is frequently the cause of sudden death. (*Footnote: Trotter on the Scurvy.)

The predisposition to corpulency varies in different persons. In some it exists to such an extent, that a considerable secretion of fat will take place, notwithstanding strict attention to the habits of life, and undeviating moderation in the gratification of the appetite. Such a disposition is generally connate, very often hereditary; and when accompanied, as it frequently is, with that easy state of mind, denominated "good humour," which, in the fair sex, Mr. Pope tell us,

"...............teaches charms at last

Still makes new conquests, and maintains the past."

Or when in men, the temper is cast in that happy mould, which Mr. Hume so cheerfully congratulates himself upon possessing, and considers as more than equivalent to a thousand a year, "the habit of looking at every thing on its favorable side" - corpulency must ensue.

Where the predisposition exists, the generally exciting causes of corpulency are a free indulgence in rich and nutritious food, which may be considered as the first and principal. On this account it is a disease, with which the lower orders of society, the poor and laborious, are seldom encumbered; it is only among those who have the means of obtaining the comforts of life without labour, that excessive corpulency is met with.

Many other causes have been adduced as co-operating. Dr. Beddoes has applied the theory of Pneumatic Chemistry to this subject, and attaches great importance, to deficiency of oxygen. But Dr. B remained inconveniently fat during his life. Dr. Malcolm Flemyng, lays great stress on the defective evacuation of fat, or oil, through the outlets of the body. The total cessation of any natural discharge - much sleep - and a sedentary life, great assist. Thus we find persons who have been long confined to their rooms, from any accident, not interfering with the digestive powers, usually grow corpulent. I lately attended a gentleman, about thirty-five years of age, of a thin spare habit, who had the misfortune to rupture the Tendo Achilles. In the course of three months he increase so much in size, that a coat which sat loosely on him, before he met with his accident, would not meet to button, by nine or ten inches.

Having given this short detail of the nature of the disease, I shall proceed to make a few remarks on the means of cure; first, taking a slight view of the various medicines, that have at different time, been recommended as specifics.

Coelius Aurelianus, to whose diligence in collecting the opinions of preceding writers, we are much indebted, mentions two ways of curing this complaint; by taking food that has little nutrition in it, or by observing certain rules of exercise. He enjoins the patient to ride on horseback, or take a sea voyage, to read aloud, and to give the limbs motion by walking quickly. He recommends the body to be sprinkled with sand, and rubbed with a coarse dry towel. Sweating is to be produced by the aid of stoves and the warm bath. Sometimes the cold bath is to be used to strengthen and invigorate the body. He orders the patient to to be covered with hot sand, and to be put into medicated waters, after having been in the sweating bath, and then to be sprinkled with salt, or rubbed with pulverized nitre. He is to drink little, and acid wines should be mixed with his liquors. His food is to be chiefly bread made with bran; vegetables of all kinds; a very small quantity of animal food, and that is to be dry and free from fat. He advises very little sleep, and positively forbids it after meals. He condemns the practice of bleeding and particularly objects to vomiting after supper, so much recommended by his predecessors.

Borrelli, recommends chewing tobacco; but this practice is objected to by Etmuller as he thinks it may be to consumption. Etmuller asserts, there is not a more efficacious remedy than vinegar of squills.

Few things have been more generally administered in the cure of corpulency than acids of various kinds. The emaciating properties of acid liquors, particularly vinegar, are very well known. It is said, that the famous Spanish General, Chiapin Vitellis, well know in the time he lived for his enormous size, reduced himself, solely by drinking of vinegar, to such a degree that he could fold his skin round his body. In countries where cyder is drank as a beverage, the inhabitants are leaner than in those where beer is the common liquor.

Soap, is strongly recommended by Dr. Flemyng, on account of its diuretic properties. After making some observations on the quantity and quality of food, and enforcing the necessity of abstinence; he considers what is the most effectual method of increasing the evacuation of animal oil, which, he says, is to be done, with the greatest safety, by diuretics. For this purpose he recommends soap, considering it as a specific. Purgative medicines, he observes, are dangerous; and little is to be done by perspiration. But where there is no morbid obstruction, mild diuretics, particularly soap, will, he thinks, effect a cure, without inconvenience or danger to the constitution.

"A worthy acquaintance of mine," says Dr. Flemyng, "a judicious and experienced physician, in his younger days had been very active, and used much exercise, both on foot and on horseback, and for many years seemed as little liable to corpulency as most people. By insensible degrees, as he diminished his daily labours, fatness stole upon him and kept increasing, insomuch, that when I met with him about six years ago, I found him in the greatest distress, through mere corpulency, of any person, not exceeding middle age, I ever knew. He was obliged to ride from house to house to visit his patients in the town where he practised, being quite unable to walk an hundred yards at a stretch; and was, in no small degree, lethargic. In other respects, he seemed pretty clear of any remarkable disease, except gout, of which he had felt some, not very violent, attacks. I warmly recommended the inward use of soap, in order to reduce his corpulency, as the safe and effectual remedy in his case, and a remedy which he might continue to use the longest; I enforced my advice by the reasonings above urged, of which he was too good to judge not to perceive their full cogency: according he began to take it July 1754, at which time he weighed twenty stone and eleven pounds, jockey weight; a vast load for him to bear, who is little above middle stature, and withal small boned - He took every night at bed time, a quarter of an ounce of common home-made castile soap, dissolved in a quarter of a pint of soft water; in about two or three months time he began to feel more freedom, and an increase of activity, which encouraged him to persevere; and that he did with success, that in August 1756 (as he informs me in a letter now lying before me) his bulk was reduced two whole stone weight, and he could walk a mile with pleasure. He had continued the use of the soap all the time between June 1754 and August 1756, with very short interruptions, in the manner and quantity above mentioned; it operated remarkably, without every producing the least troublesome effect. And now, while I am sending these plates to the press (April 1760) I am certainly informed that he is hearty and well."

The author of "*Zoonomia*" is of opinion, that the eating of much salt, or salted meat, is more efficacious than soap, as it increases perspiration, and produces thirst, by which, if the patient can bear it, the absorption of his fat will be greatly increased, as in fever. He advises that one entire meal should be omitted, as supper; to drink as little as possible of any fluid, but aerated alkaline water, which he recommends from an idea of its rendering fat more fluid. * (*Footnote: *Zoonomia*, v.II.c.1.23.)

Dr. Cullen, however, well observes, "that the inducing a saline and acrid state of the blood," (which are supposed to be the effect of vinegar and soap) "may have worse consequence than the corpulency it was intended to correct, and that no person should hazard those while he may have recourse to the more safe and certain means of *abstinence* and *exercise*. "The diet," he adds, "must be sparing, or rather, what is more admissible, it must be such as affords little nutritious matter; it must therefore be chiefly or almost only of vegetable matter, and at the very utmost, milk. Such a diet should be employed and generally ought to precede exercise, for obesity does not easily admit of bodily exercise, which, however, is the only mode that can be very effectual." * (*Footnote:. - *Prac. Of Physic*, v.IV.p.131.)

The theory of the celebrated Brown, naturally led him to prefer and recommend the free use of animal food in our general diet; but he agrees with Dr. Cullen in the chief points, "that as animal food is the principal noxious power, the quantity should be reduced, and more exercise taken. These mean," he observes, "sufficient for the cure."

Dr. Fothergill, to whom we are indebted for two curious cases of corpulency, holds the same language. "A strict vegetable diet," says the doctor, "reduces exuberant fat more certainly than any other means I know. Perhaps a reasonable use of wine, not a generous one, should here be allowed, lest the strength should be diminished too much in proportion. All the means of increasing the thinner secretions, are evidently pointed out as necessary, if to these we joint small doses of chalybeates, or other medicines; and an abstinence from animal food, as far as the patient's health, situation, and manner of life, will admit of it; we are, perhaps, rendering all the reasonable assistance we can, till future discoveries make us better acquainted with the real causes of this singular distemper." * (*Footnote: *Med. Obs. And Inq. V.V.* p.251.)

The cure of this disease, according to the opinion of the late Dr. Beddoes, consists, in giving to the constitution a greater quantity of oxygen, independent of the mechanical effects of exercise, which increases absorption. The doctor asks, "may it not also, by introducing more oxygen into the system, by diffusing it more widely, check the formation of a substance containing little oxygen, while the fat, with the other fluids and solids, is absorbed?" * (*Footnote p 28 – *Observations on Calculus.*)

Salivation, decoction of guaicum with sweating, + (Footnote: *Med. Obs. and Inq. V.III.* p.69) have been proposed; and in cases of enlarged omentum, a bandage has been recommended, that might be tightened and relaxed at pleasure.

These, I believe, are the principal articles that have been resorted to in the medical treatment of this disease; and the person who depends solely on the benefit to be derived from the use of any of them, will, I fear, find himself grievously disappointed.

Soap has been tried, and not answered the expectations Dr. Flemyng's conjectures gave rise to. The emaciating properties of vinegar are well known; but the experiments of modern chemists, particularly Mr. Pilger, are decisive of its highly deleterious effects on the organs of digestion, when taken in sufficient quantity to effect the diminution of fat.

Nor will any of the other medicaments proposed afford better prospects of success. As auxiliaries they may occasionally be useful, but the only certain and permanent relief, is to be sought in a rigid abstemiousness, and a strict and constant attention to diet.

It has been well observed by an experienced surgeon, that in hereditary disease, "more dependence is to be had upon diet than medicine; and that the whole constitution may be changed by a proper choice of aliment."* (*Footnote: *Kirkland's Surgery*, v.II.p.456)

The truth of this opinion will not, I presume, be doubted, and in no instance is it more applicable than in the present. Unfortunately however, the continued perseverance necessary to render such a plan effective, makes it one of the most difficult tasks that can be imposed on corpulent persons, whose habits are generally connected with great inactivity of body and indecision of mind, and who are consequently, little inclined to administer to themselves.

Many would willingly submit to any violent remedy, so that an immediate benefit could be produced; but unless the disease speedily gives way, they despair of success; consider it as unalterably connected with their constitution, and of course, return to their former habits. This feeling is too often encouraged by the ill-judged advice of friends, who thereby perhaps, become unthinking accomplices in the destruction of those whom they esteem and regard.

The beneficial alteration capable of being produced in the human body by a strict course of abstemiousness, cannot be more remarkably exemplified than in the history of Mr. Wood's case (the Miller of Billericay) as given by the late Sir George Baker in the *Medical Transactions of the Royal College of Physicians*.

Mr. Wood had arrived at his forty-fourth year, before his complaints were sufficiently serious to attract his attention, when the life of Cornaro fortunately suggested to him the salutary course of living he afterwards pursued, by which, to use his own words, "he was metamorphosed from a monster, to a person of moderate size; from the condition of an unhealthy, decrepit old man, to perfect health, and the vigour and activity of young."

He began by using animal food, sparingly, and leaving off malt liquor, and by degrees, he brought himself to do without any liquor whatever, excepting what he took in the form of medicine; and latterly the whole of his diet consisted of a pudding made of sea biscuit; by this plan it is supposed he reduced himself ten or eleven stone weight.

The salutary effect of vegetable diet and rigid abstemiousness, is further corroborated by Dr. Fotherbill, under whose direction a case of obesity, in a person thirty years of age, was completely cured. Another greatly relieved, but afterwards terminated fatally from the interference of friends, who dissuaded the patient from continuing the plan. As they are related in a medical work * (*Footnote: *Medical Observations and Inquiries*) that may not fall in the way of many of my readers, and as the account is short, I will take the liberty of quoting them in this place.

"A country tradesman, aged about thirty, of a short stature, and naturally of a fresh sanguine complexion, and very fat, applied to me for assistance. He complained of perpetual drowsiness and inactivity; his countenance was almost livid, and such a degree of somnolency attended him, that he could scarce keep awake whilst he described his situation. In other respect he was well."

"I advised him immediately to quit all animal food, to live solely on vegetables, and every thing prepared from them, allowed him a glass of wine or a little beer occasionally, but chiefly to confine himself to water. He pursued the plan very scrupulously, lost his redundant fat, grew active as usual in about six months. I recommended a perseverance for a few months longer, then to allow himself light animal food once or twice a week, and gradually to fall into his usual way of living. He grew well and continued so."

"A young unmarried woman, about twenty-three years of age, of a low stature, and very fat, applied to me for assistance, in a great difficulty of breathing, somnolency, and incapacity for any exercise. It was a hardship to her to be obliged to go up stairs, and at last to cross the floor of her apartment."

"It seemed to me that mere obesity was her principal malady: indeed she had no other complaint, but such as apparently might be accounted for from this supposition. She was ordered to pursue a vegetable diet, and, in the summer, to drink the waters at Scarborough. She conformed to these directions, became more agile, less sleepy, less averse to exercise: she walked up the steps at Scarborough from the Spaw, a task of no little difficulty to people much less incumbered. I urged a continuance of the same diet; she was dissuaded from it by her friends, and died of fat in the twenty-seventh year of her age."

These cases afford strong evidence of the efficacy of vegetable diet, and at the same time prove the necessity of attending to *quantity*. Some writers however have been of opinion, that the basis of fat was a slight nutritious oil, principally extracted from vegetables, and Lorry considers the *abundant* use of succulent vegetable aliment, as an irresistible cause of corpulence.

The following case is a singular instance of the *facility* with which succulent nutritious vegetable matter, will increase bulk.

A few years ago, a man of about forty years of age, hired himself as a labourer, in one of the most considerable Ale-breweries in the City: at this time he was a personable man; stout, active, and not fatter than a moderate sized man in high health should be. His chief occupation was to superintend the working of the new beer, and occasionally to set up at night to watch the wort, an employment not requiring either activity or labour; of course at these times he had an opportunity of tasting the liquor, of which, it appears, he always availed himself; besides this, he had a constant access to the new beer. Thus leading a quiet inactive life, he began to increase in bulk and continued to enlarge, until, in a very short time, he because of such a unwieldy size, as to be unable to move about, and was too big to pass up the brewhouse staircase; if by any accident he fell down, he was unable to get up again without help. The integuments of his fat hung down to the shoulders and breast: the fat was not confined to any particular part, but diffused over the whole of his body, arms, legs, &c. making his appearance such as to attract the attention of all who saw him. He left this service to go into the country, being a burthen to himself, and totally useless to his employers. About two years afterwards he called up his old masters in very different shape to that above described, being reduced in size nearly half, and weighing little more than ten stone. The account that he gave of himself was, that as soon as he had quitted the brewhouse he went to Bedfordshire, where having soon spent the money he had earned, and being unable to work, he was brought into such a state of poverty, as to be scarcely able to obtain the sustenance of life, often being a whole day without food: he drank very little, and that was generally water. By this mode of living he began to diminish in size, so as to be able to walk about with tolerable ease. He then engaged himself to a farmer, with whom he staid a considerable time, and, in the latter part of his service, was able to go through very hard labour, sometimes being in the field ploughing and following various agricultural concerns, for a whole day, with no other food than a small pittance to bread and cheese. This was the history he gave of the means by which this extraordinary change was brought about. He added, his health had never been so good as it then was.* (*Footnote: There is a remarkable contrast to this case, in the person of a French prisoner of war, who was extremely lean, though the following was his general consumption of one day.

Raw Cow's Udder ......4 lb
Raw Beef..................10 lb
Candles ....2 lb
Total................16 lb
Besides five bottles of porter.

Vide letter from Dr. Johnson to Dr. Blane, *Medical and Physical Journal*, v. III.p.211)

The approach of most chronic diseases is so gradual, that it is not till they are far advanced that they become an object of attention. This is particularly the case with corpulence. Many even congratulate themselves on their comely appearance, and consequently do not seek to remedy for what they do not consider an evil.

From the account given by Mr. Lambert, it appears, that at the age of twenty-three, he weighed thirty-two stone. At this period it is related that he walked from Woolwich to the Metropolis, with much less apparent fatigue than several middle-sized men who accompanied him. It is clear therefore that he was a strong active man, long after the disease had made great progress; and I think it may fairly be inferred, the he would not have fallen a sacrifice so early in life, if he had, encouraged by the success of former cases, had fortitude enough to have met the evil, and to have opposed it with determined perseverance.

CLASSICS IN OBESITY

MEDICO-ACTUARIAL MORTALITY INVESTIGATION

REPORT OF THE JOINT COMMITTEE ON THE MEDICO-ACTUARIAL MORTALITY INVESTIGATION

INFLUENCE OF BUILD ON MORTALITY AMONG MEN

The material supplied by the [Insurance] Companies for the study of the influence of build on mortality consisted of–

(a) General Build cards, for all policies on standard lives in the United States and Canada issued in January of the odd years and July of the even years 1885 to 1900, inclusive.

(b) Special Build cards, for policies issued in the other months of these years and in all months of the years 1901 to 1908 inclusive on lives whose weight came within the groups 3, 4, 5, 7, 8 and 9 of the table adopted by the Committee for the purpose of obtaining data on overweights and underweights (Vol. I, pp. 120-121). The Height and Weight Table contained in the instructions issued to the Companies at the beginning of the investigation is for age 37; groups 0, 1, 2 and 6 comprise those between 15% below the scale and 25% above it; groups 3, 4 and 5 those more than 25% heavier; and groups 7, 8 and 9 those more than 15% lighter than the average weight for age 37 at entry.

The object in calling for the Special Build cards was to secure sufficient material among the insured who were distinctly overweight or underweight. As the table used in distinguishing the Special Build cases for all ages at entry was based on the weight of men aged 37, the material supplied by the Companies included a large number of cases at the younger ages less than 15% underweight, and at the old ages at entry less than 25% overweight. Both the General Build and the Special Build cards called for the height and weight of the insured, and the mortality investigations have been based upon the statistics of height and weight according to the ages of the insured at entry. Therefore, the use of a Height and Weight table based on age 37 at entry, for determining whether or not any policy should be included in the data supplied by the Companies, did not invalidate in any way the deductions drawn from the data, but had the advantage of securing additional material where it was most needed. To repeat, neither the manner of securing the material, nor the different proportion of overweights and underweights at young and old ages respectively, has had any effect on the mortality, measured according to degree of departure from the average weight, because the true average weight *for age at entry* has been used in classifying the cases. General Build cards for issues subsequent to 1900 were not called for, as the additional material would have been confined to entrants varying little from the average weight, and exhibiting no marked departure from normal mortality. The exclusion of these recent issues has slightly affected the results for the groups at or near the average weight.

There were received, in all, the records on 812,221 policies on the lives of men, but it was deemed advisable to eliminate the cases at the extremes of height and of ages at entry. The Committee, therefore, dealt with policies on men whose ages at entry were from 20 to 62 inclusive, and whose heights ranged from 5 feet 3 inches to 6 feet 2 inches, representing 744,672 cases, or 92% of the data submitted. With regard to the insured above age 62 at entry, it was thought that the adverse effect of self-selection by the applicants at these advanced ages

Compiled and published by The Association of Life Insurance Medical Directors and The Actuarial Society of America.
The Association of Life Insurance Medical Directors and The Actuarial Society of America. *Medico-Actuarial Mortality Investigation*. New York:1913;2:5-9,44-47.
Reprinted with permission from The Society of Actuaries, 475 N. Martingale Rd., Suite 800, Schaumburg, IL 60173-2226, and The American Academy of Insurance Medicine, P.O. Box 545939, Surfside, FL 33154.
Special thanks to Judy Roberts of the Pennington Information Center for help in acquiring this document.

MEN

AVERAGE PERIOD OF EXPOSURE

Height 5 Feet 3 Inches to 6 Feet 2 Inches inclusive. Ages at Entry 20 to 62, inclusive.

Ages at Entry	Number Entering	Years of Exposure	Average Period of Exposure in Years
20-24	152,862	948,394	6.20
25-29	175,155	1,223,743	6.99
30-34	149,016	1,093,268	7.34
35-39	109,762	805,614	7.35
40-44	73,934	537,156	7.27
45-49	44,530	312,055	7.01
50-53	20,855	142,896	6.85
54-56	9,792	67,632	6.91
57-59	5,850	39,275	6.71
60-62	2,916	19,265	6.61
Total	744,672	5,189,298	6.97

on the one hand, and on the other, the greater care in selection exercised by the Companies, had disturbed the normal mortality sufficiently to render any investigation into the influence of build of little value.

The group insured at ages 15 to 19 was also excluded for several reasons. These ages mark the transition period from boyhood to manhood. There is a wide difference between the average weight at age 15 and the average weight at age 19, and deductions made from investigations based on a variation of 5, 10, 15 etc., pounds from the average weight in the group would be of little value. More than three-quarters of the data were on lives from 10 to 20 pounds under the average weight, and statistics for other weight-groups were too meagre to be of value. In this connection it may be explained that the average weight was derived from the General Build cards, while, as already mentioned, the present statistics include the Special Build cards, much the greater part of the latter for age-group 15-19 being on light weights. Furthermore, the methods of selecting risks at these young ages probably differed widely among the Companies.

The extent of the material and the average period of exposure to risk may be seen from the [above] table.

METHOD OF HANDLING THE DATA

The Committee desired information on two main points:

1. The variation of the mortality according to the degree of departure from the average weight;

2. The build at which the lowest mortality was experienced for the various ages at entry.

The cards under each age-group and height were first sorted into weight-groups, the unit figure 0 or 5 of the weight being the central figure in each group. For example, the weights 123, 124, 125, 126, and 127 formed one group, and the weights 128, 129, 130, 131 and 132 the next group. The 5-pound groups in which the average weights (see p. 37, Vol, I) for each age-group and height were located constitute the average-weight groups. The overweight and underweight groups were then classified as follows:

UNDERWEIGHT GROUPS	OVERWEIGHT GROUPS
- 5 pounds	+ 5 pounds
- 10 pounds	+ 10 pounds
- 15 pounds to - 20 pounds	+ 15 pounds to + 20 pounds
- 25 pounds to - 30 pounds	+ 25 pounds to + 30 pounds
- 35 pounds to - 45 pounds	+ 35 pounds to + 45 pounds
- 50 pounds and more	+ 50 pounds to + 60 pounds
	+ 65 pounds to + 80 pounds
	+ 85 pounds and more

The group "+ 5 pounds" is the next higher 5-pound group to that in which the average weight is found. Thus, if the average weight were 126 pounds, the "average-weight group" would contain all persons of 123 to 127 pounds, and the "+ 5 pounds group" would contain all persons from 128 to 132 pounds. Similarly, if the average weight were 124 pounds, the "average-weight group" would be the group from 123 to 127 pounds, and the "+ 5 pounds group" the group containing those from 128 to 132 pounds.

Consideration was given to dividing the statistics into one-pound or two-pound groups, but this was deemed inadvisable, especially in view of the considerable proportion of estimated weights, and of the fact that 60% of the stated weights of the insured ended with 0 or 5 (Vol. I, p. 16). It is believed that the plan adopted of 5-pound groups will give as accurate results as may be obtained from the statistics.

TABLE A
MEN
ALL POLICY YEARS COMBINED

Ages at Entry	Number Entering	Actual Deaths	Expected Deaths	Ratio
20-24	152,862	4,982	4,362	114%
25-29	175,155	6,496	6,008	108
30-34	149,016	6,617	6,117	108
35-39	109,762	6,209	5,614	111
40-44	73,934	5,801	5,115	113
45-49	44,530	4,598	4,180	110
50-53	20,855	3,082	2,746	112
54-56	9,792	1,796	1,752	103
57-59	5,850	1,334	1,317	101
60-62	2,916	802	827	97
Total	744,672	41,717	38,038	110%

ALL AGES AT ENTRY COMPARED

Policy Years	Actual Deaths	Expected Deaths	Ratio
1	3,258	3,214	101%
2	3,462	3,221	107
3	3,340	3,023	110
4	3,129	2,835	110
5	2,975	2,681	111
1–5	16,164	14,974	108
6–10	12,862	11,500	112
11–15	8,299	7,365	113
16–24	4,392	4,199	105
1–24	41,717	38,038	110%

The data were then combined into three sections according to height:

(a) Short men–5 feet 3 inches to 5 feet 6 inches inclusive

(b) Men of average height–5 feet 7 inches to 5 feet 10 inches inclusive

(c) Tall men–5 feet 11 inches to 6 feet 2 inches inclusive.

The expected deaths were then determined under each age-group for each of the three sections of height and according to the fifteen subdivisions already described–namely, the average-weight group, the six underweight groups, and the eight overweight groups.

The expected deaths were calculated by the select table of mortality known as the M.A. Table, which appears on pages 89 and 90 of Volume I. Full details appear in Table I (not shown).

Attention is especially drawn to the fact that in all the exhibits hereafter given, and in all the comparisons of actual and expected deaths the grouping is based upon the average weight *according to the ages at entry*. The table appearing in the Instructions, which was based on the average weight at age 37, has not been used in determining the influence of build on mortality, nor in any way other than to ascertain which entrants came within the Special Build limits.

SYNOPSIS OF RESULTS

In Table II (not shown), the three divisions of height are combined, the number entering, the actual and expected deaths and the ratio being given under each age-group for each weight-group. A synopsis of table II by ages at entry and by policy years is given in Table A. In these and the succeeding tables the statistics include only the data of heights from 5 feet 3 inches to 6 feet 2 inches inclusive, at ages at entry 20 to 62 inclusive.

TABLE B
MEN
ALL AGES AT ENTRY AND POLICY YEARS COMBINED

Variation from Average Weight in Pounds	Number Entering	Actual Deaths	Expected Deaths	Ratio
-50 and more	1,685	165	160	103%
-35 to -45	57,737	4,199	4,375	96
-25 to -30	207,486	9,873	9,442	105
-15 to -20	209,805	7,997	7,481	107
-10	28,894	1,574	1,637	96
-5	26,186	1,480	1,529	97
Average	24,525	1,381	1,422	97
+5	20,412	1,176	1,188	97
+10	16,453	970	999	97
+15 to +20	22,363	1,497	1,443	104
+25 to +30	14,520	1,267	1,122	113
+35 to +45	54,295	5,061	3,876	131
+50 to +60	46,417	3,697	2,563	144
+65 to +80	12,119	1,144	695	165
+85 and more	1,775	236	106	223
Total	774,672	41,717	38,038	110%

The foregoing tables show that the aggregate mortality is only 10% in excess of the expected deaths by the select mortality table adopted by the Committee, the maximum variation of any age-group being 14% from the standard. In view of the fact that fully one-half of the cases are more than twenty pounds over or under the average weight (see Table B), some excess of actual over tabular mortality was to be expected.

The next table is a synopsis of the results according to various weight-groups for all ages and policy years combined.

The mortality from 10 pounds underweight to 10 pounds overweight, inclusive, is about 97% of the expected deaths, and from 20 pounds underweight to 20 pounds overweight, 102%, these percentages indicating the reliability of the M. A. Table. There is an apparent steady advance in relative mortality with increasing weight, but only a slight increase in the mortality among underweights compared with those of average weight. It would be unwise to base conclusions on this synopsis without further analysis, because all ages are combined and the effect of underweight at the young ages is obscured.

It will be seen from Table II (not shown), that the relatively large numbers in the weight-group -15 to -20 pounds, and in the weight-group -25 to -30 pounds, are found chiefly at the younger ages at entry, and are due to the use of a table of height and weight based on age 37 at entry in determining Special Build cases. The distribution of overweights has been affected by the same cause.

INFLUENCE OF BUILD ON MORTALITY AMONG WOMEN

There were two sets of statistics on women collected from the companies:

(a) Data intended to be the basis of the height and weight table.

(b) Data for the study of the four classes of women.

The cards for the former contained the height and weight in each case, but did not differentiate among spinsters, married women and widows; while the cards for the latter did not give the height and weight. The investigation into the four classes of women showed that there was a substantial difference in the mortality between spinsters and married women; but, in the hope that something of value would be obtained towards determining the influence of build on mortality, the Committee thought it advisable to make an investigation of the data on the cards under *(a)* together with additional homogeneous data supplied by four representative companies. The cases were divided into three height-groups:

(1) 4 feet 11 inches to 5 feet 2 inches, inclusive
(2) 5 feet 3 inches to 5 feet 6 inches, inclusive
(3) 5 feet 7 inches to 5 feet 10 inches, inclusive.

These divisions were selected because the average

WOMEN

HEIGHT 4 FEET 11 INCHES TO 5 FEET 10 INCHES INCLUSIVE.

ALL POLICY YEARS COMBINED

	Ages at Entry 20 to 29 Inclusive			Ages at Entry 30 to 39 Inclusive		
Variation from Average Weight in Pounds	Actual Deaths	Expected Deaths	Ratio of Actual to Expected Deaths	Actual Deaths	Expected Deaths	Ratio of Actual to Expected Deaths
−15 to −30	742	647.36	115%	953	920.25	104%
−10 to +10	826	733.10	113	474	507.99	93
+15 to +30	142	114.38	124	154	168.18	92
+35 to +60	33	35.68	92	145	117.10	124
Total	1743	1530.52	114%	1726	1713.52	101%

	Ages at Entry 40 to 49 Inclusive			Ages at Entry 50 to 67 Inclusive		
Variation from Average Weight in Pounds	Actual Deaths	Expected Deaths	Ratio of Actual to Expected Deaths	Actual Deaths	Expected Deaths	Ratio of Actual to Expected Deaths
−15 to −30	393	474.61	83%	273	267.09	102%
−10 to +10	296	311.21	95	264	240.61	110
+15 to +30	174	152.53	114	205	165.88	124
+35 to +60	214	183.68	117	222	168.05	132
Total	1077	1122.03	96%	964	841.63	114%

TOTAL

Variation from Average Weight in Pounds	Actual Deaths	Expected Deaths	Ratio of Actual to Expected Deaths
−15 to −30	2361	2,309.31	102%
−10 to +10	1860	1,792.91	104
+15 to +30	675	600.97	112
+35 to +60	614	504.51	122
Total	5510	5207.70	106%

height of the women was found to be 5 feet 4 1/4 inches. All women shorter than 4 feet 11 inches or taller than 5 feet 10 inches were excluded; and also those under age 20 or over age 62 at entry, irrespective of height. The average weight is taken from the table given in Vol. I, p. 66, based on the weight of women at the various ages at entry. The treatment of all weight-groups is the same as for men (see p. 7)

In Table XI (not shown) appears a synopsis of the results for the various groups of ages at entry for all policy years combined.

The percentages of actual to expected deaths are irregular, and do not exhibit any decided tendency. To ascertain whether a further grouping might show the trend of the mortality, the (above) exhibit was prepared.

In interpreting these results and for purposes of comparison it should be remembered that the relative mortality in the four classes of women combined was 114% of the M.A. Table for ages at entry 20 to 29, 104% for ages 30 to 39, 98% for ages 40 to 49 and 99% for ages 50 to 62. A comparison of these percentages for women with those of weight-group from 10 pounds underweight to 10 pounds overweight follows:

WOMEN
HEIGHT 4 FEET 11 INCHES TO 5 FEET 10 INCHES INCLUSIVE
ALL POLICY YEARS COMBINED

Variation from Average Weight in Pounds	Ages at Entry 20 to 39 Inclusive			Ages at Entry 40 to 62 Inclusive		
	Actual Deaths	Expected Deaths	Ratio of Actual to Expected Deaths	Actual Deaths	Expected Deaths	Ratio of Actual to Expected Deaths
−25 to −30	459	455.83	101%	433	497.76	87%
−15 to −20	1236	1111.78	111	233	243.94	96
−10 to +10	1300	1241.09	105	560	551.82	101
+15 to +30	296	282.56	105	379	318.41	119
+35 to +60	178	152.78	117	436	351.73	124
Total	3469	3244.04	107%	2041	1963.66	104%

TOTAL

Variation from Average Weight in Pounds	Actual Deaths	Expected Deaths	Ratio of Actual to Expected Deaths
−25 to −30	892	953.59	94%
−15 to −20	1469	1355.72	108
−10 to +10	1860	1792.91	104
+15 to +30	675	600.97	112
+35 to +60	614	504.51	122
Total	5510	5207.70	106%

RATIO OF ACTUAL TO EXPECTED DEATHS

	20-29	30-39	40-49	50-62
−10pounds to +10 pounds..	113%	93%	95%	110%
All women.......	114	104	98	99

The differences at ages 30-39 and 50-62 appear to indicate that the data are not free from accidental fluctuations.

At ages 20 to 29 the ratio of actual to expected deaths for those from 10 pounds underweight to 10 pounds overweight is 113% of the M.A. Table, while for those from 15 to 60 pounds overweight the ratio is only 117%. At ages at entry 30 to 39 the lowest mortality is among those from 10 pounds underweight to 30 pounds overweight. For ages at entry 40 to 49 there is a gradual increase with increased weight in the ratio of actual to expected deaths, the most favorable group being those from 15 to 30 pounds underweight. At the oldest ages at entry the mortality is probably lowest with those markedly underweight.

There is evidently little reliable information regarding the influence of build on longevity that can be obtained from the foregoing table, and accordingly another table has been prepared of more comprehensive groupings.

The foregoing table brings out more clearly the markedly better quality of the distinctly underweight risks at the older ages at entry but in other respects does not afford any conclusive results.

EFFECT OF HEIGHT ON MORTALITY

A brief synopsis is given of the subdivision of the statistics into three sections by height, and as the results were exceedingly irregular when narrow groups by weight were employed, the following table contains only those from 20 pounds underweight to 20 pounds overweight, inclusive.

It is evident that no satisfactory deductions can be drawn from the foregoing table.

WOMEN
EFFECT OF HEIGHT ON MORTALITY
From 20 Pounds Underweight to 20 Pounds Overweight Inclusive

	Height 4 Feet 11 In. to 5 Feet 2 In.			Height 5 Feet 3 in. to 5 Feet 6 In.			Height 5 Feet 7 In. to 5 Feet 10 In.		
Ages at Entry	Actual Deaths	Expected Deaths	Ratio of Actual to Expected Deaths	Actual Deaths	Expected Deaths	Ratio of Actual to Expected Deaths	Actual Deaths	Expected Deaths	Ratio of Actual to Expected Deaths
20–29	399	328	122%	893	820	109%	225	195	115%
30–39	324	305	106	756	745	101	138	144	96
40–49	141	149	95	337	349	97	70	62	113
50–59	140	119	118	229	221	104	37	27	137

CONCLUSION

In the investigations of the four classes of women it was shown that the mortality among married women was about 50% greater than among spinsters, and it would therefore be quite possible to have a lower mortality among a group of spinsters greatly overweight than among a group of married women of average weight. The statistics on build were of a heterogeneous nature on account of the variation in the mortality of the four classes. As already pointed out, the mortality under Endowment policies was very much lower than under Ordinary life, and the proportion of Endowment insurance was twice as great among spinsters as among married women. On account of the large amount of labor involved, and the problematical value of the results, the Committee did not deem it advisable to investigate separately the influence of build on the mortality of spinsters or of married women.

While the statistics on the influence of build on mortality of women have enabled the Committee to deduce little of substantial value, the following conclusions are suggested by the synoptical tables:

1. The effect of underweight or overweight, particularly at the younger ages, is less than among men, though exhibiting the same general tendencies.

2. At the older ages, underweight to the extent of at least 30 pounds (below which weight statistics are too meagre to draw conclusions from) is an advantage, and overweight is a disadvantage, increasing with the degree of overweight.

BODY BUILD AND LONGEVITY

Louis I. Dublin
Statistician, Metropolitan Life Insurance Company, New York

The very expression "well built" has become a part of our language. It implies that persons of a particular build or structure are better coordinated or somehow can function better than other people and may, therefore, be expected to have a greater life span. Variations in the structure of individuals are marked and serve to distinguish fairly definite types. Insurance experience has crystallized into a number of fairly definite conclusions with regard to the relative longevity of certain of these types. Extremes of stature, for example, are decided handicaps. Extreme overweight and underweight carry with them increased mortality and correspondingly shorter life. Very heavy people are more likely to succumb prematurely to such conditions as diabetes, organic heart disease, renal impairment, hardening of the arteries, and very light persons, particularly at the younger ages, are more likely to develop tuberculosis. Insurance experience has confirmed the popular judgment that the individuals who approach the mean of these body measures are better able to withstand the hazards of life and to round out a fairly full expectation.

Another observation of great importance is that certain measures of the human body, such as stature, body surface, weight, height sitting, chest measurement and vital capacity, are closely related in their variability. In our current terminology, we say that they are highly correlated, some pairs being more closely related to each other than others. As long ago as 1846, Dr. John Hutchinson considered some of these relationships and especially those existing between standing height, weight, circumference of the chest, and the vital capacity. More recently, Dreyer of Oxford, following up the clues of Hutchinson, thought he could establish definite norms of build and relate these to physical fitness.

Dublin, LI. Body Build and Longevity. In: *DeLamar Lectures 1925-1926*. Maryland: The Williams & Wilkins Company; 1927:113-127.
Reprinted with permission from The Williams & Wilkins Company, 428 E. Preston St., Baltimore, MD, 21202.
Special thanks to Judy Roberts of the Pennington Information Center for help in acquiring this document.

I have already intimated that the experience of the life insurance companies has shown that overweights as a group have a below-average duration of life. Generally speaking, it has been the custom of the medical directors of the life insurance companies to be guided in their selection of risks by a table of average weights which was constructed from the heights and weights of a large number of persons insured on standard policies. Their practice has been to consider as normal, weights within a range of 20 per cent above and 20 per cent below the average. Beyond these limits, applicants for insurance were considered as possibly subnormal as to build and expected to give a higher mortality, depending upon the extent of the departure from the average weight.

For a long time, there has been the suspicion among insurance executives that there were in fact several types of overweights and that these would show different mortality experiences. Chest as compared with abdominal girth, and especially the length of the spine have been considered important characters which might determine the mortality of overweights. Or, to put it more definitely overweights with large chests and long trunks have been expected to show a much more favorable subsequent mortality than those with a relatively narrow chest and short trunk. In a number of companies, overweights have been selected on this basis for some time. To determine the truth of these suspicions, a Committee of the Association of Life Insurance Medical Directors was appointed to study the question, and the problem was assigned to my office for investigation. Fortunately, the Union Central Life Insurance Company of Cincinnati had for many years recorded the length of the spine for all of its applicants for insurance, together with the other body measurements that are usually taken, total height and weight, chest and abdominal girth, etc. There thus became available for this investigation the very complete records of more than 38,000 overweights, together with their subsequent survival his-

TABLE 1
Number of overweight men in specified build and height classes, Union Central Policy Issues, 1887 to 1907

BUILD CLASS	ALL MEN		SHORT MEN		MEN OF MEDIUM HEIGHT		TALL MEN	
	Number	Per cent of total over-weights	Number	Per cent of total over-weights	Number	Per cent of total over-weights	Number	Per cent of total over-weights
All overweights..........	38,062	100.0	6,567	100.0	22,888	100.0	8,607	100.0
Build class:								
1..........	25,932	68.1	4,390	66.8	15,866	69.3	5,676	65.9
2..........	9,495	24.9	1,670	25.4	5,560	24.3	2,264	26.3
3..........	2,323	6.1	450	6.9	1,279	5.6	594	6.9
4..........	304	0.8	55	0.8	180	0.8	69	0.8
5..........	9		2		3		4	

tory, covering the period of years from the date of their entry between 1887 and 1907 to the anniversary of their policies in 1922. Here was obviously the material necessary for the solution of the question whether this particular character, that is, the length of spine, either alone or in combination with other body measurements, played a part in determining the subsequent mortality of overweights.

Table 1 presents the facts for the constitution of this group of 38,062 overweight men according to build-class. Class I consists of those who showed an excess of 16 pounds and less than 32 pounds over an assumed norm; Class II, an excess of 32 pounds and less than 48 pounds; Class III, 48 pounds and less than 62 pounds;

TABLE 2
Characteristics of relative spine length (percentage spine length of total height) for overweight men in respective build classes according to height groups

CHARACTERISTICS; BUILD GROUP	HEIGHT GROUP		
	Short men	Men of average or medium height	Tall men
Mean relative spine length:			
Build group:			
All overweights..........	37.650 ± 0.026	37.404 ± 0.013	37.131 ± 0.021
1..........	37.493 ± 0.031	37.268 ± 0.015	37.033 ± 0.025
2..........	37.948 ± 0.052	37.661 ± 0.026	37.242 ± 0.042
3..........	38.022 ± 0.101	37.821 ± 0.053	37.544 ± 0.079
4..........	37.991 ± 0.293	38.469 ± 0.145	37.878 ± 0.237
5..........	*	41.100 ± 3.312	38.800 ± 2.551
Standard deviation:			
Build group:			
All overweights..........	3.080 ± 0.018	2.867 ± 0.009	2.873 ± 0.015
1..........	3.030 ± 0.022	2.872 ± 0.011	2.835 ± 0.018
2..........	3.146 ± 0.037	2.825 ± 0.018	2.950 ± 0.030
3..........	3.183 ± 0.072	2.824 ± 0.038	2.868 ± 0.056
4..........	3.225 ± 0.207	2.887 ± 0.013	2.925 ± 0.168
5..........	*	8.505 ± 2.342	7.564 ± 1.804

*Only two cases in classification.

TABLE 3

Comparison of actual and expected mortality among overweights, 1887-1908. By height class and relative spine length. White male issues of Union Central Life Insurance Company*

All build classes

BUILD CLASS AND RELATIVE SPINE LENGTH	ALL HEIGHT CLASSES			OVERWEIGHT SHORT MEN†			OVERWEIGHT MEN OF MEDIUM HEIGHT‡			OVERWEIGHT TALL MEN§		
	Actual deaths	Expected deaths	Ratio, actual to expected	Actual deaths	Expected deaths	Ratio, actual to expected	Actual deaths	Expected deaths	Ratio, actual to expected	Actual deaths	Expected deaths	Ratio, actual to expected
All build classes¶...	4,571	4,299.2	106.3	786	760.7	103.3	2,683	2,582.5	103.9	1,102	956.0	115.3
Relative spine length:												
Above limit of S.D. + from mean..........	493	468.2	105.3	117	108.4	107.9	286	271.0	105.5	90	88.8	101.4
Within limits of S.D. + or - from mean.....	3,573	3,334.3	107.2	596	575.7	103.5	2,107	1,998.2	105.4	870	760.4	114.4
Below limit of S.D. - from mean...........	505	496.7	101.7	73	76.6	95.3	290	313.3	92.6	142	106.8	113.0

*Select and ultimate, by M.A. Table.
†Short men 66 inches and under.
‡ Men of medium height, 67 to 70 inches.
§Tall men, 71 inches and over (Page 7, Vol. II, Medico-Actuarial Investigation).
¶For build classification see pp. 120-121, Vol. I, Medico-Actuarial Investigation also p. 173, Proceedings 34th Ann. Meeting, Association of Life Insurance Medical Directors, 1924.

Class IV, 62 pounds and less than 78 pounds and Class V, 78 pounds or more in excess of the assumed norm. More than two-thirds of the overweights were in Class I, approximately one-fourth were in Class II, and Class III contained a little more than 6 per cent of the total. Classes IV and V were negligible for our purposes. These proportions, moreover, did not vary markedly in each one of the three sub-groups of short men, men of medium height and tall men.

We next computed for each of our height-build classes the average relative spine length, that is, the percentage spine length of total height. [Table 2] shows these averages vary but little from 37 to 38 per cent of the total height. The standard deviation from the average for each one of the build groups is, moreover, close to three units. This classification makes it possible to divide each one of the height and build groups into three parts: first, those who are within the limits of the standard deviation, plus and minus, from the average spine length; second, those whose spine length is above the standard deviation from the mean spine length; and third, those below the standard deviation from the mean spine length. The first of these three classes are obviously those with average spines, the second, with long spines, and the third, those with short spines. The material was then ready to tabulate for the actual mortality experienced as contrasted with the expected mortality according to the Medico-Actuarial Table, with due regard to the effect of medical selection during the first five years of insurance.

The resulting mortality tables are shown herewith.

The first of these is for all build-classes combined. The 38,062 overweight entrants who were classified in this table gave an aggregate of 400,331 years of life exposed to risk, or an average of 10.5 years. There were 4,571 actual deaths and 4,299 expected deaths according to the M.A. table (Select and Ultimate), or a ratio of 106.3 per cent actual to expected mortality. The entire group gave a mortality similar to that of other groups of overweights carefully selected by insurance medical directors. A further examination of Table 3 will show that short overweights and those of medium height have a lower mortality than those who are tall, the two former groups giving a ratio of 103.3 actual to expected and 103.9, respectively, as contrasted with a ratio actual to expected of 115.3 per cent for overweight tall men. This likewise is in accord with expectation. Tall men, as a group, especially at the younger ages, give higher mortality than the average. Those who are five feet, eleven inches or taller and under age 40 have a mortality

TABLE 4

Comparison of actual and expected mortality among overweights, 1887-1908. By height class and relative spine length. White male issues of Union Central Life Insurance Company Build Class I

BUILD CLASS AND RELATIVE SPINE LENGTH	ALL HEIGHT CLASSES			OVERWEIGHT SHORT MEN			OVERWEIGHT MEN OF MEDIUM HEIGHT			OVERWEIGHT TALL MEN		
	Actual deaths	Expected deaths	Ratio, actual to expected	Actual deaths	Expected deaths	Ratio, actual to expected	Actual deaths	Expected deaths	Ratio, actual to expected	Actual deaths	Expected deaths	Ratio, actual to expected
Build Class I.....	2,786	2,840.9	98.1	467	484.4	96.4	1,687	1,741.5	96.9	632	615.0	102.8
Relative spine length:												
Above limit of S.D. + from mean..........	251	265.8	94.4	58	61.7	94.0	150	155.5	96.6	43	48.6	88.5
Within limits of S.D. + or - from mean.....	2,198	2,224.0	98.8	361	369.1	97.8	1,334	1,360.1	98.1	503	494.8	101.7
Below limit of S.D. - from mean...........	337	351.1	96.0	48	53.6	89.6	203	225.9	89.9	86	71.6	120.1

See footnotes for Table 3. These apply also to this table.

in excess of the standard mortality tables even under the most favorable conditions of weight.

Our chief interest in this study, however, was to determine the mortality ratios according to spine length. In the entire group, that is, all build-classes combined, those with short spines, namely, those who are below the limit of the standard deviation from the mean, have the lowest mortality, 101.7 per cent of the M.A. Table. This condition is particularly striking for the overweight short men (95.3 per cent) and overweight men of medium height (92.6 per cent). Among tall overweights, on the other hand, those with long spines have a much better mortality (101.4 per cent) than those with short spines (133.0). It would appear, therefore, from this preliminary survey at least, that only among tall men was the suspicion of the medical directors confirmed as to the advantage of a long trunk. Among short men and among men of medium height, the very reverse condition prevailed.

A similar relationship is found in each one of the build-classes. Thus, Build-Class 1 (table 4), that is, those who are moderately overweight, and who constitute the bulk of this experience, showed a mortality of only 98.1 per cent ratio of actual to expected. The tall men in this group showed a somewhat higher mortality than the short men and the men of medium height but not materially so. But, the very lowest mortality is found among those with short spines among short men and men of medium height; whereas, among the tall men of this class, the best mortality was found among those with relatively long spines. In Build-Class 2 (table 5), a parallel situation was found, all of the figures being proportionately higher because of the increased mortality with added weight. Unfortunately, Build-Class 3 (table 6) was not large enough to give significant figures in each one of the sub-divisions. But, the figures that are available, show essentially the same conditions.

We may summarize the findings of this investigation to this point as follows: A fundamental difference between tall men, on the one hand, and short and medium height men, on the other, exists with relation to relative spine length and mortality. Among tall men, those who have above average relative spine lengths, that is, those who have short legs, have a very much better mortality than those who have below average relative spine length, that is, those who have long legs. Among short overweights and overweights of medium height, this particular relationship is reversed.

Possibly, these results indicate that relative spine length is not of itself a sufficient criterion of physical fitness among overweights. For this reason, we thought it would be desirable to bring into the picture the additional measurement of chest capacity to see whether this added factor would not clarify the results of the investigation of spine length and mortality.

Let us first examine the statistical constants of chest-girth in relation to height and relative spine length. These are a necessary preliminary to a classification of the materials for the mortality investigation on these items.

The first point of interest is that chest-girth increases with total height. Within a given height class, there is no important variation of chest-girth with an increase in relative spine-length. It is also observed that with

TABLE 8

Percentage, actual to expected mortality among overweight white males. By height, relative spine length, and chest measurement groups. (All build classes combined.) Union Central Policy Issues 1887 to 1908, experience carried to policy anniversary in 1921*

Select and ultimate basis by M.A. Table

RELATIVE SPINE LENGTH: CHEST GIRTH	ALL HEIGHT CLASSES			SHORT MEN*			MEDIUM HEIGHT MEN			TALL MEN*		
	Actual deaths	Expected deaths	Ratio, actual to expected with P.E. †	Actual deaths	Expected deaths	Ratio, actual to expected with P.E. †	Actual deaths	Expected deaths	Ratio, actual to expected with P.E. †	Actual deaths	Expected deaths	Ratio, actual to expected with P.E. †
Totals..........	4,571	4,298.6	106.3 ± 1.1	786	761.4	103.2 ± 2.5	2,683	2,579.3	104.1 ± 1.3	1,102	957.9	115.0 ± 2.4
All spine lengths combined:												
Chest below mean.	1,999	2,132.6	93.7 ± 1.4	318	334.1	95.2 ± 3.6	1,232	1,326.5	92.9 ± 1.8	449	472.0	95.1 ± 3.0
Chest above mean	2,572	2,166.0	118.7 ± 1.6	468	427.3	109.5 ± 3.4	1,451	1,252.8	115.8 ± 2.1	653	485.9	134.4 ± 3.5
Relative spine length:												
Below limit of S.D. (- from mean):												
Chest below mean	230	255.1	90.2 ± 4.0	35	39.1	89.5 ± 10.2	138	161.1	85.7 ± 4.9	57	54.9	103.8 ± 9.3
Chest above mean	275	244.3	112.6 ± 4.6	38	38.0	100.0 ± 10.9	152	153.8	98.8 ± 5.4	85	52.5	161.9 ± 11.9
Within limits of S.D. (+ or - from mean):												
Chest below mean	1,564	1,662.6	94.1 ± 1.6	230	244.5	94.1 ± 4.2	976	1,043.1	93.6 ± 2.0	358	375.0	95.5 ± 3.4
Chest above mean	2,009	1,666.6	120.5 ± 1.8	366	331.0	110.6 ± 3.9	1,131	949.8	119.1 ± 2.4	512	385.8	132.7 ± 4.0
Above limit of S.D. (+ from mean):												
Chest below mean	205	214.9	95.4 ± 4.5	53	50.5	105.0 ± 9.7	118	122.3	96.5 ± 6.0	34	42.1	80.8 ± 9.3
Chest above mean	288	255.1	112.9 ± 4.5	64	58.3	109.8 ± 9.2	168	149.2	112.6 ± 5.9	56	47.6	117.6 ± 10.6

*Height Groups were: Short men–66 inches and under; medium height men–67 to 70 inches; tall men–71 inches and over.
†P.E. = "probable error."

increase in height there follows an increase in the variability of chest-girth, that is to say, short men adhere more closely to the average chest-girth than do tall men. Within each height class (i.e., overweight short men), there is no change in the variability or dispersion of chest-girths with increase in spine-length. These findings suggest therefore that the chest-girth factor does not account for the peculiar mortality showing of the relative spine-length classes reported above. Chest-girth is an independent factor and within chest-girth classes the showing with respect to relative spine-length is approximately the same as for all chest-girth groups combined; the short men and men of medium height have the lower mortality ratios in the lower spine-length classes and tall men give the more favorable readings in the high relative spine-length group.

For the purpose of this study, we established two chest-girth classes: (1) Chest-girths below the mean; (2) chest-girths above the mean; and distinguished these two groups in each one of our previous classifications of relative spine-length. The mortality results of this classification are shown in Table 8. Regardless of the classification by chest-girth, tall overweights still show lower mortalities in the long spine-length class, and short men and men of medium height show the lower mortality readings in the long spine-length classes, quite irrespective of whether the chest measure is below or above the mean.

The classing of the material by chest-girth brings out another surprising conclusion. Invariably, the lower mortality is shown in the chest-girth groups *below* the mean. Combining the chest-girth and relative spine-length readings, we may say that the best mortalities are found among overweight short men and men of medium height with *short* relative spine-length and with chest-girths *below* average. For overweight tall men, the mortality is best among *long* relative spine groups and with chest-girths *below* average!

The above results indicate that we cannot depend upon the original Dreyer tables, neither for practical life insurance underwriting nor for general use in clinical medicine. The assumptions of Dreyer led us to believe that the more favorable mortality ratios would be found among persons with relatively long spines and with chests above average. But, in general, the results of this investigation show a contrary indication, except in a minor way for tall overweights. It is possible, of course, that some of these results reflect medical selection. But this can be at best only a minor item. There is still much in this study that calls for further examination, and it is hoped that additional investigations of the material will be made as time proceeds.

AN EXPERIMENT WITH THE SPECIALIZED INVESTIGATION.

RUFUS W. WEEKS

The recent Specialized Mortality Investigation has presented to the actuarial world a vast mass of valuable material arranged in systematic form. Various lines of inference and experiment are suggested by the mere possession of this material. One of these lines concerns the matter of a standard for measuring the mortality in the various classes contained in the investigation.

Doubtless the ideal standard would have been a set of mortality tables for successive years of insurance, representing the entire experience of the companies during the thirty years, including the classes actually investigated as well as all the other insurances issued and in force within the same years. This, however, would have meant handling something like five times the amount of material included in the task actually undertaken; so colossal an undertaking was never contemplated for a moment by the Society or by the Committee. The Committee used, for the purpose of measuring the degrees of mortality, an artificial standard, corresponding to the impressions of its members as to what the normal mortality rates among the average of American insured lives have been; and upon this standard are based the published ratios of actual to expected deaths in the respective classes.

Another possible method of treating the matter of a standard for comparison will suggest itself, upon a mere restating of the main facts of the investigation in the form of a list of the classes, arranged in the order of their mortality-quality on the standard of the Committee; a list in which the best class is put first, and the others follow successively, ending with the worst. Such a list is given below. In preparing this list classes seventy-seven to ninety-eight, which consist of persons insured in certain selected counties of the United States, have been omitted.

Weeks RW. An experiment with the specialized investigation. In: Actuarial Society of America. *Transactions.* 1904;8:17-23.
This article is under the auspices of The Society of Actuaries, 475 N. Martingale Rd., Suite 800, Schaumburg, IL 60173-2226.
Special thanks to Judy Willis of the Pennington Information Center for help in acquiring this document.

What first strikes the eye, on looking at this list, is the great number of classes which show a mortality better than the assumed standard. Out of the seventy-six classes no less than thirty-two present this favorable appearance, and they embrace 65,992 deaths out of the total of 140,622. Of these thirty-two, twenty-two embracing 37,189 deaths show a mortality less than ninety per cent of the standard, and of the twenty-two, four embracing 1,443 deaths, show a mortality less than eighty per cent of the standard.

It is noteworthy, also, that the aggregate deaths of the entire seventy-six classes are slightly less than the aggregate number expected according to the assumed standard. The inference is that the standard assumed is on the whole the equivalent of such mortality tables as the aggregated data of these seventy-six classes would have produced. It would not seem, *a priori*, a natural assumption, that the combined data of seventy-six classes, selected as these were, would give the same results as the entire business of the companies would have given if attainable. On the contrary, it would seem to be a safe proposition that since everyone of these seventy-six classes was supposed in advance to represent a blemish, it must follow that if the data of a large number of the best of the classes are combined, the tables deduced from such data could not, to any considerable extent, show a lighter mortality than would the ideal tables which would have been brought out from the entire business of the companies, good, bad and indifferent. To put the statement in another form, it is not likely that any large section of the impaired or classified business would show a lighter mortality than the total "accepted" business of the various companies. With this idea I have taken the first twenty-seven classes of the above table, those which show less than ninety-five per cent. of the standard mortality, and have combined the exposures and deaths of these twenty-seven classes by insurance years and ages of exposure. The total number of deaths contained in this body of experience is 57,596, being over forty per cent. of the entire number

LIST OF SEVENTY-SIX CLASSES. ARRANGED IN ORDER OF COMMITTEE'S PERCENTAGES OF ACTUAL TO EXPECTED DEATH.				
Class	Description	Committee's Expected Deaths	Actual Deaths	Per-centage
66	Weight C, parent dead below 70 of kidney of Bright's disease	1,796	1,475	82.1
67	Weight C, parent dead below 70 of heart disease	3,858	3,269	84.7
65	Weight C, parent dead below 70 of consumption, phthisis or tuberculosis	6,198	5,382	86.8
70	Weight C, both parents reached 75	9,060	8,020	88.5
72	Weight D, not included under 58 or 71	13,602	12,452	91.5
62	Weight B, neither parent noted as dead below 70	2,345	2,312	98.6
74	Height below five feet	93	93	100.0
71	Weight D, parent dead below 70 of any lung disease	1,864	1,869	100.3
59	Weight A, neither parent noted as dead below 70	899	1,060	117.9
63	Weight B, one parent, or both dead below 70	549	5,465	120.1
64	**Weight B, girth of abdomen greater than chest expanded**	403	536	133.0
61	**Weight A, girth of abdomen greater than chest expanded**	276	419	151.8
49	Has had gout	109	168	154.1

*This is a partial list of the 76 classes. The bold are the groups with abdominal girth greater than chest girth and increased mortality.

of deaths in the seventy-six classes.

The first question undertaken to be answered in connection with this mass of data was — How many distinct mortality tables for successive periods of duration of the insurances are necessary in order to present a true picture of the facts? In other words, at what rate and how soon does the selection wear off? To answer this question the expected mortality according to the American Table has been calculated upon the exposures for each policy year separately, from the 1st to the 15th, then for the 16th to the 20th combined, and for the 21st to the 30th combined, and then the total number of the tabular deaths so found for each insurance year or group of years has been compared with the total number of actual deaths. The results of this preliminary comparison are given in the table below.

If we may assume that the percentages in the foregoing tables approximately represent the true movement we should have to conclude that the normal mortality relatively to tabular goes up by steps for four years only, then remains upon a level from the fifth to the ninth years inclusive, and then takes another upward step and remains upon the level so reached from the tenth year to the fifteenth year inclusive, then takes one more upward step, finding its permanent level from the sixteenth year on.

I should interpret these figures as giving a fair picture of the normal Endowment mortality of the combined companies — the deterioration at the tenth year being due to the disappearance of the ten-year Endowments (the high death rate in the tenth year itself being presumably an accident), and the further deterioration at the fifteenth year being due to the disappearance of the fifteen-year Endowments.

The foregoing material suggests seven distinct mortality tables, representing successive stages in the lifetime of the insurances, as follows:

1st insurance year.
2d insurance year.
3d insurance year.
4th insurance year.
5th to 9th insurance years.
10th to 15th insurance years.
16th to 30th insurance years.

Mr. Arthur Hunter has undertaken for me the construction of these select tables, and furnishes the following statement:

"After the data were collected the ungraduated rate of mortality was obtained. This was then graduated by means of Mr. G. F. Hardy's method of using Woolhouse's formula. This method has not received the attention it deserves, as it appears only in the form of an actuarial not in Vol. XXXII of the *Institute Journal*. The method is so simple that it does not require a high grade of help to carry it out. The rule is as follows:

"Sum three times successively in groups of five, subtract three times the central second differences of the result so obtained, divide by 125, and the result is the we have refrained from carrying the work further because we thought it advisable not to eliminate irregularities which might be characteristic. It will be noticed that the mortality decreases with advancing years at the young ages. The same peculiarity may be noticed in the select tables prepared by Dr. Sprague from the H^M Experience. In those tables the mortality for the first calendar year decreases from age twenty to age twenty-seven, and does not exceed that mortality at age twenty until age thirty-six. Also, in the second, third and fourth calendar years the same condition is observed, although it does not cover so many ages. Even Dr. Sprague's rate of mortality for the fifth and subsequent calendar years is higher at age twenty-four than at any subsequent age until age thirty-eight is reached. In the first policy year in our experiment there is a steady increase in the rate of mortality from the earliest years, but in the second to the ninth years inclusive the same conditions are seen as in Dr. Sprague's tables although not to the same marked extent. The grouping of the data for the tenth to the fifteenth, and from the sixteenth to the thirtieth policy ears shows an increasing mortality for each successive age, with slight exceptions.

ACTUARIAL SOCIETY OF AMERICA.

TRANSACTIONS.

NEW YORK, MAY 20, 1903.

The undersigned, composing the Committee in charge of the present mortality investigation, have the honor to present their final report.

The work has been completed, except that of printing the resulting tables, which will be ready before the meeting of the Congress of Actuaries, as originally proposed. The cost is less than two-thirds of the original maximum estimated, thanks chiefly to the aid of the Prudential Insurance Company of America, whose entire organization, as far as necessary, has been placed at the disposal of the Committee, without charge except the actual outlay of the company.

The following percentage of the mortality by the standard table have been employed for obtaining the expected number of death losses during the first five years of insurance:

Ages at Entry.	Year I.	Year 2.	Year 3.	Year 4.	Year 5.
15 to 28	45	64	79	90	97
29 to 42	50	68	82	92	98
43 to 56	55	72	85	94	99
57 to 70	60	76	88	96	100

It will be remembered that the standard table employed for comparison is Farr's Healthy English Male Table, modified at certain ages, and that the table as modified was given in the report presented by this Committee one year ago and printed on page 277 of Vol. VII of the *Transactions*. The reasons for choosing this table appear on pages 274 and 275. It is unnecessary to re-state them. The standard table is believed to represent fairly and adequately the mortality to be expected upon American insured lives, after the first five years of insurance, and, modified by the percentages above indicated, during the first five years. It is, however, to be understood that the standard now employed must itself be modified from time to time as circumstances change and experience increases.

As will be seen by comparison of the percentages of mortality at different ages between this standard table and the American Table and other tables used for premium and reserve calculations, the differences are in some cases quite notable. If it be desired by anyone to compare the results of the present investigation with the expected mortality by the American or any other table, the detailed facts shortly to be published will enable such a comparison to be made. It has appeared to us more important at present to compare the experience upon the 98 special classes of risks with what we believe to represent the average experience upon good business, and thus to carry out the chief object of the investigation, namely, to supply to those officers who have to decide upon the acceptance of risks the materials for ascertaining whether a particular class is better or worse than the average of good business. A company is entitled to be protected by the selection of risks in such a manner as to prevent the intrusion of more than a minimum proportion of under-average risks, at whatever age.

In particular, the American Table differs from the standard table chiefly at the old ages, for which it shows an exceptionally high mortality. This effect was produced designedly by the author of the table, partly because of the scantiness of his materials at those ages, partly for safety. The assumption at old ages, for reserve purposes, of a mortality above the normal becomes especially useful whenever there arises, for any cause, among risks long in force, an abnormal "selection against the company" by the withdrawal of good risks in excessive proportion. The American table is therefore, at the older ages, more useful for reserve calculations than as a guide for the selection of fresh normal risks. In the present investigation the old entrants of a few classes exhibit a mortality slightly

Actuarial Society of America. *Transactions.* 1901-1903;492-497.
This article is under the auspices of The Society of Actuaries, 475 N. Martingale Rd., Suite 800, Schaumburg, IL 60173-2226.
Special thanks to Judy Willis of the Pennington Information Center for help in acquiring this document.

above the normal, while on the other hand, as compared with the American table, the same facts would exhibit a mortality slightly less than the expectation.

Before proceeding to indicate the results which have been secured relating to the individual classes under consideration, we cannot express too strongly one necessary warning. It must not be forgotten that the facts about to be given relate to the respective classes of risks among lives selected for insurance, and do not relate to the same classes among the general population. For example, it is not conceivable that, among the general population, those who have had at least one parent dying of consumption are above the average of the others in vitality. If this is found to be the case as regards that particular class of insured lives, it indicates only that such persons of that class as have actually been accepted for insurance have been selected so carefully as to secure for acceptance only those who are peculiarly good representatives of the class. If, on the other hand, the results appear only moderately bad upon a class of risks heretofore accepted with great circumspection, it is to be inferred that, had such circumspection not been exercised, the results would have been still worse. We trust earnestly that this warning may be borne in mind as applying, and intended to apply, to each one of the classes under consideration.

In presenting to the Society at this time a brief outline of some of the more important results of this investigation, we shall indicate the group of persons entering upon their insurance at ages from 15 to 28 inclusive as "young entrants;" those entering at ages from 29 to 42 inclusive as "mature entrants;" those entering at ages from 43 to 56 inclusive as "elderly entrants;" and those entering at ages from 57 to 70 inclusive as "old entrants."

Class 1 consists of persons insured for $20,000 or more on one application. Notwithstanding the care always taken in the selection of such risks, the result is unfavorable except upon young entrants, and increasingly so with the increase of the ages of entry. The old entrants are by far the worst, and the inference is that insurances for large amounts should be made with extreme care upon old lives. The experience after five years was almost equally unfavorable with that within five years after entry.

Class 2, consisting of cases in which insurances granted were for amounts smaller than those applied for, comprises, as would be expected; a bad class of risks.

Class 3 consists of persons insured on a plan different from that which they had asked for, so as to require the payment of a higher rate of premium. The results here are much nearer the normal than in Class 2, and this again was to be expected.

Class 4, men born in Germany, shows well for those insured in early life, but badly for those insured at the higher ages.

Class 5, persons born in Ireland, is decidedly unsatisfactory. The one favorable feature, the good results after five years on those insured at young ages, would indicate that the difficulty is not necessarily one of race, but may be due to circumstances. The matter needs further investigation, but the warning thus given by existing experience should not be lightly overlooked.

Class 6, born in Sweden or Norway, is excellent.

Class 7, persons of the colored race, shows well after five years, though badly within the first five years of insurance. It has been supposed in the past that colored people have less vitality than whites, but the somewhat scanty facts here available do not prove it. It must be recollected that great care has been taken in the selection of this class of risks.

Class 8, army risks in time of peace, is not satisfactory, though the improvement after five years may indicate that due care was not always exercised in the selection of the risks. As insurance officers consider themselves to have exercised more than usual prudence in the acceptance of army risks, the doubt heretofore felt concerning this class cannot be said to have been removed.

Class 9, officers in the navy, has been unprofitable at all ages of entry, in accordance with prior experience, as well as with the results upon other classes of seafaring risks.

Class 10, comprising civil officers such as marshal, sheriff, police, constable, etc., shows unfavorable results through the term of insurance, except upon old entrants.

Class 11, consisting of members of paid fire departments in cities, shows unfavorably.

Class 12, physicians, indicates an improvement over earlier statistics. Those insured below age 43 have proved themselves to be good risks, while the result has been unfortunate upon physicians insured at ages above 42. These remarks apply both to the earlier and later years of insurance.

Most interesting facts have been developed concerning certain kinds of occupation frequently supposed to be dangerous. Classes 13 (exposed to electricity), 14 (engaged in sawmills), 16 (working in iron or steel at high temperatures), 19 (house painters), 20 (printers), 21 (tailors), 22 (butchers and meat dealers,) 26 (traveling salesmen), such of them as have heretofore been accepted for life insurance, are good risks.

On the other hand, Class 15, steel grinders, though accepted only in small numbers, have proved unprofitable, and the same is true of Class 17, glass workers.

The results in Class 18, potters, are on the whole favorable.

Class 23, laborers, shows heavy mortality, except upon young entrants.

Class 24, contractors, comprises good risks in the younger age groups and poor risks in the older, for all durations of insurance.

Class 25, of theatrical occupations, exhibits a very high mortality.

Class 27, cattle dealers and drovers, risks which one or two companies have found unsatisfactory, must be regarded as no worse than the average, excepting the old entrants.

Classes 28 and 29 are bad in each one of the age groups. They comprise two classes of dealers in liquors, often supposed to be good risks. Class 28 consists of hotel keepers not giving personal attention to their barrooms, and Class 29 consists of dealers in wines or liquors who have stated, and warranted it to be true, that they are total abstainers.

Still worse, on the whole, is Class 30, sellers of wines or liquors, who have not represented themselves as total abstainers.

Again still worse, on the whole, is Class 31, brewers and their employees.

On the other hand, Class 32, distillers and their employees, may almost be regarded as good risks, at least during the early years of insurance, the experience being less favorable after five years.

Railway passenger conductors, Class 33, show a mortality only slightly above the expectation. Class 36, railway express messengers, exhibits results which are favorable as regards the younger risks, but quite unfavorable for those insured later in life. On the other hand, the railway mail clerks, Class 35, have been excellent risks.

In gathering the statistics of Class 34, railway passenger trainmen, it was determined to exclude all risks taken prior to 1890, in order to see whether it is true, as has sometimes been supposed, that risks of this class, all young and hardy men, ought to be fairly good risks, now that modern appliances for safety are so generally in use. The results may not seem conclusive, as they comprise only 2,523 years of exposure; but they are uniformly bad for each of the three groups of ages at entry.

Locomotive engineers, Class 37, show bad results, while locomotive firemen, Class 38, are still more unprofitable risks. As regards these and all other classes, the warning must not be forgotten that the statistics now collected relate only to persons actually selected for insurance by prudent companies, from among those prudent individuals who have shown themselves able and willing to take out insurance on their lives.

Bad results have been experienced upon Class 39, officers of ocean steam vessels; while the losses upon officers of sailing vessels, Class 40, have been still more heavy. On the other hand, contrary to expectation, the loss upon Class 42, seamen and fishermen, has not been excessive, though insurances effected at young ages have resulted in considerable loss.

The comparatively small class of pilots, Class 41, develops the interesting fact that these risks have, in each of the four groups of ages at entry, been particularly good risks during the first five years of insurance and particularly bad risks thereafter.

Those who have been accepted for insurance notwithstanding an intermittent or irregular pulse, Class 43, have proved themselves to be good risks when insured at the younger ages, but not so good when insured at the older ages.

Those who have been accepted, with more or less doubt, notwithstanding a pulse rate below sixty per minute, Class 44, have proved themselves to be extraordinarily good risks at all ages of entry and for all durations of insurance.

Those who have been insured after having reformed from intemperate habits, Class 45, show bad results, notwithstanding the extreme care usually taken in the acceptance of such cases.

Asthmatics, Class 46, show well, except the group of elderly entrants, who have proved themselves bad risks.

The care with which medical selection has discriminated against risks giving a recent history of inflammatory rheumatism is witnessed by the results. Class 47 comprises those who had had inflammatory rheumatism once before entrance, and Class 48 those who had had it oftener than once. Both classes show good results upon young entrants, and Class 47 shows good results for mature entrants. The other groups are not quite satisfactory. On the whole, Class 47, which is much the larger, has done well except as regards old entrants, while Class 48 has not been satisfactory except as regards young entrants.

Class 49, those showing a record of gout, exhibits results which are seriously disappointing to those who had hoped that earlier adverse reports on this class of cases might be overborne by wider and later experience. The mortality on this class is only slightly excessive within the first five years of insurance, but is afterwards nearly double the expectation.

Applicants showing a history of syphilis, Class 50, exhibit an almost equally bad record.

Contrary to expectation, those who have had otorrhoea, Class 51, appear to be good risks.

Three age groups of those who state that they have had hepatic colic, Class 52, show a favorable mortality, but for elderly entrants the results are unsatisfactory.

Class 53 comprises persons whose applications indicate that they have had renal colic, calculus or gravel. The young entrants have proved good risks: the mature and elderly entrants are below the average in vitality, after the first five years of insurance, and the old entrants are bad risks.

Somewhat similar, but much more remarkable, indications are afforded by the experience upon Class 54, where there is a history of inflammation of the bowels, peritonitis or appendicitis. The youthful entrants show an astonishingly good record; the mature entrants have been distinctly good risks; the elderly but little worse than the average, and the old decidedly worse.

An opposite tendency is indicated in Class 55, where there is a record of blood-spitting. The old entrants of this class have been good risks; the mature and elderly rather bad, and the young decidedly bad.

Persons insured who have had disease of the hip joint, Class 56, have been bad risks at all ages at entrance.

Old entrants of Class 57 and Class 58, dyspeptics, have been moderately bad risks. All other groups of dyspeptics show good results, except the young entrants of Class 58, dyspeptics of light weight.

Classes 59, 60 and 61 consist of persons of extraordinarily heavy weight, called Weight A. With the exception of the young entrants, all these classes of extra heavy risks have proved most unsatisfactory. The young entrants of Class 59, the class comprising those whose parents are noted either as living or as dying above 70 years of age, are distinctly good. The young entrants of Class 60, for whom one parent at least has been noted as dying below 70, and those of Class 61, having a greater girth of the abdomen than of the chest expanded, appear to be fair average risks. All three classes, for ages at entrance above 28, are notably bad risks, those of Class 60 being on the average about as bad as those of Class 61, contrary to the common expectation. Omitting the young entrants, Classes 60 and 61 have had a mortality slightly greater than fifty per cent. above the expectation. Taking the classes during the first five years of insurance, Class 60 shows the worse results, the contrary being the case after that period.

Classes 62, 63 and 64 are precisely similar to the three classes just mentioned, except that the weight of the individuals, though still excessive, is not so great, these risks being noted as of Weight B. The young entrants of all these classes have done well, except that after five years of insurance those of class 63, having a parent dying below 70, show unsatisfactory tendencies. The same is true of the mature entrants of Class 62, for whom there is no record of a parent dying below 70. The older entrants of this class are bad risks, though not so bad as those of Class 59. The older entrants of Class 63 are very bad risks, though not so bad respectively as those of class 60. Finally, the several groups of Class 64, having excessive abdominal girth, excluding the young entrants, are very bad risks, though not so bad respectively as the corresponding groups of Class 61.

Classes 69 and 70 consist of persons of ordinary weight, Weight C, those in 69 having had both parents dying below 60, and those in 70 having had both parent attain the age of 75. In Class 69, the two younger groups of entrants are fairly satisfactory, while the two older groups show unfavorably, the oldest the worst. On the other hand Class 70 consists of excellent risks, with the exception of one very small group, consisting of the children of aged parents. The young entrants, both of whose parents were at the time living at 75 or upwards, have had a favorable mortality experience during the first five years of insurance, but the mortality has been excessive after that period. This result may be explained by the smallness of the group or may possibly indicate some constitutional weakness.

Classes 65 to 68 consist of those cases which have been accepted, notwithstanding what has customarily been considered an unfavorable family record. They include only persons of ordinary weight. Class 65 comprises those who have had at least one parent dying below 70 of a disease distinctly stated as consumption, phthisis or tuberculosis. This class shows excellent results both before and after five years from the data of insurance. The same is true of Class 66, where at least one parent has died below 70 of some form of kidney disease, except that the elderly entrants of this classes have not done well after five years. Class 67, consisting of persons having at least one parent dying of heart disease below 70, shows well for all groups except that the elderly and old entrants of this class appear to be worse after five years. Class 68 comprises those who have had one parent at least dying below 70 of apoplexy or paralysis. The two younger groups of entrants show well, the two older groups less favorably.

Classes 71 and 72 consist of persons of positive light weight, Weight D. Class 71 includes only those of light weight who have had at least one parent dying below 70 of any kind of disease of the lungs. The young entrants of this class have been decidedly bad risks, but all the others good. Class 72, a very large class, includes all other light weight risks of every description, not already considered under Classes 58 or 71. These risks are uniformly good, for all ages at entrance, and for all durations of the insurance.

Class 73 consists of unusually tall men, those above six feet three inches in height. The younger entrants have been good risks, and the older bad.

Class 74 consists of unusually short men, those below five feet in height. These have been good risks, except that the results have been remarkably bad upon the comparatively small number of old entrants of this class.

Class 75 comprises persons who have had any near

relative die of cancer. The results are very good on young entrants, almost equally good on mature entrants, fairly good on elderly entrants, but not good on old entrants.

Class 76 comprises persons who have had any near relative develop insanity. These risks are very good, except that the elderly entrants show an excessive mortality after five years.

The remaining classes, 77 to 98, consist of persons insured in selected counties of the United States. On the whole, a gratifying change has taken place since the experience of the Thirty American Companies was collected nearly thirty years ago. In order to ascertain the amount of benefit obtained from recent improvements in hygienic science, all persons entering before the year 1890 were excluded from consideration in the present investigation. So far as appears from the materials at hand, the total deaths have been less than the number expected in the following counties: Jefferson and Phillips in Arkansas, Arapahoe in Colorado, Monroe in Florida, Chatham in Georgia, McCracken in Kentucky, Dallas and Travis in Texas. The number of deaths has been about equal to the number expected in the counties of Duval in Florida, Adams and Warren in Mississippi, New Hanover in North Carolina and Harris in Texas. Moderately bad results have appeared in the counties of Mobile in Alabama, Charleston in South Carolina, Galveston in Texas, and Norfolk in Virginia. The most unsatisfactory experience has been found in the counties of Montogomery in Alabama, Orleans in Louisiana, Santa Fe in New Mexico, Shelby in Tennessee and Bexar in Texas.

EMORY MCCLINTOCK,
B. J. MILLER,
J. G. VAN CISE,
RUFUS W. WEEKS,
D. H. WELLS,
JOHN K. GORE.

SEXUAL DIFFERENTIATION.

A DETERMINANT FACTOR OF THE FORMS OF OBESITY

By Jean Vague. Marseilles.

Experience of obesities and their treatment reveals the variety of their clinical aspects, in other words of their morphological and functional assessment and their resistance to therapy. The question then arises as to the reasons why this assessment is so variable from one subject to another. It can be advanced that investigation of obesities from the point of view of sexual differentiation could throw some light on their mechanism and consequently their treatment could be improved.

A - THE MORPHOLOGICAL AND FUNCTIONAL ASSESSMENT OF OBESE PERSONS

The classical divisions into endogenous and exogenous obesities, those with endocrine origin and those due to overfeeding and insufficient movement do not provide a key to the problem. Among the most long standing conceptions only the separation into plethoric and anemic obesities envisages the question from the fruitful metabolic standpoint. The essential fact of obesity is the predominance of anabolism over catabolism whatever the absolute value of these latter may be - increased, normal or decreased in comparison with mean values. This predominance of anabolism concerns above all fat and circulating and interstitial humours. However it may also - according to circumstances - attain the muscle tissue and the various metabolisms. Howbeit the nutritive disturbances show up - in totality - on the biotype in its three aspects: morphological, physiological and psychological.

Habitually we establish an assessment - as complete as possible - of these three closely linked aspects of obese subjects. A predominant part is attributed to topography of excess fat and muscular development.

Two groups of measurements in selected points - chosen after many experiments - provided us with practical diagram of fat distribution and relative development of fat and muscle.

There are:

a) Caliper measurement of skinfold thickness of the nape at the atlas level and that of the lower part of the retro-sacral area, while the subject standing;

b) Measurement of the perimeter of the limbs at their base, with the limb extended and in lying position, and that of the skinfold on the same perimeter at the 4 cardinal points, in front, behind, and on the 2 sides.

The ratio of N^2/S^2 between the skinfold of the nape of the neck and the sacral skinfold, both squared, provides a precise measurement of the relative development of fat in these 2 regions.

After measurement of the perimeter and thickness of the cell tissue at the base of the limbs - on alive persons and on corpses - it can be stated that the section of the limb at this level is more or less circular and that the unequal distribution of fat at the 4 cardinal points is also more or less equalized by the mean of its measurement in these 4 points. Consequently an approximate calculation of the surface occupied by fat and muscle on the limb section can then easily be made. Our measurements revealed that the surface occupied by the bony, vasculonervous and interstitial tissues amounted to approximately 1/10 of the total surface decreased by that of the peripheral fat, and that the deep, muscular and interstitial fat increased the surface of the paniculus adiposis section by about 1/5.

Where r is the radius of the limb section, r' the radius of this same section decreased by the thickness of the adipose tissue, that is to say half the skinfold, F the surface of the superficial and deep fat section, M the

Vague J. La différenciation sexuelle facteur déterminant des formes de l'obésité. *Presse Medicale.* 1947;55:339-340.

surface of the muscle tissue section, F' and M' these same surfaces corrected with regard to height H, mean height being 170 cm in men and 160 cm in women, we obtain:

a) $$F = \pi r^2 - \pi (r')^2 + \frac{\pi r^2 - \pi (r')^2}{5}$$

$$M = \pi r'^2 - \frac{\pi r^2 - \pi (r')^2}{5} - \frac{\pi (r')^2}{10}$$

where π can be suppressed in the calculation of the ratios only, and

$$F' = \left(r^2 - r'^2 + \frac{r^2 - r'^2}{5}\right) \quad \frac{170^2 \text{ or } 160^2}{H^2}$$

$$M' = \left(r'^2 - \left(\frac{r^2 - r'^2}{5}\right) - \frac{r'^2}{10}\right) \quad \frac{170^2 \text{ or } 160^2}{H^2}$$

b) $\frac{F}{M} = \frac{F'}{M'}$ = the adipomuscular ratio, AMR, which is thus obtained for the 2 limbs.

c) The relation of the brachial AMR to the femoral AMR provides the brachiofemoral adipomuscular ratio, BFAMR, an index on the limbs, like the nucho-sacral ratio on the trunk, of distribution of fat with regard to height;

d) Finally, the mean of these 2 values

$$\frac{BFAMR + \frac{N^2}{S^2}}{2}$$

gives us the fat distribution index, FDI.

The systematic study of obesities according to this method has induced us to oppose:

1°Obesities which prevail on the upper half of the body, and which are hypersthenic, hypermetabolic, hyperemic and orthohydropexic; the fat overload there is accompanied by muscular hypertrophy generally linked to a robust skeleton. The predominance of the aqueous anabolism concerns the blood much more than it does the interstitial plasma. Vital prognosis is above all linked to the circulatory consequences of the plethora: red hypertension, premature atherosclerosis, cardiorenal and cerebral failure etc. Red hypertension is indeed a usual manifestation, precocious and parallel to the extent of fat overload. Hyperglycemia and diabetes are frequent and then also follow the development of adipose hypertrophy. The very small role of hydropexia of interstitial tissue and the absence or weak extent of cellulitis renders the dietetic treatment efficient and therapeutic action on the panniculus adiposis unnecessary.

2°Obesities which are predominant on the lower half of the body and which are orthosthenic or hyposthenic, orthometabolic or hypometabolic, orthohemic or hypohemic and hyperhydropexic. The circulatory system there is secure from plethora as aqueous hyperanabolism is not effected towards the circulating blood but towards the interstitial plasma. Hypertension there is rare, contingent, independent of the degree of obesity and then identical - in its determination and evolution - to the pale hypertension of thin persons and subjects of normal weight. Glycoregulation disturbances are also rare and independent of the fat overload. Complications are directly linked to this latter and to its mechanical consequences. Due to considerable hydropexia and cellulitis dieting is often illusory, treatment is difficult and local actions on adipose tissue are advisable.

3°Between these two extreme varieties there are mixed ones, where the degree of orientation in either direction can be measured.

B - FAT TOPOGRAPHY AND SEXUAL DIFFERENTIATION

It seemed to us that these relations between muscular development, excess or insufficiency of metabolism, the direction of hydric anabolism - towards the blood or the interstitial plasma - and fat topography, were constant. Now it is well known to all that subcutaneous fat distribution is one of the main morphological features of sexual differentiation. The relative independence of each of these features in relation to each other is, indeed, equally classical. However our study of the FDI - both in normal subjects of different ages and in patients of all types - showed that fat topography was without doubt one of the most faithful signs - not to say the most - of total sexual differentiation, as if the various elements of this latter were all more or less reflected there. Moreover this is the opinion of Maranon and Pende. Measurement of the FDI provides this topology with a mathematical value applicable to all cases; and systematic comparison with the other sexual, morphological and functional features has shown - with perfect regularity - that any elevation of this index corresponded to a stressing of all android features and any lowering a decrease of these features and an exaggeration of the gynoid features.

As the FDI therefore seems; firstly, to translate regularly the sexual differentiation and secondly to evolve concurrently - in the relative hyperanabolism of obesity - with muscular development, intensity of metabolic assessment and blood plethora, we believe that we are entitled to apply - in both sexes - the epithet android to obesities of the first groups and the qualificative gynoid to those of the second group.

Using the mean value of the FDI adult obesities can then be classed as follows:

The extreme forms in both sexes notably include grave tumorous obesities, Cushing type syndromes

	HYPER-ANDROID	0 ANDROID	MIXED	GYNOID	HYPER-GYNOID
In men :					
FDI...	> 3	2 to 3	1 to 2	0.70 to 1	< 0.70
In women :					
FDI	> 1	0.81 to 1	0.61 to 0.80	0.40 to 0.60	< .40

through tumour of the androgen apparatus and obesities of Babinski-Froelich type whose androgen insufficiency and gynoid features are grossly evident.

Apart from the symptoms and evolution already known, android obesity in men is generally associated with considerable genital capacity. In women it is above all observed during the menopause, where Maranon was the first to isolate it under the name of plethoric adiposis of the female climateric and to mention its relations with climateric virilization. Women who show this type of obesity and whose android orientation is constitutional are frequently characterized, from the genital point of view, by their tendency towards the syndrome known as hyperfolliculinemia, a virile active type of libido and orgasm and weak maternal sense.

Whereas android obesity of women only exceptionally coincides - before the natural or artificial menopause - with distinct, ovarian insufficiency, gynoid obesity can be associated with all degrees of ovarian functioning. This phenomenon is partly explained by female homozygous sex of the human species, as of all mammals; the male - heterozygous - sex being more labile. It is for this reason that castration always decreases masculine differentiation, in the same way that it accentuates the primary tendency of the metabolism. This can lead to leanness; more frequently to obesity and - always according to the constitutional predisposition of the woman - to an android or gynoid state.

Infantile and prepubertal obesity is more often gynoid and is then always accompanied by sexual retardation in boys and various pubertal disturbances in girls. On the other hand precocious puberty in both sexes - grave and tumorous or benign and functional - is always correlative, this has indeed been emphasized by Maranon, with an android state and most often with an obesity of this type.

C - ETIOLOGICAL RELATIONS OF SEXUAL DIFFERENTIATION AND OBESITY

It seems to be beyond debate that sexual differentiation imposed on obesities all their morphological and functional features apart from their intensity and certain contingent complications. The etiological relations which unite these two phenomena of sexual orientation and relative hyperanabolism remain to be defined. From this point of view, the sexological and metabolical study of normal or abnormal subjects reveals two groups of facts:

1°There is no constant relation between sexual differentiation and metabolism - all types of combinations can be observed between the normal and pathological aspects of these two phenomena. For example castration - in both men and women - can increase body weight, decrease it, or maintain it at its initial figure, according to the previous orientation of the metabolism

2°However this independence is tempered by the two following relations:

a) Although suppression of the genital apparatus may not affect weight or even determine leanness, it more often leads to obesity.

b) A certain number of endocrine affections and foremost of which the two lesional types of android and gynoid obesities. Cushing and Babinski-Froelich type syndromes, but also multiple, functional and benign alterations, determine both obesity and genital disturbances.

We believe that it can be concluded from these data that:

1°Connected with an alteration, most often genetic and increased by occasional factors of the diencephalo-pituitary region, the predominance of anabolism over catabolism - which constitutes obesity - is determined in its form and not in its initiation by the previous sexual differentiation and that of the moment. In other words relative hyperanabolism and sexual differentiation combine to produce an android, gynoid or mixed obesity.

2°The independence and probable proximity of the "centres" which are responsible for the greater part of the sexual differentiation, and of those which assume control of the metabolism, accounts for the possibility that they be injured separately and also the frequency of their common injury.

REFERENCES

The details of our investigations are to be found in three personal articles:

Les obésités: Etude biométrique: Biologie Médicale. January 1947. Le traitement des obésités: Marseille Médical. May 15th 1946. Diagnostic étiologique des obésités: Marseille Médical. January 1st 1947 and in the thesis of our pupils J. BRIAN, G. FAVIER, R. POUGAUD, S. MAIGROT, P. ROMAIN, H. CONILH, J. RASCLE: MARSEILLE, 1944-45, 1946-47.

The Degree of Masculine Differentiation of Obesities:

A Factor Determining Predisposition to Diabetes, Atherosclerosis, Gout, and Uric Calculous Disease

By Jean Vague, M.D.*

From the standpoint of their frequency, as well as from that of their chemical and especially hormonal mechanisms, the complications of obesity are much better known to us today than they were just a few years ago. All are agreed in recognizing the frequency of diabetes, atherosclerosis, gout, uric calculous disease, disturbances due to circulatory changes, emphysema, sudden cardiac collapse, and premature aging due to corpulence. On the other hand, the hormonal mechanisms of lipid metabolism are only gradually becoming clearer, although the origin of the lipid hyperanabolism itself remains to be discovered.

If, instead of considering excess adiposity as an isolated and always identical phenomenon, varying only in intensity, one investigates the frequency of its complications according to its chief clinical characteristics, one is immediately confronted with invaluable etiologic relationships.

Experience proves, in fact, that what is important in the evolution of obesities is not so much excess adiposity per se but the activity of this excess, which is dependent on the subjacent musculature and blood supply, controlled, in turn, by neurohormonal mechanisms.

Although the means of evaluating these phenomena are available, their utilization on a large scale is still somewhat impractical. Therefore, for the past ten years, we have preferred to utilize an anthropometric method which is simple to carry out and which gives numerical values that are easily handled.

One aspect of excess adiposity which immediately attracts the clinician's attention is the distribution of subcutaneous fat in the upper portion of the body of hypersthenic obese persons, but in the lower portion of the body in others.

In studying the distribution of subcutaneous fat tissue in healthy individuals, one notices considerable differences between the male and female by simply pinching the fat masses with calipers. This fat is thicker in the female all over the body except over the first three cervical vertebrae. At normal weight, the fat of the male all over the body is less than that of the female; and it is thicker in the upper portion of the body than in the lower portion. The reverse is true in the female, infant, and the adolescent. Therefore, it seemed useful to obtain a numerical value for this localization of fat.

UTILITY AND MEASUREMENT OF THE INDEX OF MASCULINE DIFFERENTIATION

Several studies along these lines have precede ours. The measurements of Neumann,[41] Batkin,[2] Peiser,[45] Hille,[16] Kading,[23] Oeder,[42] in Germany; of Richer[50] in France; of Pende[46] and Oppenhein[43] in Italy; of Tchoutchoukalo[59] and of Bounak[6] in the U.S.S.R; and the recent radiographic measurements of Reynolds and Grote,[48] Stuart, Hill, Shaw and Swinell,[56 57] and Wilmer[62] in the United States have contributed to the tracing of the thickness of fatty tissue on the surface of the body. More recently, Edwards,[11] in London, has resumed this topographic investigation, simultaneously with ourselves. A systematic study of the thickness of fat as measured by calipers in the various regions of the

Vague J. The degree of masculine differentiation of obesities: A factor determining predisposition to diabetes, atherosclerosis, gout, and uric calculous disease. *Am J Clin Nutr.* 1956;4:20-34.

Editor's Note: Only certain figures have been included in this reproduction.

*Professor, Faculty of Medicine of Marseille; Physician to the Hospitals; 19, Rue Fontange, Marseille, France.

body has led us to select certain sites which are particularly suggestive.[61]

Two groups of sites have thus been selected: (1) the nape of the neck, and the sacrum; (2) the four proximal attachments of the limbs. At these ten points, the fatty mass is pinched in such a way that it is completely mobilized in the aponeurosis without being compressed; thus it is possible to measure its double thickness, plus the negligible thickness of the skin. We believe it is preferable not to use a measured, uniform pressure, as several authors have done, for in order to obtain a fold corresponding as exactly as possible to a double thickness, the pressure must be varied according to the consistency of the fatty tissue and the elasticity of the skin, both variable from one area to another. For this reason, in subjects who have recently lost weight, the minimum of pressure should be exerted in detaching the fatty tissue from the deep layer, and the thickness measured is apt to be less than it actually is. If, however, the fatty tissue is taut, hard, and only slightly movable, strong pressure must be exerted in order to avoid obtaining too high a figure. With a little practice, the hand easily and immediately judges the degree of tension of the fatty tissue and so regulates the pressure which must be brought to bear on the calipers. With the exception of a few rather unusual cases and the presence of scars or deep spontaneous adhesions, this method is not difficult.

(1) Fat on the Trunk

The region situated between the first three cervical vertebrae and particularly over the atlas, is the only site where, at equal weights, fat is normally more abundant in the male than in the female. Conversely, the contrast between the thickness of the fat in the female and its thinness in men is most marked in the retrosacral region.

Consequently, the relationship of *the thickness of the fold of the nape of the neck to that of the sacral fold is much greater than unity in the normal male, but much less in the female.*

The development of the underlying muscles has only a negligible influence on the importance of these fatty localizations. On the other hand, variations in weight considerably modify their relationship. As weight increases the relationship of the thickness of fat on the nape of the neck to the fat of the sacral region decreases. A study of this ratio during the course of weight gain and loss has permitted us to trace the very regular curve of its variations and to formulate the normal nape-to-sacrum ratio in the adult man as a function of the thickness of the adipose tissue in these two regions.

(2) Fat on the Limbs

In marked contrast, variations in weight do not noticeably modify the relationship of the thickness of the fat on the arm to that of the thigh, measured at the four main points of their proximal attachment. The concomitant measurement of the perimeter of the arms or legs at the same level enables one to estimate the fatty area on a particular section of the arm or leg. Sections from cadavers demonstrate that the fat in interstitial muscle is equivalent to one-fifth of the subcutaneous fatty tissue, and that the area occupied by the osseous, vascular and connective tissues varies slightly, measuring about one-tenth of the total area, minus the surface of the peripheral fat.

This relationship of the fatty area to the muscle area is the *adipo-muscular ratio; it is higher on the arm than on the thigh in the normal adult man, while the inverse is true in the female. We may say that the brachio-femoral adipo-muscular ratio is above unity in men, below unity in women.*

The average of the nape: sacrum ratio (corrected in terms of the total thickness of the fat in the two regions) and the brachio-femoral adipo-muscular ratio gives an index of masculine differentiation (IMD). Calculated according to the method used for determination of basal metabolism, this gives a value of "0" for the male and "-60" for the female, for subjects between 30 and 50 years of age; according to age groups, the average quadratic deviation ranges from 13 to 17, and approximates 15.

It is thus possible to establish five delimited groups with about $+1\sigma$ as their average. All subjects of either sex fall into one of these groups (Table I).

To understand and utilize this index, one must have a knowledge of its average evolution with age and its distribution at each age in both sexes. Our study has revealed the following facts (Figs. 1 and 2):

(1) From the age of 5 years, the IMD curve is con-

TABLE I

Classification of Masculine Differentiation on the Basis of the IMD Scale (see text)

IMD scale	Group
>+15 +15	hyperandroid
0	android
-15 -45	intermediate
60	gynoid
-75 <-75	hypergynoid

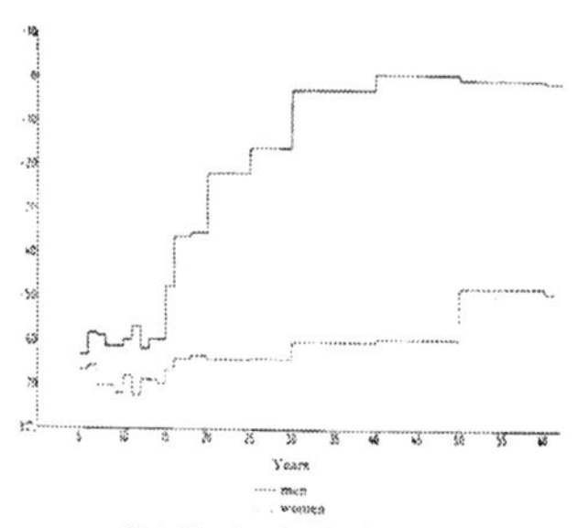

Fig. 1 Index of masculine differentiation (IMD)

(1) The IMD curve is always higher in men than in women, from the age of 5 years on.

(2) This minimal difference, which is more or less the same up to age 15, is then suddenly accentuated. The IMD rises markedly and progressively in men, reaching its maximum at 40 to 50 years of age and diminishing very slightly thereafter.

In women, it rises very slowly up to 50 years of age, at which time it climbs about 12 per cent (to the IMD level of a 15-year-old boy), and then reaches its maximum, descending only 5 per cent afterwards.

Index on the ordinate. Age on the abscissa

stantly higher in the male than in the female.

(2) Up to the age of 15 years, the IMD is very low, about -60 in boys, -70 in girls.

(3) At about 15 years, the difference between the two sexes is suddenly accentuated, the IMD rising to -47 in boys. It will reach -36 in the male at 16 years, -22 at 20 years, -16 at 25 years, -2 at 30 years, and 0 at 40 years, where it is subsequently maintained; however, in the female, the figure of -60 at 15 years of age remains unchanged up to 50 years, at which age the IMD will reach -47, identical to that of a boy of 15 years.

(4) A number of facts emerge from the study of the overlapping of the degrees of masculine differentiation measured by fat distribution in both sexes at successive ages. We may note three principal facts:

(a) The proportion of males whose differentiation is that of the normal or hypergynoid woman (about -60) reaches 44 per cent at 18 years of age, then falls to 15 per cent at 20 years, and 7 per cent-the minimum figure-between 30 and 50 years.

(b) The percentage of android and hyperandroid females (by our classification) reaches only 6 per cent between 40 and 50 years of age and never exceeds 12 per cent at its highest level, after 50 years.

(c) The intermediate degree of masculine differentiation, which includes 51 per cent of males at 20 years of age, and 23 per cent at 50 years, is only seen in 12 per cent of females from 20 to 40 years of age, but in 34 per cent after the fiftieth year.

These figures thus illustrate a double concept: fat distribution is very definitely a sexual characteristic, but there is a high percentage of overlapping between one sex and the other, especially at the two extremes of life.

These measurements applied to the study of excess adiposity, and particularly its complications, provide us with the means of objectively distinguishing two extreme types of obesity, and of exactly locating the intermediate forms in relation to them.

The obesities which we have called *gynoid* and *hypergynoid* (Figs. 3 and 4) are characterized by the elective localization of fat on the lower part of the body, the poor development of musculature, reduced activity and function of the arterial circulation, the basal metabolism being usually normal but the luxus consumption retarded,* a usually moderate appetite and digestive capacity, a tendency to water retention and venous circulatory insufficiency. Obesity of this hyposthenic, anemic, hypometabolic, hyperhydropexic type is more frequent in women and may become more acute at each phase of the reproductive life. It is also seen in children of both sexes, and is not rare in the adult male, in whom it is always accompanied by other signs which reveal inadequate masculine differentiation. It can become quite serious, and by the immobility to which it condemns the patient it creates a vicious pathogenic circle which contributes to its aggravation. The heart, surrounded and infiltrated with fat, may suddenly collapse, for example, in the course of an infectious disease, generally without any signs of arterial involvement having been evidences.

The *android* and *hyperandroid* obesities (Figs. 5 and 6) are the opposite of the preceding types, with elective localization of fat on the upper part of the body, great development of the musculature and arterial circulation both in strength and activity with a tendency to hypertension, plethora, and hyperalbuminemia,[8] a strong appetite and digestive capacity, a normal basal metabolism and an increased luxus consumption, less hydropexy of the cellular tissues that in gynoid obesity and a usually normal venous circulation. Obesity of this hypersthenic, hyperemic, hypermetabolic type is more frequent in the male, but is also seen in the female, particularly at the menopausal age, where it is always accompanied by other elements of virilization, especially in the sphere of behavior. The woman afflicted with android obesity often gives birth to large infants, successive children sometimes being larger and larger. This phenomenon must alert one to the ultimate appearance of diabetes, as has been demonstrated by Miller,[37-39] Kriss,[27] Gilbert,[12] and Hoet.[17] We have shown that this does not occur in gynoid-obese women. Jackson[18] has likewise revealed that pre-diabetes, associated with android obesity of the father, can be the cause of excessive neonatal weight, which indicates a hereditary factor

*The theory of "Luxus Konsumption" (Grafe) states that there is an increase in metabolism when a normal person ingests excess food. In this way body weight tends to remain constant. The "constitutionally" obese person was thought to lack this homeostatic mechanism and to have no means of disposing of excess food. Proof of the validity of this concept is still lacking.-ED.

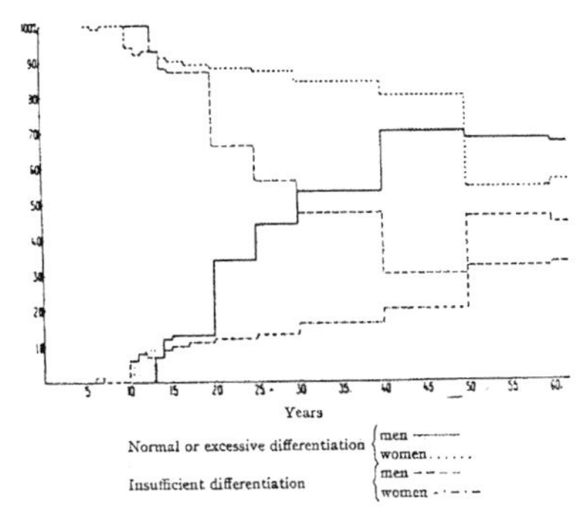

Fig. 2. Percentage of normal or excessive differentiation, on the one hand, and of insufficient differentiation, on the other, in both sexes, according to age.
Normal differentiation: IMD between +1 and −1σ about the average:
for men: $<+15>-15$
for women: $<-45>-75$
Excessive differentiation: deviation from the IMD $>1\sigma$ in the direction of the deviation:
for men: $>+15$
for women: <-75
Insufficient differentiation: deviation from the IMD $>1\sigma$ in the opposite direction to that of the differentiation:
for men: <-15
for women: >-45
Percentage on the ordinate. Age on the abscissa.

predisposing to macrosomia and to diabetes.

Patients with android obesity may attain considerable weights, but they do not develop the monstrous appearance sometimes seen in gynoid obesity. The development of android obesity almost always carries with it a tendency to vascular accidents proportional to the degree of masculine differentiation and to the degree of obesity. There is also frequently a tendency to diabetes. Treatment by weight reduction may ward off these complications for a long time, or may even combat them.

Opposite to each other in their extreme types, the android and gynoid obesities are connected by intermediate forms. The measurement of fat distribution by the IDM method has always indicated to us the exact position of these forms in our classification and, in addition, has provided prognostic data.

When one is not making a statistical study, this somewhat lengthy measurement of the IMD can by avoided. A satisfactory indication for ordinary purposes may be obtained merely by estimating between thumb and fingers the thickness of the fat over the trochanter, and over the deltoid. The latter is greater than half the retrochanteric fat in normal men, but is definitely less than half the retrochanteric fat in normal women.

THE RELATIONSHIP BETWEEN ANDROID OBESITY AND DIABETES

The influence of the degree of masculine differentiation of obesity and its complications is particularly clear for diabetes. All the statistics, of which the most important are those of Joslin *et al.*,[20] are in accord in recognizing that infantile and juvenile diabetes does not seem to be under the influence of excessive adiposity, but that beginning with the twentieth year, even more from the thirtieth on, and especially after the fortieth, diabetes occurs most often among obese persons: it was found in 70 per cent of those between 20 and 30 years of age, and in from 80 to 90 per cent afterwards. It is quite evident, as the recent experience of the last war has clearly shown, that weight reduction almost always improves, and often "cures," diabetes in the adult.

The frequency of diabetes in the population as a whole according to Boulin,[5] and also Joslin,[20] is about one per cent. It is more difficult to establish the frequency of diabetes among the obese. The available figures range between 3 and 12 per cent. Our last survey (600 cases) gives us, for hyperandroid, android, intermediate, gynoid, and hypergynoid obesities after 20 years of age, percentages of diabetes of 60, 33, 4, 0, and 0, respectively, in the male; 35, 25, 7, 2, and 1 in the female. These statistics are valueless as far as the absolute figures are concerned; they are certainly too high, since many patients who consulted us especially for their diabetes we should never have seen for their obesity alone. But it is clearly demonstrated that gynoid and hypergynoid obesity in no way represent a predisposition to diabetes, for its incidence is no greater in these groups than in the general population, while its frequency in obesity increases in proportion to the degree of masculine differentiation.

There is no doubt, therefore, that if obesity is at the origin of four-fifths of the cases of adult diabetes, it is through the obligatory mediation of a pronounced masculine differentiation. Thus the calculation from the opposite standpoint-that of the masculine differentiation of diabetics-becomes necessary, in order to establish the place occupied by this differentiation in the origin of diabetes as a whole. The figures show not only that diabetes does not occur in obesity except when it is associated with a pronounced masculine differentiation, but also that the majority of cases of adult diabetes occur when these two conditions are realized, that is, in obesity of a more or less android type, in women as well as in men.

Just as thinness is generally associated with a slightly lower masculine differentiation, the majority of obese persons have, in both sexes, a higher masculine differentiation than normal subjects. There is, in other words, a general android tendency in obese persons of both sexes; this tendency is more pronounced than that in subjects of normal weight, which, in turn, is greater than that in thin people. Adjusting for age, we can estimate the average IMD in diabetics, in the obese as a whole, and in subjects of normal weight. We ascertained then that the three masculine curves are higher than the feminine curves, but that in each sex the diabetic curve in the adult is by far the highest; it is definitely above the curve of the obese, which is itself higher than that of subjects of normal weight (except for men between 20 and 40 years of age, where a considerable number of gynoid-obese subjects lowers the average masculine differentiation of the obese total). Thus the average IMD after 50 years of age for diabetic men is +40 instead of +15 in obese men as a whole, or 0 in men of normal weight. At the same age, it is -15 in diabetic women, instead of -38 in obese women as a whole and -47 in women of normal weight (Fig. 7).

If, therefore, diabetes in the infant and adolescent escapes the influence of weight and masculine differentiation, adult diabetes, especially after 40 years of age, develops in 80 to 90 per cent of the cases in the presence of an obesity in which the degree of masculine differentiation is far higher than average, for each sex and age.

The glucose tolerance test studies the sensitivity of the gluco-regulatory function. Labbe[28] and Boulin[5] thirty years ago pointed out the frequency of induced "paradiabetic" hyperglycemia in obese subjects. Resuming this study with Benoit, in terms of the IMD, we have confirmed that hyperglycemia (after glucose ingestion) is not high in obese subjects unless the masculine differentiation is equally pronounced. It was also confirmed that gynoid obesity is no more conducive to prandial hyperglycemia that to diabetes.

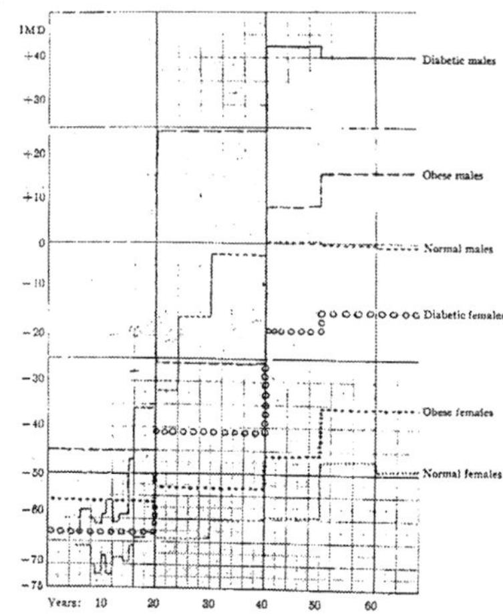

Fig. 7. Averages of the index of masculine differentiation in terms of age in diabetic, obese, and normal subjects.

RELATIONSHIP OF ANDROID OBESITY TO GOUT AND URINARY AND BILIARY CALCULOUS DISEASE

Renal and biliary lithiasis and gout are generally favored by excessive adiposity. But her again, it is proper to make distinctions according to the type of this excess. All our gouty subjects, without exception, are obese, with an average IMD of +16 for men, and of -20 for women, which is definitely higher than normal. The same holds for uric acid calculus (an IMD of +15 in men). Contrariwise, the average weight and IMD of our patients with phosphatic and oxalic calculi do not deviate from the normal. These two forms of renal lithiasis do no appear to be influenced either by weight or by masculine differentiation.

The case of biliary calculus is more complex:

(1) The majority of women with painful-or at least annoying-calculi are, on the average, obese. This fact is in agreement with the improvement of a large number of cases of biliary calculus by spontaneous or forces weight loss.

(2) This obesity assumes all degrees of masculine differentiation, with a slight predilection for increased differentiation. The frequency of intermediate or android obesity in case of biliary calculus is especially noted in lithiasis with large cholesterol calculi.

(3) In the male, the influence of weight on biliary calculus is less important than in the female, and the influence of the degree of masculine differentiation is almost nil.

We can, therefore, conclude that biliary calculus is extremely common in the female, since certain statistics indicate its presence in 25 per cent of women after 50 years of age, and is, if not more frequent, at least more often manifest, in obese women, with a slight predilection for the android-obese woman. The clinically android-obese woman is generally hypertensive, arteriosclerotic, frequently diabetic, and with one or sever large calculi of cholesterol in her gallbladder. In all cases, whatever the degree of masculine differentiation, weight loss facilitates tolerance of the calculi.

RELATIONSHIP BETWEEN ANDROID OBESITY AND ATHEROSCLEROSIS

In this area, too, statistics agree in recognizing the greater frequency of hypertension and atherosclerosis with its various localizations in obese persons, considered as a whole. But the same distinction must be made as for diabetes and precipitating diseases. The results of our investigations with Jouve,[22,60] show that atherosclerosis is even more influenced by the degree of masculine differentiation than by excessive weight. The mean IMD of patients with coronary artery disease is higher by an average of 15 per cent in the male, and 22 to 45 per cent, depending on age, in the female.

With Favier we have noted in hyperandroid, android, intermediate, gynoid, and hypergynoid obese subjects over 40 years of age, respective percentages of coronary artery disease of 100, 42.1, 9.5, 4.7, and 0 in men; 100, 100, 50, 10.6, and 1.7 in women.

The implications of these facts seem to us to be very clear. Gynoid obesity leads to direct mechanical complication: trophic disturbances of the venous-lymphatic circulation, respiratory difficulty, and rapid circulatory decompensation in banal circumstances such as a bronchopulmonary infection; but this form of obesity does not exercise any influence on the metabolic disorders, such as diabetes, gout, uric calculous disease, and atherosclerosis. On the other hand, the development of the latter four conditions is very strongly favored by android obesity, especially when weight and the index of masculine differentiation are very high.

MECHANISM BY WHICH ANDROID OBESITY GIVES RISE TO COMPLICATIONS

In contrast to gynoid obesity, all the anatomical characteristics of android obesity-that is, the predominance of fat deposits over the upper portion of the body, the great muscle-blood development, the biologic characteristics, the activity of its metabolism and consequently the rapid lipolysis and liposynthesis-are observed facts which are easy to check.

The hormonal causes of these phenomena are more obscure and hypothetical. Nevertheless, more suggestive that the measurement of urinary steroids, the excretion of which is not significantly abnormal in ordinary diabetes or in atherosclerosis, the example of severe cases of basophilic hyperplasia of the pituitary and of the adrenal cortex strongly warrants the supposition that this type of obesity is related to an absolute or relative overactivity of the pituitary-adrenal axis, with growth hormone, corticotropin (ACTH), cortical steroids, and epinephrine being either secreted in greater abundance or merely exerting a stronger action than in the average individual.

Furthermore, this concept accounts for a great many of the complications which are exclusively characteristic of android obesity and from which gynoid obesity is free,

A. Eight- to nine-tenths of cases of adult diabetes are of the android-obese type. In the light of these facts, the causes of diabetes may be conceived today in the following manner:

(1) In the child and the adolescent, we are almost entirely ignorant of the causes of the disease, other than genetic predispositions.

(2) In the adult, these genetic predispositions are also clear. On these are superimposed etiologic factors favoring or triggering diabetes.

(a) In the first group of cases, weight and masculine differentiation are without effect. These include:

(i) Visceral and especially pancreatic hemochromatosis, a genetic disease which is perhaps more frequently involved in the origin of diabetes than is classically supposed.

(ii) Acquired pancreatic lesions: pancreatitis, lithiasis, etc.

(iii) Certain cases in which, as in the young person, no factor other than heredity is demonstrated.

(b) Eight- to nine-tenths of cases of diabetes after 20 years of age, and especially after the thirtieth year, are the consequence of android obesity. The terms "fat diabetes" of Lancereaux,[29] "lipiplethoric diabetes" of Lawrence,[30] "diabetes through adipose obstruction" of Darnaud,[9,10] recall this idea.[31] But, as we have demonstrated since 1945, and as the work of Maranon[35] on climacteric adiposity, and of Pavel and Anghelesco[44] on the hyperpituitary constitution had enabled us to foresee, only android obesity is involved here.

So it is that Lawrence,[30] discussing the origin of lipoplethoreic diabetes, invokes the inability of the excess adipose tissue to facilitate liposynthesis at the expense of glucose, which would thus remain in circulation. But then why does not gynoid obesity, which is often much more serious than android obesity, have the same effect?

According to Sherlock, Bearn and Billings,[53] the fatty infiltration of the liver which is frequent in the obese diabetic inhibits the action of insulin, the more so as the diabetic is fatter. But neither does this hypothesis explain why gynoid obesity has no effect here.

Several recent ideas may perhaps supply this explanation. Insulin is indispensable to liposynthesis from carbohydrates.[7,54,55] It is equally necessary for protein synthesis by growth hormone.[4,34,40] The initial effect of this latter substance is to increase insulin secretion[4,49,36,19] and later to exhaust it,[63] while it augments that of glucagon and, together with the glucocorticoids, perhaps opposes the action of insulin on hexokinase.

The metapituitary diabetes of Young[63] seems then to involve a first phase in which insulin secretion is increased, favoring liposynthesis, and a second phase of pancreatic depletion. Long[3] believes that obesity leads to diabetes by thus exhausting the insulin available for liposynthesis. This is the hypothesis which is most in harmony with experimental facts and clinical data.

Pituitary-adrenal overactivity, responsible for the increase in appetite, digestive capacity, and protein and lipid synthesis, as well as for an accelerated metabolism with marked gluconeogenesis (perhaps at the expense of lipids as well as proteins, in any case certainly with a pronounced lipolysis[25,51]) leads at first to uncomplicated android obesity. The enhanced utilization of insulin by liposynthesis which rapidly replaces lipolysis, the anti-insulin effect of most of the pituitary and adrenal hormones, and perhaps the secretion of glucagon and the glycogenolytic action of ephinephrine, explain how diabetes is evolved if the least genetic fragility of the islets exists. However, gynoid obesity, in which the circulation of lipids is effected more slowly, does not result in the same disorders.

The fact that diabetes does not occur on an average in more than a third of android-obese individuals allows us to suppose that two genes or groups of genes, at least, are involved in ordinary diabetes, one of constitutional pituituary-adrenal overactivity, and one of fragility of the islets.

B. The rather more obscure mechanism of the effects of android obesity on gout and on uric calculous disease seems to be of the same order. In these genetic disturbances of purine metabolism, doubled in the case of gout by an equally hereditary tendency to allergic symptoms, pituitary-adrenal overactivity, acting on a large protein-lipid capital, is perhaps the cause of the hyperuricemia and its critical manifestations. The break-up of an attack of gout and of urate calculous precipitations by corticotropin, cortisone, and various other agents, and the transient pituitary exhaustion which results therefrom, argues in favor of this thesis without, however, proving it.

The relationship of excessive obesity, especially of the android type in women, to biliary cholesterol calculus is more obscure. Perhaps the activity of lipid metabolism plays a role here.

C. The definite clinical relationships between atherosclerosis and android obesity also pose a complex pathogenic problem. Let us note, however, that in contrast to the gynoid-obese individual, who has a tendency to immobilize his too heavy body, the android-obese individual is driven by his temperament to ceaselessly move around the extra burden of his excess weight, thus exerting an excessive strain on his circulatory system-a cause of premature wear and tear. Let us add that epinephrine,[21,32] desoxycorticosterone,[52] and anterior pituitary extract[52] have an arteriosclerogenic action, and that the movement of lipids from fatty tissue toward the liver through the action of growth hormone, glucocorticoids, desoxycorticosterone, and epinephrine, induces the passage into the blood of large lipoprotein molecules[13-15] and their precipitation in the arterial endothelium, if phosphorylation is inadequate. A whole series of facts thus accounts for the mechanism (which is undoubtedly even more complex and in which the kidney plays an important part) by which android obesity leads to atherosclerosis, whereas the gynoid-obese person will generally die without his arteries undergoing premature aging.

The common mechanism of atherosclerosis and diabetes explains for the most part the frequency and the peculiarities of their association. The inconstancy of diabetes in the course of atherosclerosis when the islets of Langerhans offer a sufficient genetic resistance to the overwork imposed by pituitary-adrenal overactivity, in contrast to the constancy of atherosclerosis in adult diabetes and its relative independence of the degree of hyperglycemia, cease to surprise us if we regard arterial lesions and diabetes as the consequences of an identical cause acting against a background which may suffer from a genetic fragility of the islets or be free from it. It goes without saying that all these concepts of pathogenesis must be entertained with the greatest prudence. Let us agree, nevertheless, that the clinical data and experimental findings are strangely coincident, and that pituitary-adrenal overactivity seems to be the most probable mechanism in android obesity and its complications.

In clinical practice, the estimation of the degree of masculine differentiation of an obese individual remains indisputably the means of predicting, and thus, it is hoped, of preventing, the complications with which he is threatened.

SUMMARY

The obesities are distinguished from each other essentially by the degree of protein anabolism, that is, muscle-blood anabolism, which is associated with adipose hyperanabolism. Anthropometry demonstrates that the degree of this muscle-blood anabolism is greater in proportion to the predominance of fat over the upper part of the body, a characteristic linked to others which indicate the degree of masculine differentiation in both sexes. The calculation of an index of masculine differentiation (which is described) enables one to distinguish android and gynoid obesities and their intermediate forms.

Gynoid obesity, with lower body predominance, with poor muscle-blood development, is menaced only by direct mechanical complications of excessive adiposity: locomotor difficulty, abdominal pressure, limitation of respiratory motion, slowing of the venous and lymphatic circulation, cellulitis, lowering of energy, and reduction of the elasticity of the fat-infiltrated myocardium-complications which are all proportional to the degree of excess fat.

Android obesity, with upper body predominance and pronounced muscle-blood development, leads to metabolic disturbances. It not only is associated with premature atherosclerosis and diabetes, but it is also the usual cause of diabetes in the adult in 80 to 90 per cent of the cases. Gout and uric calculous disease generally appear in this form of obesity.

Overactivity of the pituitary-adrenal axis appears to be the most probable cause both of android obesity and its complications.

BIBLIOGRAPHY

1. Barret, H. M., Best, C. H., and Ridout, S. H.: The source of liver fat. *J. Biol. Chem.* 123: 3, 1938.
2. Batkin, S.: Die Dicke des Fettpolsters bei gesunden und kranken Kindern. *Jahrb. f. Kinderheilk.* 82: 103, 1915.
3. Bornstein, J., Reid, E., and Young, F. G.: The hyperglycemic action of bliid from animals treated with growth hormone. *Nature* 168: 903, 1951.
4. Best, C. H., Campbell, J., Haist, R. E., and Ham, A. W.: The effect of insulin and anterior pituitary extract on the insulin content of the pancreas and the histology of the islets. *J. Physiol.* 101:17, 1942.
5. Boulin, R.: Les troubles de la gluco-regulation dans l'obesite. These Medecine. Paris 1924, Lecon inaugurale. *Presse Méd.* 62: 559, 1954.
6. Bounak, V. V.: Anthropometria. Praktitchieskii Kours. 1 vol. 368 p. Bosoudarstviennoie outchiebno-pedagogitchieskoie izdatielistvo Narkomprosa RSFSR. Moscow, 1941 (in Russian).
7. Boxer, G. E., and Stetten, D., Jr.: Studies in carbohydrate metabolism. II-The glycogenic response to glucose and lactate in the previously fasted rat. *J. Biol. Chem.* 155: 237, 1944.
8. Broustet, P., and Marty, J.: *Plethore et hypertension.* 29e Congres francais de Medecine. Masson edit. Paris 1953, pp. 259-288.
9. Darnaud, C., Ferret, P., Denard, Y., Moreau, G., and Verez, P.,: L'etat fonctionnel et histologique du foie au cours du diabete par encombrement adipeux. *Arch. App. Dig.* 42: 1360, 1953.
10. Darnaud, C., Denard, Y., and Moreau, G: Le diabete par encombrement adipeux. *Rev. Internat. d'Hepatologie* 3: 525, 1953.
11. Edwards, D. A. W.: Observations on the distribution of subcutaneous fat. *Clin. Science* 9: 259, 1950.
12. Gilbert J. A. L: The association of maternal obesity, large babies and diabetes. *Brit. M.J.* 1: 702, 1949.
13. Gofman, J. W., Lindgren, F., Elliott, H., Mantz, W., Hewitt, J., Strisower, B., Herring, V., and Lyon, T. P.: the role of lipids and lipoproteins in stherosclerosis. *Science* 111: 166, 1950.
14. Gofman, J. W., Jones, H. B., Lindgren, F., Lyon, T.P., Elliott, H.A., and Strisower, B." Blood lipids and human atherosclerosis. *Circulation* 2: 161, 1950.
15. Gofman, J. W., Jones, H. B., Lyon, T. P., Lindgren, F., Strisower, B., Colman, D., and Herring, V." Blood lipids and human atherosclerosis. *Circulation* 5: 119, 1952.
16. Hille, G.: Die Fettpolsterdicke bei der Beurteilung des Ernahrungszustandes von Kindern. *Archiv. F. Kinderheilkunde* 73: 134, 1923.
17. Hoet, J. P.: Les grossesses prediabetiques. ler Congres international du diabete. Leyden, July 1952. *Presse Med.* 60: 1407, 1952; *Diabete et grossesse. Less acquisitions medicales recentes.* Flammarion edit. Paris, 1953, pp. 51-57.
18. Jackson, W. P. U.: The prediabetic syndrome. Large babies and the (pre) diabetic father. *J. Clin. Endocrinol.* 14: 177, 1954.
19. De Jongh, S. E.: Insulin and growth hormone. *Experimental Diabetes.* Symposium 1953. Blackwell Scientific Publication, Oxford, 1954, pp. 243-258.
20. Joslin, E. P., Root, A. F., White, P., Marble, A., and Bailey, C.: *The Treatment of Diabetes Mellitus.* Lea and Febiger, Philadelphia, 1948.
21. Josue, A.: Atherome aortique experimental par injections repetees d'adrenaline dans les veines. *Compt. rend. Soc. de biol.* 55: 1374, 1903.
22. Jouve, A., Vague, J., and Mongin, M.: La differenciation sexuelle en pathologie cardio-vasculaire. *Arch. Mal. de Coeur.* 44: 893, 1951.
23. Kading, H.: Alter und Fettpolsterdicke als alleiniger Maastab fur den Ernahrungszustand. *Munchen. med. Echnschr.* 69: 433, 1922.
24. Kayser, C., and Dell, P.: Signification et variation du quotient respiratoire en fonction de la temperature du milieu chez le Hamster reveille. *Compt. rend. Soc. de Biol.* 126: 698, 1937.
25. Kayser, C.: Les lipides assurent preferentiellement la thermogenese de rechauffement chez le cobaye. *Compt. rend. Soc. de Biol.* 126: 701, 1937.
26. Kinsell, W. L., michaels, G. D. et al: The case for cortical steroid hormone acceleration of neoglucogenesis from fat in deabetic subjects. A summary of five years' investigation work. *J. Clin. Endocrinol.* 14: 161, 1954.
27. Kriss, J. P., and Futcher, P. H.: The relation between infant birth weight and subsequent development of maternal diabetes mellitus. *J. Clin. Eodocrinol.* 8: 380, 1948.
28. Labbe, M.: L'epreuve d'hyperglycemie provoquee; son application a la clinique. *Annales de Med.* 17: 116, 1925.
29. Lancereaux, E.: *Lecons de clinique medicales* (2 vol.). Bahe edit., Paris, 1892-1894, vol. 1, p. 416.
30. Lawrence, R. D.: Human and experimental diabetes. In *Experimental Diabetes.* Blackwell Scientific Publications, Oxford, 1954. p. 304-308; *Ciba Foundation Colloquia on Endocrinology. VI. Hormonal factors in Carbohydrate Metabolism.* Churchill, London, 1953. pp. 243-249.
31. Lederer, J., and Delfosse, J.: Obesite et deabete. *Journees du diabete de Vals.* Habauzit edit. Aubenas, 1952, pp. 203-217.
32. Loeper, M.: L'action de l'adrenaline sur l'aprenale. *Compt. rend. Soc. de Biol.* 55: 1453, 1903.
33. Long, C. N. H.: *Experimental Diabetes.* Symposium 1953. Blackwell Scientific Publicaitons, Oxford, 1954, pp. 305-308.
34. Lukens, F. D. W.: Hormaonal control of the interconversion of carbohydrate, protein and fat. Hormonal influences in the synthesis of fat from carbohydrate. *Ciba Foundation Colloquia on Endocrinology.* VI. Churchill, London, 1953, pp. 55-67.
35. Maranon, G.: L'adipose climacterique. *Rev. fr. d'Endocrinologie* 14P 467, 1936; *Prediabetisch. Zustande* (1 vol.) Novak, Budapest, 1927.
36. Marx, W., Herring, V. V., and Evans, H. M.: Hypoglycemic effect of growth hormone in fasting hypophysectomized rats. *Am. J. Physiol.* 141:88, 1944.

37. Miller, G., and Wilson, H. M.: Macrosomia, cardiac hypertrophy, erythroblastosis and hyperplasia of the islets of Langerhans in infants born to diabetic mothers. *J. Pediatrics* 23:251, 1943.
38. Miller H. C., Hurwitz, D., and Kuder: Fetal andnoenatal mortality in pregnancies complicated by diabetes mellitus. *J.A.M.A.* 124: 271, 1944.
39. Miller, H. C.: The effect of the prediabetic state on the survival of the fetus and the birth weightof the newborn infant. *New England J. Med.* 233: 376, 1945.
40. Mirsky, I. A.: The influence of the anterior pituitary gland on protein metabolism. *Endocrinology* 25: 52, 1939.
41. Neumann, H.: Die Dicke des Fettpolsters bei Kindern. *Jahrb. f. Kinderheilk.* 75: 481, 1912.
42. Oeder, G.: Korperwagung und Fettpolstermessung. *Fortschr. der Med.* 13: 1289, 1913.
43. Oppenheim, M.: Evaluation des proportions des parties molles et du squelette des membres chez les differents types morphologiques. *Biotypologie* 5: 93, 1939; Distribution de la graisse souscutanée et constitution morphologique. *Biotypologie* 7: 192, 1939.
44. Pavel, I., and Anghelesco, A.: Recherche sur le type constitutionnel dans le diabete. Role du type constitutionnel du parent sain. *Presse Méd.* 57: 725, 1949.
45. Peiser, J.: Uber objecktive Beurteilung des kindlichen Ernahrungszustandes. *Jahrb. f. Kinderheik.* 95: 195, 1921.
46. Pende, N.: *Trattato di Biotipologia umana,* Vallardi, Milan, 1939.
47. Pollack, A.: Transport et métabolisme des lipides dans le foie sous l'action de l'adrénaline. *Compl. rend. Soc. de Biol.* 130: 149, 1939.
48. Reynolds, E. L., and Grote, P.: Sex differences in the distribution of tissue components in the human leg from birth to maturity *Anat. Rec.* 102: 43, 1948.
49. Richardson, K.C., and Young, F. G.: The "pancreatropic" action of anterior pituitary extracts. *J. Physiol.* 91: 352, 1937.
50. Richer P.: *Nouvelle anatomie artistique du corps humain. I. Cours pratique. Eléments d'anatomie. L'homme. II. Cours supérieur Morphologie. La Femme.* Plon édit., 1920.
51. Schaeffer, G., and Pollack, A.: Parallélisme entre l'augmentation des oxydations au niveau du métabolisme de base et la chute de la lipémie apres injection d'adrénaline chez le lapin. *Compt. rend. Soc. de Biol.* 127: 1925, 1938.
52. Selye, H.: *Textbook of Endocrinology,* University of Montreal, 1947.
53. Sherlock, Bearn, and Billings: *Liver Injury.* 10th Conference. Josiah Macy, Jr. Foundation, F.W. Hoffbauer, New York, 1951.
54. Stetten, D., Jr., and Boxer, G.E.: Studies in carbohydrate metabolism I - The rate of turnover of liver and carcass glycogen studied with the aid of deuterium. *J. Biol. Chem.* 155: 231, 1944; Studies in carbohydrate metabolism III - Metabolism defects in alloxan diabetes. *J. Biol. Chem.* 156: 271, 1944.
55. Stetten, D., and Salcedo, J.: The source of the extra liver fat in various types of fatty liver. *J. Biol. Chem.* 156: 271, 1944.
56. Stuart, H. C., and Dwinell, P. H.: The growth of bone, muscle and overlying tissues in children 6 to 10 years of age as revealed by studies of roentgenograms of the leg area. *Monogr. Soc. Res. Child Development* 13, 195, 1942.
57. Stuart, H. C., and Dwinell, P. H.: The growth of bone muscle and overlying tissues in children 6 to 10 years of age as revealed by studies of roentgenograms of the leg area. *Child Devlopment* 13, 195, 1942.
58. Stuart, H. C.: The thickness of the skin and subcutaneous tissue y age and sex in childhood. *J. Pediat.* 28: 637, 1946.
59. Tchoutchoukalo, G. I.: Le développement du tissu souscutané et du systeme musculaire chez les enfants et les adultes et les méthodes de leur appréciation objective. *l'Anthropométrie de l'Ukraine* 1: 49, 1926 (in Russian, summary in French).
60. Vague, J., Jouve, A., and Teitelbaum, M.: La place de la différenciation sexuelle dans les syndromes coronairens. *Arch. Mal. du Coeur.* 48:. 377, 1955.
61. (a) Vague, J.: Le traitement des obesities. *Marseille Med.* 83: 210, 1946.
(b) Les obésities. *Biologie Médicale.* 36: 33, 1947.
(c) La différenciation sexuelle facteur déterminant des formes de l'obésité. *Press Méd.* 55: 339, 1947.
(d) Les aspects cliniques des obésities *La Vie Médicale* 31:8, 1950.
(e) Diagnostic étiologique des obésitiés. *Marseille Méd.* 84: 45, 1947.
(f) Le diabete de la femme androide. *Presse Méd.* 57: 835, 1949.
(g) *La différenciation sexuelle humaine. Ses incidences en pathologie* Masson édit., Paris, 1953.
(h) Le régime dans les variétés des diabetes et dans les états prédiabétiques. *Journées du diabete de Vals.* Habauzie édit., Aubenas, 1952, pp. 294-309.
(i) Obésité, artériosclérose et diabete. *Sud Méd et chirurg.* 87: 3162, 1954.
(j) Les relations entre la forme et le degré de l'anabolisme et les précipiations tissulaires et cavitaires. *Congres du centenaire de Vittel,* 1954, pp. 279-286.
(k) Comment la surcharge adipeuse favorise-t-elle le développement de l'artériosclérose et du diabete? *Sem. Hop. Paris.* 30: 3244, 1954.
(l) Apres la fragilité génétique des ilots, l'obésite androide parait la cause principale du diabete de l'adulte. Quelles sont ses relations avec la suractivité hypophysosurrénale? *Folia Endocrinolgoica* 8:1, 1955.
62. Wilmer, H.: Changes in structural components of the human body from 6 lunar months to maturity. *Proc. Soc. Exper. Biol. & Med.* 43: 545, 1940; Quantitative growth of skin and subcutaneous tissue in relation to human surface area. *Proc. Soc. Exper. Biol. & Med.* 43: 386, 1940.
63. Young, F. S.: Permanent experimental diabetes produced by pituitary (anterior lobe) injections. *Lancet* 2: 372, 1937; Growth hormone and experimental diabetes. *J. Clin. Endocrinol.* 11: 531, 1951.

A Case of Polysarka, in Which Death Resulted from Deficient Arterialisation of the Blood

James Russell

Under the care of James Russell, M.D.

The following case indicates a somewhat unusual mode in which an excessive tendency to the production of fat in the general cellular tissue may cause death. So far as I am aware, the tendency to death in cases of this description is usually through the heart. My present case exhibits this tendency taking place through the lungs.

Under ordinary circumstances, death takes place in consequence of the heart participating in the abnormal growth of fat in the tissues. Fat becomes deposited upon the exterior of that organ as a part of the general growth of fat in the system, constituting the fatty growth of Dr. Quain. By degrees the quantity of fat augments; and, in the process of time, the fat-globules begin to intrude themselves between the muscular fascicles, and gradually effect their destruction.

It may, however, be noted in passing, that this process of wasting of the muscular fascicles is not a necessary consequence of the growth of fat upon the exterior of the heart. Fat may exist there in preternatural quantity, whilst the fibre retains its healthy condition; but wasting is always liable to occur, and such liability constitutes one of the chief dangers of the state of corpulence. Under the former circumstances a sharp line of demarcation is seen on section, separating the fat from the muscular tissue; but, in proportion as this line becomes indistinct, and the fat tissue merges gradually into the muscular, is the destructive tendency, of which we are speaking, being developed.

In the advanced stages of the disease, such scanty remains of muscular fibre are found in the heart, that the observer finds it difficult to explain how the heart could possibly have carried on its work; and thus death takes place emphatically through the heart, sometimes very suddenly, at other times by a more gradual but very painful process of cardiac apnoea.

In the case which I am about to relate, a condition of complete cyanosis was established some time before death, evidently by very gradual stages. Venous blood had been evidently circulating through the vessels for a considerable length of time, and the patient died poisoned by carbonaceous matter. This tate of cyanosis seemed attributable to want of pulmonary capacity, sufficient to meet the increased demand for oxygen created by the highly carbonised state of the tissues and of the blood. The disproportion between the size of the lungs and that of the entire body, enlarged as it was by excessive growth of fat, was most striking after death. The lungs were manifestly unequal to the requirements of the case.

The amount of fat upon the heart was comparatively small; and the fascicles of the organ were nearly healthy. But the heart was generally and considerably enlarged; and this enlargement of the heart coincides with the explanation already given. As is well known during asphyxia, the circulation of the blood highly charged with carbon, through the capillaries of the lungs, is retarded and finally arrested; but Dr. John Reid has established that a similar obstruction to the capillary circulation is present at the same time through the entire body, and for a like reason. He found that the mercury in the hæmadynamometer connected with one of the large arteries "actually stood higher...and the large arteries became more distended and tense for about two minutes after the animal had become insensible...than when the animal was breathing atmospheric air freely." This phenomenon Dr. Reid explained by "an impediment to the passage of the venous blood through the capillaries of the systemic circulation, similar to that pointed out in the capillaries of the pulmonary circulation, by which the force of the left ventricle was principally concentrated in the arterial system." (*Researches*, 1848, p. 26.)

Russell J. Illustrations of hospital practice: metropolitan and provincial. Birgmingham General Hospital. A case of polysarka, in which death resulted from deficient arterialisation of the blood. BMJ. 1866:220-221.
Reprinted with permission from the British Medical Journal Publishing Group, BMA house Tavistock Square, London. Special thanks to Judy Roberts and Sandra Graves of the Pennington Information Center for help in acquiring this document.

In the case under consideration, a gradual process of asphyxia, so far as the blood was concerned, was slowly established during life; and consequently the condition proper to asphyxia was set up in the capillaries of the lungs and also of the system at large. Hence the equal hypertrophy of the pulmonary and systemic ventricles was established in order to overcome the obstacle. Hence also, at the period of decease, when the capillary obstruction was complete, all the cavities of the heart were alike loaded with dark blood. No doubt, the renal disease, which appeared to be secondary to the other morbid processes, would also contribute in causing hypertrophy of the systemic ventricle, in accordance with what is usually observed in Bright's disease of the kidneys.

It is worthy of observation that, with so extensive and general a production of fat, the secreting cells of the liver and kidneys did not at all participate; in fact, the liver-cells were unusually destitute of oil. The question suggests itself, whether the unusual absence of fat from the cells of the liver does not indicate that the latter organ was wanting in the discharge of its proper function, and had thereby thrown more work upon the lungs.

CASE. Mrs. W., aged 45. Her family presents a marked tendency to corpulence, both parents being very stout, especially her father, and one sister likewise. She declared herself to have been a hearty eater, but not to have cared for meat. These two particulars she repeated several times. She had drunk a good deal of tea; and had been fond of fats, of bacon, and of vegetables, and had eaten largely of bread. She had not been intemperate, and had let an active life until the last nine or ten years.

She had been increasing much in corpulence during the last three years especially; and, for this term or longer, she had suffered from shortness of breath, but she had never had cough nor any expectoration of importance.

For two years, she had been exceedingly drowsy. To such an extent had this been the case, that she had been afraid to sit near the fire; and, whilst attending as an out-patient, she requested to be dismissed speedily, lest she should fall asleep in the hall. She had not had much headache, but considerable vertigo for five months.

She was a very corpulent woman, with abundant deposit of fat; she had a copious double chin, and extensive abdomen, and such full breasts, that it was impossible to percuss the cardiac region. Her face was injected with dark blood, and she stated that the lividity was often very intense; the jugulars were not distended. Her urine was loaded with albumen and presented a large number of hyaline and waxy casts, small and of full size.

She continued to attend as an out-patient for some weeks, and then was admitted into the hospital. At this time she was very dull and tropid; her face was completely livid. There was general but not copious anasarca of the trunk and lower extremities. Yet she was able to lie down easily; and presented no important symptoms of chest-disturbance. Her appetite continued very good; even on the last day of her life, she applied for an increase in the ordinary hospital allowance.

She lived for fifteen days, becoming gradually more torpid, and soon fell into a state of low delirium. Her death seemed to be hastened by an attack of livid erysipelatous inflammation, which attacked her legs and extended to her trunk. Her pulse varied between 104 and 132. Her respiration rose, with some variations, from 32 to 64.

The temperature of the axilla attained 103.2° for a single day, with the setting in of the erysipelas; but, with this exception, it only once rose so high as 98°, and twice-viz., six days and one day before death-sank to 95°.

SECTIO CADAVERIS. Two inches of fat existed beneath the integuments of the abdomen, and more than one inch over the thorax. The peritoneal folds were also loaded with fat. The lungs were gorged with blood; they were partially emphysematous at their edges. The bronchial tubes were very livid, and contained some mucus. The lungs looked surprisingly small when compared with the magnitude of the body. The disproportion struck us at first sight. It would even have been apparent even had no increase of size been contributed by the fat. The heart weighed nineteen ounces; its cavities were loaded with dark coagula. Its ventricles were uniformly dilated, and were hypertrophied to a corresponding extent. No important amount of fat existed upon its surface. The coronary arteries were healthy; the valves nearly so. The pulmonary artery was free. The muscular tissue was firm and healthy; the fascicles were nearly healthy; those of the right ventricle only falling a little short of the normal standard, by reason of some fine mottling apparent in several of them. Two or three of the external muscles of the body were examined, but were only found to present a tendency to fine mottling in particular fascicles. The liver weighed five pounds; its cells were abnormally free from oil; the gall bladder was small, and contained a small quantity of dark bile. The spleen weighed ten ounces and a half; it was healthy. The two kidneys weighed fifteen ounces and a half. The tufts and intertubular capillaries were loaded with blood, and the former were very opaque. The cells were small and imperfectly formed; but few well developed cells presented themselves. The renal tissue was generally very opaque, especially around the tufts, rendering the use of acetic acid necessary for a satisfactory examination; but hardly any oil was discovered. Many separate tubes were loaded with cells, and quite opaque. The shape and size of the tubes were normal. Several of the small arteries were hypertrophied; the matrix was thickened.

Narcolepsy

Richard Caton

Clinical Society of London
Friday, February 8th, 1889
Christopher Heath, FRCS, President, in the Chair

Narcolepsy–Dr. R. Caton (Liverpool) described this case. P. S., aged 37, was admitted to the Liverpool Royal Infirmary on January 12th, 1888, complaining of extreme drowsiness. He had been a very healthy man until his thirtieth year, when he became rapidly stout, and the drowsiness, which had troubled him more or less ever since, first came on. Unless in active exercise he found it impossible to keep awake, and even when walking in the streets sleep had come on. During sound sleep a convulsive closure of the glottis occurred, during which entrance or exit of air was entirely suspended, and violent inspiratory and expiratory efforts were made. Respiration was suspended for a minute, or a minute and a half, or even longer, and the most marked cyanosis occurred: at length the spasm yielded, respiration was re-established, and the cyanosis disappeared. Attacks of this kind occurred at short intervals, all night, and in the day also, during sound sleep. During sleep there was considerable salivation, none during the waking condition. The patient suffered from psoriasis, but was otherwise healthy. The symptoms were attributed to excess of poisonous extractives, leucomaines, or ptomaines in the blood. Salmi, Gautier, Bouchard, and others had demonstrated the existence of such bodies having narcotic, convulsant, and salivating action. Treatment consisted in the administration of naphthalin, iodoform, and charcoal, under which the asphyxiating spasms and the salivation entirely subsided and the drowsiness decreased greatly. – The President alluded to the classical case of the fat boy in *Pickwick* and mentioned a case quoted by Dr. Guy of a woman who used to sleep so heavily that her husband had connection with her without awakening her. He observed that many persons, who slept whilst reading or in church, suffered from a modified form of narcolepsy. He inquired whether the position of the head had not to do with the snoring, and whether by "salivation" was meant an augmented flow of saliva or merely a dribbling from the open mouth during sleep. –Dr. Savill alluded to a patient, a curate, who had applied to him on account of his inability to remain awake during his rector's sermons. He had examined the man thoroughly, and came to the conclusion that the fault was not entirely the rector's. He attributed the somnolence to a species of lithæmia. By restricting the diet and giving him bark and acids he had been enabled to resist the somnolent tendency.–Dr. Sidney Phillips asked whether Dr. Caton's patient had ever had syphilis, as in tertiary forms of that affection prolonged hypnotism was often present. – Dr. Hale-White observed that most cases of prolonged sleep were associated with increase in weight, and fat people were generally sleepy.–Dr. DeHavilland Hall mentioned the case of a very stout gentleman, aged 29, whose height was 5 feet 9 inches, but who weighed 20 st. 4 lbs., who also suffered from constant drowsiness. He reduced his allowance of alcohol, and advised him to take from a pint to a pint and a half of hot water daily. In three weeks he lost a stone in weight, and the somnolence was decreasing. The patient then had to go abroad and so passed out of sight. – Dr. Arkle was reminded of a case under Dr. Bastian. The patient was always to be seen sound asleep. He had had syphilis. He was known in the hospital as "the sleeping man," and could sleep at any time, even when walking about. He had the dribbling of the saliva like Dr. Caton's patient, but no spasm of the glottia. No improvement took place under treatment, and no signs of disease of the nervous system could be made out. He gradually lost ground and died, and during his last days always had a very low temperature; on post-mortem examination, they only found some wasting of the surface of the brain and some thickening of the membranes.–Dr. Caton, in reply, explained that there was no real snoring, but absolute temporary closure of the glottis, which supervened after the patient had been asleep a short time, and placed the patient apparently in great danger, as he became quite cyanosed. The flow of saliva was very greatly increased: it saturated the pillow, and was itself a source of great inconvenience. The patient had never had syphilis. At the time the sleepiness came on the patient was gaining weigh at great speed, but when first seen by Dr. Caton, although the weight was diminishing, the sleepiness had continued for a short time. Dr. Caton considered that the case mentioned by Dr. Arkle more closely resembled his own than any other he had ever heard of. Dr. Bouchard had found that if the urine of a healthy man was injected into the system of a rabbit it produced many symptoms, amongst which was an increased flow of saliva. He thought this fact suggestive.

Caton R. Clinical Society of London. Narcolepsy. BMJ. 1889:358-359.
Reprinted with permission from the British Medical Journal Publishing Group, BMA house Tavistock Square, London. Special thanks to Judy Roberts and Sandra Graves of the Pennington Information Center for help in acquiring this document.

Somnolence with Cyanosis Cured by Massage

Alexander Morison

Somnolence as a morbid symptom has a wide distribution in the territory of disease, and occasionally, as in the "sleeping sickness" of the West Coast of Africa, appears to sum up all that is known of a disorder which is usually fatal (*Quain's Dictionary*, p. 1438). It is rare however in this country to meet with cases in which an excessive somnolence of obscure origin, and extending over a prolonged period, is all the diagnosis at which it is possible to arrive after a careful examination of the patient. The following is such a case; and it is the more interesting because it ultimately yielded so directly to a certain line of treatment as to leave little doubt that the cure was immediately consequent upon the means adopted to effect it.

S.G., aged 43 years, a diamond merchant, tall, stout, married, and the father of a healthy family, who in early life had travelled in South America, where he had fever, and somewhat later contracted syphilis, suffered for at least fifteen years from drowsiness, and during the last two years became deeply somnolent. He would fall asleep while interested in and playing a game of cards, the cards suddenly dropping out of his hands on to the table, and he beginning to snore, and his face becoming darkly engorged until his companions succeeded in rousing him. On one occasion he fell asleep while standing on a door-step waiting for the door to be opened, to the imminent peril of his neck, but for the aid of a bystander. I have myself observed him asleep in bed with an intensely cyanotic countenance, a condition from which he was roused after a snorting and choking sound had issued from his respiratory passages, the cyanosis then gradually disappearing. The patient has been more or less under my care for this condition for about two years, during which time he has been treated almost without result by antisyphilitics, antilithatics, a limited nitrogenous dietary, the injunction of exercise, and abstinence from or great moderation in the use of alcohol and tobacco; a diet necessary to a free liver, and the son of a free liver, who had eaten, drunk, and smoked, without any knowledge of or regard for consequences.

Morison A. Somnolence with cyanosis cured by massage. Practitioner. 1889;42:277-281.
Reprinted with permission from The Practitioner, 30 Calderwood Street, London, England.
Special thanks to Judy Roberts and Sandra Graves of the Pennington Information Center for help in acquiring this document.

During the two years he was under my care his urine was free from albumen, and his other organs were free from gross lesion. Within this period he also consulted two other physicians, one of whom considered his case malarial and prescribed quinine; and another, an authority on tropical diseases, excluded malarial infection and prescribed Epsom salts. Neither the quinine nor the salts however had any effect upon the somnolent condition.

After an interval of nearly twelve months, the patient again consulted me in *November* 1988, his friends being alarmed for his life on account of his insuperable drowsiness and the accompanying livid turgescence of his countenance. I then found that in addition to his previous symptoms, his urine had become albuminous, and the muscles of his legs and to a less extent those of his arms had become subject to involuntary clonic contractions. The heart's impulse was weakened, its action without bruit, his pulse 90, and his body free from apparent œdema, though his countenance was somewhat swollen, and his whole physique was gross. His respirations numbered 18 per minute, and his temperature was subnormal (97.4°). His tongue was large and pale, and his bowels constipated. His urine was, as I have stated, albuminous (about 1/12 of albumen), and its quantity greatly diminished. He was also incapable of taking exercise, having soon to desist from a sense of feebleness and breathlessness.

Medicinally, he was treated mainly with alkalies, including carbonate of ammonium combined with digitalis and nux vomica. On one occasion antipyrin was prescribed. Two to three grains of calomel with compound rhubarb pill were also prescribed, and acted as an efficient purgative. As however this line of treatment had proved futile on previous occasions, I advised a systematic course of massage at the hands of a person trained to that manœuvre.

On *November* 19 I have a note that two days previously he fell fast asleep during vigorous massage, and note also that his drowsiness had diminished, and that he complained greatly of thirst and dry tongue. About a fortnight later (*December* 7), I note that his pulse was 84 and his heart regular, that he was passing large quantities of urine, and that his somnolence had almost entirely disappeared. His wife remarked on this occasion that he was better in this respect than he had been for five years. He could also walk farther and with less breathlessness. On January 11, 1889, he remarks that he feels "1,000 per cent. better." His muscular twitchings had disappeared, and his difficulty now was to fall asleep. He continued to pass large quantities of urine, and although I have not noted at this date the absence of albumen, this disappeared soon after the commencement of treatment, coincidently with the increased secretion. He mentioned the fact however that at the end of the year he drank one tumbler of champagne, which sent him off to sleep immediately, and in his own words "he got as blue as could be again." Until the beginning of *January* 1889, the patient had undergone massage daily for five weeks, and had lost, so far as could be ascertained, 15 pounds in weight, for, whereas his present weight was 17st. 6lbs., he had weighed 18st. 7lbs. six weeks before treatment. As an evidence of his improvement I have also a note at this date, that on *January* 9 he went to "a party" and stayed till 3 A.M. on the 10th, that notwithstanding he rose at 6 A.M., walked during the day about ten miles, did his day's work, went the same evening to a musichall, whence he returned home at midnight and felt no drowsiness, in spite of his having taken a glass of champagne.

The specific gravity of his urine at this date was 1025, and the urine was free from albumen. In the general blunting of his sensibility I should have mentioned that his sexual appetite was almost abolished, and returned with his general improvement.

My final note of his case on *February* 9, 1889, is that he had recently had occasional sudden attacks of giddiness, but notwithstanding felt "perfectly well, " as he expressed it; that he had no abnormal sleepiness; that his bowels acted regularly; and that his urine was copious and free from albumen and sugar. His pulse on this occasion was 78 and regular, and his cardiac and respiratory sounds normal.

I may mention that I have since seen the patient, and that notwithstanding an occasional lapse as regards prohibited articles of diet, he continues to feel well, takes exercise without undue fatigue, and undergoes occasional massage "to keep himself right."

Remarks – At a meeting of the Clinical Society of London, held on *February* 8, 1889, Dr. Caton, of Liverpool, related a case which had many features in common with this one. He proposed to term the condition "narcolepsy," meaning to indicate thereby a cyanotic fit, due apparently to closure of the glottis, and coupled with deep sleep. But, as this event must be regarded, in my opinion, merely as an incident in the general somnolent state, the name appears to me inapt.

The failure of iodide of potassium and of quinine to benefit this patient weaken if they do not remove the probability of his early specific, and possibly malarial, infections being important factors in the production of his somnolent state, while the absence of any organic lesions entirely attributable to such causes likewise serves to exclude them. I was inclined to think at one time that some cigarettes, of which he smoked a large number, might be operative in producing his sleepiness; but on enquiry there is no evidence to suspect that the tobacco employed in making these was in any way drugged. I am therefore inclined to regard the condition as one of the protean manifestations of gout, begotten of excessive and injudicious aliment, coupled with insufficient exercise.

Whatever points of interest the etiology of the case may present, however, they are thrown into the shade by the marvellous effects of massage upon the patient. It will be remembered that cardiac and general tonics, evacuants, and a corrected dietary, had little influence upon him. It is probable that had he been able to take sufficient exercise, there would have been no necessity for massage; but a patient with puffing respiration and a feeble heart, palpitating in a large and flabby body, may be excused if he finds he cannot take as much exercise as might, from a therapeutic point of view, be desirable. If such an one, moreover, persisted in the endeavour to carry out any stringent instructions on this head, both he and his adviser might find the remedy worse than the disease. Under such circumstances massage finds an appropriate place, and it succeeded beyond all expectation in the present case. A fortnight's use of this manœuvre removed a somnolence of long standing, steadied an enfeebled circulation, cured an albuminuria, and established an abundant in place of a scanty urinary secretion.

The *rationale* of the action of massage differs in different classes of cases, and this is not the place to enter more fully into a consideration of the subject , but I may be permitted to mention incidentally the two great classes (1) in which nutriment has to be attracted to, and assimilated by, an impoverished part, and (2) in which tissue-respiration has to be promoted, and waste-products carried away, by a peripheral and central stimulation of the nervous system, leading to a more active absorption by the lymphatic and blood-vascular systems. Dr. Lauder Brunton has published a very striking example of the former class in his *Lettsomian Lectures on Digestive Disorders*, in which a veritable living skeleton, under the use of massage and forced feeding, assumed proportions which, Dr. Brunton remarks, would have justified their owner in joining a Highland regiment, and wearing a kilt without being ashamed. Of the other class, I have met with no more notable instance than the case I have just related.

Case XXII. Excessive Sleepiness

Byrom Bramwell

The next patient is a boy, aged seventeen. He complains of excessive sleepiness. He presents in a minor degree a condition similar to the Fat Boy in *Pickwick* – whenever he sits down he seems to go to sleep. He seems to be quite well otherwise. He is a post-boy by occupation, and while driving he often goes to sleep on the box. His master naturally thinks this a somewhat serious matter, and has sent him here to get our opinion regarding the nature of the case.

I have carefully examined him, and with the exception of a slight systolic murmur in the aortic region I can find nothing abnormal; this murmur does not appear to me to be of any great significance.

The patient states that he sleeps ten hours at night, and if he sits down on a chair after breakfast he immediately goes to sleep, and, his mother says, will sleep on indefinitely; she has never, however, timed him.

The patient is a squat, big, heavy-looking boy. The possibility of acromegaly, in which excessive sleepiness not unfrequently occurs, suggests itself, but I cannot detect any definite evidence of that disease.

Excessive sleepiness is, as you perhaps know, sometimes seen in cases of intracranial tumour; I have seen it in cases of tumour of the pituitary and in tumours of the frontal lobe, it is also met with in some cases of tumour involving the corpus callosum. In this case there has been no headache and no other symptoms or signs suggestive of intracranial disease.

The chief interest in this case, from his master's point of view, is the possibility of accident. The patient falls asleep, as I have already told you, sometimes when he is driving; if an accident occurred under these circumstances, his employer might have an action for damages brought against him. He is probably insured against such risks; but the insurance company, if they knew that his employer was aware of the fact that the patient is apt to go to sleep on the box, might naturally dispute the claim. When you get into practice you will meet with all sorts of compensation cases. This is the first case which has come under my notice in which excessive sleepiness might be the cause of such a claim.

As regards treatment, I do not know that a great deal can be done. I propose to put him on a spare diet; to give him a tonic; and to tell his mother never to let him sit down and go to sleep in the daytime.

Bramwell B. Clinical Studies. A quarterly journal of clinical medicine. Edinburgh: R&R Clark, Ltd.; 1910:276-277.
Reprinted with permission from T & T Clark, Ltd, Edinburgh, Scotland.
Special thanks to Judy Roberts and Sandra Graves of the Pennington Information Center for help in acquiring this document.

Extreme Obesity Associated with Alveolar Hypoventilation – A Pickwickian Syndrome*

C. Sidney Burwell, Eugene D. Robin, Robert D. Whaley, †Albert G. Bickelmann

The purpose of this article is to consider the association of obesity, somnolence, polycythemia and excessive appetite. A careful study of one patient will be used to illustrate the discussion.

Review of Literature

The association of these characteristics has long been recognized. Medical texts of the early nineteenth century accept the association of these signs and symptoms as well established. The following quotation from Wadd (1) is an example. "A country tradesman aged about thirty, of a short stature and naturally of a fresh, sanguine complexion and very fat applied to me for assistance. He complained of perpetual drowsiness and inactivity. His countenance was almost livid and such a degree of somnolency attended him that he could scarce keep awake whilst he described his situation. In other respects he was well."

A classic description of the association of signs and symptoms under discussion was written by Charles Dickens (2). The author refers to "a fat and red-faced boy in a state of somnolency." This boy was subsequently addressed as "Young Dropsy," "Young Opium-Eater" and "Young Boa-Constrictor" – no doubt in reference to his obesity, his somnolence and his excessive appetite, respectively. A characteristic of these patients is an extraordinary degree of somnolence in which sleep may overcome the patient while he is sitting up or even while he is engaged in conversation of other muscular activity. The somnolence of his character was described by Mr. Dickens in the following words:

"A most violent and startling knocking was heard at the door; it was not an ordinary double knock, but a constant and uninterrupted succession of the loudest single raps, as if the knocker were endowed with the perpetual motion, or the person outside had forgotten to leave off.

"Mr. Lowton hurried to the door...The object that presented itself to the eyes of the astonished clerk was a boy – a wonderfully fat boy –...standing upright on the mat, with his eyes closed as if in sleep. He had never seen such a fat boy, in or out of a traveling caravan; and this, coupled with the utter calmness and repose of his appearance, so very different from what was reasonably to have been expected of the inflicter of such knocks, smote him with wonder.

" 'What's the matter?' inquired the clerk.

"The extraordinary boy replied not a word; but he nodded once, and seemed, to the clerk's imagination, to snore feebly.

" 'Where do you come from?' inquired the clerk.

"The boy made no sign. He breathed heavily, but in all other respects was motionless.

"The clerk repeated the question thrice, and receiving no answer, prepared to shut the door, when the boy suddenly opened his eyes, winked several times, sneezed once, and raised his hand as if to repeat the knocking. Finding the door open, he stared about him with astonishment, and at length fixed his eyes on Mr. Lowton's face.

" 'What the devil do you knock in that way for?' inquired the clerk, angrily.

" 'Which way?' said the boy, in a slow, sleepy voice.

" 'Why, like forty hackney-coachmen,' replied the clerk.

" 'Because master said I wasn't to leave off knocking till they opened the door, for fear I should go to sleep' said the boy."

Figure 1 represents Thomas Nast's drawing of Mr. Wardle's boy, Joe (3). This masterful description by Charles Dickens of a patient with marked obesity and

---

*From the Department of Medicine, Harvard Medical School and the Medical Clinics, Peter Bent Brigham Hospital; supported in part by a research grant (H-2243) from the National Heart Institute of the National Institutes of Health, Public Health Service and in part by a grant from the Massachusetts Heart Association; presented in part before the Opening General Assembly of the Boston Clinical Meeting of the American Medical Association on November 29, 1955. †Present address, Buffalo, New York.

Burwell CS, Robin ED, Whaley RD, Bickelmann AG. Extreme obesity associated with alveolar hypoventilation–a Pickwickian Syndrome. *Am J Med.* 1956;21:811-818.

Reprinted with permission from Cahners Publishing Co, Inc., publishers of the *American Journal of Medicine*, Morris Plains, NJ.

Special thanks to Judy Roberts and Sandra Graves of the Pennington Information Center for help in acquiring this document.

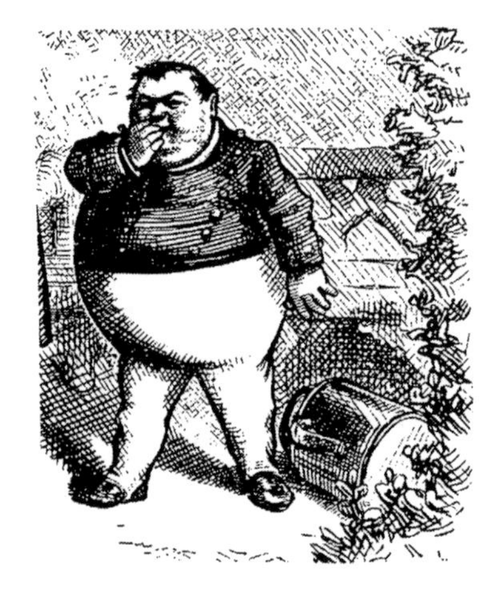

Figure 1: Thomas Nast's drawing of the fat boy in "The Pickwick Papers."

somnolence is the first complete description of this syndrome that we have been able to find in the literature. For this reason we have called it the Pickwickian syndrome. (Table I)

Attention may be drawn to a few recent publications which are also relevant to the particular patient to be presented. In our own laboratories at the Peter Bent Brigham Hospital and at the Boston Lying-In Hospital pertinent observations on pulmonary function in obesity and in pregnancy have been made by Woodbury and by Merriman (4). Cugell and his colleagues at the Boston City Hospital (5) have made systematic studies of pregnant women and comparable studies of patients with ascites have been made by Abelman et al. (6).

Table I
Clinical Features of the Pickwickian Syndrome

1. Obesity, marked
2. Somnolence
3. Twitching
4. Cyanosis
5. Periodic respiration
6. Polycythemia, secondary
7. Right ventricular hypertrophy
8. Right ventricular failure

In general the observations of these workers have indicated that increasing abdominal girth, whether from an enlarging uterus, ascites or obesity, is accompanied by a decreasing expiratory reserve and that when the increase in girth is extreme, it may lead to a state of relative ventilatory insufficiency.

In 1954 Sicker and his colleagues (7) reported on four patients who exhibited extreme obesity and in whom somnolence, periodic respirations, intermittent cyanosis polycythemia and right axis deviation were also noted. Ventilatory studies showed decreased total lung volume, decreased functional residual capacity and decreased expiratory reserve volume. The study by Sieker et al. is the first modern and scientific description of this syndrome which they named "obesity heart disease." This term appears inaccurate if the heart disease in this group of patients is, as it seems to be in our patient, secondary to pulmonary disease of an unusual variety. This concept will be discussed at greater length. Among the important additions to our knowledge made by these workers was the demonstration that many aspects of this syndrome could be reversed by a sufficient loss of body weight.

A patient similar in many respects to ours was described by Auchincloss et al. (8). This patient was an obese young man who exhibited many of the phenomena presented by our patient. A weight loss of 24 pounds and multiple phlebotomies were followed by a decrease in the dyspnea and edema but not by a disappearance of physiologic abnormalities. Alveolar hypoventilation, arterial hypoxia and hypercapnia were still present.

Weil (9) reported on two patients in whom obesity and polycythemia were associated and in whom weight reduction was accompanied by a return of the hematocrit to normal. It is probable that most cases in which the association of polycythemia and obesity is present are examples of the Pickwickian syndrome.

Case Report

An example of the syndrome under discussion is presented in the following patient. He was a fifty-one year-old business executive who entered the hospital because of obesity, fatigue and somnolence. This patient reported that he had been overweight all his remembered life and for many years had weighed approximately 200 pounds. When this weight was maintained, he was alert, vigorous and able to work long hours. The patient was accustomed to eating well but did not gain weight progressively until about one year before admission. At this time driven, as he said, by anxieties and frustrations he increased his intake of food and began progressively to gain weight. As the patient gained weight his symptoms appeared and became worse. He was unable to give the specific date of the onset of his symptoms but he reported that during the year preceding admission he had often fallen asleep while carrying on his daily routine; indeed, during the latter part of the year he sometimes found it difficult to distinguish between reality and dreams. He noticed that dyspnea which he had long associated with vigorous exercise was produced by less exertion than formerly and that his breathing was often rapid and shallow even when he was resting. On several occasions he suffered brief episodes of syncope. Persistent edema of the ankles developed. These symptoms which continued in spite of treatment with digitalis, mercurial diuretics and phlebotomy gradually became worse. Finally an experience which indicated the severity of his disability led him to seek hospital care. The patient was accustomed to playing poker once a week and on this crucial occasion he was dealt a hand of three aces and two kings. According to Hoyle 12 this hand is called a "full house." *Because he had dropped off to sleep he failed to take advantage of this opportunity.* A few days later he entered the Peter Bent Brigham Hospital.

Physical examination revealed an extremely obese man, 5 feet 5 inches tall who weighed 263 pounds. He was florid and had cyanosis of the face and nailbeds but no clubbing of the fingers. He was extremely somnolent and several times fell asleep in the middle of a conversation. His eyes would close and he would snore. When roused, however, his mind was clear and his intelligence was obvious. If the patient sat down in a chair, he usually fell asleep promptly and on several occasions fell asleep while standing.

Irregular twitching movements of many muscle groups were observed while the patient was sleeping and during his more active hours. His respirations were variable but generally were shallow and rapid and exhibited a definite tendency to periodicity. This periodic respiration differed from the usual Cheyne-Stokes breathing in that periods of apnea alternated with periods of tachypnea rather than hyperpnea. His general contour was strikingly similar to that of the boy shown in Figure 1.

It was notable that this man in whom cyanosis and abnormal respirations were present had no abnormal physical signs in his lungs. Observation of the patient's chest movements suggested that the extent of these movements was less than normal but the percussion note over the lungs was resonant; the breath sounds although distant were not otherwise abnormal and no rales were heard. The heart was entirely normal on physical examination although the patient's extreme obesity made the examination difficult. The neck veins appeared to be somewhat distended. The liver was demonstrably enlarged, the edge being felt 5 cm. below the right costal margin. The abdomen was extremely obese. Definite edema of the ankles was noted.

A routine neurologic examination revealed no abnormalities of reflexes or of sensation. Electroencephalograms and roentgenograms of the skull were normal. The extreme somnolence was the only abnormal manifestation of the central nervous system. At the time of observation this was so marked that more than once the patient fell asleep in the middle of a sentence.

Laboratory studies were informative. Urine analysis was normal. The hematocrit was 65 per cent. The white cell count, the differential count and the blood smear were normal. Blood chemistry studies indicated no fundamental abnormality of renal or of hepatic function.

The circulation was studied by usual methods. The arterial pressure was 120/90 and the venous pressure was 165 mm. of water. The circulation time (decholin®) was 23 seconds. The electrocardiogram at the time of admission showed auricular premature beats, low voltage and an incomplete right bundle branch block.

X-rays of the chest were interesting. Both sides of the diaphragm were elevated; this was expecially marked on the right side. The heart was somewhat enlarged in transverse diameter but did not exhibit specific enlargement of any chamber. A curious rounded shadow closely connected with the lower pole of the right hilum was observed. This raised the possibility of a pulmonary arteriovenous fistula but despite laminagrams and angiograms no more accurate definition could be made of this shadow. For approximately six months this shadow has been observed with no evidence of alteration.

Preliminary investigations indicated definite abnormalities of pulmonary function in that this patient had arterial oxygen unsaturation and marked hypercapnia. Therefore further studies were made of pulmonary function to isolate the physiologic disturbances present and to elucidate their mechanism.

Methods

Standard methods were used for the determination of lung volumes, functional residual capacity, index of pulmonary mixing, arterial oxygen saturation and carbon dioxide content, one-second vital capacity and maximum breathing capacity (11).

The alveolar—arterial oxygen gradient was determined by means of the Riley technic (12). Pulmonary diffusion was also studied by means of the carbon monoxide single breath method (13). Physiologic dead space and alveolar ventilation were calculated from the Bohn equation, using arterial PCO_2 as equal to alveolar PCO_2. The sensitivity of the respiratory center to carbon dioxide inhalation was studied by a modification of the

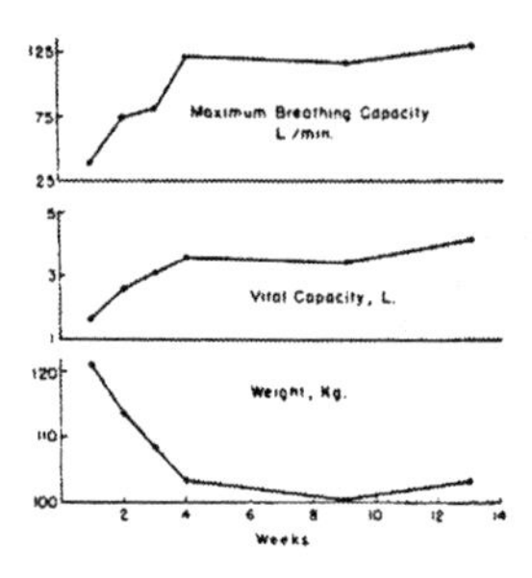

Figure 2: Changes in pulmonary function with changes in weight.

technic of West et al. (14). The results of these studies are tabulated in Table II. The various pulmonary functions and related figures are reported (1) at the patient's original weight, (2) after loss of 17.8 kg and (3) as values predicted for the patient's height and weight after reduction. The results will be discussed herein. Successive values for some of these measurements during weight reduction are shown in Figures 2 and 3.

Therapy consisted chiefly of enforced weight reduction by means of an 800-calory diet. On this regimen the patient's weight fell from 121.4 to 103.6 kg in a period of three weeks. As he lost weight his somnolence, twitching, periodic respiration, dyspnea and edema gradually subsided and his physical condition became essentially normal.

Interpretation of Data

During weight reduction the total vital capacity increased from 1.6 to 4.2 L. However, the most striking change in lung volumes was in the expiratory reserve volume which increased during weight loss from 0.46 to 1.8 L. It is noteworthy that the residual volume was low (1.66 L) rather than high and changed insignificantly, rising only to 1.8 L. after weight reduction. This indicated that no significant degree of pulmonary emphysema was present. The functional residual capacity changed from 2.1 to 3.6 L. and the total lung volume from 3.3 to 6.0 L. The physiologic dead space, which is normally between 150 and 225 ml., was calculated as 372 ml. when the patient entered the hospital and as 147 ml. after weight reduction.

The observations on ventilation are perhaps the most significant. With weight reduction the tidal volume increased from 315 to 365 ml. The total minute volume altered only from 6 L. per minute to 7.3 L. per minute. The significant and perhaps most important finding was an alteration in alveolar ventilation from 2.7 L. per minute to 4.4 L per minute.

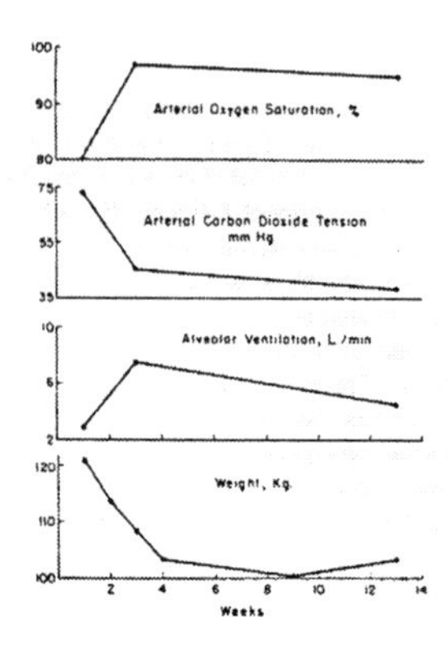

Figure 3: Changes in arterial blood gas and alveolar ventilation with changes in weight.

Distribution within the lungs was found to be normal by determination of the index of pulmonary mixing. The diffusion capacity of the lungs by the alveolar-arterial oxygen gradient and by the carbon monoxide single breath method was within normal limits.

The study of arterial blood gases was more revealing. When this patient was first studied, the oxygen saturation of the arterial blood while breathing room air was 80 per cent and after weight reduction was 98 per cent. These studies were repeated after the inhalation of 100 per cent oxygen for 15 minutes. When the patient was first studied in the obese state, the oxygen saturation rose only from 80 to 97 per cent. It thereby failed to reach the predicted value of 105 per cent; this suggested the possibility of a right-to-left shunt within the heart or lungs.* When this test was repeated after weight reduction, the observed saturation of 106.5 per cent was equal to the predicted value and thus was a strong argument against the presence of a right-to-left shunt.

In view of this observation and the hilar shadow on x-ray it is necessary to consider the possibility that a right-to-left shunt was present before weight reduction and was absent after weight reduction. Considering all the evidence this appears unlikely.

One of the most striking observations concerned the PCO^2 in the arterial blood which was 73 mm. Hg when first observed during the patient's obese state. It fell

*The failure to achieve full saturation on the inhalation of 100 per cent oxygen for 15 minutes has been reported as indicating the presence of an anatomic right-to-left shunt (15). This is usually the case but it has been our experience that patients with severe pulmonary disease may also exhibit undersaturation on 100 per cent O_2 inhalation for 15 minutes. With improvement in the pulmonary status full saturation may then be attained. Our patient is an example of this phenomenon.

progressively during weight reduction as shown in Figure 3 and at the end of the period of observation was 37 mm. Hg, a normal figure. While this was taking place the PO^2 in the arterial blood was rising from a low of 52 mm. Hg to a high of 110 mm. Hg, a high normal figure. The pH was slightly below normal when the patient was in the obese state but thoroughly normal after weight reduction.

The changes in the mechanics of breathing were also striking. The spirogram showed no air trapping at any time in either state and the one-second vital capacity was a normal percentage of the total before and after weight reduction. The maximum breathing capacity, however, showed a striking change. It was 41.5 L. per minute before weight reduction and rose progressively to the essentially normal figure of 133 L. per minute after weight reduction.

The sensitivity of the respiratory center to carbon dioxide stimulation was studied shortly after admission and again after weight reduction. The effects of increased tensions of carbon dioxide on alveolar ventilation are shown in Figure 4. It is clear that at the time of admission when the patient had a high arterial PCO^2 the sensitivity of the respiratory center was far below the normal level. However, after weight reduction this patient responded in an essentially normal manner.

These observations are of importance for three reasons: (1) They rule out a central lesion involving the respiratory center as the cause of this patient's hypoxia and hypercapnia. (2) They demonstrate the fact that prolonged exposure to high levels of carbon dioxide produces adaptation so that an increase in arterial PCO^2 no longer produces a normal augmentation of ventilation. This response to increased arterial PCO^2 has been categorized as a "diminished respiratory center sensitivity." (3) They illustrate that this diminished respiratory center sensitivity can be reversed by decreasing arterial PCO^2 to a normal level (16).

These studies enable us to rule out for all practical purposes such a chronic pulmonary diseases as fibrosis, emphysema or chronic bronchial disorder. Against the presence of any one of these we cite the following points: (1) the absence of cough, sputum and wheezing, (2) the normality of the lungs on physical examination, (3) the absence of signs associated with emphysema on the x-ray film, (4) the fact that the lung volumes and the pattern of ventilation do not fit the diagnosis of emphysema or pulmonary fibrosis, (5) the normal level of pulmonary diffusion when studied by the carbon monoxide single breath method and by the alveolar-arterial gradient and (6) the normal level of the index of pulmonary mixing.

These findings enable us also to rule out a pulmonary arteriovenous shunt as a major factor in the situation, since the alveolar ventilation is low rather than high and the arterial carbon dioxide tension is high rather than low.

We can conclude at this point that the major physiologic abnormality demonstrated was an inadequate alveolar ventilation.

Physiologic Mechanisms

A low alveolar ventilation leads to a low alveolar oxygen and a high alveolar carbon dioxide and therefore explains the arterial blood gas tensions in this patient. It seems reasonable to conclude that inadequate alveolar ventilation caused this patient's chronic hypoxia and chronic hypercapnia. These in turn could produce cyanosis and the resultant polycythemia, somnolence, periodic breathing, and the outer symptoms and signs present in this patient.

If, as appeared possible, the hypoventilation of the alveoli was due to the increase in weight, then the final test would be the effect of weight reduction on the pulmonary functions and the general status of the patient. It does appear from a study of Table II and Figures 2, 3 and 4 that weight-reduction was followed by an improvement in the level of alveolar ventilation and by a restoration of the various values relating to pulmonary function to essentially normal levels.

It is now necessary to consider whether or not there

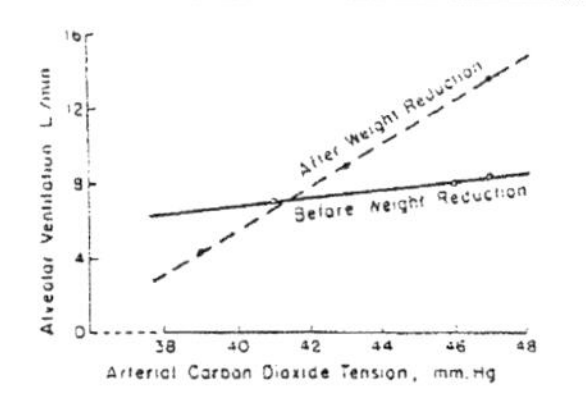

Figure 4: Respiratory center "sensitivity" to carbon dioxide before and after treatment. Each point represents the alveolar ventilation at an observed arterial carbon dioxide tension.

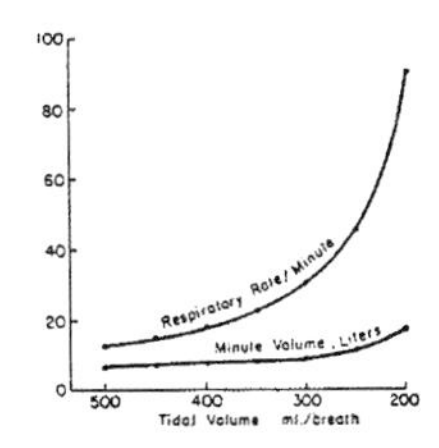

Figure 5: The effect of decreasing tidal volume on alveolar ventilation, assuming a constant minute volume and a constant dead space.

Table II
Pulmonary Function Studies

	Before Weight Reduction	After Weight Reduction	Predicted After Reduction
Weight (kg)	121.4	103.6	....
Lung Volumes (BTPS)			
Inspiratory capacity, L.	1.20	2.40	3.60
Expiratory reserve volume, L.	0.46	1.80	1.20
Vital capacity, L.	1.64	4.20	3.80
Residual volume, L.	1.66	1.83	1.80
Functional residual capacity, L.	2.12	3.63	2.40
Total lung volume, L.	3.32	6.03	6.00
Dead space, physiologic, ml.	372	147	150-225
Ventilation (BTPS)			
Tidal volume, ml./breath	315	365	....
Frequency, breaths/min	19	20	....
Minute volume, L./min	6.0	7.3	....
Alveolar ventilation, L./min	2.7	4.4	4.5
Oxygen consumption, resting, ml./min.STPD	405	242	....
Distribution			
Pulmonary mixing index, % nitrogen in expired gas	1.49	0.37	<1.5
Diffusion			
Alveolar-arterial oxygen gradient, mm.Hg	0	....	0-15
Carbon monoxide, single breath, ml. CO/min./mm.Hg	23	....	15-40
Arterial Blood			
Oxygen saturation, %, air	80	98	>95
Oxygen saturation, %, 100% oxygen	97	106.5	105
Carbon dioxide tension, mm.Hg	73	37	35-40
Oxygen tension, mm.Hg	52	110	100
pH	7.31	7.41	7.35-7.45
Mechanics of Breathing			
Maximum breathing capacity, L./min	41.5	133.0	122.0
Air trapping	None	None	None
Vital capacity, one sec., % of total	81	83	>75
Respiratory Center Sensitivity			
Increase in alveolar ventilation per unit increase in arterial carbon dioxide tension L./min./mm.Hg	0.065	1.32	1.30

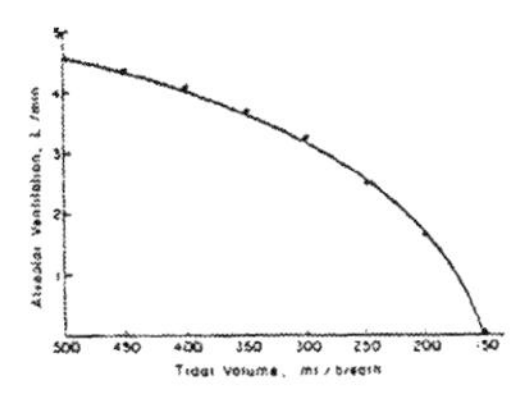

Figure 6: Calculated respiratory rate and minute volume necessary to maintain a constant alveolar ventilation as tidal volume decreases.

is any reason to believe that extreme and progressive obesity can lead to subnormal alveolar ventilation and so set in motion the complicated course of events and the results observed in this patient. It is known that obesity leads to a low expiratory reserve volume and to a diminished functional residual capacity. These changes have certain practical disadvantages in that they deprive the patient of certain buffer mechanisms normally available and permit unusual fluctuations in the blood gases. It has been observed (4) that, by some mechanism in patients with a high degree of obesity there is a tendency to shallow respiration. The precise mechanism by which obesity leads to shallow respiration is not known. Butler and Arnott (18) have shown that below the usual level of respiration, that is, as the lung approaches the expiratory position, the work of breathing increases. Therefore the obese man with a diminished expiratory reserve volume will do more work than is normally required to maintain his alveolar ventilation. Such an increase in work may conceivably lead to a change in the type of breathing. If this work demand or some other change associated with obesity can lead to shallow respiration, then the rest of the sequence leading to alveolar hypoventilation is not difficult to explain.

Shallow breathing leads to alveolar hypoventilation because ventilation of the anatomic dead space must occur before alveolar ventilation can take place. By the Bohn equation: alveolar ventilation per breath = tidal volume – dead space ventilation per breath. Therefore at a constant minute volume any reduction of tidal volume will mean an automatic reduction of alveolar ventilation. This is shown graphically in Figure 5. An anatomic dead space of 150 ml. and a constant minute volume of 6.5 L. are assumed. Despite the maintenance of a constant minute volume by an increased respiratory rate, alveolar ventilation falls as tidal volume falls, that is, as breathing becomes more shallow.

When the reduction of tidal volume reaches a critical point, the maintenance of alveolar ventilation by means of increased respiratory rate becomes impossible. (Fig. 6.) In this figure the respiratory rate and minute volume necessary to maintain normal alveolar ventilation have been calculated on the assumptions that anatomic dead space is 150 ml. and that alveolar ventilation is 4.55 L. per minute. As tidal volume becomes less than 250 ml. respiratory rates greater than 40 per minute become necessary. Although it has been shown that even at tidal volumes which are smaller than dead space volume some alveolar ventilation takes place* (18) it can be seen that continued shallow respiration means eventual alveolar hypoventilation. For example, it is generally accepted that when patients in tank respirators are forced to rapid and shallow breathing alveolar hypoventilation develops, resulting in high levels of carbon dioxide and low levels of oxygen.

It is suggested that periods of shallow breathing may develop under the mechanical conditions existing in obese patients, and that such periods of shallow breathing may in some patients set off a progressive and vicious cycle which in extreme cases may lead to the pitiable state in which this patient presented himself. At any rate, there is accumulating evidence that in some individuals there is a critical degree of obesity at which ventilatory insufficiency appears.

The heart disease manifested by this patient was clearly related to his underlying pulmonary disease. The peripheral edema, venous hypertension, hepatomegaly and even the incomplete right bundle branch block disappeared as the patient lost weight and his pulmonary status improved. Thus this form of heart disease is properly classified as a form of cor pulmonale. The return to normal of this patient's pulmonary and cardiac status makes this syndrome an example of curable heart and lung disease.

Summary

The association of alveolar hypoventilation with obesity is described. The literature relating to the clinical manifestations of this association is reviewed.

A patient is presented in whom these phenomena are illustrated. The physiologic defects present were isolated by means of pulmonary function tests. Reversal of these defects was achieved by means of weight reduction.

References

1. **Wadd W.** *Cursory remarks on corpulence: by a member of the Royal College of Surgeons.* London; 1810.

*Maintenance of alveolar ventilation when tidal volume is less than dead space volume is accomplished by two mechanisms: (1) centrally placed alveoli with a dead space less than 150 ml., (2) inspired air travelling as a cone front rather than as a square front.

2. **Dickens C.** *The posthumous papers of the Pickwick Club.* London: Chapman & Hall; 1837.
3. **Nast T.** *Drawing from an American edition of the posthumous papers of the Pickwick Club.* New York: 1873.
4. **Woodbury J, Merriman J.** Personal communication.
5. **Cugell DW, Frank NR, Gaensler EA, Badger TL.** Pulmonary function in pregnancy. I. Serial observations in normal women. *Ann Rev Turbec.* 1953;67:755.
6. **Abelman WH, Frank NR, Gaensler EA, Cugell DW.** Effects of abdominal distension by ascites on lung volume and ventilation. *Arch Int Med.* 1954;93:528.
7. **Sieker HO, Estes EH, Jr., Kelser GA, McIntoch HD.** A cardiopulmonary syndrome associated with extreme obesity. *J Clin Inves.* 1955;34: 916.
8. **Auchincloss JH, Jr, Cook E, Renzetti AD.** Clinical and physiological aspects of a case of obesity, polycythemia and alveolar hypoventilation. *J Clin Invest.* 1955; 34:1537.
9. **Weil MH.** Polycythemia associated with obesity. *JAMA.* 1955;159:1592.
10. **Hoyle E.** *Hoyle's Standard Games.* Racine. Whitman Pub; 1949.
11. **Comroe JH, Jr.** *Methods in medical research.* Chicago: Year Book Publishers; 1950;2:74-244.
12. **Riley RL, Lilienthal JL, Proemmel DD, Franke RE.** On the determination of the physiologically effective pressures of oxygen and carbon dioxide in alveolar air. *Am J Physiol.* 1946;147:191.
13. **Forster RE, Ogilvie CM, Morton JW, Blakemore WS.** A single breath measurement of pulmonary diffusing capacity. *J Clin Invest.* 1955;34:917.
14. **Alexander JK, West JR, Wood JA, Richards DW.** Analysis of the respiratory response to carbon dioxide inhalation in varying clinical states of hypercapnia, anoxia, and acid-base derangement. *J Clin Invest.* 1955;34:511.
15. **Dow J.** Personal communication.
16. **Robin ED, Whaley RD, Bickelmann AG.** To be published.
17. **Biscoe WA, Forster RE, Comroe JH.** Alveolar ventilation at very low tidal volumes. *J Appl Physiol.* 1954;7:27.
18. **Butler J, Arnott WM.** The work of pulmonary ventilation at different respiratory levels. *Clin Sci.* 1955;14:703.

ON CONGENITAL OBESITY SYNDROME WITH POLYDACTYLY AND RETINITIS PIGMENTOSA

(A CONTRIBUTION TO THE STUDY OF CLINICAL FORMS OF HYPOPHYSEAL OBESITY)

Thesis, for the degree of Doctor of Medicine

Georges Bardet

PREAMBLE

The origin of this thesis is the observation of an obese girl that we have had the good fortune to follow under Monsieur le Docteur Garnier at the Medical Consultation Service of Maternity Hospital. She was first observed during the semester preceding WWI then at the hospital Lariboisiere during the course of these last few months.

This little girl was presented with hexadactyly and congenital ocular malformation (retinitis pigmentosa) that had developed during the first months of infancy. Having at this time also a considerable obesity, we believe this case must be attached to a very special clinical variety of hypophysis obesity that we will individualize during the course of this modest work (thesis). But we cannot begin this subject without addressing first of all to our revered master docteur Garnier as the inspiration for this thesis. To him we owe the expression of our deepest sentiments for the kind sympathies that he has continuously showed as master of our course of studies. All our thanks also go to the other eminent specialists, Dr. Chaillous, ophthamologist of Quinze-Vingts, and Messieurs Vailliant and Béclère, radiologists on whom we have so largely depended to complete our observations.

Bardet G. *Sur un Syndrome d'Obésité Congénitale avec Polydactylie et Retinite Pigmentaire (Contribution a l'etude des formes clinique de l'Obésité hypophysaire).* Paris: 1920. Thesis (Faculté de Médeciné de Paris).

Special thanks to Judy Willis of the Pennington Information Center for help in acquiring this document.
Translated by Dr. George Bray and Ms. Pamela Gay, Baton Rouge, LA.

Chapter I.
Generalities of obesity – the pituitary and its problems related to a classification of pituitary obesity

The pathogenesis of obesity, and in particular of infantile onset obesity has found considerable rationale in the works of the last 30 years which have illuminated the important role, perhaps the primary role, stemming from the problems of internal secretions. These are involved in the origin of all diseases of nutrition in general and of obesity in particular. However, if the alteration or functional troubles with certain glands or internal secretions often appears to be responsible for the dystrophic state, obesity cannot be considered as a definite clinical entitiy but as a complex, pathogenic syndrome which can only be understood in these terms. It is not from the antagonism between glandular and diasthetic theory that obesity appears as one of the causes in clinical manifestations. A large role must be given to a form described as exogenous obesity which occurs from overeating; indeed super alimentation is sufficient, even necessary, before beginning the pathologic process of obesity. The predisposition must necessarily be of this diasthetic state in particular, which with the bone changer evokes a combination difficult to define. Of the complex causes occuring at the basis of all nutrition, however, a capital role revolves around all varieties of gastro-patho-pancreatic dyspepsia disease and intestinal problems. Thus at the base of oxygenation is the considerable action of the systemic nervous system. Imperative also is the auto pathogenisis of the autonomic system of toxic forms of obesity or toxic infection forms which, at least, must be admitted that infections and intoxications produce a dystrophiant action diffused through the body. It is not illogical to think that these can only interfere with organic alteration or functional alteration of the vascular glands. Whatever may be, the considerable role involved in the regulatory action by nutrition of the vascular glands, it is the thyroid and the pituitary of which we are going to concern ourselves at this time.

I. THE PITUITARY AND ITS PATHOPHYSIOLOGY

The hypophysis or pituitary of man is a small organ, the size of a walnut, weighing only a small few demigrams, which sits at the base of the brain in the cella tursica and which is connected to the floor of the third ventricle by a short peduncle, the infundibulium (Schafer).

It can be differentiated microscopically into two lobes: a larger anterior part and a smaller posterior lobe, largely enshrined in the former. These two differ in their development, their structure, and their function.

The pituitary has a double embryologic origin, being both epithelial and neural. The epithelial portion arises from the germ cells in the pharynx (Rathke's pouch) which forms the anterior globe, also called the glandular lobe and by the pars media which constitutes the glandular part of the posterior lobe. This lobe is a posterior prolongation of the floor of the third ventricle which has an embryologic central cavity that is obliterated in the adult.

The two lobes, anterior and posterior, are separated from one another at one height by a linear vent filled with a glarous liquid. In front of this vent is the glandular anterior lobe formed by masses of tribecular of epithelial cells which are clear and glandular, between which circulate the ramifications of a very rich arborization of blood capillaries affecting the relations between and in which diverse hormones of the anterior pituitary reside.

The posterior lobe is vascularized to a small degree. On the contrary, it is nearly entirely formed of neurologic cells where the name neurohypophysis is justified. The anterior face in effect is covered up with a epithylial covering that separates the intraglandular vent and constitutes the pars intermedia of which the role will be central in the pathophysiology of the posterior pituitary lobe.

This pars intermedia is of the same embryonic origin as the anterior lobe but it is much less vascularized and its cells are less granular. It is not limited by definite tissue from the side of the posterior lobe in the cords of cells of the pars intermedia and the cords of cells of the pars intermedia can under an extending circumvariable penetrate between the fibers of the nervous part. The globular hyaline bodies or granular derivitives of these cells penetrate very far into the interior of the neural lobe to the prolongation of the third ventricle in the peduncle of the gland. A test has shown conclusively that the hyaline substances and granular products of the transformation and the dissociation of the cells of this intermediary part constitute the secretion of this portion of the hypophysis. In addition Cushing and Goetsch have experimentally demonstrated that this secretion passes into the cerebral spinal liquid. This understanding is important for the comprehension of the glandular role of the posterior lobe of the pituitary.

From the functional point of view the hypophysis has ceased to be considered as a rudimentary form being thus of morphologic interest but without importance physiologically and its role in growth and nutrition is always discussed even though the different active principles of the pituitary have not been yet isolated for certain.

Our knowledge of the *pathophysiology* of the hypophysis and each of its lobes thus results in clinical understanding that experimentation has tentatively verified.

Because of its situation in effect, the pituitary is a difficult gland to access because one can not study the effects of its ablation without difficult manipulations, multiple lesions of the sinus and neighboring nerves and of the cerebral substance and when the accidents of nature occur it is important to attribute the operation those related to the pituitary glandular insufficiency (P Roger). Thus a remark to Messieurs Garnier and Thaon illustrates the hypopysectomy is always a difficult operation to interpret and the experimental pituitary insufficiency remains yet to be studied. With these reservations we can say the following:

1) *a complete ablation of the pituitary*, in most of the experiments, carries a high mortality (Palulesco, Livon, Ascoli, Cushing) while for others, on the contrary, (Aschner, Horsely, Camus, Roussy) extirpation of the pituitary is not compatible with life.

2) *Total extirpation of the anterior lobe* gives the same results as extirpation of the entire gland. After partial ablation it often produces immediate and temporary glycosuria that Cushing attributes to the operative pressure and to the resorption of the accumulated secretions. Appearing later principally in young animals are troubles of growth and development characterized by the cessation of growth, delay of the ossification process, and retardation in the development of sexual organs (experiences of Caselli, Gemalli, Aschner, Ascoli, Legnani).

3) After *total extirpation of the surviving animals posterior lobe* and after a transent glycasuria and polyuria, a fatness appears with a considerable and per-

manent elevation in the limit of assimilating sugars. The subcutaneous injections of an extract of the posterior lobe can diminish or cause the intolerance to carbohydrate to disappear (Goetsch, Cushing, Jacobson). This activity of the extracts of the posterior lobe was, according to the authors, due to the products of secretion of the paris intermedia which have diffused into the texture of the neural lobe.

4) As for the tentative *experiment on hyperpituitarism* performed by grafts of the gland they have only resulted in repeated disappearance or rapid degeneration of the organ.

CLINICAL PITUITARY SYNDROMES

A. –Clinical syndromes of the anterior lobe

The anterior lobe of the hypophysis presides over the skeletal development and the clinical syndromes which result from functional troubles of this anterior lobe are well known today.

a) Classic syndromes of *gigantism* and of acromegly of Pierre Marie depend on hyperfunctioning by hyperplasia ; "Gigantism is the acromeglia of the period of growth and acromegly the gigantism of the period of adult growth. One and the other are different expressions of one and the same morbid state" in following the perhaps too exact formulation of Brissaud and Meige. True acromegly does not correspond to a hyperfunctioning of the hypophysis by simple hyperplasia of the organ but from a dysfunctional state due to an adnomatous lesion or neoplasia (Roussyn).

b) The *hypofunctional* state of pituitary infantilism was established by indisputable means by Chauvet in his thesis on the complete superposition of experimental and clinical facts, of which certain have been obtained with anatomic verification and histologic control.

B. –Clinical syndromes of the posterior lobe

The posterior lobe can thus be considered as a neural conjunctive residual (Joris) to have been designated by physiological interest to reveal the important bodily functions (actions of the vascular system, the urinary secretion, and the muscles of tissue fibers). The two clinical syndromes of diabetes insipidus and of pituitary obesity thus give etiologic basis for the functional troubles of this part of the hypophysis.

a) The existence of the *polyuria with and without polydipsia* after diverse lesions in the region of the pituitary has been known for a long time and has been attributed to hyperfunction of the posterior lobe of the pituitary by Schafer and Herind, and to a hypofunctional state by van der Velden, Romer, and Motzfeld. This hypothesis seems confirmed by the therapeutic action of an ingestive extract of the posterior lobe by Msrs. Jean Camus and G. Rosse who have demonstrated by experimentation that it is neither the lesion nor ablation of the hypophysis which determines polyuria but a superficial lesion at the base of the brain. It can thus in effect raise the hypophysis of the dog without provoking polyuria and on the other hand provoke polyuria without touching the hypophysis.

Thus for them, facts concerning the self-proclaimed pituitary diabetic observed in clinic stem from a lesion or an irritation in the optical peduncle region (infundebulum for Claude Lhermiten), the polyuria being not a pituitary symptom properly but a related symptom.

b) *Pituitary obesity*.– Besides, in that which concerns obesity attributed to a pituitary lesion, these authors seem to revere the ancient theory already defended by Erdheim and Pick of the cerebral origin of this obesity. For us the constituitive elements of the adiposeo genital syndrome seem much less conditioned by lesions of the hypophysis than by damage to the base of the brain. Furthermore, the polyuria will be due to a central regulatory problem of water retention by the organism. The obesity of the adiposo-genital syndrome results from a change in the central nervous system of the regulation and assimilation of carbohydrates; these nervous centers being placed not in the nervous fragment that is the posterior lobe of the pituitary but higher at the base of the brain in the gray substance of the third ventricle. However this hypothesis by Erdheim of a mesencephlic regulation of the fat and adipolytic functions and which appears to be caused either by a compression (tumor of the hypophysis or neighboring areas) or by a toxic infection without resting on a solid experimental basis and existing against all clinical data to date. The absence of obesity in marked compression and diffuse masses in the brain appears to be disagreement with this theory which explains just as poorly cases of infectuous obesity and thus cannot explain small, atrophied pituitary glands. Thus the adiposo-genital syndrome must be semi-constant and at its maximum degree in agromegly where the tumor always appears outside of the sella tursica, irritating consequently the base of the brain. In reality the obesity rarely accompanies acromegly and is never very noteable when it does exist.

Recalling from memory the theory of Marburg attributing obesity in the case of tumors of the pituitary region less to the localization than to the nature of the tumor (teratome) and knowing that the present glandular theory actually attracts the largest number of supporters to the adiposo-genital syndrome.

Adiposity seems due not to a functional insufficiency of the anterior lobe, as certain authors have suggested (Jameson, Evans and Rose), but to the posterior lobe (Fischer); and it is to this theory that Cushing has given all the authority by means of his numerous clinical and experimental researches.

For him the posterior lobe regulates the metabolism of carbohydrates. Its hypofunctional state, whatever may be the cause, determines 1) adiposity by exaggeration of the tolerance of carbohydrates, 2) the tendancy of subnormal temperature 3) the synergy with abolition of the sexual glands and hypotrichosis which is a consequence thereof.

Even the clinical facts plead in favor of this theory and the optometrist furnish arguments which are not without value.

Cushing, Borchardat, and other experimenters have shown that the injection of an extract of the posterior lobe of the pituitary, and of the posterior lobe only, retards the appearance of experimentally produced adiposo-genital syndrome and it attenuates its manifestations.

In the experimentally operated animal with hypopituitarism, even as in the clinical state of pituitary obese, if individual injection of an extract of the posterior lobe lowers glucose to the limit of tolerance of carbohydrates and lowers it nearly to the lower limits of normal tolerance for carbohydrates.

Thus injection of an extract of the posterior pituitary lobe from pituitaries of obese subjects as with obese hypophisectomized animals provokes an increased temperature that one never observes in the normal subject and Cushing attaches a very great importance to this *thermo-reaction of Frankl-Hochwart* which he considers as characteristic of the pituitary insufficiency of the low posterior lobe.

2. CLASSIFICATION OF CLINICAL FORMS OF PITUITARY OBESITY

The adiposo genital syndrome of Frohlich-Launois is today considered the only unique representative of pituitary obesity. The symptomology which translates the insufficiency of the posterior lobe is not particularly uniquely evoked in cerebral signs, eye signs or radiographic signs.

And the clinical forms which result from the posterior lobes lesion contain certain common features which differ. Between them in the same way as the processes of the posterior lobe lesion. On the one hand they follow the same formula which destroyed the posterior lobe and on the other hand they follow the glandular deficiencies which are initiated.

Thus we arrive at the following classification:

Alpha congenital obesity is congenital pituitary obesity due to a lesion of the pituitary beginning during intra-uterine life.

Beta hypophysis obesity is acquired during the course of extra-uterine life; formed in many ways with the most frequent and best known being a practical division following the information furnished by radiography: Acquired obesity with a large sella turcica due to a pituitary tumor; Acquired obesity with a small sella turcica. Acquired obesity with an unchanged sella turcica in which the symptomatology will be very variable as we are going to see.

Chapter II.
Congenital hypopituitary obesity

Pituitary obesity manifesting itself at birth or in the first months of life constitutes, in certain cases, a very special clinical type of pituitary obesity that we are going to try and individualize. This particular clinical type is characterized by the development from birth of a progressive obesity and by the association of this obesity with congenital malformations carrying alterations in the visual apparatus (retinitis pigmentosa) and on the extremities (polydactyly).

The obesity in this form seems to be a true congenital malformation. The digital malformations associated with its presentation to our notice are a very great value semeologically in truly locating the pituitary as the morbid process which engenders the obesity and the event where this pituitary alteration is produced.

It is the clinical form of the obesity of the little sick child that we have observed in the service of our master Dr. Garnier.

OBSERVATION I

Odette P..., aged 11 years, is a perfect example of infantile obesity associated with the two congenital malformations: hexadactyly of the right foot and retinitis pigmentosa.

Hereditary Antecedents – nothing especially important. No cases of obesity malformation or of diabetes in the family. The father was aged 40 years, he's of medium height and of good constitution and presents no signs of endocrine disease.

No history of alcoholism or syphilis but a very suspect right apex of the lung from a tubercular point of view.

The mother, age 40 years, is of normal height and weight but did have an episode of infectious illness as part of two episodes of rheumatic arthritis which were not part of any cardiac lesion. No stigmata of tuberculosis or syphillis – the Wassermann done on two occasions remains normal in the mother as in the daughter. A small enlargement of the thyroid gland was noted, marked only at the edge of the right lobe but without signs of hyper or hypo thyroidism. Menstruation began late at age 17 but has since been regular and normal. No abortions, only one normal pregnancy without incident but which terminated itself by a premature delivery at 7 1/2 months from a cause which we do not know.

Personal history. –Odette P... was thus born before term in January 1909 weighing only 1,750 grams at birth and during the first two and a half months was raised in a sheltered environment. Before being taken home by her mother at age 6 months she was given basic nourishment and bottle fed.

Malnourished from the earliest beginnings she very rapidly began to gain weight, and was even well above the normal limits in pounds for a child of her age. Her mother said even at that age she had weighed 14 to 15 kg and her size and weight were a subject of marvel in the neighborhood. Dentition was normal; by six months she had the two inferior medium incisors and the other incisors followed at 8 and 10 months and the baby teeth were achieved at a little less than 2 years of age. She was not retarded in her walking, which first occurred at 12 months. She walked alone and without support within one to two months. This was followed by a very severe case of bronchitis which left her unable to walk for several months and she did not begin to walk again normally until 18 months.

She began speaking at 2 years. Her childhood illness included measles at 5 years of age, and a whooping cough at 6 years following complications.

History of the present illness.– It was for her history of obesity that Odette P was examined for the first time at age 5 years by Dr. Garnier in his consultation suite at the maternity hospital in the spring of 1914. She had been seen by Msr. Chailous, an ophthalmologist from Quinze-Vingts who the parents had consulted because they had noted for a long time that the child's vision appeared bad and, in the evening in particular, Odette had difficulty guiding herself. After dilitation of the pupil and examination of the fundii which was very difficult because of the age of the child no lesion was apparent. In addition to the visual troubles, Odette presented a truly pathological obesity which began, according to her mother, in the early months after birth and which attracted the attention of others since the child's height was very small for her age. The precise details of her weight and of her measurements from this time unfortunately cannot be obtained as this part of the observation occurred during the war (WWI). Even though her obesity was already considerable by this age. The infant was begun on thyroid therapy without a noticeable change in her weight. The war supervened and the infant was lost to follow up for 5 years until April 1919 when the parents of Odette came to consult Dr. Garnier anew on the state of their child.

Medical status (April 1919). - Odette was 10 years and 3 months of age and had become more and more obese, and her height of 1.24 m was below the normal. She attained a weight of 42 kilograms (being 17 kg more than she should weight) and this was particularly striking when one undressed the child. It is this considerable obesity shown in the photograph in Figure 1 (for whom we are obliged to Msr. Vaillant radiologist at the hospital Lairboisiere who rendered a more complete description of her). The adiposity was generalized to all the body but spared somewhat the extremities and thus the hands and feet are chubby. Thus of the first phalanges the two last phalanges of the fingers and toes are respected. The abdominal paniculus was firm, hard, and non-painful and developed in the skin at the base of the arms which held a cylindrical aspect on the trunk skin region in the mammillary region but it is principally at the pubis and on the abdomen that the fat had accumulated most abundantly. The abdomen was substantially protuberant giving a classic roundness. The neck was very short and nearly proconsulor and the thyroid was buried in the fat and could not be felt. The face was large and puffy with coloration of the skin and showing a double chin. Yet the facial features were agreeable and nearly fine and in all cases Odette did not present the round face of myxedema. Her face was not inexpressive, she did not have a flat nose the lips were wide her eyelids swollen and the axillary and pubic hair totally absent, the eyebrows and the lashes are well defined and the hair growth is thick, long, and abundant.

The skin is dry and cold to the touch and the extremities present a little cyanotic appearance which is exaggerated in the resting position. This cyanosis is more marked on the skin of the hands and of the ankles. On examination of the hand and foot the existence of a supplementary digit is noted between the fourth and fifth digit of the right foot.

The fingernails are small and thin and lunleua are missing at the base.

There are no abnormalities of the skin and the pictures of the skeleton or parts of the head. The cranium is notably regular and symetric and does not appear altered in its dimensions (52 cm around the head). There are no signs of hydrocephaly or symptoms of intracranial hypertension. The ocular troubles persist and are even augmented. And it is especially on this subject that the parents came for consultation.

They are concerned that their infant sees less and less and has begun to be worried herself. At school Odette cannot distinguish the desks and the chairs and she recognizes only the large letters of the alphabet. She cannot see children.

They stated that their child saw less and less and this disturbed them. At school Odette did not distinguish the lines (furrows) of the books and if she recognized the large letters of the alphabet she could not see the small ones. One could not make her do the courses and towards the end of the day she was incapable of distinguishing them. She advanced hands in front of each other towards the sun with the feet to guide her as a beggar.

Monsieur Chaiolus performed a new practical examination which showed a divergent strabismus but no nystagmus. The pupils were equal and reacted normally. The vision from each eye appeared to be a tenth. The middle of the eyes were transparent. The two pupils appeared to be lightly decolorized only on their temporal segment. Examination of the periphery at the depth of the eye showed the presence of pockets of disseminated choreoretinitis which joined to the existence of the hemorolopsia observed by the parents justified the diagnosis of *retinitis pigmentosa*.

The information furnished by the ophthalmoscopic examination made the existence of a tumor of the hypophysis improbable. A very beautiful radiogram of the skull at Lariboisiere by Monsieur Vaillant in April 1919 showed the sella tursica to be absolutely normal and there were no abnormalities noted in the bones at the base of the skull. Six months later a second radiogram was performed by Monsieur Henri Beclere. It is reproduced in figure 3 and shows no less clearly that the sella tursica was entirely normal in form and dimension. There is thus clearly no tumor of the hypophysis.

General Examination.– Examination of different organs (lungs, heart, liver) revealed nothing abnormal. The pulse was regular beating at 84 beats per minute. The arterial blood pressure after pachon was one-four maximum and nine minimum. Examination of the GI track showed the child to have a good appetite, even to the point of being a gourmet, but that she was not "a big eater." She was very fond of meat and of fatty foods and had a marked taste for sweets. She tended to be constipated. Her urine did not contain albumin or sugar. There was no polyuria. Carbohydrate tolerance was evaluated after the ingestion of 100 grams of glucose. There was no glycusuria.

Intellectually, Odette has a slow, somnolent intelligence endormie. After having been at school since age 6 she does not yet read or reads only imperfectly. As a result of the visual difficulties she often guesses the letters that she doesn't read.

She is affectionate with sentiments, passive of character and indolent. The child makes little movements and has a very marked tendency to somnolence.

The cutaneous and tendon reflexes are normal. There are no difficulties with sensation or from the other organs of sense (apart from the visual troubles) nor of the sphincters.

Basal motor troubles already noted of the extremities au pommettes (need translation).

She never perspires. She is very sensitive to the cold; frilosite (need translation); frequent injuries to the hands and feet, no motor troubles.

There are no stigmata of rickets. The only skeletal anomaly is the hexadactyly of the right foot. This supernumerary toe is little, being formed with the three phalanges and the nail. It is articulated to the head of the fifth metatarsal, and it sits on the dorsal surface of the foot in the fourth interdigital space. The skull is symmetric and normally formed. There is no prognathism and no frontal bossing; the nostrils are not closed the soft palate is not abnormal and there are no Hutchinson's teeth nor tubercles of carabelli. The teeth are well developed with enough space and are of a slightly triangular form. Tonsils are a little large and the adenoids show no abnormalities.

The contrast of the large stubby base of the feet and hands with the relative brevity of the feet, hands and fingers is worth noting.

Besides, this shortening is also evident in the distal segments as is shown by the measurements of the upper limbs. The arm measures 22 cm from the acromion to the inter-line of the elbow and of the forearm and measures 15 cm from the interline of the elbow to the interline of the radial carpal with an index of RH of 68 which is shorter than normal. All opposite to the consequences of the index in the micromelia, risomelia a chondroplasia which is larger than normal.

The hypopyseal test of Poraik has been practiced in January 1920; after a meal studied by Claude Baudoin (100 grams of bread, 75 cL of milk, 8 morceaux of sugar) one gives an intramuscular injection of 0.5 cc of a posterior hypophysis extract. The appearance of glucose in the urine over the course of the next 12 hours was followed. Immediately after the injection the pulse accelerated, rising from 110 to 120 to 124; it returned to 110 at the end of one hour and a half; a drop in the arterial blood pressure, the minimum passing from 8 to 7 1/2 and the maximum from 14 to 12.5 before returning to 14 at the end of 1 1/2 hours. An increase in the temperature to 38 degrees was noted in the evening after the injection.

Evolution.– The child was first treated with thyroid but she responded badly to this and the treatment was followed only intermittently; the development of obesity continued with the weight rising from 42 kg in April to 45.3 kg on the first of October.

The thyroid replacement was completed at the end of June; the child was put on a reconstituted treatment which caused the appearance on the skin over the last dorsal vertebrate of non-painful protuberances of the prickly apophyses.

The child was put on pituitary replacement from the end of October 1919 to January 1920 and the weight fell from 45 kg to 42.3 kg; but this fall of weight did not prevent the evolution of a Potts disease of the dorsal lumbar spine for which the child was finally seen at Berck in February 1920.

In summary.– Two congenital malformations (hexadactyly and retinitis pigmentosa) in a child who became obese from birth. What is the gland which can be incriminated? An epiphyseal or superrenal origin can be eliminated immediately. One can think of the possibility of thyroid insufficiency but our little sick child presented no symptoms of myxedema and no signs of a forme fruste of hypothyroidism on which M.L. Leevy insisted; moreover the replacement with thyroid was manifestly ineffective in curing her. The absence of ocular symptoms or radiologic findings of the syndrome of Frohlich eliminates an hypophysis tumor. Also the absence of any symptoms is not consistent with insufficiency of the pituitary by compression. We shall see in the following, where we review, the other clinical forms of hypophysis obesity that it is a pituitary lesion beginning during the period of embryonic development that we believe was producing the obesity of our sick child.

We are basing this diagnosis, on the one hand, on the actual character of this obesity, and on the other, on the presence of the digital malformation which co-exists with obesity in our infant. This is not for us a simple coincidence due to chance. We have been content to find in the medical literature an entirely superimposable observation of a case similar to the one that we have reported containing a triad of symptoms: polydactyly, retinitis pigmentosa, and obesity manifesting itself at birth. The case of the Italian author is perhaps more demonstrative than ours; the triad exists, in effect, in full force, the polydactyly existing on two feet and on one hand of the child. Thus, this malformation is consistent with our observation.

OBSERVATION II

Bertolotti. – *Polydactyly arrested in development of members and concomitant hypophysis dystrophy in the Journal de la Academie de Medicine de Torrino* 1914, p. 6.

Marguerite Catt, 39 years old; no hereditary illnesses of ancestors; no consanguinity in the parents. Three brothers and sisters are normally developed. Was born at term and nourished by her mother. There was a nodal retardation in her teeth and of her first words.

The obesity dated from infancy; the visual troubles caused the child not to go to school. At age 39 she had outwardly a considerable child-like fatness with the distribution on the neck, the mammillary region, the abdomen, and the maleolar region. She weighed 89 kg. This adiposity was accompanied by an impaired glucose tolerance and no glycosuria after ingestion of 200 g of glucose a hypothermia which developed after the injection of pituitrin (Park Davis) with the rectal temperature rising from 36 to 38 degrees (thermal reaction of Cushing).

On the genital side there were few troubles. Menstruation appeared to begin at age 12 years and was regular. The author noted the very slight development of the lesser lips and of the uterus. There was trouble with hair, the nails were poorly developed and very friable and the skin was dry.

There was bilateral blindness, slight divergence strabisnus, slight nystagmus. Examination of the fundus revealed only traces of papillary stasy but complete atrophy of the optic nerve and *retinitis pigmentosa.*

Along with this obesity and ocular troubles there was an associated series of teratolgic stigmata; dental abnormalities, a malformation of the liver, abnormality of the inferior lip, a malformation of the skull (very pronounced occipital platycephaly) and arrest in the development of the limbs; She can barely touch her large trocanter with the extremity of her hand. *Accromelia was very evident on the disal extremities*; and the hand was notably very reduced in length in contrast with the largness of the digits.

In addition to these diverse malformations there was *polydactyly* of the right hand and of both feet. An X-ray of the right hand showed that the fifth metacarpal was markedly augmented in volume and presented as a protuberance a centimeter long in the transverse direction which articulated with true small phalanges. On the left foot the anomaly was a little less evident. On the right foot the fifth metatarsal has a volume twice normal and bifurcates at the level of its superior two ramifications, each of which articulates with a toe.

One can state that the bones of the tarsal joints are profoundly altered and that the second and third cuneiform bones are reduced in the dimensions of the little toe. There is nothing noterworthy of the other organs, apart from the smallness and the irregularities of the pulse. The reflexes and other sense organs were normal.

Radiography of the skull. The sella tursica was not enlarged or abnormal. The posterior clinoids tended to approach one another. The author attributed this to the pressure of a suprasellar tumor in the diaphragm sellae of the hypophysis which inserts into the clinoids which he believed to produce an opacity on the radiograph.

These two typical cases can be related to two other less complete observations where the symptomatic triad is incomplete partial (congenital obesity, polydactyly co-existing with visual troubles that without express mention of retinitis pigmentosa).

OBSERVATION III

De Cyon (*Bulletin of the Academy of Medicine of Paris, 22 Nov. 1898*)

A 12-year-old boy *afflicted since early infancy* with an excessive development of his skeleton and *obesity* accentuated since his weight has increased 54 kg and for his height of 1.15 m. Dystrophy accompanied by intense headaches, by intellectual apathy, and by frequent slowing and irregularities of the pulse and visual problems (slight ptosis, myosis, and nystagmas).

Despite of the absence of nervous tissue inherited from both parents, this youth has two brothers, one aged 7 1/2, the other aged 5 1/2, both of whom are afflicted to varying degrees. All three pre-sent with two feet having six well-developed toes corresponding to four metatarsals.

The author notes a disappearance of headache, improvement of intellectual ability, a regularity and slowing down of pulse and a weight from 54 to 45 kg, with height increasing from one meter 1.15 to 1.80 m.

This curious and dated observation is of interest in view of a family profile of digital malformations and problems with the pituitary gland. It is very similar to the case reported by Rozabal Farnes of which we regret having but a brief account at our disposition.

OBSERVATION IV

Rozabel Farnes (*Clinical review of Madrid, June 1st,* 1913) (Analysis in *Neuro Review*, 1913, p. 439)

Typical adiposo-genital syndrome in two brothers aged 11 and 14 accompanied by significant visual problems.

Skull X-rays revealed only some excess of depth in sella turcica.

The author points out the existence of six *toes on each foot in each of these two brothers, but notes a curious shortening of the fingers in the eldest.*

Also, through additional observation, we have concluded that one of the three integral components of the triad was lacking, either retinitis pigmentosa or polydactyly.

It is true from the recently-published opinion of Variot that we are in the process of restating that no examination of the fundus was performed. In view of the absence of visual problems which might have drawn attention to the eye, but in view of the child's young age, these might have been difficult to detect.

OBSERVATION V

Variot and Bouquier. *In The Hospital Gazette,* April 27, 1920.

Pierrette B., 15 months old, is the oldest child of young parents who were in good health. No history of syphilis, and no malformations in the family history. The mother had a very difficult pregnancy afflicted with profoundly violent emotional swings. Nevertheless, the child was carried to term without intervention although labor lasted 33 hours. The child presented with a number of congenital malformations on both the skull and as skeletal malformation.

The child experienced normal growth, but at the age of six weeks and nine months, suffered serious attacks of torpor without convulsions, which lasted three to four days.

At the age of 15 months, the child is truly *polysarsic* (her weight is 12 kg instead of 10). She is also still short measuring 73 cm instead of 78 cm.

She presents a *syndactyly with polydactyly* on four extremities. The fingers of her hands are joined at their respective extremity, giving to each hand the appearance of "midwife's hand". A sixth finger is attached to the fifth, having only one phalanx. In contrast both feet contain six toes with complete skeleton visible on X-ray.

The skull and facial dysostosis was very prominent. The heightr of the anterior region of the skull was especially noticeable. The forehead measures 7.5 centimeters whereas the bi-temporal diameter is only 11.5 centimeters. The bregma and the anterior region of the sagital suture have undergone early synostosis with perceptible protuberance to the touch. This is nevertheless less perceptible than the medial-frontal suture which continues without demarcation along the base of the nose. The face is enlarged, the eyes protrude and the nasal cavity exists on a posterior plane. The two frontal lumps are replaced with a depression.

The X-ray revealed a significang decrease of the anterior region at the base of the skull in the leve'dium sphenoidal region with pronounced flattening from front to back. *The sella turcica although not exceptionally small, was severely diminished in the anterior-posterior dimension.*

In the following observations, two elements of the symptomatic triad coexist: retinitis pigmentosa and the adiposo-genital syndrome. Polydactyly was absent, however.

OBSERVATION VI

J. Madigan and Thomas Verner Moore. *In the Journal of the American Medical Association,* March 9, 1918, p. 669

A ten-year old boy is born of sane parents. Congenital malformations had been noted in the family of the maternal grandfather.

The child was born at term following a normal pregnancy. He did not walk or speak until the age of 5. He bedwet until age 9. From age 2 to age 9 he was afflicted with bronchial-pneumonia, with chicken-pox, with whooping-cough, and with mumps. At the age of 10, he was hospitalized for mental retardation. *His obesity and visual problems appear to have been present since birth.* Actually, the child is 6 cm taller than average and presents with feminine obesity. with genital aplasia. His penis is rudimentary, his testicles are ectopic. The mons Veneris protrudes and his mammary glands are hypertrophied. Hair growth is abundant; there are no axillary and public hairs. His physiognomy is fine with delicate skin and *tapering toes.*

There is no hydrocephalus the circumference of the head is 50 cm nor are there signs of cranial hypertension. There are prominent ocular problems, dating from birth. His mother had noted nystagmus when the child was only 3 months old.

There was nearly total blindness. He can still see some light. During the ophthtalmoscopic exam, a slow lateral nystagmus was noted with no papillary edema. There was a white atrophy of the optic nerve with vascular atresia. The retina revealed a mosaic appearance with small masses of pigmentation scattered irregulary (*retinitis pigmentosa*).

The X-ray reveals a non-enlarged but nevereless deformed sella turcica. This was flattened, primarily at the posterior clinoids. The author presents the hypothesis of a sella turcica compressed by an overlying tumor. The intelligence of the child was diminished. He speaks poorly and possesses nasal hydrorrhea. There is a marked prognathism of the superior maxilla.

In addition to the above observations in which retinitis pigementosa and abnormalities of the extremities exist either conjointly or in isolation, we are able to cite through documentation two prior observations where retinitis pigmentosa accompanies digital malformations. In these cases, however, there is no mention of obesity.

In both cases in question, we can ask if obesity is truly absent. This is possible, but we are also led to believe that this fact has been omitted, especially if it was not pronounced. Indeed, we draw from two poorly-detailed and very old observations which date from a period where the role of the pituitary gland on nutrition and development was not known. Perhaps the authors of each of these clinical cases considered obesity as common knowledge, without importance and thus not worth mentioning.

THE OBSERVATION OF DARIER

(*Observation #6 of Darier) in Opthalmological Archives,* 1887, p. 174

A child, aged 12, born of sane parents without inbreeding, presents with visual problems of hemeralopia which began at age 5. Upon ophthalmoscopic examination, the presence of *retinitis pigmentosa* was noted. In addition, the child had *six digits on each foot and hand.*

THE OBSERVATION OF ED. FOURNIER

These de Paris, 1898, Case #328

Retinitis pigmentosa, with normal papilla, is present in the case of a young patient with hereditary syphilis. He presented with multiple skull malformations, including a frontal meningocoele and a *syndactyly of the toes and fingernails.*

The six cases we have just considered can now be summarized in light of these two congenital malformations, one ocular, the other digital, with obesity dating from birth. Perhaps obesity coincided with these two malformations, as in Observations #1 and #2 (and perhaps #3 and #4). Or perhaps it coincided with only one of these two conditions (re: Observations #5 and #6).

Our remaining task is to examine which findingss actually do exist among the three arms of this symptomatic triad: obesity, anomalies of the extremities, or retinitis pigmentosa. We can either perceive these congenital malformations in these cases or, on the contrary, a causal relationship common to all three which can explain their coexistence.

***

As concerns obesity and digital malformations, the answer can hardly be more obvious. In view of our findings on the role of the pituitary gland on nutrition and the development of the skeleton (in reference to the first chapter of this thesis) the coexistence of polydactyly and obesity can be easily explained. The common origin of both malformation and dystrophy result from a pituitary lesion affecting both the anterior and posterior lobes during the period of foetal development.

This hypothesis of a possible pituitary origin for polydactyly is not new. Polydactyly is no longer regarded as an anomaly of simple reversion. The atavistic theory that Poirier defended in his doctoral thesis no longer has support. No longer can malformations such as the polydactyly of the four extremities or syndactyly really be said to result from an exterior trauma invoked by the amniotic theory. Clearly, the pathogenic explanation of these malformations can be found in problems which set in during the normal embryonic evolution of limb formation.

In a communication to The Academy of Sciences of 1904 on similar cases of symmetrical anomalies of the four extremities, Babes reports having constantly found "specific or trauma-produced inflammatory lesions" at the base of the skull. According to his findings, it appeared that the main lesions developed on the level of the sphenoidal bone and of the *pituitary gland which he had found to be "poorly developed, cystic, or even completely lacking."* From these findings he deduced that "at the level of the base of the skull a region exists where in the early stages of embryonic development, a disorder determines the transformation of all extremities in the sense of an excess, or of a default or modification." He concludes that a center governing the normal formation of the extremities must necessarily be supposed to exist in this region of the skull.

In 1906, Apert used the term acrocephalosyndactyly to describe a teratology compatible with life and well-characterized by the coexistence of syndactyly of the four extremities and a particular skull malformation with increased height of the cranial cavity – at the expense of its antero-posterior dimensions, flattening of the occipital bone, and a crest formation of the frontal bone. The autopsy performed in two of these cases revealed an arrest of development and precocious synostosis of bones at the base of the skull. Apert, rallying around the theory of Babes, admits that in these cases a trophic relation exists between the base of the skull and the development of the four extremities.

In 1911, Fumarola put forth the hypothesis that "the region at the base of the skull described by Babes is capable, through the influence exerted on it by sphenoidal lesions, of causing the origin of congenital deformities of the extremities of the skeleton and that this is nothing other than the *pituitary.*

Recently, Bertolotti, discussing the pathogenisis of the clinical case (Obs. #2), attributes the pathological origin of the polydactyly and its dependancy on a *pituitary change which sets in during the embryonic period.*

Indeed, and in a general manner, if the importance of the role of the endocrine glands is great for the adult, it is even more so for the child during its period of development. It is logical to conclude that this role is no less important during the life of the foetus and embryo, "at the period of edification of the new being." (Parhon).

The teratology may only consist of a chapter in foetal pathology. Already, in several congenital bone dystrophies, such as achondroplasia or cleido-cranial dysostosis (which, it should be noted, is frequently accompanied by obesity), we tend more and more to invoke a dysendocrinie pathogenesis.

As concerns the pituitary gland more particularly a hitherto indisputable fact exists concerning the close relationship between the functions of the anterior lobe and the development of the bony system in the child as in the adult. This has been shown by the study of pituitary infantilism on one hand, and gigantism and acromegaly, on the other.

Another well-known fact concerns the selective localization on the extremities of bony formations. In acromegaly, these are explained by a distrubance in the function of the anterior lobe of the pituitary gland. It is of interest to contrast the malformations of the extremity in acromegalics with the anomalies, which are observed in the distal areas of the skeleton in a number of cases of the adiposo-genital syndrome.

In this manner, both in Bertelotti's case and in our own case, insufficient function of the two pituitary lobes could result in the obesity and the short stature. We noted a curious shortening of the distal segments of the limbs, and small, short hands and feet.

This tinyness of the extremities with short, tapered fingers, called *"acromicria"* by W. Timme's, frequently accompanies pituitary obesity. We find this mentioned in a number of cases of acquired pituitary obesity stemming from diverse clinical types. English language authors--notably Cushing and his pupils, insist on the tinyness of the extremities. They attribute a true diagnostic importance to their existence. Indeed, it would seem that the same morbid process (of tumor, infection, etc.) that determines functional insufficiency through a lesion of the posterior lobe of the pituitary gland sustained during childhood, causes the obesity and, at the same time, the arrest in the development of the terminal extremities of the limbs.

The primary role played by the hypophysis during the intra-uterine lifespan on the morphological and statural role of the skeleton, in general, and on the development of the extremities, in particular, makes it likely that the pituitary plays a primary role on the normal ontogenesis of the extremities during this lifespan. And it is also logical to think that a pituitary lesion commencing during the embryonic or foetal period can impede the regular evolution of developing members and, more particularly, the histogenesis of the extremities, even to the extent of producing malformations such as polydactyly and syndactyly.

In addition, congenital malformations of the extremities are of prime importance for the diagnostic pathogenesis of obesity itself when they are noted in young children. In these cases, polydactyly --- more than the obesity itself --- will attract the pediatrician's attention to the pituitary and will reveal to him the functional problem of the pituitary system "in utero."

In our opinion, in these cases of infant obesity, polydactyly "signals" the pituitary origin of the concomittant obesity and *"dates"* the glandular lesion which conditioned the dystrophy.

***

If the relationship between obesity of pituitary origin and polydactyly or syndactyly is evident in these arguments, the possible relationship of retinitis pigmentosa to a pituitary problem is much less clear and can only be surmised.

In our observations, we have seen retinitis pigmentosa coincide two times with polydactyly and obesity (obs. 1 and 2). Once, it coexisted with obesity alone (obs. 6). Twice it coexisted with polydactyly or with syndactyly alone in the observations of Darier and of Ed. Fournier (1).

The existence of retinitis pigmentosa is now perceived to be frequent in cases of pituitary dystrophy as we have seen. But does a cause and effect relationship exist between fetal pituitary lesions and the congenital ocular malformation? It is plausible but cannot actually be shown. On the one hand, we lack knowledge of the etiological mechanism of pigmentary retinosis. On the other hand, we do not know the anatomical state of the pituitary and of the para-pituitary region in cases of retinitis pigmentosa associated with pituitary dystrophy.

We limit ourselves then to pointing out facts and to posing the problem, leaving the task of its resolution to those more qualified than ourselves.

***

In the course of fetal development, pituitary lesions that determine functional problems of the anterior and posterior lobes of the hypophysis remain to be defined, especially given the absence up to now of autopsy proof in cases of this kind. Let us note however, in cases of polydactyly, Babes has found "the cystic gland poorly developed or even completely lacking" (2).

Even causes of "dyspituitarism" remain hypothetical; whether one invokes an atrophy or a sclerosis of the gland, a teratoma or a subcelluar tumor, as Bertolotti and Madigan (obs. 2 and 6) thought, or a malformation of the bony sphenoidal seat, as in the case of Variot (obs.5). In the case we have reported, the unpublished observation (obs.1), the etiological cause has not yet been determined.

***

Whatever may be the cause, the clinical observations we have presented and the preceding considerations justify, in our opinion, the naming of the syndrome as "*obesity by fetal dyspituitarism,*" which we propose for this particular form of pituitary obesity that we have attempted to define. This naming in no way anticipates the nature of the process which has caused the total disintegration of the pituitary gland during *its intra-uterine existence*, thus engendering obesity along with congenital malformations.

(1) Let us note that lesions of sella turcica have been detected by X-ray in "familial optical atrophy," Leber's disease. – James Taylor, in The British Journal of Ophthalmology, May, 1919.

(2) As another example of the complete absence of the pituitary, cf. the observation of J. Charpentier and Jabouille. L"Encephale, July 10, 1911. "Nanism myxedematal. Adiposity. Absence of thyroid and pituitary."

Chapter IV
Elements of positive and differential diagnosis of diverse clinical forms of pituitary obesity

In the diverse clinical forms of pituitary obesity that we have just reviewed, the diagnosis of pituitary problems – which always necessitates the collaboration of doctor, ophthalmologist and X-ray technician – can be posited with variable difficulty according to each case undertaken. There exists, in the first case, a series of clinical forms which are relatively easy to link to a pituitary etiology. This is notably the case for congenital pituitary obesity in its typical form, with the triad: obesity, polydactyly, and retinitis pigmentosa, all of which we have attempted to individualize and seem easily linked to its cause. (Obs. 1 to 6).

It is also the case concerning acquired pituitary obesity which has shown itself in the adiposo-genital syndrome of the Frohlich type (obs. 7 to 13) or even that which accompanies acromegly or gigantism (obs. 14 to 18) with its ocular and radiographic symptoms. These are truly pathognomonic of a pituitary tumor (concentrical shortening of the visual field, bi-temporal hemianopsla, and a large sella turcica). In addition this is true of cases of obesity without ocular problems, but accompanied with a very pronounced infantile state, accompanied on X-ray by an abnormally small sella turcica (obs. 19-20).

Conversely, this is not the case with other forms of pituitary obesity where clinical examination reveals no accentuated problem of skeletal development --- pointing to a lesion associated with the anterior lobe of the pituitary --- and where X-ray examination shows no characteristic change of the sella turcica. In these cases, there is no proof of pituitary lesion and the diagnosis can only be very inconclusive. The presence of a para-pituitary tumor (obs. 24-35) or of a hydrocephaly, with their accordant symptoms (obs. 36-43) can be rendered probable by the presence of cerebral and ocular symptoms-- (signs of intra-cranial hypertension, optic atrophy, papillary stasis).

A diagnosis can be rendered ever the more delicately in cases of post-infectous pituitary obesity (obs. 50-62) where ocular symptoms or positive radiology are difficult to diagnose. The clinical presentation often results in adiposity and identical genetic problems to Frolich's syndrome both in sequence and in type. The diagnosis will be even more difficult with "rough cases" which are summarized in several cases (obs. 63-82). A case is difficult to diagnose as due to the adiposo-genital dystrophy "tending to produce a breadth permitting it to embrace a large number of cases of *essential obesity* since childhood. (Mouriquand).

Whatever may be the reservations concerning our interpretation of a number of these cases, given the knowledge at hand, a pituitary etiology can often be presumed by the clinical similarity of these cases to those of the Frohlich variety and also by the presence of other small signs of a pituitary problems that a complete, attentive physical examination of the subject often uncovers: diabetes insipidus; excess growth; marked tinyness of the extremities). In certain cases nervous problems frequently associated with a pituitary lesion even outside of glandular tumors may also be present, according to Cushing).

It is especially in these cases that one can use the "*thermo-reaction*" test to which Cushing attaches such great importance for diagnosis --- as well as the *research on carbohydrate tolerance* (I.) Increased tolerance for carbohydrates in itself is not present in hypopituitarism, and for Garod (I) and Knoepfelmacher (2), it could equally be observed in thyroid obesity by the lowering of carbohydrate tolerance. This state is only produced with injections of posterior lobe extract (of the pituitary gland in the case of pituitary obesity whereas it would only be produced, under the influence of thyroid treatment in cases of obesity related to thyroid insufficiency).

Whatever the case may be and in waiting for the results of "*biological tests*" which would be indispensable to uncover simple secretory disturbances of the endocrine glands, pituitary obesity, in a practical sense, presents a sufficiently defined clinical type to be often most easily linked to its cause. These diverse clinical forms, otherwise variable, are always linked by a certain number of points in common to this type of obesity. From this obesity stems various types found in the clinical setting. This rapidly progressive obesity, generalised and always respecting the extremities even when it attains collosal proportions, differs from other types of glandular obesity and notably thyroid obesity.

Confusion is impossible with the special subcutaneous infiltration which consitutes *myxoedema* which is ablsolutely not reported with obesity. The diagnosis may not be made exept in the case of *obesity accompanying an untreated hypothyroid condition*, especially in the case of a child. The obesity offers a florid type, its exterior forms possessing no disharmony, the face remaining round without a "lunar" appearance and the intelligence being normal. But it is still possible to discern several traits of myxoedema facies: the nose is lightly flattened, the eyelids sometimes a little puffy. In the pituitary patient, hairgrowth is never affected. Sometimes it is even very abundant. The hypothyroid patient has less abundant and often even sparase growth. His eyebrows are sparse, especially in their external third (sign of Hertoghe's eye). However the analogy to pituitary obesity can be as great and the confusion as easy as in the case of hypothyroidism. At the approach of puberty, signs of genital insufficiency will often appear. The genital organs are rudimentary, the body is without hair, the voice keeps its childlike timbre and "predominantly localized obesity" tending to erase the sexual classification." With obese children, the diagnosis of hypothyroidism does not become easily evident so that one must carefully evaluate "minor signs of thyroid insufficiency" on which Hertoghe, L. Levi and H. de Rothschild (obesity accompanied by rarification of the pilous system, notably of hair growth, coldness, cooling of the extremities, sleep walking, rapid fatigue, facial rashes, vague and transitory arthralgias, late fusion of the epiphyses, hytpotension), have insisted. These symptoms are important as a grouping, for their juxtaposition enables the diagnosis of thyroid insufficiency --- a true test in these cases --- permitting the confirmation and differentiation as well of pituitary obesity which, in its true form, often had many symptoms in common.

This diagnosis with obesity of thyroid origin is certainly the diagnosis that will be far more often made in practice, and which will sometimes present the most difficulties. It is only in very exceptional cases that one thinks of pituitary or adrenal obesity.

Obesity due to an epiphyseal tumor is a childhood obesity hardly ever found in females. In males it constitutes an inconstant symptom of epiphysic tumors since it is only found in a fourth of all cases (Nathan) and is probably only a borrowed symptom. It appears clinically to resemble Frohlich's syndrome. In half of all cases, it is accompanied by very marked and precocious genital development, as much from a functional point of view as from a constant cerebral syndrome, both complex and polymorphous and constituted with general symptoms of cerebral tumor (blindness, vertigo, nausea, psychic problems, papillary stasis) and neighboring ones as well, (such as the paralysis of diverse cranial nerves).

Adrenal obesity is even rarer. It is also infantile but always uniquely observed in the female sex. It is an obesity which evolves rapidly with monstrous development often accompanied by a hypertrophy of the genital organs, of generalized hypertricosis (underdevelopment) of masculine characteristics but differing from epiphyseal obesity through the absence of all symptoms of cerebral compression. When an adrenal tumor develops in a female child at puberty, it can determine an evolution toward "pseudo virility" as much physical as psychic. At the same time that obesity develops, menstrua-

(1) GARROD.– The Lancet. fév-mars 1912.
(2) KNOEPFELMACHER.– Wienes Klein, Wochens., ...

tion ceases, and the young girl looses her female physionomy, her allure, and her psychology. Her face puts on flesh and becomes hairy. A mustache and beard appear and her body is covered with abundant fleece. Her voice assumes a lower timbre. Her personality becomes imperious and violent. Following this first hypersthenic period, a depression with asthenia sets in. Progressive cachexia sometimes coincides with the appearance of an abdominal or lumbar tumor.

These two forms of glandular obesity, otherwise rare, are rarely confused with pituitary obesity. One might have better recourse to consider *obesity of genital origin*, the oldest known form of glandular obesity which can be particularly observed at the onset of puberty, marriage, maternity or menopause. In the case of a child, this obesity will not assume pronounced or decisive clinical characteristics. Let us also note that in cases of adiposo-genital syndrome due to pituitary problems all the more often thyroidian, genital lesions do not represent the "primary cause." Furthermore genital insufficiency is secondary to thyroidal or pituitary lesions ---- and nothing better demonstrates this than the classic observation of Madelung, an observation which has the value of a true experience. (Obs.)

Obesity and polyglandular syndromes. In young subjects as in adults it is possible to observe outside of typical forms of well individualized syndromes, atypical forms of the fundamental constituant symptoms. Sometimes several can be subdued or even suppressed following simultaneous trouble with other endocrine organs.

In such a way, obesity has been described by an entire series of polyglandular syndromes of which polymorphism defies all efforts at classification. We are content to point this out without insisting on the fact. The question of reciprocal actions of endocrine glands is one of the most complex and "at the actual hour we are only suspecting their synergy without, in fact, being able to pinpoint their laws."

Mr. Roussy, remarking that nothing proves the simultaneousness of noted lesions in pluriglandular syndromes, concluded that "a considerable unknown exists, whose field of observation and experimentation remains open" in all instances of these problems.

This is true in the case of the pituitary. In spite of the abundance of works published in the course of recent years, our knowledge of the pituitary [gland] is still very imprecise. A pathological histology of the posterior lobe, notably, remains almost entirely to be undertaken. Its physio-pathology remains obscure. The pituitary merits then a renewed attraction on the part of physiologists and clinicians by virtue of the more and more considerable importance attributed to this gland on bodily development and nutrition.

CONCLUSION

1. Among clinical forms of pituitary obesity, it is possible to distinguish a discerning feature of congenital origin manifested from the first months of the life cycle.

2. This variety is accompanied by malformations of the extemities (polydactyly or syndactyly) and by retinitis pigmentosa.

3. We are reporting two observations of this clinical type (one of which interests us personally) but we have been able to call attention to several other observations in the medical literature where the triad is incomplete, whether a case of missing ocular lesions or of malformations of the extremities.

4. Today, the role played by the pituitary gland in nutrition and in skeletal development of the extremities is well-known, permitting us to attribute this syndrome to a pituitary lesion occuring during intra-uterine life.

FOUR CASES OF "RETINITIS PIGMENTOSA" OCCURRING IN THE SAME FAMILY, AND ACCOMPANIED BY GENERAL IMPERFECTIONS OF DEVELOPMENT.

REPORTED BY J. Z. LAURENCE,
SURGEON, AND
ROBERT C. MOON,
HOUSE-SURGEON, TO THE OPHTHALMIC HOSPITAL, SOUTHWARK.

Marian T., age 7, 3 feet 8 inches in height, is a fat, flat-featured, heavy-looking child, with light auburn hair and grey irides. The father, who brought her to the Ophthalmic Hospital, Southwark, on Feb. 10, 1865, stated that her sight had been defective for about two years. What he had principally observed was, that instead of looking straight at an object, she always looked to one side of it; and on being told to place her hand upon anything, she would be unable to direct it at once to the object, but felt about until she came in contact with it. He also remarked that she appeared to see worse as evening approached. In daylight she was rather slow in her movements; but at night and by artificial light she walked with evident caution, always groping her way about with a degree of uncertainty. She also had a great objection to going out of doors at night, fearing that she should be "run over."

Upon examination, one of the first things remarked was a slight lateral oscillation of each eye, combined with very imperfect power of fixation. Her acuteness of vision with either eye, so far as could be ascertained, was reduced to about 1/5.

It was impossible, in consequence of her want of intelligence and imperfect power of fixation, to determine accurately by lenses the refractive condition of the eyes; but it might be inferred from the conformation of the globes, and the subsequent ophthalmoscopic examination, that she was hypermetropic.

It was with some interest that we proceeded to take her field of vision, and were not a little surprised to find that, to all appearances, it was perfectly normal. Objection might, however, be made to this result, in consequence of the child's imperfect power of fixation. We would, therefore, remark that care was taken to observe that each eye in turn was pretty constantly fixed upon the center of the board. For the purpose of testing the accuracy of the child's statement that she could see the piece of chalk when it was moved to the utmost limit of the board, we at different times suddenly moved it away altogether, when she at once remarked its disappearance.

Ophthalmoscopic Examination after complete mydriasis.– Scattered over the fundus oculi, but especially aggregated towards its periphery, were several irregular figures of a deep black colour. None were visible either in the situation of the macula lutea or its immediate neighborhood. Their forms were exceedingly various, some being flakes or streaks of pigment, whilst others appeared as black oblong or oval spots, with fine dark lines extending from them, very closely resembling bone corpuscles in shape.

The pigment-spots were apparently situated in the substance of the retina, on a level with its vessels – in some places interrupting these in their course, and at others running for a short distance closely by their sides. They were distinctly on a plane anterior to the choroid. The vessels of this latter structure could everywhere be most beautifully seen, even to their minutest ramifications, excepting at those parts where the pigment

Laurence JZ, Moon RC. Four cases of "Retinitis Pigmentosa," occurring in the same family, and accompanied by general imperfections of development. *Opthalmol Rev.* 1866;2:32-41.
Reprinted with permission from John Sheratt and Son Ltd., Manchester, England.
Special thanks to Judy Willis of the Pennington Information Center for help in acquiring this document.

obscured them from view. The spaces between these vessels were of a paler colour than the vessels themselves.

Each optic papilla was of a reddish pink-colour, with a rather bright stippled center; its margin softly defined, and surrounded by a narrow pale zone.

The direct image was well seen without an eye-piece (hypermetropic refraction) when the ophthalmo-scope-mirror was held close to the patient's eye; and yet at about a foot distance the indirect image was also distinctly visible without the objective. This phenomenon was remarked by two independent observers.

Observations have been made by Professor von Gräfe in reference to the hereditary occurrence of Retinitis pigmentosa; and Dr. Liebreich has directed attention to the fact that many of the subjects of this disease are the offspring of marriages of consanguinity. In the present case, however, no hereditary tendency can be traced, nor do the parents appear to be in any way related by blood. For three years the mother resided in the West Indies, whence she returned to England at the age of twenty. Soon after reaching England she became acquainted with her present husband, to whom she was previously "a perfect stranger." They were married in a few months afterwards, and have had in all ten children. Two of these died in infancy – the one of small-pox, the other of "consumption."

The father is tall and well-built. He is active, intelligent, and remarkably healthy; and has never experienced any imperfection in his sight. His acuteness of vision, and the accommodation of both eyes, are perfectly normal. On examination with the ophthalmoscope (with fully dilated pupils) nothing abnormal could be discovered in either fundus oculi, excepting a small palish spot behind the right upper retinal vein, close to its exit from the disc. No pigmentary deposits could be seen in either retina.

The mother is of an average height, and has never had any serious illness, excepting the small-pox, which she took from the child she was suckling at the time, and who eventually died from it. Her sight is quite perfect, she being able to read No. 1 (diamond) type, and "thread a needle without glasses." Both eyes were examined with the ophthalmoscope, after complete mydriasis by atropine. Each fundus oculi yielded a dullish red reflex, contrasting remarkably with the light orange red-coloured fundi of her daughter Marian and the rest of her children, to be hereafter described. Both entrances were bright and stippled in their centres, and normally defined. No deposit of pigment was visible in either retina, and no abnormal condition of either eye was observed, beyond a decidedly hypermetropic refraction.

The parents were very willing to afford any information we desired in reference to their eight surviving children.

The following is a list of all the children now living, arranged in the order of their respective ages, with the description given of each by their father and mother:

1. Richard Nelson, age 24 - "A fine young man, healthy in every respect."
2. Arthur Robert, age 22- - "A fine young man, healthy in every respect."
3. Harry, age 20 - "Afflicted, and has bad sight."
4. Frederick, age 18 - "Afflicted, and has bad sight."
5. Charles, age 15 - "Afflicted, and has bad sight."
6. Edwin, age 13 - "Healthy in every respect, very sharp at learning."
7. Willie, age 9 - "Healthy in every respect."
8. Marian, age 7 - "Very quiet, slow child, and has bad sight."

It will be seen from the above enumeration, that the patient Marian, whose case has been above described, is the youngest, and the only girl of the family. It was very remarkable that the first, second, sixth, and seventh should have escaped any bodily or visual defect; and that the boys Harry, Frederick, and Charles, the third, fourth, and fifth on the list, should be the subjects of an impairment of vision, accompanied by certain imperfections of the bodily organs to be presently referred to. An opportunity was afforded for the personal examination of these three "afflicted" boys, who were brought to the hospital on a subsequent day.

Harry S., age 20, is short for his age – measuring only 5 feet 3 1/4 inches in height. He walks with a slouching, heavy gait, "as if he were tipsy." He appears to have hardly sufficient power to drag his legs along, and cannot walk far without taking hold of a person's arm, or something near at hand, to support himself by. He goes up and down stairs with considerable difficulty and slowness, appearing rather to pull himself up by his hands than to make much use of the muscles of his lower extremities.

An examination of his back showed that the series of dorsal vertebrae ran perfectly straight downwards, leaving a rather deep depression between the scapulae. The curve of the lumbar vertebrae was, however, very considerable, causing the trunk to be thrown forward from the hips, and the buttocks to appear more prominent than usual. His lower extremities were rather short, and the muscles flabby.

He has a stolid, heavy countenance, and appears to be rather obtuse and unintelligent. He answers questions slowly, but with tolerable accuracy.

He has always been observed to have defective sight, and, from his earliest years, "in trying to read a book, he would hold it quite close to his eyes." He sees very imperfectly in the daytime, and is unable to find his way about at all when in a place he is not well acquainted with. he sees still worse by gas-light, and habitually feels and gropes his way about the house after dusk.

His power of fixation is very imperfect, and his eyes are continually moving from side to side, but not so rapidly as to constitute – what is generally understood by the term – an oscillation. The eyeballs are externally of normal conformation. His hair and irides are of a light brown colour. The pupils are moderately contracted, and act briskly under the stimulus of light.

His acuteness of vision with either eye is not more than 1/10, and as in the case of his sister, the visual field is not at all diminished.

Ophthalmoscopic Examination.– Both optic papillae are bright and stippled in their centres, reddish around this center, their margin softly defined. Around the discs is a narrow pale halo. The superficial stratum of the choroid is considerably atrophied, allowing the choroidal vessels to be everywhere beautifully seen, with blackish, finely granular interspaces – which are, probably, the remains of the epithelial pigment-layer. A few isolated dark black pigment-spots are scattered over the fundi; none, however, being visible in the neighborhood of either yellow spot, although the choroid at this part seems to be more atrophic than at any other portion of the fundus.

This young man presents the same refractive (?) phenomena as his sister.

Frederick, age 18, measuring 4 feet 6 1/2 inches in height, is a fattish, heavy-looking boy, deeply pitted from small-pox, with light brown hair and irides. Like his brother Harry, he walks with a slouching, helpless gait, dragging his legs from the hips. His eyesight was first observed to be defective 11 or 12 years ago, from which time it has gradually become worse. He says he can only read in the sun-light, and his parents state that after dusk he gropes his way around the house, seeming afraid to walk about at night.

His acuity of vision is reduced to 1/15; the visual fields of both eyes, however, appear to be perfectly normal. He fixes very imperfectly, and, like his brother and sister, has a slight lateral oscillation of both eyes. His eyeballs are hypermetropic in form, and sunken in the orbit.

Ophthalmoscopic Examination.– Exactly the same appearance as in Marian's eyes; only that the process is more advanced, especially in the right eye, where, at parts, the fundus has the appearance of a diffused staphyloma posticum – all vessels having disappeared, and nothing but a stippled yellowish-white ground being visible. The interspaces of the choroidal vessels, as in Harry's case, are finely granulated. On and around the macula lutea are several small pigmentary deposits. The refractive (?) phenomena noted in the two previous cases were also well seen in Frederick.

Charles, age 15, measures 4 feet 4 1/2 inches. He is dull and inanimate, like the two other youths, and has a slouching gait, but not at all to the same extent as his brothers. His hair and irides are of a light-brown colour.

The parents have observed his sight to be defective for the last three years. He sees badly at night, and has imperfect fixing power, combined with a constant but slight lateral movement of the eyes.

His acuity of vision is about 1/10, the visual field is apparently normal in both eyes.

Ophthalmoscopic Examination.– The ophthalmoscopic description given of Harry applies to this boy, with the addition that in the macula lutea are a few granular pigment-spots. The refraction is like that of his sister, but rather less marked.

In the above report the height of each patient has been given for the purpose of directing attention to the dwarfish stature of the boys for their age. The organs of generation are also strikingly implicated in the general want of development. The penis and scrotum of the eldest boy are not larger than those of an infant at twelve months old. Only the left testicle – and that an exceedingly small one – can be felt in the scrotum. A few short bristly hairs are to be seen on the pubes. In the second boy (Frederick) the penis is somewhat larger, and two small testicles can be distinctly felt in the scrotum. There are a few fine scattered hairs on the pubes. In the third boy (Charles) no testicles at all can be discovered, his penis and scrotum being about the same size as those of his brother Harry.

The two younger boys have no malformation of the spine, nor has either of them any tenderness of the vertebrae. The mother states that the girl is perfectly formed and well developed.

In all these cases the hemeralopic symptoms, so characteristic of Retinitis pigmentosa, were very prominently marked. It was worthy of note that, notwithstanding the imperfect power of fixation they all possessed, there did not appear to be any limitation of the field of vision in any case.

None of these children had every suffered any pain in the eyes, and in no case was any opacity observed in the refractive media.

The aetiology of Retinitis pigmentosa is at present enveloped in considerable mystery, and the structure primarily affected, as well as the process by which pigment becomes deposited in the retina, are as yet debated questions. Dr. Mooren, in his very comprehensive paper, reproduced in a former number of this journal (vol. i. pp. 46-57), has given at some length the opinions held by several very eminent pathologists. Some are of opinion that the pigment is developed in the retina itself, whilst others consider that it originates in the choroid, and that the retina becomes secondarily infiltrated by the morbid product. Both these views are no doubt individually correct in reference to the eyes which have been examined by different observers; but a large number of accurately observed and faithfully reported cases are yet needed, in addition to confirmatory anatomical examinations, to complete our knowledge of the pathology of this disease.

It would, however, appear that there are some cases in which the retinal changes are the only ones to be observed, and others in which both the retina and choroid are simultaneously implicated.

It would be interesting to determine, if possible, the precise influence the changes in the retina and choroid respectively exert on the diminution of the field an acuity of vision.

In the present cases the impairment of vision was proportionate to the choroidal atrophy – not to the comparatively insignificant deposits of pigment. Mooren, in this paper already referred to, says:"Although on the whole there exists a certain correspondence between the amount of pigment and the diminution of the field of vision, still this latter appears to precede the deposition of pigment. We have several times had the opportunity of observing, that in families whose elder children were affected with confirmed Retinitis pigmentosa, there existed in the younger members, along with hemeralopic evils, so deficient a power of localization as was only to be explained by a high degree of contraction of the field of vision; and yet the ophthalmoscopic examination did not disclose event he least trace of pigmentary deposition." Our cases agree with this statement in the occasional disproportion between the hemeralopia and the pigmentary deposition, but differ from it in referring the former to any contraction of the field of vision.

In calling these cases by the name of "Retinitis pigmentosa," we have been guided rather by usage than by the intimate nature of the cases. Had we have taken the latter view, we should rather have entitled our paper "Four Cases of Arrest of Development and Atrophy of the Eye;" or we might have gone even a step further in the generalization of our title, as the arrest of development was by no means confined to the eye, but affected several other organs of the body. In this later point of view, and more especially when we regard the general imperfection of the mental faculties, these patients may in a certain sense be not unaptly compared to cretins in a mild degree.* In no member of the entire family, however, was there any bronchocele. Mr. Little has kindly supplied us with the following additional notes on these cases:

"Of the four children, the one, aged 18, seems to present the abnormal symptoms in the most marked degree. His body is well developed (the muscles appearing quite of the average size), though exceedingly short, his height being only four feet six inches, whilst some of his brothers are six feet.

There is no contraction and no paralysis of any muscles; but the influence of the will over all of them seems defective. He can, it is true, put any muscle into action, but only slowly and not with the ordinary force. This is most marked when he walks: then the knees bulge out, or the joints are never quite extended, so that he rolls about and takes hold of a table, chairs, etc, to steady himself; he also stoops considerably The genital organs are those of a boy of five years old.

The mother says that two of her children were partially asphyxiated at birth; she does not know which. I see no signs of rickets, scrofula, or syphilis."

---

* Watson ("On the Principles and Practice of Physic," 4th ed. vol. i. p. 800) says: - "Cretinism . . . is a strange and melancholy disease: a sort of idiocy, accompanied by (and doubtless dependent upon) deformity and imperfection of the bodily organs. The mental affection exists in all degrees, from mere obtuseness of thought and purpose to the complete obliteration of intelligence. Many of the cretins are incapable of articulate speech; some are blind, some deaf, and others labour under all these privations. They are mostly dwarfish in stature, with large heads, wide vacant features, and goggle eyes, short crooked limbs, flabby muscles, and tumid bellies. The worst of them are insensible to the decencies of nature, and obey, without shame or self-restraint, every animal impulse. In no other class of mortals is the empress humanity so pitiably defaced."

Fodere says: "Le crétin deviet pubère plus tard que les autres, et alors les organes de la génération acquièrent un grand volume" ("Traité du Goître et du Crétinisme," p. 124). Further on (p. 126) he says, "Le seul sens de la vue paraît intact." Dr. Ed. Wells, in his Essay upon Cretinism and Goitre (p. 16), states that in this disease "the eyes are small and weak, the pupils dilated, and generally affected with strabismus." It will be remembered that in our cases the eyes possessed a hypermetropic (strabismic) conformation. Dr. Twining states that where cretinism is endemic, the characters of the Cretin and the Albino may be seen united, although the peculiarity of the white hair may not exist. He lays stress upon the visual imperfection, which, he says, may go on to entire blindness, and he considers the whole series of phenomena in these cases as "an imperfect development of the entire being." Guggenbuhl and Baillarger, before Twining, took the same view of the question. Mooren (Op. cit., p. 56) calls attention to the concurrence of mutism and cretinism with many cases of Retinitis pigmentosa.

A Pair of Siblings with Adiposo-Genital Dystrophy

Artur Biedl

Biedl showed a pair of siblings with adiposo-genital dystrophy next to the illustration of a third case. Alteration in the hypophysis as well as signs of a brain tumor or pathological brain pressure are completely absent and congenital deformations (retinitis pigmentosa, polydactyly, and anal atresia), as well as characteristic signs of an obstruction of cerebral development, of which the main point expresses itself in the existence of an unusual intellectual torpidity. In one case in particular the reduced principle of the gas exchange is detectable. Strikingly unusual indigestion. This new symptom complex will be traced back to a primary developmental obstacle of the brain and especially of the metabolic center of recovered brain region. It will be placed as a pathogenetic extreme of the pure hypophyses and pure cerebral form. For among the greater number of cases of adiposo genital dystrophy, it will be accepted that the pathogenetic momen, is a tumor of the hypophyses or in that neighborhood, or a pathological brain pressure of the hypophyses on one side, and of the mid brain on the other side. The same malfunction takes place when the irritant of the intermediary secretions doesn't unleash its effect on the mid-brain center or when this center itself becomes disrupted in its operation. An analogous assessment demands also that the diabetes insipidus can occur, as purely hypophyseal or purely cerebral, through the disruption of the realm of the Tubercle cinereum which regulates water centers.

An excerpt from Prag, Verein deutscher Aerzte: Biedl A. Geschwisterpaar mit adiposo-genitalier dystrophie. 16. VI. 1922. *Dtsch. med. Wschr.* 48;(1922):1630. Reprinted with permission from Georg Thieme Verlag, Rudigerstrasse 14, D-70469, Stuttgart, FRG.
Translated by Scott R. Houghton, Baton Rouge, LA.

CLASSICS IN OBESITY

The Fröhlich Syndrome Report of the Original Case

Hilde Bruch, M.D.
New York

The term "Fröhlich Syndrome" is so frequently used as a diagnosis for obesity in childhood and adolescence that it has almost entirely lost the specific, well defined significance which it originally possessed. One reason for the vague and indiscriminate application of this diagnosis seems to be that many physicians are not familiar with the clinical picture which Fröhlich reported in 1901.[1] Since his paper is not readily accessible, the present report is written with the intention of reconstructing the clinical picture of this case. The original publication was given in the form of a lecture; most of the data were recorded in incomplete sentences. This style is not well suited to a verbatim translation. The present report follows the original description as closely as possible. The quotations from the older literature, which Fröhlich discussed in detail in his paper, have been omitted. The order in which the material was presented has been rearranged.

Report of the Case described by Fröhlich

R.D., a boy, was born in 1887. Information concerning the family history and the early development of the patient is not recorded. The child was apparently normal and healthy until the onset of the condition which brought him to the outpatient department of Dr. Nothnagel on Nov. 4, 1899.

The mother stated that since April the boy had been complaining of severe headaches about twice a week on coming home from school. Sometimes the interval between headaches was as long as two weeks. He had to go to bed, and he vomited about two hours later; occasionally he vomited immediately after he came home. The headaches were usually on the left; sometimes they were bilateral, being localized in the frontal region. The boy had continued to do good work at school; his memory was unimpaired, and he showed no signs of nervousness or hysteria. There was no history of previous disease or preceding trauma. His eyesight was good. Except for headaches and vomiting, he had no complaints. The functions of the bladder and the rectum were normal.

The physical examination failed to reveal any pathologic feature. Notwithstanding this, a detailed record was kept. The optic fundi presented no abnormality. They had been examined previously by Professor Königstein and had been found to be normal.

In view of the negative findings, it was felt that the patient suffered from hemicrania, and therapeutic advice was given accordingly.

On Aug. 19, 1901, he returned to the clinic with a number of serious complaints. The mother gave the following information: Since March 1899 the patient, who previously had been slim, had been rapidly gaining weight. In January 1901 he complained about diminishing eyesight on the left; not much attention was given to the complaint. In July the headaches recurred, and subsequently they increased in severity. The boy tired easily and vomited repeatedly, mostly after meals. Visual acuity diminished progressively until complete blindness in the left eye ensued. Later, vision in the right eye also began to fail.

On September 9 treatment with thyroid tablets was begun. After this, subjective improvement was noted. The body had fewer headaches and did not complain of dizziness. He had not felt nauseated for ten days prior to the date on which this improvement was recorded. The appetite and sleep were good, but he lost some weight. His weight had been 54 Kg. (118.8 pounds) in August and was 51.5 Kg. (113.3 pounds) on September 23.

Results of the examination on this date were recorded in detail. Intelligence and speech appeared normal. All movements of the head were free. Only the left tem-

Brusch H. The Fröhlich Syndrome: Report of the Original Case. Am J Dis Child 1939;58:1281-1289.
Reprinted with permission from the American Journalof Diseases of Children, December 1939, Volume 58

1. Fröhlich, A.: Ein Fall von Tumor der Hypophysis cerebri ohne Akromegalie, Wien, klin. Rundschau 15:833 and 906, 1901.

poral region was sensitive to percussion. Examination of taste, smell and hearing gave normal results. There were no disturbances in the other cranial nerves except for the optic nerve. Motility and sensation of the extremities and of the trunk were entirely normal. The tendon reflexes, especially the patellar reflex, were active. No ankle clonus was observed; Romberg's phenomenon was not elicited. The function of the sphincters was normal. Examination of the visceral organs revealed no abnormalities. The urine was free from sugar and albumin.

The eyes were examined by Dr. Kuhn. The pupils were equal and 4 mm. in diameter. The left pupil did not react to light but reacted well in accommodation. The right pupil reacted immediately to light and in accommodation. Both eyeballs moved freely; no nystagmus was observed.

The left eye was amaurotic. The vision on the right was 5/20 (the measuring unit is not stated); it was not improved by glasses. There was right temporal hemianopia.

On general examination the patient, now 14 years old, appeared to be well developed and excessively well nourished (fig. 1). The body was 54 Kg. (118.8 pounds) in August 1901. The average weight of a boy of the same age and height was recorded by Fröhlich as 39 to 40 Kg. (The height of the patient is not recorded. From the average weight and the age of the patient, the height can be assessed as approximately 145 cm. [58 inches], which corresponds to the average height of a 13 year old boy. The excess of weight is approximately 36 per cent.) The adiposity had developed simultaneously with the appearance of the other symptoms. The chronologic connection was emphasized by Fröhlich. Under thyroid treatment the patient had lost 2.5 Kg. (5 1/2 pounds) in three weeks, and as previously stated he weighed 51.5 Kg. (113.3 pounds) on September 23. The fingers, with the exception of the terminal phalanges, were plump; the hands appeared to be well padded. The bony structures did not in any way take part in the increase in volume. The largest accumulation of fat was in the subcutaneous tissue of the trunk, particularly on the abdomen and in the neighborhood of the genitals. There the accumulation of fat was so enormous that it protruded markedly around the genitals. The penis, which was normally developed, appeared so deeply embedded in

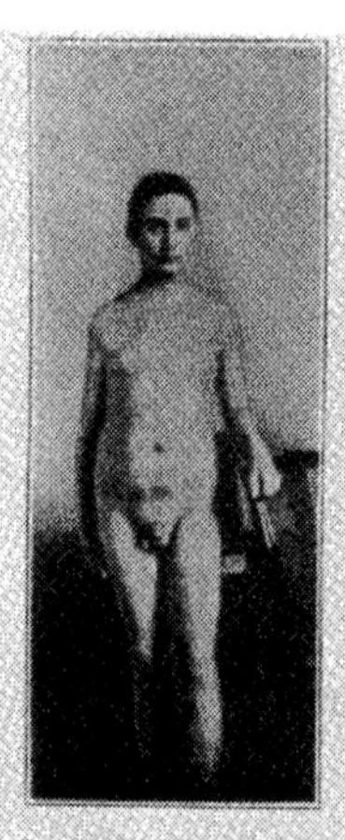

Figure 1

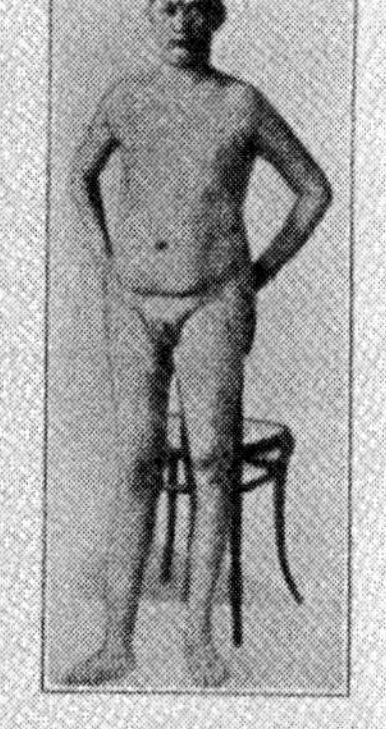

Figure 2

Fig. 1.—The patient at 14 years of age. The plate is reproduced from Fröhlich's publication.[1]

Fig. 2.—The patient after operation; the age was not stated. The plate is reproduced from Biedl's book.[4]

the fat tissue that the genitals approached the feminine type. The testes were small but were palpable in the depth of the masses of fat. Another considerable accumulation of fat tissue was observed in the mammary regions. A few small nodules could be felt in the mammary glands; no fluid could be expressed. Axillary hair was absent; at the genitals a few fine hairs were noted.

The hair of the skull was brittle, short and scanty; it had been falling out since the beginning of the disease. The skin was dry and scaling in many places. Over the trunk it could be lifted in thick folds together with the subcutaneous fat tissue. In other regions, especially over the fingers and wrists, the skin gave the impression of being somewhat thickened. The nails had been growing rapidly; the patient stated that even though he cut them every three days, they grew to a considerable length during that period.

On the basis of the clinical course and findings, Fröhlich made the diagnosis of neoplasm of the hypophysis. The arguments by which he supported this diagnosis will be reported in the discussion.

The patient was demonstrated in Vienna at a meeting of the Society for Psychiatry and Neurology on October 12. In a footnote of the publication, a subsequent examination of the eyes is recorded. On November 12 the inner half of the right papilla showed marked reddening; it was opaque and slightly swollen. The diagnosis of neuritis nervi optici was made.

Tumor of the Body of the Pituitary without Acromegaly and with Arrest of Development of the Genital Organs

Joseph P. Babinski

The anatomical and clinical observation that I report here succinctly is incomplete and thus subject to criticism; it seems to me appropriate to be related in spite of these imperfections.

The case is of a young girl, 17 years of age, that I observed 10 years ago. She complained of headaches, which appeared about three years before presentation, which increased in intensity little by little to become very violent. For several months she was subject to epiliptiform crises and her vision diminished.

One is struck after having undressed the patient by excess adipose tissue on the body and the infantile

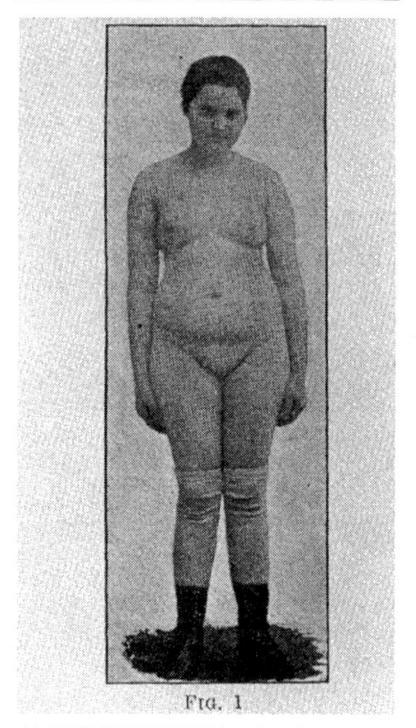

FIG. 1

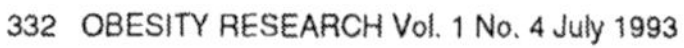

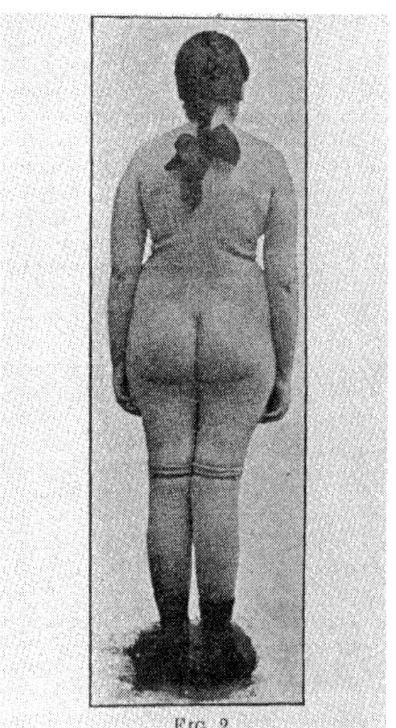

FIG. 2

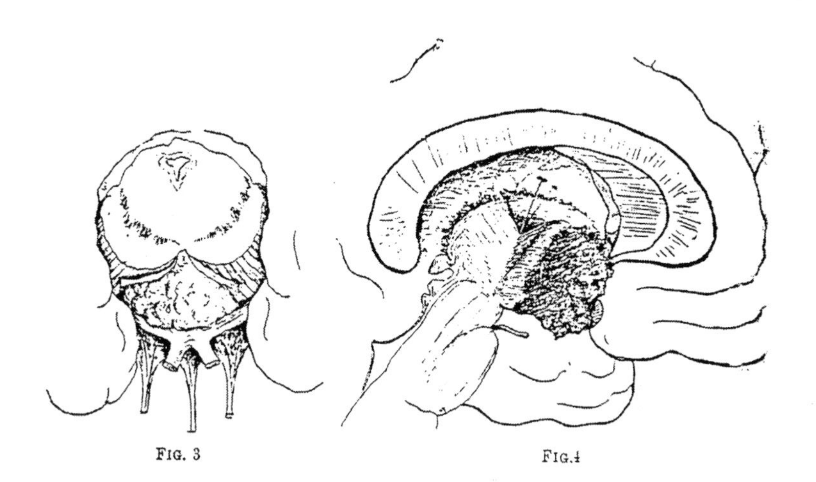

FIG. 3

FIG. 4

nature of the genital organs (Figures 1 and 2) which contrasted with her median height; the patient had not begun to menstruate. Her intelligence appeared normal, but her memory had diminished a lot for some time. There was no localized paralysis. The tendon reflexes were exaggerated and there was an epiliptiform trepidation of the foot. The ophthalmoscopic examination showed edema of the papilla in both sides. These are the objective findings which were noted.

The patient succumbed a short time after the first examination.

The autopsy showed the existence of a tumor which occupied the sella turcica adhering to the body of the pituitary and engulfing the tuber cinereum (See Figure 3 and 4 executed after a drawing of my friend or M Meige.) This neoplasm was examined histologically by Mr. Onanoff, who used this study material as the basis of his thesis (1). It appeared to Mr. Onanoff that an epithelioma developed from the epithelium of the pituitary gland. The epithelioma was of Malpigian type. The growth was taking place by indirect division in the conjunctival stroma which showed myxedematous degeneration.

The ovaries and uterus were very small; based on their dimensions they seemed to represent those of a girl age 8-10 years.

This observation is interesting from two points of view. First, there was an absence of acromegaly or gigantism in spite of the presence of a large tumor of the pituitary body; but in truth for this observation to be instructive, it would be necessary to know to what extent the gland had been altered. The other observation of interest was the coexistence of the pituitary lesions and of infantilism, characterized by the arrest of genital organ development. It is true that given the thyroid gland had not been examined one might suppose that this gland was altered and that the infantilism was under the dependence of the presumed thyroid lesion. However, it seems to me that the idea of a cause and effect relationship between the tumor of the body of the pituitary and infantilism is very acceptable. One knows, in effect, that the lesions of the hypophysis which appear in adults can bring on troubles with the genital organs, the suppression of regels and atrophy of the uterus. It thus seems very natural to believe that the appearance of the lesions in childhood produced an arrest in the development of the genital organs.

(1) ONANOFF. Sur un cas d'épithélioma. Thèse de Paris. 1892.

Babinski MJ. Tumeur du corps pituitaire sans acromegalie et avec arret de developpment des organes genitaux. Rev Neurol 1900;8:531-533.
"I am indebted to Dr. Andrea Spurti (Pennington Biomedical Research Center, Baton Rouge, LA) for translating this paper." –Dr. George A. Bray. Special thanks to the Pennington Biomedical Research Center Information Center, Baton Rouge, LA, for help in acquiring this document.

Neuropathology Communication from Dr. Mohr, Privat Docent in Würzburg

Bernard Mohr

4. Hypertrophy (myelin degeneration?) of the *hypophysis* and its pressure on the ventral *brain* surface, particularly on the optic tract and *chiasm* and the left hemisphere.

Moser, Elisa, 57 years old, wife of a gardener, was admitted to the hospital on October 22, 1839. From the patient herself, little information was obtained for anamnesis because of her poor memory, but from her friends and family members the following information was secured. M. has been suffering for 6 years (possibly the cessation of her *menses*?) from dizziness and periodic headaches. Three years ago she fell into a condition of mental disruption, which disappeared with a few weeks of bloodletting and cathartic-therapy. However, periodic memory loss, difficulty in her movements, impaired vision, headaches, and dizziness became more and more pronounced, so that the patient could only incompletely take care of housework. A few times she was found in a state of semiconsciousness lying on the floor. Further, the patient had become uncommonly obese over the last few years, and exhibited an immature, childish behavior not noticed in her earlier years. About five weeks before her admission, she was treated at the clinic for the symptom of pre-apoplexie.

Present Status. Large, round, dark-reddish face; joyful face expression; glossy "flimmery" eyes; dizziness; some ear noise; weakness in upper and lower extremities, more pronounced on the right side, with a sensation of tingling in the finger tips. Decreased sensations on the right half of her body, including face; involuntary urination; fairly regular, weak pulse; distant heart sounds with slightly increased impulse; normal digestion. Uncommonly extreme obesity. Inconsequent replies, at times with quite good grasp of surrounding, at times with mixing up everything around her.

These symptoms remained the same for weeks, only infrequently interrupted by paroxysms and the signs of strong cerebral congestion (head congestion), like weak pulse, slow respiration and memory loss. After four weeks, these signs appeared more frequently (1-2 times per week), and the patient cried out and was unconscious for periods of 15 minutes, at the end of which she fell into a long stupor. At the same time, the weakness in the right body, particularly the right arm, became more and more pronounced, and vision of the right eye decreased rapidly. Involuntary defecation and urination were also present. The behavior of the patient is now very childish, immature, with almost complete loss of memory.

Without a clear prior prodrome, she experienced an apoplectic event of insult at 5 a.m. on December 19th, with the following ensuing picture: total unconsciousness and speechlessness, dark red, hot face, closed eyes (right eyeball was retracted and pulled upwards, the left eyeball was protruding outward and pointed upwards, both were insensitive to stimulation); tetanic stretching of both upper extremities (hands turned inwards, particularly the thumb, all very stiff, particularly the left hand); stertcrous, slow, intermittent respiration; very slow, weak pulse; repeated vomiting. After a few hours, the right hand stopped moving, involuntary defecation, and continuous absence of consciousness. This condition remained more or less the same until the evening, only respiration became more intermittent and stertcrous, the extremities cool, the pulse diminished, and the patient passed away, lying on her back at 5:30 a.m.

Autospy on December 21st, 45 hours after death. Body of medium size; diminished stature; extremely obese; short and large neck; Thorax short and wide, moderately arched; abdomen of extreme dimensions due to fat tissue in the subcutis (thickness 3-1/2 inch).

Head. Cranium with round shape and thick wall, deep grooves along the sagittal suture to hold the strongly developed, collection of glands that perforate the meninges. *Dura lightly* stretched over the voluminous hemisphere which seem too large for the cranium. Inner surface of dura is unusually dry, like a serous membrane that had been exposed to air for considerable time. Convex surface of hemispheres strongly arched, *planum convexum* without noticeable extrusions and crevassed (the gyri were completely flat, the *sulci* were only imprinted by the venous blood vessles of the inner meninges), like it was covered by a dried out fat layer. Above the *sella turcica,* there was an elliptoid, slightly uneven, soft tumor that was: 1) covered by the inner meninges 2) showed a red-brown cutting surface; 3) was infiltrated by numerous blood-rich new blood vessels; 4) expelling a greyish-yellow, pus-like fluid that turned more and more red with blood mixing in; and 5) that shrunk considerably after emptying the fluid. The degenerated pituitary gland was connected to the ventral brain surface by some gelatinous infiltrated tissue and a cylindrical appendix (the *infundibulum*), which was expanded by water, but at the same time much shorter.

Through an incision of the latter, several ounces of serous fluid emptied rapidly, so that the convex surface of the hemispheres collapsed noticeably. On the sella turcica, the tumor had produced a more or less circular impression of 1 1/4 inches in diameter, with partially denunded bones that felt rough to the touch. On the other side, the tumor produced an impression on the corresponding parts of the ventral brain surface with an anterior posterior diameter of 3 1/2 inches, a maximal width of 2 1/2 inches and a maximal depth of 2 inches. The cavity occupied the space between the anterior rim of the "Varolsbruke" and the anterior border of the hemispheres, with a considerably larger impingement on the left hemisphere. The left ventricle as well as the optic nerve and chiasm, was enlarged on the left side and showed signs of pathological deformation.

Examination of the upper brain surface showed the following results. Neuropil generally soft, but at the same time being dough-like tough, rich in blood, towards the ventricles more dense. Ventral surface of Corpus callosum was covered by apparently serous membrane, which was smooth to the touch and watery glossy. Anterior horn of lateral ventricles, particularly the left one, enlarged. Straitum almost as wide as normal, almost completely flattened; thalamus somewhat widened, less than normally arched. The descending and posterior horns of the lateral ventricles were normal. Fornix somewhat flattened, anterior and posterior commissure torn. The bottom of the third ventricle was removed together with the tumor. Colliculi apparently normal, as well as pineal gland, aqueduct and forth ventricle. Cerebellum somewhat soft, but otherwise normal.

Thoracic cavity. Lungs completely free, strong crackling sound when cut, in the right lower lobe full with foamy blood. Heart heavily infiltrated with fat tissue, large (1/3 larger than normal), relaxed, in the walls of its left half, in presence of moderately enlarged ventricle.

Abdominal cavity. Liver large, brown-red, cut surface shows fatty gloss, mallow, friable, with little blood. Gallbladder contains more than hundred, tetrahedric, polished, green-yellow, very dense gallstones, that had the size of between pinheads and cherry stones, and were connected by a stringy cement-like substance. Gallbladder mucosa was thickened, tough, at places lively reddish, with fact-like crevasses. Rest of abdominal viscera with very uncommonly large fat deposits in the folds of the peritoneum, particularly in the mesenterium (which was several fingers thick).

Mohr B. Hypertrophie der Hypophysis cerebri und dadurch bedingter Druck auf die Hirngrundflache, insbesondere auf die Sehverven, das Chiasma derselben und den linkseitigen Hirnschenkel. Wschr ges Heilk 1840;6:565-571.

"I am indebted to Dr. Hans Berthoud (Pennington Biomedical Research Center, Baton Rouge, LA) for translating this article." –Dr. George A. Bray.
Special thanks to the Pennington Biomedical Research Center Information Center, Baton Rouge, LA for help in acquiring this article.

The Basophil Adenomas of the Pituitary Body and Their Clinical Manifestations (Pituitary Basophilism)[1]

Harvey Cushing, M.D.
Professor of Surgery, Harvard Medical School

Introduction. In a long since superseded monograph on the pituitary body and its disorders, published in 1912, a section was devoted to a group of cases which showed peculiar and sundry polyglandular syndromes. It was stated at the time that the term "polyglandular syndrome" implied nothing more than that secondary functional alterations occur in the ductless-gland series whenever the activity of one of the glands becomes primarily affected; and further, that the term, as employed, was restricted to those cases in which it was difficult to tell where the initial fault lay.

That a primary derangement of the pituitary gland, whether occurring spontaneously or experimentally induced, was particularly prone to cause widespread changes in other endocrine organs was appreciated even at that early day, and it was strongly suspected that this centrally placed and well protected structure in all probability represented the master-gland of the endocrine series. The multiglandular hyperplasias of acromegaly, so evident in the thyroid gland and adrenal cortex, were already known, and the no less striking atrophic alterations in these same glands brought about by the counter state of pituitary insufficiency were coming to be equally well recognized. But in spite of these hopeful signs, we were still groping blindly for an explanation of many other disorders, obviously of endocrine origin, like those associated with pineal, parathyroid or suprarenal tumors. Out of this obscurity, those seriously interested in the subject have, step by step, been feeling their way in spite of pitfalls and stumbling blocks innumerable.

Cushing H. The basophil adenomas of the pituitary body and their clinical manifestations. Pituitary basophilism. *Bull Johns Hopkins Hospital.* 1932;L:137-195.

Reprinted with permission from The Johns Hopkins University Press, 2715 N. Charles Street, Baltimore, MD 21218-4319.

All figures from this reprint which relate to Case 1, except for figure 4, have been deleted. Additional illustrative material on Case 1 from Cushing's 1912 monograph (original ©J.B. Lippincott) have been included at the end of the article.

Thanks to Judy Roberts and Sandra Graves of the Pennington Information Center for help in acquiring this document.

The usual method of progression has been somewhat as follows. A peculiar clinical syndrome has first been described by someone with a clarity sufficient to make it easily recognizable by others. This syndrome in course of time has been found to be associated either with a destructive lesion or with a tumefaction primarily involving one or another of the organs in question. These tumefactions have proved in most cases to be of an adenomatous character and it was finally recognized (first in the case of the thyroid) that adenomata of this kind were functionally active structures that produced hypersecretory effects. It then gradually came to be realized that the tumor need not necessarily be bulky but, quite to the contrary, striking clinical effects might be produced by minute, symptomatically predictable adenomas. So *it is the degree of secretory activity of an adenoma*, which may be out of all proportion to its dimensions, *that evokes the recognizable symptom-complex in all hypersecretory states.*

The pituitary adenomas. The anterior-pituitary body, as distinct from the neuro-hypophysis, is a compact of cellular elements of three recognizable sorts, divided by histologists, on the basis of their staining reactions, into two principal types: [1] those having a non-granular cytoplasm, and [2] those with a cytoplasm which is distinctly granular. Cells of the former type are known as neutrophil (chromophobe) elements and of the latter–the granular type–as chromophil elements of which there are two sorts: (a) those whose granules show an affinity for acid dyes (acidophil cells) and (b) those with an affinity for basic dyes (basil or cyanophil cells). Each of these three cellular types–chromophobe, acidophil and basophil–is capable of producing its own peculiar adenomatous formations.

Whether these three types of cells are fixed in char-

[1] The subject matter of this paper was ventilated at the New York Academy of Medicine, January 5, 1932; at the Yale Medical School, February 24, 1932, and at the Johns Hopkins Hospital Medical Society, February 29, 1932.

acter or whether they represent different stages in activity of the same original cell is a matter of dispute. The most recent advocate of the unitarian view is Remy Collin of Nancy who, purely on anatomical grounds, presents[2] a convincing argument to show that the non-granular cell (*cellule principlae*: mother-cell) represents the primitive stage of activity of an element which in the process of ripening acquires a granular cytoplasm that is primarily acidophilic (eosinophillic) but which may in turn become basophilic (cyanophilic). When the ripened granular cytoplasm comes to be discharged, little is left but the nucleus and membrane of the cell which may then either degenerate or, in a renewed cycle, once more pass through these same stages to be again discharged under proper stimulus.[3] But if this is actually what takes place, the fact that each of these varieties of cells is capable of forming adenomata whose elements appear to be of fixed rather than of a changing type is highly peculiar. What is more, one would naturally expect that adenomata composed of the non-granular mother-cells (*Hauptzellen: cellules principales*) would be more likely to show evidences of cell division than would adenomata composed of elements in the more advanced stages of secretory activity. But just the opposite occurs; the elements composing the common chromophobe adenomata rarely if ever show cell division, whereas those of a chromophil adenoma, whether acidophilic or basophilic, are frequently multinuclear and show numerous mitotic figures.[4]

Meanwhile, experimental pathology has provided us with some fairly definite facts concerning the function not only of the anterior pituitary considered as a whole, but, in turn, of its different cellular constitiuents. When its frequent association with a pituitary tumor came to be recognized, it was at first supposed that acromegaly was an expression of glandular deficiency and theoretically should be reproducible by experimental extirpation of the gland. This, however, in the majority of cases led to early death, at least of adult animals (chiefly dogs), whereas younger animals when hypophysectomized, though they might recover for long periods, ceased to grow and remained sexually infantile.

It had already been observed that tumors, grossly indistinguishable in situation and type from those associated with acromegaly, were of far greater frequency and provoked a syndrome, so far as its endocrinological manifestations were concerned, of a wholly different character. Individuals affected by these tumors when of adult age, instead of a tendency to overgrowth, showed on the contrary a tendency to become adipose, to lose their secondary sex-characters, and to become impotent, in company with recognizable atrophic changes in the sexual organs. When altogether comparable changes were seen occasionally to occur in animals (dogs) after incomplete experimental hypophysectomy, it became evident that the syndrome represented a deficiency state which was termed *hypo*pituitarism; and this furnished an added reason to assume–what had already been conjectured–that acromegaly almost certainly represented the counter state of *hyper*pituitarism.[5]

The final experimental proof of the correctness of this assumption was delayed until Evans and Long,[6] by daily parenteral injections of an alkaline anterior-lobe extract, succeeded in producing experimental overgrowth (gigantism) in the rat, an animal whose epiphyses do not close throughout life; and subsequently in the dog, whose epiphyses like those of man normally do unite. Putnam, Benedict and Teel[7] produced a condition of overgrowth comparable in all respects to that characterizing acromegaly.

But this is only half the story. There was evidently a complicating element in these experiments. If only a single pituitary principle (hormone) had been involved in experimental hyperpituitarism of this kind, one might well enough have expected increased growth to go hand in hand with increased activation of the reproductive functions. But quite to the contrary, while the injections unmistakably served to promote growth, they at the same time checked the normal ovulatory cycle of the animals. In consequence of this observation, Dr. Evans was led to suspect the presence of dual glandular hormones and he came to believe, indeed, that they were in some peculiar way opposed in their action.

[2]Collin R. La neurocrinie hypophysaire. *Etude histophysiologique du complexe tubéro-infundibulo-pituitaire*. Paris: G. Doin et Cie; 1928:102 pp.

[3]Nothing of precisely this same sort, to be sure, occurs in other glands of internal secretion; but this need not unduly disturb us, for the pituitary body, whether taken from a morphological or functional aspect, is a tissue of surprises. It is now recognized by histologists that secretory cells discharge in three different ways. They may merely extrude their accumulated granules without particular change in form, as in mammary secretion; or the entire cell may be cast off, as in sebaceous secretion–and this apparently is what takes place more particularly in the neurohypophysis from whose epithelial envelope (pars intermedia) degenerating cells are cast off which migrate through the pars nervosa where they become transformed into the hyaline bodies that presumably represent the active principle of this part of the gland.

[4]It would seem that the only possible way this question of fixity or changeableness of the elements composing pituitary adenomas could be conclusively answered would be by cultivating the cells of the different types to determine whether they breed true to their original form or whether their cytoplasm undergoes progressive alteration. Efforts in this direction have so far proved uncovincing owing largely to technical difficulties due to want of experience with the artificial growth of neoplastic tissues.

[5]Cushing H. The hypophysis cerebi: clinical aspects of hyperpituitarism and of hypopituitarism. *JAMA*. 1909;*53*; 249-255.

[6]Evans HM, Long JA. The effect of the anterior lobe administered intraperitoneally upon growth, maturity, and oestrous cycle of the rat. *Anat Record*. 1921;21:62-63.

[7]PutnamTJ, Benedict EB, Teel HM. Studies in acromegaly. VIII. Experimental canine acromegaly produced by injection of anterior lobe pituitary extract. *Arch Surg*. 1929;18:1708-1736.

[8]Teel HM, Cushing H. The separate growth-promoting and gonad-stimulating hormones of the anterior hypophysis: an historical review. *Endokrinologie (Leipzig)*. 1930;vi:401-420.

At another time and place a review has been given[8] of the steps leading to the disclosure that the growth-provoking and sex-maturing principles–the former almost certainly elaborated by the acidophil and the latter presumably[9] by the basophil elements of the lobe–are chemically separable hormones. Hence the former working conception of hyperpituitarism *versus* hypopituitarism as an indication on the one hand of secretory over-activity leading to acromegaly or gigantism, and on the other hand of secretory underactivity leading to a counterposed syndrome, wholly falls to the ground. Or, if not quite so bad as this, it at least must be replaced by hyperpituitary *versus* hypopituitary states due to excessive or insufficient secretion not only of the acidophil elements concerned with growth but also of the basophil elements chiefly concerned, presumably, with the ovulatory mechanism.[10]

In an attempt to interpret in terms of human pathology the highly informing later-day disclosures of experimental biologists, we may properly review, with necessary brevity, the development of the idea that the adenomas which affect the organs of internal secretion are not mere static conglomerations of cells but represent lesions possessing an incredible degree of physiological activity, those which have most recently attracted attention being the tiny adenomas of the parathyroid glandules and those of the pancreatic islets.

The common tumors of the anterior pituitary– first looked upon merely as a local expression of acromegalic overgrowth, and subsequently as a sarcomas or "strumas" of the gland–were first clearly differentiated by Benda in 1900 as varieties of adenoma; and we have slowly come to understand with some degree of definiteness the clinical pictures produced by those whose cells possess a granular and acidophilic cytoplasm and those with a non-granular or chromophobe cytoplasm. The former, even when so small that they may easily escape postmortem detection, are productive of unmistakable acromegaly or gigantism or a combination of the two. The more common chromophobe adenomas, on the other hand, usually attain a size sufficient to distort the chiasm before they give appreciable clinical symptoms, and it is quite probable that the cells which comprise them possess no secretory activity–that is, produce no hormone. They nevertheless cause their own peculiar constitutional disorder, this being a deprivation syndrome[11] brought about in all probability through compression of the residual acidophil and basophil elements which no longer are able to produce their peculiar secretory product.

This in general terms at least approximates the truth. It must, however, be admitted that there are certain borderline syndromes in which a primary wave of pathological overgrowth appears to have been succeeded by a hypopituitary state–a condition which for lack of a better term has been called "fugitive acromegaly,"[12] the adenoma in these states proving to be of a mixed cellular type. Though the cells of these mixed adenomas are predominantly chromophobe, a few of them show a peripheral disposition of acidophil granules suggesting the functional retrogression of previously mature acidophil elements; and since these cells resemble the hypoacidophilic ("hypoeosinophilic") stage of development as described by Collin, the observation might be construed as an argument favoring his views. In other words, the supposed functional immutability of the cells of an anterior-pituitary adenoma may prove to be a misconception; but this need not particularly concern us here.

Two examples of a third type of anterior-pituitary adenoma, composed of basophil elements, were first described twenty years ago by Erdheim [13] the tiny lesions having been looked upon as curiosities of morbid anatomy rather than as findings of any conceivable clinical significance. In one instance a small basophil adenoma, 1.5 mm. in diameter, was found in a woman forty years of age supposedly the victim of Basedow's disease. The other example was found in a 43-year-old acromegalic whose relatively small pituitary body was chiefly occupied by a fair-sized eosinophil adenoma, the minute basophil adenoma measuring only 1 mm. in diameter having been regarded as an accessory finding.[14]

[9]The evidence of this is suggestive rather than conclusive. It is based on the facts: (1) that following castration, at least in the rat though not definitely in other species, there is an increase in the basophil elements; and (2) that the extracts of the pituitary glands of castrates of all species are more active than normal glands in their gonad-stimulating properties. PE Smith showed, moreover, that the central portion of the bovine anterior-pituitary which is particularly rich in basophil elements has a more pronounced effect in stimulating the thyroid to activity than the more eosinophilic cortical portion of the gland. The effect of these injections on the adrenal cortex and the genital system unfortunatley was not noted.

[10]Time has shown that *hyper*pituitarism and *hypo*pituitarism are long words whose distinguishing syllable is easily misread and misprinted. And now that it becomes necessary or advisable to recognize two hypersecretory states, the terms *pituitary acidophilism* and *pituitary basophilism* are suggested as less unwieldy and more easily interpreted than acidophilichyperpituitarism (for acromegaly) and basophilic hyperpituitarism (for the syndrome under discussion).

[11]*Cf.* Henderson WR. Sexual dysfunction in adenomas of the pituitary body. *Endocrinology.* 1931;15:11-127.

[12]Bailey P, Cushing H. Studies in acromegaly. VII. The microscopical structure of the adenomas in acromegalic dyspituitarism (fugitive acromegaly). *Am J Path.* 1928;4:545-564.

[13]Erdheim J. Zur normalen und pathologischen Histologie der Glandula thyreoidea, parathyreoidea und Hypophysis. *Beitr f path Anat u Path.* 1903;33:158-234.

[14]It is quite conceivable that acidophil and basophil adenomata may not infrequently coexist in cases of acromegaly, but I know no other example than this in the literature. Such a coincidence might account for the differing syndromes shown by acromegalic patients some of whom exhibit disturbances which in the past we have been inclined to ascribe to the effects of secondary hyperplasia or adenoma-formation in the adrenal cortex.

PRESUMPTIVE EXAMPLES OF BASOPHIL HYPERPITUITARISM

After this explanatory digression, let us return to a consideration of the peculiar polyglandular syndrome to which allusion was made in the introductory paragraph. The original example of the syndrome around which the present discussion hinges was described in my monograph (Case XLV, page 217) as having shown *a syndrome of painful obesity, hypertrichosis and amenorrhoea with overdevelopment of secondary sexual characteristics.* Whether these symptoms were chiefly attributable to disordered pituitary, adrenal, pineal or ovarian influences was uncertain.

Case 1. (JHH Surgical No. 27140) Minnie G., an unmarried Russian Jewess, aged 23, referred by Dr. Stetten of New York, was admitted to the Johns Hopkins Hospital on December 29, 1910.

Clinical history. One of a numerous and healthy family, though slight and undersized, she was well until 16 years of age, having escaped the customary children's ailments.

Her menses which started at the age of 14 were regular for two years and then suddenly ceased. She began to grow stout and in the two years prior to admission her weight had increased from 112 to 137 pounds. She suffered greatly from headaches, nausea and vomiting sometimes accompanying the more severe attacks. She complained also of aching pains in the eyes which latterly had become prominent, and there had been occasional periods of seeing double.

Other noteworthy symptoms were insomnia, tinnitus, extreme dryness of the skin, frequent sore throats, shortness of breath, palpitation, purpuric outbreaks, recurring nose-bleeds, and marked constipation accompanied by bleeding piles. A definite growth of hair had appeared on the face with thinning of hair on the scalp. She had become increasingly round-shouldered. Muscular weakness had become extreme and there was constant complaint of backache and epigastric pains.

Physical examination. This showed an undersized, kyphotic young woman 4 feet 9 inches in height (145 cm), of most extraordinary appearance. Her round face was dusky and cyanosed and there was an abnormal growth of hair, particularly noticeable on the sides of the forehead, upper lip and chin. The mucous membranes were of bright colour despite her history of frequent bleedings. Her abdominous body had the appearance of a full-term pregnancy. The breasts were hypertrophic and pendulous and there were pads of fat over the supra-clavicular and posterior cervical regions. The cyanotic appearance of the skin was particularly apparent over the body and lower extremities which were spotted by subcutaneous ecchymoses. Numerous purplish striae were present over the stretched skin of the lower abdomen and also over shoulders, breasts and hips; and a fine hirsuties was present over the back, hips and around the umbilicus. The skin which everywhere was rough and dry showed considerable pigmentation, particularly around the eyelids, groins, pubes and areolae of the breasts. The peculiar tense and painful adiposity affecting face, neck and trunk was in marked contrast to her comparatively spare extremities.

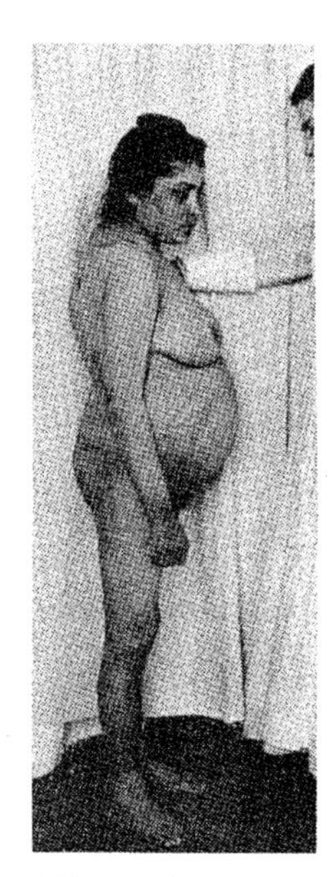

Figure 4. Case 1. The original example (1902) of basophil (unverified) obesity.

From a neurological aspect nothing was notable other than what at the time were taken to be signs of intracranial pressure: namely, headaches, slight exophthalmos, diplopia, puffiness of the eyelids and congestion of the optic discs [due, as would now appear, to deposition of introrbital fat]. The cranial x-ray showed what for the day was regarded as a normal sella turcica. The epiphyseal lines (radial and phalangeal) were still roentgenologically visible. Not only did the skin bruise easily but spontaneous ecchymoses frequently appeared. Lumbar puncture, pricking of ear, etc., caused subcutaneous extravasations. Blood examination showed 5,300,000 erythrocytes and 12,000 leucocytes (polymorphonuclears 77 per cent), with a haemoglobin of 85 per cent. The systolic blood pressure was consistently high, averaging 185 mm. Hg.

There were no clear therapeutic indications and she was discharged. She reentered the hospital again in July 1911, at which time, owing to the assumption that her continued cephalalgia might be due to intracranial pressure, an oldtime subtemporal decompression was performed, a wet brain being disclosed without subsequent protrusion at the site of the bone defect. She also at this time complained so greatly of backache and pain in the left side that an exploration of the kidney and adrenal gland was under contemplation.

It was at this stage of the story that the case was first reported. Its most striking feature was the rapidly acquired adiposity of peculiar distribution in an amenorrhoeic young woman. At the time, Dercum's adiposis dolorosa (usually a menopausal disorder), Bartel's and Fröhlich's adiposogenital dystrophy (commonly associated with hypophysial-duct tumors), and the adipositas cerebralis of Aschner and Erdheim (due to hypothalamic lesions) were but vague terms; and the possible relation of the basophilic elements in the anterior pituitary to the reproductive functions was not even suspected.

In commenting on the case at the time, it was pointed out that a somewhat similar polyglandular syndrome had previously been recorded not only in association with pinealomas but with adenomatous or hyperplastic adrenal tumors. A chance remark that we might be on the way toward the recognition of the consequences of hyperadrenalism may possibly have inclined some of those, who soon reported similar cases, to believe that the source of the trouble in all probability lay in the adrenal gland. To this I shall return.

The case of Minnie G. further: Because of her continued complaints with an increase of weight up to 151 pounds, on Dr. Stetten's recommendation she again came under observation for a period of two months from May to July, 1913, at the Brigham Hospital in Boston.

Her symptoms and general condition at this time were found to essentially unadulterated. Though there was no protrusion at the site of the old decompression, the optic discs were still hyperaemic and congested with hazy margins, while the fields of vision were contracted and the acuity considerably reduced. Her blood pressure fluctuated around 180/110, on one occasion reaching 210/140. She was still somewhat polycythemic, the erythrocytes slightly exceeding five million, the highest count having been 5,248,000 with a haemoglobin estimation of 105 per cent. Several differential blood counts were essentially within normal limits.

She was for a time studied by my medical colleague, Dr. Christian. On the basis of a defective excretion of phenolsulphonephthalein and the presence in the urine of a slight trace of albumin with occasional hyaline casts, he felt that a vascular type of nephritis was the probable cause of her hypertension. She was again discharged with no therapeutic recommendations.

On November 15, 1922, after an interval of nine years, she was for the second time admitted to the Brigham Hospital. It was then learned that her menses, after complete cessation for ten years, had late in 1913 again become irregularly re-established; also that in 1917 she had had an exploratory operation for a stone in the left kidney, but she was uncertain whether a calculus had actually been found.

The blood-pressure at this time averaged in the neighborhood of 160/95; the blood-count showed 5,240,000 erythrocytes; the basal metabolism was minus nine. Her general appearance was much as before, though she had lost some weight. The cranial roentgenograms taken at this time show [as subsequently reread] an unmistakable diffuse decalcification of the bones. Renal pyelograms were made, no trace of stone or other renal abnormality being disclosed. There was no evidence of advancing nephritis and on the whole she seemed at least no worse than in 1913. She accordingly was discharged once more without further light having been thrown on the nature of her disorder.

From correspondence it may be gathered that she at present (1932) is in reasonably good health though some of the stigmata of her malady still persist.

In the intervening years six other examples of the same or a highly similar disorder have been carefully studied at the Brigham Hospital. The patients were all comparatively young women who, in association with a more or less abrupt amenorrhoea, had become rapidly obese with a peculiar tense and more or less painful adiposity chiefly affecting head, neck and trunk. They were all plethoric in appearance, all had become abnormally hirsute, all but one showed purplish cutaneous striae. Vascular hypertension with a high red blood count and haemoglobin percentage was usually present, and all complained of aches and pains and general enfeeblement. In some of the cases the acuteness of the condition appeared to subside, and only one, so far as known, succumbed to her malady.

Meanwhile, soon after the case of Minnie G. had been reported in 1912, descriptions of polyglandular syndromes closely resembling hers began to appear in the literature; and in a few instances, owing to the fatal outcome of the disorder, a systematic study of the organs was made possible. Such of these case as have come to my attention may be given in the chronological order in which they appeared in print. The first of them was recorded in 1913 by Dr. H. G. Turney of London.[15]

Case 2. [Dr. Turney's patient.] *Amenorrhoea.*

[15]Turney HG. Discussion on disease of the pituitary body. *Proc Roy Soc Med.* (Sec Neurol and Ophth). 1913;6:lxix-lxxviii.

Acute plethoric obesity with hypertrichosis. Spinal kyphosis from skeletal decalcification. Vascular hypertension. Polycythaemia. Duration 7 years. Autopsy.

Miss A. O., a previously healthy and normal young woman, in 1907 when 20 years of age, suddenly ceased menstruating and began to grow obese. Three years later, she observed a tendency for her extremities to bruise easily. She gradually became increasingly round-shouldered (kyphotic) thereby losing two and a half inches (6.4 cm.) in height. Her chief complaints were of pain in the back.

The face was extremely fat and florid and the texture firm. The hair of the head was dry and somewhat scanty, as was the pubic and axillary hair, but there was a growth of fine short hair over the back and upper legs. Notable were the large pendulous mammae and the great obesity of the abdomen, which had the contour of a full-term pregnancy.

The obesity of the trunk was in marked contrast to the somewhat thin extremities which below the knee were of a dark brownish color, interspersed with recent ecchymoses. The skin had a parchment-like texture. Numerous broad, red, atrophic striae were present over the abdomen and thorax. An apparent partial absorption of the posterior clinoid processes was shown by cranial roentgenograms. A glistening subretinal exudate was present in the right eye, probably from an absorbed haemorrhage. The systolic blood-pressure was high, varying between 200 and 185 mm. Hg. There had been a tendency to polycythemia, the erythrocytes on one occasion having been counted at eight million and on another at six million. The urine contained no albumin. Carbohydrate tolerance was normal.

The subsequent history of this patient was briefly given in a later article by Dr. Parkes Weber.[16] Several spontaneous fractures occurred from time to time, involving sternum, clavicle, and ribs. Multiple ulcers and subcutaneous abscesses developed, and in May 1914, seven years from the symptomatic onset of the disorder, death ended the story.

An *autopsy* was performed. The body was that of an hirsute woman with "abundant hair on the chin" and multiple subcutaneous abscesses and ulcers. There was found a chronic nephritis, an hypertrophic ventricle of the left heart, a fatty infiltrated liver, and an enlarged left suprarenal gland of "bulky cortex." The ovaries were small. The bones showed calcareous deficiency ("fibrous osteitis") and were so soft they could be easily cut with scissors. "Nothing abnormal was found in the pituitary and thyroid glands." [How thorough an examination of the former was made is not stated.]

Dr. Turney at the time of this report, while the patient was still living, apparently favored a pituitary origin for the symptoms, but this opinion may have been modified by the postmortem findings; Dr. Parkes Weber, on the other hand, in his subsequent discussion of the case appears to have regarded it as unquestionably due to a primary adrenal disorder. The next example of which I have knowledge was reported two years later (1915) by Dr. John Anderson of Glasgow.[17]

Case 3. [Dr. Anderson's patient.] *Amenorrhoea. Plethoric obesity. Hypertrichosis. Vascular hypertension. Asthenia. Duration 5 years. Autopsy: osteomalacia; adenoma of anterior pituitary and of adrenal cortex.*

A women, at the age of 23, in association with a menstrual irregularity which in two years was followed by total amenorrhoea, became increasingly obese, the adiposity sparing the limbs. The adipose areas were tender on palpation. She suffered much from headaches, pains in the chest and eyeballs, the eyes having become somewhat exophthalmic. She acquired a reddish complexion and facial hirsuties, developed a tendency to petechial haemorrhages and purpuric outbreaks on her arms and legs, the slightest contusion provoking ecchymoses. The systolic blood-pressure was 185 mm.; the red blood count approximated five million. Muscular weakness became extreme, and she finally died from increasing asthenia. The whole course of the malady was something over five years.

At the *postmortem examination*, arteriosclerosis with "chronic interstitial nephritis" was found. The ribs were brittle and easily fractured. the ovaries and uterus were senile in character; the thyroid was slightly enlarged; the parathyroids were normal, the thymus atrophic. In the medulla of one of the suprarenal glands which were "slightly enlarged" was a small pea-sized tumor, microscopically resembling the structure of the zona fasciculata. The anterior pituitary contained a small adenoma [type unrecorded] the size of a millet seed close to the pars intermedia. In the rest of the anterior lobe "the basophil cells were apparently increased at the expense of the eosinophil cells."

In his discussion of this case, Dr. Anderson expressed the belief that it was primarily a pituitary disorder, his interpretation being that it was an example of hypopituitarism [*sic*] with secondary hyperfunctioning of the suprarenal glands (hyperadrenalism) accounting for the development of the secondary male sexual characteristics. Needless to say, it was not well known at the time that true hypopituitary states are associated with atrophy rather than hyperplasia of the adrenal cor-

[16] *Cf. infra.*, Brit J Dermat. 1926.

[17] Anderson J. A case of polyglandular syndrome with adrenal hypernephroma and adenoma in the pituitary gland–both of small size. *Glasgow MJ.* 1915;83:178-192.

tex, a similar dystrophy likewise affecting the thyroid and reproductive organs.

In 1919, another example of a syndrome which appears to be related to the disorder under discussion was reported by Dr. Reichmann[18] from the Medical Clinic of Jena. Apart from a swollen and plethoric face, the patient was not adipose but on the contrary was rather emaciated. She showed vascular hypertension with negative urine. There was bowing of the back and she had lost several centimeters in height. Because of the prominence of the eyes and fullness of the lids she was supposed to have Basedow's disease. This was excluded as was also cardio-renal hypertension; and under the belief that the condition was ascribable to a sympathico-adrenal disorder the left adrenal gland was surgically removed with a fatality a few days later from a generalized peritonitis. The autopsy showed a cardiac hypertrophy, hyperplastic arteriosclerosis, skeletal osteoporosis with spinal curvature, the bones being easily cut with a knife. The pituitary body, while macroscopically normal, was found on section to contain within a compressed mantle chiefly composed of basophilic elements a tumor "resembling a small-celled sarcoma." This was found to be an adenoma composed of chromophobe cells some of which contained eosinophilic [*sic*] granules. The thyroid was small; the remaining adrenal was hyperplastic; the ovaries fibrotic.

In his discussion of the case, the author, if correctly understood, was inclined to regard it as a form of acromegaly, the hyperpituitary changes being confined to the thickened and cyanotic face; the other symptoms were ascribed to a secondary adrenal origin.[19]

Chronologically the next fairly unmistakable case of which I have knowledge was described in Professor Zondek's monograph (1923) on the ductless glands[20] among other examples of so-called pluriglandular insufficiency.

Case 4. [Dr. Zondek's patient.] *Amenorrhoea. Acute adiposity. Facial hirsuties. Spinal kyphosis. Glycosuria. Duration 5 years. Autopsy: Skeletal osteoporosis; pituitary tumor (adenoma?).*

This concerned a 24-year-old Russian woman who had previously been normal in all respects and in good health. At the age of 19, amenorrhoea set in and she began rapidly to grow adipose, accumulations of fat being limited to the head and trunk, while the extremities remained thin. She began to lose the hair of her head, whereas on the cheeks and upper lip a somewhat definite beard began to appear; and as time passed she became increasingly round-shouldered.

Glycosuria was found and the urine at one time showed as much as 3 per cent of sugar. The skin became pigmented, suggesting an adrenal disorder. The cutaneous dryness from lack of normal secretion strongly suggested myxoedema. Hence there were polyglandular disturbances which appeared to affect the function of the adrenals, thyroid, ovary and pancreas. She finally died of an intercurrent erysipelas.

An *autopsy* was performed. A marked osteoporosis of the skeleton was found, it being easily possible to cut the vertebral bodies with a knife, the spongy part of the bone having largely disappeared. There was follicular atresia of the ovaries, marked lipomatosis of the *pancreas*, an increase of colloid in the abnormally small *thyroid*, hypoplasia of the *thymus*, and capillary dilation of the *parathyroid glandules*. [The adrenal glands are not mentioned and presumably would have been had they shown any change.]

The *pituitary body* showed no apparent abnormality until examined microscopically when it was found: "that the anterior lobe was enormously reduced and diminished mesially to a narrow ledge. As contrasted with this finding, the intermediary layer, as well as the posterior lobe, was rather more than normally developed. Between the gliomatous fibres of the posterior lobe, there were enlargements of the intermediary spaces, the exact nature of which, whether hydropical enlargements or myxomatous degenerations, could not be determined. In the vicinity of the diminished anterior lobe a tremendously developed fibrous tissue was encountered, into which the glandular elements of the anterior lobe gradually passed over. As to the kind of destroying process, involving particularly the anterior lobe, no definite decision was possible, this being the more difficult, as there were nests of an adenomous-like structure enclosed in the masses of fibrous tissue. The identity of these cells with the anterior-pituitary cells could not with certainty be determined, but Professor Benda, who saw the specimens, favored more the diagnosis of a tumor arising from the hypophysial duct."

This briefly reported case, in which some clinical details are unfortunately lacking, was, properly enough, regarded as one of pluriglandular nature, the most significant postmortem findings seemingly having been the lesion of somewhat obscure nature in the anterior pituitary. The adrenal glands at least we may assume to have shown no abnormality. Attention may be drawn to the fact that, as in the two preceding cases, the bones were described as being markedly softened and fragile, so much so indeed, that in his discussion of osteomala-

[18] Reichmann V. Ueber ein ungewöhnliches Krankheitsbild bei Hypophysenadenom. *Deutsch Arch f klin Med.* 1919;130:133-150.

[19] It may be assumed from the postmortem findings that this was a typical example of pituitary basophilism. The case has not been counted because of the absence of adiposity of the trunk which is so marked a feature of all the others. It suggests that the disorder may not necessarily be accompanied by abdominous obesity.

[20] Zondek H. Die Krankheiten der Endokrinen Drüsen. Berlin: Julius Springer;1923: 287.

cia Zondek refers to this case (loc. cit., p. 235) as illustrating one type of the disease.

In the following year, 1924, Drs. B. S. Oppenheimer and A. M. Fishberg of New York published a paper[21] in which the association of non-nephritic hypertension with suprarenal tumors was under discussion. Two illustrative cases were given. The first of them was that of a man said to have had an acromegalic appearance who was found after death to have had a tumor of the suprarenal cortex associated with cardiac hypertrophy. It is merely stated that the head and neck organs were negative, no specific mention being made of an histological examination of the pituitary body. It need scarcely be said that adenomas of the adrenal and cardiac hypertrophy are common in acromegaly. However, I have no wish to pick possible flaws in this highly interesting paper but rather to call attention to the authors' second case which bears a close resemblance to those under discussion. The essentials of the clinical history are as follows:

Case 5. [Patient of Drs. Oppenheimer and Fishberg.] *Plethoric obesity. Facial hirsuties. Cardiac hypertrophy. Vascular hypertension. Glycosuria. Cutaneous pigmentation and abscesses. Duration 5 years. Death without autopsy.*

S. G., an undersized child, 12 years of age, was admitted to the Montefiore Hospital complaining of weakness and adiposity. In her sixth year she suddenly began to put on flesh and became disproportionately adipose, gaining about 75 pounds (34kg). She was seen by many physicians and treated symptomatically with various glandular preparations. About a year prior to her admission the parents noticed a change in coloration of the skin and the patient developed a tendency to fall asleep. A routine urine examination revealed 4 per cent of sugar. Polyuria and nocturia developed about this time. At the age of 11, hair began to grow on the face, axilla and pubis. The patient had never menstruated.

Physical examination. An undersized child, appearing many years older than her actual age. (figs. 10-12) She was exceedingly obese and had a very red, plethoric facies. There was a well marked growth of hair on the chin and lower cheeks; pubic and axillary hair was abundant. The skin was dry and on the abdomen were pigmented striae. There were abscesses on the back and neck, a mycotic infection of the nails, and ulcers on the legs. There was no oedema whatever.

The heart was enlarged to the left. The sounds were of good quality, the second sound being accentuated over the aortic area. There were no murmurs. The blood pressure was 190 systolic, 130 diastolic.

The urine contained sugar but no acetone bodies. There was a heavy cloud of albumin but neither casts nor cellular elements were found. Phenol sulphonephthalein elimination, 45 per cent (after intravenous injection). The basal metabolic rate was normal. The blood showed 260 mg. of sugar per hundred cubic centimeters; erythrocytes, 4,500,000; white cells 11,800 with 78 per cent polymorphonuclears; haemoglobin, 90 per cent (Sahli). Roentgenologically the sella turcica was slightly larger than normal and showed bone absorption in the neighborhood.

The patient was placed on an anti-diabetic diet and digitalized. The urine rapidly became normal; the sugar and albumin disappeared completely. At one time signs and symptoms of broncho-pneumonia appeared but cleared up. The abscesses of the neck and back finally healed. At this juncture, the parents insisted on removing her from the hospital and she died three weeks later. Though no postmortem examination was obtained, the clinical picture, in the author's words, "was so characteristic of suprarenal hyperplasia as to leave little doubt of the diagnosis."

It can be seen that the syndrome presented by this patient, though it was of preadolescent onset, bore a close resemblance to that of the others so far presented: viz., a rapidly acquired adiposity sparing the extremities, a plethoric facies with pigmented abdominal striae, an exaggeration of the secondary sexual characters accompanied by a growth of hair on cheeks and chin, vascular hypertension, and glycosuria. Her precocious secondary sex-characters were unaccompanied by any signs of menstruation.

The close resemblance to the original case of Minnie G. shown by these last four patients, in their symptomatic history, in their physical appearance, and in their clinical findings, is unmistakable. They are examples unquestionably of a highly similar polyglandular disorder the interpretation of which to this point remains highly obscure in spite of three postmortem examinations. A tendency to chronic nephritis with cardiac hypertrophy probably secondary to the hypertension was noted in Cases 2, 3 and 5. A peculiar softening of the bones was mentioned in all three autopsied cases. The adrenal glands showed a unilateral enlargement in Case 2, a pea-sized adenoma in Case 3, and are not mentioned in Case 4. The pituitary body was said to be normal in Case 2, to show a minute adenoma (type undesignated) in Case 3, and an "adenomatous-like structure" of undetermined nature in Case 4.

We now come to a particularly well recorded example of the disorder published in 1926 from which something more definite can be learned. I have taken the liberty of quoting fully from the author's vivid descrip-

[21] Oppenheimer, BS, Fishberg AM. The association of hypertension with suprarenal tumors. *Arch Int Med.* 1924;34:631-644.

tion[22] of the case.

Case 6. [Dr. Parkes Weber's case.] *Plethoric obesity. Amenorrhoea. Purpuric ecchymoses and cutaneous striae. Facial hirsuties. Exophthalmos. Vascular hypertension. Duration 4 years. Autopsy: cardiac hypertrophy; nephritis; pituitary adenoma (basophilic.)*

"The patient, Mrs. E. B., aged 28 years, an Englishwoman, suffers from a 'coarse' plethoric-looking type of obesity, chronic purpura, and large 'striae cutis distensae' ('striae atrophicae') of the trunk and limbs. The purpura recurs from time to time in the form of 'crops' of cutaneous petechiae and ecchymoses. Constriction of the veins of the arm at once produces ecchymoses. The 'striae' are of different dates and vary correspondingly in color, the newer ones being purplish, the older ones paler. The face is coarsely hyperaemic. The obesity is shown chiefly in the trunk, by the large fatty pendulous breasts and the corpulent projecting abdomen.

"The limbs are not specially large, and the legs below the knees are relatively thin and have a striking appearance. They show transverse 'striae' (like the thighs do), and besides petechiae and ecchymoses there is a peculiar brownish discoloration, especially over the anterior surface, resulting probably from previous multiple haemorrhages. Moreover, a good deal of the skin in front of both legs has become shiny or parchment-like owing to some atrophic change. In spite of the obese appearance of her trunk, her body-weight is actually only 54e kgrm. [119 pounds], her height being 159 cm. [5 ft. 3 in.].

"The blood-pressure is high, the brachial systolic blood-pressure ranging from 205 to 230 mm. Hg.[23] The urine contains a little albumin, but is practically free from tube-casts. The administration of 100 grm. of sugar causes the appearance of a little sugar in the urine. The blood-sugar, when fasting, is within normal limits, but the curve after the administration of sugar by the mouth reaches its maximum height only after two hours. The blood-count shows nothing special, excepting a moderate polymorphonuclear leucocytosis, possibly connected with pyorrhoea alveolaris; the thrombocytes are 180,000 to the c.mm. of blood. Ophthalmoscopic examination (Dr. C. Markus, June 5th, 1925): In both eyes there is optic neuritis with white foci surrounding the optic discs; no haemorrhages; no mascular changes. No tumour can be felt by abdominal palpation and no enlargement of the spleen or liver can be made out; by vaginal examination the uterus is like that of nulli-para; there is no sign of any intra-thoracic disease. By rontgen-ray examination the dorsum sellae turcicae gives only an extremely faint shadow, but the pituitary fossa appears of normal size. There is slight bilateral exophthalmos. The basal metabolic rate is 20 per cent above the normal....There is slight hairiness of the chin and upper lip. The Wassermann reaction is negative...

"The *history* is that the patient was a twin, her fellow twin being born dead. Her father and mother are both living, aged 56 and 49 respectively, and the blood-pressure of each of them is high. They have had eleven children, of whom only four are living....She was married in December, 1922, and has never been pregnant. Her menstrual periods ceased suddenly about September, 1921, but she had three slight periods again after her marriage. Since then (March, 1923) there has been complete amenorrhoea. About March 1922, she already began to get fatter, especially in the face and abdomen. But it is only since about March, 1923, *with the onset of permanent amenorrhoea*, that her chief symptoms have gradually developed; headaches, pains in her whole body, attacks of dyspnoea (accompanied by a sensation of suffocation), feelings of sickness (for which she sometimes induces vomiting by putting her finger in her mouth), frequent slight, epistaxis, the 'coarse' type of obesity already mentioned, the cutaneous 'striae,' the purpura, the slight exophthalmos.

"The patient died on July 4th, 1925, in an attack clinically resembling acute pulmonary oedema. She had had a similar attack previously in the hospital, relieved apparently by blood-letting."

At the *postmortem examination*: There was no tumour in either *adrenal gland*, but the medullary substance was apparently rather in excess. The left ventricle of the heart was hypertrophied. There was slight chronic interstitial nephritis (slight renal sclerosis). In the anterior lobe of the *pituitary gland* was a minute adenoma consisting of basophil cells. There was no evidence of disease in the *thyroid gland* or in the *ovaries*; the latter were said to have been rather small but histologically normal.

Microsopical examination "The *pituitary gland*: Its three parts can be easily distinguished. In the anterior part is a rounded nodule (3 x 4 1/2 mm. in the hardened sections) of basophil cells, in alveolar arrangement (with some minute calcareous spots), contained in a thin connective-tissue capsule; it is evidently a basophil adenoma. The remainder of the anterior part and the middle and posterior parts of the pituitary gland are of normal appearance. In the anterior lobe-spur of the pedicle of the pituitary gland there are many relatively large epithelial islands (Erdheim) [cf. Case 4]. This is

[22] Parkes Weber F. Cutaneous striae, high blood-pressure, amenorrhoea and obesity, of the type sometimes connected with cortical tumours of the adrenal glands, occurring in the absence of any such tumour–with some remarks on the morphogenetic and hormonic effects of true hypernephromata of the adrenal cortex. *Brit J Dermat.* 1926;38:1-19.

[23] On May 31st, when the brachial systolic blood-pressure was 220 mm. Hg., the brachial diastolic blood-pressure was 170 mm. Hg.

remarkable, but must not be considered pathological. No special immigration of cells from the middle lobe into the posterior lobe can be made out."

Dr. Weber states in conclusion: "In my opinion it belongs to a group of cases characterized by complete amenorrhoea and by symptoms [given in the title of his paper] sometimes connected with cortical adrenal tumours, occurring in the absence of any such tumour. The main features cannot be explained by the small adenoma of the pituitary gland found at the post-mortem examination."

In search of further information regarding this important case, Dr. Weber was written to and he obligingly forwarded the original paraffin block from which further sections of the tumor have been made. He also referred me to Professor Herbert M. Turnbull of the London Hospital who first recognized the nature of the lesion as a basophil adenoma and who kindly sent me the accompanying photographs from the single section in his possession.

Much has been learned since 1926 concerning the influence of the pituitary body on the development and regulation of the genital system,[24] and Dr. Weber would have been more likely to-day than at that time to suspect the probable influence on his patient's syndrome of a pituitary adenoma which was then so easily explained away in favor of an adrenal influence even in the absence of any definite microscopical abnormality in these latter glands.

It was at about this time that it had become possible by crude chemical methods to separate the growth and sex hormones from bovine hypophyses and though Dott and Bailey in a study of the pituitary adenomas in Brigham collection had stated in 1925[25] that basophil adeniomata occur only in the form of minute intraglandular nodules that give rise to no known clinical manifestations, some of us soon began to suspect that this was probably a matter of not knowing what to look for.

This at least was the conclusion arrived at as the result of a survey of the then known facts regarding the dual anterior pituitary hormones which, chiefly for our own information, my junior co-worker, Dr. Harold Teel, and I shortly afterward came to put together.[26] The prepared mind was what enabled Dr. Teel during his house officership at the Lakeside Hospital in Cleveland for the first time to predict the presence of a basophil adenoma, as will be told, was confirmed at autopsy.[27]

[24] Cf. Smith PE, Engle ET. *Am J Anat.* 1927;40:159-217. Also: Zondek B. Aschheim S. *Klin Wchnschr.* 1927;6:248-252.

[25] Dott NM, Bailey P. Hypophysial adenomata. *Brit J Surg.* 1925;13:314-366.

[26] Teell HM, Cushing H. Theseparate growth-promoting and gonad-stimulating hormones of the anterior hypophysis: an historical review. *Endokrinologie* (Leipzig). 1930;6:401-420.

[27] Teel HM. Basophilic adenoma of the hypophysis with associated pluriglandular syndrome. *Arch Neurol Psychiat.* 1931;26:593-599.

The case history, which unfortunately is lacking in many details, may be briefly summarized as follows:

Case 7. [Dr. Teel's patient.] *Obesity. Hypertrichosis. Menstrual irregularity. Meningitis. Autopsy: basophilic adenoma.*

An exceedingly obese and abundantly hirsute young woman, 20 years of age, admitted to hospital in a comatose condition due to a meningococcal meningitis, was under clinical observation for only three days before she died.

Owing to her physical condition, a personal history was not obtainable, but it was learned that at the age of nine she had a continuous menstrual flow lasting four months. Subsequently, at the age of 14, she was said to have attained a normal adolescence, but her periods were subsequently most irregular. From the age of 15 she had grown exceedingly stout, the maximum weight of 206 pounds (93.4 kg) having been recorded seven months before her hospital admission. Because of excessive fatigability she had consulted a physician at about that time, and when he found she had a basal metabolic rate of +33, her enlarged thyroid was roentgenologically radiated. This was said to have caused little or no symptomatic improvement.

At *autopsy*, a suppurative meningococcic leptomeningitis was found to be the obvious cause of death. The pituitary body appeared to be of normal size, but suspecting from the patient's general appearance what might be found, Dr. Teel had the gland serially sectioned and a small though unmistakable basophil adenoma measuring 2.5 mm. in diameter was disclosed. There was a persistent thymus, a slight enlargement of the thyroid, questionable enlargement of the pancreatic islets, and a definite enlargement (20 gm.) of the suprarenals with no histological change of structure, no definite secondary adenomata being present in any of these organs. The ovaries were enlarged apparently from increase in stroma; there was a single large corpus luteum with a small central haemorrhagic area and several smaller ones in various stages of organization. The only true neoplastic growth was the small anterior-pituitary adenoma to which the other endocrine changes were regarded as purely secondary.

THE SYNDROME AS IT OCCURS IN THE MALE

To this point, examples have been presented of this peculiar polyglandular syndrome as it occurs in women who seem to be more commonly victimized than do men. Why this should be so, if it is actually so, is not fully apparent. It is perhaps reasonable to assume that the combination of amenorrhoea, adiposity and heterosexual hirsuties may excite the attention of physicians and be recorded as a freakish disorder more often than would corresponding maladies in men.

However this may be, five cases of the same or a comparable disturbance, three of them with and two without autopsy, can be cited in the male. The first case, unfortunately unaccompanied by photographs of the patient, was briefly reported after careful study by Dr. E.D. Friedman of New York.[28] The essentials only need here be given.

Case 8. [Dr. Friedman's case.] *Obesity. Hypertrichosis. Vascular hypertension. Glycosuria.*

E. C., a student, 19 years of age, complained of obesity, hypertension and recurrent pains in the region of the spine for six months.

He was an undersized young man who at the age of ten in the course of two months had grown rapidly stout. Treatment with thyroid extract was without avail. His abdomen became pendulous and face ruddy. More recently he had been having shooting pains in the region of the spine, chest, and abdomen. He was thought to have "kidney trouble." There was shortness of breath, palpitations and tremor on exertion, dimness of vision and occasional headaches with impairment of memory. Nycturia was present; libido absent.

Physical examination. The patient was round shouldered and short (136.5 cm.: 4 ft. 7 in.), obese (46.4 kgm.: 102 lbs.), with an erythematous face and a pendulous, distended abdomen. The mammae were well developed, the genitals small, and the fat distribution was of feminine type. There was an overgrowth of hair at the bridge of the nose and the body was covered with a fine lanugo. The heart was somewhat enlarged to the left. The skin, which was dry, showed ringworm in the axillae and pubes; erythema and telangiectasis of the face; and "striae distensae" on the abdomen and thighs.

Blood-pressure was 198/110 and there were two minute haemorrhages in the outer side of the left optic disc. The basal metabolic rate was –5 per cent. The urine showed glycosuria with a faint trace of albumin; the phenolsulphonephthalein excretion was diminished. The blood showed 95 per cent haemoglobin, 4,860,000 erythrocytes, 13,400 white cells of which 76 per cent were polynuclears. Chemical examination disclosed, in mgm. per cent, an excess of non-protein nitrogen (46.6); of cholesterin (308); and of sugar (240).

Roentgenograms: of the skull, showed markedly atrophic and thin bones of sella and sphenoid; of the hands, "a development of bones such as is usually seen in persons about 13 years of age."[Dr. Friedman informs me that the patient died of pneumonia in November of the year in which his report was made: there was no autopsy.]

It was recognized that this boy's syndrome had no relation to hyperpituitarism (acromegaly) nor to hypo pituitarism (syndrome of Fröhlich). This condition nevertheless was thought to be of pituitary origin though the tendency to hypertrichosis and high cholesterin content of the blood suggested an involvement of the adrenals.

In the same year as the forgoing (1921) a highly suggestive example with a detailed postmortem examination was recorded by Dr. Hermann Mooser from the Pathological Institute of Zurich then under the direction of Professor Busse.[29] Though the protocol specifically states that the pituitary body was normal, the case so definitely fits into the polyglandular syndrome under consideration it cannot properly be neglected any more than can examples of acromegaly without gross changes in the pituitary body be excluded in a general consideration of acromegaly.

Case 9. [Dr. Mooser's case.] *Acute painful obesity sparing extremities. Cutaneous pigmentation. Spinal deformity from osteoporosis. Duration three years. Autopsy: osteomalacia with multiple fractures; cardiac hypertrophy; atheromatous vessels; contracted kidneys; acute pancreatic necrosis; testicular atrophy. Pituitary body large but said to be normal.*

Clinical history. The patient, aged 27 (born in 1890), the eldest of eleven children, one of them a pituitary [?] dwarf, was an unmarried merchant, a polylinguist, and fond of sport. Previously spare and of slight build at the age of 24, while in military service during the autumn of 1914, he began to grow so stout as scarcely to be recognizable. The adiposity was so rapidly acquired that broad striae atrophicae appeared over the trunk and extremities. The tension of the skin was such it gave the disagreeable feeling of being electrically stimulated. Ere long, he began having pain in his spine, which the military surgeon thought indicated a tuberculous spondylitis and he was sent to a sanitarium. There his disorder was diagnosed as adiposo-genital dystrophy of pituitary organ.

The adiposity, which was confined to face, neck and trunk, progressively increased and the suffering from his tense skin which greatly disturbed his sleep became scarcely endurable. In the course of the next six months he became so weak he could scarcely hold a pencil or feed himself. He was given heliotherapy, which he bore badly, as it provoked alternating attacks of hyperaemia, cyanosis and sweating lasting from a few minutes to half an hour.

At first, there was little complaint of headache, but this for a time became more marked and later on again subsided. He was made sleepless by trembling of the body, noises in the ears, dreams and visions. He also

[28]Friedman ED. An usual hypophyseal syndrome. *NY MJ*: 1921;114:113.

[29]Mooser Hermann. Ein Fall von endogener Fettsucht mit hochgradiger Osteoporose. Ein Beitrag zur Pathologie der inneren Sekretion. *Virch Arch.* 1921;229:247-271.

complained of visual disturbances on moving his head. Ophthalmoscopic investigation, apart from a slight lessening of visual acuity, showed no abnormality. He had a marked polydipsia which obliged him to get up three or four times at night. The genitalia became dystrophic. The urine examination showed during 1916-1917 a slight trace of albumin with a few hyaline casts and no sugar; amount was not recorded.

His height diminished from 165 cm. in 1914 to 158 cm. in 1917. The body circumference increased from 91 cm. in November 1915 to 96 cm. in January 1917, with a gain in weight from 52 to 63.9 kgm.

Roentgenological studies in 1916 showed that the contours of the sella turcica were scarcely visible, the bones porous. An examination a year later showed these conditions to be still more advanced. There was apparent destruction of the bodies of the mid-thoracic vertebrae associated with a gibbus which was diagnosed in 1915 as osteitis vertebralis; in 1916 as spondylitis tuberculosa; in 1917 recognized as part of a non-tuberculous generalized porosity or decalcification of the skeleton.

Following a brief period of asthmatic dyspnoea and haemoptysis, he died on November 27, 1917, three years from the onset of symptoms.

Postmortem examination.[30] The body was that of a man whose head, neck and body were exceedingly adipose in marked contrast to his relatively thin extremities. The abdomen was likened to a pillow, the circumference being 99 cm. at the level of the navel. The color of the skin was everywhere strikingly brown, the region of the pelvis being of a lighter color, presumably from the fact that during his periods of heliotherapy this region was protected by swimming tights. Radiating scars were present on inner surface of thigh and upper arm. The hairiness of the lower body was normal in distribution.

Head: The inner part of the calvarium showed sharply circumscribed red spots, the largest of which had a diameter of 5 to 3 cm. The cerebral vessels were markedly atheromatous. The sella turcica was not enlarged. The hypophysis measured 14 by 8 by 7 mm. The neurohypopyhysis was plainly evident. The organ was put immediately in formalin. The base of the sella turcica was of red but smooth bone. Thorax: Subcutaneous fat 3.5 cm. thick. The ribs were found to be greatly softened; the upper part of the sternum greatly thickened. The heart was enlarged; the aorta atheromatous; the thymus not to be identified in the abundant mediastinal fat. The thyroid gland was fibrotic, difficult to cut, and contained but little colloid.

Abdomen: Panniculus 4.5 cm. thick; omentum exceedingly large and fat; perirenal fat abundant. The adrenal glands, though buried in fat, were of average size and of normal appearance. In the pancreas was found an area of central necrosis. The testes were small.

The investigation, particularly of the bones, showed that the thickened sternum was due to the callus of a healing fracture; several ribs also showed old healed fractures. The manubrium was intensely red and soft, and contained great holes of soft marrow. The ribs were easily cut, as was true of the spinal column, part of which was removed. The greatly compressed bodies of the vertebrae, in places only 1 cm. thick, were so soft they could easily be cut with a knife.

The gross *pathological diagnosis*: lipomatosis; osteomalacia (seu rachitis tarda); multiple fractures of the ribs; vertebral collapse; hypertrophy of the cardiac ventricles; atheromatosis of aorta and of the cerebral vessels; encephalomalacia of the right occipital lobe; fibrino-purulent peritonitis; necrosis of the pancreas; hypoplasia of the thymus; granular atrophy of the kidneys.

The principal histological findings of note were those relating to the peculiar structure of the softened bones. The kidneys showed slight glomerular fibrosis; the cerebral vessels an endarteritis proliferans. No abnormality was found in the adrenals, pineal or pituitary glands.

The small [from a Swiss standpoint] thyroid showed an increase of intralobar connective tissue with small and atrophic intermedial follicles; the single parathyroid detected was closely attached to the capsule of the thyroid, measured 4 by 3 by 2 mm., and showed an increase of connective tissue. The thymus could scarcely be identified in the mediastinal fat. The pancreatic islets were relatively few and atrophic in the part of the gland that had escaped necrosis. The testes also showed fibrosis with atrophic changes, though some active spermatogenesis was still present.

The outstanding symptomatic features of this remarkable case were: [1] The suddenly acquired, and peculiarly disposed, painful obesity; [2] The softening of the bones affecting the entire skeleton but more particularly the vertebrae, leading to multiple fractures (cf. Case 2); [3] The ultimate enfeeblement with fatality at the expiration of three years. In view of the slightly contracted kidneys, the enlarged heart and the arteriovascular changes found after death, vascular hypertension was probably present during life. Plethora was not particularly emphasized nor purplish abdominal striae, but pigmentation of the skin was noted by the pathologist.

The author, in his analysis of the case, comes to the conclusion that the disorder represents a polyglandular deficiency, and ascribes the skeletal decalcification to sclerosis of the parathyroid glandules; the adiposity was taken to be chiefly thyroidal in origin though something

[30]Professor Busse's detailed protocol is herein greatly abbreviated.

was to be said in favour of a pancreatogenous insufficiency. A possible pituitary origin was discussed only insofar as to point out the lack of resemblance of the syndrome to that of adiposo-genital dystrophy. Whether the gland was scrutinized for the possible presence of an adenoma is not apparent. The gross measurements were certainly in the upper limits of normal.

The next case, also with autopsy, figures in a report made from Professor Biedl's clinic in Prague in 1924 by Dr. William Raab[31] on the general topic of hypophysial and cerebral adiposity, or what is commonly called adiposo-genital dystrophy. The subject was approached largely from its roentgenological aspects, and it was a mere chance that in 1920 when preparing for my Lister Lecture[32] I happened to hit upon the fact in reading this paper that in one of the patients (Case 2) a basophil adenoma had been disclosed at autopsy. The photographs of the patient were so striking and bore such a close resemblance to the appearance of a patient at the time under observation in my own wards (*cf.* Case 11) that I felt little doubt but that they had been afflicted in all certainty with the same disorder. The translation of Dr. Raab's brief note of his case is as follows:

Case 10. [The Raab-Kraus case.] *Acute recent plethoric obesity, sparing extremities. Purplish striae. Backache with kyphotic spine. Death from infection. Autopsy: osteoporosis of skeleton; testicular atrophy; basophil adenoma of pituitary body.*

"Karel W., a man aged 31, showed gigantism of moderate degree (192 cm.), with very long extremities, externally well-developed genitalia and distribution of hair of normal masculine type. Patient complains of suffering from headaches for the past two weeks previous to his admission into the clinic and claims to have taken on 10 kgm. in weight during the same *[sic]* short period. This was confirmed by the family doctor.[33] The libido had always been rather low; he had been impotent for the past fortnight.

"There is a marked obesity of the face which appears, therefore, considerably disfigured when compared with former photographs (slit-eyes), and a marked adiposity of the abdomen. There is no adiposity of the long, slender extremities and of the nates. The abdomen is tremendously prominent and shows flame-shaped striae of dark-red color which are, in part, more than 2 cm. broad. The hips reveal the same feature. Weight 96 kgm. [211 pounds]. The X-ray plate shows a sella which, while not being excessively large, reveals nevertheless the characteristic deconfiguration produced by a process enlarging the intrasellar space. *Diagnosis:* tumor hypophyseos.

"The headaches improving and the weight remaining unchanged, the patient left the clinic, but returned in a few weeks, feverish and suffering from excessive pains in the lumbar vertebral column. Shortly afterwards he acquired a streptococcal phlegmon of the hand and died from acute sepsis in spite of generous incisions and amputation of his arm.

"The *autopsy* revealed an operculum sellae which was, as usual, concave; the pituitary body was scarcely enlarged; the posterior lobe was softened supposedly by postmortal changes. The pathologist emphatically denied the presence of a growth. Histologically, however, a small basophil adenoma was discovered which had almost entirely replaced the posterior lobe and showed central softening–a verification of the clinical diagnosis. An osteoporosis of extreme degree involving the vertebral column and the long bones accounted for the vertebral pain."

Further details of the postmortem examination of this case were given in a separate report in the same year (1924) by Professor E. J. Kraus[34] of Prague who has been kind enough to send me sections of the pituitary body for study, and whose personal description is translated as follows:

"The *autopsy* reveals besides signs of a general septic infection a marked enlargement of the pituitary body which, however, does not protrude out of the pituitary fossa. There was, in addition to these findings, a definite osteoporosis of the vertebral column, sternum and ribs, there being a slight degree of kyphosis of the thoracic spine. There was a small diffuse colloid struma of the *thyroid.* The *testes* were strikingly small. The thickness of the fat layer was on the neck 1.3 cm., on the upper arm 2 cm., above the sternum 2 cm., on the abdomen 3.5 cm., and the upper leg 2 cm.

"The *morphological examination* of the endocrine organs reveals: *hypophysis* 0.93 gm. In the posterior lobe there is an infiltrating basophil adenoma, situated especially in its anterior two-thirds, having destroyed about two-thirds of the adjacent substance of the anterior lobe. In the non-affected third of the lobe there are several small cysts as big as hemp-granules. The tumor, almost in its entirety, is sharply demarcated, slightly compressing the adjacent glandular parenchyma, and infiltrating the neurohypophysis. Furthermore, the tumor sends a pointed process into the stalk of the pituitary body, thus replacing about half of its cross-cut

[31]Raab W. Klinische und röntgenologische Beiträge zur hypophysären und zerebralen Fettsucht und genital Atrophie. (Case 2) *Wien Arch f inn Med.* 1924;7:443-530.

[32]Cushing H. Neurohypophysial mechanisms from a clinical standpoint. *Lancet* (Lond.). 1930;2:119-127; 175-184.

[33]In view of the postmortem findings of advanced testicular atrophy and decalcification of the skeleton, the disease presumably was of longer duration than this statement would indicate.

[34]Kraus EJ. Zur Pathogenese der Dystrophia adiposogenitalis. (Case 3) *Med Klinik.* 1924;20:1290-1292; 1328-1330.

area. The numerous eosinophil cells on an average are somewhat smaller in size than normal. There are strikingly few ripe basophil cells. Many cells which have lost their granules *(Entgranulierte)* represent former basophil elements. There are many mother-cells *(Hauptzellen)*, augmented apparently in relation to the diminished number of basophil cells. The pharyngeal-hypophysis could not be found in the many histological slides.

"The *pineal body* is of normal size and also histologically normal. The slightly enlarged *thyroid gland* contains much colloid, reveals enlarged vesicles, a partly cubic, partly flat epithelium, and a delicate interstitial tissue. Three *parathyroid glands* (weight together 9.16 gm.!) are strikingly infiltrated by fat tissue, and here and there occur rather large nests of oxyphil cells. The *pancreas* (weight 94 gm.) shows marked postmortal autolysis as do also the *adrenal glands*. The two *testes* (without the epididymes) weigh 18.3 gm. The canalicules of the testes have a delicate tunica propria. Spermatides, spermatoblasts and spermatozoa are wanting; only heads of spermatozoa are found in a very few canalicules. The epithelium for the most part shows four or five rows; the amount of lipoid is somewhat diminished. The interstitial cells are definitely diminished; the epididymes histologically normal."

Professor Kraus, if I understand him correctly, looked upon the hypophysial tumor as "an incidental finding" without relation to the clinical features shown by the patient, whereas Dr. Raab believed that the adenoma in some way influenced the secretory activities of the posterior lobe, the relation of which (pituitrin) to adiposity he has made the special object of study.[35] With neither of these views do I find myself in accord; and inasmuch as Professor Kraus not only was one of the first to describe basophilic adenomas,[36] but has since made other important contributions to the subject,[37] his seeming reluctance to correlate the adenoma with the clinical syndrome is the more surprising. This may be explained by the fact that only in later years, largely through the work of P. E. Smith and his collaborators, has the functional importance of these cells been pointed out. However this may be, I quite agree with Professor Kraus' opinion that the adiposal syndrome presented by this case was something wholly different from that seen in adiposo-genital dystrophy, which is a deprivation syndrome due usually to inactivation of the hypophysis by compression. The adipose disorder under consideration, on the contrary, is almost certainly due to a hypersecretory influence of some kind, and since the adrenal glands, apart from their postmortal change, were supposedly normal in this case whereas an adenoma was found in the pituitary body, the latter would seem to be the most probable primary seat of the trouble.[38]

We may now turn to the next of the male patients whose syndrome bears so close similarity to the foregoing case that even without a postmortem examination it may safely be ascribed to a lesion of the same primary sort. Fortunately the somewhat meagre clinical record for the preceding case, in which many details are missing, can now be supplied.

Case 11. (P.B.B.H. Surgical No. 37076) *Rapidly acquired and painful adiposity, sparing limbs. Purplish striae. Vascular hypertension. Glycosuria with azoturia. Progressive weakness till bedfast. Clinical diagnosis: basophilic adenoma. Radiotherapeusis of pituitary gland. Marked improvement.*

E. G. F., a dentist 30 years of age, referred for therapeutic recommendations by Drs. R. T. Woodyatt and A. R. Colwell of Chicago, entered the Brigham Hospital August 11, 1930, with the principal complaints of painful obesity, loss of strength, irritability, polyuria and polyphagia.

Family and personal history. The patient was one of twelve children of healthy parents, both living and well, none of this large family having had any known endocrinological disorders. He had been married for ten years and was the father of two children, the first of whom died following an instrumental delivery at birth, the second being a healthy girl one year of age. Until the past year the patient had always enjoyed excellent health. He was a tall man, standing over six feet, his normal average weight having been 160 pounds.

Present illness. This, he thinks, started five years before admission, when he began slowly to grow round-shouldered and stout. In the course of the next three years he gained 25 pounds and during the fourth year there was a more rapid gain of 35 pounds, his weight reaching 220 pounds (100 kgm.). He then began limiting his diet and finally succeeded in losing a few pounds, but under this régime he soon found himself without energy, easily fatigued, unable to concentrate

[35]Raab W. Das hormonal-nervöse Regulations-system des Fettstoffwechsels. *Ztschr f d ges exper Med.* 1926;49:179-269.

[36]Kraus EJ. Die Beziehungen der Zellen des Vorderlappens des menschlichen Hypophyse zeuinander unter normalen Verhältnissen und in Tumoren. *Beitr z path Anat u z allg Path.* 1914;58:159-210.

[37]Kraus EJ. Über die Bedeuting der basophilen Zellen des menschlichen Hirnanhangs auf Grund morphologischer Studien. Med Klinik. 1928;24:623-662.

[38]Kraus has pointed out, particularly in relation to hypertension, that whenever there is an hyperplasia of the adrenal cortex an increased number of basophilic cells are found in the anterior pituitary, and the reverse is true–namely, an adrenal hypoplasia is accompanied by few basophils. He suggests that the "hypercholesterinämie" of hypertension may be the common basis or at least play an important role.

his mind on his work, and fits of unnatural irritability alternated with periods of depression.

At this juncture he consulted a physician who resotred some carbohydrates to his self-imposed dietary restrictions. He immediately felt better but his weight quickly increased, his abdomen became prominent, and for the first time he noticed a peculiar disposition of localized masses of fat on his face and neck. These fat deposits, which appeared in symmetrical regions over the head (cheeks, temples, orbital region, supramental and suprasternal regious, as well as over the cervicodorsal spine), were at first soft, but tended to become increasingly firm and tense. They moreover were accompanied by most uncomfortable "drawing sensations," presumably from stretching of the cutaneous nerves. The tense skin over these swellings acquired a peculiar florid reddish-bronze color and showed telangiectases so altering his appearance that he was scarcely recognizable to his friends.

At about this time (December 1929) he began to have an excessive thirst associated with a polyuria which was more marked at night when he would be obliged to void from four to six times. He experienced also susceptibility to fatigue, forgetfulness, restlessness, palpitation on slight exertion, swelling of the feet and ankles, generalized weakness, and impotence. A distinct loss of body hair was observed.

In January 1930, he was found to have a glycosuria and this led to his admission to the Presbyterian Hospital in Chicago where, by Drs. Woodyatt and Colwell, his condition was carfully investigated at various periods during the course of the next six months. They found, to make the story short:

[1] "A slight *leucocytosis* of from 10 to 18 thousand, with some preponderance of neutrophilic polymorphonuclear elements; erythroctes in normal limits.

[2] "A variable *glycosuria* and hyperglycaemia, together with increased nitrogen excretion. On a diet with a daily glucose value of 201 grams, there was a daily excretion of 5.7 grams sugar (glucose) which was controlled by 50 units of insulin daily. This glycosuria was looked upon as a truly diabetic phenomenon, but it was accompanied by an unexpectedly great and wholly unrelated polydipsia and polyuria, the largest daily excretion observed having been 6720 cc. Attempts to modify this polyuria by pituitrin injections up to a dosage of 3 cc. in twelve hours were wholly ineffective.

[3] "*Azoturia.* On a diet containing 81 gm. of protein daily (13 gm. nitrogen), there was a daily nitrogenous excretion of 20-24 gm. despite approximate caloric balance. This loss was later balanced by increasing the protein intake. Since then there has been a continuous excretion in the urine of 20 to 30 gm. daily.

[4] "*Blood chemistry:* urea N. 19.0; uric acid 3.8; creatinine 1.1; total N.P.N. 36.0; chlorides 466; calcium 7.1-8.9; cholesterol 147.5 (all values in mg. per 100 cc. blood); CO_2 77.7 vol. per cent. Wassermann reaction negative.

[5] "*Basal metabolic rate:* minus 10% to plus 1% on repeated readings.

[6] "A moderate degree of *vascular hypertension,* from 165/70 to 178/100, without evidences of arteriosclerotic change.

[7] "The administration of iodine was without effect. One of the *fat pads* on the front of the neck was removed for study and proved to be fatty tissue of customary pannicular type."

Finally, when a suspicious *enlargement of the pituitary fossa* was roentgenologically detected suggesting a possible pituitary or hypothalamic disorder, he was referred to the Brigham Hospital for an opinion.

Physical examination (on admission). This showed a tall (184.2 cm.), extremely abdominous, and somewhat round-shouldered man with patchy adiposity of the face, neck and trunk, and comparatively spare extremities (weight 86.8 kgm.) All his movements, such as those incidental to rising from a chair, were obviously made with great effort, as though his limbs were scarcely strong enough to support his huge body. His face was peculiarly florid and dusky, and on forehead, cheek bones, temples, and chin were deposits of fat which were tender to the touch and covered by tense, glistening skin. Similar accumulations of fat were present on the anterior aspect of the neck and over the cervico-thoracic region in the back.

Owing to the puffiness of his face and eyelids, the palperbral slits were narrow, the eyes being injected and somewhat prominent. Vessels of the fundus oculi were exceedingly tortuous and the edges of the discs were blurred, but there was no measurable swelling. The fields of vision were normal.

Wide purplish striae radiated from the groins over the abdomen and smaller striae were present over medial aspects of both thighs. There was some pitting oedema about the ankles and some swelling of the hands, so that he was unable to remove a ring. He was partially bald and the hirsuties of the extremities and axillae was scanty, but there was abundant hair on the chest which was normal in deposition and texture. The skin of the axillae, groins and crotch was pigmented and scaly.

He was free from headache, but complained greatly of discomforts associated with the adiposity and also of variable pain in the back and shoulders. Roentgenograms were made of the entire skeleton, which in Dr. Sosman's opinion showed no evidence of decalcification. The pituitary fossa was not enlarged but the posterior clinoids appeared to show some absorption. No acromegalic changes were present. The spine and pelvis, so far as could be seen, were normal.

The blood examination, frequently repeated, averaged 4,600,000 red cells, 16,700 white cells, 85 per cent of them being polymorphonuclears. Haemoglobin was variously estimated at 90 to 100 per cent. The basal metabolic rate was −10 per cent; a specific-dynamic test with a 200 gm. steak-breakfast showed (possibly because of his nitrogen imbalance) a rise only to +4 per cent at the end of a four-hour period. The systolic blood-pressure was over 170 mm. of Hg., indicating a moderate vascular hypertension. There were no renal elements or albumin in the urine.

Blood Studies	August 18, 1930, Diet Unrestricted	August 22, 1930, Diet Restricted
Erythrocytes	4,600,000	4,260,000
White cells	13,000	9,200
Haemoglobin	13.88 gm.	13.32 gm.
Cells	40.9%	36.6%
Plasma	59.1%	63.4%
Individual cell volume	8.8×10^{-11} cc.	8.5×10^{-11} cc.
Blood iron	43.5 mgm. %	41.6 mgm. %
Blood sugar	219 mgm. %	164 mgm. %
Non-protein nitrogen	36.8 mgm. %	45.8 mgm. %
Amino-acid nitrogen	17.0 mgm. %	6.8 mgm. %
Blood urea nitrogen	9.0 mgm. %	18.0 mgm. %
Creatinine	2.2 mgm. %	2.4 mgm. %
Uric acid	5.9 mgm. %	3.88 mgm. %
Whole-blood chlorides	255 mgm. (NaCl)	290 mgm. (NaCl)
Calcium	10.0 mgm. %	10.0 mgm. %
Cholesterol	246 mgm. %	190.8 mgm. %
Total protein	7.05 gm. %	6.94 gm. %
Albumin	3.98 gm. %	3.02 gm. %
Globulin	2.91 gm. %	3.53 gm. %
Fibrinogen	0.16 gm. %	0.39 gm. %

When admitted to hospital, he was still on the somewhat restricted diet which finally had been worked out by Dr. Woodyatt as most effective in caring not only for the diabetes but also for the increased nitrogen output. In order to balance this and to keep up the patient's strength, it had been found necessary to increase the protein in the diet from 200 to 475 grams. He was taking in addition 65 units of insulin daily, divided into two doses, 40 in the morning and 25 at night. This, however, had been found in Chicago, as it was found here, to be most variable in its effect. His polyphagia was most striking. He was hungry all the time, and even when allowed a full meal, of which he would partake greedily, he would feel ravenous again after an hour's interval.

Laboratory studies. During his long hospital sojourn of 71 days, his condition was investigated from every angle, both when under dietary restrictions and when free from them. Various authorities on diabetes and the blood, among them Dr. Reginald Fitz, Dr. W. P. Murphy, and Dr. E. P. Joslin, saw him in consultation but had no therapeutic suggestion to make. Under the supervision of one or another of them frequent detailed studies were made of the blood and during the entire period daily record was kept of the total protein, total nitrogen, total uric acid, and total sugar elimination in the urine, both diurnal and nocturnal.

Soon after his administration, a study of the fasting blood was made in Dr. Murphy's laboratory the morning after he had been on a wholly unrestricted diet for comparison with the findings after a period of dietary restriction, with the results shown in the subjoined table of blood studies.

Plasma lipids

	Cholesterol	Total Fatty Acids	Lecithin	Total Lipins
	mgm. per 100 cc.	*mgm. per 100 cc.*	*mgm. per 100 cc.*	*mgm. per 100 cc.*
Normal average	230	390	210	680
The patient, E.G.F.	326	575	344	901
Controls:				
Patient's brother	189	259	230	448
A 9-year diabetic	391	286	330	667

During the 24 hours prior to the test on the morning of August 18th, the diet was estimated to contain 412 gm. carbohydrate, 188 gm. protein, and 256 gm. of fat with an approximate glucose value of 546 gm. The corresponding urinary output had been 5410 ccm. containing: 58.4 gms. sugar; 20.4 gms. total nitrogen (127.5 gms. total protein); and 855 mgm. uric acid.

During the 24-hour period preceding the August 22nd test, the diet contained 92 gm. carbohydrate, 178 gm. protein, and 177 gm. fat with a glucose value of 212 gms. The corresponding urinary output had been 4550 ccm., containing: 15.5 gm. sugar; 36.4 gm. total nitrogen (227.5 gm. total protein); and1595 mgm. uric acid.

During the month of August, also, acting on the assumption that a basophil adenoma might conceivably show a sex-maturing substance in the urine similar to that present during pregnancy, a series of observations was made by Mr. D. W. Gaiser to test this point. The urine was highly toxic for immature rats but the survivors showed no change in ovaries or seminal vesicles at the end of 120 hours. Similar tests on immature mice were equally without result.

On September 12, 1930, during a period when he was again on a restricted diet without insulin [he showed on this particular day a fasting blood sugar 0.214, with the elimination of 4300 cc. of urine containing 24.4 grm. sugar, 183 grm. total protein, 29.2 grm. total nitrogen, and 1495 mgm. total uric acid], an estimation in Dr. Joslin's laboratory was made of his plasma lipids (the patient's brother and an insulinized case of diabetes of nine years' duration serving as controls), with the following results:

Though the patient's fatty acids and total lipids were considerably in excess of the controls, they were regarded as "approximating those seen in cases of mild or moderate diabetes in the days before the introduction of insulin."[39]

As weeks passed, he became increasingly more feeble, was reluctant to get out of bed, and appeared rapidly to be going downhill, the progressive loss of strength causing him great concern. Not only did he suffer from pain in his hips and shoulders but from such extreme sensitiveness of his face he could not bear the pressure of a pillow against it. It was very difficult to make him comfortable in bed, recourse being finally had to an air mattress. He ceased to take an interest in his surroundings; became so feeble he was unable even to turn in bed; and he finally acquired a carbuncular infection at the lower end of his spine which began rapidly to spread. Knowing that other patients with this syndrome had died either from or with ulcerative cutaneous infections (cf. Case 10), it was feared that his end was near.

From the outset, he had been pleading for an exploratory operation which was considered impracticable, but in view of the growing conviction that his trouble must be due to a basophil adenoma, which might conceivably be amenable to radiation, he was given, between October 14th and 17th, four x-ray treatments. During their course, he felt particularly miserable, but by the 19th his downward progression for the preceding month was unmistakably checked. The improvement in his general condition was so striking it must have been something more than coincidence. He felt stronger, began to show an interest in his surroundings, to make efforts to move himself about, was conscious of a diminution in thirst, and of lessening in his discomforts. The carbunclar infection of the lower spine began to show improvement, and though he was unable as yet to get out of bed, he at this juncture (October 21, 1930) insisted on being taken home. There he continued rapidly to improve and the infected area on his back and hip soon healed.

According to his frequent letters he continued to complain of the backaches and of the painful sensations in the tense, adipose areas; and on March 6, 1931, he reported a further gain in weight up to 235 pounds. But on the whole, he made steady progress and by July 1931, was able to walk a half-mile or more at a time without over-fatigue. In October 1931, he stated that the "tumorous growths" of his head had nearly disappeared, and two months later he wrote from Florida, where he had gone for the winter, stating that he was still improving and no longer showed sugar on an ordinary diet, even without insulin.

The sudden improvement following radiation of the patient's pituitary body was looked upon as something more than mere coincidence. As will be pointed out in the next section, the average duration of life of the fatal cases had been in the neighborhood of five years and all the patients succumbed to progressive enfeeblement associated in most of the cases with terminal infections, a happening which in this particular instance there was every reason to anticipate when recourse was finally had to radiotherapeusis.

The exhaustive laboratory studies of the blood and urine gave no information of value though attention may be called to the consistently high non-protein nitrogen percentages and to the high cholesterol reading, on a single occasion, of 246 mgm. per cent. In this connection it is interesting that Professor Kraus, after the painstaking enumeration of the number and condition of the basophilic elements in the anterior pituitary in various pathological states, expresses the conclusion in a recent paper (loc. cit., 1928) that a definite relationship exists between the number of these cells, those of the adrenal, the blood pressure and cholesterin metabolism.

Another matter to which attention may be called is the fact that the patient's diabetes, like that complicating cases of acromegaly, was far more difficult to regulate and control by insulin than is the diabetes primarily of pancreatic origin. What, if anything, this may have to do with the known counter-effect of posterior lobe extract (pituitrin) on the action of insulin needs further ventilation.

Another unmistakable example of this same disorder, recently reported by Dr. Wieth-Pedersen from the Rigshospital of Copenhagen, has been called to my attention by a Danish student in our Medical School. The author gives a detailed report[40] of two cases both of which showed marked striae distensae cutis to which

[39] Attention may be drawn to two recently published papers by Anselmino and Hoffman (*Klin. Wchnschr.*, 26 Dec. 1931, pp. 2380-86) in which the presence in the anterior pituitary of what is called a metabolizing (*Stoffwechsel*) hormone is claimed. This appears to be related to but is separable from the gonad-stimulating hormone. Its injections increase the acetone-body content in the blood by accelerating fat combustion.

[40] Wieth-Pedersen G. Et Tilfaelde af Binyretumor og et af Hypofysetumor med Binyrehyperplasi, begge med Striae distensae cutis. *Hospitalstidende.* 1931;74:1231-1244.

factor attention is particularly drawn. One of the patients had a malignant adrenal tumor with metastases, the other a pituitary tumor associated with adrenal hyperplasia, the syndrome in both having been ascribed to the adrenal factor.

The first case was that of a woman, 158 cm. in height, with headaches, puffy skin (without hypertrichosis), dimness of vision, increase of 16 kg. in weight, with reddish-blue striae distensae, hypertension 245/150, cardiac enlargement and polydipsia. She died a year after the onset of symptoms. An adrenal tumor 12 by 6 cm. with metastases was found at autopsy. The pituitary body was said to be normal but was not examined microscopically. An abbreviated report of the second case follows:

Case 12. [Dr. Wieth-Pedersen's patient.] *Delayed adolescence. Plethoric adiposity with striae. Albuminurnia, Hyperglycaemia. Glycosuria. Vascular hypertension. Cardiac hypertrophy. Duration 4 years. Autopsy: pituitary adenoma (type unverified); adrenal hyperplasia.*

Clinical history. A young man, 24 years of age, entered the hospital May 6, 1930, and died there three months later. He had always been well but his puberty was delayed until the age of 20 when he began to grow abdominous and the color of his face and hands became bluish red. He had polyphagia, polydipsia, and polyuria. He perspired freely when at work. He needed to shave only twice weekly. There was no headache or dizziness. His vision had become impaired in later years and he had lost some weight under treatment during the nine months prior to admission.

Physical examination. The appearance was that of a man older than his age. He was of slight stature. Height 161.5 cm. (5 ft. 3 in.); weight 61.3 kg. (135 lbs.). There was quite marked adiposity, localized around abdomen, thorax and face, the extremities not being affected. No dyspnoea while resting. The teeth were carious. The thyroid gland was covered by a cushion of fat, but not enlarged. No peripheral adenitis. No cardiac enlargement was detected. There were numerous pigmented naevi on the chest.

On both sides of the abdomen were reddish striae distensae, 1 cm. in width and 5 to 6 cm. in length.; otherwise nothing abnormal. The external genitalia were not hypoplastic. The face and hands showed a deep red-blue color. There was cyanosis of the lower legs with spots of light brownish pigmentation which contrasted with the varices which were present. At the time of the examination there was a four days' growth of beard which amounted to 2 mm. at the most. The hair on the head, eyebrows, axillae and pubis was normal.

The urine contained sugar and albumin with a few hyaline casts. Blood-pressure 190/170: haemoglobin 93 per cent (Sahli). Wassermann negative. The cranial roentgenograms showed no abnormality; the sella was normal (10 by 12 mm.) with no evidence of a destructive process. The epiphyseal lines in both knees and wrists were open, corresponding with 16 to 17 years of age. No signs of atherosclerosis.

The basal metabolic rate was approximately normal. Renal function was unimpaired. The eyes were normal, except for a polar cataract visible in both of them. Blood urea [non-protein nitrogen ?] 44 mgm.%; fasting blood sugar, highest estimate 263 mgm.%. No ketonuria observed. Only on days of fasting was it possible to make the patient sugar-free; even on an anti-diabetic diet with greatly reduced calories the urine still showed sugar. Insulin was not used.

Course of disease. There was considerable variation from day to day, not only in the hypertension, but in the albuminuria and in the percentage of sugar in the blood. The patient complained of headache, of pains in the ears, and became dull and sleepy. On one occasion, he had subjective dimness of sight, marked dizziness, and vomited, the blood-pressure registering 185/120 with a rapid pulse. The abdominal striae grew more pronounced and finally reached all the way up to the axillae on both sides. Ecchymoses occurred from time to time on the legs and arms; his left hand became oedematous. On August 1st, the patient became dyspnoeic and cyanotic and died that evening.

Autopsy: August 2nd. the extremities were lean compared with the trunk. There were striae distensae on the abdomen, running longitudinally to thorax and even the axillae. The skin was without oedema, apart from that on the left forearm and back of hand. The growth of the hair was natural, except the beard, which was scanty. Broncho-pneumonia was found, also marked hypertrophy of the left ventricle and atheroma of the aorta and common iliacs. The mesentery was exceedingly fat. The kidneys were slightly granular.

The *thyroid gland* was small (each lobe measuring 3 by 1.3 cm) and firm. The right adrenal was normal, but the left was hyperplastic, weighting 27 grams; the tissue on fresh section appeared normal, but the medullary portion was oedematous and of a brownish-green color. The *pituitary gland*, on removal of the brain, was found to be replaced by a soft tumor-like growth of reddish color, which measured 3 by 2 by 2.5 cm. The brain itself was oedematous, the ventricles moderately dilated.

Microscopical examination. The *thyroid gland* showed changes like those found in a colloid struma, the epithelial lining of the follicles being low cuboidal, with no proliferation and no increase of connective tissue. The *pancreas* showed slight increase of connective tissue, with an unusual number of islets. The *left adrenal gland* had a normal structure without oedematous cell proliferation. Toward its centre, there was some oedema and congestion of the vessels without cell degeneration. The hyperplasia was evenly distributed between cortex and marrow, the two structures being indefinitely contrasted with indistinct arrangement of cell columns. The *kidneys* showed no definite change, though casts were found in the tubules.

Hypophysis: "The tumor tissue consists of a coarse network of rather delicate connective tissue, often containing thin-walled, wide, congested vessels. Although there are postmortem changes, one is of the impression that the network of connective tissues with its branches all throughout has been covered by cells of epithelial nature. These cells are polygonal, at times somewhat extended, and containing a nucleus of varying sizes and shape with a dark nucleolus. Quite often there are seen large plump complexes of nuclei, a few mitoses. These cells form, as a rule, a quite dense layer and line irregularly-shaped vacuoles which are filled with granular material consisting of necrotic and degenerative cells. Thus, the tumor tissue appears papillomatous in structure. The connective tissue, which is increased in amount in the periphery of the tumor, is also infiltrated with tumor cells. There is no evidence of sarcoma. The endothelium of the vessels appears normal."

Pathological diagnosis: Tumor of the hypophysis. Hyperplasia of the suprarenal glands, of the thyroid and of the pancreas. Hypertrophy of the left hear, Chronic glandular nephritis. Compression of the left optic nerve. Hydrocephalus internus. Oedema of pia and arachnoid. Dilation of sella turcica. Atheromatosis of mitral valve and aorta. Oedema of face and back of hand. Striae distensae cutis. Pigmentation and ecchymoses of the skin.

In his interesting discussion of the two cases, the author naturally ascribed the polyglandular disorder in the first of them to the adrenal tumor. In the second case, he laid chief emphasis (as did Dr. Parkes Weber in Case 6) upon the unilateral adrenal hyperplasia. He however ascribed the delayed puberty, retarded ossification and the adiposity to a pituitary effect as an example of dystrophia adiposo-genitalis [sic].

COLLATION OF SYMPTOMATIC AND PATHOLOGICAL DATA

The twelve patients whose case histories have been presented, as will have been noted, were all relatively *young adults*. Their *average age* at the onset of the malady, so far as can be estimated (Case 10 being eliminated for want of information) has been 18 years; the youngest was six (Case 5) and the oldest 25 (Case 11).

In *stature*, the female patients all appear to have been definitely undersized. Where heights were given, the tallest (Case 6) was 159 cm. (5 ft. 3 in.), the shortest (Case 1), 145 cm. (4 ft. 9 in.). Two of the male patients, on the other hand, were tall: Case 9, 192 cm. (6 ft. 1 1/2 in.); Case 11, 184.2 cm. (6 ft. 1/2 in.).

The *average duration* of the disease of the disease from onset to death in the cases where definitely stated (Case 10 again eliminated) has been slightly over five years, the extremes being three (Case 9) and seven [?] years (Case 8).

The following features are characteristic of all cases: (1) A rapidly acquired, peculiarly disposed and usually painful *adiposity* (in one instance representing a 40 per cent gain in weight) confined to face, neck and trunk, the extremities being spared; (2) A tendency to become round-shouldered (kyphotic) even to the point of measurable loss of height (*cf.* Cases 2 and 9) associated with lumbo-spinal pains; (3) A sexual dystrophy shown by early *amenorrhoea* in the females and ultimate functional *impotence* in the males; (4) An alteration in normal hirsuties shown by a tendency to *hypertrichosis* of face and trunk in all the females as well as the preadolescent males (Cases 8 and 12) and possibly the reverse in the adult males; (5) A dusky or plethoric appearance of the skin with *purplish lineae atrophicae*; (6) *Vascular hypertension*, present in all cases except Cases 4, 7 and 9 where no mention was made of blood-pressure; it varied from the highest recorded in Case 6 of 230/170 to the lowest in Case 11 of 178/100; (7) A tendency to *erythraemia*, a count exceeding five million having been present in five of the nine cases in which blood counts were recorded; (8) Variable *backaches, abdominal pains, fatigability* and ultimate extreme *weakness*.

Other features less consistently recorded have been as follows: *Acrocyanosis* (e.g., Cases 1, 12); *Purpura-like ecchymoses*, whether from bruising or occurring spontaneously (Cases 1, 2, 3, 6, 12); *Aching pains in the eyes*, associated with slight exophthalmos (Cases 1,3,6,11), with transient diplopia (Case 1), with suggestive papilloedema (Cases 1, 6, 11), with dimness of vision (Cases 8, 9, 12), with subretinal exudate (Case 2) and retinal haemorrhage (Case 8); Extreme *dryness of skin* (e.g., Cases 1, 2, 4, 6, 8), with pigmentation (e.g., Cases 1, 4 ,6, 11, 12); *Polyphagia*, polydipsia and polyuria (e.g., Cases 11, 12); *Oedema of the lower extremities* was noted in several cases and in Case 12, of the hand; A *susceptibility to pulmonary infections* (Cases 5, 6, 8, 9, 12); *Albuminuria* of slight degree with occasional casts was found in six patients (Cases 1, 5, 6, 8, 9, 12); A *sense of suffocation* and difficulty in swallowing were occasionally noted (Cases 1, 6); *Insomnia* was a not uncommon complaint; An increase of non-protein nitrogen and of cholesterin in the blood was recorded in the only patients (Cases 8, 11 and possibly 12) in which it was estimated; A *polymorphonuclear leucocytosis* was noted in Cases 1, 5, 6, 8, 11.

Secondary endocrine disturbances conceivably affecting the *adrenal glands* were suggested not only by the hypertension, by the pigmentation (particularly noted in Cases 1, 4, 9, 12) but by the terminal extreme weakness; on the part of the *pancreatic islets*, by the glycosuria (Cases 4, 5, 8, 11, 12); conceivably on the part of the *thyroid gland*, by the increased metabolic rate (Cases 6, 7), though this was once recorded as low (Case 11) and in most cases was not noted; of the *parathyroid glandules*, possibly by the osteoporosis from decalcification, either roentgenologically apparent (Case 1) or demonstrated at autopsy, and to which the marked upper thoracic kyphosis (e.g., Cases 1, 2, 4, 9, 10, 11) and the spontaneous fractures (Cases 2, 9) are attributable. There was no increase of blood calcium in Case 10; in no instance was calcium elimination estimated.

Postmortem findings. The malady appears to leave the patients with a definite *susceptibility to infections*. Death in the nine fatal cases, eight of which came to postmortem examination, was ascribable to, or associated with, multiple cutaneous abscesses and ulcers (Cases 2, 5), intercurrent erysipelas (Case 4), acute pulmonary complications (Case 5, 6, 12), intercurrent meningitis (Case 7), a streptococcal phlegmon (Case 10), pancreatic necrosis (Case 9). *Chronic nephritis* of mild degree was found, in the absence of any definite clinical signs, in Cases 2, 3, 6, 9 and 12; *hypertrophy of the cardiac ventricle* in Cases 2, 6, 9 and 12; and vascular atherosclerosis was noted in Cases 3, 9, 12. An *osteoporosis of the skeleton* most marked in the spine was specifically described in six (Cases 2, 3, 4, 6, 9, 10) of the eight autopsies, Cases 7 and 12 being the exceptions and in these it may have escaped notice.

The ductless glands. A *basophilic adenoma of the pituitary body* was found in Cases 6, 7 and 10; an undifferentiated adenoma in Cases 3 and 12; what was described as an adenomatous-like structure in a fibrosed area of the anterior pituitary was noted in Case 4; and in Cases 2 and 9, the gland was said to be "normal." The *thyroid* was described as slightly enlarged (colloidal) in Cases 3, 7, 10, 12; as small in Case 4; as fibrotic in Case 9. The *parathyroids* were described as normal in Case 3; to have shown capillary dilatation in Case 4; to be fibrotic in Case 9; and infiltrated with fat in Case 10. The *suprarenal glands* in Cases 2 and 6 showed a cortical hyperplasia; in Case 3, a small adenoma; while in Cases 4, 7, 9 and 10, no abnormality was noted. The *ovaries* and uterus were said to be senile in Case 3; in Case 4 to show atresia; in Case 6, to be small but normal; and in Case 7, to show hypertrophy with signs of increased functional activity. The *testes* in Cases 9 and 10 showed atrophy of the spermatogenous epithelium.

DISCUSSION AND RECAPITULATION

In ascribing this obscure polyglandular syndrome to a pituitary rather than to an adrenal source, I am aware that much might be said in favour of the latter seat of origin. Indeed, it was my original belief in the case of Minnie G. that her malady was in all probability associated with an adrenal tumor. What light the contemporary literature served to shed on the subject was strongly in favour of such an interpretation, containing, as it did, numerous examples of precocious sexual development in children or of the masculinization of women who were found to have large suprarenal tumors. A striking example was that reported in 1911 by Launois, Pinard and Gallais[41] of a bearded and amenorrhoeic woman who showed plethoric adiposity with an abundance of purplish lineae over the trunk. A suprarenal tumor of cortical type with metastases to liver and lungs was found at autopsy in association with what was said to be a normal pituitary body, though the sella turcica was said to have measured 18 mm. in its largest diameter which, to say the least, is at the upper limit of normal for her age, this being 14.4 mm. according to Erdheim and Stumme's measurements.

About this same time, twenty years ago, I had the opportunity in London to see with Dr. Gordon Holmes a striking example of masculinization or heterosexual virilism in a woman from whom an adrenal tumor was subsequently removed by Sir Percy Sargent with prompt restoration of the patient's original normal feminine appearance and reactions.[42] This woman had a lean, mannish habitus quite unlike the highly plethoric and adipose individuals herein depicted, and the case may possibly have unduly coloured my impressions of hyperadrenalism of which, to be sure, several differing types have been described. Primary adrenal tumors, therefore, may cause striking constitutional transformations, but there nevertheless is justification in again emphasizing the fact that all known primary pituitary disorders inevitably cause marked secondary changes in the adrenal cortex, a pathological observation which is amply supported by what occurs after experimental pituitary dwarfism or gigantism. And if the acidophilic adenomas of acromegaly inevitably cause hyperplasia not infrequently associated with actual adenomata of the adrenal cortex,[43] it is reasonable to assume that basophilic adenomas may well enough do the same.

[41] Launois P-E, Pinard M, Gallais A. Syndrome adiposo-génital avec hypertrichose, troubles nerveux et mentaux d'origine surrénale. *Gaz d hop.* 1911;84:649-654.

[42] Holmes G. A case of virilism associated with a suprarenal tumour: recovery after it removal. *Quart J Med.* 1924-25;18:143-152.

An excess or deficiency of anterior-pituitary hormones, in other words, secondarily affects the function of the adrenal cortex with established certainty, whereas nothing comparable to this occurs in the reverse direction. Hence, if further study should prove that adrenal tumors in the absence of any demonstrable change in the pituitary body may cause a polyglandular syndrome in many respects similar to that under discussion, it may well enough be assumed that when the same features characterize the syndrome of a basophilic adenoma, they in all probability are secondarily ascribable to a hypersecretory influence of adrenal cortex even in the absence of any histologically appreciable abnormality as exemplified by the Parkes Weber and by the Raab-Kraus cases cited above.[44]

The disorders under discussion in all probability are much more common than would appear from the present assembly of twelve examples which with four exceptions have been restricted to case in which a postmortem examination has been held. Acromegaly was once looked upon as a rare disease, and in its extreme form may still be so considered. However, one encounters on every hand persons with unmistakable traces of pituitary acidophilism (acromegalic overgrowth) so mild in its effects medical advice has not been sought; and the same is probably true of persons affected by transitory or mild degrees of pituitary basophilism.

I am quite aware that in ascribing the disorder to the basophilic elements, even were their association with maturation and the ovulatory mechanism established beyond peradventure, many questions arise which are at present unanswerable. For example: [1] If the sex-maturing principle, which during pregnancy appears to spill over into the urine, is excreted by the basophilic cells, should it not be found (cf. Case 11) in the urine of patients with basophilic adenomas if the polyglandular disorder under consideration is actually due to the hypersecretory effect of such a lesion?[45] [2] Whereas premature sexual maturity appears to characterize the disorder in children of either sex, why, in adult women, should amenorrhoea occur together with an apparent reversal of the secondary characters of sex? [3] If in this syndrome we are actually dealing with an oversecretion of the gonad-stimulating factor, why should atretic ovaries be found in the females instead of over-follicularized or over-luteinized ("mulberry") ovaries such as occur in immature or adult female rats after repeated injections with extracts containing one or the other gonad-stimulating factors?[46] [4] If the polyglandular features of the disorder are partly due, as premised, to a secondary hyperplasia of adrenal cortex, why has this not been observed in rats after injection with the gonad-stimulating extracts whereas it is a striking effect of injecting growth-promoting extracts?[47] An answer to these and other questions will doubtless in time be forthcoming.

A *chronological recapitulation* of the facts that have chiefly served to throw light on this subject during the past twenty years are as follows: [1] Primary anterior-pituitary disorders are commonly produced by adenomas; [2] Adenomas of the endocrine series are as a whole functionally active lesions; [3] Even minute adenomatous tumors of parathyroid glandules and pancreatic islets may lead to serious constitutional derangements of hypersecretory type; [4] Pituitary adenomas are of three principal varieties–neutrophil, acidophil and basophil, no constitutional disorder heretofore having been definitely ascribed to the last; [5] There is experimental evidence to suggest that the basophilic elements of the anterior pituitary secrete the sex-maturing hormone; and finally, [6] A polyglandular syndrome hitherto supposed to be of cortico-adrenal origin characterized in its full-blown state by acute plethoric adiposity, by genital dystrophy, by osteoporosis, by vascular hypertension, and so on, has been found at autopsy in six out of eight instances to be associated with a pituitary adenoma which in the three most carefully studied cases (Cases 6, 7, 10) has been definitely shown to be composed of basophilic elements, the lesion in one instance (Case 7) having been clinically predicted before its postmortal verification.[48]

Conclusions. Of all subjects that engage the attention of the profession at the present day, that of endocrinology particularly lends itself to the temptation of impressionistic speculation. During the past ten years, innumerable syndromes of so-called polyglandular type, some of them bearing a certain resemblance to that under consideration, have often been described in print. Examples of "diabetes in bearded women," of rapidly acquired obesity, of hypertension, of masculinization in the female and of sexual precocity in children

[43]Cushing H, Davidoff LM. The pathological findings in four autopsied cases of acromegaly with a discussion of their significance. *Monogr Rockefeller Inst M Research.* 1927;22:109.

[44]Smith and Engle, as may be recalled, found that pituitary transplants in the immature female rat produced precocious sexual maturity even after bilateral adrenalectomy. *Loc cit.* 1927.

[45]The hypophysial hyperplasia which occurs in pregnancy, described by Erdheim and Stumme (1909), is composed of modified chief cells which are nongranular. One would assume that this means the cells are not advancing to secretory maturity. The source of the gonad-stimulating substance in the urine, unless it is provided by the placenta (*cf.* Collip), is therefore not clear.

[46]*Cf.* Fevold HL, Hisaw FL, Leonard SL. The gonad-stimulating and the luteinizing hormones of the anterior lobe of the hypophysis. *Am J Physiol.* 1931;97:291-301.

[47]*Cf.* Smith and Engle. 1927. *loc cit.*

[48]Since Erdheim and Stumme's classical paper (Uber die Schwangerschaftsveränderung der Hypophyse. [III. Adenome der Hypophyse.] *Ziegler's Beitr.* 1909;46:1-132), no one appears to have made a systematic search for the presence of adenomata in supposedly normal pituitary glands. These authors found adenomas in approximately one out of ten of the glands that were serially sectioned.

of either sex, often associated with hyperplasias or tumors of one sort or another of the suprarenal glands, have been so many and varied as to baffle analysis.

Some of these syndromes have unquestionably been due to cortico-adrenal tumors and in not a few instances, indeed, such a tumor has been removed at operation with definite amelioration of symptoms. What is more, in similar states suprarenal tumors have been found after death in the absence of any recognizable abnormality in the pituitary body, though all too often the protocol refers to the examination of this structure either in the briefest terms or not at all.

While there is every reason to concede, therefore, that a disorder of somewhat similar aspect may occur in association with pineal, with gonadal, or with adrenal tumors, the fact that the peculiar polyglandular syndrome, which pains have been taken herein conservatively to describe, may accompany a basophil adenoma in the absence of any apparent alteration in the adrenal cortex other than a possible secondary hyperplasia, will give pathologists reason in the future more carefully to scrutinize the anterior-pituitary for lesions of similar composition.

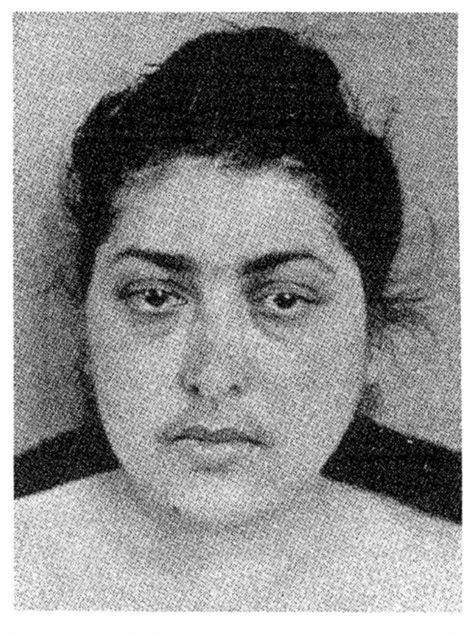

FIG. 281–Case XLV. Showing hirsuties of lip and forehead.

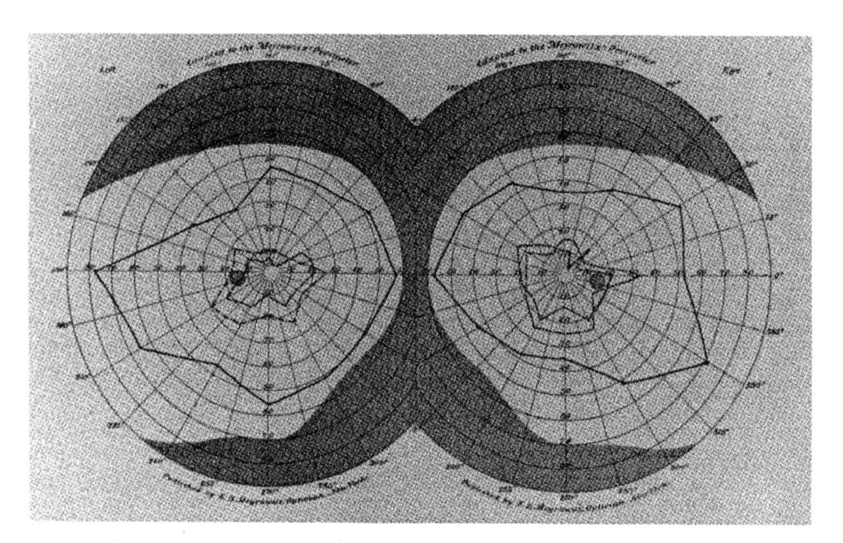

FIG. 282.–Case XLV. Fields with constriction and color interlacing.

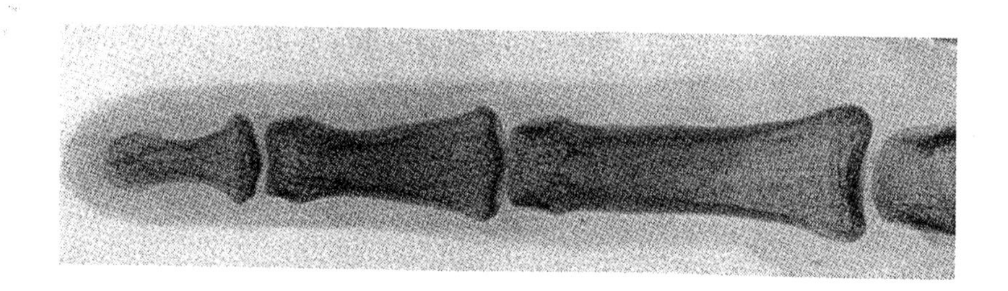

FIG. 284–Case XLV. X-ray of middle finger (unreduced) showing traces of epiphyseal lines.

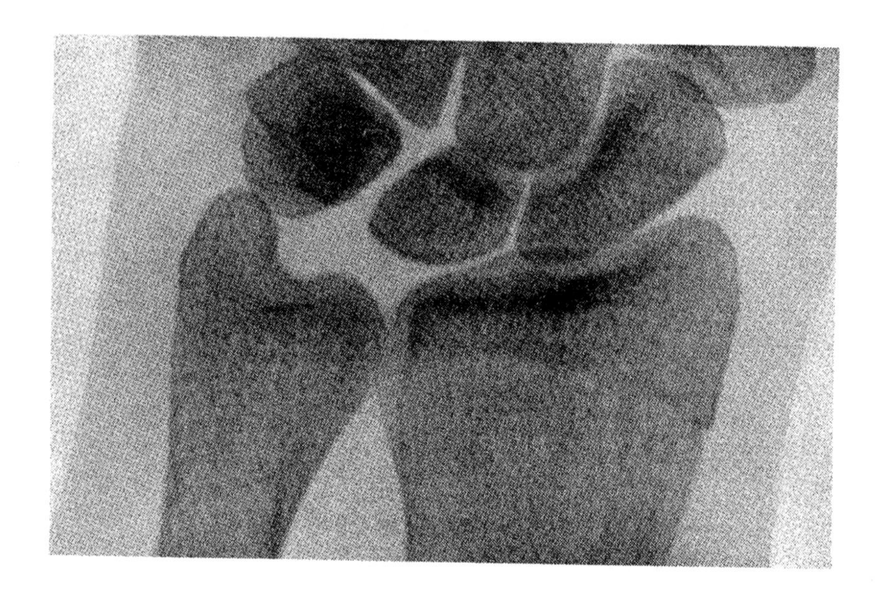

FIG. 285.–Case XLV. X-ray of wrist showing incomplete epiphyseal ossification.

Letter on Corpulence, Addressed to the Public

Third Edition

William Banting

Preface to the Third Edition

THE second edition of this pamphlet (consisting of 1,500 copies) being exhausted, and the result being very gratifying to my mind, in the large amount of satisfaction and benefit which I am able to report from evidence of others (*beyond my most sanguine expectations*), considering the hitherto limited circulation, I have felt impelled to publish, advertise, and sell this third edition, at cost price, which I am informed must be sixpence a copy. If this small charge, however, should yield any profit, I shall devote it to the Printer's Pension Society, or som other benevolent institution; but I have no such expectation, or would very gladly reduce the charge at starting.

The first and second editions were no very serious expense to me, scarcely three pence a copy, but the circulation of them, and the correspondence involved, have cost me far more; yet, I saw no way of securing my motives from misconception except by gratuitously presenting the pamphlet to the public.

The truthful tale has, however, made its way into a large circle of sufferers with marvellous effect; and I can now believe the public will rather prefer to purchase the third edition at a reasonable charge than be under obligation to me for a gratuitous supply. I therefore humbly trust, and fully believe, that by this means the useful knowledge will be distributed twenty-fold to benefit of suffering humanity, which, indeed, is my sole object.

Third edition reprinted with permission from the private collection of Dr. George A. Bray, M.D., Baton Rouge, LA., Mr. Harvey's Remarks reprinted with permission from the National Library of Medicine, Bethesda, MD., and the Letters from Mr. Banting to the owner of the 1869 edition reprinted with permission from the Boston Medical Library Francis A. Countway Library of Medicine, Boston, MA. All works part of public domain. Special thanks to all of these contributors.

KENSINGTON
***December*, 1863.**

This letter is respectfully dedicated to the Public simply and entirely from an ernest desire to confer a benefit on my fellow creatures.

W.B.

Corpulence

OF all the parasites that affect humanity I do not know of, nor can I imagine, any more distressing than that of Obesity, and, having just emerged from a very long probation in this affliction, I am desirous of circulating my humble knowledge and experience for the benefit of my fellow man, with an earnest hope it may lead to the same comfort and happiness I now feel under the extraordinary change,–which might almost be termed miraculous had it not been accomplished by the most simple common–sense means.

Obesity seems to me very little understood or properly appreciated by the faculty and the public generally, or the former would long ere this have hit upon the cause for so lamentable a disease, and applied effective remedies, whilst the latter would have spared their injudicious indulgence in remarks and sneers, frequently painful in society, and which, even on the strongest mind, have an unhappy tendency; but I sincerely trust this humble effort at exposition may lead to a more perfect ventilation of the subject and a better feeling for the afflicted.

It would afford me infinite pleasure and satisfaction to name the author of my redemption from the calamity, as he is the only one that I have been able to find (and my search has not been sparing) who seems thoroughly up in the question; but such publicity might be construed improperly, and I have, therefore, only to offer my personal experience as the stepping stone to public investigation, and to proceed with my narrative of facts, earnestly hoping the reader will patiently peruse and thoughtfully consider it, with forbearance for any fault of style or diction, and for any seeming presumption in publishing it.

I have felt some difficulty in deciding on the proper and best course of action. At one time I thought the Editor of the Lancet would kindly publish a letter from me on the subject, but further reflection led me to doubt whether an insignificant individual would be noticed without some special introduction. In the April number of the *Cornhill Magazine* I read with much interest an article on the subject–defining tolerably well the effects, but offering no tangible remedy, or even positive solution of the problem–"What is the Cause of Obesity?" I was pleased with the article as a whole, but objected to some portions, and had prepared a letter to the Editor of that Magazine offering my experience on the subject, but again it struck me that an unknown individual like myself would have but little prospect of notice; so I finally resolved to publish and circulate this Pamphlet, with no other reason, motive, or expectation than an earnest desire to help those who happen to be afflicted as I was, for that corpulence is remediable I am well convinced, and shall be delighted if I can induce others to think so. The object I have in view impels me to enter into minute particulars as well as general observations, and to revert to bygone years, in order to show that I have spared no pains nor expense to accomplish the great end of stopping and curing obesity.

I am now nearly 66 years of age, about 5 feet 5 inches in stature, and, in August last (1862), weighed 202 lbs., which I think it right to name, because the article in the *Cornhill Magazine* presumes that a certain stature and age should bear ordinarily a certain weight, and I am quite of that opinion. I now weigh 167 lbs., showing a diminution of something like 1 lb. per week since August, and having now very nearly attained the happy medium, I have perfect confidence that a few more weeks will fully accomplish the object for which I have laboured for the last thirty years, in vain, until it pleased Almighty Providence to direct me into the right and proper channel–the "tramway," so to speak–of happy, comfortable existence.

Few men have led a more active life–bodily or mentally–from a constitutional anxiety for regularity, precision, and order, during fifty years' business career, from which I have now retired, so that my corpulence and subsequent obesity was not through neglect of necessary bodily activity, nor from excessive eating, drinking, or self-indulgence of any kind, except that I partook of the simple aliments of bread, milk, butter, beer, sugar, and potatoes more freely than my aged nature required, and hence, as I believe, the generation of the parasite, detrimental to comfort if not really to health.

I will not presume to descant on the bodily structural tissues, so fully canvassed in the *Cornhill Magazine*, nor how they are supported and renovated, having no mind or power to enter into those questions, which properly belong to the wise heads of the faculty. None of my family on the side of either parent had any tendency to corpulence, and from my earliest years I had an inexpressible dread of such a calamity, so, when I was between thirty and forty years of age, finding a tendency to it creeping upon me, I consulted an eminent surgeon, now long deceased,–a kind personal friend,–who recommended increased bodily exertion before my ordinary daily labours began, and thought rowing an excellent plan. I had the command of a good, heavy, safe boat, lived near the river, and adopted it for a couple of hours in the early morning. It is true I gained muscular vigour, but with it a prodigious appetite, which I was compelled to indulge, and consequently increased in weight, until my kind old friend advised me to forsake the exercise.

He soon afterwards died, and, as the tendency to corpulence remained, I consulted other high orthodox authorities (*never any inferior adviser*), but all in vain. I have tried sea air and bathing in various localities, with much walking exercise; taken gallons of physic and liquor potassæ, advisedly and abundantly; riding on horseback; the waters and climate of Leamington many times, as well as those of Cheltenham and Harrogate frequently; have lived upon sixpence a–day, so to speak, and earned it, if bodily labour may be so construed; and have spared no trouble nor expense in consultations with the best authorities in the land, giving each and all a fair time for experiment, without any permanent remedy, as the evil still gradually increased.

I am under obligations to most of those advisors for the pains and interest they took in my case; but only to one for an effectual remedy.

When a corpulent man eats, drinks, and sleeps well, has no pain to complain of, and no particular organic disease, the judgment of able men seems paralyzed,–for I have been generally informed that corpulence is one of the natural results of increasing years; indeed, one of the ablest authorities as a physician in the land told me he had gained 1 lb. in weight every year since he attained manhood, and was not surprised at my condition, but advised more bodily exercise–vapour-baths and shampooing, in addition to the medicine given. Yet the evil still increased, and, like the parasite of barnacles on a ship, if it did not destroy the structure, it obstructed its fair, comfortable progress in the path of life.

I have been in dock, perhaps twenty times in as many years, for the reduction of this disease, and with little good effect–none lasting. Any one so afflicted is often subject to public remark, and though in conscience he may care little about it, I am confident no man labouring under obesity can be quite insensible to the sneers and remarks of the cruel and injudicious in public assemblies, public vehicles, or the ordinary street traffic; nor to the annoyance of finding no adequate space in a public assembly if he should seek amusement or need refreshment, and therefore he naturally keeps away as much as possible from places where he is likely to be made the object of the taunts and remarks of others. I am as regardless of public remark as most men, but I have felt these difficulties and therefore avoided such circumscribed accommodation and notice, and by that means have been deprived of many advantages to health and comfort.

Although no very great size or weight, still I could not stoop to tie my shoe, so to speak, nor attend to the little offices humanity requires without considerable pain and difficulty, which only the corpulent can understand; I have been compelled to go down stairs slowly backwards, to save the jarr of increased weight upon the ancle and knee joints, and been obliged to puff and blow with every slight exertion, particularly that of going up stairs. I have spared no pains to remedy this by low living (*moderation and light food* was generally prescribed, but I had no direct bill of fare to know what was really intended), and that, consequently, brought the system into a low impoverished state, without decreasing corpulence, caused many obnoxious boils to appear, and two rather formidable carbuncles, for which I was ably operated upon *and fed into increased obesity*.

At this juncture (about three years back) Turkish baths became the fashion, and I was advised to adopt them as a remedy. With the first few I found immense benefit in power and elasticity for walking exercise; so, believing I had found the "philosopher's stone," pursued them three times a-week till I had taken fifty, then less frequently (as I began to fancy, with some reason, that so many weakened my constitution) till I had taken ninety, but never succeeded in losing more than 6 lbs. weight during the whole course, and I gave up the plan as worthless; though I have full belief in their cleansing properties, and their value in colds, rheumatism, and many other ailments.

I then fancied increasing obesity materially affected a slight umbilical rupture, if it did not cause it, and that another bodily ailment to which I had been subject was also augmented. This led me to other medical advisers, to whom I am also indebted for much kind consideration, though, unfortunately, they failed in relieving me. At last finding my sight failing and my hearing greatly impaired, I consulted in August last an eminent aural surgeon, who made light of the case, looked into my ears, sponged them internally, and blistered the outside, without the slightest benefit, neither inquiring into any of my bodily ailments, which he probably thought unnecessary, nor affording me even time to name them.

I was not at all satisfied, but on the contrary was in a worse plight than when I went to him; however he soon after left town for his annual holiday, which proved the greatest possible blessing to me, because it compelled me to seek other assistance, and, happily, I found the right man, who unhesitatingly said he believed my ailments were caused principally by corpulence, and prescribed a certain diet,–no medicine, beyond a morning cordial as a corrective,–with immense effect and advantage both to my hearing and the decrease of my corpulency.

For the sake of argument and illustration I will presume that certain articles of ordinary diet, however beneficial in youth, are prejudicial in advanced life, like beans to a horse, whose common ordinary food is hay and corn. It may be useful food occasionally, under peculiar circumstances, but detrimental as a constancy. I will, therefore, adopt the analogy, and call such food human beans. The items from which I was advised to abstain as much as possible were:–Bread, butter, milk, sugar, beer, and potatoes, which had been the main (and, I thought, innocent) elements of my existence, or at all events they had for many years been adopted freely.

These, said my excellent adviser, contain starch and saccharine matter, tending to create fat, and should be avoided altogether. At the first blush it seemed to me that I had little left to live upon, but my kind friend soon showed me there was ample, and I was only too happy to give the plan a fair trial, and, within a very few days, found immense benefit from it. It may better elucidate the dietary plan if I describe generally what I have sanction to take, and that man must be an extraordinary person who would desire a better table:–

For breakfast, I take four or five ounces of beef, muton, kidneys, broiled fish, bacon, or cold meat of any kind except pork; a large cup of tea (without milk or sugar), a little biscuit, or one ounce of dry toast.

For dinner, Five or six ounces of any fish except salmon, any meat except pork, any vegetable except potato, one ounce of dry toast, fruit out of a pudding, any kind of poultry or game, and two or three glasses of good claret, sherry, or Madeira–Champagne, Port and Beer forbidden.

For tea, Two or three ounces of fruit, a rusk or two, and a cup of tea without milk or sugar.

For supper, Three or four ounces of meat or fish, similar to dinner, with a glass or two of claret.

For nightcap, if required, A tumbler of grog
–(gin, whisky, or brandy, without sugar)
–or a glass or two of claret or sherry

This plan leads to an excellent night's rest, with from six to eight hours' sound sleep. The dry toast or rusk may have a table spoonful of spirit to soften it, which will prove acceptable. Perhaps I did not wholly escape starchy or saccharine matter, but scrupulously avoided those beans, such as milk, sugar, beer, butter, & c., which were known to contain them.

On rising in the morning I take a table spoonful of a special corrective cordial, which may be called the Balm of life, in a wine-glass of water, a most grateful draught, as it seems to carry away all the dregs left in the stomach after digestion, but is not aperient; then I take about 5 or 6 ounces solid and 8 of liquid for breakfast; 8 ounces of solid and 8 of liquid for dinner; 3 ounces of solid and 8 of liquid for tea; 4 ounces of solid and 6 of liquid for supper, and the grog afterwards, if I please. I am not, however, strictly limited to any quantity at either meal, so that the nature of the food is rigidly adhered to.

Experience has taught me to believe that these human beans are the most insidious enemies man, with a tendency to corpulence in advanced life, can possess, though eminently friendly to youth. He may very prudently mount guard against such an enemy if he is not a fool to himself, and I fervently hope this truthful unvarnished tale may lead him to make a trial of my plan, which I sincerely recommend to public notice,–not with any ambitious motive, but in sincere good faith to help my fellow–creatures to obtain the marvellous blessings I have found within the short period of a few months.

I do not recommend every corpulent man to rush headlong into such a change of diet, *(certainly not)*, but to act advisedly and after full consideration with a physician.

My former dietary table was bread and milk for breakfast, or a pint of tea with plenty of milk and sugar, and buttered toast; meat, beer, much bread (of which I was always very fond) and pastry for dinner, the meal of tea similar to that of breakfast, and generally a fruit tart or bread and milk for supper. I had little comfort and far less sound sleep.

It certainly appears to me that my present dietary table is far superior to the former–more luxurious and liberal, independent of its blessed effect–but when it is proved to be more healthful, comparisons are simply ridiculous, and I can hardly imagine any man, even in sound health, would choose the former, even if it were not an enemy; but, when it is shown to be, as in my case, inimical both to health and comfort, I can hardly conceive there is any man who would not willingly avoid it. I can conscientiously assert I never lived so well as under the new plan of dietary, which I should have formerly thought a dangerous extravagant trespass upon health; I am very much better, bodily and mentally, and pleased to believe that I hold the reins of health and comfort in my own hands, and, though at sixty-five years of age, I cannot expect to remain free from some coming natural infirmity that all flesh is heir to, I cannot at the present time complain of one. It is simply miraculous, and I am thankful to Almighty Providence for directing me, through an extraordinary chance, to the care of a man who could work such a change in so short a time.

Oh! that the faculty would look deeper into and make themselves better acquainted with the crying evil of obesity–that dreadful tormenting parasite on health and comfort. Their fellow men might not descend into early premature graves, as I believe many do, from what is termed apoplexy, and certainly would not, during their sojourn on earth, endure so much bodily and consequently mental infirmity.

Corpulence, though giving no actual pain, as it appears to me, must naturally press with undue violence upon the bodily viscera, driving one part upon another, and stopping the free action of all. I am sure it did in my particular case, and the result of my experience is briefly as follows:–

I have not felt so well as now for the last twenty years.

Have suffered no inconvenience whatever in the probational remedy.

Am reduced many inches in bulk, and 35 lbs. in weight in thirty-eight weeks.

Come down stairs forward naturally, with perfect ease.

Go up stairs and take ordinary exercise freely, without the slightest inconvenience.

Can perform every necessary office for myself.

The umbilical rupture is greatly ameliorated, and gives me no anxiety.

My sight is restored–my hearing improved.

My other bodily ailments are ameliorated; indeed, almost past into matter of history.

I have placed a thank-offering of £50 in the hands of my kind medical adviser for distribution amongst his favourite hospitals, after gladly paying his usual fees, and still remain under overwhelming obligations for his care and attention, which I can never hope to repay. Most thankful to Almighty Providence for mercies received, and determined to press the case into public notice as a token of gratitude.

I have the pleasure to afford, in conclusion, a satisfactory confirmation of my report, in stating that a corpulent friend of mine, who, like myself, is possessed of a generally sound constitution, was labouring under frequent palpitations of the heart and sensations of fainting, was, at my instigation, induced to place himself in the hands of my medical adviser, with the same gradual beneficial results. He is at present under the same ordeal, and in eight weeks has profited even more largely than I did in that short period; he has lost the palpitations, and is becoming, so to speak, a new made man–thankful to me for advising, and grateful to the eminent counsellor to whom I referred him–and he looks forward with good hope to a perfect cure.

I am fully persuaded that hundreds, if not thousands, of our fellow men might profit equally by a similar course; but, constitutions not being all alike, a different course of treatment may be advisable for the removal of so tormenting an affliction.

My kind and valued medical adviser is not a doctor for obesity, but stands on the pinnacle of fame in the treatment of another malady, which, as he well knows, is frequently induced by the disease of which I am speaking, and I most sincerely trust most of my corpulent friends (and there are thousands of corpulent people whom I dare not so rank) may be led into my tramroad. To any such I am prepared to offer the further key of knowledge by naming the man. It might seem invidious to do so now, but I shall only be too happy, if applied to by letter in good faith, or if any doubt should exist as to the correctness of this statement.

WILLIAM BANTING, Sen.,
Late of No. 27, St. James's Street, Piccadilly, Now of No. 4, The Terrace, Kensington
May, 1863

Addenda

HAVING exhausted the first Edition (1,000 copies) of the foregoing Pamphlet; and a period of one year having elapsed since commencing the admirable course of diet which has led to such inestimably beneficial results, and, "as I expected, and desired," having quite succeeded in attaining the happy medium of weight and bulk I had so long ineffectually sought, *which appears necessary to health at my age and statue*–I feel impelled by a sense of public duty, to offer the result of my experience in a second Edition. It has been suggested that I should have sold the Pamphlet, devoting any profit to Charity as more agreeable and useful; and I had intended to adopt such a course, but on reflection feared my motives might be mistaken; I, therefore, respectfully present this (like the first Edition) to the Public gratuitously, earnestly hoping the subject may be taken up by medical men and thoroughly ventilated.

It may (and I hope will) be, as satisfactory to the public to hear, as it is for me to state, that the first Edition has been attended with very comforting results to other sufferers from Corpulence, as the remedial system therein described was to me under that terrible disease, which was my main object in publishing my convictions on the subject. It has moreover attained a success, produced flattering compliments, and an amount of attention I could hardly have imagined possible. The pleasure and satisfaction this has afforded me, is ample compensation for the trouble and expense I have incurred, and I most sincerely trust, "as I verily believe," this second Edition will be accompanied by similar satisfactory results from a more extensive circulation. If so, it will inspirit me to circulate further Editions, whilst a corpulent person exists, requiring, as I think, this system of diet, or so long as my motives cannot be mistaken, and are thankfully appreciated.

My weight is reduced 46 lbs., and as the very *gradual reductions* which I am able to show may be interesting to many, I have great pleasure in stating them, believing they serve to demonstrate further the merit of the system pursued.

My weight on 26th August, 1862, was 202 lbs.

On 7th September,	it was	200,	having lost	2
27th "	"	197	"	3 more.
19th October	"	193	"	4 "
9th November	"	190	"	3 "
3rd December	"	187	"	3 "
24th "	"	184	"	3 "
14th Jan. 1863	"	182	"	2 "
4th February	"	180	"	2 "
25th "	"	178	"	2 "
18th March	"	176	"	2 "
8th April	"	173	"	3 "
29th "	"	170	"	3 "
20th May	"	167	"	3 "
10th June	"	164	"	3 "
1st July	"	161	"	3 "
22nd "	"	159	"	2 "
12th August	"	157	"	2 "
26th "	"	156	"	1 "
12th September	"	156	"	0 "
	Total loss of weight.. ..			46 lbs.

My girth is reduced round the waist, in tailor phraseology, 12 1/4 inches, which extent was hardly conceivable even by my own friends, or my respected medical adviser, until I put on my former clothing, over what I now wear, which was a thoroughly convincing proof of the remarkable change. These important desiderata have been attained by the most easy and comfortable means, with but little medicine, and almost entirely by a system of diet, that formerly I should have thought dangerously generous. I am told by all who know me that my personal appearance is greatly improved, and that I seem to bear the stamp of good health; this may be a matter of opinion or friendly remark, but I can honestly assert that I feel restored in health, "bodily and mentally," appear to have more muscular power and vigour, eat and drink with a good appetite, and sleep well. All symptoms of acidity, indigestion, and heartburn (with which I was frequently tormented) have vanished. I have left off using boot hooks, and other such aids which were indispensable, but being now able to stoop with ease and freedom, are unnecessary. I have lost the feeling of *occasional faintness*, and what I think a remarkable blessing and comfort is that I have been able safely to leave off knee bandages, which I had worn *necessarily* for 20 past years, and given up a truss almost entirely; indeed I believe I might wholly discard it with safety, but am advised to wear it at least occasionally for the present.

Since publishing my Pamphlet, I have felt constrained to send a copy of it to my former medical advisers, and to ascertain their opinions on the subject. They did not dispute or question the propriety of the system, but either dared not venture its practice upon a man of my age, or thought it too great a sacrifice of personal comfort to be generally advised or adopted, and I fancy none of them appeared to feel the fact of the misery of corpulence. One eminent physician, as I before stated, assured me that increasing weight was a necessary result of advancing years; another equally eminent to whom I had been directed by a very friendly third, who had most kindly but ineffectually failed in a remedy, added to my weight in a few weeks instead of abating the evil. These facts lead me to believe the question is not sufficiently observed or even regarded.

The great charm and comfort of the system is, that its effects are palpable within a week of trial, which creates a natural stimulus to persevere for a few weeks more, when the fact becomes established beyond question.

I only intreat all persons suffering from corpulence to make a fair trial for just one clear month, as I am well convinced, they will afterwards pursue a course which yields such extraordinary benefit, till entirely and effectually relieved, and be it remembered, by the sacrifice merely of simple, for the advantage of more generous and comforting food. The simple dietary evidently adds fuel to fire, whereas the superior and liberal seems to extinguish it.

I am delighted to be able to assert that I have proved the great merit and advantage of the system by its result in several other cases, similar to my own, and have full confidence that within the next twelve months I shall know of many more cases restored from the disease of corpulence, for I have received the kindest possible letters from many afflicted strangers and friends, as well as similar personal observations from others whom I have conserved with, and assurances from most of them that they will kindly inform me the result for my own private satisfaction. Many are practising the diet after consultation with their own medical advisers; some few have gone to mine, and others are practising upon their own convictions of the advantages detailed in the Pamphlet, though I recommend all to act advisedly, in case their constitutions should differ. I am, however, so perfectly satisfied of the great unerring benefits of this system of diet, that I shall spare no trouble to circulate my humble experience. The amount and character of my correspondence on the subject has been strange and singular, but most satisfactory to my mind and feelings.

I am now in that happy comfortable state that I should not hesitate to indulge in any fancy in regard to diet, but if I did so should watch the consequences, and not continue any course which might add to weight or bulk and consequent discomfort.

Is not the system suggestive to artists and men of sedentary employment who cannot spare time for exercise, consequently become corpulent, and clog the little muscular action with a superabundance of fat, thus easily avoided?

Pure genuine bread may be the staff of life as it is termed. It is so, particularly in youth, but I feel certain it is more wholesome in advanced life if thoroughly toasted, as I take it. My impression is, that any starchy or saccharine matter tends to the disease of corpulence in advanced life, and whether it be swallowed in that form or generated in the stomach, that all things tending to these elements should be avoided, of course always under sound medical authority.

WILLIAM BANTING.

Concluding Addenda

It is very satisfactory to me to be able to state, that I remained at the same standard of bulk and weight for several weeks after the 26th August, when I attained the happy natural medium, since which time I have varied in weight from two to three pounds, more or less. I have seldom taken the morning draught since that time, and have frequently indulged my fancy, *experimentally*, in using milk, sugar, butter, and potatoes–indeed, I may say all the forbidden articles *except beer*, in moderation, with impunity, but always as an exception, not as a rule. This deviation, however, convinces me that I hold the power of maintaining the happy medium in my own hands.

A kind friend has lately furnished me with a tabular statement in regard to weight as proportioned to stature, which, under present circumstances and the new movement, may be interesting and useful to corpulent readers:–

STATURE.				WEIGHT				
5	feet	1	should be	8	stone	8	or	120 lbs.
5	"	2	"	9	"	0	"	126 "
5	"	3	"	9	"	7	"	133 "
5	"	4	"	9	"	10	"	136 "
5	"	5	"	10	"	2	"	142 "
5	"	6	"	10	"	5	"	145 "
5	"	7	"	10	"	8	"	148 "
5	"	8	"	11	"	1	"	155 "
5	"	9	"	11	"	8	"	162 "
5	"	10	"	12	"	1	"	169 "
5	"	11	"	12	"	6	"	174 "
6	"	0	"	12	"	10	"	178 "

This tabular statement, taken from a mean average of 2,648 healthy men, was formed and arranged for an Insurance Company by the late Dr. John Hutchinson. It answered as a pretty good standard, and insurances were regulated upon it. His calculations were made upon the volume of air passing in and out of the lungs, and this was his guide as to how far the various organs of the body were in health, and the lungs in particular. It may be viewed as some sort of probable rule, yet only as an average,–some in health weighing more by many pounds than others. It must not be looked upon as infallible, but only as a sort of general reasonable guide to Nature's great and mighty work.

On a general view of the question I think it may be conceded that a frame of low stature was hardly intended to bear very heavy weight. Judging from this tabular statement I ought to be considerably lighter than I am at present: I shall not, however, covet or aim at such a result, nor, on the other hand, feel alarmed if I decrease a little more in weight and bulk.

I am certainly more sensitive to cold since I have lost the superabundant fat, but this is remediable by another garment, far more agreeable and satisfactory. Many of my friends have said, "Oh! you have done well so far, but take care you don't go too far." I fancy such a circumstance, with such a dietary, very unlikely, if not impossible; but feeling that I have now nearly attained the right standard of bulk and weight proportional to my stature and age (between 10 and 11 stone), I should not hesitate to partake of a fattening dietary occasionally, to preserve that happy standard, if necessary; indeed, I am allowed to do so by my medical adviser but I shall always observe a careful watch upon myself to discover the effect, and act accordingly, so that, if I choose to spend a day or two with Dives, so to speak, I must not forget to devote the next to Lazarus.

The remedy may be as old as the hills, as I have since been told, but its application is of very recent date; and it astonishes me that such a light should have remained so long unnoticed and hidden, as not to afford a glimmer to my anxious mind in a search for it during the last twenty years, even in directions where it might have been expected to be known. I would rather presume it is a new light, than that it was purposely hidden merely because the disease of obesity was not immediately dangerous to existence, nor thought to be worthy of serious consideration. Little do the faculty imagine the misery and bitterness to life through the parasite of corpulence or obesity.

I can now confidently say that *quantity* of diet may be safely left to the natural appetite; and that it is the *quality* only, which is essential to abate and cure corpulence. I stated the quantities of my own dietary, because it was part of a truthful report, but some correspondents have doubted whether it should be more or less in their own cases, a doubt which would be better solved by their own appetite, or medical adviser. I have heard a graphic remark by a corpulent man, which may not be inappropriately stated here, *that big houses were not formed with scanty materials*. This, however, is a poor excuse for self indulgence in improper food, or for not consulting medical authority.

The approach of corpulence is so gradual that, until it is far advanced, persons rarely become objects of attention. Many may have even congratulated themselves on their comely appearance, and have not sought advice or a remedy for what they did not consider an evil, for an evil I can say most truly it is, when in much excess, to which point it must, in my opinion arrive, unless obviated by proper means.

Many have wished to know (as future readers may) the nature of the morning draught, or where it could be obtained, but believing it would have been highly imprudent on my part to have presumed that what was proper for my constitution was applicable to all indiscriminately, I could only refer them to a medical adviser for any aid beyond the dietary; assuring them, however, it was not a dram but of an alkaline character.

Some, I believe, would willingly submit to even a violent remedy, so that an immediate benefit could be produced; this is not the object of the treatment, as it cannot but be dangerous, in my humble opinion, to reduce a disease of this nature suddenly; they are probably then too prone to despair of success, and consider it as unalterably connected with their constitution. Many under this feeling doubtless return to their former habits, encouraged so to act by the ill-judged advice of friends who, I am persuaded (from the correspondence I have had on this most interesting subject) become unthinking accomplices in the destruction of those whom they regard and esteem.

The question of four meals a-day, and the night cap,

has been abundantly and amusingly criticized. I ought perhaps to have stated as an excuse for such liberality of diet, that I breakfast between eight and nine o'clock, dine between one and two, take my slight tea meal between five and six, sup at nine, and only take the night cap when inclination directs. My object in naming it at all was, that, as a part of a whole system, it should be known, and to show it is not forbidden to those who are advised that they need such a luxury; nor was it injurious in my case. Some have inquired whether smoking was prohibited. It was not.

It has also been remarked that such a dietary as mine was too good and expensive for a poor man, and that I had wholly lost sight of that class; but a very poor corpulent man is not so frequently met with, inasmuch as the poor cannot afford the simple inexpensive means for creating fat; but when the tendency does exist in that class, I have no doubt it can be remedied by abstinence from the forbidden articles, and a moderate indulgence in such cheap stimulants as may be recommended by a medical adviser, whom they have ample chances of consulting gratuitously.

I have a very strong feeling that gout (another terrible parasite upon humanity) might be greatly relieved, if not cured entirely, by this proper natural dietary, and sincerely hope some person so afflicted may be induced to practice the harmless plan for three months (as I certainly would if the case were my own) to prove it; but not without advice.

My impression from the experiments I have tried on myself of late is, that saccharine matter is the great moving cause of fatty corpulence. I know that it produces in my individual case increased weight and a large amount of flatulence, and believe, that not only sugar, but all elements tending to create saccharine matter in the process of digestion, should be avoided. I apprehend it will be found in bread, butter, milk, beer, Port wine, and Champagne; I have not found starchy matter so troublesome as the saccharine, which, I think, largely increases acidity as well as fat, but, with ordinary care and observation, people will soon find what food rests easiest in the stomach, and avoid that which does not, during the probationary trial of the proposed dietary. Vegetables and ripe or stewed fruit I have found ample aperients. Failing this, medical advice should be sought.

The word "*parasite*" has been much commented upon, as inappropriate to any but a living creeping thing (of course I use the word in a figurative sense, as a burden to the flesh), but if fat is not an insidious creeping enemy, I do not know what is. I should have equally applied the word to gout, rheumatism, dropsy, and many other diseases.

Whereas hitherto the appeals to me to know the name of my medical adviser have been very numerous, I may say hundreds, which I have gladly answered, though forming no small item of the expense incurred, and whereas the very extensive circulation expected of the third edition is likely to lead to some thousands of similar applications, I feel bound, in self-defence, to state that the medical gentleman to whom I am so deeply indebted is Mr. Harvey, Soho Square, London, whom I consulted for deafness. In the first and second editions, I thought that to give his name would appear like a puff, which I know he abhors; indeed, I should prefer not to do so now, but cannot, in justice to myself, incur further probable expense (which I fancy inevitable) besides the personal trouble, for which I cannot afford time, and, therefore, feel no hesitation to refer to him as my guarantee for the truth of the pamphlet.

One material point I should be glad to impress on my corpulent readers–it is, to get accurately weighed at starting upon the fresh system, and continue to do so weekly or monthly, for the change will be so truly palpable by this course of examination, that it will arm them with perfect confidence in the merit and ultimate success of the plan. I deeply regret not having secured a photographic portrait of my original figure in 1862, to place in juxta position with one of my present form. It might have amused some, but certainly would have been very convincing to others, and astonishing to all that such an effect should have been so readily and speedily produced by the simple natural cause of exchanging a meagre for a generous dietary under proper advice.

I shall ever esteem it a great favour if persons relieved and cured, as I have been, will kindly let me know of it; the information will be truly gratifying to my mind. That the system is a great success, I have not a shadow of doubt from the numerous reports sent with thanks by strangers as well as friends from all parts of the kingdom; and I am truly thankful to have been the humble instrument of disseminating the blessing and experience I have attained through able counsel and natural causes by proper perseverance.

I have now finished my task, and trust my humble efforts may prove to be good seed well sown, that will fructify and produce a large harvest of benefit to my fellow creatures. I also hope the faculty generally may be led more extensively to ventilate this question of corpulence or obesity, so that, instead of one, two, or three able practitioners, there may be as many hundreds distributed in the various parts of the United Kingdom. In such cases, I am persuaded, that those diseases, like Reverence and Golden Pippins, will be very rare.

Appendix

SINCE publishing the third edition of my Pamphlet, I have earnestly pressed my medical adviser to explain the reasons for so remarkable a result as I and others have experienced from the dietary system he prescribed, and I hope he may find time to do so shortly, as I believe it would be highly interesting to the Faculty and the public generally. He has promised this at his leisure.

Numerous applications having been made to me on points to which I had not alluded, in which my correspondents felt some doubt and interest, I take this opportunity of making some few corrections in my published dietary:–

I ought, "it seems," to have excepted veal, owing to its indigestible quality, as well as pork for its fattening character; also herrings and eels (owing to their oily nature), being as injurious as salmon. In respect to vegetables, not only should potatoes be prohibited, but parsnips, beetroot, turnips, and carrots. The truth is, I seldom or ever partook of these objectionable articles myself, and did not reflect that others might do so, or that they were forbidden. Green vegetables are considered very beneficial, and I believe should be adopted at all times. I am indebted to the "Cornhill Magazine" and other journals for drawing my attention to these dietetic points. I can now also state that eggs, if not hard boiled, are unexceptionable, that cheese, if sparingly used, and plain boiled rice seem harmless.

Some doubts have been expressed in regard to the vanishing point of such a descending scale, but it is a remarkable fact that the great and most palpable diminution in weight and bulk occurs within the first forty-eight hours, the descent is then more gradual. My own experience, and that of others, assures me (if medical authority be first consulted as to the complaint) that with such slight extraneous aid as medicine can afford, nature will do her duty, and only her duty: firstly, by relieving herself of immediate pressure she will be enabled to move more freely in her own beautiful way, and secondly, by pursuing the same course to work speedy amelioration and final cure. The vanishing point is only when the disease is stopped and the parasite annihilated.

It may interest my readers to know that I have now apparently attained the standard natural at my age (10 stone 10, or 150 lbs.), as my weight now varies only to the extent of 1 lb., more or less, in the course of a month. According to Dr. Hutchinson's tables I ought to lose still more, but cannot do so without resorting to medicine; and, feeling in sound vigorous health, I am perfectly content to wait upon nature for any further change.

In my humble judgment the dietary is the principle point in the treatment of Corpulence, and it appears to me, moreover, that if properly regulated it becomes in a certain sense a medicine. The system seems to me to attack only the superfluous deposit of fat, and, as my medical friend informs me, purges the blood, rendering it more pure and healthy, strengthens the muscles and bodily viscera, and I feel quite convinced sweetens life, if it does not prolong it.

It is truly gratifying to me to be able now to add that many other of the most exalted members of the Faculty have honoured my movement in the question with their approbation.

I consider it a public duty further to state, that Mr. Harvey, whom I have named in the 43rd page as my kind medical adviser in the cure of Corpulence, is not Dr. John Harvey, who has published a Pamphlet on Corpulence assimilating with some of the features and the general aspect of mine, and which has been considered (as I learn from correspondents who have obtained it) the work of my medical friend. It is not.

I am glad, therefore, to repeat that my medical adviser was, and is still, Mr. WILLIAM HARVEY, F.R.C.S., No.2, Soho Square, London, W.

WILLIAM BANTING.

April, 1864.

Mr.Harvey's Remarks

"My patient, Mr.Banting having published for the benefit of his fellow sufferers, some account of the diet which I recommended him to adopt with a view to relieve himself of a distressing degree of hypertrophy of the adipose tissue. I have been frequently urged by him to explain the principles upon which I was enable to treat with success the inconvenient and in some instances distressing condition of the system.

"The simple history of my finding occasion to investigate the subject is as follows: when in Paris in the year 1856, I took the opportunity of attending a discussion on the views of M. Bernards who was at that time propounding his now generally admitted theory of the liver functions. After he had discovered by chemical processes and physiological experiments, which it is unnecessary for me to recapitulate here, that the liver not only secreted bile, but also a peculiar anyloid or starch-like product which he called glucose, and which in its chemical and physical properties appeared to be nearly allied to saccharine matter, he further found that this glucose could be directly produced in the liver by the ingestion of sugar and its ally starch and that in diabetes it existed there in considerable excess.

It had long been well known that a purely animal diet greatly assisted in checking the secretion of diabetic urine; and it seemed to follow, as a matter of course, that the total abstinence from saccharine and farinaceous matter must drain the liver of this excessive amount of glucose, and thus arrest in a similar proportion the diabetic tendency.

Reflecting on this chain of argument and knowing too that a saccharine and farinaceous diet is used to fatten certain animals, and that in diabetes, the whole of the fat in the body rapidly disappears, it occurred to me that excessive obesity might be allied to diabetes as to its cause, although widely diverse in its development: and that if a purely animal diet was useful in the latter disease, a combination of animal food with such vegetable matter as contained neither sugar nor starch, might serve to arrest the undue formation of fat. I soon afterwards had an opportunity of testing this idea. A dispensary patient who consulted me for deafness, and who was enourmously corpulent, I found to have no distinguishable disease of the ear. I therefore suspected that his deafness arose from the great development of adipose matter in the throat, pressing upon and stopping up the eustachian tubes. I subjected him to a strict non-farinaceous and non-saccharine diet, and treated him with the volatile alkali alluded to in his Pamphlet, and occasional aperients and in about seven months he was reduced to almost normal proportions, his hearing restored and his general health immensely improved. The case seemed to give substance and reality to my conjectures, which further experience has confirmed.

"When we consider that fat is what is termed hydrocarbon, and deposits itself so insidiously and yet so gradually amongst the tissues of the body it is at once manifest that we require such substances as contain a superfluity of oxygen and nitrogen to arrest its formation and to vitalize the system. That is the principle upon which the diet suggested in his pamphlet works, and explains on the one hand the necessity of abstaining from all vegetable roots which hold a large quantity of saccharine matter, and on the other beneficial effects derivable from those vegetables, the fruits of which are on the exterior of the earth, as they lose, probably by means of the sun's action a large proportion of their sugar.

"With regard to the tables of Dr. Hutchinson, referred to in his Pamphlet, it is no doubt difficult, as he says, to determine what is a man's proper weight, which must be influenced by various cases. Those tables, however, were formed by him on the principle of considering the amount of air which the lungs in their healthy state can receive and apply to the oxidation of the blood. I gave them to Mr. Banting as an indication only of what the approximate weight of persons in proportion to their stature should be, and with the view of proving to them the importance of keeping down the tendency to grow fat; for, as that tendency increases, the capacity of the lungs, and consequently the vitality and power of the whole system must diminish. In conclusion, I would suggest the propriety of advising a dietary such as this in diseases that are in any way influenced by a disordered condition of the hepatic functions as they cannot fail to yield in some degree to this simple method of treatment if fairly and properly carried out; it remains for me to watch its progress in a more limited sphere.

WILLIAM HARVEY, F.R.C.S.
Surgeon to the Royal Dispensary for Diseases of the Ear
2, Soho Square
April, 1864

Mr. Banting's :Letters to the Owner of the 1869 Edition which Is at Countway Library at Harvard Medical School

18 October 1870
4, The Terrace
Kensington.W.

To: James H. Brown, Esq.

My dear Sir

I have the pleasure to acknowledge the receipt of your letter "dated 30th September." This morning, nothing you could possibly have sent me from America or any other part of the World could have been more gratifying. I thank you heartily for it as well as for the newspaper scraps which accompanied it showing your kind, noble, and generous vindication of the Banting system. I assure you I am quite delighted that you and some of your friends have found benefit from a trial of it. I am constantly still receiving gratifying letters and the medical men in England; or at least some of the most important of them, have written to compliment me on what I have done. Hundreds regret they did not inaugurate it and indeed I for one am sorry they did not for I do not like notoriety. They all knew that my advice was right for attaining muscular strength for boating, cricket, and all athletic sports but just stopped short of applying it to the corpulent invalid. So, I have won a T'ams which I never thought of and they have lost it but I surely believe if any Medical Man had written the Pamphlet no one would have cared to read or pursue the plans which hundreds and thousands of people have pursued beneficially in all parts of the World.

It matters very little and certainly nothing to me what jest ridicule or abuse is bestowed upon the system for the great and simple fact remains uncontroversial and I am beyond suppression of any kind and simply highly pleased and delighted that I have aided in waking up Medical Men and others to a proper state of reflection.

Like you, I do not vary more than a pound during the year. I am now close on 74, have general good health, mentally and bodily, which I had not when I had to carry 50 lbs additional useless fat. I thank you for good and kind wishes. I and mine are all well and quite happy and all beyond the reach of want or poverty. It will be our own fault if we ever fall into worse circumstances, not at all likely.

With reiterated and hearty thanks and every good wish

I remain
Dear Sir
Yours sincerely
W. Banting

Let me beg of you to read thoughtfully and carefully D. Meinigers lecture published (translated from the German) in my 4th Edition. He is the most eminent Professor and Physician in Germany and it is well worthy careful notice. the medical men in England; or at

England
4, The Terrace,
Kensington.W.
30 July 1869

Dear Sir

I am very much gratified by your highly interesting letter just received-much obliged to you for sending to me, very much pleased to acknowledge and reply to it with my hearty congratulations that you have found benefit from the even partial practice of the dietary system which it was my privilege to disseminate for the advantage and benefit of my fellow man in all parts of the civilized world. I am very glad you have obtained my fourth edition on account of the confirmatory proof of the correction of my own humble testimony. You have done so much and so well that I have not a word to add in the way of advice. You may now feel you have the reins of your own health in your own hands and can slacken or tighten them as you think proper. I am sure you will disseminate your experience to our fellow men as I have endeavoured to do and I hope that in time when skepticism is quite abated we may drive undue corpulence out of the civilized world.

With every good wish I remain
Dear Sir
Yours sincerely
William Banting

4 The Terrace
Kensington, London
31 Jan 1870

Dear Sir

I beg to acknowledge the receipt of your kind letter and the articles from the Philadelphia Daily Evening Telegraph of the 8th. I think it a very able and highly interesting article. It is particularly gratifying to me to have the matter so noticed, not for any feeling as regard myself personally, but I think it will much aid in disseminating the system for the benefit of our fellow men. I heard of it last week and have written to the Editor today how much I was pleased. I was gratified to learn that my 3rd Edition had gone through 5 or 6 in Philadelphia and that it had gone through several in New York as well as being published in its entirety in one of their Journals.

Niemeyer's lecture in my 4th Edition is a most interesting and valuable testimonial to the utility of the system properly considered and judiciously followed and I thank you on the part of our fellow men for doing all you can to bring it fully into public consideration. I heartily thank you for the letter and the article, remaining with every good wish to you and yours.

Dear Sir
Yours faithfully
William Banting

I continue in good bodily and mental health, am in my 76th year - have lost 50 lbs in weight - 13 inches in girth and maintain my normal condition - Few men of my age more active - I cannot expect this will last much longer.

My 3rd Edition reached 63,000 copies when I published the result and since that 3 or 4 hundred copies have been sold.

CLASSICS IN OBESITY

A DEPARTURE FROM THE USUAL METHODS IN TREATING OBESITY

By Frank A. Evans, M.D.
Attending Physician, Western Pennsylvania Hospital
and James M. Strang, M.D.
Assistant to the Attending Physician, Western Pennsylvania Hospital
(From the Medical Service of the Western Pennsylvania Hospital, Pittsburgh, PA)

Obesity, in degrees worthy of comment, has for sometime been appreciated by physicians as a menace to continued health. It has not been so considered by most patients, even when constituting a frankly pathologic condition. Any rational treatment demands intelligent cooperation of patients, and for these reasons, in the past, satisfactory results were not always obtained. Recently, however, since people have become more interested in preventive medicine, from a personal point of view, overweight is being taken more seriously. More patients than formerly are presenting themselves to physicians complaining of obesity alone, and of these a gratifying percentage make the necessary sacrifices for relief and cooperate willingly.

The apparent paradox that some people get fat and others do not on what appears to be equivalent diets has invited much speculation. In a few cases, of course, a lowered metabolic rate and increased sugar tolerance is associated with endocrine disorders. These are outspoken cases of endocrine disease and are rare. In the vast majority of persons no such disorders are demonstrable. One might expect that these people have normally a lower metabolic rate, but we have ample evidence that when calculated by the usual methods, it is within normal limits: (Jones;[1] Preble;[2] Means;[3] Strouse, Wang and Dye;[4] Lauter;[5] Labbé and Stèvenin[6]). In normal persons, combustion is speeded up after protein ingestion due to the specific stimulative effect of certain amino-acids on the oxidative processes of the organism. It has been suggested that in the obese this so-called specific dynamic action of protein is not so marked (Gibbons;[7] Strouse, Wang and Dye[4]). Recently some observers (Wang, Strouse and Saunders;[8] Hagedorn, Holten, Becht;[9] Wang and Strouse[10]) not only postulate a diminished specific dynamic action of protein in the obese but also some abnormality of fat metabolism by which it is spared and thus becomes available for storage. These patients are said to use protein and especially carbohydrate more easily than normal, so much more easily than fat that as long as any protein and carbohydrate is available no fat will be used. If these suggested disorders of metabolism in the obese do exist they are, possibly, dependent upon an endocrine cause imbalance varying in some minor degree from the accepted normal. But it is none that is now recognized and, therefore, not a condition which can be treated by any rational endocrine therapy. No person, whatever his endocrine function may be, will gain in weight if his caloric intake balances or is less than his energy output. And, except in those rare cases in which obesity is associated with the true endocrine disorders too widely known to need description here, in which endocrine therapy should be instituted for the endocrinopathy itself, endocrine products should not be thought of in connection with obesity. The treatment should be dietary, and dietary alone.

One hears all sorts of fads and fancies in diet suggested for reducing weight. No special article of food has any merit in this regard. Total calories must be reduced. Folin and Denis[11] tried, apparently with good results, alternate periods of complete fasting and absolute freedom of diet. Most régimes, however, merely state that sufficient protein be given to keep the patient in nitrogen equilibrium and total calories be reduced by a lowered intake of carbohydrate and fat, reducing the caloric intake cautiously and the weight gradually. This is safe, rational, and may frequently be carried through.

If we thought of this problem with the same metabolic insight as used in the dietary treatment of diabet-

Evans FA, Strang JM. A departure from usual methods in treating obesity. *Am J Med Sci.* 1929;177:339-348.
Reprinted with permission from J.B. Lippincott Co., 227 E. Washington Square, Philadelphia, PA 19106.
Special thanks to Judy Roberts of the Pennington Information Center for help in acquiring this document.

ics, could we not with safety be somewhat more radical? Instead of cautiously reducing the diets of the obese to 14 or 15 calories per kilogram with resulting weight losses of 6 to 8 pounds a month, would it not be safe in some cases to give them half as may calories, say 6 to 8 per kilogram, and get a more rapid reduction? It was tried and found satisfactory.

The method used has been to calculate the correct diet for the ideal weight or whatever weight is desired. Different from diabetes, more than enough protein has been given to keep the patient in nitrogen equilibrium, 1 gm. of protein per kilogram, because in the treatment of obesity the specific dynamic action of protein probably was desirable. With a gram of protein per kilogram, enough carbohydrate and fat was calculated to give 25 calories per kilogram, the carbohydrate and fat in such proportion that the ketogenic-antiketogenic ration was 1 1/2 to 1. Having obtained the figures for protein, fat and carbohydrate, the menu was made up to fit the figures for protein and carbohydrate, and as much of the fat was omitted as could be, while allowing the patient the desired amount of protein.

For example: A woman, married, aged thirty-four years, 64 inches tall, should have an ideal weight of 60 kg. The diet for her ideal weight was calculated with 1 gm. of protein and 25 calories per kilogram and carbohydrate and fat in such proportion that the ketogenic-antiketogenic ratio was 1 1/2 to 1. The figures obtained were:

	Grams	Calories
Protein................	60	240
Carbohydrate........	45	180
Fat....................	120	1080
		1500

The menu made up and given to this patient contained:

	Grams	Calories
Protein...............	60	240
Carbohydrate.......	45	180
Fat..................	29	261
		681

The patient weighed 176 pounds or 80 kg. She was, therefore, getting in this diet 8.5 calories per kilogram.. Assuming that she needed, not 25 calories as calculated in her reduction diet, but 30 calories per kilogram to maintain her weight, there was a deficit of 21.5 calories per kilogram. She was, therefore, getting in the diet given 1720 calories per day less than she needed to maintain her weight. If these calories were supplied from her own fat she was using 185 gm. of fat, which is equivalent to 212 gm. of her own fatty tissue (12) each day, 1500 gm. per week. She might be expected to lose, therefore, not 6 to 8, but 12 to 14 pounds a month.

The possibility of the development of acidosis on this diet does not appear to be great. The maximum possible ketogenic-antiketogenic ratio, according to Woodyatt's formula, may be estimated by assuming that the entire caloric deficit is supplied by fat alone and that the stored fat metabolizes in the same manner as the fat in the diet. If this assumption is correct the caloric deficit of 1720 is equivalent to 185 gm. of fat. In addition to the 60 gm. of protein and 45 gm. of carbohydrate, the menu supplied 29 gm. of fat. The total amount of fat utilized is, therefore, 214 gm. The glucose equivalent is 101, the fatty acid equivalent 221, a ratio of less than 2.2 to 1. We know that ketogenic-antiketogenic ratios of 2 to 1 are well tolerated, and, under certain circumstances, ratios as high as 3 1/2 to 1 have been used with safety even in diabetic patients. In view of the possibility of a transformation into glucose of some fraction of the endogenous fat metabolized,[13] the actual ratios are probably much lower.

The diet was maintained for ten weeks, during which time the patient lost 42 pounds. She suffered no unpleasant symptoms until the end of this period, when she began to feel tired. The diet was increased until she had gained 4 pounds. The diet was then changed to maintain this weight and she remained so for over one year. The following year she gave birth to her second child, normal in all respects, and since then she has been heavier, but never, over a period of three years, more than 150 pounds.

More radical reduction with higher theoretical ketogenic-antiketogenic ratios have been used in many cases with nothing but the most gratifying results. For example: An unmarried woman, aged forty-six years, 59 1/2 inches tall had an ideal weight of less than 50 kg. The diet for her ideal weight was calculated with 1 gm of protein and but 20 calories per kilogram and carbohydrate and fat in such proportion that the ketogenic-antiketogenic ratio was 1 1/2 to 1. The figures obtained were:

	Grams	Calories
Protein................	50	200
Carbohydrate........	26	104
Fat....................	77	693
		997

The menu made up and given to this patient contained:

	Grams	Calories
Protein................	50	200
Carbohydrate........	26	104
Fat....................	27	243
		547

This patient weighed 178 pounds or 80 kg. She was, therefore, getting in this diet 6.81 calories per kilogram. If we assume that she needed as much as 30 calories per kilogram to maintain her weight, there was a deficit of 23.2 calories per kilogram. She was, therefore, getting in this diet 1856 calories per day less than she needed to maintain her weight. If this was made up from her own fat she was using 199 gm. a day. With the same assumptions as above for the calculation of this menu, we get a glucose equivalent of 78 and a fatty-acid equivalent of 226. This is a ketogenic-antiketogenic ratio of slightly less than 3 to 1.

This diet was maintained for ten weeks, during which time the patient lost 37 1/4 pounds, and suffered no discomfort or inconvenience. It has now been twelve months since she stopped dieting and she has at no time weighed more than 140 pounds. During this period, no evidence of organic or functional damage has presented itself and there has been no diminution of energy or vitality.

The menu given to this patient and the instructions appended to all menus given out are as follows:

Breakfast: 1 egg, 1 ounce bread.

Lunch: 1 egg, 4 ounces vegetables as listed.

Dinner: 1 cup bouillon (if desired) 3 ounces lean meat (weighed after cooking), 4 ounces vegetables as listed.

Acceptable vegetables: Lettuce, cucumbers, spinach, asparagus, endive, celery, mushrooms, tomatoes, brussels sprouts, watercress, cauliflower, radishes, cabbage, onions-very sparingly.

1. If the bread is eaten as toast, it must be weighed before toasting.
2. Eggs may be taken boiled, poached, or raw.
3. Meat may be boiled, broiled, or roasted.
4. No fried foods may be eaten.
5. No lard or butter may be used in cooking.
6. Vegetables must be prepared without milk, oil, or egg dressing.
7. Water may be taken as desired.
8. Salt, pepper and vinegar (not lemon juice) may be used as desired.
9. It is just as important that all this be eaten as that nothing not on the list be taken.
10. Take a level teaspoonful of soda in half glass of water twice each day.

No thought was given to vitamin or salt content of the diet, the menus given being considered satisfactory in these regards for the limited periods of dieting required. The patients were urged to eat preferably the salad vegetables which could be taken raw. With salt, pepper, vinegar, and egg when listed, and mineral oil, many patients developed salad dressings to satisfy the most exacting.

Using this method for metabolic orientation, a number of patients have been kept for weeks on diets containing less than 8 calories per kilogram. This report is based on 111 patients who are either completed cases or have been dieting four weeks. These patients averaged 47.5 per cent overweight. Among them 5 patients were 100 per cent overweight, 11 were 75 to 100 per cent overweight, and 27 were 50 to 75 per cent overweight.

Ninety-eight patients are completed cases. Their data may be summarized as follows:

98 patients in 858 weeks lost a total of 2590 pounds.

Average time on diet, 8.75 weeks.

Average loss per patient, 26.4 pounds.

Average loss per week, 3.02 pounds.

The data for the 11 patients at the end of the first week summarized is:

111 patients lost 714 pounds.

Average loss per patient, 6.43 pounds.

Figures are available for exactly four weeks on 75 patients. This data summarized is:

75 patients lost 1209 pounds in four weeks.

Average loss per patient in four weeks, 16.1 pounds.

Average loss per week, 4.03 pounds.

Forty-seven patients were weighed exactly at the end of eight weeks. This data in summary is:

47 patients lost 1265 pounds.

Average loss per patient, 26.9 pounds.

Average loss per week, 3.36 pounds.

This rapid reduction is satisfactory only if the patient is not damaged by it. All the patients thus treated have at the end of a week felt much better and, at the end of two weeks, were quite enthusiastic. Statements such as "I am sleeping better than for years," are common throughout the entire period of dieting. During the first two to three days there was sometimes headache, dizziness, weakness, occasionally nausea; but this had passed by the fourth day. A bad taste in the mouth lasted very often a week, but no longer. All these patients had acetone in the urine at first, sometimes for weeks, but still were enthusiastic in their expressions of well-being.

So far, there have been no disasters or even minor misfortunes. The hemoglobin and red-cell counts have either remained the same or increased, and there has been no acidosis. Eighty-eight of these patients have been followed for six months or more after being thus radically reduced and none have shown a floating kidney, splanchnoptosis, hernia, or, where varicose veins were present, anything but improvement in them.

All the cases were thoroughly examined for contraindications before the treatment was undertaken. No doubt a tuberculous lesion would be a contraindication, but the list of others has been growing smaller as experience increases. Patients with myocardial lesions are supposed to be poor subjects for reduction, and they probably are. Among these patients there were 8 with definite evidence of myocardial damage and many with symptoms, such as dyspnea, swelling of the feet, and palpitation, suggesting minor grades of myocardial insufficiency. These patients were dieted exactly as the others and, with one exception, the results were just as gratifying. The exception was a case shown, six months after dieting, to be complicated by a psychopathic lesion leading to moral turpitude of a criminal nature for which he was convicted and confined.

Adolescents and the elderly are thought to bear reduction cures poorly. There was one twelve-year-old girl in the series, who reduced from 208 1/2 to 164 1/2 pounds –44 pounds– in twenty weeks, with nothing but marked improvement in her physical and mental equipment. Another girl, aged sixteen years, was reduced from 223 to 143 pounds–80 pounds–in twenty weeks and she not only improved mentally and physically but a dysmenorrhea of three years' standing disappeared and has not returned in three years.[12] At the other extreme of life, one patient, aged sixty-seven years, came into the office walking with difficulty. She was having 15 to 18 extrasystoles a minute and her blood pressure was 240 systolic, 110 diastolic. She was reduced from 278 to 182 pounds - in twenty-four weeks, an average of 4 pounds a week. After the first two weeks, the extrasystoles disappeared. Her blood pressure after four weeks dieting was 135 systolic, 80 diastolic, and for the last two years has not been above 150. After four weeks, she began doing housework and marketing with ease and comfort. The age range of this short series, twelve to sixty-seven years, would seem to cast doubt on adolescence and senescence as contraindications to the reducing cure, if sound metabolic principles are followed.

The reaction of the blood pressure to this method of dieting is interesting. If it is normal, it remains so. If it is high, in a gratifying number of cases it comes down. In this series of 111 patients, there were 33 with systolic blood pressures above 150. All but one of them showed a lowered systolic pressure after a period of dieting. In some, this was remarkable. One patient with a systolic reading of 215 at the beginning had 135 after eight weeks dieting. Another came down from 260 to 170. The elderly patient mentioned above, whose systolic pressure of 240 was reduced to 135 in four weeks, was seen later after a period of careless eating during a trip to California, 22 pounds heavier than on discharge. In spite of this weight increase her systolic blood-pressure reading was 150. Among 23 patients who had systolic blood pressures between 150 and 200, there were 16 who attained normal figures. For the entire group of 33 patients, the average systolic blood pressure was 189 at the beginning, and 146 after dieting. This is in accord with the findings of Preble[2] and Terry[15] who reduced their cases much more gradually than was done in this series.

Before dieting, a surprising number of these patients complained bitterly of headaches, which in 9 of them were so severe and so frequent as to suggest migraine. In every one, remarkable relief was obtained. One patient under observation at present who previously had two prostating headaches each week, had one the first and second day of dieting and none since, now six weeks. Another, equally bad, had one headache during two months of dieting and another in the succeeding three months. A dull, heavy feeling in the head, complained of by so many, has been completely relieved in all.

A caution about the development of wrinkles and a drawn expression of the face was given to about the first 25 of these patients. It is now no longer given because it was found unnecessary. Except for an occasional deepening of the nasolabial fold and flabbiness resulting from the removal of a "double chin," no wrinkles developed. These patients looked better and younger because of clearer skin and a more animated expression. These features, in contrast to those often found heretofore on reducing patients, suggest that the drawn expression was due to starvation and not to removal of subcutaneous fat of the face.

Minor skin disorders were frequently relieved. Intertrigo disappeared or became easy to control in every case in which it was found. One case diagnosed epidermophytosis, and another with such annoying pruritus vulvae that oxyuris infestation was seriously considered, obtained complete relief in three and six weeks respectively. It cannot be stated yet that this relief is permanent, for these patients are still dieting.

With the exception of the patient with the psychopathic trend mentioned above, the mental attitude of these patients has been excellent. The appreciable weight loss during the first week and the feeling of well-being experienced during the second week, which showed them that a rapid weight loss could be obtained without making them sick or interfering with their usual activities, put them in a cheerful frame of mind. The irritability of starvation was entirely absent, indicating that these patients were not being physiologically starved.

These patients were not selected, all presenting being treated the same way, whether of the alimentary or the so-called endocrine type. No difference was found in the reaction of the two types of cases except possibly in the speed of reduction. The symptom obesity, of the cases of "endocrine obesity," can be treated with success by dietary measures alone. Indeed it appears that other symptoms in these cases of "endocrine obesity" yield to this method of dieting, especially menstrual disorders.[12] In many of these patients the flow was scanty, the period prostrating. Most were relieved. Six of these patients had menstrual disorders of pathologic proportions. All but one were relieved. These will be reported in detail later, but one especially interesting case may be presented briefly here. A woman, unmarried, aged twenty-three years, weighed 150 pounds at the age of eighteen years. Menstruation began when she was fourteen years of age and was normal for eight years. From eighteen until twenty-two years of age she gained 50 pounds. Menses then stopped. The patient presented herself, not having menstruated for eleven months, during which time she had gained 50 pounds. She weight 259 pounds. She had a marked hypertrichosis of the upper lip, chest, forearms, and legs with a masculine distribution of the crines. During twenty-eight weeks' dieting, with a loss of 86 pounds, she menstruated six times without discomfort.

The diets were begun suddenly. All of the patients complained of hunger during the first day, many during the second, and a few for as long as three days. There were only 4 patients in this series who complained of hunger during the entire period of restricted diet. In 2 of these, there was strong suspicion that they kept tempting themselves by nibbles. Many of the patients expressed contentment with the diet. Others lost their appetites and became indifferent to eating, even when active around the kitchen. For this reason, the ninth instruction given them was found necessary and it was always emphasized. None of the patients developed an aversion to food.

Practically all of these patients suffered from constipation, and in some it was really troublesome. This symptom was met in the usual manner and disappeared with resumption of a more generous diet. Agar and bran were not given because with 6 or 7 ounces of 5 per cent vegetables in the diet, it seemed that the constipation was not caused by a diminution of bulk or too refined foodstuffs. The cause of this constipation has not been determined. Possibly the limited carbohydrate of the diet is a factor.

The weight loss was not regular from week to week. In some weeks it would be double that in others. Over a longer period it averaged closely to the calculated figures, however, and after a week with little or no loss one could reassure the patient that in the next she would make up the deficit. This irregularity is due in large part to variations in water balance. Studies on this factor will be reported in detail in a later paper.

When the patients had reached the desired weight, the diet was changed as suddenly as at the beginning. They were put on a weighed diet calculated to maintain them at their present weight and asked to be just as accurate as with the restricted menu. After one month's observation, any corrections necessary were made and they were dismissed for one month. At the end of the second month they were weighed, told to weigh each week and to eat as they desired and could without gaining, and discharged to report in six months. A number of these patients came back saying they had found they could eat as they wanted without gaining. Enquiry revealed that they were eating by choice, after this period of gustatory discipline, just about the proper food.

All these patients continued to lose, and at an increased rate, for one or more weeks after being put on the more generous diet. That this should happen when the diet was suddenly increased so much – often from 600 to 2000 calories – is interesting. The cause of this has been investigated and will be presented in a subsequent report.

Many patients presented themselves for reduction who, when they found out what was necessary, did not go through with it. Practically all those who were faithful for two weeks went to the end. The need for accuracy was emphasized strongly at the beginning and these patients were handled somewhat more firmly than one would care, perhaps, to deal with all his private patients. None of these patients were put in the hospital, all being private patients seen in the office who prepared and weighed their own food at home. It was tried with dispensary patients but did not succeed, these patients being either unwilling or incapable of giving the necessary cooperation.

Conclusion. 1. The importance of metabolic orientation in the treatment of the obese is emphasized.

2. If sound metabolic principles are followed, obese patients can be kept for weeks on diets containing less than 7 calories per kilogram.

3. One hundred and eleven patients, so treated and here reported, lost weight rapidly with nothing but the most gratifying results. They were not hungry. They were cheerful. Headaches were relieved and elevated systolic blood pressures were reduced. Minor disorders of different kinds showed improvement. A sense of wellbeing while on the diet – often as low as 600 calories – was obtained which was in sharp contrast to the irritability and cachexia seen with more generous diets not carefully planned on metabolic principles.

4. The obesity of "endocrine obesity" yields to dietary measures as well as that of the alimentary type. Endocrine products are, therefore, not indicated in the treatment of this symptom of these patients.

5. Most of the menstrual disorders so common in the obese are corrected by proper diet alone.

BIBLIOGRAPHY.

1. Jones, H.M.: Basal Metabolic Rate in Simple and Pathologic Obesity, J. Lab. and Clin. Med., 1926, 11, 959.
2. Preble, W.E.: Obesity: Observations on One Thousand Cases, Boston Me. and Surg. J., 1923, 188, 617.
3. Means, J.H.: The Basal Metabolism in Obesity, Arch. Int. Med., 1916, 17, 704.
4. Strouse, S., Wang, C.C., and Dye, M.: Studies on the Metabolism of Obesity, J. Am. Med. Assn., 1924, 82, 2111.
5. Lauter, S.: Genesis of Obesity, Deutsch. Arch f. klin. Med., 1926, 150, 315.
6. Labbé, M., and Stévenin, H.: Basal Metabolism in the Obese, Compt. rend. Soc. de biol., 1923, 88, 9.
7. Gibbones, R.: Specific Dynamic Action of Proteins in Dogs, Am. J. Physiol., 1924, 70, 26.
8. Wang, C.C., Strouse, S., and Saunders, A.D.: Metabolism of Obesity, Arch. Int. Med., 1924, 34, 573.
9. Hagedorn, H.C., Holten, C., and Becht, J.: Pathologic Metabolism in the Obese, Hospitalstidende, Copenhagen, 1926, 69, 853.
10. Wang, C.C., and Strouse, S.: Metabolism of Obesity: IV. Distribution of Energy Production after Food, Arch. Int. Med., 1915, 36, 397.
11. Folin, O., and Denis, W.: On Starvation and Obesity, with Special Reference to Acidosis, J. Biol. Chem., 1915, 21, 183.
12. Bozenraad, quoted by Du Bois, E.F.: Basal Metabolism in Health and Disease, Philadelphia, Leas & Febiger, 1927, p. 235.
13. Thannhauser, S.J.: Can the Organism form Carbohydrate from Fat, Deutsch. med. Wchnschr., 1927, 40, 1676.
14. Evans, F.A.: A Radical Cure of Simple Obesity by Dietary Measures Alone, Atlantic Med. J., 1926, 29, 240.
15. Terry, A.H.: Obesity and Hypertension, J.Am. Med. Assn., 1923, 81, 1283.

THE CONTROL OF EATING

BY CHARLES B. FERSTER, JOHN I. NURNBERGER, AND EUGENE B. LEVITT
Indiana University Medical Center

Although many investigators have described patterns of eating behavior and reported a wide range of factors related to obesity (1,2,5,9,10,11), specific techniques for changing an individual's eating behavior are given little or no attention in published reports, and programs of weight control based on behavioral principles are virtually non-existent. This report is an account of the application of some elementary general principles of reinforcement theory (7) to the analysis of the behavior of the human eater. This theoretical framework of reinforcement was used to analyze actual performances in eating, and particularly self-control of eating. Supplementing the account of this system are descriptions of experimentally developed techniques which should illustrate practical applications of the theoretical principles of self-control.[1]

The theoretical analysis begins with the simple observation that the act of putting food in one's mouth is reinforced and strongly maintained by its immediate consequences: the local effects in the gastro-intestinal system. But excessive eating results in increased body-fat and this is aversive to the individual. The problem in therefore to gain control of the factors which determine how often and how much one eats. An individual will manipulate these variables if the control of eating is reinforcing to him — if he escapes from or avoids the ultimate aversive consequences of eating (UAC). Unfortunately for the overeater, the long-term or ultimate aversive consequences of obesity are so postponed as to be ineffective compared with the immediate reinforcement of food in the mouth. Alcoholism is a similar example in which hangover symptoms and the full impact of asocial activity are not suffered until considerable time has elapsed. Realization of self-control, then, demands an arrangement that will bring the influencing conditions into closer association with the reduction of eating behavior.

The analysis and development of self-control in eating involves four steps:

1. *Determining what variables influence eating.* Almost every known behavioral process is relevant to this. Among these are control of eating by stimuli, effect of food deprivation, chaining, avoidance and escape, prepotent and competing behaviors, conditioned alimentary reflexes, and positive reinforcement (2).
2. *Determining how these variables can be manipulated.* Specification of performances within the repertoire by which the individual can manipulate these variables. One example would be the choice of foods which are weak reinforcers, yet rewarding enough to maintain the behavior of eating them at some low level.
3. *Identifying the unwanted effects (UAC) of overeating.* Avoidance of these is the basic motive for developing the required self-control.
4. *Arranging a method of developing required self-control.* Some of the required performances may call for so drastic a change of behavior that it may be necessary to produce the required repertory in stages by reinforcing successive approximations.

Self-control requires for our purposes a more precise definition than is conveyed by the term "will-power." It refers to some specific performances which will lower the disposition to emit the behavior to be controlled. These performances involve the manipulation of conditions influencing this behavior. A convenient datum for our analysis is the frequency of the behavior's occurrence. The strength, durability or persistence of the behavior is measured by its frequency. Frequency has the measurement advantage of being a continuous variable. Similarly, the disposition to eat can vary from small to large. The various conditions which the individ-

Ferster CB, Nurnberger JI, Levitt EB. The control of eating. J Mathetics. 1962;1:87-109.
Reprinted with permission of Marilyn B. Gilbert, The Mathetics Foundation. Special thanks to Ms. Gilbert and Dr. Paul Siegel.

[1] The experiments are still underway and will be reported separately by the second and third authors.

ual himself can manipulate to lessen the frequency of the controlled behavior will be presented in detail in the next section, Avenues of Self-Control. The technical problem of generating the self-control performance and maintaining it in strength will be dealt with in the section Shaping and Maintaining the Self-Control Performance.

AVENUES OF SELF-CONTROL

The Ultimate Aversive Consequences

Avoidance of the ultimate aversive consequences (UAC) of uncontrolled eating is essential in developing performances with which a person may regulate his eating behavior. Self-control is needed because of the time lapse between the act of eating and its UAC. To overcome this time lapse, techniques were sought which would derive a conditioned stimulus from the UAC and apply it at the time the disposition to eat was strong. This is based on the principle that almost any event may become aversive when paired with a known aversive event. Such a conditioned stimulus may be the person's own verbal behavior, if specific training procedures are applied. It is not enough for the subject to know what the aversive effect of overeating is, for such knowledge by itself leads only to verbal responses weaker than the food-maintained behavior and may not lessen the strong disposition to eat. Therefore an extensive repertoire must be established so that the subject has under his control large amounts of verbal behavior dealing with the consequences of eating. The continued intensive pairing of facts about the UAC with various kinds of eating performance will make the performances themselves conditioned aversive stimuli. Once a given performance such as eating a piece of pie acquires conditioned aversive properties, any approach to it will produce aversive stimuli. These stimuli will reinforce any self-control because the self-control terminates the aversive stimulus and prevents the uncontrolled act. By such a process, certain foods like pies, cakes, cokes, doughnuts or candy may become conditioned aversive stimuli, at least until other avenues of control became available.

Before the unwelcome consequences of overeating can be used in developing self-control, they must be identified and developed for the individual. It cannot be assumed that an obese person already has a repertoire about the UAC of eating. In the application of the principles to human subjects being studied, the development of the UAC was one of the major parts of the practical program. However, developing a repertoire by which the subjects could create an aversive state of affairs for themselves presents serious technical problems. First, to establish this repertoire, the actual aversive events must be identified for the subject in terms that are meaningful for his daily life. Second, the subject must learn an active verbal repertoire with which he can translate caloric intake into ultimate body fat.

We first disclosed, in great detail, the consequences of uncontrolled eating for each individual. After each subject described anecdotes about UAC in group sessions, we helped each one to develop fluent verbal repertoire about the relevant aversive consequences. We found that simply recognizing the various aversive consequences did not give these subjects an active verbal repertoire which could be invoked immediately and whenever needed. To develop an active repertoire about the UAC, we arranged rehearsals, frequent repetitions, and written examination. In general, the subjects were unaware of their inability to verbalize the relevant aversive consequences, and were surprised by the poor results of the early written and oral examinations. Verbal descriptions of aversive consequences the subjects had actually experienced were far more compelling than reports of future and statistically probable consequences, such as diabetes, heart disease, high blood pressure, or gall bladder disorder. In other words, descriptions of actual or imagined social rejection, sarcastic treatment, extreme personal sensitivity over excess weight, demeaning inferences concerning professional incompetence or carelessness, or critical references to bodily contours or proportions were much more potent. All of our subjects found their constant and unsuccessful preoccupation with dieting aversive, and any ability to control their own habits highly rewarding.

All of the exercises in this area were designed to develop a strong and vivid repertoire that could be introduced promptly in a wide variety of situations intimately associated with eating and despite a strong inclination to eat. The actual aversive effects of being overweight are largely individual matters which differ widely from person to person. We therefore used group discussions as an aid for each person to discover how her body weight affected her life. The discussion was guided toward explicit consequences and anecdotes rather than general statements such as "I want to lose weight because I will feel better." We found that after only four or more group sessions, subjects shifted from vague statements such as "I'll look better in clothes" to specific ones such as "My husband made a sarcastic remark about an obese woman who crossed the street as we were driving by." Perhaps, the verbalization of the UAC was too aversive before we had demonstrated that self-control was possible.

Amplifying the Aversive Consequences of Overeating.

To establish the bad effects of eating more than one's daily requirements, it is necessary that the individual know the metabolic relationships between different kinds of food, general level of activity, and gain or loss of weight. Phrases like "Everything I eat turns to fat" illustrate that the required repertoire is frequently absent. Thorough training should be given in the caloric properties of all of the kinds of foods which the individual will encounter. The aversive effects of eating certain undesirable foodstuffs can be amplified by generating verbal repertories which describe the full consequences of eating them. For example, the subject should be made to recognize that a 400-calorie piece of pie is the caloric equivalent of a large baked potato with butter plus a medium-size steak. The pie is equivalent to one-tenth of a pound of weight gained, and so forth. Again, knowing these facts is not at issue. The issue is that a strong-enough repertoire be established, and with enough intraverbal connections, that the UAC behavior will occur with a high probability in a wide enough variety of situations.

An important exercise early in the weight-control program is the identification of the individual's actual food intake. The subject's casual summaries of his daily food intake are likely to be grossly inaccurate. His ability to recognize his actual food intake is improved by an interview technique in which the interviewer probes and prompts him: "What did you have for breakfast?" "How many pieces of toast?" "How many pieces of bread?" "What did you do between ten and eleven in the morning?" "Were you at a snack bar or a restaurant at any point during the day?" "Were you offered any candy at any point?" and so forth.

With the pilot subjects, we leaned most heavily on a written protocol which we used as a basis for individual interviews about their diets. Each subject kept a complete written account of everything she had eaten, along with calculations of fat, carbohydrate, protein, and numbers of calories. A large part of the early sessions was devoted to problems in recording food intake, such as difficulties in estimating mixed foods like gravies, stews, or sauces.

For the first four weeks of the program, when some simpler kinds of self-control were developed, the subjects' caloric intake was set to maintain a constant weight. We overestimated the maintenance levels, and all subjects gained weight during this month. However, the weight increase proved the relationship between caloric intake and weight change in a situation where the caloric intake was carefully defined. In spite of the weight gain, however, some measure of self-control emerged, particularly in changes in the temporal pattern and regularity of eating.

Deprivation

The effect of food deprivation may be observed in a pigeon experiment in which the frequency of a pigeon's key pecking, maintained by producing food, is measured as a function of changes in the level of food deprivation. Changes in the level of food deprivation produce continuous changes in the bird's performance over an extremely wide range if we can measure the frequency of the bird's pecking. This frequency of pecking is intuitively close to notions like the bird's disposition to eat, probability of action, or motivation. When a wide range of frequency response can be measured sensitively, the level of deprivation affects the bird's performance continuously, from free-feeding body weight to as low as 65 to 70 per cent of normal body weight. Food deprivation of the order of six to twenty four hours constitutes a very small part of the effective range. The magnitude of food deprivation therefore continues to increase the organism's disposition to emit responses, reinforced by food, long after no further changes occur in gastrointestinal reactions (e.g., hunger pangs) and other conditioned effects of food in the mouth. The hunger pangs, which are ordinarily taken as symptoms of hunger (from which the effect of food deprivation is inferred), are more closely related to the conditioned stimuli accompanying past reinforcements of eating than to the level of food deprivation. The conditioned reflexes involving the gastrointestinal system occur at relatively low levels of deprivation compared with the effective range of food deprivation in respect to the changes in frequency of operant behavior. There may be a similar lack of correspondence between the tendency to verbalize, introspectively, reports of hunger and the actual disposition to eat. For purposes of developing self-control, the actual performances resulting in food in the mouth are more relevant than the introspective reports of "hunger."

Controlling the rate at which the subject loses weight proves to be a major technique of self-control. For any degree of establishment of a self-control repertoire, there is probably some level of food deprivation which will cause the subject to eat in spite of the self-control behavior. Therefore, a major principle of self-control would be to pace the rate of the subject's weight loss so that the effect of the weight loss on the disposition to eat would be less than the given stage of development of self-control. Many avenues of self-control may be learned without causing any weight loss. Placing the eating behavior under the control of specific stimuli or breaking up the chain of responses usually present in the compulsive eater are examples of this. The former will be discussed below. Breaking up a chain causes the eating performance to become a series of discrete acts which are more easily interrupted than a continuous performance in which each chewing response of each swallow occasions placing the next bit of food on the fork.

If the self-control performances which may be

developed are to be useful, they must be maintained by conditions which will be present continuously, even after the weight-control therapy procedures are discontinued. Many unsuccessful crash diet programs illustrate the way in which too rapid a loss of weight produces a level of deprivation and a disposition to eat exceeding the existing self-control. The usual diet involves some program which taps the motivation of the dieter temporarily. For example, slight aversive pressure from the husband or family doctor may produce a rapid loss in weight, perhaps on the order of three to five pounds a week. The effect of the rapid weight loss is a large increase in the disposition to eat which then overcomes the subject's temporary motive.

Limiting the diet to one specific food, such as protein, probably will produce a heightened disposition to eat other food stuffs regardless of the general weight level. These are the traditional specific hungers. An all-protein diet, for example, even if taken without limit of calories, would probably generate an enormous disposition to eat carbohydrates, sugars, and fats. Therefore, a balanced diet should be maintained and a weight loss brought about by a uniform reduction in amount rather than kind of food.

Although the major effects of food deprivation appear when weight losses are of the order of pounds, the time elapsed since eating would have local effects on the disposition to eat. Local satiation effects may best be used as a limited avenue of self-control by arranging the eating schedules so that the subject ingests a meal or a significant amount of food just before a situation in which the disposition to eat might be unusually strong. An example is a social situation in which eating has frequently occurred in the past or when preferred foods are present. The housewife who eats continuously while preparing dinner can control the disposition to nibble the foods being prepared by shifting the preparation of the dinner meal to the period of time immediately following lunch, when her disposition to eat is lower because she has just eaten.

In the application of the self-control principles to actual exercises, we specified a weight loss of one pound per week and insisted that our subjects adhere to this rate of weight loss even though each of them wanted to cut her diet more stringently in order to lose weight at a greater rate. Different rates of weight loss might possibly be arranged at different stages of development of self-control after more is known about the effectiveness of different avenues of self-control and about the relative effects of weight loss depending upon the initial level.

The continued ingestion of food during a meal provided another variation in level of food deprivation which was used to provide a gradual transition to the final self-control performances. Exercises, such as brief interruptions in eating, were first carried out toward the end of the meal when some satiation had occurred. After the subjects began to learn how to use auxiliary techniques to stop eating and their existing eating patterns began to break down, the exercises were moved progressively toward the early part of the meal, when their levels of deprivation were higher so that the exercises had to be more difficult.

Self-control by Manipulating Stimuli

The characteristic circumstances when an individual eats will subsequently control his disposition to eat. The process is illustrated by the pigeon whose key pecking produces food only when the key is green and not when it is red. The frequency with which the pigeon pecks the key (reinforced by food) will later depend upon which color is present. Thus, changing the color of the key can arbitrarily increase or decrease the frequency of pecking independently of the level of food deprivation. A frequent factor in the lack of self-control in the obese person may be the large variety of circumstances in which eating occurs. In contrast, a much narrower range of stimuli is present during the more infrequent eating periods of the controlled person. Therefore, the disposition to eat possibly could be decreased by narrowing the range of stimuli which are the occasions for the reinforcement by food. By proper choice of the actual stimuli controlling the eating behavior, it should also be possible to increase the individual's control over these stimuli. There are circumstances when even the pathologically compulsive eater will have a considerably lower disposition to eat for periods of time simply because the environment is novel enough so that eating has never occurred then. Consider, for example, walking in an isolated forest area.

The first step in the development of self-control in this category is to narrow the range of existing stimuli which control eating. The overweight individual eats under a large variety of circumstances. Thus, the problem of self-control is made difficult by the large number of daily occasions which bring the tendency to eat to maximal levels because in the past they have been the occasions when eating has occurred. Two kinds of behavior need to be brought under stimulus control. The first is the elicited reflex effects of food, such as salivation, gastric secretion, and other responses of the gastrointestinal tract. The other involves operant behavior, or the behavior involving the striated musculature of the organism — walking, talking, reaching, cooking, and so forth. In the so-called voluntary behaviors, the major datum is the frequency of the behavior rather than the magnitude of an elicited reflex, as with the smooth-muscle response of the digestive system. Although these two types of behavior control are inevitably tied together, their properties are different and they must be distinguished both dynamically and statically. In order to break down the control of eating by the stimuli which have been the characteristic occasions on which eating has been reinforced in the past, the stimuli must occur without the subsequent reinforcement by the food. The process is a direct extrapolation from the extinction of a Pavlovian conditioned response. If the dog is to discontinue salivation on the occasion of the bell, the bell must be presented repeatedly in the situation in which the food no longer follows. The amount of saliva the bell elicits then declines continuously until it reaches near-zero. Similarly, the stimuli characteristic of the preparation of a meal will cease to control large amounts of gastric activity if these stimuli can be made to occur without being followed by food in the mouth. Initially, the stimuli will elicit large amounts of gastric activity; but with continued exposure to these stimuli, the amount of activity will decline continuously until low levels are reached.

Delimiting existing stimulus control of eating may take considerable time because (1) the loss of control by a stimulus is a gradual process, requiring repeated exposure to the relevant stimuli; and (2) it may be a long time before the individual encounters all of the situations in which he has eaten in the past. The sudden temptation of the ex-smoker to light a cigarette when he meets an old friend is an example of the latter kind of control.

Self-control developed under procedures involving very special situations and foods (for example, liquid diets, all-protein diets, or hard-boiled eggs and celery) will be difficult to maintain when the diet circumstances return to normal. The very abrupt shift in eating patterns, kinds of food eaten, and characteristic circumstances surrounding eating will weaken the self-control performances as well as strengthen eating behaviors which were previously in the person's repertoire under the control of the more normal environment. Hence, self-control performances must be developed under circumstances and with foods which are to be the individual's final eating pattern.

Temporal Control of Eating

The time of day is an important event controlling eating. With the individual who characteristically eats at regular intervals, gastric activity comes to precede these occasions very closely, and is at low levels elsewhere regardless of levels of deprivation. The same can be said for operant behavior associated with eating, although the order of magnitude of some of the parameters may be different. After the conditioned responses associated with eating are brought closely under the control of a strict temporal pattern, feelings of hunger should disappear except just before meal-time. However, many individuals have no such routine patterns of eating, so that the temporal pattern of eating does not limit the amount of gastro-intestinal activity. The obese person frequently eats in the absence of any gastric activity. A technique of self-control in this category would rigidly specify a temporal pattern of eating and find conditions for adhering to it. As with the gastrointestinal reflexes, this general disposition to engage in operant behaviors reinforced by the ingestion of food can be brought under the control of a temporal pattern of eating, with a resulting lower disposition to eat during the intervals between regular meals. In the early stages of learning self-control, the development of a rigid temporal pattern perhaps should be carried out under conditions in which no weight loss is to be expected and the amount of food, ingested at specified meals, is large enough to minimize the disposition to eat on other occasions. The subsequent maintenance of this temporal pattern of eating when the subject begins to lose weight will depend upon the concurrent action of other categories of self-control performances. The control of eating by temporal factors can also be developed for situations other than the normal routine meals, as, for example, at social gatherings and parties. Because the availability of food is predictable here, early stage of self-control can include arranging a specific time when the eating will occur rather than indeterminate consumption of whatever foods happen to be available.

The Eating Situation

As with the temporal properties of eating, the actual characteristics of the eating situation may be used to control the disposition to eat. However, the stimuli here are clearer and probably exert control of an even larger order of magnitude than that of the temporal pattern. This application of the principle of stimulus control is the same as in the temporal contingency: to arrange that eating occur on limited and narrowly circumscribed occasions and never otherwise. To simplify the development of the stimulus control, eating situations should be associated with stimuli which occur infrequently in the individual's normal activities. For example, an eating place in the home should be chosen so that it is maximally removed from the routine activities of the day. Nor should eating occur together with any other kind of activity such as reading. If reading occurs frequently enough while the subject is eating, then reading will increase the disposition to eat because it has been an occasion on which eating has been reinforced.

Emphasizing the Stimulus Control

The occasions characterizing eating can be emphasized by deliberately arranging very obvious stimuli. For example, the subject always eats sitting down at a table which has a napkin, a place setting, and a purple table cloth. The latter makes the situation even more distinctive. In the extreme case, a specific item of clothing might be worn whenever the subject eats. Narrowing the range provides another form of stimulus control. By eating only specific foods in specific places, the disposition to eat when other foods are available will be minimized. This factor will also be discussed under chaining; but the aspect emphasized here is the effect of the foods eaten as one of the elements in the occasion associated with eating. If a subject has eliminated ice cream, candy, and cake from his diet, the sweet shop will have little control over his behavior.

In the actual procedures with subjects, stimulus control was the first avenue of self-control developed. The subjects learned to keep daily diet protocols during the first few meetings and to determine the number of calories necessary to maintain their weight. We restricted eating to three meals a day, eliminated concentrated fats and sugars from the diet, and attempted to bring about an increase in the amount of food taken in at meals, particularly at breakfast, to bring about a normal pattern of eating without any expected weight loss. For individuals having difficulty in restricting their eating to meals, we arranged a specific and routine extra feeding, as, for example, a glass of milk and a few crackers at bedtime. The extra feeding was to be taken routinely, however, so it did not become a reinforcer for increasing the probability of eating on a wide variety of occasions. No weight loss was attempted until the subjects were successful in eating a normal range of food at meals without any eating at other times. We attempted to create an eating pattern which could be carried out without interruption after the weight-control program was terminated. Our major problems were insufficient protein or excess fat in the diet. None of the subjects ate excessive amounts of carbohydrate except perhaps as candy. However, all subjects had trouble eating a full meal. It was paradoxical that women who joined the program because they could not limit their eating had difficulty in ingesting a maintenance diet at mealtimes. One complained of nausea, another of chest pains, and a third of discomfort from overeating. All of the complaints disappeared in a week, however.

Chaining

Eating is a rough designation for a chain of behavioral sequences culminating in swallowing and the subsequent gastrointestinal reflexes. An illustrative sequence might be as follows: Dressing makes possible leaving the house; leaving the house leads to walking to the store; entering the store is followed by the selection of foods, a basket of food is the occasion for paying the clerk and leaving the store; a bag of groceries at home leads to storing the food; stored food is the occasion for cooking or otherwise preparing the food; the prepared food is the occasion for setting the table and sitting down; the sight of food is the occasion for cutting it with a fork or knife; the dissected food leads to placing food in the mouth; food in the mouth is followed by chewing; and chewing is followed by swallowing. The sequence differs from individual to individual and from time to time, but any selected elements illustrate the process.

Because the frequency of occurrence of the final member of the chain depends on the nature of the earlier members of the eating sequence, some degree of self-control can be arranged by dealing with the dynamic properties of the eating sequence. The length of the chain of responses leading to swallowing will markedly influence the frequency with which the eating sequence is carried out. The longer the sequence of behaviors in the chain, the weaker will be the disposition to start the chain. This property of chaining suggests a technique of control which could be useful if used in conjunction with the other avenues of control. By arranging that all of the foods available or accessible require a certain amount of preparation or locomotion, the tendency to eat can be reduced simply because the chain of responses leading to swallowing was lengthened. Keeping food out of areas normally entered, shopping on a day-to-day basis (at a time when the disposition to eat is low), buying foods which are not edible without cooking or other preparation, and placing food in less accessible places are some techniques for weakening the disposition to eat by lengthening a chain. As in some of the avenues of control, this technique would be inadequate under extreme levels of deprivation without additional support from other types of control. The chain must not be lengthened too much, or it might become so weakened that prepotent eating behaviors would occur or the chain short-circuited.

The actual form of the eating chain in the latter members just before swallowing may be rearranged to reduce the rate of eating. The behavior of swallowing is so strongly reinforced that it could occur very soon after food enters the mouth, without very much chewing. Similarly, the behavior of placing food in the mouth (reinforced by the taste of food) has high strength and occurs as soon as the mouth empties. Many eaters carry out this sequence at a very high rate by reaching for additional food just as soon as food is placed in the mouth and by swallowing while the fork is in transit to the mouth. This analysis is confirmed by the high rate with which many obese people eat compared with that of nonobese eaters.

To reduce the rate of eating and to make it possible for the subject to stop eating at any point, we designed simple exercises to break the chain, particularly the near-final members, so that the occasion for placing food on the fork is swallowing rather than chewing. The new sequence was: food on the fork only after other food is swallowed and the mouth is empty. These exercises depended on ancillary techniques of control already developed by other techniques of self-control. At the start, the interruptions were only a few seconds; then, they were gradually increased to several minutes. The ability to stop eating at any point represents the final effect of nearly all of the other avenues of control; nevertheless, it constitutes a separate technique of control demanding special exercises. In later, more difficult exercises, the subject holds food on a fork for various periods of time without eating. Similarly, chewing is prolonged before swallowing for increasing periods. These exercises are carried out initially at the end of a meal, when the deprivation level is low.

The type of food eaten is of major importance in how reinforcing it would be, and hence how long a chain of responses can be maintained by the food reinforcement. The disposition to eat could be somewhat regulated by a selection of foods in the individual's diet that are sufficiently reinforcing (appetizing, caloric, etc.) to be eaten, but minimally reinforcing so as to minimize the resulting disposition to eat. A certain balance must be achieved; if the foods chosen are so unappetizing or unappealing that their reinforcing effect is negligible, the subject will simply switch to other foods. Also relevant here are the dynamic effects of food deprivation. Foods which are maximally reinforcing should be eaten when the individual is less deprived, and minimally reinforcing foods should be eaten under stronger conditions of deprivation. In other words, the effect of the highly reinforcing foodstuffs on the disposition to eat would be minimized by a lower level of deprivation so that the subject can stop eating more easily. In special cases, the food intake could be increased temporarily in order to minimize the highly reinforcing effect of certain foods. For example, if an individual who is highly reinforced by caloric pastries knows she will be in a situation where such pastries are being served, she could lessen the probability of eating them by increasing her food intake during the preceding meal or by a glass of milk before entering the situation.

Prepotent Repertoires

One way to lessen the disposition to eat is to supplant it by establishing other activities incompatible with eating. In an extreme case, an apparently large disposition to eat is often due to a behavioral repertoire in which eating appears strong because the rest of the repertoire is weak. Some degree of self-control should be possible if some activity could be maintained at a potentially high strength and circumstances arranged so that the subject could engage in this activity whenever the disposition to eat was strong. An example of such an activity might be telephoning a friend just after breakfast instead of indulging in the customary between-meal nibbling. The use of prepotent repertoires as a technique of control implies a certain amount of control over the prepotent repertoire. In order for these substitutive repertoires to be effective, special attention must be given to methods for strengthening them, particularly when they are needed. For example, instead of reading the newspaper as soon as it arrives, it could be put aside until some time when the peak tendency to eat occurs. Similarly, the telephoning of friends could be postponed in order to keep this behavior at high strength. Such activities occur initially because of independent reinforcement. Another kind of prepotent repertoire may be established by starting some strongly reinforced activity whose reinforcement occurs only if the behavior occurs uninterrupted for a period of time. Examples are washing a floor, going to a movie, taking a bus ride, reading a short story, or going for a walk. Such performances will be prepotent over eating because of the temporary aversive consequences resulting from their interruption. In many cases, the prepotent repertoires physically remove the individual from the place where eating can occur.

The effective use of prepotent repertoires depends upon the development of other avenues of control. Probably no one of these "prepotent" performances would be effective by itself if the disposition to eat were strong. For example, the individual going for a walk could simply stop at a restaurant to eat. Nevertheless, there is still a net advantage, because the supplementary types of self-control needed are relatively easy. For example, compare the disposition to stop at a restaurant during a walk with the disposition to eat in the normal situations when eating usually occurs. If the individual usually eats at home, the tendency to stop at a restaurant and eat will be considerably less than the tendency to eat at home. No explicit training was required in the pilot experiment to establish self-control by the use of prepotent repertoires; but all of the subjects used them during several phases of the experiment.

Prepotent repertoires may be affected by emotional factors. For example, many persons eat when depressed, affronted, thwarted, or frustrated. In the terms of the functional analysis of eating used here, emotional factors may weaken behaviors other than eating so that eating becomes relatively stronger. Putting food in one's mouth remains a highly reinforcing activity even if the remainder of the individual's repertoire is severely depressed. Eating then occurs because it is less disrupted by the emotional variables depressing the rest of the individual's repertoire.

Eating may interact with emotional factors in more subtle, but nonetheless important, ways, as a mechanism by which a person might escape or avoid emitting verbal behavior which is highly aversive, e.g., thinking about impending circumstances which are highly aversive. Because of its very strong and immediate reinforcement, eating will be prepotent over thinking about anxiety-evoking occurrences. Thus, eating comes to acquire two sources of strength: The immediate reinforcement from food in the mouth, and the reinforcement from postponing or avoiding the aversive consequences of emitting the verbal behavior which the eating supplants. Emotional disturbances will also disrupt the performances by which the individual controls himself, as will any general depression or disturbance of the individual's over-all repertoire. Self-control performances will be especially liable to disruption early in their development, before they become strong and maintained.

The manipulation of factors to minimize the effects of emotional disturbances is a separate topic, involving self-control of variables different from those in eating and thus requiring a separate analysis. The main avenue of control in eating lies in increasing the strength and durability of the self-control performances so that they will remain intact during emotional disturbances. For example, a person who has acquired an active and extensive verbal repertoire about all of the personal aversive consequences of being overweight will be able to emit these behaviors even during some general depression of his behavioral repertoire. The behavior about the ultimate aversive consequences of eating will be even more durable during possibly disrupting situations if it has already been effective in producing self-control, that is, if the behavior about the UAC has been reinforced effectively by suppression of the disposition to eat.

If existing levels of self-control are certain to break down because of an emotional disturbance, the individual should be trained to plan a controlled increase in food intake. The advantage of explicitly increasing the level of food intake would be that the food would be eaten under controlled conditions, so that stimulus control and other factors of self-control already developed would be maintained, and the effects of absence of progress in self-control would be minimized. Overeating under planned conditions would probably weaken the already developed self-control repertoires less than unplanned or uncontrolled eating.

In many situations, the general depression of an individual's repertoire occurs only for a limited time. Here, the necessary self-control performances would be a manipulation of the physical environment so that food is not available then, or would be the creation of a prepotent environment. The depressed individual who wishes to control his eating goes to a movie, takes a ride on a bus, or goes for a long walk. These activities give time for the emotional states to disappear and simultaneously provide an environment in which eating has not been reinforced very frequently in the individual's past experience. Of course, applications of these techniques of control depend upon the prior achievement of a certain amount of self-control, and probably are some of the most difficult areas of self-control to acquire. Such items would not be attempted at an early stage of the self-control program.

Shaping and Maintaining the Self-Control Performance

Self-control is a very complex repertoire of performance which cannot be developed all at once. If self-control consists of items of behavior with the same dynamic properties as those of the rest of human behavior, the self-control performance, as a complicated repertoire, must be developed in slow steps. These would begin with some performance already in the individual's repertoire and proceed in successive stages to more complicated performances. With each gain in self-control, the individual has a repertoire from which a new degree of complex behavior may emerge. Simply "telling" the subject the nature of the performances required for the development of self-control is not a sufficient condition for their development. The situation is analogous to that of a complicated motor or intellectual activity. One cannot explain to the novice how to differentiate an equation in calculus without first establishing a repertoire in algebra. Similarly, as most golfers have learned, no amount of verbal instruction will take the place of slow development of behavior reinforced by its effect on the golf ball. The actual disposition to emit the self-control behavior builds up because it was emitted successfully to reduce the long-term aversive effects of the behavior to be controlled. What is required here is to begin with some performance very close to one in the individual's repertoire, and to arrange circumstances so that those performances have at least some effect on the disposition to eat. The early reinforcement of this initial repertoire by a discernible movement in self-control provides the basis for the subject's continued attendance to the self-control program.

In the development of self-control, the concern is

not simply the presence or absence of a self-control performance. A group of behaviors must be built constituting a repertoire that will occur with a sufficient degree of certainty to be maximally effective.

Just as the disposition to eat can vary from near-zero to very large values, the behaviors involved in self-control can also be weak or strong. Whether the individual "knows" what the potential techniques of self-control are, or even can emit them, is not so important as the durability of the self-control repertoire. A set of performances is needed which will occur with high-enough probability despite competition from the individual's other repertoires. The maintaining event for the self-control performance is the reduction in the disposition to eat. The effect of the reinforcement is not an all-or-none matter, and the reinforcing effect of gains in self-control repertoires can be variously small, large, or even intermittent. Uncontrolled eating should not be viewed as a failure in control, but simply as the absence of progress. If the positive aspects of the program are emphasized, as well as the development of specific performances to control the disposition to eat, each small increment in the ability of the subject to control himself will reinforce further participation in the self-control program. A failure of a self-control performance to prevent eating defines an intermittent schedule of reinforcement of the self-control behavior. It may still continue to maintain the performances, just as any other act that is intermittently reinforced.

Some types of self-control require that old performances disappear rather than a specific repertoire, as, for example, the development of stimulus control, be built. The development of this kind of self-control is largely a function of the number of exposures, without eating, in situations when the individual has eaten in the past. Verbal behavior has only limited relevance here, since it can be little more than a report of what is taking place. Recognizing that the preparations for dinner are increasing the disposition to salivate and eat is of little use in controlling these effects. Extinguishing the effects of these stimuli is an orderly process requiring only exposure to the stimuli and passage of time. However, knowledge of the process might be of use in conjunction with the various avenues of self-control, particularly in respect to emphasizing the stimuli involved. Once the subject recognizes that the extinction of the stimulus control is a slow process, even minor decrements in the extent of the control by the stimuli will provide reinforcements for maintaining the self-control, as, for example, when several days are required for extinction. In the absence of knowledge of the order of magnitude of the course of the process, weakly maintained self-control behaviors might extinguish. In the actual self-control program, noting reductions in the strength of eating behavior during its extinction provides interim reinforcement for the self-control performances.

Discussion

Traditionally, the development of self-control has been in a framework of classical psychoanalytic and dynamic psycho-therapeutic approaches to human behavior. These approaches view self-control in terms of its developmental and dynamic origins and the inner-directed, private forces which sustain, direct, or distort its external manifestations. Prior life experiences are considered in detail through interviewing and related techniques, including analyses of current actions and attitudes (transference and counter-transference). The focus is on the past to assist the individual in discovering those formative experiences and relationships which have functioned to establish current attitudes and current modes of alleviating anxiety and guilt. A major structural goal of this system is the development of effective insight with increased intellectual freedom and more realistic self-appraisal. A major symptomatic goal is the ultimate reduction of anxiety and guilt, with a resultant diminished need to exploit heroic or uneconomic measures in the control of either or both. A fundamental assumption here is that the human being who becomes sufficiently aware of his personal developmental behavioral determinants and who is sufficiently relieved of neurotic anxiety of guilt, will, by virtue of this achievement, progressively lose his dependence on irrational and restrictive defenses. A corollary is that a healthy behavioral repertoire is potentially available at any time the individual gains relief from the guilt and anxiety of his deviant developmental history. These assumptions are not at all unreasonable for many problems encountered by the clinician, and sometimes appear to be convincingly supported by satisfactory therapeutic outcome. However, there are outstanding exceptions, characterized by certain common behavioral elements. Among these are (1) elaborately ritualized performances; (2) long-standing maintenance of such patterns; and (3) large amounts of strongly maintained and sustained activity. These are the symptoms present in many alcoholic individuals, in all obsessive-compulsive neurotics, in many patients with neurotic depressive reactions, in drug addicts, in a variety of schizophrenic patients, and in many individuals with eating disturbances (obese as well as anorexic). Successful and sustained therapeutic improvement is exceptional for all, including the obese (8), however prolonged and insightful the therapeutic experience may be. The kind of functional analysis of behavior proposed here may provide a conception of human behavior as an alternative to the classical psychoanalytically oriented systems.

The terms in such an analysis are the actual performances of the patient and their exact effects on his environment. The frequency of occurrence of the performance is studies as a function of its effect on the environment, and every attempt is made to observe and deal with the relevant performances rather than with inferred processes. The specificity of the analysis does not mean that the patient must have an intact repertoire by which he deals with the world, and attention can be focused on creating whatever repertoire is necessary. Most of the present report is a presentation of certain practical techniques which can be applied to the problem of uncontrolled eating. The preliminary results of this pilot program are not included as a record of even mediocre success, but rather as a description of the medium within which the specific techniques of control were imparted. A much longer follow-up period and a larger number of cases are necessary to develop a successful program as well as test it. Nor can we now designate these aspects of the program which were effective or ineffective. This report is intended to provide a theoretical and practical model for more structured programs of self-control in eating. We have shown eating habits can be changes in a short-term, small-group-therapy program by the use of the basic principles outlined here. Whether or not the weight losses reported during the first 15 sessions are primarily due to the application of the principles outlined can be determined only by appropriately controlled study experiments. We are not concerned whether one or another program can effect weight loss, since many pharmacologic individual- and group-therapy programs lead to temporary loss of weight, as is generally known. The central issue is the development of self-control in eating which will endure and become an available part of the individual's future repertoire. Most conventional programs do not focus on the eating patterns available to the subject after he has lost weight, nor do they present recognizable techniques for developing such future control. Possible exceptions are in individual programs of psychotherapy which are directed toward an exploration and resolution of the unconscious determinants of eating behavior, and in certain of the conditioned-reflex techniques. Yet, even in these programs, this question remains: Do proper eating habits exist after the individual is free of the relevant disability? The program outlined here has the special advantage of focusing directly and specifically on future eating behavior and of presenting even more specific techniques for bringing this behavior under control. Application of the basic principles requires no special instrumental or technical training and is relatively economical. Slow and controlled weight loss under relatively high-caloric intake levels minimizes medical and psychological problems.

We cannot state whether the program we carried out is suitable for severely obese individuals (particularly those who have medical or psychiatric complications). Nor can we specify how the technical principles and procedures can be applied to subjects of low educational level or of limited intelligence. A major problem here would undoubtedly be the difficulty of daily and accurate caloric-intake records. Some of these fundamental questions are subjects for future study.

REFERENCES

1. BRUCH, H. The importance of overweight. New York: W. W. Norton, 1957.
2. CAPPON, D. Obesity. Canadian Medical Association Journal, 1958, 78, 568-573.
3. FERSTER, C. B. Reinforcement and punishment in the control of human behaviro by social agencies. Psychiatric Research Report, 1958, 10, 101-118.
4. FERSTER, C. B., and SKINNER, B. F. Schedules of reinforcement. New York: Appleton-Century-Crofts, 1957.
5. GALVIN, E. P., and MCGAVACK, T. H. Obesity, its cause, classification and care. New York: Hoeber-Harper, 1957.
6. SKINNER, B. F. The behavior of organisms. New York: D. Appleton Century Co., 1938.
7. SKINNER, B. F. Science and human behavior. New York: Macmillan, 1958.
8. SKINNER, B. F. Cumulative record. New York: Appleton-Century-Crofts, 1959.
9. STUNKARD, A. The results of treatment for obesity. Archives of Internal Medicine, 1959, 103, 79-85.
10. STUNKARD, A. Eating patterns and obesity. Psychiatric Quarterly, 1959, 33, 284-295.
11. STUNKARD, A. Obesity and the denial of hunger. Psychosomatic Medicine, 1959, 21, 281-289.

Received March 15, 1961

BEHAVIORAL CONTROL OF OVEREATING

RICHARD B. STUART

School of Social Work, University of Michigan

(*Received* 12 *May* 1967)

Summary – A behavioral treatment for overeating, utilizing operant and respondent conditioning techniques is described. To date, all eight patients with whom this treatment has been employed have been successfully treated and no negative secondary reactions have been observed.

OBESITY is well-recognized as a major health hazard. Only two common characteristics have been observed in obese persons: a tendency to overeat and a tendency to under-exercise (U.S. Public Health Service, undated). While obesity has been ascribed to various causes (Bychowski, 1950; Hamburger, 1951; Deri, 1955; Stunkard, 1959; Mendelson, 1966), the treatment of overeating has been successful when it is based solely upon a functional analysis of the maladaptive response (Ferster et al., 1962). The present paper presents Ferster's approach in somewhat modified form and reports upon the clinical results to date.

SELF-CONTROL

Man clealry controls his own behavior so as to achieve his own objectives. The source of this control is commonly ascribed to central adaptive mechanisms ranging from the ego to the conscience. From a behavioral point of view, self-control is an inference drawn from the functional relationships among observable responses (Bijou and Baer, 1961). The behavioral processes involved in a person's control of himself are the same as those one would use in controlling the behavior of others (Skinner, 1953).

Stuart RB. Behavioral control of overeating. *Behav Res Ther.* 1967;5:357-365. Reprinted by permission of Behaviour Research and Therapy, Elsevier Science Ltd., The Boulevard, Langford Lane, Kidlington, Oxford OX5 1GB, England. Special thanks to Judy Willis of the Pennington Information Center for help in acquiring this and reference documents.

The first step in self-control is a precise analysis of the response to be controlled and its antecedent and consequent conditions. An anlysis of overeating would naturaly include a precise description of the topography of the response, the conditions under which it occurs, and its consequences. The second step is the identification of behavior which facilitates eating a proper amount of food (including behavior which interferes with overeating). The third step is the identification of positive or negative reinforcers which control these behavior patterns. A reinforcer can be identified for every response, using Premack's principle ("Of any two responses, the more probable response will reinforce the less probable one;" Premack, 1965). Thus a reinforcer is always available for any desired response, independent of the topography of that response. The fourth step requires the application of the reinforcement to alter the probability of the preselected response (Homme, 1965). The outcome of self-control can be termed "contingency management" and is designed to increase the frequency of desired overt or covert responses while decreasing the frequency of undesired responses.

Treatment sessions are scheduled three times per week, usually last for approximately 30 min, and extend over a 4- to 5-week period. Subsequent sessions occur as needed, but usually at intervals of 2 weeks for the next 12 weeks. "Maintenance" sessions are scheduled as needed, while follow-up sessions occur on a planned monthly basis. The logic of scheduling frequent sessions at the start of treatment is that it is assumed that learning can occur most efficiently when teaching occurs in massed trials. As sessions become less frequent, more relevant experience is accumulated than can be fully discussed, and too much irrelevant or competing experience is accumulated. Massed sessions at the start also increase the opportunity for monitoring the patient' performance, which helps to make success more likely. It is essential that the patient encounter immediate success, for "if the self-contingency manager does not get reinforced for self-management, extinction will occur" (Homme 1965).

INITIAL INTERVIEW

The initial interview combines the processes of behavioral assessment with the establishment of a working therapeutic contract. All techniques utilized in each session are explained to the patient, along with a discussion of their rationale. In this way, the patient is able to focus his attention upon a particular routine and can work with the therapist in finding ways of achieving greater success. He is also trained in a new method of describing his own behavior. "Rather than telling him to modify them (something which he may have already told himself), he is trained in the experimental analysis of behavior, and also in the variables which maintain it, or which he can recruit to modify it" (Goldiamond, 1965). No diagnostic formulations are entertained unless they are relevant to the current therapeutic contract, and all such formulations are communicated to the patient. A record is kept of all phases of the treatment, and this record is reviewed by the patient periodically. In addition to an anecdotal record of the treatment maintained by the therapist, two daily records are kept by the patient throughout therapy.

1. *Food Data Sheets*

These records account the time, nature, quantity and circumstance of all food and drink intake. Time is important as a means of determining the pattern of between-meal eating as well as the duration of scheduled meals. The nature and quantity of food consumed is important because of its obvious bearing upon weight gain. This entry includes the mode of preparation, e.g. broiled, fried, etc., often as much a source of unnecessary weight gain as the nature of the foodstuffs themselves. Describing the precise weight or volume of foods is useful not only as a monitoring procedure, but because it requires a slight interruption in the normal chain of eating responses. Finally, knowledge of the circumstances under which eating occurs provides clues to the ways in which it can be controlled, through identification of the current controlling conditions. Such factors as tension, solitude, cleaning up, reading or watching television are commonly associated with excessive eating. When this is known, it is possible to take steps to change the responses to these stimuli.

2. *Weight Range Sheets*

The patient's weight range is important because it consists of a running record of fluctuations in gross body weight. Weight is to be recorded before breakfast, after breakfast, after lunch, and before bedtime. There is a natural reduction of weight during the night as energy is expended in maintaining body functions such as breathing, temperature regulation and heartbeat, while food and liquid consumption are almost nil. This weight is gradually regained during the day as caloric intake exceeds caloric expenditure. Obesity occurs because the amount of food consumed is in excess over that which is needed for energy. This gross weight is the target of the therapeutic program. Having the patient weigh himself four times daily serves as four daily reminders of the therapeutic program. In addition, the patient is provided with direct evidence of the effect of food and drink intake upon his weight. This serves as a periodic, mildly aversive stimulus associated with overeating.

Additional data is gathered in two areas. First, the patient is asked to list high probability behavior patterns, free operant responses which occur with high frequency and which, by implication, are positively reinforcing. For some patients, activities such as reading, talking to friends, watching television or reading the newspaper are readily available. For other patients, those suffering from a "behavioral depression," eating may be the only readily available high probability behavior. It may be necessary to help the patient to cultivate a reservoir of positively reinforcing responses. For example, two patients were helped to develop intense interests in caged birds and growing African violets. While these responses are not to be used until the fifth step in the treatment, it is essential to gather the necessary information at the beginning to allow time for the development of new interests. A second type of data, with the same eventual application, deals with the patient's most urgent, weight-related fears. For some patients, these fears concern ultimate physical consequences of overeating, such as cardiovascular disease or death from infection because surgery is impossible. For other patients, these fears concern social consequences, such as the loss of a mate or the total cessation of sexual experiences.

A weight-loss goal of from 1 or 2 lb/week is set during the initial interview. Greater loss of weight poses certain physiological hazards and creates the risk of food deprivation, while loss of less than 1 lb/week is not sufficiently reinforcing and is relatively ineffective. Finally, treatment recommendations are made in the first as well as all subsequent sessions, as needed.

Behavioral curriculum — Step One. Behavioral therapy, as an action therapy, emphasizes patient activity as a means of goal attainment. The first step in treatment, following introduction of the recording procedures, requires the patient to interrupt his meal for a predetermined period of time, usually 2 or 3 min which is gradually increased to 5 min. He is instructed to put down his utensils and merely sit in his place at the table for a specified period of time.

Rationale. The logic of this maneuver is that the patient is given an early experience of control over one aspect of his eating, however small, and learns that eating is a response which can be broken down into components which can be successively mastered. The reinforcement for success is immediate, and consists of the knowledge that the patient has taken his first step toward overcoming his compulsion. It is important that the patient be successful in his first step, and he is instructed to telephone the therapist if he encounters any difficulty. In such instances, the interval would be reduced to the point at which the patient can meet with success. The therapist is available by telephone at all times, in order to guard against any failure by the patient which might adversely affect his expectation of success.

SECOND INTERVIEW

Each interview following the first has the same general format: The Food Data and Weight Range Sheets are discussed; the patient's progress with the behavioral curriculum is discussed with abundant praise for success; and new steps are planned and put into operation with the patient's full participation. Patients are asked to anticipate any forthcoming stressful events in their lives, and this is followed by planning how to minimize the possibility of compensatory overeating.

As the Food Data Sheets are reviewed, the patient is asked if he sees any obvious changes which might be made. There are often suggestions for changing the mode of food preparation or for the substitution of a less-fattening substance for a particularly harmful one, such as sherbet in place of ice-cream. Changes are rarely suggested by the therapist, as self-dosing is an important prerequisite for complete self-control. At times, patients have been cautioned to be more temperate in their deletion of foods so as to reduce the possibility of deprivation.

Behavioral curriculum — Step Two. The patient is instructed to remove food from all places in the house, other than the kitchen. He is also instructed to keep in the house only those foods which require preparation, other than salad greens and the like, and he is instructed to prepare only one portion at a time.

Rationale. Much compulsive eating is "automatic," in the sense that the patient may be unaware of the fact that he is eating. If a series of actions is required prior to eating, the patient is forced to become aware of his behavior. Therefore, a trip to the kitchen and the task of food preparation are both reminders that eating is about to occur. This may be an effective deterrent. If not, the need for preparation of individual portions may serve as an effort which outweighs the reward of eating.

Behavioral curriculum — Step Three. The patient is instructed to make eating a "pure experience," that is, he is instructed to pair eating with no other activity, such as reading, listening to the radio, watching television or talking on the telephone or with friends.

Rationale. If the patient reads while he eats, he is most likely to want to eat while he reads, etc. If eating can be held separate from other behavior, it will not continue as a conditioned response to the occurrence of this other behavior.

Confinement of the food to the kitchen and the elimination of other responses associated with eating are means of promoting stimulus control of the response. These are stimuli which set the occasion for eating. Additional steps, such as controlling the interval during eating, are designed to promote control of the proprioceptive or mediating stimuli inherent in the complex response of eating.

It should be noted that the rigors of steps two and three, no direct limitation of the type of quantity of food has been suggested. The goal of these steps is not the immediate reduction of food intake. Instead, it is to so manipulate the eating response as to make it more readily self-controlled, first by bringing it to awareness and then by disrupting its chaining to other behavioral responses.

THIRD INTERVIEW

No new steps are suggested in the third interview, to avoid "overloading" the patient with behavioral prescriptions. Instead, following a review of his experiences, the patient's help is elicited in refining the steps which have been taken.

FOURTH INTERVIEW

The first week of treatment will have been accomplished by this time. The Weight Record is therefore reviewed, and the first entry is made on a chart recording weekly weight changes. This chart is retained by the patient and serves as a reminder of progress. It should be noted that weight loss may be greater during the first 2 weeks of treatment than it will be subsequently. This is probably related to the "honeymoon effect" of treatment and to the fact that the patient has a greater amount of voluble fat which is convertible to energy during this time. Accordingly, the patient is forewarned to anticipate a more gradual weight loss of between 1 and 2 lb weekly.

Behavioral curriculum — Step Four. Obese patients have been observed to eat very rapidly whenever they eat, so that large quantities of food are consumed in very brief periods. To slow the process of ingestion, the patient is instructed to put a small amount of food in his mouth, and to replace his utensils on the table until he has swallowed.

Rationale. This step is aimed directly at manipulation of the eating response, and success with this step is tantamount to direct control over the response. In addition to its control value, this step also helps the patient to derive more enjoyment from his food so that he can replace quantity with quality in his eating. Rapid eating not only leads to indigestion, but it also obviates the possibility for full enjoyment of the taste and aroma of food. By eating more slowly, the patient can improve his digestion and learn to savor his food. He may eventually achieve a normal state of satiation with less food intake. This step is easily followed at all meals, including those eaten socially, and has the added value of making the patient a more tolerable eating companion.

FIFTH INTERVIEW

Following all of the normal interview procedures, the therapist enlists the patient's aid in identifying "danger periods" of between-meal eating. These are times of high arousal when "the probability of the most practiced response appearing is increased" (Pyke et al., 1966). As eating is the most practiced response, it is highly likely to occur at these times. Training the patient in controlling eating under high arousal circumstances is tantamount to training him in temporal control of eating.

Behavioral curriculum — Step Five. The patient is instructed to engage in one of the previously identified high probability behaviors at times when he would normally eat. This is analogous to a procedure developed for the control of smoking: "If a response other than smoking can be conditioned to stimuli which ordinarily lead to smoking and the link between these stimuli and the response of smoking weakened, then it should become easier for the individual smoker to cut down his consumption or to quit entirely. That is, the smoker now has at his disposal an alternative response to smoking" (Pyke et al., 1966). The patient is instructed to read the newspaper or to call a friendly neighbor at exactly 10:00 a.m. if eating occurs consistently at this hour. Similar alternative responses are planned for other times of the day which have been identified as periods of high arousal. Before embarking upon the substitute behavior, the patient is instructed to repeat the phrase: "I can control my eating by engaging in other activities which I enjoy."

Rationale. Between-meal eating is understood to be an important source of positive reinforcement for patients who overeat. They cannot be expected to forego this reinforcement without a substitute. The substitute has inherent reinforcing value (it is a high probability behavior) and it implies the occurrence of self-control which is reinforcing. Specifically, the patient learns a new response to stimuli which previously set the occasion for eating. In order to set the occasion for the emission of the alternate response, the patient is trained to verbalize the rationale for the procedure. Since this behavior is in the service of the patient's goal attainment, following the prescription adds a measure of reinforcement for the new behavior.

SIXTH INTERVIEW

This session, like the fourth, is used to consolidate gains made to date. There is considerable discussion of ways of refining behavioral steps so as to maximize their effectiveness. By this time, patients are often active in planning their own curricula and have been ingenious in devising procedures of great value to themselves. For most patients, the behavioral curriculum is complete at this point, with subsequent sessions being devoted to refinement of the program, and with patient decisions about dietary changes. At the request of one patient, the service of a dietitian was contracted for an hour in which professional advice was obtained in careful food selection. This service is of help, but not essential.

SEVENTH THROUGH TWELFTH INTERVIEWS

These sessions further refine the curriculum and reinforce progress. Two patients who encountered difficulty with the control of between-meal eating were offered one additional therapeutic step.

Behavioral curriculum — Step Six. Joseph Cautela (1966) has described the process of "coverant sensitization" in which the patient is trained to relax, then to imagine that he is about to indulge in a compulsion, then to imagine the occurrence of an aversive event.* One patient found considerable difficulty in controlling the eating of a particular kind of cookie at specific times during the day. She was first trained in vivid imagery and then her lips, hearing her teeth crunch as the cookie crumbles, tasting its sweetness, etc.), and she was finally instructed to immediately switch to the detailed image of her husband in the interview. This process proved highly successful in both instances of its use (requiring one session with one patient and two with the

*In the original work done with the patients discussed in this report, patients were told to imagine that they were actually tasting the forbidden food before then being told to imagine the aversive condition. In a personal communication, Dr. Cautela correctly labeled this a punishment procedure. It lacks the forward conditioning advantage of an escape or avoidance conditioning procedure in which the aversive condition is applied before commission of the compulsive act.

TABLE 1. AGE, MARITAL STATUS, WEIGHT LOSS AND NUMBER OF THERAPEUTIC SESSIONS OF EIGHT FEMALE PATIENTS RECEIVING BEHAVIOR THERAPY FOR OVEREATING

Patient	Age	Marital status	Weight loss over 12 months	Therapeutic sessions to date
1	37	M	46	19
2	21	S	38	24
3	41	S	29	30†
4	30	M	26	28
5	24	M	35	16
6	28	M	35	21‡
7	43	M	46	30
8	30	M*	47	41

*Divorced during treatment.
†One covert sensitization session.
‡Two covert sensitization sessions.

other) in reducing between-meal eating, without any disturbance of normal food intake. In short, it proved highly specific and powerful in its effect.

Rationale. In this treatment, the image of a forbidden object (CS) is paired with the image of an aversive stimulus (also a CS). The imagined aversive CS then forestalls the occurrence of the forbidden CS and ultimately interferes with eating. Two aspects of this procedure are of note. First, the patient demands the occurrence of a thought, or coverant (Homme, 1965). The reinforcement for the occurrence of the thought is the removal of the aversive stimulus. Second, salivation and the so-called "gustatory responses" are respondent behaviors. In this treatment, operant behavior (a thought) elicits fear which, in turn, prevents the elicitation of salivation.

DISCUSSION

There are several differences between the approach described by Ferster and his associates and the procedure which has been presented here. Ferster's treatment is a purely operant procedure, while this treatment combines operant and respondent techniques. Ferster worked with his patients in groups, while the treatment described here is conducted entirely on an individual

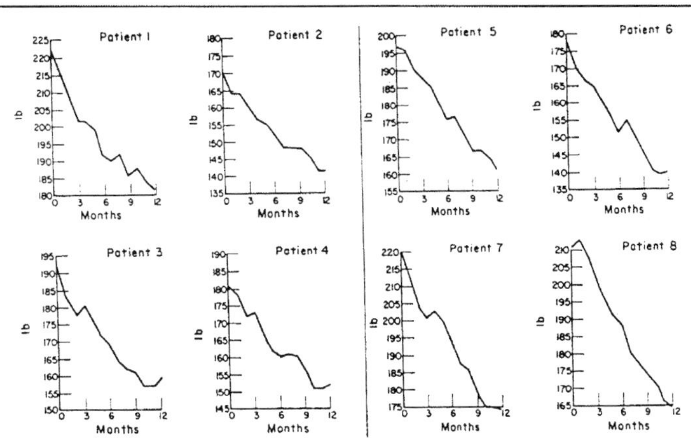

FIG. 1. Weight profile of eight women undergoing behavior therapy for overeating.

basis. Finally, Ferster stressed the ultimate aversive consequences of obesity, while reference to these consequences was only incidental in the treatment described here.

The treatment is aimed at building the skill of the patient in being his own contingency manager. This is a self-control procedure which is reinforced through the patient's experience of success in the control of his own behavior, the reduction of the aversive consequences of a lack of self-control, and through considerable reassurance by the therapist. More occurred in the interaction between therapist and patients than the presentation of the curriculum and a review of progress. Reassurance was given as an antecedent to each new step and praise was given for success. More tightly controlled research is needed in order to isolate the contribution of the non-specific interaction effect to total therapeutic outcome.

There are two essential features of this approach. First, treatment is offered specifically for the problem of overeating. No effort is made to distinguish the historical antecedents of the problem and no assumptions are made about the personality of the overeater. This is comparable to the treatment of anorexia described by others (Ayllon et al., 1964; Bachrach et al., 1965). Second, the specific format of the approach is based upon verbal behavioral assignments to be followed by the patient. These assignments can be translated into techniques of self-control because the patient receives both didactic discussion of the rationale and training the analysis of his own behavior so that he can discern opportunities for the subsequent application of the techniques.

TREATMENT RESULTS

This report covers all eight patients who received the therapy for whom 12 month follow-up data is available. Long-term data is a necessity, for the essential therapeutic problem is not the reduction of overeating but the stabilization of a reduced level of eating. Two patients began but did not complete treatment, and they have been excluded from this report. One woman became pregnant while the other, a probable psychotic, wanted another type of therapy and was dropped from this project following the second session. In general, all of these patients can be classified at the least disturbed points along the continua proposed by Mendelson (1966) and Hamburger (1951).

All of the patients are women, six of whom are married (see Table 1). Of the married patients, two have children. All are voluntary patients who were referred for private treatment. The patients initially weighed from a low 172 to a high of 224 lb, and all were judged by their physicians to be obese.

Figure 1 presents the data covering the gross weight for each patient during the 12 months for which data is available. While the figures present an almost linear line of decrease, it should be noted that the time intervals cover 4-week periods during which fluctuations were common. In actuality, weight loss varied from as little as 6 oz to as much as 5 lb/week for individual patients. Most patients showed either diminished weight loss or slight weight gains during the weeks prior to menstruation and slightly exaggerated weight losses following menstruation. This is probable attributable to water retention associated with menstrual periods. An average overall weight loss of somewhat less than 1 lb/week was accomplished, and this is regarded as a reasonable expectation.

During the follow-up interviews at 9, 32 and 52 weeks, patients were asked to describe their current situations. Only one unusual situation was noted, one patient having obtained a divorce for which procedures were begun 1 yr prior to the start of treatment. Seven of the eight patients reported having an increased range of social activities, and three of the six married patients reported more satisfying relationships with their husbands. Three of the eight who were also compulsive smokers reported that they had self-applied the same general curriculum to smoking and either substantially reduced or eliminated smoking. While this evidence is in no sense conclusive, it suggests that "symptom substitution" has not occurred. Follow-up sessions were scheduled will in advance and undoubtedly served both as monitoring experiences and as added reinforcement for continuing the program. All patients knew of their inclusion in this clinical-research sample.

REFERENCES

AYLLON T., HAUGHTON E. and OSMOND H.O. (1964) Chronic anorexia: a behavior problem. Can. psychiat. Ass. J. 9, 147-154.

BACHRACH A.J., ERWIN W.J. and MOHR J.P. (1965) The control of anorexia by operant conditioning techniques. In Case Studies in Behavior Modification (Eds. ULLMANN L.P. and KRASNER L.). Holt, Rinehart & Winston, New York.

BIJOU S. and BAER D. (1961) Child Development I: A Systematic and Empirical Theory, p. 80. Appleton-Century-Crofts, New York.

BYCHOWSKI G. (1950) On neurotic obesity. Psychoanal. Rev. 37, 301-319.

CAUTELA, J.R. (1966) Treatment of compulsive behavior by covert sensitization. Psychol. Rec. 16, 33-41.

DERI, S.K. (1955) A problem in obesity. In Clinical Studies of Personality (Eds. BURTON A. and HARRIS R.E.). Harper, New York.

FERSTER C.B., NURENBERGER J.I. and LEVITT E.B. (1962) The control of eating. J. Math. 1, 87-109.
GOLDIAMOND I. (1965) Stuttering and fluency as manipulatable operant response classes. In Research in Behavior Modification (Eds. KRASNER L. and ULLMANN L.), p. 153. Holt, Rinehart & Winston, New York.
HAMBURGER W.W. (1951) Emotional aspects of obesity. Med. Clins. N. Am. 35, 483-499.
HOMME L.E. (1965) Perspectives in psychology: XXIV control of coverants, the operants of the mind. Psychol. Rec. 15, 501-511.
MENDELSON M. (1966) Psychological aspects of obesity. Int. J. Psychiat. 2, 599-610.
PREMACK D. (1965) Reinforcement theory. In Nebraska Symposium on Motivation (Ed. LEVINE D.), p.132. University of Nebraska Press, Lincoln
PYKE A., AGNEW N. M. and KOPPERUD J. (1966) Modification of an overlearned response through a relearning program: a pilot study on smoking. Behav. Res. & Therapy 4, 197-203.
SKINNER B. F. (1953) Science and Human Behavior. Macmillan, New York.
STUNKARD A.J. (1959) Eating patterns and obesity. Psychiat. Quart. 33, 284-295.
U.S. Public Health Service (undated) Obesity and Health. Public Health Service Publication Number 1485, Washington, D.C.

CLASSICS IN OBESITY

Human Autonomic Pharmacology

XVI. Benzedrine Sulfate as an Aid in the Treatment of Obesity

Mark F. Lesses, Abraham Myerson†*
Boston

When energy intake in the form of food is greater than energy output, the excess potential energy is stored as body fat. If imbalance between food intake and energy output occurs, a change in weight must take place; whether it is to be a gain or a loss depends on the direction of the imbalance. From this point of view, the cause of obesity may be a defect of the appetite-regulating mechanism, rather than an alteration of metabolism. The perfect appetite mechanism will adjust itself to all changes of energy output, or metabolism, by a corresponding change in energy, or food intake, and thus the body will maintain its usual weight. Defect of the appetite mechanism will create imbalance in the energy output-intake relation, and a change in weight will result.

The factors which govern the appetite may be divided into the following groups: 1) physical status, particularly with reference to the endocrine glands; 2) social habits; and 3) psychologic influences. The effect of physical status on the appetite may be considered under the two aspects of disturbances due to acute or chronic organic disease, and disturbances due to metabolic abnormality as mediated through the endocrine glands. With regard to the former, little comment is needed, as the appetite disturbance of the sick is a matter of common knowledge. With regard to metabolic abnormalities, the bulimia of hyperthyroidism and the anorexia of Addison's disease may be mentioned as contrasting pictures. A more subtle disturbance of metabolism, mediated especially through the pituitary gland, has been invoked by many writers from von Norder onward, and has given rise to the concept of exogenous versus endogenous obesity (1).

In this connection, the work of Newburgh and his associates (2) shows that energy exchange is in no way different in a proved case of pituitary disease (Cushing's Syndrome) from what it is in normal persons. The loss in weight caused by any given reducing diet may be predicted for any period with great exactness. Furthermore, in patients suffering from myxedema, where the depression in energy metabolism is greater than it is in any other disease, striking obesity is the exception.

All visceral functions, including the appetites, are strongly modified by social habits. The appetite for food and eating have become almost as much social as they have physiologic and psychologic. People eat without particular desire under the influence of social feeling, as at parties and banquets. They are also forced to defer eating when the desire for food is very great, because of social conventions as to the serving of meals. In addition, the social and economic environment makes food and drink easily accessible to many without physical exertion (3,4).

The relation of physiologic, pathologic, and sociologic phenomena to the causation and maintenance of obesity having been pointed out, there remains for discussion the effect on the appetite of numerous psychologic influences. In previous papers (3,4,5), one of us (A.M.) has described a syndrome as part of the neurosis known as anhedonia. This symptom complex consists in a diminution, even to the point of disappearance or antagonism, of satisfactions normally obtained from life activities, and in a loss or distortion of the appetites and desires. The appetites involved are hunger, thirst and sex, desire for rest and recuperation, and desire for social relations, work and entertainment.

When satisfaction becomes impaired and there is no corresponding diminution in appetite, as is the case in the earlier stages of anhedonia, there is a restless seeking for stimulation in order to secure the longed-for satisfaction. The mood becomes unpleasant, and the expression of it may take many forms. One of such expressions, commonly seen in sedentary persons, is

From the Division of Psychiatric Research, Boston State Hospital, Boston, aided by grants brom the Commonwealth of Massachusettes and the Rockefeller Foundation. *Research associates, Boston State Hospital. †Director of research, Boston State Hospital.
Lesses MF, Myerson A. Human Autonomic Pharmacology XVI. Benzedrine Sulfate as an Aid in the Treatment of Obesity. *N Engl J Med* 1938:218:119-124. Massachusettes Medical Society. Reprinted with permission from the *New England Journal of Medicine*, 1440 Main St., Waltham, MA 02154-1649.

frequent eating. People who are restless because their lives are unsatisfied may be seen nibbling candy, nuts, crackers or the like. The ingestion of food becomes in a certain measure an escape. Food is easily obtained, and eating is often merely a something-to-do which has become a prime need.

The etiology of obesity and treatment of the obese person therefore appear to involve a careful consideration of the anhedonic syndrome, since in many such patients there is an associated neurosis of varying degree. A similar concept has been elaborated by Newburgh and his associates (6), who have pointed out that obesity is in the main outcome of a perverted habit and that there is "dulling of the acuity of the sensations...weak will and a pleasure-seeking outlook upon life."

To attack the syndrome of anhedonic obesity through the psychologic mechanisms involved, in an effort to cut down the unphysiologic desire for food, seems more rational than the usual therapeutic efforts, which are largely aimed at increasing the metabolism through drug administration–for example, thyroid extract or dinitrophenol– or exercise, or decreasing the food intake by strenuous dieting. The latter methods are successful, but do nothing to eliminate the cause, that is, the anhedonia. This neurotic relation is shown by the easy fatigability of the obese, which is, we believe, due not so much to the excessive weight that must be carried as to the neurotic factors which have produced and are sustaining the obese state. This is well attested by the fact that in many of the cases to be described the fatigue was not that seen after physical effort, unusual or customary, as in normal persons, but was the characteristic "morning tiredness," occurring even without the expenditure of energy, which is seen in the neurotic and the physically sick. Thus, the excess food ingestion of the anhedonic obese person rarely occurs in the morning, when desire and mood are especially low, but comes later in the day and in the evening.

Benezedrine sulfate (phenlisopropylamine) is an advantageous drug with which to attack the problem. Its action is primarily that of a sympathetic stimulant; chemically speaking, it is an adrenergic drug. Thus, on the eye and the vascular system is has the classic effects of sympathetic stimulation; it relaxes the spasm of the gatrointestional tract (8), and tends to decrease the gastric juice while increasing its acidity (9). Its effects on the mood, on the sensation of energy and its output, and on the gastrointestinal tract offered the desired psychophysiologic action. Given in small doses, below the point where it produces marked changes in the visceral activities, benezedrine sulfate prevents sleepiness and drowsiness; this is the basis for its use in narcolepsy (10). The dissipation of the feeling of fatigue and the beneficial influence on state of mind effected by this drug in both normal and neurotic persons have been established by recent reports (11,12,13). Because of these psychologic effects the urge to eat as a means of filling out an empty existence is lessened.

The direct effect of benzedrine sulfate on the appetite for food is of primary importance in the group of cases to be discussed. That it seems to cause a loss in weight has already been noted by Nathanson (12). Evidence of its availability to reduce the appetite will be adduced below.

A group of 17 unselected and consecutive private patients, with a primary complaint of obesity, were placed after initial study on a measured, unweighed diet of about 1400 calories, with an approximate composition of protein 69 gm and iron 0.014 gm. No further instructions as to the diet were given after the first visit. No patient was urged to follow the diet, or to do otherwise than obey his natural desire. All patients were observed at intervals of from seven to fourteen days, and at each visit the weight, blood pressure and pulse rate were observed. All reported symptoms were noted, and leading questions which might obscure the subjective effect of the drug were avoided. Prolonged observation by Myerson and his associates (14) indicated that in man the elevation of the blood pressure was the most toxic effect of benzedrine. This hypertensive effect was rarely associated with an increase in the pulse rate. The dosage of benzedrine utilized never caused blood-pressure elevation, even in patients with hypertension. Subjectively, the more important criteria of benzedrine toxicity were nervousness, a jittery sensation and nocturnal insomnia. Here again, careful regulation of the dosage prevented these reactions.

Benzedrine sulfate is distributed in 10 mg. tablets, which are scored so that they may be broken into quarters, each representing 2.5 mg. The most satisfactory plan of treatment was to give three doses daily–a large dose in the morning immediately on waking or rising, a moderate dose at noon, and small or moderate dose in the late afternoon. As a rule, we started with 7.5 mg on arising, 5 mg at noon, and 2.5 mg at 5 p.m. This dosage was gradually increased from week to week as the need arose, but the dosage was stopped well short of the point at which nervousness or nocturnal insomnia was produced. Ordinarily, an increase of 5 mg weekly caused no untoward symptoms. The largest dose given any patient was 30 mg. daily, divided into three unequal doses (12.5 mg. on arising, 10 mg. at noon and 7.5 mg. at 5 p.m.)

This dosage schedule accomplished two desirable results: the largest dose was given in the morning, when the feeling of energy was at its lowest, and the smallest was given in the afternoon, when the energy output was increasing and the time for sleep was approaching. In occasional cases, where the appetite for excess ingestion of food during the evening was uncontrollable, the plan of giving a large dose in the morning, a small dose at noon, and a moderate or large dose at 5 p.m. was tried with some success, particularly if insomnia did not follow. All patients were supplied with only enough tablets to last until the next visit, in order to prevent dangerous self-medication. No patient was given a prescription for the drug or was told its name.

Tolerance to the drug, so far as its effect on the appetite was concerned, did not seem to develop, for substitution of placebo tablets or omission of the drug always caused a return of increased appetite, even after months of administration.

Out of the group of 17 cases, the complete histories of 8 are given below. Table 1 gives the factual data for the entire group. Although we here stress the utilization of benzedrine in cases of obesity which are associated with varying degrees of anhedonia and neurosis, the drug was found to be of as much benefit in cases of obesity without any obvious neurotic background, such as a case associated with narcolepsy and several cases with endocrine stigmas.

Table 1. *The Effect of Benzedrine Sulfate as an Aid in the Treatment of Obesity.*

Case No.	Sex	Initial Weight	Period of Observation	Total Weight Loss	Average Weekly Weight Loss	Maximum Daily Dose of Benzedrine
		lb.	*weeks*	*lb.*	*lb.*	*mg.*
1	F	171	17	29	1.7	22.5
2	F	210	15	17	1.1	27.5
3	F	194	23	26	1.1	22.5
4	F	216	6 1/2	11 1/2	1.7	25.0
5	F	145	10	11	1.1	13.0
6	F	217	6	7 3/4	1.3	22.5
7	M	316	12 1/2	54	4.3	30.0
8	F	189	20 1/2	32	1.5	20.0
9	F	150	19	27	1.4	22.5
10	F	231	25	48	1.9	27.5
11	F	157	10	18	1.8	20.0
12	F	176	10	0	0	22.5
13	F	135	12	13	1.1	22.5
14	F	145	14	9	0.6	30.0
15	F	151	10 1/2	20 1/4	1.9	17.5
16	F	207	10	10	1.0	27.5
17	F	179	10 1/2	13 1/2	1.3	15.0

Case Reports

Case 1 (obesity and psychoneurosis). A housewife of 24 complained of being overweight and of abnormal fatigability. She had gained 25 lb. since the birth of her baby 7 months before. For over a year she had noted increased fatigue, particularly on wakening in the morning. The past history was otherwise negative.

The height was 62 in. and the weight 169 lb. (50 lb. overweight). There was no deviation from normal except for the generalized obesity. The blood pressure was 110/64. The urine was free of albumin, sugar and abnormalities of the sediment.

The patient was placed on the standard low-calorie diet. She did not return again until 11 months later, when she weighted 171 lb. She stated that she felt tired and sleepy all the time, had become very nervous and had frequent crying spells. Examination at the time revealed no change from the previous one. The blood pressure was 110/60.

In view of the fact that the patient was suffering from a psychoneurosis, she was given both stimulating and sedative therapy. She was placed on benzedrine sulfate, 5 mg. on arising, 5 mg. at noon and 2.5 mg at 5 p.m., and Amytal (isoamylethyl barbituric acid), 15 mg at noon, supper and bedtime. In addition, she was given the standard low-calorie diet. During the course of the next month she was seen at weekly intervals and showed a weight loss of 16 lb. Her nervousness gradually decreased, her crying spells disappeared, and she stopped munching between meals. She had no difficulty in getting a satisfactory night's sleep. She stated, "I am not hungry any more." For the first time in her life, however, she became slightly constipated. During this period the blood pressure and pulse rate remained unaltered.

At the close of the 1st month of therapy the patient was given a 2 weeks' supply of the tablets and told to return at that time. This she was unable to do, so that she was not seen again until 6 weeks later. At this visit she stated that following the omission of the benzedrine tablets she had had a marked increase in appetite: "I kept nibbling all day. When I take the tablets [of benzedrine] I have to force myself to eat." Whereas she had lost 16lb. in her 1st month of treatment, during the subsequent 6 weeks she lost only 5 lb. During the period of benzedrine therapy, she finally attained a dosage of 10 mg on rising, 7.5 mg at noon, and 5 mg at 5 p.m. The tablets of isoamylethyl barbituric acid were omitted when the nervous symptoms disappeared. Following the resumption of benzedrine therapy the loss in weight continued, and in the final 6 weeks she lost 8 lb. During 2 of these weeks she again missed an appointment and was without benzedrine for 2 weeks. Upon cessation of the benzedrine her appetite became "tremendous," and she ate so much that there was a temporary gain in weight. At her last visit she stated that she felt perfectly well, and physical examination disclosed no abnormality. She lost 29 lb. during the 17 weeks of observation.

Case 2 (obesity with psychoneurosis). A housewife of 32 complained of being overweight and of weakness, easy fatigability and tiredness. She had always been overweight, but since her marriage 8 years previously her weight had increased from 165 to 212 lb. without apparent cause. Her appetite had always been very good, and she ate a great deal between meals. She had had weakness and easy fatigability for the past year. Six and a half years previously, following the birth of her first child, she had had a "nervous breakdown." During that period she lost 35 lb., so that her weight dropped to 140 lb. Since then her weight had increased to its present figure. The cause of the breakdown was not known to her. She said that at that time, "I could not eat...I could not look at food...I had terrible and crazy thoughts; nothing interested me...I did not care for anything...I had frequent ideas of falling." She was ill for about a year with this condition, and then gradually improved. She had always slept well but awoke every morning with a tired feeling and without a normal sensation of restfulness. During the day her fatigue occurred without relation to exertion. The rest of the history was irrelevant.

The height was 61 in. and the weight 210lb. (87 lb. overweight). The patient showed a centripetal obesity, the fat being chiefly over the buttocks, thighs, abdomen and upper arms. The hands and feet were small and in proportion to the height. The blood pressure was 120/80. The rest of the examination was normal. The hemoglobin was 60 per cent (Sahli) with 4,100,000 red blood cells per cu. mm. The blood smear showed moderate hypochromia of the red cells, but no abnormalities of the white cells. A sugar-tolerance test, following the ingestion of 100 gm. of dextrose in 20 percent solution, showed no glycosuria up to 2 hours. The blood sugar at the end of the second hour was 72 mg. per cent (Folin-We method).

This patient was placed on the standard low-calorie diet and was given benzedrine sulfate, 7.5 mg. on rising, 5 mg. at noon and 5 mg. at 5 p.m. This was gradually increased to 10 mg on rising, 10 mg. at noon and 7.5 mg at 5 p.m. The patient was observed at weekly intervals for 15 weeks, during which time she lost 17 lb. Her fatigue disappeared, although her sense of well-being was not particularly improved. There was a significant decrease in the appetite. The blood pressure remained within normal limits. This patient is still under observation.

Case 3 (obesity with psychoneurosis). A housewife of 38 complained of being overweight and of nervousness. She had been overweight most of her life. Seventeen years previously, at the time of her marriage, she had weighed 140 lb., and since then had gradually gained in weight. One year previously she had undergone a tonsillectomy, and had gained 15 lb. shortly thereafter. Her appetite had always been excellent, but she was not accustomed to eating between meals. She stated that she had always done her own cooking and did do a good deal of tasting. Recently she had become accustomed to sleeping 10 or 11 hours at night. She had been nervous and easily irritable since her husband had been diagnosed as having heart trouble. Her father had died of Bright's disease at the age of 52, and one brother had diabetes and heart trouble. The rest of the history was negative.

The height was 64 in. and the weight 194 lb. (62 lb. overweight). Except for generalized obesity, the physical examination was negative. The blood pressure was 126/80. The urine was free of albumin, sugar and abnormalities of the sediment. The hemoglobin was 78 per cent (Sahli). The basal metabolic rate in a satisfactory test was–15 percent (Mayo standards).

The patient was placed on the standard low-calorie diet and given benzedrine sulfate, 2.5mg. on rising, 2.5 mg. in mid-morning and 2.5 mg. at noon. The dosage was gradually increased until she was taking 10 mg. on rising, 7.5 mg. at noon and 5 mg. at 5 p.m. This patient was seen at weekly intervals for a period of 23 weeks and in that time lost 26 lb. The craving for food was lost; the nervousness and irritability became markedly decreased. She slept well, was free of all unpleasant subjective symptoms and in fact had a sense of well-being. Benzedrine was omitted and placebo tablets were given for 2 weeks during the period of observation; during that time, she spontaneously stated, she had had a return of her nervousness and craving for food. During this period there was a gain in weight of 2 lb.

Case 7 (obesity with narcolepsy). A 34-year-old salesman complained of being overweight and of sleepiness. His birth weight was 16 lb. and he had been continuously overweight since birth. At the age of 16 he weighed 140 lb.; at the age of 19, 200 lb. His weight gradually increased until at the age of 29 he weighed over 300 lb. The weight had been stationary for the last 4 years. His appetite had always been very good, and he ate continuously throughout the day. In addition to sleeping 9 or 10 hours at night, he found himself continually falling off to sleep throughout the day whenever the opportunity presented itself. In the past history there was nothing of importance except that he had had gonorrhea 18 years before, which had apparently never cleared up, as since then he had noted a slight penile discharge intermittently. He had also had nocturia during the last 7 or 8 years, but apparently no daytime frequency or polyuria. There was no impairment of sexual desire or potency.

The height was 69 in. and the weight 316 lb. (158

lb. overweight). The blood pressure was 104/80. The patient was very obese, with the excess adiposity concentrated about the abdomen. There were a few red striae over the lower abdomen. The fundi showed clear and well-outlined nerve heads, normal arteries and slightly engorged veins. The mouth, throat, neck, heart, and lungs were normal. The genitalia were normal. All reflexes were normal. The urine had no albumin or sugar, but the sediment showed 10 white blood cells per high-power field, and the stained urinary sediment showed many extracellular cocci. The prostatic smear showed many pus cells and cocci. The basal metabolic rate was +8 and +10 percent (Mayo standards) in two fairly satisfactory determinations. The blood Hinton test was negative. Blood sugars taken 1 and 2 hours after the ingestion of 100 gm. of dextrose in 20 percent solution showed values of 174 mg. percent and 95 mg. percent respectively. A 24-hour urine was measured to exclude the possibility of diabetes insipidus and showed a volume of 3000cc.

This patient presented two clinical problems: lethargy almost to the point of narcolepsy, and a huge appetite, present since birth. He was placed on the standard low-calorie diet and given benzedrine sulfate, 10 mg. on rising, 10 mg. at noon and 5 mg. at 4 p.m. This dosage was later changed to 12.5 mg. on rising, 10 mg. at noon and 7.5 mg at 5 p.m. He was seen at weekly intervals for the next 12 1/2 weeks, during which period he lost 54 lb. He followed the diet with ease, and stated voluntarily that his appetite was markedly decreased, and that he had become more active physically and felt very well. His daytime drowsiness disappeared, although he continued to sleep well at night. No unusual symptoms presented themselves, except for slight constipation. He stated that he was seldom hungry and was satisfied with the amount of food allowed in the diet. For 1 week during the period of observation he did not take the benzedrine tablets, and during that period there was no loss in weight and the narcolepsy returned. Upon resumption of the benzedrine tablets the drowsiness disappeared and the loss in weight continued. Later on the patient stopped all treatment for 1 month and regained 11 lb. in that time. Upon resumption of benzedrine the loss in weight continued as before.

Case 8 (obesity with hypomenorrhea). A housewife of 27 complained of being overweight and of irregular menstruation, shortness of breath, backache and nervousness. In the 6 months preceding her first visit she had gained 40 lb. For many years before that her weight had been constant. She did not know the cause of her gain in weight, and felt sure it was not due to overeating or any change in activity. Careful inquiry disclosed one significant change in her daily habits which was a factor. Shortly before the onset of her gain in weight, her 5-year-old son had started to attend school. Whereas previously, having once risen in the morning she was accustomed to staying up, she had now developed the habit of going back to bed for several hours after sending her son to school. Since her regular sleeping habits had not changed in any way, this gave her several hours more of rest every day. She had always been a light sleeper, accustomed to going to bed late and rising early because of her children.

During the period of gain in weight, her menses, which had previously occurred at 28-day intervals, came form 1 to 3 weeks late and were of short duration, with a more scanty and painful flow. During that time she had also noted some low-back pain, usually made worse by prolonged sitting. She had consulted a gynecologist, who found no pelvic abnormality. The shortness of breath was of only a few months' duration and occurred following the gain in weight. Her past history showed that she had been pregnant twice and on each occasion had developed hypertension, which was said to have disappeared at the end of the pregnancy.

The height was 65 in. and the weight 189 lb. (53lb.overweight). Except for generalized obesity, the examination was negative. The blood pressure was 126/84. The urine showed no albumin, sugar or abnormalities of sediment. The hemoglobin was 70 percent (Sahli); the red blood cells numbered 4,000,000 per cu. mm., and the smear showed normal red and white blood cells.

This patient was placed on the standard low-calorie diet. She was given a mild hypnotic (sodium bromide) to aid her in securing sound sleep, and a fairly large dose of benzedrine in the morning immediately on rising in order to break up the habit of returning to sleep. On this regimen she showed a weight loss of 32 lb. in 21 weeks. The blood pressure ranged from 140/90 to 106/76, tending to drop during observation. During the course of treatment she found it very easy to follow the diet. Moreover, the morning benzedrine tablet eliminated the desire to go back to bed at that time. She had no difficulty in falling asleep at night, and after a few nights omitted the hypnotic entirely. Her feeling of energy was markedly increased, and her appetite was noticeably less. She became slightly constipated. There were no untoward symptoms, except occasional headaches, which were no more frequent than those she had occasionally had before taking the benzedrine, and were of the same nature. Toward the end of the period of study the patient developed an increase in appetite during the evening. To counteract this, the benzedrine medication was rearranged so that she took 5 mg. on rising, 2.5 mg. at noon and 7.5 mg. at 5 p.m. This rearrangement did not seriously interfere with sleep and it helped in decreasing the excessive evening appetite.

During a 2-week period the patient was given placebo tablets and gained 4 lb. She noted a return of sleepy spells and marked increase in appetite.

Case 9 (obesity following subtotal thyroidectomy). A houseworker of 38 complained of being overweight. Two years before her first visit she had had a subtotal thyroidectomy for hyperthyroidism, from which she had completely recovered. In the 2 years following the operation she had gained 35 lb., mostly in the first year. The rest of the history was irrelevant.

The height was 61 in. and the weight was 150 lb. (27 lb. overweight). There was generalized obesity. The eyes were prominent but showed no lid lag. The skin over the elbows and over the posterior surfaces of the upper arms was somewhat dry and rough. The hair was slightly course. The neck showed a well-healed thyroidectomy scar, with a small amount of thyroid tissue palpable in both lobes. There was slight puffiness under the eyelids. The urine was free of albumin, sugar and abnormalities of the sediment. The hemoglobin was 78 percent (Sahli); the red-blood-cell count was 4,650,000; the smear was normal; the basal metabolic rate was –3 percent (Mayo standards) in a satisfactory test; the blood pressure was 110/80.

There was an apparent disturbance in the appetite-regulating mechanism, as evidenced by a constant craving for food. There was no clear-cut clinical evidence of myxedema, and the basal metabolic rate bore out this negative impression. She was therefore placed on the standard low-calorie diet and was given benzedrine sulfate, 5 mg. on rising, 5 mg. at noon and 2.5 mg. at 5 p.m. Her highest blood-pressure reading during the course of treatment was 126/84. The pulse rate was always within normal limits. She was seen at biweekly intervals during the next 19 weeks, during which time she lost 27 lb. There were no untoward symptoms throughout the course of observation. Her sleep was not interfered with and she found it very easy to follow the diet. Her appetite was good, but she lost the craving for food. She was discharged after 19 weeks of treatment because she had attained her normal weight. The final physical examination showed no abnormalities.

Case 10 (obesity). A housewife of 45 complained of being overweight and of easy fatigability. She had been overweight all her life. Twenty year previously, at the time of her marriage, she weighed 170 lb. Her appetite had always been unusually good. She had dieted many times but without any success, and in fact within the preceding months had gained 5 lb. The rest of the past marital and family histories was irrelevant.

The height was 65 in. and the weight 231 lb. (95 lb. overweight). There was generalized distribution of the excess fat except for the breasts, which were normal in size. The blood pressure was 152/78. The heart was not enlarged, but a barely audible systolic murmur was heard over the apex. The rest of the examination was normal. The urine was free of albumin, sugar, and abnormalities of sediment.

The patient was placed on the standard low-calorie diet and was given benzedrine, 5 mg. on rising, 2.5 mg. in mid-morning and 2.5 mg. at noon. This dosage was gradually increased and the time of administration was rearranged, so that eventually she was taking 12.5 mg. on rising, 10 mg. at noon and 5 mg. at 5 p.m. She was seen at intervals of 10 days over a period of 25 weeks, and during that time lost 48 lb. The initial blood pressure, which was somewhat elevated, showed a normal reading on subsequent visits, and on several occasions went as low as 104/70. During the period of observation she noted a decreased appetite and an increased feeling of energy. There were no other subjective changes. She found it easy to follow the diet. For several weeks the rate of loss in weight was so marked that the diet had to be increased. At no time was there interference with the ability to fall asleep or stay asleep. During one 10-day interval blank placebo tablets were substituted for the benzedrine sulfate. The patient gained weight in that period and noted a marked return of appetite and "extreme hunger."

Case 12 (obesity–failure of benzedrine to aid in reducing weight). This patient, a student of 20, had been under intermittent observation for a period of 3 years. She had undergone a previous course of reducing with diet and thyroid extract quite satisfactorily, attaining a final weight of 135 lb., 2 1/2 years before the present period of study. In the interim she had gradually gained weight to a maximum of 177 lb. This gain occurred while she was working as a cook.

The height was 63 in. and the weight 176 lb. (48 lb. overweight). Examination showed centripetal obesity, the excess adiposity being largely confined to the middle third of the body, and most marked over the buttocks and upper thighs. The breasts were small and pubescent. The hair distribution was normal. The rest of the examination was normal. The basal metabolic rate in two determinations was ±0 percent (Mayo standards). The blood pressure was 94/60.

The patient was placed on the standard low-calorie diet and was given benzedrine sulfate, 7.5 mg. on rising, 5 mg. at noon and 2.5 mg at 5 p.m. The dosage was gradually increased to 10 mg. on rising, 7.5 mg. at noon and 5 mg. at 5 p.m. Over a period of 10 weeks there was no change in weight. Numerous unpleasant symptoms were complained of–inability to breathe deeply, marked nervousness, constipation, dry cough, increased irritability with difficulty in falling asleep and marked fatigue. Further study of the emotional background disclosed that just before coming under observation the patient had gone through an unhappy love affair, which had left her quite depressed. She stated that during her periods of greatest depression she ate large amounts of food in an effort to compensate for her disturbed emotional state. The benzedrine in this instance had of course failed to restore the feeling of well-being and of increased energy, which is often essential to its action in reducing the appetite. Appropriate psychotherapy in this patient eventually restored some degree of emotional calm, and the administration of benzedrine during this phase effected moderate loss in weight without unpleasant symptoms.

Benzedrine sulfate is an important aid in the treatment of obesity of any type; on the one hand it decreases the appetite, and on the other so increases the sense of well-being and of energy that physical activity is spontaneously increased. Its proper place in the treatment of obesity is as an adjuvant. In associated with a properly selected low-calorie diet, it helps the patient to follow the diet with greater ease by abolishing the neurotic and ill-timed craving for foods which plays so important a role in the genesis and maintenance of obesity. Our experience, however, shows that benzedrine will not so readily effect weight reduction when it does not lift the patient's mood and increase the sense of well-being. In the more profound neuroses where elevation of mood is not in any permanent way affected by the drug and where the appetite is already absent, benzedrine sulfate is not indicated. Its use in the neurotic obese, therefore, is largely limited to those cases associated with what we have here termed a mild anhedonic state.

Summary and Conclusions

1. Obesity is often due to a defect in the mood which upsets the appetite-regulating mechanism. In such cases increased eating, which does not represent true hunger, takes place in order to offset and compensate for the disturbed mood.
2. The commonest cause of this disturbance in appetite is the anhedonia associated with psychoneurosis.
3. Benzedrine sulfate, by improving the anhedonic state, acts as an aid in obese neurotic persons.
4. Benzedrine sulfate has a direct effect in depressing the appetite and in increasing physical activity, and is therefore useful in any type of obesity
5. In a group of obese patients suffering from associated psychoneuroses, endocrine disease and narcolepsy, benzedrine sulfate has been used as an adjuvant to weight reduction without development of any toxic signs or symptoms, during periods ranging from six to twenty-five weeks.

At the time of going to press benzedrine sulfate has been used in the treatment of 40 obese patients over periods of from three to nine months. The above conclusions are substantiated with regard to benefit and lack of toxicity in the indicated dosage.

371 Commonwealth Avenue

References

1. **Means JH.** Obesity. In: *Cecil's Text-Book of Medicine.* 3rd ed. Philadelphia and London: W.B. Saunders Company; 1933:666.
2. **Freyberg RH, Newburgh LH.** Obesity and energy exchange in a verified case of pituitary basophilism. *Arch Intern Med.* 1936; 58:229.
3. **Myerson A.** The social conditioning of the visceral activities. *N Engl J Med.* 1934;211:189.
4. **Myerson A.** *Social Psychology.* New York: Prentice-Hall Co; 1934.
5. **Myerson A.** Neuroses and neuropsychoses; the relationship of symptom groups. *Am J Psychiatry.* 1936;S3:263.
6. **Newburgh LH, Johnston MW.** The nature of obesity. *J Clin Invest.* 1930;8:197.
7. **Myerson A, Thau W.** Human autonomic pharmacology; the effect of cholinergic and adrenergic drugs on the eye. *Arch Ophthalmol.* 1937;18:78.
8. **Myerson A, Ritvo M.** Benzedrine sulfate and its value in spasm of the gastrointestinal tract. *JAMA.* 1936;107:24.
9. **Myerson A, Rinkel M, Dameshek W.** The autonomic pharmacology of the gastric juices. *N Engl J Med.* 1936;215:1005.
10. **Prinzmetal M, Bloomberg W.** The use of benzedrine for the treatment of narcolepsy. *JAMA.* 1935;105:2051.
11. **Myerson A.** Effect of benzedrine sulfate on mood and fatigue in normal and in neurotic persons. *Arch Neurol Psychiatry.* 1936;36:816.
12. **Nathanson MH.** The central action of beta-aminopropylbenzene (benzedrine): clinical observations. *JAMA.* 1937;108:528.
13. **Davidoff E, Reifenstein EC, Jr.** The stimulating action of benzedrine sulfate: a comparative study of the responses of normal persons and of depressed patients. *JAMA.* 1937;108:1770.
14. **Myerson A, Loman J, Demeshek W.** Physiologic effects of benzedrine and its relationship to other drugs affecting the autonomic nervous system. *Am J Med Sci.* 1936;192:560.

CLASSICS IN OBESITY

Metabolic Observations in Patients with Jejunocolic Shunts*

J. HOWARD PAYNE, M.D., LOREN T. DEWIND, M.D. AND ROBERT R. COMMONS, M.D.,†
Los Angeles, California

From the Departments of Medicine and Surgery, University of Southern California, School of Medicine, Los Angeles, California. *Aided in part by a grant from the Foundation for Surgical Research.*

Most surgeons have been confronted with many interesting, and, as yet, unanswered problems of the patient who has a major portion of their small intestine resected in an uncontrolled situation. The usual reasons for the uncontrolled bowel resections are mesenteric artery occlusion with infarcted intestine, volvulus, extensive neoplastic disease, ileitis and adhesions. An enormous amount of clinical and laboratory experience has been accumulated that man can survive the sacrifice of most of his intestine (1-5).

In 1954, Kremen, Linner and Nelson (2) reported a careful study in dogs of the consequence of bypassing various portions of the small intestine. The significant conclusion of their study was that "sacrifice of the distal 50 per cent of the small intestine produces a profound interference with fat absorption associated with loss of weight." Doctor Philip Sandblom of Lund, Sweden, in discussion of the paper stated that "this questionable method of controlling obesity will have the necessary experimental foundation." He also mentioned that Dr. V. Henrikson of Gothenberg has resected "an appropriate amount of small intestine" because of obesity and had induced weight loss, but created a situation of difficult nutritional balance.

In the course of continuing studies of the basic nature and treatment of the obese state, opportunity arose in 1956 to study the metabolic effects on patients who had a planned controlled intestinal bypass operation. The purpose of this paper is to present the clinical observations and laboratory findings in these patients.

METHODS AND MATERIALS

The clinical study included ten patients who had planned jejuno-colic shunts bypassing some jejunum, the entire ileum and the right colon. Partial or complete intestinal continuity was re-established when the ideal weight was reached or before if a valid reason presented itself.

Patients selected for surgical therapy were considered to have uncontrolled obesity. In our opinion, uncontrolled obesity exists when the patient is at least 125 pounds overweight, all other methods to control weight have been tried and failed, and life was endangered by an associated disease such as cardiopulmonary failure (Pickwickian syndrome), diabetes, hypertension and liver disease. All of our patients willingly agreed and seemed to understand the serious nature of the undertaking. The indications for surgery were rigid and limited to a very few extremely obese patients. The study was divided into seven phases. (Table I).

CASE REPORTS

Case 1. L. M. was chubby during her childhood. At age sixteen, during a period of continuous hospitalization on a measured 1,000 calorie diet she lost weight from 240 pounds to 145 pounds. One year later she weighed 240 pounds. At age twenty-five, she was 5 feet 2 inches tall and weighed 294 pounds with a blood pressure of 250/160 mm. Hg. At this time, metabolic studies were consistent with the clinical diagnosis of "Cushing's syndrome." In May 1954 an exploratory celiotomy, ovarian biopsy and left adrenalectomy were done. Pathologic report of the

Reprinted by permission of the publisher from
Payne JH, DeWind LT, Commons RR. Metabolic observations in patients with jejunocolic shunts. *Am J Surgery*. 1963;106:273-289.

Editor's note: Only selected figures have been reproduced.
Special thanks to Judy Willis of the Pennington Information Center for help in acquiring this document.

*Presented at the Annual Meeting of the Pacific Coast Surgical Association at Palm Springs, California, February 3-6, 1963.
† Deceased, December 8, 1961.

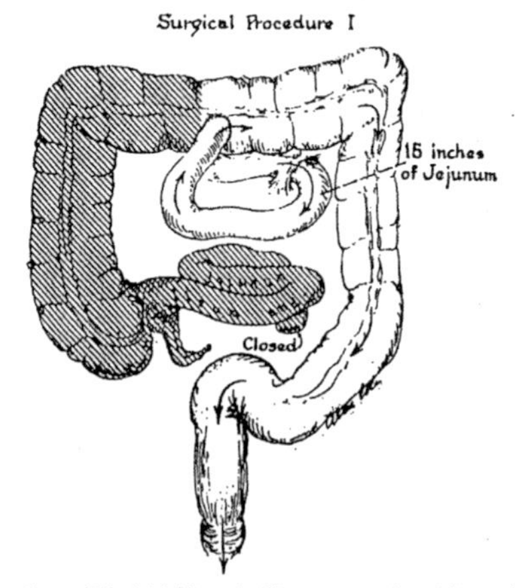

FIG. 1. The initial intestinal bypass operation. Jejuno-colic anastomosis.

resected adrenal did not confirm the diagnosis. In 1956, her weight was 292 pounds and her blood pressure 260/150 mm Hg. She was in cardiopulmonary failure spending most of her time in bed either eating or sleeping. It was the internist's impression that she represented the classical Pickwickian syndrome. After preparation in May 1956, a controlled jejuno-colic shunt was created. (Fig. 1.) A small wound seroma was the only complication. She was discharged on her fifteenth postoperative day. Her only complaint was anal irritation from six to ten semisolid stools per day. Six months later, she still had five or six bowel movements a day when she overate food of high fat or carbohydrate content. In excess, these foods produced intestinal cramps and prolonged diarrhea for thirty or forty minutes after each meal.

In May 1957, the intestinal shunt was abolished and normal intestinal continuity was established. A gallbladder filled with stones was removed; biopsy specimens were taken of the liver, kidney and intestine. She weight 120 pounds (Fig. 2) with a blood pressure of 120/70 (Fig. 3.) She was weak, but otherwise had no complaints. Photographs before and after the intestinal shunt are presented. (Fig. 4.)

CASE II. B. E., a twenty-five year old 4 feet 11 inch Caucasian married woman, weighed 242 1/2 pounds. Since age twelve, she gained weight steadily in spite of a "very low intake." She tried various diets on numerous occasions. In addition, she consulted several "obesity specialists" including a psychiatrist, but without any improvement. She had menstruated infrequently and scantily during the past three years. There was no family history of excess weight. After careful evaluation (Table 1), she was referred for surgical therapy. On April 23, 1957, a controlled jejuno-colic shunt was created. She was discharged on her eleventh postoperative day. Only complaint was anal irritation from six stools per day.

Her recovery was satisfactory with a weight loss which averaged five pounds per month. By the fifth month, her menstrual periods became regular. She did report thinning of scalp hair. In August 1958, she weighed 134 pounds; then, the rate of weight loss slowed down. It was ten months later before she weighed 118 pounds (Fig.2) with a blood pressure of 120/70 mm. Hg (Fig. 3.)

On June 15, 1959, fifteen inches of jejunum was anas-

TABLE I

SEVEN PHASES IN THE EVALUATION AND TREATMENT OF AN OBESE PATIENT

Phase One

Clinical, psychologic screening and laboratory examinations includes: complete blood cell count and morphologic study, urine analyses, serum proteins, serum protein bound iodine, serum cholesterol, blood urea nitrogen, total protein, fasting blood sugar, electrocardiogram, twenty-four hour excretion of creatinen, 17 keto-steroids, and 17 ketogenic steroids excretion.

Phase Two

Preparation for surgery includes: glucose tolerance test on high carbohydrate diet (oral and intravenous), bromsulphalein excretion test, serum sodium, CO2, potassium, calcium, phosphorus, alkaline phosphatase, and bowel preparation with Neomycin.

Phase Three

Initial surgery includes: jejuno-colic shunt, panniculectomy, intestinal biopsy, liver biopsy and kidney biopsy. Umbilical hernioplasty and an appendectomy if indicated.

Phase Four

Postoperative follow-up study includes: careful clinical observation, laboratory studies as done in preoperative studies, and serum carotenoid levels.

Phase Five

Second preoperative study and preparation for surgery (Phases One and Two).

Phase Six

Surgical revision of shunt, including kidney, liver and jejunal biopsies with panniculectomy. Remove any pathologic organs.

Phase Seven

Postoperative follow-up study includes: careful clinical observation and serial laboratory studies as indicated.

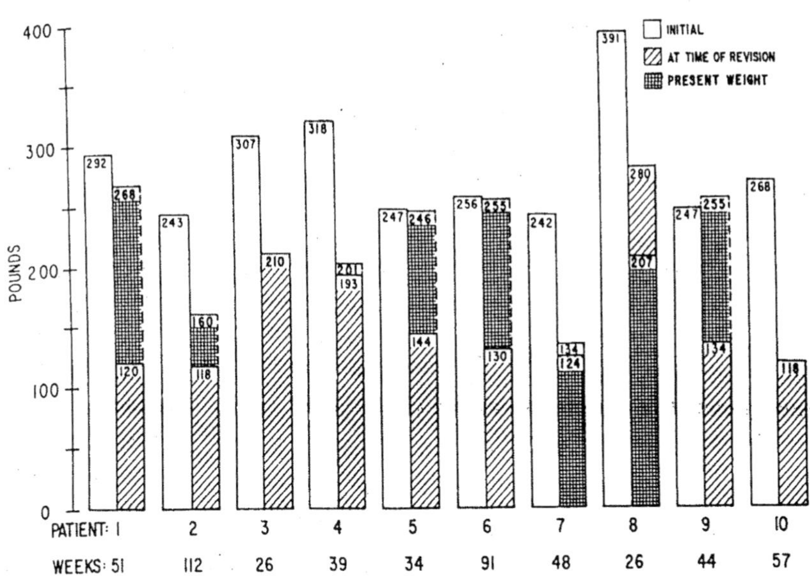

FIG. 2. Changes in weight caused by a controlled intestinal bypass operation. The number of weeks the intestine was bypassed is shown.

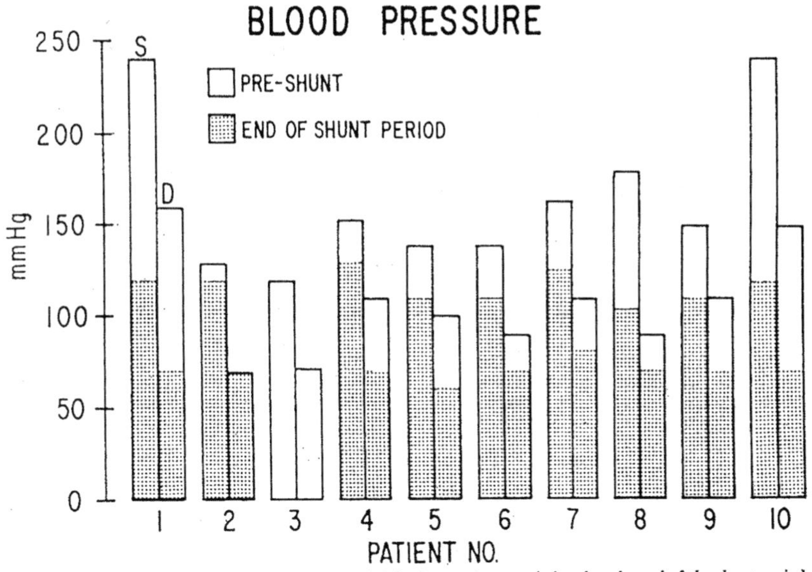

FIG. 3. Systolic and diastolic blood pressure recorded in the preshunt period and at the end of the shunt period. Note Cases I, VIII and X.

tomosed to 20 inches of ileum. (Fig. 5.) She was discharged eight days later weighing 112 pounds. Her calculated ideal weight was 111 pounds. Within two months, she became pregnant. With this pregnancy she gained to 170 pounds. Since that time, she has had three children, the latest on January 17, 1963, at which time she weighed 160 pounds and was eating everything she wanted.

CASE III. W. H., a twenty year old 5 feet 3 1/2 inches Caucasian woman, weighed 307 pounds, para II gravida II. History of being fat since age six in spite of "I have tried everything to lose weight, but can't." After careful evaluation, (Table 1) a controlled jejuno-colic shunt was created on June 25, 1957. (Fig. I.) In addition, a liver biopsy, appendectomy, umbilical hernioplasty and panniculectomy were done. (Table II and III.) Except for an initial fall in blood pressure, the patient tolerated the procedure well and made an uneventful recovery. She was discharged on her ninth postoperative day. She was seen at regular intervals for observation, the last time was December 12, 1957. She was in excellent condition, in electrolyte balance and weighed 204 pounds. On December 23, 1957, she died suddenly of a pulmonary embolism. The origin of the embolus was from the pelvic veins, established at postmortem examination.

CASE IV. C. L., a forty-two year old, 5 feet 8 inches Caucasian woman, weighed 318 pounds with a blood pressure of 154/110 mm. Hg; her father is a Doctor of Medicine. She has been fat since early childhood and all measures to reduce her weight were either temporary or failed. After the usual preoperative evaluation (Table I), she was referred for surgical therapy. In June 1957 a controlled jejuno-colic shunt was created. (Fig. I.) An appendectomy, umbilical hernioplasty, paniculectomy and liver biopsy were also accomplished. (Table II and III.) Her postoperative course was complicated by thrombophlebitis and she was discharged on the twentieth postoperative day. She was seen at regular intervals and was losing weight on an average of three pounds per week. However, this patient became unreliable and failed to keep her appointments, was drinking heavily which we learned now as not being new for her, became hostile and had a myriad of complaints. Consequently, we were unwilling to continue with the intestinal shunt. Therefore, on March 25, 1958 intestinal continuity was completely re-established before the ideal weight was reached. Her weight was 193 pounds; she had lost 126 pounds in thirty-nine weeks. (Fig. 2.) Her blood pressure was 130/70 mm. Hg. (Fig. 3.) She was discharged on her tenth postoperative day with no complaints. She was last seen in May 1958 when she weighed 201 pounds. We have not seen or heard from her since that time.

TABLE II

INITIAL SURGICAL PROCEDURES

Data	No.
Jejuno-colic shunt	10
Panniculectomy	10
Liver biopsy	10
Intestinal biopsy	10
Renal biopsy	3

TABLE III

ADDITIONAL SURGICAL PROCEDURES

Appendectomy	5
Umbilical hernioplasty	3
cholecystectomy	1
Hysterectomy	1

CASE V. R. G., a 5 foot 8 inch thirty year old Caucasian woman, weighed 247 pounds. She gave the usual history of these obese women. Her blood pressure was 140/11 mm. Hg. After the usual preoperative evaluation (Table I), she was referred for surgical therapy. On July 2, 1957, a controlled jejuno-colic shunt was created. (Fig. I.) In addition, an appendectomy, umbilical hernioplasty, panniculectomy and liver biopsy were done. (Table II and III.) She was discharged on the tenth postoperative day after an uncomplicated recovery. She had eight to ten stools per day with anal irritation. Except for modest loss of hair and a complaint of weakness, her convalescence was satisfactory. On February 28, 1958, normal intestinal continuity was re-established in addition to panniculectomy, renal and liver biopsy. Her weight reached a low of 144 pounds (Fig. 2) and her blood pressure was 110/60 mm. Hg (Fig. 3) when she was discharged on her seventeenth postoperative day. In spite of "really trying" she regained her weight to 250 pounds. Last seen on January 28, 1963, at age thirty-six, her weight was 244 pounds. She came in asking to have the operation done agian, "Please give me just one more chance."

CASE VI. E. L., a 5 foot 2 inch forty year old Caucasian woman, weighed 255 pounds. She gave the usual history as recorded previously. Her blood pressure was 140/90 mm. Hg. After the usual preoperative evaluation, she was referred for surgical therapy. On July 9, 1957, a controlled jejuno-colic shunt was created. (Fig. I.) In addition, an appendectomy, panniculectomy and liver biopsy were done. Itables II and III.) She was discharged on her eighth postoperative day after an uncomplicated convalescence. It was necessary to rehospitalize her on April 22, 1959, because of symptoms which suggested potassium and calcium depletion, in spite of normal serum levels (calcium, 4.3 mEq. per L.; potassium, 4.8 mEq. per L.). It was apparent that we were unable to control her electrolyte balance by oral medicine. Consequently, on April 30, 1959 intestinal continuity was partially re-established. Eighteen inches of jejunum was anastomosed to 42 inches of distal ileum. Biopsy specimens of the liver and intestien were taken. She was discharged on her ninth postoperative day after an uncomplicated recovery, weighing 130 pounds (Fig. 2) and a blood pressure of 110/70 mm. Hg. (Fig. 3.) She was seen during the postoperative period on ten occasions. When last seen on November I, 1961, we were back where we started at 254 pounds with a very unhappy, unstable woman.

CASE VII. D. L., a twenty-six year old 5 foot I inch Caucasian woman, weighed 242 pounds. Blood pressure 164/110 mm. Hg. Until seven years ago, she was of average weight, 120 pound. Since her marriage, there was a gradual increase in her weight. After this, her historical review is identical to the other obese women. After the usual work-up (Table I), she was referred for surgical therapy. On July 19, 1957, a controlled jejuno-colic shunt was created. In addition, a panniculectomy and liver biopsy were done. After an uncomplicated postoperative course, she was discharged on her eighth postoperative day. She had only one stool after each meal. After six months, she was having trouble with profuse menstruation for protracted periods of time up to seven weeks. On June 20, 1958, at the weight of 134 pounds (Fig. 2) and blood pressure of 126/82 mm. Hg (Fig. 3), her intestinal continuity was re-established to normal. In addition, a total hysterectomy, panniculectomy, liver and renal biopsies were done. She was discharged after an uncomplicated recovery, weighing 128 pounds on her eleventh postoperative day. Since discharge, she was seen at regular intervals. Her weight was last recorded at 124 pounds in 1961.

CASE VIII. I. L., a thirty-two year old 5 foot 2 inch Caucasian woman, weighed 391 pounds with a blood pressure of 180/90 mm. Hg. she is a teacher of abnormal psychology. Since childhood, she has been fat. Her mother is heavy, but her father is not. Other than this, she gave the usual history of the obese woman. After evaluation (Table I), she was referred for surgical therapy. On July 19, 1959, using two operating tables to support the patient, a controlled jejuno-colic shunt was created. (Fig. I.) In addition, a panniculectomy and liver biopsy were done. She had an uneventful recovery and was discharged on her eighth postoperative day. This patient had a great deal of difficulty maintaining her serum protein, calcium and potassium levels. She had to be admitted to the hospital on three occasions for intravenous therapy because of inability to control her serum electrolytes by oral medication. (Tables V and VI.) Therefore, on January 14, 1958, normal gastrointestinal continuity was re-established. On her tenth postoerative day she was discharged feeling well and weighing 280 pounds (Fig. 2), with a blood pressure of 104/70 mm. Hg. (Fig. 3.) It was necessary to do bilateral thigh lipectomies (twenty-five pounds each) in October 1961 to enable her to walk. At this time, she was still teaching abnormal psychology daily and would like to have the operation again.

CASE IX. D. F., a 5 foot 2 inch twenty-five year old Caucasian woman, weighed 247 pounds with a blood pressure of 160/90 mm. Hg gave a history similar to the other patients in this series. After the usual work-up (Table I), she was referred for surgical therapy. On July 23, 1957, a controlled jejunocolic shunt was created. (Fig. I.) In addition, an appendectomy, panniculectomy and liver biopsy were done. She made an uncomplicated recovery and was discharged on the seventh postoperative day. Her only complaint was constipation. During the following seven months, she was admitted to the hospital because of pain in the left lower quadrant of her abdomen, dehydration and a low serum potassium (3.8 mEq. per L.). On March 27, 1958, when she weighed 134 pounds (Fig. 2) with a blood pressure of 110/70 mm. Hg (Fig. 3), normal intestinal continuity was re-established. In addition, biopsy specimens were taken from the liver and intestinal tract. After an uncomplicated convalescence, she was discharged on her seventh postoperative day. With increasing domestic problems, she promptly regained her weight to 255 pounds by April 1961.

CASE X. L. B., a 5 foot 2 inch thirty-one year old Caucasian woman, weighed 268 pounds. Her blood pressure was 250/150 mm. Hg. She gave the same history as the other obese patients in this group. After thorough evaluation, she was referred for surgical therapy. On November 4, 1961, a planned jejunocolic shunt was done. Twenty inches of jejunum was anastomosed to the transverse colon. In addition, the liver and intestine were biopsied. Her recovery was uneventful and she was discharged on her seventh postoperative day. She had five stools per day. It soon became apparent that she had an incisional hernia. After losing 147 pounds, she was admitted for revision at the weight of 119 pounds (Fig. 2) and her blood pressure was 118/70 mm. Hg. (Fig. 3.) On December 10, 1962, 15 inches of jejunum was anastomosed to the side of the ileum to inches from the ileocecal valve. Biopsies were taken of the liver and intestine. Her postoperative course was uneventful. At the time of discharge on her tenth postoperative day, she weighed 118 pounds and her blood pressure was 120/70 mm. Hg. Except for a mild weakness, she was in good condition. The patient was last seen on February 1, 1963. Her weight was 123 pounds and she is clinically well.

SURGICAL PROCEDURE

The operation was done exactly the same in the first nine patients. (Fig. I.) The tenth operation varied in one respect. The jejunum was divided 20 inches from the ligament of Treitz instead of 15 inches. A transverse elliptical incision was used excising the fatty abdominal apron and the umbilicus. The average depth of the subcutaneous fat was 6.4 cm. (the largest 11 cm. and the smallest 3 cm.); the average weight of the panniculus was 1,971 gm. (the largest 2,388 gm. and the lightest 230 gm.). Both rectus abdominis muscles were divided transversely and the celomic cavity entered. An exploratory celiotomy was performed. Biopsy specimens were taken from the liver, kidney and jejunum. (Table II.) If the appendix was present, it was removed. Any pathologic organ was excised. If an umbilical hernia was present, it was repaired. (Table III.)

The jejunum was divided 15 inches from the ligament of Treitz. Measurement was made on the mesenteric border. The distal end was closed in two layers, using 4-0 catgut for the inner row and 4-0 silk in the outer layer. The end of the proximal jejunum was anastomosed to the side of the transverse colon, to the right of the midline. A two layer anastomosis was done using 4-0 catgut for the inner layer and interrupted 4-0 silk for the outer row. The abdominal wound was closed with chromic 0 catgut in the peritoneum and transversalis fascia; interrupted No. 24 cotton in the fascia; No. 26 steel wire retention sutures were used down to, but not through, the peritoneum; and interrupted 3-0 silk in the skin. Penrose drains were brought out at each end of the long transverse incision. Spinal anesthesia was used, in all but one patient who had a general anesthetic. No significant anesthetic problems were encountered.

REVISION

The first six patients requiring revision had their intestinal tract restored to normal continuity. The other three have had less than normal lenth left in continuity. E. L. (Case VI), had 15 inches of jejunum anastomosed to the ileum 42 inches from the ileocecal valve. B. E. (Case II), had 15 inches of jejunum anastomosed to the ileum 20 inches from the ileocecal valve. L. B. (Case X), had 15 inches of jejunum anastomosed to the ileum, 10 inches from the ileocecal valve (Fig. 5.)

We have not resected any small bowel except for biopsy purposes. The gut has been merely bypassed. To date we have not had any symptoms or pathologic changes to suggest the "blind loop" syndrom. Mr. Tanner [6] states he prefers and did, indeed, resect the intestine int he two cases he reported to us. (Table IV.)

RESULTS

Blood Pressure. Eight of the ten patients had elevated blood pressure recorded when they were obese.

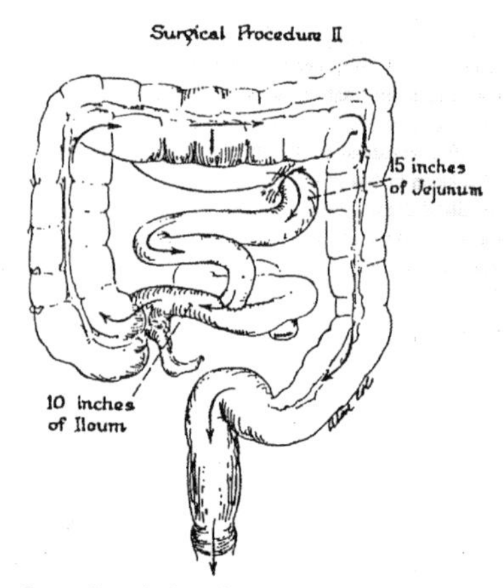

Fig. 5. Intestinal continuity only partially restored. Jejuno-ileal anastomosis.

In each instance the blood pressure returned to normal when significant weight loss had occurred. (Fig. 3.) Cases I and X were considered to be examples of the classic pickwickian syndrome. Both patients were in cardiopulmonary failure with blood pressure recordings of 240/160 and 240/150 mm. Hg, respectively. They responded in a gratifying manner. Their symptoms of cardiopulmonary failure were relieved after they had lost approximately fifty pounds. Patient (Case I) remained symptom free until she regained most of her weight. Patient (Case X) has remained clinically well.

Electrolytes. No consistent or unphysiologic changes were observed in the serum levels of sodium, carbon dioxide combing power, phosphorus, alkaline phosphatase, urea nitrogen, creatine or iron.

Potassium. In spite of large supplemental oral intake, the serum potassium levels fell in all ten patients. (Table V.) five patients were symptomatic and required intravenouis therapy at various times to restore their well being.

Calcium. Because calcium is primarily absorbed in the upper gastrointestinal tract, we did not expect to see hypocalcemia. It soon became apparent with the decreased transit time and diarrhea that not enough calcium was being abdorbed. (Table VI.) All patients, after the third, were given supplemental calcium. Four patients had symptoms suggesting calcium deficiencies. Two had to be hospitlaized to receive intravenous potassium and calcium to restore their well-being. A deficiency in Vitamin D absorption may be a factor in the low serum calcium levles. Numerous roentgenograms were taken of these patients; no evidence of demineral-

TABLE IV
OTHER INVESTIGATORS INTERESTED IN THE INTESTINAL BYPASS OPERATION

Doctor	Cases	Institution
A. K. Kremen	8	University of Minnesota
C. D. Sherman, Jf.	4	University of Rochester Medical Center, Rochester, New York
J. C. Drye	3	University of Louisville
N. C. Tanner	2	Charing Cross Hospital London, England
R. B. Turnbull, Jr.	2	Cleveland Clinic

TABLE V
HIGHEST SERUM POTASSIUM LEVEL ON PRESHUNT PERIOD; LOWEST LEVEL IN SHUNT PERIOD

Case No. and Patient	Preshunt Period	Shunt Period	Symptomatic
I, L. M.	4.8	3.7	...
II, B. E.	4.7	3.9	...
III, W. H.	4.3	...	...
IV, C. L.	4.4	3.3	X
V, R. G.	4.4	3.5	...
VI, E. L.	5.1	3.8	X
VII, D. L.	4.3	3.4	...
VIII, I. L.	3.9	2.7	XX
IX, D. F.	4.5	3.8	X
X, L. B.	4.8	4.0	X

NOTE: Normal = 4.1 to 5.6 mEq. per L.

ization of the bones was noted. Because the serum levels of patassium and calcium could not be maintained except in the hospital, two patients (Cases IV and VIII) had their intestinal continuity re-established before the calculated ideal weight had been obtained.

Cholesterol. During the shunt period the serum cholesterol levels fell into the normal range. (Fig. 6.) Similar results were recorded by Lewis, Turnbull and Page (7). Measurements in three of our patients in the postshunt period, after significant weight gain had occurred, revealed they all had raised to higher levels. The changes subsequently to be described in the liver may also be a factor by affecting the endogenous synthesis of cholesterol by the liver.

Carotenoids. Serum carotene levels were measured only during the shunt period. Each measurement was below the normal range. Our observations are in accord with others who have found that the serum carotene levels are extremely valuable in the diagnosis of the malabsorption syndrome. (Fig. 7.)

Adrenal Steroids. It was possible in four patients to study urinary excretion of 17 ketosteroids and 17 ketogenic steroids prior to and during the shunt period. Three patients had a significant reduction in the 17 ketosteroid and 17 ketogenic steroid levels during the period of intestinal bypass. One only had a minor rise in excretion levels of both substances. (Fig. 8.)

Blood Studies. Many blood counts and stained smears were done in all ten patients. All had a slight fall in number of erythrocytes. Also, the hemoglobin content gradually fell. This was especially true in the "Pickwickian" (Case I) in which the hemoglobin content fell from 17.4 gm. to 14.2 gm. The leukocyte counts and distribution of cells remained within the normal range. In only one instance, Case IX, was there a report of slight anisocytosis and poikilocytosis during the shunt period. Serum iron levels were measured in only one patient (Case X), and they were in the low normal range during the shunt period. Therefore, she was treated with intramuscular injections of iron.

Protein. In all ten patients there was a fall in the levels of serum protein bound iodine. This can be correlated with the low serum protein levels also seen in our patients and may represent a drop in the thyroid binding globulin. Predigested proteins (hydrolysates) were poorly handled. Their ingestion produced an increase in distressing diarrhea. A high carbohydrate diet contain-

TABLE VI
HIGHEST SERUM CALCIUM LEVEL IN PRESHUNT PERIOD; LOWEST LEVEL IN SHUNT PERIOD

Case No. and Patient	Preshunt Period	Shunt Period	Symptomatic
I, L. M.	...	...	...
II, B. E.	...	50	...
III, W. H.	...	...	...
IV, C. L.	3.3	5.2	...
V, R. G.	5.1	4.7	...
VI, E. L.	4.3	3.8	X
VII, D. L.	5.2	5.0	...
VIII, I.L.	7.0	2.6	XX
IX, D. F.	4.9	4.7	X
X, L. B.	4.4	4.1	X

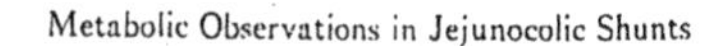

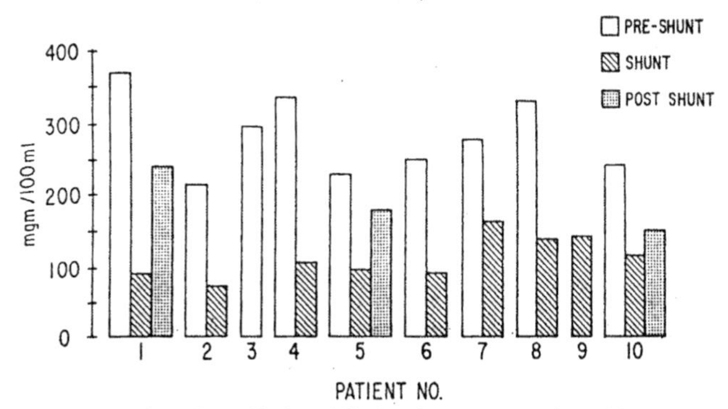

FIG. 6. Serum cholesterol levels recorded in the preshunt, shunt and postshunt periods.

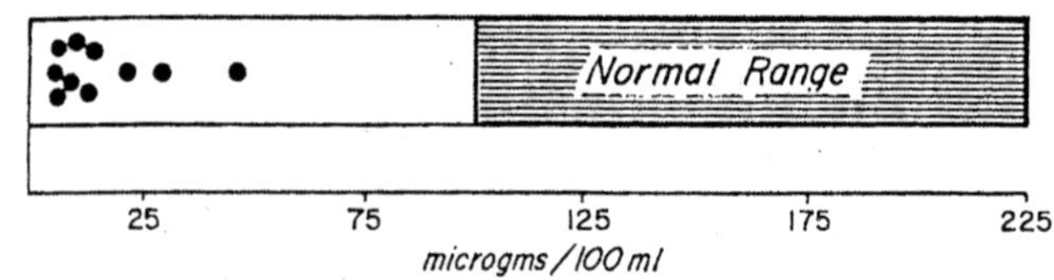

FIG. 7. Ten measurements of serum carotenoids during the shunt period.

ing a modest amount of protein and fat will provide the lowest fecal nitrogen and fat excretion (5). Although we attempted to regulate their diets in this manner, these patients were not able or willing to follow our instructions.

In all but two instances (Cases II and V), serum protein paper electrophoresis measurements were recorded at the end of the shunt period. There was a modest reduction in the total proteins. The albumin content was slightly lower than normal in two patients. The greatest changes were seen in the globulin fraction. $Alpha_1$ was elevated in threee patients; $alpha_2$ low in two patients; $alpha_3$ was present in two patients; and beta was normal in all. The gamma fraction was slightly elevated in three patients.

Carbohydrate. The carbohydrate metabolism appeared to be altered during the shunt period as evidenced by the flat glucose tolerance curves observed in this series. (Fig. 9.) Another indication of disturbed carbohydrate metabolism in our series was that several patients complained of distnetion and excessive flatulence.

Fat and Body Weight. The most significant finding in these patients was their failure to absorb fat. The amount of fat absorbed varied with the individual person and amount of fat eaten, amount of intestine in contact with the ingested fat, and transit time. It was certain that if they ate a large, faty meal, they would pay for it in diarrhea and anal irritation. The subsequent diarrhea made the electrolyte control more difficult. Fat requires digestion before it can be absorbed. Although some is absorbed in the jejunum, absorption is not normally complete until it passes through the ileum. Failure to absorb fat produced a relentless weight loss. (Fig. 2.) The average weight loss at fifty-two weeks was 123 pounds. Although variable with occasional plateaus, the patients lost weight on an average of 2.36 pounds per week. An interesting comparison is the 2.5 pounds per day weight loss recently reported during periods of total fasting (8). Photographs of a patient in the pre- and post-shunt periods are shown in Figure 4A and B. With both 15 inches and 20 inches of jejunum in use, weight loss was noted until gastrointestinal continuity was either partially or completely restored. One patient (Case II) went 112 weeks before revision. Her weight stabilized between 125 and 130 pounds for almost one

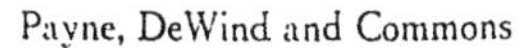

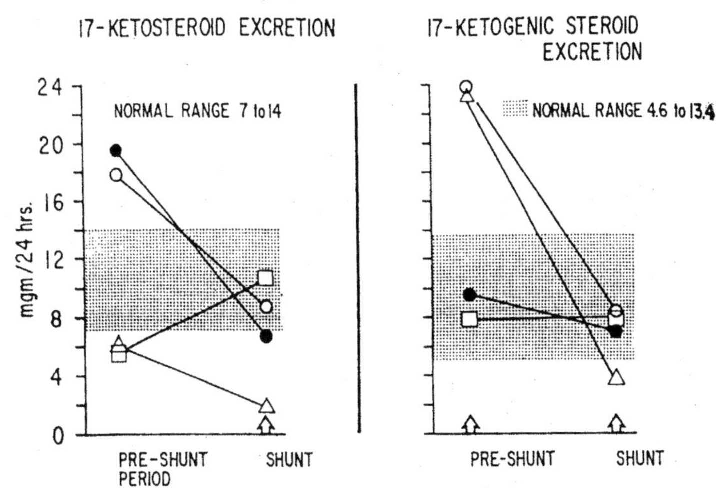

FIG. 8. Changes recorded in the 17 ketosteroid and 17 ketogenic steroid excretion.

year. Then her weight suddenly dropped to 118 pounds. At the time, intestinal continuity was partially restored.

Renal. Needle biopsies of the kidney in three cases id not reveal any pathologic process.

Intestine. Biopsies of the jejunum were done at the time of the inital surgery in all ten patients. No gross or microscopic abnormalities were seen. When the intestinal shunts were revised, a biopsy was taken from the proximal and the bypassed jejunum. Again no gross or microscopic pathologic condition was identified. We did not observe any objective or symptomatic evidence of the blind loop syndrome.

Liver. Liver function was estiamted by bromsulphalein (BSP) retention tests. (Table VII) Five of the seven patients studied prior to the intestinal shunt had abnormal BSP retention. The remaining two had borderline elevations. At the end of the shunt period, four ofthe seven had abnormal BSP tests, one was normal and two had borderline elevation. In five patients in whom comparison was possible between the pre- and postshunt periods, the BSP was unchanged or slightly elevated in three and significantly elevated in two. The latter two had significant morphologic change in the liver during the shunt period. In the other three, there was no positive correlation between the BSP and the fatty changes is the liver. All patients in our series had liver biopsies done at the time of the initial surgery. In four, the fatty change was absent or slight. The other ˙x showed a moderate degree of fatty change. (Figs. 10 .id 11.) When slight, the fatty change was irregularly focal in distribution. When moderate, fatty deposits were controlobular. In three patients, slight periportal fibrosis was noted; and in several, periportal inflammatory change was present. No alcoholic hyalin, necrosis, fatty "cysts," nodular hyperplasia or frank cirrhosis were present. Nine patients had liver biopsies at the time of revision. All showed a varying degree of fatty change, either moderate or sever. There was only one patient in whom the fatty change remained the same or diminished at the end of the shunt period. Significantly, there was no increase in fibrosis or other pathologic changes noted after the shunt period.

Two cases (V and VII) were of particular interest in that the appearance of the liver changed from normal or only slightly fatty change to one of rather severe change. (Figs. 12 and 13). Where the fatty change was pronounced and associated with slight periportal fibrosis, the histologic picture was similar to that of an early stage of Laennec's or nutritional cirrhosis. There was no evidence of reversibility of the fatty change in the period of study despite the striking weight loss.

COMPLICATIONS

Surgical complications were minimal. (Table VIII.) In fact, we were delightfully surprised to see how well these enormous persons tolerated major surgical procedures. There has been no surgical mortality. All patients had diarrhea with and discomfort of variable degrees. Most started out with ten to twelve stools per day. By the time they left the hospital, this had been

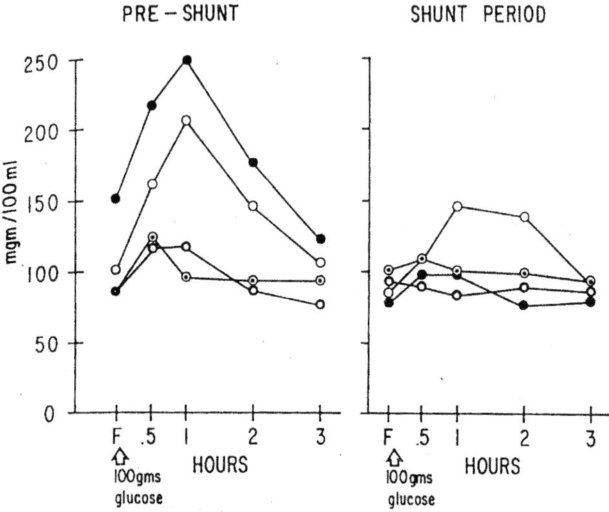

FIG. 9. Flattening of the glucose tolerance curves during the shunt period as recorded in four patients.

reduced to three to five stools per day. After discharge, the number of stools per day was governed by the nature of food and liquid intake. If they went on a carbohydrate or fat binge, they paid for it by spending most of the day on the toilet with distressing rectal symptoms, such as pain and bleeding. One patient had an incisional hernia, one a wound seroma, two reported thinning scalp hair, one had a thrombophlebitis and five had difficulty maintaining their serum potassium and calcium levels in spite of oral supplementation.

COMMENTS

The clinical and laboratory details of ten morbidly obese female patients who had planned, controlled jejuno-colic shunts have been presented. The physiologic and emotional aspects of obesity as related to mental health have been partially studied in man; the published report has clarified several facets of this intriguing problem (9). The scope of this paper does not permit a comprehensive review of the reasons why these patients were obese, and with one exception unable to maintain their ideal weight. Suffice to say that they were not able to remain thin and regained their original weight, almost to the pound. The later observation may be significant. The theory that slimness resolves all problems of the obese patient is seriously challenged by our results. One patient (Case 11) had her regular menstrual cycle restored. After this she has been able to have three pregnancies and three children.

The blood pressure was lowered during the shunt period in every instance, dramatically so in two. It is our impression that the lowered levels of blood pressure were salutary and not the result of adrenal insufficiency, dehydration or electrolyte imbalnce.

No consistent or pathologic changes were observed in the serum electrolyte levels except potassium and calcium. Oral supplementation with potassium and calcium were required. It was necessary to re-establish intestinal continuity in two patients before the ideal calculated weight had been obtained because adequate serum levels of potassium and calcium could not be maintained except in the hospital.

Initial high levels of the serum cholesterol fell to normal during the shunt period. These observations indicate that when a smaller absoptive area is present, smaller amounts of cholesterol and cholesterol precursors are absorbed. The extremely low serum corotene levels we recorded during the shunt period may reflect an inadequate transport vehicle as suggested by Cornwell, Kruger and Robinson (10) and Lewis, Turbull and Page (7).

The change in urinary excretion of 17 ketosteroids and 17 ketogenic steroids during the shunt period are interesting. The significant reduction in three patients during the shunt period is consistent with the hypothesis that obesity represent physiologic stress. Better support for this concept could be provided by demonstrations of consistently lowered levels at stabilized weights. Increased excretion of adrenal steroids in obesity makes it difficult to exclude Cushing's syndrome in some subjects (11). An additional source of difficulty is the presence of facial hair and abdominal striae.

The drop below normal in Case IX should probably not be considered significant without confirmation, but it alerts us to the possibility of adrenal failure, particularly in the presence of disturbed electrolyte balance. The flat glucose tolerance curves most likely are a reflection of a shortened time of exposure to the absorptive surface of the duodenum and jejunum. Studies in animals and man show that glucose is absorbed in the upper part of the intestinal tract and should be complete before the ileum is reached. There is excellent evidence that the frequency of diabetes in the obese adult is three to four times as great as in the nonobese adult (12). Similar observations in the controlled and uncontrolled intestinal shunt have been reported by other invesitgators (4,5).

Failure to absorb fat produced a variable but relentless weight loss. However two patients had to have normal intestinal continuity restored before calculated ideal weights were achieved because of serious metabolic disturbances created by the intestinal shunt. It is significant that only one of the seven patients who had complete intestinal continuity restored was able to maintain an ideal weight. It is extremely interesting to note that the patient (Case VI) was able to regain her original weight of 255 pounds with only 15 inches of jejunum and 42 inches of ileum. Also, the patient (Case 11) was able to gain to 160 pounds with only 15 inches of jejunum and 20 inches of ileum. Patient (Case X) has 15 inches of jejunum and 10 inches of ileum. Her weight is now 118 pounds on a generous American diet. However, the period of observation has been too short for this to be a valid observation. At the present time, she is clinically well.

TABLE VII
LIVER CHANGES*

Patient	Liver Biopsy	Brom-sulph-alein Per cent†	Liver Biopsy	Brom-sulph-alein Per cent†	No. of Weeks
I	+++	...	+++	...	51
II	0-+	...	++	0	112
III	+++	23	++++	...	26
IV	+++	7.5	+++	6	39
V	0-+	5	+++	5	34
VI	++	10	++	5.5	91
VII	0-+	5	+++	30	48
VIII	0-+	11.5	...	...	26
IX	0	16	++++	29	44
X	+++	...	++++	9	57

*Results of the bromsulphalein retention tests, and an estimation of the degree of fatty changes seen in the liver biopsies.
†Normal 4 per cent or less

The changes that we observed in the peripheral blood picture were minor and were not consistent with the report of Booth (I) that in these patients a megaloblastic anemia from Vitamin B12 deficiencyshould develop. However, it is entirely possible that our patients did not have their intestinal shunts long enough to exhaust the body stores of Vitamin B12. It must be remembered that most of our patients had some degree of abnormal liver function. Patient (Case X) only received parenteral Vitamin B12. Evidence has been recorded indicating that if any patient has been permanently deprived of the ileum, he will require Vitamin B12 treatment indefinitely (I). Our observations were consistent with the fact that no signs or symptoms to suggest a blind loop dyndrome were seen in any of our patients.

Protein require digestion before it can be absorbed. Consequently, much of the protein ingested is absorbed by the ileum. Therefore, with the ileum bypassed, relatively small amounts of protein will be absorbed. In spite of excessive loss of nitrogen in the feces, these patients can be kept in positive nitrogen balance if given a high protein diet. Clinical evidence to substantiate this has been reported by Christensen, Musgrove and Wallaeger (13).

Renal biopsies did not produce any signifcant changes.

No significant gross or microscopic changes were seen in the jejunum in continuity or in the bypassed segment.

The occurrence of fatty change in the liver in the

TABLE VIII
COMPLICATIONS

Data	No.
Incisional hernia	1
Wound seroma	1
Electrolyte problems	5
Scalp hair loss	2
Thrombophlebitis	1

obese patient is well known. The pathogenesis of these changes has not been established.

Bromsulphalein retention tests were useful as a measure of hepatic function in this group of patients, but did not consistently correlate with the severity of fatty changes as found in the biopsy. Fatty changes were present in most of the obese patients in our series and varied from mild to moderate. The shunt procedure, although causing weight loss, did not reverse the fatty changes in the liver. There was some evidence that the pathologic changes were increased. Two cases are of particular interest in this regard, since although obese, they had little or no fatty liver changes prior to the shunting procedure. (Fig. 13.) Paradoxically, although the shunt led to dramatic weight loss in these two patients (as in the others), liver changes of considerable severity appeared in both. In addition to fatty changes, slight fibrosis and periportal inflammatory changes were present in severl of the patients. The changes described were not appreciably altered by the shunt procedure. True Laennec's cirrhosis did not appear in any of our patients during the period of observation.

Whether these changes in the patients with intestinal shunts will subside or prove more serious must await further follow-up observations over a longer period of time.

Complications were minimal. The most important complication was the disturbance in the potassium and calcium balalce. Diarrhea and anal irritation was a distressing situation. The serious metabolic disturbances, which are created, are not completely understood.

The minimum amount of small itnestine required to support life has not been established, but our studies indicate it will be very little. Survival plus clinical well-being has been reported in a patient with only 18 inches of small bowel remaining (3). A very complete study on the normal functions of different segments of the small bowel and the metabolic effects of intestinal resection has been published by Booth (1).

There are other investigators and clinicians who are interested in these unfortunate, obese patients. Controlled intestinal bypass procedures have been done in their institutions for control of obesity. The number of cases each man has had is shown on Table IV. In addition, we are grateful to them for the moral support and encouragement given us to publish this report (2,4,6,7,15)

REFERENCES

1. BOOTH, C. C. The metabolic effects of intestinal resection in man. *Postgrad. M. J.*, 37: 7, 1961.

2. KREMEN, A. N., LINNER, J. H., NELSON, C. H. Experimental evaluation of the nutritional importance of proximal and distal small intestine. *Ann Surg.* 140: 439, 1954.

3. MEYERS, H. W. Acute superior mesenteric artery thrombosis: recovery following extensive resection of small and large intestine. *Arch. Surg.*, 53: 208, 1954.

4. SHERMAN, C. D., JR. A review of clinical and experimental data of possible significance in bowel bypassing procedures in obese patients. Personal communication.

5. WECKESSER, E. C., CHINN, A. B., SCOTT, M. W., JR. and PRICE, J. W. Extensive resection of small intestine. *Am. J. Surg.*, 78: 706, 1949.

6. TANNER, N. C. Personal communication.

7. LEWIS, L. A., TURNBULL, R. B., JR. and PAGE, I. H. "Short-circuiting" of the small intestine. *J. A. M. A.*, 182: 77, 1962.

8. DUNCAN, G. G., JENSEN, W. K., FRASER, R. I. and CRISTOFORI, F. C. Correction and control of intractable obesity. *J. A. M. A.*, 181: 309, 1962.

9. MOORE, M. E., STUNKARD, A., SROLE, L. Obesity, social class, and mental illness. *J. A. M. A.* 181: 962, 1962.

10. CORNWELL, D. G., KRUGER, F. A. and ROBINSON, H. B. Studies on absoption of beta corotene and distribution of total corotenoid in human serum lipoproteins after oral administration. *J. Lip. Res.* 3: 65, 1962.

11. SIMKIN, B. Urinary 17-ketosteroid and 17-ketogenic steroid excretion in obese patients. *New England J. Med.*, 264: 974, 1961.

12. HANDLEY, J. H. Diabetics; overweight: U. S. problems. *J. Am. Dietet. A.*, 32: 417, 1956.

13. CHRISTENSEN, N. A., MUSGROVE, J. E. and WALLAEGER, E. E. Extensive resection of bowel for occlusion of superior mesenteric artery: report of case with postoperative studies of function of gastrointestinal tract. *Proc. Staff Meet. Mayo Clin.*, 25: 499, 1950.

14. SCHIFF, L. Diseases of the Liver, p. 432. Philadelphia, 1956. J. B. Lippincott Co.

15. DRYE, J. C. Personal communications.

Gastric Bypass in Obesity

EDWARD E. MASON, M.D., PH.D., F.A.C.S.

CHIKASHI ITO, M.D.

An ideal operation for control of obesity should limit ability to overeat and yet should allow normal nutrition. Subtotal gastric resection would satisfy these objectives but is too radical and irreversible.

Gastric bypass is an operation exactly like Billroth II gastric resection except that nothing is removed. A 15 to 30 per cent fundic segment is anastomosed to the upper jejunum. The distal segment of stomach is closed and sutured to the surface of the fundic pouch.

EXCLUSION OPERATIONS

Antral exclusion was used early in the history of ulcer operations in order to avoid closing a badly diseased duodenal stump. The operation was abandoned because of stomal ulceration. The procedure was resurrected by McKittrick, Moore, and Warren as the first stage of a two-stage operation. At the second stage the antrum was removed. Waddell and Bartlett performed 50 hemigastric exclusion operations with vagotomy. The inclusion of vagotomy with antral exclusion eliminated the high risk of stomal ulceration.

D. W. Kay theorized that if sufficient acid-secreting mucosa were excluded with the antrum, the acid gastric juice bathing the antrum would inhibit gastrin release. He reported 23 patients with 50 per cent gastric exclusion, three of whom developed stomal ulcers.

A. W. Kay reported 20 patients treated with hemigastric exclusion and eight of these developed stomal ulcers between one and 18 months after the operation.

The failure of hemigastric exclusion does not seem surprising in view of the failure of hemigastrectomy in the treatment of ulcer.

ANIMAL EXPERIMENTS

Litter-mate dogs approximately six weeks of age were divided into three experimental groups and subjected to either a sham operation, 85 per cent gastric bypass of 85 per cent gastric resection. Only one of six resected dogs survived for one year and this dog's weight remained unchanged. Gerwig and Zimmerman have shown that there is a hormone in the stomach which is necessary for survival of dogs. This is an added argument for an operation which preserves the stomach even if it is taken out of the food stream. Three sham operated dogs doubled their weight in one year.

Three dogs with 85 per cent bypass gained 15, 17 and 46 per cent in body weight in one year and a fourth dog doubled its body weight in ten months. None of these dogs developed stomal or duodenal ulcers. Intravenous glucose tolerance tests one year after gastric bypass revealed normal blood glucose removal rates. The resected dog after one year had a subnormal removal rate. Gastric bypass decreased the rate of weight gain as compared with sham operated dogs but the animals did grow at a normal rate as far as their skeletal development was concerned.

Stomal Ulcer

Two experiments have been performed to determine whether two-thirds gastric bypass would prevent stomal ulcer. In the first experiment several different procedures were used for ulcer production while two-thirds gastric bypass and two-thirds gastric resection were compared. Fifty-two dogs were used. In three groups the experimental variable was an increasing length of the proximal loop with a maximum length of 48 inches. With this longest loop the average number of ulcers appearing in the jejunum in both bypass and resection was six per dog. These were all rather small erosions observed at the time of sacrifice after three weeks. Weight loss averaged 16 per cent in the bypass dogs and 14 per cent in the resection animals. This was too mild an ulcerogenic procedure.

In a fourth group the dogs were subjected to a

Mason EE, Ito C. Gastric bypass in obesity. *Surg Clin North Am.* 1967; 47:1345-1351.
Reprinted by permission of W.B. Saunders Co., Curtis Center, Independence Square W, Philadelphia, PA 19106.

Mann-Williamson type of operation. These animals lost an average of 27 per cent body weight. This caused too severe a disturbance in nutrition to be of use in comparing the effects of bypass and resection upon ulcer production.

There were two experimental groups wherein a comparison could be made regarding stomal ulceration. In group five, half of the antrum was transplanted to the colon, and the bypass dogs developed an average of three ulcers whereas the resection dogs developed an average of nine ulcers. Weight loss averaged 10 per cent in bypass and 19 per cent in resected dogs. In group six, 12 dogs with 10-inch proximal loops were given 30 mg. of histamine in beeswax once a day for three weeks. The six bypass dogs developed an average of three ulcers and the six resection dogs an average of five ulcers. Weight loss was 9 per cent in bypass and 17 per cent in resection dogs.

On the basis of these results, a second experiment was undertaken with histamine in beeswax given for four weeks and with comparisons between gastric bypass, gastric resection, antrectomy-vagotomy, and sham operations. The results of this experiment confirmed the earlier results, namely, that two-thirds gastric bypass was as effective preventing stomal ulceration as gastric resection. Gastric bypass proved to be superior to antrectomy-vagotomy.

Parietal cell counts were performed before and after four weeks of histamine in beeswax in the last experiment. Parietal cells were increased in the bypassed gastric segment after four weeks of histamine. It is concluded from these results that the excluded portion of the stomach does secrete increased acid under the stimulation of histamine in beeswax and that the acid juice washing over the antrum and duodenum could have an inhibitory effect in bypass animals.

Bypass Physiology

There is increasing evidence that both the antrum and duodenum contain mechanisms for inhibition of gastric secretion which are activated when there is sufficient acid in the area. Brackney et al. showed that either the removal of the duodenum or the interposition of a segment of small bowel between the stomach and duodenum was followed by an increase in gastric secretion. The amount of acid secreted after gastric bypass probably depends upon a balance between the amount of acid bathing the blind loop and the amount of bile and food which regurgitates into the antrum.

Avoidance of vagotomy would seem to be in line with the thesis of preserving normal inhibitory mechanisms while at the same time diverting food from the antrum and thereby reducing stimulation. Secretin inhibits the intestinal phase of gastric secretion when the vagus is intact but, after vagotomy, secretin augments the intestinal phase.

Evaluation of bypass by pouch secretion followed a plan similar to one suggested by Gregory in which the fundic stomach, pouch, and gastroenterostomy were maintained constant and the excluded stomach was varied. Six dogs were prepared with Pavlov pouches. After recovery they were tested in four different ways: (1) maximum histamine stimulation, (2) histamine in a dose predicted to give approximately a half maximum secretion rate, (3) half maximum histamine plus a standard meal, and (4) a standard meal. After completion of these tests the stomachs were divided, leaving an estimated 60 per cent of the stomach in the excluded pouch. The four secretory tests were repeated. Then the acid-secreting portion of the excluded stomach was removed and the tests were repeated. Finally, the antrum was removed, converting each animal to a two-thirds gastric resection and the secretion tests were repeated.

The results showed that the various stages of resection had very little effect upon maximum response to histamine. There was likewise little effect on submaximal histamine stimulation with or without feeding. Andersson et al. and Passaro and Gossman observed that the inhibition by acid in the duodenal bulb was specific for gastrin and not for histamine.

The only secretory experiments which revealed a distinct difference among the various stages were the feeding experiments, and these are shown in Figure 1. There was wide variability in the response of the six dogs and one additional dog to a test meal with just the Pavlov pouch. Most of this response was eliminated by two-thirds gastric bypass and the inhibition was sustained for the three and one-half hours of the experiment. By contrast, when the acid-secreting mucosa was removed, converting the preparation to an antral exclusion operation, there was a steady rise in secretory rate throughout the three and one-half hours of the feeding experiment, suggesting that the retained antrum was releasing gastrin and that the late intestinal phase was active. Finally, when the antrum had been removed it was possible to compare gastric resection with gastric bypass and to observe that resection caused the greatest inhibition of secretion of the fundic pouch.

These results are consistent with the recent literature on the effect of acid in inhibiting gastric secretion by antral and duodenal mechanisms and with the thesis that antral gastrin must be released in order to have an intestinal phase of gastric secretion. These secretory experiments are also consistent with our failure to produce chronic stomal ulcers in dogs with 60 per cent gastric bypass subjected to histamine in beeswax. It appears that subtotal gastric bypass in normal or obese patients should not cause stomal ulcers and that, in fact, a 60 per cent or greater bypass might be satisfactory for the treatment of peptic ulcer.

EXPERIENCE IN MAN

The first patient subjected to this operation was operated upon May 10, 1966:

This was a 50-year-old woman. An appendectomy had been performed at age 16 and at age 21 an incisional hernia appeared. Five attempts at repair failed. Repeated efforts at weight reduction were unsuccessful. At age 35 the uterus was found to be in the hernial sac and was removed. At age 48 the hernia became tender. There was increasing constipation suggesting some partial bowel obstruction and finally the skin over the more dependent portion of the hernial sac became ulcerated. At the time of admission the patient was 4 feet 10 inches tall and weighed 208 pounds. Her blood pressure was 150/88 mm. of mercury and the pulse 92 per minute. A large hernia arose in the right lower abdomen, as can be seen in Figure 2.

Gastric bypass was performed through a midline upper abdominal incision, leaving an estimated 20 per cent of the fundus anastomosed to the jejunum at a point 24 inches beyond the ligament of Treitz. A Polya gastroenterostomy was performed anterior to the colon. The distal closed segment of stomach was sutured to the anterior surface of the fundic segment.

When the patient was seen two months later she had only two complaints. She could not eat as much as she like and sweet things made her sick to her stomach. Within nine months a 60-pound weight loss had occurred. The patient was readmitted to the hospital and pneumoperitoneum instituted. Sixteen liters of air were introduced in 1- to 4-liter doses over a period of three weeks. The hernia was then repaired. The immediate postoperative appearance of the patient is shown on the right of Figure 2. It is our plan to leave the gastric bypass as a permanent arrangement, since re-establishment of normal gastric capacity would undoubtedly be followed by weight gain and recurrence of the hernia.

Eight patients, including the first patient, have been subjected to gastric bypass. None of the patients has lost weight at a dangerous rate. Five of the patients have had hernias as their added indication for an operation. In two the operation was performed through the hernial sac, extending the incision superiorly sufficient to reach the fundus of the stomach. The hernial defect was then repaired with Marlex mesh with the intention of carrying out a more definitive repair after normal weight has been reached and after the use of pneumoperitoneum. So far the Marlex has been well tolerated and a second operation may not be necessary.

Three patients have been operated upon primarily because of their extreme obesity. These patients have been maintained in the hospital on a 600-calorie diet for a sufficient period to achieve a safe operative weight. A normal diet is then provided for several weeks immediately before the operation. Two patients have had a supracostal incision which makes the operation easier to perform.

One 65-year-old man with a previous perforation of a duodenal ulcer has submitted to gastric bypass. He was asymptomatic and had a normal hemoglobin eight months later. His preoperative weight was 125 pounds and his eight-months' weight 131 pounds. This patient does not complain of any symptoms after eating. Several of the obese patients do, however, have mild weakness and sweating if they eat excessively or if they eat foods that are too rich. One patient has loose stools if she overeats and on several occasions has vomited after overeating. None of the patients has asked to have the stomach returned to normal. All have lost weight. It appears that most will remain at a normal or high normal weight. With this limited experience it now seems advisable to leave only a small fundic pouch.

Remaining Questions

Further evaluation of the effect of bypass is being directed along five main lines: (1) the long-term effects on lipid metabolism, (2) early and late effects on carbohydrate metabolism, (3) bacteriology of the blind loop, (4) further evaluation and perhaps modification of the operation to assure safe control of obesity, and (5) evaluation of the potentialities of gastric bypass in the treatment of peptic ulcer.

Gastric bypass is not recommended for general use at the present time because of the questions which still need to be answered. There may be selected patients such as the one presented above in the case report who might be managed justifiably in this way. The operation should not be performed without preoperative weight reduction except in emergency. Because of the type of patient, this preparation must be made in a hospital or under strict supervision. Patients with peptic ulcer should not be subjected to gastric bypass until more is known about the effects in animals and man through controlled studies in research centers.

REFERENCES AND SUGGESTED READING

1. Andersson, A., and Uvnas, B.: Inhibition of postprandial gastric secretion in Pavlov pouches by instillation of hydrochloric acid into the duodenal bulb. Gastroenterology 41:486-490, 1961.
2. Andersson, S., Nilsson, G., and Uvnas, B.: Inhibition of gastric secretion by acid in ¡ x-x-o ¡proximal and distal duodenal pouches. Acta Physiol. Scand. 65:191-191, 1965.
3. Atkinson, M., and Henley, K. S.: Levels of intragastric and

intraduodenal acidity. Clin. Sci. 14:1-14, 1955.
4. Brackney, E. L., Thal, A. P., and Wangensteen, O. H.: Role of duodenum in the control of gastric secretion. Proc. Soc. Exp. Biol. & Med. 88:302-306, 1955.
5. Gerwig, W. H., Jr., Zimmermann, B., Mendoza, C. B., Hooton, T. E., and Payan, H. M of nutrition through endocrine activity of specialized gastric mucosal cells. Ann. Surg. 164:635-641, 1966.
6. Goldstein, F., Wirts, W., and Kramer, S.: Relationship of afferent limb stasis and bacterial flora to the production of postgastrectomy steatorrhea. Gastroenterology 40:47©54, 1961.
7. Gregory, R. A.: Secretory Mechanisms of the Gastrointestinal Tract. London, Edward W Arnold Ltd. 1962, p.30.
8. Harrison, R. C., Lakey, W. H., and Hyde, H. A.: Production of an acid inhibitor by the gastric antrum. Ann. Surg. 144:441-447, 1956.
9. Hay, L. J., Varco, R. L., Code, C. F., and Wangensteen, O. H.: The experimental production of gastric and duodenal ulcers in laboratory animals by the intramuscular injection of histamine in beeswax. Surg. Gynec. & Obst. 75:170-182, 1942.
10. Kay, A. W.: The pyloric antrum and peptic ulceration. Gastroenterologia 89:282-286, 1958.
11. Kay, D. W.: Hemi-gastric exclusion in the treatment of duodenal ulcer. J. Roy. Col. Surg. Edinb. 2:54-60, 1957.
12. Kelly, K. A., Nyhus, L. M., and Harkins, H. N.: The vagal nerve and the intestinal ¡ x-x-Q ¡phase of gastric secretion. Gastroenterology 46:163-166, 1964.
13. Konturek, S., and Grossman, M. I.: Effect of perfusion of intestinal loops with acid, fat, or dextrose on gastric secretion. Gastroenterology 49:481-489, 1965.
14. Mason, E. E.: Pneumoperitoneum in the management c giant hernia. Surgery 39:143151, 1956.
15. McKittrick, L. S., Moore, F. D., and Warren, R.: Complication and mortality in subtotal gastrectomy for duodenal ulcer. Report on a two-stage procedure. Ann. Surg. 120:531-554, 1944.
16. Passaro, E. P., and Grossman, M. I.: Effect of vagal innervation on acid and pepsin response to histamine and gastrin. Am. J. Physiol. 206:1068-1076, 1964.
17. Rheault, M. J., Semb, L. S., Harkins, H. N., and Nyhus, L. M.: Acidification of the gastric antrum and inhibition of gastric secretion. Ann. Surg. 161:587-591, 1965.
18. Shay, H., Gershon-Cohen, J., and Fels, S. S.: A self-regulatory duodenal mechanism for gastric acid control and an explanation for the pathologic gastric physiology in uncomplicated duodenal ulcer. Am. J. Dig. Dis. 9:124-128, 1942.
19. Sircus, W.: Studies on the mechanisms in the duodenum inhibiting gastric secretion. Quart. J. Exp. Physiol. 43:114-132, 1958.
20. Uvnas, B., Andersson, S., Elwin, C., and Malm, A.: Influence of exclusion of the antrum-duodenum passage on the HCl secretion in Pavlov pouch dogs Gastroenterology 30:790-803, 1956.
21. Vasko, J. S.: Valuable approach to upper abdominal cavity. Surg. Gynec. & Obst. 122:844-845, 1966.
22. Waddell, W. R., and Bartlett, M. K.: Antral exclusion with vagoltomy for duodenal ulcer. I. Acid secretory studies on 50 patients. Ann. Surg. 146:3-11, 1957.
23. Wormsley, K. G., and Grossman, M. I.: Inhibition of gastric acid secretion by secretin and by endogenous acid in the duodenum. Gastroenterology 47:72-81, 1964.

University Hospitals
Iowa City, Iowa 52240

List of Figures and Tables

Index of Subjects

Index of Personal Names

Page numbers in *Italics* indicate location of a biographical sketch; those in **bold type** indicate the location of a classic paper.